Handbook of Veterinary Drugs

THIRD EDITION

Handbook of Veterinary Drugs

THIRD EDITION

Dana G. Allen, DVM, MSc, Diplomate ACVIM (Internal Medicine)
Professor, Department of Clinical Studies
Ontario Veterinary College, University of Guelph
Guelph, Ontario, Canada

Patricia M. Dowling, DVM, MS, Diplomate ACVIM (Internal Medicine) and ACVCP
Professor, Veterinary Clinical Pharmacology
Director, Canadian gFARAD
Western College of Veterinary Medicine
Veterinary Biomedical Science
Saskatoon, Saskatchewan, Canada

Dale A. Smith, DVM, DVSc
Professor, Department of Pathobiology
Ontario Veterinary College, University of Guelph
Guelph, Ontario, Canada

With

Associate Editor
Kirby Pasloske, DVM, DVSc, Diplomate ACVCP
Research Programme Manager
Jurox Pty. Ltd.
Veterinary Pharmaceuticals Manufacturer
Rutherford, New South Wales, Australia

Assistant Editor
J. Paul Woods, DVM, MSc, Diplomate ACVIM (Internal Medicine)
Ontario Veterinary College, University of Guelph
Guelph, Ontario, Canada

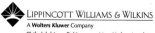
LIPPINCOTT WILLIAMS & WILKINS
A **Wolters Kluwer** Company
Philadelphia · Baltimore · New York · London
Buenos Aires · Hong Kong · Sydney · Tokyo

Acquisitions Editor: David B. Troy
Managing Editor: Rebecca A. Kerins
Marketing Manager: Christen DeMarco
Production Editor: Bill Cady
Designer: Doug Smock
Compositor: Circle Graphics
Printer: R. R. Donnelley & Sons

Printed in the United States of America

First Edition, 1993
Second Edition, 1998

Library of Congress Cataloging-in-Publication Data

Allen, Dana G. (Dana Gray)
    Handbook of veterinary drugs / Dana G. Allen, Patricia M. Dowling, Dale A. Smith with associate editor, Kirby Pasloske, assistant editor, J. Paul Woods.—3rd ed.
        p. cm.
    ISBN 0-7817-4126-2
    1. Veterinary drugs—Handbooks, manuals, etc. I. Dowling, Patricia M. II. Smith, Dale A. III. Title.

SF917.A44 2004
636.089'51—dc22

2003066092

To purchase additional copies of this book, call our customer service department at **(800) 638-3030** or fax orders to **(301) 824-7390.** International customers should call **(301) 714-2324.**

Visit Lippincott Williams & Wilkins on the Internet: http://www.LWW.com. Lippincott Williams & Wilkins customer service representatives are available from 8:30 am to 6:00 pm, EST.

04 05 06 07 08
1 2 3 4 5 6 7 8 9 10

PREFACE

In undertaking the revision of *Handbook of Veterinary Drugs,* we endeavored to provide readers with the same useful and practical data, dosing information, and a user friendly format that made the first two editions a success. *Handbook of Veterinary Drugs* serves as a useful reference for commonly used drugs in veterinary medicine.

We designed *Handbook of Veterinary Drugs* to be a practical aid to both veterinary students and busy practitioners. To provide readers with rapid access, the book is divided into three sections: Small Animals (dogs and cats), Large Animals (horses, ruminant species, and miniature pigs), and Exotics (avian species, ferrets, reptiles, rodents, and rabbits). Each section begins by listing common drug dosages and routes of administration. The reader then finds practical tables listing antimicrobial agents in dogs and cats, antiparasitics in dogs and cats, analgesics for acute pain in dogs and cats, analgesics for chronic pain in dogs and cats, chemotherapeutic protocols for dogs, and chemotherapeutic protocols for cats (Small Animals section). In the Large Animals section, the reader finds tables outlining pathogens and useful antimicrobials and parasites and useful anthelmintics. The second part of each section describes those drugs listed in drug doses under the following headings:

INDICATIONS: A description of the drug and its use(s) is listed. Where available, serum drug levels are given. Common trade names in Canada ♣ and the United States ★ are included to facilitate acquisition of the drug.

ADVERSE AND COMMON SIDE EFFECTS: Emphasis is placed on information as it pertains to veterinary medicine and the species under discussion. When these data are not available, reference to human experience with the drug is given. Management of drug toxicity is discussed in cases where appropriate data are available.

DRUG INTERACTIONS: Where such information is available for animals, it is provided. Some of the data, however, are derived from experience in human medicine.

SUPPLIED AS: This section provides common drug formulations. As in other sections, veterinary-specific information is listed where available, with human medicine filling in some of the gaps. Note that available formulations may change over the course of this publication and may differ between Canada and the United States.

OTHER USES: This segment discusses extralabel uses including drug dose(s), where available. Although we generally do not condone extralabel use when approved veterinary drugs are available, such uses may be necessary in practice, especially when treating exotic species. Much of the information contained herein has been derived from empirical use and not from scientifically controlled studies. In those cases in which conventional therapy has been unsuccessful or has not been established for the condition present, alternative drug therapy is supplied for the reader's information. Informed consent must be obtained from owners or agents before such use of the drug is employed.

Additional features of *Handbook of Veterinary Drugs* include a chart for conversion of body weight to body surface area, located at the front of the Small Animals section. We have added a description of the idiosyncrasies of drug use in the various exotic species. A list of abbreviations is provided to clarify areas of possible confusion. Along with drugs licensed for use in the stated species, some drugs not licensed for specific use are listed. This book makes no attempt to validate reports of drugs for extralabel use. Practitioners are urged to follow manufacturers' recommendations concerning the use of any drug. In the Large Animal section, dosage regimens for aerosol medications are also included. In the Exotic Animals section, drug dosages derived from scientific studies are distinguished from dosages derived from empirical use alone. Readers will not find data pertaining to pharmacokinetic studies unless that information is important to the practitioner's use of the drug. To keep the book practical and portable, references have been omitted. References are available on request to the editor(s).

Handbook of Veterinary Drugs is also available electronically on PDA. This product allows the user to search by species and locate a selected drug, problem or condition, or table. We hope that both media will be useful resources for veterinarians in training and in practice.

D. G. Allen
Guelph, Ontario, Canada

ACKNOWLEDGMENTS

We thank the following individuals for their assistance in reviewing material for this book: Meredith Gauthier, BA, DVM (Part I: Small Animals); Ulrike Helvoigt, DVM, Cranbrook, British Columbia (Part II: Large Animals); Kymberley Mcleod, DVM, Toronto, Ontario (Part II: Large Animals); Michael Taylor, DVM, Service Chief, Avian/Exotic Medicine, Veterinary Teaching Hospital, Ontario Veterinary College, University of Guelph, Guelph, Ontario (Part III: Exotics); and Marc H. Kramer, DVM, Avian & Exotic Animal Medical Center, Miami, Florida (Part III: Exotics).

CONTENTS

ABBREVIATIONS

♣—Canadian usage
★—U.S. usage

bid—twice daily
q—every
qid—four times daily
qod—every other day
tid—three times daily

IC—intracardiac
IM—intramuscular
IP—intraperitoneal
IV—intravenous
PO—per os
PRN—as required
SC—subcutaneous

BUN—blood urea nitrogen
D_5W—5% dextrose in water
g—gram
gr—grain
IU—international unit
L—liter
mL—milliliter
lb—pound
m^2—square meter (body surface area)
µg—microgram
mEq—milliequivalent
OD—right eye
OS—left eye
OU—both eyes
w/v—weight (of solute) per volume (of solvent)
w/w—weight (of solute) per weight (of solvent)

Part I

Small Animals

Conversion of Body Weight to Body Surface Area in Dogs

Body Weight (kg)	Body Surface Area (m^2)	Body Weight (kg)	Body Surface Area (m^2)
0.5	0.06	29.0	0.94
1.0	0.10	30.0	0.96
2.0	0.15	31.0	0.99
3.0	0.20	32.0	1.01
4.0	0.25	33.0	1.03
5.0	0.29	34.0	1.05
6.0	0.33	35.0	1.07
7.0	0.36	36.0	1.09
8.0	0.40	37.0	1.11
9.0	0.43	38.0	1.13
10.0	0.46	39.0	1.15
11.0	0.49	40.0	1.17
12.0	0.52	41.0	1.19
13.0	0.55	42.0	1.21
14.0	0.58	43.0	1.23
15.0	0.60	44.0	1.25
16.0	0.63	45.0	1.26
17.0	0.66	46.0	1.28
18.0	0.69	47.0	1.30
19.0	0.71	48.0	1.32
20.0	0.74	49.0	1.34
21.0	0.76	50.0	1.36
22.0	0.78	51.0	1.38
23.0	0.81	52.0	1.40
24.0	0.83	53.0	1.41
25.0	0.85	54.0	1.43
26.0	0.88	55.0	1.45
27.0	0.90	56.0	1.47
28.0	0.92	57.0	1.48

From Ettinger SJ. Textbook of Veterinary Internal Medicine. Vol. I. Philadelphia: WB Saunders, 1975:146.

Conversion of Body Weight to Body Surface Area in Cats

Body Weight (kg)	Body Surface Area (m²)
2.3	0.165
2.8	0.187
3.2	0.207
3.6	0.222
4.1	0.244
4.6	0.261
5.1	0.278
5.5	0.294
6.0	0.311
6.4	0.326
6.9	0.342
7.4	0.356
7.8	0.371
8.2	0.385
8.7	0.399
9.2	0.413

Handbook of Veterinary Drugs, Third Edition, edited by Dana Allen,
Lippincott Williams & Wilkins, Baltimore. © 2005

Section 1

Drugs in Small Animals

Highlighted drugs denote that additional dosing information is available in
Description of Drugs for Small Animals

Drug	Dog	Cat
Acemannan	1 mg/kg weekly IP for up to 6 weeks, followed by monthly injections for 1 year plus, 2 mg intratumor prior to surgery for up to 6 weeks; surgical excision of tumor at 4th to 7th week, then radiation treatment started (fibrosarcoma)	Same **OR** FeLV- or FIV-induced syndromes; 2 mg/kg once weekly; IV, SC, IP for 6 weeks (FeLV) or 12 weeks (FIV) followed by 2 mg/kg once monthly (FIV)
Acepromazine	0.55 to 2.2 mg/kg; PO 0.025 to 0.200 mg/kg; IV (maximum of 3 mg) **OR** 0.10 to 0.25 mg/kg; IM, PO (restraint, sedation)	1.1 to 2.2 mg/kg; PO 0.05 to 0.10 mg/kg; IV, IM, SC (maximum of 1 mg) (restraint, sedation)
Acetaminophen	15 mg/kg tid; PO	None

Drug	Dog	Cat
Acetaminophen with Codeine	Follow dosing as per Codeine	None
Acetazolamide	10 mg/kg qid; PO (metabolic acidosis) 2 to 5 mg/kg tid; PO (glaucoma)	Same 50 mg/kg once; IV 7 mg/kg tid; PO (glaucoma)
Acetylcysteine (10% and 20% solutions available)	50 mL/hour for 30 to 60 minutes bid; by nebulization (respiratory disease)	140 mg/kg PO, then 70 mg/kg qid; PO, IV q 4 hours for 5 doses (acetaminophen toxicosis)
Albendazole	25 mg/kg bid; PO for 10 days (*Paragonimus*) *Giardia:* 4 doses at 25 mg/kg	Same *Giardia:* 10 doses at 25 mg/kg
Albuterol	0.02 to 0.04 mg/kg 1 to 3 times daily; PO	Unknown
Aldactazide	2 mg/kg once to twice daily; PO	Same
Allopurinol	10 mg/kg bid to tid for 1 month then reduce to 10 mg/kg daily **OR** 15 mg/kg bid; PO; if poor response increase dose by 10% to 25% (urate calculi)	None
Alpha Keri	1 capful to 1 to 2 quarts of water for final rinse or spray aerosol onto wet coat and rub well	Same
Aluminum hydroxide	30 to 90 mg/kg 1 to 3 times daily; PO (hyperphosphatemia) **OR** 2 to 10 mL q 2 to 4 hours; PO (antacid)	30 to 90 mg/kg per day; PO (hyperphosphatemia)

Drug	Dog	Cat
Amikacin	5 mg/kg tid; IM, IV, SC	Same
Aminophylline	10 mg/kg tid; PO, IM, IV	5 mg/kg bid to tid; PO **OR** 4 mg/kg bid; PO, IM
Amitraz	10.6 mL in 2 gallons of water; dip every 2 weeks for 3 to 6 treatments; let dry on coat **OR** 0.125% applied half-body daily; topically	0.0125% applied weekly; topically (demodex)
Amitriptyline	2.2 to 4.4 mg/kg once daily; PO **OR** 2.2 mg/kg once to twice daily; PO (separation anxiety) **OR** 1 to 6 mg/kg once to twice daily; PO 1 mg/kg bid; PO (pruritus)	5 to 10 mg once daily; PO **OR** 0.5 to 1 mg/kg per day; PO
Amlodipine	2.5 mg/dog; PO **OR** 0.1 mg/kg per day; PO	0.065 to 0.125 mg once daily **OR** 0.18 mg/kg once daily; PO
Ammonium chloride	200 mg/kg divided tid; PO	20 mg/kg bid; PO
Amoxicillin	10 to 20 mg/kg bid; PO, SC, IV **OR** 11 to 22 mg/kg bid to tid; PO	10 to 20 mg/kg bid; PO, SC, IV **OR** Same
Amphotericin B	0.15 to 1 mg/kg dissolved in 5 to 20 mL D_5W; rapidly IV; 3 times weekly for 2 to 4 months (not to exceed 2 mL/kg) **OR**	Same

Drug	Dog	Cat
Amphotericin B (continued)	0.25 to 0.5 mg/kg in 0.5 to 1.0 L D_5W; IV over 6 to 8 hours; qod to total dose of 8 to 10 mg/kg or BUN and creatinine increase	
Ampicillin	22 mg/kg tid; PO **OR** 11 to 22 mg/kg tid to qid; SC, IV, IM	Same
Amprolium	100 to 200 mg/kg once daily; PO in food or water for 7 to 10 days	Unknown
Apomorphine	0.04 mg/kg; IV 0.08 mg/kg; IM, SC 0.07 to 0.1 mg/kg	0.04 mg/kg; IV **OR** 0.08 mg/kg; IM or SC
Ascorbic acid	100 to 500 mg/day; PO (maintenance) 100 to 500 mg 1 to 3 times daily; PO (urine acidification)	100 mg/day; PO (maintenance) 100 mg 1 to 3 times daily; PO (urine acidification) 30 mg/kg qid; PO for 7 treatments (acetaminophen toxicosis)
Asparaginase	10,000 to 30,000 IU/ m^2; IM weekly (lymphocytopenia) **OR** 400 U/kg; IM once (thrombocytopenia)	10,000 IU/m^2; IM, SC every 1 to 3 weeks (neoplastic disease)
Aspirin	10 mg/kg bid; PO (antipyretic) 25 to 35 mg/kg tid; PO (musculoskeletal pain) 10 mg/kg once daily; PO **OR** 0.5 mg/kg bid (antithrombotic therapy)	6 mg/kg q 48 to 72 hours; PO (antipyretic) 40 mg/kg q 72 hours; (antirheumatic) 25 mg/kg twice weekly; PO (antithrombotic therapy)

Drug	Dog	Cat
Aspirin (continued)	5 to 10 mg/kg once daily; PO (heartworm therapy) 10 to 25 mg/kg bid to tid; PO (analgesia)	10 mg/kg q 48 to 72 hours; PO **OR** 10 to 20 mg/kg q 48 hours; PO (analgesia)
Atenolol	6.25 to 12.5 mg bid; PO **OR** 0.25 to 1 mg/kg once to twice daily; PO	6.25 to 12.5 mg once daily; PO **OR** 5 mg once to twice daily; PO **OR** 3 mg/kg bid; PO
Atracurium	0.22 mg/kg; IV; give 1/10th to 1/6th initially as a priming dose, then 4 to 6 minutes later, the remainder with a sedative or hypnotic agent (induction dose) 0.11 mg/kg; IV (intraoperative dose)	Same
Atropine	0.022 to 0.044 mg/kg PRN; IM, IV, SC or 0.04 mg/kg tid to qid; PO (sinus bradycardia, sinus block, AV block) 0.02 to 0.04 mg/kg; SC, IM (preanesthetic) 0.2 to 2 mg/kg;1/4th dose IV, rest SC, IM (cholinergic toxicity)	Same Same
Auranofin	0.05 to 0.2 mg/kg bid; PO	Unknown
Aurothioglucose	1st week: 5 mg; IM, 2nd week: 10 mg; IM, then 1 mg/kg once weekly; IM decreasing to once monthly	1st week: 1 mg; IM, 2nd week: 2 mg; IM, then 1 mg/kg once weekly; IM decreasing to once monthly

Drug	Dog	Cat
Azathioprine	2 mg/kg once daily; PO initially then 0.5 to 1 mg/kg qod	1 mg/kg qod; PO (with caution)
Azithromycin	10 mg/kg once q 5 days; PO **OR** 3.3 mg/kg once daily for 3 days **OR** 5 to 10 mg/kg per day for 1 to 5 days; PO	5 mg/kg qod; PO **OR** 5 to 10 mg/kg per day; PO for 1 to 5 days
BAL: Dimercaprol	4 mg/kg q 4 to 6 hours until recovered; IM	Same
Benazepril	0.25 mg/kg once daily; PO (dose may be doubled as indicated)	Same
Benzoyl peroxide	Bathe every 3 to 4 days to once every 1 to 2 weeks; leave on skin for 10 minutes and rinse	Same
Betamethasone	0.15 mg/kg once; IM	Unknown
Bethanechol	5 to 25 mg tid; PO 2.5 to 10 mg tid; SC	2.5 to 5 mg tid; PO
Bisacodyl	5 to 20 mg once daily; PO	5 mg once daily; PO
Bismuth subsalicylate	10 to 30 mL q 4 to 6 hours; PO **OR** 2 mL/kg tid to qid; PO	1 to 2 mL/kg q 4 to 6 hours; PO
Bleomycin	0.2 to 0.6 mg/m^2; SC or IV daily for 5 days, then twice a week for 5 weeks	Same
Bromide; Potassium	Initially 70 to 80 mg/kg once daily; PO (used as a single agent) 22 to 30 mg/kg once daily; PO (those also on phenobarbital) 22 to 40 mg/kg per day; PO	Same **OR** 30 mg/kg per day; PO

Drug	Dog	Cat
Bromide; Potassium (continued)	**OR** 10 mg/kg bid; PO as a 100 mg/mL solution diluted in water with food	
Budesonide	2 mg/dog per day; PO	1 mg/cat per day; PO
Buprenorphine	0.005 to 0.02 mg/kg q 4 to 8 hours; IV, IM	0.005 to 0.01 mg/kg q 4 to 8 hours; IV, IM
Buspirone	2.5 to 10 mg bid to tid; PO **OR** 1 to 2 mg/kg 1 to 3 times daily; PO (behavioral problems)	2.5 to 5 mg bid to tid; PO 5 mg bid; PO. If no response increase to 7.5 mg bid; PO (urine spraying) 0.5 to 1 mg/kg 1 to 3 times daily; PO (behavioral problems)
Busulfan	3 to 4 mg/m^2 per day; PO	Same
Butorphanol	0.55 mg/kg bid to qid; PO to a maximum of 5 mg/4.5 kg **OR** 0.5 to 1 mg/kg bid to qid; PO **OR** 0.05 to 0.12 mg/kg bid to tid; PO (antitussive) 0.2 to 0.4 mg/kg q 2 to 5 hours; IM, IV **OR** 0.4 mg/kg; SC, IM **OR** 0.2 to 0.8 mg/kg q 1 to 3 hours; IM, IV, SC (analgesia)	0.5 to 1 mg/kg bid to qid; PO (antitussive) 0.1 to 0.4 mg/kg; IV, IM, SC (lasts 2 to 5 hours) **OR** 0.8 mg/kg; IV (lasts 2 hours) **OR** 0.2 to 1.0 mg/kg q 4 to 6 hours; PO (analgesia)
Calcitonin-salmon	4 to 7 U/kg tid to qid; SC **OR** 4 to 6 IU/kg q 2 to 3 hours; SC, IM until serum calcium stabilizes **OR**	Unknown

Drug	Dog	Cat
Calcitonin-salmon (continued)	4 U/kg; IV initially followed by 4 to 8 U/kg once to twice daily; SC	
Calcitriol	0.02 to 0.03 µg/kg once daily; PO (loading dose) followed by 0.005 to 0.015 µg/kg per day (maintenance)	Same
	2.5 mg/kg once daily; PO (chronic renal failure)	Same
Calcium carbonate	1 to 4 g/day; PO **OR** 100 to 150 mg/kg divided bid to tid; PO	Same
Calcium chloride (10% solution)	1 mL per 10 kg; IV (ventricular asystole)	Same
	0.1 mL/kg (100 mg/mL solution); IV (hyperkalemia or hypocalcemia)	
Calcium EDTA	100 mg/kg per day for 5 days; make a solution of 1 g versenate per 100 mL D$_5$W, divide total quantity into 20 aliquots at 1 dose; SC qid for 5 days (lead poisoning)	Same
Calcium gluconate (10% solution)	0.5 to 1.5 mL/kg over 20 to 30 minutes; IV; may repeat tid to qid **OR**	Same **OR** 5 to 10 mL/cat; IV
	10 to 15 mg/kg per hour; IV infusion	
Calcium lactate	0.5 to 2 g; PO **OR** 130 to 200 mg/kg tid; PO	0.2 to 0.5 g; PO **OR** Same

Drug	Dog	Cat
Captopril	0.5 to 2 mg/kg bid to tid; PO	2 mg bid to tid; PO
Carbenicillin	15 mg/kg tid; PO, IV	Same
Carboplatin	300 mg/m² q 21 days; IV	Unknown
Carnitine	2 g bid to tid; PO **OR** 100 mg/kg bid; PO **OR** 220 mg/kg per day; IV, or divided daily; PO (cardiomyopathy)	250 to 500 mg once daily; PO **OR** 50 to 100 mg/kg; PO (hepatic lipidosis)
Carprofen	4 mg/kg; IV initially Then 2.2 mg/kg; IV, SC, PO, IM Repeat in 12 hours if needed	Same 2 mg/kg bid; PO (2 days maximum)
Carvedilol	Up to 0.25 mg/kg bid; PO—start at 1/4th of this and assess	Unknown
Cefaclor	4 to 20 mg/kg tid; PO	Same
Cefadroxil	22 mg/kg bid; PO	Same
Cefamandole	6 to 40 mg/kg tid to qid; IM, IV	Same
Cefazolin	5 to 15 mg/kg tid to qid; IM, IV	Same
Cefotetan	30 mg/kg tid; IV, or bid; SC	30 mg/kg q 5 to 8 hours; IV
Cefixime	5 mg/kg once daily; PO	Unknown
Cefotaxime	20 to 80 mg/kg tid; IM, IV, SC 25 to 50 mg/kg tid; IM, IV, SC	20 to 80 mg/kg qid; IM, IV, SC Same
Cefoxitin	6 to 20 mg/kg tid; IM, IV, SC **OR** 6 to 40 mg/kg tid to qid; IV **OR** 30 mg/kg q 5 hours; IV and 30 mg/kg tid; SC	22 to 30 mg/kg tid; IM, IV, SC
Ceftazidime	25 mg/kg bid to tid; IM, SC	Same

Drug	Dog	Cat
Ceftazidime (continued)	30 mg/kg q 4 hours; SC or as constant IV infusion— loading dose 4.4 mg/kg; rate 4.1 mg/kg per hour (*P. aeruginosa*)	
Cephalexin	20 to 40 mg/kg bid to tid; PO	Same
Cephalothin	20 to 35 mg/kg tid to qid; IM, IV, SC	Same
Cephapirin	20 to 30 mg/kg tid; IM, IV, SC	Same
Cephradine	20 to 40 mg/kg tid; PO, IV, IM	Same
Charcoal (activated)	1 g/5 mL water; give 10 mL slurry/kg; PO	Same
Chlorambucil	2 to 8 mg/m^2 once daily; PO for 3 weeks beyond remission, then 1.5 mg/m^2 once daily; PO; for 15 days, then every 3rd day	1.5 mg/m^2 once daily; PO then as for dog 0.2 mg/kg per day; PO (immune-mediated anemia)
Chloramphenicol	50 mg/kg tid; PO, IM, IV, SC	50 mg/kg bid; PO, IM, IV, SC
Chlorhexidine (1%)	Apply ointment after cleansing area; repeat PRN	Same
Chlorothiazide	20 to 40 mg/kg bid; PO	Same
Chlorpheniramine	0.5 to 1 mg/kg bid to tid; PO 0.22 mg/kg tid; PO (pruritus)	1 to 2 mg bid to tid; PO 2 to 4 mg bid; PO (pruritus)
Chlorpromazine	3.3 mg/kg 1 to 4 times daily; PO **OR** 1.1 to 6.6 mg/kg 1 to 4 times daily; IM **OR** 0.55 to 4.4 mg/kg 1 to 4 times daily; IV	Same

Drug	Dog	Cat
Chlorpromazine (continued)	0.5 mg/kg tid; IM (antiemetic)	Same
	3 mg/kg bid; PO **OR**	Same **OR**
	0.5 mg/kg bid; IM, IV (sedative, restraint)	0.5 mg/kg once daily; IM, IV
	Up to 1.1 mg/kg; IM 1 to 1.5 hours prior to surgery (pre-anesthetic)	Same
	0.5 to 3.3 mg/kg 1 to 4 times daily; PO (behavioral problems)	Same
Chlorpropamide	10 to 40 mg/kg once daily; PO	Unknown
Cimetidine	5 to 10 mg/kg tid to qid; PO, IV, IM (chronic gastritis, GI ulcer)	5 mg/kg tid to qid; PO, IV **OR** 10 mg/kg bid; PO, IM, IV **OR** 2.5 to 5 mg/kg bid; PO, IV
Ciprofloxacin	10 to 15 mg/kg bid; PO **OR**	Unknown
	5 to 11 mg/kg bid; PO	Same
Cisapride	0.1 to 0.5 mg/kg bid to tid; PO	Same **OR** 2.5 mg tid; PO <4 kg 5 mg tid; PO >4 kg **OR** 1 mg/kg tid; PO **OR** 1.5 mg/kg bid; PO
Cisplatin	60 mg/m^2 slowly IV over 20 minutes q 3 weeks; pretreat with IV fluids 4 hours before (20 mL/kg per hour) and 2 hours after **OR**	None
	70 mg/m^2 q 21 days; IV over 20 minutes; saline given for 3 hours before cisplatin at 25 mL/kg per hour and after at same rate for 1 hour	

Drug	Dog	Cat
Clavamox	13.75 mg/kg bid; PO	62.5 mg bid; PO
Clemastine	0.05 to 0.1 mg/kg bid; PO	0.68 mg bid; PO **OR** 0.1 mg/kg bid; PO
Clindamycin	11 mg/kg bid; PO **OR** 22 mg/kg per day; PO	5.5 mg/kg bid; PO **OR** 11 mg/kg per day; PO (*Staphylococcus*) 11 mg/kg bid; PO **OR** 22 mg/kg per day; PO (anaerobes) 12.5 mg/kg bid; PO for 4 weeks (toxoplasmosis)
Clofazimine	Unknown	1 mg/kg to a maximum of 4 mg/kg per day; PO
Clomipramine	1 to 2 mg/kg bid; PO **OR** 1 to 3 mg/kg	0.5 mg/kg
Clonazepam	1 to 10 mg 1 to 4 times daily; PO **OR** 1.5 mg/kg divided tid; PO 0.1 to 0.5 mg/kg bid to tid; PO (behavioral problems)	0.016 mg/kg 1 to 4 times daily; PO (behavioral problems)
Clorazepate	2 mg/kg bid; PO 0.55 to 2.2 mg/kg once to twice daily; PO or PRN (behavioral problems)	Same (behavioral problems)
Clotrimazole	Apply to lesions bid for 2 to 4 weeks; continue treatment 1 week beyond clinical cure	Same
Cloxacillin	10 to 15 mg/kg qid; PO, IM, IV	Same
Coal tar shampoos	May be used daily or less often; leave in contact with skin for 10 minutes, then rinse	None

Drug	Dog	Cat
Codeine	0.1 to 0.3 mg/kg tid to qid; PO **OR** 1 to 2 mg/kg tid; PO (cough) 0.5 to 1 mg/kg tid to qid; PO **OR** 1 to 4 mg/kg q 1 to 6 hours; PO (pain) 0.25 to 0.5 mg/kg tid to qid; PO (diarrhea) 1 to 2 mg/kg bid to tid; PO (acetaminophen and codeine)	1 to 2 mg/kg bid; PO (with caution) 1 to 2 mg/kg tid; PO (cough)
Colchicine	0.03 mg/kg tid; PO, SC **OR** 0.025 to 0.03 mg/kg per day; PO	None
Cyclophosphamide	50 mg/m^2 once daily; PO for 4 days a week for 3 to 4 weeks (immune thrombocytopenia) 2 mg/kg per day 4 days of each week; PO (immune-mediated anemia) 1 mg/kg per day for 4 days of each week; PO (polymyositis)	10 mg/kg weekly; IV 100 mg/m^2; PO q 3 weeks [with doxorubicin] (mammary cancer) 1.5 mg/kg per day **OR** 10 mg/kg once weekly; PO (immune-mediated anemia)
Cyclosporine	20 mg/kg once daily; PO 10 mg/kg once to twice daily; PO (immune-mediated anemia) **OR** 10 to 20 mg/kg per day; IM, PO for 5 days, stop for 2 days, resume at 5 mg/kg per day on a 5 days on, 2 days off regimen as clinical signs warrant	10 mg/kg bid; PO **OR** 8 to 10 mg/kg per day; PO (immune-mediated anemia)

Drug	Dog	Cat
Cyproheptadine	1.1 mg/kg bid to tid; PO (antihistamine) 5 to 20 mg once to twice daily; PO (appetite stimulant)	2 to 4 mg once to twice daily; PO (appetite stimulant) **OR** 8 mg 1 to 3 times daily; PO
Cytarabine	5 to 10 mg/kg once daily for 2 weeks **OR** 30 to 50 mg/kg once a week; IV, IM, SC **OR** 100 mg/m^2 once daily; IV, IM for 4 days, then 150 mg/m^2	Same
Dacarbazine	200 mg/m^2 once daily; IV for 5 days; repeat q 3 week **OR** 800 mg/m^2 via 8-hour continuous infusion q 3 week	Same
Dactinomycin	0.015 mg/kg once daily for 3 to 5 days; IV, wait 3 weeks for marrow recovery 1.5 mg/m^2 once weekly **OR** 0.5 to 1.1 mg/m^2 q 2 to 3 weeks; IV **OR** 0.6 to 0.7 mg/m^2 q 3 weeks; IV	Same Same
Danazol	5 mg/kg bid; PO **OR** 5 mg/kg tid; PO **OR** 10 to 20 mg/kg per day divided bid to tid; PO (immune-mediated anemia)	5 mg/kg bid; PO for 2 to 4 weeks (immune-mediated anemia)
Dantrolene	3 to 15 mg divided bid to tid; PO **OR** 1 to 5 mg/kg bid; PO (urethral obstruction)	Same **OR** 0.5 to 2.0 mg/kg tid; PO (urethral obstruction)

Drug	Dog	Cat
Dapsone	1.1 mg/kg tid to qid; PO **OR** 1 mg/kg tid; PO (sub-corneal pustular dermatosis)	Same **OR** 50 mg bid; PO (mycobacteriosis)
Dehydrocholic acid	10 to 15 mg/kg tid; PO until urine negative for bilirubin	Same
Demeclocycline	6 to 12 mg/kg bid to qid; PO (human dose)	Unknown
Deracoxib	3 to 4 mg/kg once daily; PO	None
Derm Caps	1 capsule per 9 kg once daily; PO	Same
Derm Caps (liquid)	To 4.5 kg give 0.35 mL To 9 kg give 0.7 mL To 13.6 kg give 1.05 mL	Same
Derm Caps ES	1 capsule per 31.5 to 40 kg	
Derm Caps ES (liquid)	To 13.6 kg give 0.5 mL To 27.2 kg give 1 mL To 40.8 kg give 1.5 mL	Same
Desmopressin acetate [DDAVP 100 µg/mL] (1 drop = 1.5 to 4.0 µg; 1 spray = 10 µg)	1 to 4 drops intranasally or in conjunctival sac once to twice daily **OR** 2 µg once to twice daily; SC (central DI) 1 µg/kg; IV, SC **OR** 0.3 µg/kg; IV (diluted in 50 mL saline and infused over 15 to 30 minutes) repeat PRN (von Willebrand's disease)	Same Same Unknown
Desoxycorticosterone pivalate (DOCP)	2.2 mg/kg q 25 days; IM	Unknown

Drug	Dog	Cat
Dexamethasone	2 mg/kg; IV, then 1 mg/kg tid to qid; SC in decreasing doses **OR**	Same
	1 to 4 mg/kg; IV followed by gradually tapering doses q 6 to 8 hours (cerebral edema)	
	2 to 3 mg/kg; IV, then 1 mg/kg bid to tid; SC, IV for 24 hours, then 0.2 mg/kg bid to tid; SC in decreasing doses for 5 to 8 days (spinal cord trauma)	
	2 to 8 mg/kg slowly; IV (shock)	
	0.25 to 0.30 mg/kg once; IV or SC, then 0.10 to 0.15 mg/kg bid for 5 to 7 days; SC or PO for 7 days then decrease oral dose by ½ q 5 to 7 days for 3 weeks, then go to alternate day therapy for 6 weeks (immune thrombocytopenia)	
	0.1 to 0.5 mg/kg q 4 to 8 hours; SC, IV (allergic reactions)	
	0.11 mg/kg q 48 hours (pruritus)	0.2 mg/kg q 48 hours (pruritus)
Dextran 40 and 70	10 to 20 mL/kg per day; IV then 10 mL/kg per day thereafter **OR**	Same **OR**

Drug	Dog	Cat
Dextran 40 and 70 (continued)	2 to 5 mL/kg per hour; IV infusion	5 to 10 mL/kg per day
Dextroamphetamine	5 to 10 mg tid; PO (narcolepsy) 0.2 to 1.3 mg/kg PRN; PO (hyperkinesis)	None
Dextromethorphan	2 mg/kg tid to qid; PO	2 mg/kg qid; PO, SC, IV
Diazepam	0.5 to 1 mg/kg; IV in increments of 5 to 10 mg to effect **OR** 0.5 mg/kg intranasally (status epilepticus) 1 to 4 mg/kg divided tid to qid; PO (seizures) 0.5 to 2 mg/kg of injectable solution per rectum (cluster seizures) 2 to 10 mg tid; PO (relax urinary sphincter)	2 to 5 mg tid; PO, IV (seizures) 0.05 to 0.15 mg/kg once to every other day; IV or 1 mg once daily; PO (appetite stimulant) 2.5 mg tid to qid; PO (relax urinary sphincter)
Diazoxide	10 to 40 mg/kg per day divided; PO **OR** 5 to 13 mg/kg bid; PO	None
Dichlorphenamide	2 to 4 mg/kg bid to tid; PO	1 mg/kg bid to tid; PO
Dichlorvos	11 to 22 mg/kg; PO repeat in 3 weeks	Same
Dicloxacillin	10 to 20 mg/kg tid; PO **OR** 50 mg/kg tid; PO	Same
Diethylcarbamazine	6.6 mg/kg once daily; PO (heartworm prevention)	None
Diethylstilbestrol	0.1 to 0.4 mg/kg per day for 3 to 5 days; PO, then once to twice weekly for maintenance (urinary incontinence)	0.05 to 0.1 mg/day; PO (urinary incontinence)

Drug	Dog	Cat
Digitoxin	0.04 to 0.1 mg/kg divided tid; PO	0.005 to 0.015 mg/kg once daily; PO
Digoxin	0.005 to 0.008 mg/kg bid; PO (elixir) 0.005 to 0.010 mg/kg bid; PO (tablet) 0.22 mg/m² bid; PO	0.003 to 0.004 mg/kg bid; PO (elixir)
Dihydrostreptomycin	5 to 10 mg/kg bid; IM, SC **OR** 12.5 mg/kg bid to tid; IM, SC	Same
Dihydrotachysterol	0.03 mg/kg once daily for 2 days then 0.01 to 0.02 mg/kg per day; PO	Same **OR** 1 to 2 drops once to twice daily; PO
Diltiazem	0.5 to 1.5 mg/kg tid; PO **OR** 0.75 to 1.5 mg/kg tid; PO	1.75 to 2.5 mg/kg bid to tid; PO **OR** 1 mg/kg tid; PO **OR** 3.5 to 7 mg tid; PO 0.2 mg/kg; IV **OR** 10 mg/kg per day; PO (long-acting form)
Dimethyl sulfoxide	Apply topically tid to qid 1 g/kg slowly (over 45 minutes); IV (increased CSF pressure from head trauma)	None
Diphenhydramine	2 to 4 mg/kg tid to qid; PO, IM, IV 2.2 mg/kg tid (pruritus)	Same Unknown
Diphenoxylate	2.5 to 10 mg qid; PO **OR** 2.5 mg bid to qid; PO	0.6 to 1.2 mg bid to tid; PO
Disopyramide	Dog >18 kg, 100 mg tid to qid; PO	None
Dobutamine	250 mg in 1 L of 5% dextrose at 2.5 µg/kg per minute; IV **OR**	2.5 to 10 µg/kg per minute constant rate infusion; IV

Drug	Dog	Cat
Dobutamine (continued)	10 to 20 µg/kg per minute constant rate infusion	
Docusate calcium	50 to 100 mg once to twice daily; PO	50 mg once to twice daily; PO
Docusate sodium	50 to 200 mg bid to tid; PO	50 mg once to twice daily; PO
Domperidone	0.05 to 0.1 mg/kg; once to twice daily; PO	Same
Dopamine	2 to 15 µg/kg per minute; IV infusion (inotrope) 2 to 4 µg/kg per minute; IV infusion in D_5W (renal vasodilator; acute renal failure)	Same
Doxapram	5 to 10 mg/kg once; IV; may be repeated in 15 to 20 minutes	Same
Doxorubicin	30 mg/m² in 150 mL D_5W once q 3 to 9 weeks; IV (not to exceed total dose of 250 mg/m²)	Same (not to exceed 90 mg/m²)
Doxycycline	5 mg/kg; PO as a loading dose followed in 12 hours by 2.5 mg/kg, then 2.5 mg/kg q 24 hours thereafter **OR** 5 to 10 mg/kg bid; PO, IV **OR** 15 to 20 mg/kg bid; PO	Same **OR** 2.5 to 5 mg/kg bid; PO (*Hemobartonella*)
Edrophonium chloride	0.1 to 0.2 mg/kg; IV (maximum of 5 mg) **OR** 0.1 to 0.5 mg; IV (puppies)	2.5 mg/cat; IV

Drug	Dog	Cat
Enalapril	0.5 mg/kg once to twice daily; PO	0.25 to 0.5 mg/kg once to twice daily; PO
Enilconazole	Apply 10 to 20 mg/kg bid topically for 10 to 14 days; (10% solution divided 50:50 with water) [aspergillosis] Wash 4 times at 3 to 4 day intervals; (0.2% solution) [dermatophytes]	Unknown
Enrofloxacin	5 to 20 mg/kg per day; PO	2.5 mg/kg bid; PO
Ephedrine	5 to 15 mg bid to tid; PO (bronchodilator) 5 to 15 mg tid; PO (urethral sphincter incompetence) 0.05 to 0.2 mg/kg; IV **OR** 0.1 to 0.25 mg/kg; IV may be repeated up to 3 times (hypotension)	2 to 5 mg bid to tid; PO (bronchodilator) 2 to 4 mg tid; PO (urethral sphincter incompetence) Same
Epinephrine (1:10,000 solution)	0.1 mL/kg; IC (cardiac arrest) 0.5 to 1.5 mL; IV, repeat in 30 minutes (anaphylaxis)	Same Same 0.1 mg q 4 to 6 hours; SC (feline asthma)
Epsiprantel	5.5 mg/kg once; PO	2.75 mg/kg once; PO
Erythromycin	10 to 20 mg/kg tid; PO (antimicrobial dose) 0.5 to 1 mg/kg tid; PO (prokinetic dose)	Same
Erythropoietin	100 U/kg 3 times weekly; SC until PCV in low normal range, then dose interval decreased to twice weekly; if adequate control	Same

Drug	Dog	Cat
Erythropoietin (continued)	not achieved with this regimen increase dose by 25 to 50 U/kg maintaining dose interval between once and 3 times weekly	
Esmolol	Loading dose 200 to 500 µg/kg; IV over 1 minute followed by CRI of 25 to 200 µg/kg per minute **OR** 0.05 to 0.1 mg/kg slowly q 5 minutes to maximum of 0.5 µg/kg **OR** Infusion of 50 to 200 µg/kg per minute **OR** 25 to 200 µg/kg per minute; IV	Loading dose 200 to 500 µg/kg per minute over 1 minute followed by CRI 25 to 200 µg/kg per minute
Estradiol cypionate	44 µg/kg; IM 3 to 5 days after onset of estrus (pregnancy termination)	250 µg 40 hours postcoitus; IM (pregnancy termination)
Etidronate	5 mg/kg per day **OR** 15 mg/kg bid; PO	10 mg/kg per day; PO
Etodolac	10 to 15 mg/kg once daily; PO	None
Famotidine	0.5 to 1 mg/kg once to twice daily; PO, IV **OR** 5 mg/kg once daily; IM, SC, PO	Unknown
Felbamate	15 to 20 mg/kg tid; PO **OR** 200 mg/day tid for small dogs and 400 mg/dog tid for larger dogs, increasing dose by 200 mg increments until seizures controlled	Unknown

Drug	Dog	Cat
Fenbendazole	50 mg/kg once daily for 3 days; repeat in 3 weeks; PO	30 mg/kg once daily for 3 to 6 days; PO
Fentanyl	0.04 to 0.08 mg/kg; IM, IV, SC (provides 2 hours analgesia) **OR** 25 µg/hour patch (<10 kg) 50 µg/hour patch (10 to 30 kg) 75 to 100 µg/hour patch (>30 kg)	(<10 kg) 25 µg/hour patch (<5 kg) cover 1/3rd to 2/3rds patch
Ferrous sulfate	100 to 300 mg once daily; PO	50 to 100 mg once daily; PO
Finasteride	5 mg once daily; PO (10 to 50 kg)	None
Florfenicol	25 to 50 mg/kg q 8 hours; PO, IM for 3 to 5 days	Same
Fluconazole	10 to 12 mg/kg per day; PO	50 mg/cat once or twice daily; PO
Flucytosine	30 to 50 mg/kg tid to qid; PO **OR** 50 to 75 mg/kg tid; PO	Same
Fludrocortisone	0.1 to 0.8 mg daily; PO, **OR** 0.02 mg/kg per day; PO	0.1 to 0.2 mg daily; PO
Flumazenil	0.1 to 0.2 mg total dose PRN; IV	Same
Flumethasone	0.06 to 0.25 mg once daily; PO, IM, IV, SC	0.03 to 0.125 mg once daily; PO, IM, IV, SC
Flunixin meglumine	0.5 mg/kg bid; IV for 1 to 2 treatments (ocular disease) 1 mg/kg once; IV (acute gastric dilatation)	0.25 mg/kg once; SC, can be repeated in 12 to 24 hours (surgical pain)

Drug	Dog	Cat
Flunixin meglumine (continued)	0.5 mg/kg once to twice daily for 3 treatments; IV (GIT obstruction) 0.5 to 1 mg/kg per day; IV (not to exceed 5 days) 0.25 to 1 mg/kg; IV, SC, IM, can be repeated in 1 to 2 treatments (ocular disease) 0.25 mg/kg; IV, SC, IM, once; can be repeated in 12 to 24 hours if needed (pyrexia) 1 mg/kg; IM, IV, SC daily (surgical pain)	
Fluorouracil	150 mg/m^2 once weekly; IV	None
Fluoxetine	1 mg/kg once to twice daily for 6 to 8 weeks; PO **OR** 0.5 to 1 mg/kg per day; PO **OR** 5 mg per dog once daily; PO **OR** 1 to 1.5 mg/kg per day; PO	0.5 to 1 mg/kg per day; PO
Folic acid	5 mg/day; PO (dietary supplement) 1 mg/day; PO (supplement to pyrimethamine)	2.5 mg/day; PO Same
Fomepizole	20 mg/kg; IV loading dose; then 15 mg/kg (12 hours), 15 mg/kg (24 hours) and 5 mg/kg (36 hours); then 5 mg/kg bid PRN	None

Drug	Dog	Cat
Fucidic acid	Apply in eye(s) once daily for 48 hours after infection resolved	Same
Furosemide	2 to 4 mg/kg bid to tid; PO, IM, IV (diuresis–heart failure)	1 to 4 mg/kg bid to tid; PO, IM, IV, SC
	1 to 2 mg/kg once to twice daily; PO, SC (ascites from liver failure)	Same
	1 to 2 mg/kg bid to tid; IV, IM (diuresis–hypercalcemia)	
	5 to 20 mg PRN; IV (initiate diuresis in acute renal failure)	
	2 to 4 mg/kg q 4 to 12 hours; PO, IM, IV (pulmonary edema)	
	1 to 2 mg/kg bid; PO (hypertension)	
Gentamicin	2 mg/kg tid; IM, SC	Same
Glipizide	0.25 to 0.5 mg/kg bid; PO	2.5 mg initially to 5 mg bid; PO
Glyburide	0.2 mg/kg once daily; PO	0.2 mg/kg once daily; PO (nonmicronized product)
Glycopyrrolate	0.005 to 0.010 mg/kg; IV, **OR**	Same
	0.01 to 0.02 mg/kg; SC, IM (sinus bradycardia, SA block, AV block)	
Gonadorelin	50 to 100 μg; SC, IV; if no response repeat in 4 to 6 days (undescended testes)	25 μg; IM after mating (stimulate ovulation)
Granulocyte colony-stimulating factor (human)	5 μg/kg once daily; SC	Same

Drug	Dog	Cat
Griseofulvin	20 to 50 mg/kg once daily for 3 to 6 weeks; PO	Same
Guaifenesin	44 to 88 mg/kg; IV **OR** 33 to 88 mg/kg; IV with 1.1 mg/kg ketamine (restraint) 110 mg/kg; IV (to cause muscle relaxation with strychnine or tetanus)	None
Halothane	Induction: 3% Maintenance: 0.5% to 1.5%	Same
Heparin	200 IU/kg; IV then 50 to 100 IU/kg tid to qid; SC (arterial thromboembolism) 75 to 100 IU/kg qid; IV (DIC) 100 IU/kg bid; SC (acute pancreatitis) 100 to 200 IU/kg for 1 to 4 treatments; IV (burns)	Same
Hetastarch	20 mL/kg per day; IV then 10 mL/kg per day; IV **OR** 25 to 30 mL/kg over 6 to 8 hours; 2nd dose immediately following 1st (severe hypoproteinemia with volume depletion, pulmonary edema, or effusion) Severe cases give concurrent crystalloids at 2/3rds daily dosing requirements	5 to 10 mL/kg per day

Drug	Dog	Cat
Hydralazine	1 to 3 mg/kg bid; PO (arterial vasodilator) 0.5 to 2 mg/kg bid to tid; PO (systemic hypertension)	2.5 mg bid; PO (arterial vasodilator and systemic hypertension)
Hydrochlorothiazide	2 to 4 mg/kg bid; PO	Same
Hydrocodone	0.22 mg/kg bid to tid; PO	2.5 to 5 mg bid to tid; PO (with caution)
Hydrocortisone sodium succinate	8 to 20 mg/kg; IV **OR** 50 to 150 mg/kg; IV (shock) 5 to 20 mg/kg q 2 to 6 hours; IV (hypoadrenocortical crisis)	Same 1 to 3 mg/kg; IV (asthma)
Hydroxyurea	50 mg/kg once daily, 3 days/week; PO	25 mg/kg once daily, 3 days/week; PO **OR** 12.2 mg/kg once daily for 16 days followed by maintenance dose every other day; PO
Hydroxyzine	2 mg/kg tid to qid; PO, IM 2.2 mg/kg tid (pruritus) 2.2 mg/kg bid to tid; PO (behavioral problems)	10 mg bid; PO Unknown Same
Imipenem-cilastatin	2 to 5 mg/kg tid; IV	Same
Imipramine	0.5 to 1 mg/kg tid; PO **OR** 1 mg/kg divided bid; PO (maximum of 3 mg/kg per day)	2.5 to 5 mg bid; PO
Immunoglobulin G	0.4 to 0.5 mg/kg per day for 5 days; IV (repeat PRN) **OR** 0.5 to 1.5 g/kg; IV as a 12-hour infusion	Unknown
Inamrinone	1 to 3 mg/kg; IV bolus followed by 30 to 100 µg/kg per minute	Unknown

Drug	Dog	Cat
Innovar-Vet (fentanyl-droperidol)	0.3 to 0.5 mL/55 kg; IV (tranquilization) 1 mL/20 kg; IM (preanesthetic)	None
Insulin		
Regular	Initially 0.2 U/kg; IM, then 0.1 U/kg hourly until glucose is less than 250 mg/dl [13.8 mmol/L] **OR**	Same
	2.2 U/kg per day; slow IV infusion (ketoacidosis)	Unknown
Intermediate-acting [NPH, Lente]	<15 kg, 1 U/kg once to twice daily; SC >25 kg, 0.5 U/kg once to twice daily; SC	0.25 to 0.5 U/kg bid; SC
Long-acting [Ultralente]	0.5 U/kg once daily; SC	1 to 3 U once to twice daily; SC
Protamine zinc	None	0.5 to 1 U/kg once to twice daily; SC
Interferon	Unknown	30 IU once daily for 7 days; PO on a 1 week on/1 week off basis
Ipecac (syrup)	5 to 15 mL; PO **OR** 3 to 6 mL; PO	Same **OR** 2 to 6 mL; PO
Iron dextran injection	10 to 20 mg/kg once; IM, followed by oral ferrous sulfate	50 mg; IM at 18 days of age (to prevent transient neonatal iron deficiency anemia)
Isoflurane	Induction: 5% Maintenance: 1.5% to 2.5%	Same
Isoproterenol	15 to 30 mg q 4 hours; PO 0.1 to 0.2 mg qid; IM, SC	Same

Drug	Dog	Cat
Isoproterenol (continued)	1 mg in 250 mL D$_5$W at 0.01 µg/kg per minute; IV **OR**	Same
	0.04 to 0.08 µg/kg per minute; IV	0.5 mg in 250 mL D$_5$W; IV to effect
Isotretinoin	1 to 3 mg/kg per day; PO	Same
Itraconazole	2.5 mg/kg bid to 5 mg/kg once daily; PO **OR**	10 mg/kg per day; PO **OR**
	5 mg/kg bid; PO for 60 days (blastomycosis) **OR**	50 mg/day cats <3.2 kg and 100 mg/day cats >3.2 kg minimum 2 months beyond clinical remission (*Cryptococcus*)
	5 to 10 mg/kg bid **OR** 10 mg/kg once daily; PO	10 mg/kg once daily; PO for 4 to 6 months (pulmonary mycoses)
Ivermectin	50 to 200 µg/kg once; PO (microfilaricide)	200 µg/kg; SC (*Otodectes cynotis*)
	6 to 12 µg/kg once monthly; PO (heartworm prevention)	400 µg/kg; SC (*Notoedres cati* and *Cheyletiella*)
Kanamycin	10 to 12 mg/kg qid; PO	Same
	5 to 7.5 mg/kg bid; IM, SC	Same
	4 to 6 mg/kg qid; IM, SC	Same
Kaolin-pectin	1 to 2 mL/kg q 2 to 6 hours; PO	Same
Ketamine hydrochloride	5.5 to 22 mg/kg; IV, IM with adjunctive sedative or tranquilizer	11 mg/kg; IM (restraint)
		22 to 33 mg/kg; IM **OR**
		2.2 to 4.4 mg/kg; IV (anesthesia)
		0.5 to 1.0 mg/kg; IM
		1.0 to 4.0 mg/kg; IV (analgesia; lasts 30 minutes)

Drug	Dog	Cat
Ketoconazole	10 to 40 mg/kg per day or divided bid; PO (fungal disease) 5 to 10 mg/kg once to twice daily (dermatophyte)	10 mg/kg once to twice daily; PO
Ketoprofen	2 mg/kg; IM, IV, SC on day 1 then continue 1 mg/kg; once daily; PO for 4 days For more severe cases give 2 mg/kg; IM, IV, SC once daily for 3 days	Same
	2 mg/kg initially; PO, then 1 mg/kg per day (chronic pain)	Same
Ketorolac	0.5 mg/kg tid up to 48 hours; IM or slowly IV; dose can be increased to 0.75 mg/kg if pain persists—if pain relief persists beyond 8 to 12 hours decrease dose by 50% 0.5 mg/kg tid; PO 0.3 to 0.5 mg/kg bid to tid for 1 to 2 treatments; IV, IM (surgical pain) Dogs 20 to 30 kg: 5 mg bid; PO for 6 treatments Dogs >30 kg: 10 mg bid; PO for 6 treatments (panosteitis)	0.25 mg/kg bid; IM, dose can be increased to 0.5 mg/kg in cases of severe pain 0.25 mg/kg bid-tid; IM for 1 to 2 treatments
Lactulose	0.5 mL/kg tid; PO (hepatic encephalopathy) 1 mL/4.5 kg tid; PO (constipation)	2.5 to 5 mL/cat tid; PO (hepatic encephalopathy) Same

Drug	Dog	Cat
Levamisole	10 mg/kg once daily for 6 to 10 days; PO (microfilaricide) 0.5 to 2 mg/kg 3 times weekly; PO (immunostimulant)	20 to 40 mg/kg qod for 5 to 6 treatments; PO (lungworm) 25 mg qod for 3 treatments; PO (plasma cell gingivitis)
Levothyroxine (T$_4$)	22 µg/kg bid; PO **OR** 0.02 mg/kg bid; PO **OR** 0.5 mg/m^2 daily; PO	20 to 30 µg/kg per day; PO once daily or divided bid **OR** 0.1 to 0.2 mg/day; PO
Lidocaine	2 to 4 mg/kg over 1 to 2 minutes; IV **OR** 25 to 80 µg/kg per minute; IV infusion	0.25 to 0.75 mg/kg; slowly IV (with caution) **OR** 10 to 40 µg/kg per minute; IV infusion 15 mg/kg topically [ELA-Max]
Lincomycin	15 mg/kg tid; PO 10 mg/kg bid; IM, IV	Same
Liothyroxine (T$_3$)	4 to 6 µg/kg tid; PO	4.4 µg/kg bid to tid; PO
Lisinopril	0.5 mg/kg once to twice daily; PO	0.25 to 0.5 mg/kg per day; PO
Lithium	10 mg/kg bid; PO	None
Lomustine	60 mg/m^2 initially; if no toxicity noted increase to 80 mg/m^2 every 5 to 8 weeks; PO (brain tumors) 90 mg/m^2 every 3 weeks (lymphoma and mast cell tumors)	50 to 60 mg/m^2 every 6 weeks; PO
Loperamide	0.08 mg/kg tid; PO	0.1 to 0.3 mg/kg once to twice daily; PO (with caution)
Magnesium hydroxide	5 to 30 mL once to twice daily; PO (antacid) 3 to 5 times antacid dose (cathartic)	5 to 15 mL once to twice daily; PO (antacid) Same

Drug	Dog	Cat
Magnesium sulfate	2 g (in 250 to 500 mL) over 1 to 2 hours; IV **OR** 300 mg qid for 7 to 10 days; PO (mild deficiency) 2 to 4 g (in 250 to 500 mL) over 4 to 6 hours; IV (moderate) 2 g in (20 mL) over 2 minutes, then 2 g (in 100 mL) over 20 minutes, then 2 to 4 g (in 250 mL) over 2 to 4 hours; IV (severe)	Unknown
Mannitol	1 to 2 g/kg q 6 hours; IV (20% solution)	Same
	0.25 to 2 g/kg; IV over 20 minutes; repeat q 3 to 8 hours for a maximum of three doses over 24 hours (25% solution) [head trauma]	Same
Marbofloxacin	2.75 to 5.55 mg/kg per day; PO for 2 to 3 days beyond remission of clinical signs	None
Mebendazole	22 mg/kg once daily for 3 days; PO (with food)	None
Meclofenamic acid	1.1 mg/kg daily for 5 to 7 days; PO. Maintain dose if effective. If signs worsen give 1.1 mg/kg q 3rd day for 7 days; if still effective give q 4th day, then q 5th day etc. until signs recur	None

Drug	Dog	Cat
Medetomidine	750 µg; IV **OR** 100 µg; IM per m^2 **OR** 30 to 40 µg/kg; IM (maximum of 50 µg/kg)	80 to 110 µg/kg; IM (maximum of 120 µg/kg)
Medium-chain triglyceride (MCT) oil	1 to 2 mL/kg per day; PO (in food)	None
Medroxyproges-terone acetate	20 mg/kg once; IM repeat in 3 to 6 months if needed (skin conditions) 10 mg/kg PRN; IM, SC (behavioral conditions)	50 to 100 mg once; IM repeat in 3 to 6 months if needed (skin conditions) 10 to 20 mg/kg PRN; SC (behavioral conditions)
Megestrol acetate	1 mg/kg per day; PO (skin conditions) 0.5 mg/kg per day for 8 days; PO (pseudocyesis) 2 to 4 mg/kg once daily; PO; reduce to half dose at 8 days (behavioral conditions)	5 to 10 mg qod; PO for 10 to 14 treatments, then every 2nd week (eosinophilic ulcers) 2.5 mg once daily for 10 days, then qod for 5 treatments, then PRN; PO (plasma cell gingivitis)
Melarsomine	2.5 mg/kg; IM twice 24 hours apart via deep lumbar injection (L$_3$ to L$_5$ only)	None
Meloxicam	0.2 mg/kg on day 1; PO then 0.1 mg/kg per day	Same for 2 to 3 days
Melphalan	1.5 mg/m^2 once daily for 7 to 10 days, then no treatment for 2 to 3 weeks **OR** 0.05 to 0.1 mg/kg once daily; PO	Same Same
Meperidine	5 to 10 mg/kg PRN; IM	1 to 4 mg/kg; IM (with caution)

Drug	Dog	Cat
Mercaptopurine	50 mg/m² once daily; PO **OR** 2 mg/kg once daily; PO	None
Meropenem	20 mg/kg tid; IV **OR** 40 mg/kg tid; IV (meningitis) 8 mg/kg bid; SC (infection)	Unknown
Metamucil	2 to 10 g once to twice daily (in moistened food)	2 to 4 g once to twice daily (in moistened food)
Methenamine mandelate	10 mg/kg qid; PO	None
Methimazole	None	2.5 mg bid to tid; PO
Methionine	0.2 to 1 g tid; PO	0.2 to 1 g once daily; PO
Methocarbamol	For relief of moderate conditions: 44 mg/kg; IV For controlling severe effects of strychnine and tetanus 55 to 220 mg/kg; IV; give half dose rapidly, wait until relaxation occurs and continue (not to exceed 330 mg/kg per day)	Same
	Initially 132 mg/kg per day divided bid to tid; PO, then 61 to 132 mg/kg divided bid to tid; PO. If no response in 5 days discontinue	Same
	15 to 20 mg/kg tid; PO (for muscle relaxation of intervertebral disc disease)	Unknown
Methohexital	11 mg/kg slowly; IV giving ½ rapidly and titrating to effect	Same **OR** With premeds give 5.5 to 6.6 mg/kg; IV, 10% to 30% given

Drug	Dog	Cat
Methohexital (continued)	**OR** With premeds 5 mg/kg, give 1/2 to 3/4ths over 10 minutes	rapidly IV, then remainder to effect
Methotrexate	2.5 mg/m^2 daily; PO (neoplasia) 5 mg/m^2 on days 1 and 5 of a weekly maintenance schedule (lymphoma)	2.5 mg/m^2 2 to 3 times weekly; PO **OR** 0.3 to 0.8 mg/m^2 q 7 days; IV (neoplasia) 2.5 to 5 mg/m^2 2 to 3 times per week; PO (lymphoma)
Methoxyflurane	Induction: 3% Maintenance: 0.5 to 1.5%	Same
Methylene blue	8.8 mg/kg (1% solution); slowly IV; repeat PRN 100 to 300 mg daily; PO (methemoglobinemia)	Same
Methylphenidate hydrochloride	5 to 10 mg bid to tid; PO (narcolepsy) 2 to 4 mg/kg PRN; PO (hyperkinesis)	None
Methylprednisolone sodium succinate	30 to 35 mg/kg; IV (shock)	Unknown
	30 mg/kg; IV, then 15 mg/kg; IV 2 hours later, then 10 mg/kg; IV, SC for 2 days, then taper dose over 5 to 7 days (spinal trauma)	Same
	Initially 30 mg/kg; IV, then 15 mg/kg; IV at 2 and 6 hours, then 2.5 mg/kg per hour for 42 hours (head trauma) **OR**	Same

Drug	Dog	Cat
Methylprednisolone sodium succinate (continued)	30 mg/kg; IV bolus followed by 5.4 mg/kg per hour infusion for 23 hours (spinal trauma)	
Metoclopramide	0.2 to 0.5 mg/kg tid; PO, SC **OR** 1 to 2 mg/kg per day; IV infusion (antiemetic)	0.2 to 0.5 mg/kg tid; PO, SC (GIT motility disorders, esophageal reflux)
Metoprolol	5 to 50 mg tid; PO	2.5 to 5 mg tid; PO
Metronidazole	25 to 65 mg/kg once daily for 5 days; PO **OR** 25 mg/kg bid; PO for 5 days (giardiasis)	10 mg/kg bid; PO **OR** 25 mg/kg once daily; PO for 5 days (inflammatory bowel disease) 12 to 25 mg/kg bid; PO for 5 days (giardiasis)
Mexiletine	4 to 10 mg/kg tid; PO	Unknown
Mibolerone	1 to 11 kg, 30 µg/day; PO 12 to 22 kg, 60 µg/day; PO 23 to 45 kg, 120 µg/day; PO >45 kg, 180 µg/day; PO (estrus prevention)	None
Midazolam	0.066 to 0.22 mg/kg; IM, IV (preoperative agent) **OR** 0.1 mg/kg; IV	Same Unknown
Milbemycin	Up to 4.5 kg, 2.3 mg 5 to 11 kg, 5.75 mg 12 to 22 kg, 11.5 mg 23 to 45 kg, 23 mg	None
Mineral oil	5 to 30 mL; PO **OR** 1 to 2 mL/kg per rectum	5 to 20 mL bid; PO **OR** per rectum

Drug	Dog	Cat
Minocycline	5 to 15 mg/kg bid; PO	Same
Misoprostol	2 to 5 µg/kg bid to tid; PO	Unknown
Mitotane	40 to 50 mg/kg per day for 7 to 10 days, then once weekly; PO	None
Mitoxantrone	5 mg/m² once q 3 weeks; IV	2.5 to 6.5 mg/m² q 3 weeks; IV
Morphine sulfate	0.5 to 1 mg/kg PRN; IM, SC 0.05 to 0.4 mg/kg q 1 to 4 hours; IV **OR** 0.2 to 1 mg/kg q 2 to 6 hours; IM, SC 0.3 to 3 mg/kg q 4 to 8 hours; PO **OR** 0.3 to 3 mg/kg bid to tid; PO (slow-release)	0.05 to 0.1 mg/kg PRN; IM, SC (with caution) **OR** 0.05 to 0.2 mg/kg q 2 to 6 hours; IM, SC
Nafcillin	10 mg/kg qid; PO, IM	Same
Naloxone	0.04 mg/kg; IM, IV, SC (opioid reversal)	0.05 to 0.1 mg/kg; IV (opioid reversal)
Naltrexone	2 to 5 mg once daily **OR** 1 to 2.2 mg/kg bid to tid; PO	25 to 50 mg/cat per day; PO
Nandrolone decanoate	1 to 5 mg/kg per week; IM (maximum of 200 mg/week) (anabolic effect)	Same (anabolic effect) 10 to 20 mg/week; IM (marrow stimulant)
Neomycin	2.5 to 10 mg/kg bid to qid; PO **OR** 20 mg/kg bid to tid; PO 3.5 mg/kg tid; IM, IV, SC	Same Same Same
Neostigmine	0.5 mg/kg bid to tid; PO (myasthenia gravis) 1 to 2 mg PRN; IM 5 to 15 mg PRN; PO	None

Drug	Dog	Cat
Nitrofurantoin	4 mg/kg tid to qid; PO	Same
Nitroglycerin ointment	1/4th to 1 inch tid to qid; topically	1/8th to 1/4th inch tid to qid; topically
Nitroprusside	1 to 10 µg/kg per minute; IV infusion	Same
Nitroscanate	50 mg/kg; PO	Same
Nizatidine	2.5 to 5 mg/kg per day; PO	Same
Norfloxacin	22 mg/kg bid; PO	Same **OR** 5 mg/kg bid; PO (urinary tract infection)
Novobiocin	10 mg/kg tid; PO	Unknown
Nystatin	100,000 U qid; PO	Same
Olsalazine	10 to 20 mg/kg tid; PO **OR** 11 mg/kg bid; PO	None
Omeprazole	0.7 mg/kg once daily; PO **OR** >20 kg, 1 capsule (20 mg) daily; PO <20 kg, 1/2 capsule (10 mg) daily; PO <5 kg, 1/4th capsule (5 mg) daily; PO	Same
Ondansetron	0.1 mg/kg; IV bid to tid **OR** 0.5 to 1 mg/kg; PO **OR** 0.5 mg/kg loading dose; IV followed by 0.5 mg/kg per hour infusion for 6 hours	0.1 to 0.2 mg/kg tid; SC 0.1 to 1.0 mg/kg once daily to bid; PO Same
Orbifloxacin	2.5 mg/kg once daily; PO **NB:** dose may be increased to 7.5 mg/kg once daily; PO if required	Same
Oxacillin	15 to 25 mg/kg tid to qid; PO 8.8 to 20 mg/kg q 4 to 6 hours; IM, IV	Same

Drug	Dog	Cat
Oxazepam	0.2 to 1 mg/kg once to twice daily; PO (behavioral problems)	0.2 to 0.5 mg/kg once to twice daily; PO (appetite stimulant)
Oxtriphylline	14 mg/kg tid to qid; PO **OR** 30 mg/kg bid; PO (sustained-release)	6 mg/kg bid to tid; PO
Oxybutynin	5 mg bid to tid; PO	1 mg/kg bid; PO
Oxyglobin	30 mL/kg to10 mL/kg per hour; once; IV	Unknown
Oxymetholone	1 mg/kg once to twice daily; PO	Same
Oxymorphone	0.05 to 0.1 mg/kg; IM, IV **OR** 0.1 to 0.2 mg/kg; IM, SC (sedation) 0.02 to 0.1 mg/kg q 2 to 4 hours; IV (analgesia) 0.05 to 0.2 mg/kg q 2 to 6 hours; IM, SC (analgesia)	0.02 mg/kg. IV (with caution) **OR** 0.05 to 0.2 mg/kg; IV, IM (analgesia; lasts 2 to 5 hours)
Oxytetracycline	22 mg/kg tid; PO 7 to 12 mg bid; IM, IV	Same **OR** 25 mg/kg tid; PO (*Hemobartonella*) Same
Oxytocin	5 to 20 U; IM once (uterine prolapse) 5 to 20 U; IM or IV infusion, may repeat in 30 to 60 minutes (uterine inertia) Spray intranasally 5 to 10 minutes prior to nursing (stimulate milk letdown)	5 U; IM once (uterine prolapse) 2.5 to 5 U; IM or IV infusion (uterine inertia)
Pancuronium	0.1 mg/kg; IV **OR** 0.03 mg/kg; IV with methoxyflurane 0.06 mg/kg; IV with halothane	0.044 to 0.11 mg/kg; IV (higher dose used initially; lower doses if drug repeated)

Drug	Dog	Cat
Pantaprozole	1 mg/kg per day; slow IV over 15 minutes (maximum of 30 mg/dog)	Unknown
Paroxetine	2.5 to 5 mg/day per dog; PO	Same
Penicillamine	15 mg/kg bid; PO (cystine urolithiasis) 10 to 15 mg/kg bid; PO (copper hepatopathy) 33 to 100 mg/kg per day divided qid for 7 days, wait 7 days, repeat; PO (lead poisoning)	None
Penicillin G (aqueous) Potassium	20,000 U/kg q 4 hours; IM, IV, SC 40,000 U/kg qid; PO	Same
Sodium	20,000 U/kg q 4 hours; IM, IV, SC 40,000 U/kg qid; PO	Same
Penicillin G (procaine)	20,000 U/kg once to twice daily; IM, SC	Same
Penicillin V	10 mg/kg tid; PO	Same
Pentastarch (10%)	10 to 20 mL/kg per day over 1 to 24 hours as indicated for up to 3 days	5 to 10 mL/kg per day over 1 to 24 hours as indicated for up to 3 days
Pentazocine	0.2 to 0.5 mg/kg PRN; IM **OR** 1 to 3 mg/kg q 30 minutes to 3 hours; IM, IV (analgesia)	2.2 to 3.3 mg/kg; IM, IV, SC (with caution) 2 to 3 mg/kg; IM, IV, SC (analgesia; lasts 2 to 4 hours)
Pentobarbital	2 to 4 mg/kg; IV (sedation) 10 to 30 mg/kg; IV (anesthesia)	Same 25 mg/kg; IV (anesthesia)

Drug	Dog	Cat
Pentoxifylline	10 mg/kg bid; PO (skin) **OR** 10 mg/kg bid to tid; PO **OR** 15 mg/kg tid; PO	100 mg/cat bid to tid; PO
Phenobarbital grain = 65 mg	1 to 2 mg/kg bid; PO [may require up to 16 mg/kg per day] (seizures) 3 to 30 mg/kg; IV to effect (status epilepticus) 2.2 mg/kg bid; PO (irritable colon)	1/8th to 1/4th grain once to twice daily; PO (seizures) 6 mg/kg bid to qid; IM, IV (status epilepticus) 1 mg/kg bid; PO (sedation)
Phenoxybenzamine	5 to 15 mg once daily; PO **OR** 2.5 to 30 mg tid; PO (urinary incontinence)	0.5 mg/kg once daily; PO **OR** 0.25 mg/kg tid; PO (urinary incontinence)
Phenylbutazone	15 to 22 mg/kg bid to tid; PO (maximum of 800 mg/day)	None
Phenylpropanolamine	12.5 to 50 mg tid; PO **OR** 1 mg/kg tid; PO (urinary incontinence) 1 to 2 mg/kg bid; PO (decongestant)	12.5 mg tid; PO (urinary incontinence) Same (decongestant)
Phenytoin	15 to 40 mg/kg tid; PO (seizure) 2 to 4 mg/kg in increments, up to 10 mg/kg total dose; IV (arrhythmias) 6 mg/kg bid to tid; PO (tumor-induced hypoglycemia)	None
Phosphate enemas (Fleet)	1 to 2 mL/kg (medium to large dogs)	None
Pimobendan	0.2 to 0.6 mg/kg per day; PO	Unknown
Piperazine	100 mg/kg; PO, repeat in 3 weeks	Same

Drug	Dog	Cat
Piroxicam	0.3 mg/kg q 48 hours; PO (degenerative joint disease/pain)	None
Plicamycin	25 µg/kg; IV (hypercalcemia)	Unknown
Polysulfated gly-cosaminoglycans [Adequan]	4.4 mg/kg twice weekly; IM (maximum of 8 injections) **OR** 5 mg/kg q 3 to 5 days; IM (repeated 5 to 10 times)	Unknown
Potassium chloride	0.5 mEq/kg per day; not to exceed 0.5 mEq/kg per hour 1 to 3 g/day; PO, IV **OR** 0.1 to 0.25 mL/kg tid; PO (dilute with water 1:1) 1.5 to 2 mEq/kg; IV (chemical defibrillation)	Same 0.2 g/day; PO
Potassium citrate	100 to 150 mg/kg per day; PO (calcium oxalate urolithiasis)	Unknown
Potassium gluconate	2.2 mEq/100 kcal of energy per day; PO **OR** 5 mEq bid to tid; PO (Kaon elixir)	Same **OR** 5 to 10 mEq divided bid to tid; PO (severe cases); decrease to 4 to 6 mEq/day with clinical improvement; 2 to 4 mEq/day; PO (maintenance) (Kaon elixir) 5 to 8 mEq once to twice daily; PO (Tumil-K)
Potassium iodide	40 mg/kg tid; PO	20 mg/kg bid; PO (with food)

Drug	Dog	Cat
Potassium iodide (continued)		**OR** 30 to 100 mg/cat daily for 10 to 14 days
Potassium phosphate	0.01 to 0.03 mmol/kg per hour; IV for 6 hours	Same **OR** 0.011 to 0.017 mmol/kg per hour for 6 to 12 hours; IV
Praziquantel	1/2 tablet per 2.5 kg; PO (maximum of 5 tablets)	Up to 1.8 kg, 1/2 tablet; PO 2.3 to 5 kg, 1 tablet; PO >5 kg, 1½ tablets; PO
Prazosin	1 mg/15 kg tid; PO 0.1 mg/kg per day divided into 3 doses; PO (detrusor-urethral dyssynergia)	0.03 mg/kg; IV in combination with dantrolene (1 mg/kg) (urethral obstruction)
Prednisolone and Prednisone	0.2 to 0.4 mg/kg once daily to qod; PO (hypoadrenocortical maintenance)	Same
	0.5 mg/kg bid; PO, IM (allergy)	1 mg/kg bid; PO, IM (allergy)
	2 to 4 mg/kg per day; PO, IM (immunosuppression)	3 mg/kg bid; PO, IM (immunosuppression)
	0.5 mg/kg bid to tid; PO, IM (allergic bronchitis)	Same
	0.5 to 1 mg/kg per day; PO (pulmonary eosinophilic infiltrates)	Same
	0.5 to 1.5 mg/kg per day divided bid; PO, taper over 3 months (eosinophilic gastritis)	Same
	1 to 3 mg/kg once daily; PO, taper to qod (eosinophilic enteritis, colitis)	Same

Drug	Dog	Cat
Prednisolone and Prednisone (continued)	1 mg/kg bid; PO (plasmacytic/lymphocytic enteritis)	Same
		2.5 to 5 mg once daily to every other day; PO (urethritis, hematuria)
	1 to 4 mg/kg per day divided bid; PO (immune hemolytic anemia)	Same
	2 to 3 mg/kg bid; PO (hypercalcemia)	Same
	Initially 10 to 30 mg/kg followed by gradually tapering doses q 6 to 8 hours (head trauma)	Same
	1.1 mg/kg q 48 hours (pruritus)	2.2 mg/kg q 48 hours (pruritus)
Prednisolone sodium succinate	11 to 25 mg/kg; IV (shock)	Same
	2 to 4 mg/kg; IV, IM (allergic bronchitis, asthma)	1 to 3 mg/kg; IV, IM (allergic bronchitis, asthma)
Primidone	11 to 22 mg/kg tid; PO	Same
Procainamide	6 to 8 mg/kg over 5 minutes; IV, then 25 to 40 µg/kg per minute **OR**	7.5 to 15 mg/kg; IM 62.5 mg/cat tid; PO (sustained-release)
	6 to 20 mg/kg q 4 to 6 hours; IM	
	8 to 20 mg/kg qid; PO (regular tablets or caplets)	
	25 to 50 mg/kg tid; PO **OR**	
	8 to 20 mg/kg tid to qid; PO (sustained-release)	
Prochlorperazine	0.13 mg/kg qid; IM **OR** 0.1 to 0.5 mg/kg tid to qid; IM, SC	0.13 mg/kg bid; IM Same
	1 mg/kg bid; PO	0.5 mg/kg tid to qid; PO

Drug	Dog	Cat
Propantheline bromide	Small dogs: 7.5 mg tid; PO Medium dogs: 15 mg tid; PO Large dogs: 30 mg tid; PO	7.5 mg tid to every 3rd day; PO
Propionibacterium acnes	<7 kg, 0.25 to 0.5 mL; IV 6.8 to 20 kg, 0.5 to 1 mL; IV 20 to 34 kg, 1 to 1.5 mL; IV >34 kg, 1.5 to 2 mL; IV given 4 times in first 2 weeks at 3 to 4 day intervals, followed by 1 injection/week until signs abate or stabilize; maintenance dose once/month	2 injections (0.5 mL) weekly; IV for 2 weeks, followed by 1 injection/week for 20 weeks or until cat tests negative by IFA and ELISA (FeLV-associated disease)
Propofol	6 mg/kg; IV slowly (induction without premedication) 10 mg (1 mL)/10 to 25 kg to maintain anesthesia **OR** 0.4 to 0.8 mg/kg per minute if anesthesia >15 minutes	Same
Propranolol	0.02 to 0.06 mg/kg over 2 to 3 minutes; IV 0.2 mg/kg tid; PO (arrhythmias) 2.5 to 10 mg bid to tid; PO (systemic hypertension)	0.25 to 0.5 mg; slowly IV followed by 2.5 to 5 mg tid; PO (arrhythmias) 2.5 to 5 mg bid to tid; PO (systemic hypertension)
Prostaglandin $F_{2\alpha}$	0.25 mg/kg once daily; SC for 5 days (pyometra)	0.1 to 0.25 mg/kg once to twice daily; SC for 3 to 5 days (pyometra)

Drug	Dog	Cat
Protamine sulfate	1 mg for q 100 IU heparin used; given over 60 minutes as IV infusion	Same
Pseudoephedrine	15 to 30 mg bid to tid; PO (urinary incontinence) 15 to 50 mg tid; PO (decongestant)	Unknown 2 to 4 mg/kg bid to tid; PO (decongestant)
Pyrantel pamoate	5 mg/kg orally after a meal; repeat in 7 to 10 days	10 mg/kg; PO, repeat in 3 weeks **OR** 5 mg/kg; PO, repeat in 2 weeks
Pyridostigmine bromide	0.5 to 3 mg/kg bid to tid; PO	1 to 5 mg; IV (administer anticholinergic first)
Pyrimethamine	1 mg/kg per day for 14 to 28 days; PO (5 days only for *Neosporum caninum*) **OR** 0.25 to 0.5 mg/kg bid for 2 weeks; PO (toxoplasmosis and *Neospora caninum*)	0.5 to 1 mg/kg per day for 14 to 28 days; PO
Quinacrine	100 mg tid; PO **OR** 6.6 mg/kg bid; PO for 5 days (*Giardia*)	10 mg/kg once daily; PO **OR** 2.3 mg/kg per day; PO for 12 days (*Giardia*)
Quinidine	6 to 16 mg/kg tid to qid; PO, IM	4 to 8 mg/kg tid; IM
Ranitidine	1 to 2 mg/kg bid; PO **OR** 0.5 mg/kg bid; PO, IV, SC	3.5 mg/kg bid; PO 2.5 mg/kg bid; IV
Rifampin	10 to 20 mg/kg bid; PO	Same
S-Adenosylmethionine	18 mg/kg per day; PO	Same
Selamectin	6 mg/kg topically to skin once a month 6 to 24 mg/kg q 2 weeks over 6-week period (nasal mites)	Same

Drug	Dog	Cat
Selegiline	1 to 2 mg/kg per day; PO (pituitary-dependent hyper-adrenocorticism) 0.5 mg/kg once daily; PO (age-related behavior disorders)	Unknown
Sevoflurane	2.36 %/vol (MAC)	2.58 %/vol (MAC)
Sodium bicarbonate	10 to 15 mg/kg tid; PO (renal failure)	Same
	0.5 to 1 mEq/kg; IV (acidosis)	Same
Sodium chloride (0.9% solution)	40 to 50 mL/kg per day; IV, SC, IP	Same
Sodium iodide	20 to 40 mg/kg bid to tid; PO for 4 to 6 weeks	20 mg/kg per day; PO for 4 to 6 weeks
Sodium polystyrene sulfonate	8 to 15 g tid; PO	Unknown
Sotalol	1 to 2 mg/kg bid; PO **OR** Start with 40 mg and increase to 80 mg if needed	1 to 2 mg/kg bid; PO
Spironolactone	1 to 2 mg/kg bid; PO	Same
Stanozolol	2 to 10 mg bid; PO, IM	1 to 2 mg bid; PO
Succimer	10 mg/kg tid; PO for 8 to 10 days	Given rectally if vomiting or orally at 10 mg/kg tid; PO for 10 days or more
Sucralfate	0.5 to 1 g bid to tid; PO **OR** 1 g/30 kg qid; PO	0.25 g bid to tid; PO **OR** 0.25 to 0.5 g bid to tid; PO
Sulfadimethoxine	25 mg/kg once to twice daily; PO, IM, IV, SC	Same
Sulfadimethoxine ormetoprim	Day 1: 55 mg/kg, then 27.5 mg/kg once daily for a maximum of 21 days; PO	None

Drug	Dog	Cat
Sulfasalazine	10 to 30 mg/kg bid to tid; PO	10 to 20 mg/kg q 8 to 24 hours for a maximum of 10 days
Sulfentanil	2 µg/kg; IV to a maximum dose of 5 µg/kg	Unknown
Tacrolimus	Apply topically bid	Unknown
Taurine	See Drug Descriptions	250 to 500 mg bid; PO
Tepoxalin	10 or 20 mg/kg; PO on 1st day, then 10 mg/kg per day; PO	None
Terbutaline	2.5 mg/dog tid; PO, SC	1.25 mg bid; PO **OR** 0.625 mg bid; PO, SC **OR** 0.01 mg/kg; SC, IM
Testosterone (methyl)	1 to 2 mg/kg once daily; PO (maximum of 30 mg/day) [anabolic effects]	Same
(cypionate)	2.2 mg/kg once q 30 days; IM	Unknown
(propionate)	2 mg/kg 3 times/week; IM, SC (urinary incontinence)	5 to 10 mg; IM (urinary incontinence)
Tetracycline	25 to 50 mg/kg tid to qid; PO **OR** 22 mg/kg tid; PO 7 mg/kg bid; IM, IV	Same
Thenium closylate	2.3 to 4.5 kg: 250 mg bid for 2 treatments; PO **OR** >4.5 kg: 500 mg once; PO, repeat in 3 weeks (maximum of 110 mg/kg)	None

Drug	Dog	Cat
Theophylline	6 to 11 mg/kg tid to qid; PO, IM, IV 9 mg/kg tid to qid; PO	4 mg/kg bid to tid; PO 0.1 mg/kg tid; IM, IV 4 mg/kg bid to tid; PO
Thiabendazole	50 mg/kg once daily for 3 days; PO, repeat in 1 month	None
Thiamine (vitamin B₁)	1 to 2 mg/kg; IM 2 mg/kg once daily; PO	Same 4 mg/kg once daily; PO
Thioguanine	40 mg/m² per day; PO for 4 to 5 days, then q 3rd day thereafter	25 mg/m² per day; PO for 1 to 5 days then repeat q 30 days PRN
Thiopental sodium	25 to 30 mg/kg; IV (to effect) 22 mg/kg; IV (after tranquilization) 11 mg/kg; IV (after narcotic premed)	Same
Ticarcillin	40 to 75 mg/kg tid to qid; IM, IV	Same
Ticarcillin/clavulanate	30 to 50 mg/kg tid to qid; IV	Same
Tiletamine-zolazepam	9.9 to 13.2 mg/kg; IM (minor procedures) 6.6 to 9.9 mg/kg; IM (diagnostic procedures) 6 to 13 mg/kg; IM (surgery lasting 30 to 60 minutes)	9.7 to 11.9 mg/kg; IM (minor procedures) 10.6 to 12.5 mg/kg; IM (castration, lacerations) Same 14.3 to 15.8 mg/kg; IM (spay, declaw)
Tobramycin	1 mg/kg tid; IM, IV, SC	2 mg/kg tid; SC
Tocainide	10 to 20 mg/kg tid; PO	None
Triamcinolone	0.05 mg/kg bid to tid; PO (anti-inflammatory) 0.88 mg/kg q 48 hours; PO (pruritus) 0.015% spray applied to skin bid for 1 week, then once daily for 1 week, then q other day for 2 weeks (pruritus)	0.25 to 0.5 mg/kg once daily for 7 days; PO

Drug	Dog	Cat
Triamterene	1 to 2 mg/kg bid; PO	Unknown
Trilostane	6.25 to 7.2 mg/kg; PO	None
Trimeprazine	1.1 to 4.4 mg/kg qid; PO	Same
Trimethoprim-sulfadiazine	15 to 30 mg/kg bid; PO, SC, IV	Same
Tylosin	5 to 15 mg/kg tid to qid; IM, IV	Same
	5 to 10 mg/kg bid to tid; PO **OR** 20 to 40 mg/kg bid; PO	Same
Ursodiol	4 to 15 mg/kg per day; PO	Same **OR** 10 to 15 mg/kg once daily; PO
Valproic acid	60 mg/kg tid; PO **OR** 75 to 200 mg/kg tid; PO **OR** 25 to 105 mg/kg per day; PO if used with phenobarbital	Unknown
Vasopressin (aqueous)	10 units PRN; IV, IM	Same
Vedaprofen	0.5 mg/kg once daily; PO	None
Verapamil	10 to 15 mg/kg per day divided bid to tid; PO	None
	0.05 to 0.15 mg/kg; slow IV	
	2 to 10 µg/kg per minute; IV infusion	
Vinblastine	2 mg/m^2 q 7 to 14 days; IV	Same
Vincristine	0.5 to 0.75 mg/m^2 q 7 to 14 days; IV (neoplasia)	0.5 to 0.75 mg/m^2 once weekly; IV
	0.02 mg/kg once weekly; IV (immune thrombocytopenia)	
Vitamin E	100 to 400 IU bid; PO	Same

Drug	Dog	Cat
Vitamin K₁	2 to 5 mg/kg per day divided bid; SC **OR** 2 to 3 mg/kg per day divided tid for 5 to 7 days; PO, then 1 mg/kg divided tid for 4 to 6 weeks; PO **OR** Loading dose of 2.5 to 5 mg/kg followed by 5 mg/kg per day divided into 2 or 3 administrations; PO	Same
Warfarin	0.1 to 0.2 mg/kg once daily; PO	0.25 to 0.5 mg once daily; PO
Xylazine	0.1 mg/kg; IV 1.1 to 2.2 mg/kg; IM, SC 0.6 mg/kg; IV, IM (sedative)	Same 0.05 to 0.2 mg/kg; IV, IM (analgesia; lasts 15 to 30 minutes) 0.44 mg/kg; IM (emetic)
Zidovudine (AZT)	None	5 to 15 mg/kg bid; PO
Zinc acetate	5 to 10 mg/kg bid; PO **OR** 100 mg bid; PO for 3 months then 50 mg bid; PO	Unknown
Zinc sulfate	220 mg once to twice daily; PO (zinc responsive dermatoses) 5 to 10 mg/kg bid; PO **OR** 2 mg/kg per day; PO (hepatic copper toxicosis)	None

Handbook of Veterinary Drugs, Third Edition, edited by Dana Allen,
Lippincott Williams & Wilkins, Baltimore. © 2005

Section 2

Antimicrobial and Antiparasitic Agents in Dogs and Cats

TABLE 2-1 **Antimicrobial Agents in Dogs and Cats**

Organism	Drug(s) of Choice	Alternative Drug(s)
Anaerobic organisms *Actinomyces* sp.	Chloramphenicol Clindamycin Penicillin	Cefoxitin
Anaerobic cocci	Penicillin	Cephalosporin (1st generation) Chloramphenicol Clindamycin
Bacteroides fragilis	Cefoxitin Chloramphenicol Clavamox Metronidazole	Ampicillin Clindamycin
Bacteroides sp.	Chloramphenicol Clavamox Metronidazole Penicillin G	Ampicillin Cefoxitin Clindamycin
Clostridium *perfringens*	Cephalosporins Chloramphenicol Penicillin	Clindamycin Erythromycin Metronidazole *(continued)*

Organism	Drug(s) of Choice	Alternative Drug(s)
Clostridium sp.	Ampicillin Chloramphenicol Metronidazole Clavamox	Clindamycin
Fusobacterium sp.	Chloramphenicol Clavamox Clindamycin Ampicillin Metronidazole	
Babesia	Imidocarb diproprionate	Clindamycin Metronidazole
Bacillus anthracis	Ampicillin Penicillin G	Cephalothin Chlortetracycline Erythromycin Oxytetracycline
Bartonella sp.	Erythromycin Azithromycin	Enrofloxacin Doxycycline
Bordetella bronchiseptica	Trimethoprim- sulfamethoxazole Enrofloxacin Doxycycline	Amikacin Chloramphenicol Gentamicin Tetracycline Tobramycin
Brucella canis	Minocycline-gentamicin	Trimethoprim- sulfamethoxazole
Campylobacter	Erythromycin	Chloramphenicol Gentamicin Neomycin Clindamycin
Chlamydia psittaci	Tetracyclines	Chloramphenicol Erythromycin Rifampin
Coccidia	Sulfonamides	Amprolium
Corynebacterium sp.	Penicillin G	Erythromycin Tetracycline
Cytauxzoon felis	Imidocarb diproprionate	

Dermatophytosis
    Microsporum
    Trichophyton
	Griseofulvin	Itraconazole

Ehrlichia	Doxycycline Minocycline	Chloramphenicol Imidocarb dipropionate

Organism	Drug(s) of Choice	Alternative Drug(s)
Escherichia coli Urinary tract Infections (UTIs)	Ampicillin Trimethoprim-sulfa Enrofloxacin	Cephalosporins Chloramphenicol Nitrofurantoin Sulfonamides Tetracyclines
Other infections	Ampicillin Chloramphenicol Tetracyclines	Aminoglycosides Polymyxin Fluoroquinolones Cephalosporin (3rd generation)
Giardia	Albendazole Fenbendazole	Metronidazole Quinicrine
Hemobartonella (see Mycoplasma)		

Hepatozoon
americanum
	Trimethoprim-sulfa +
	  clindamycin + pyri-
	  methamine, followed
	  by decoquinate
		Toltrazuril

Klebsiella/Enterobacter	Gentamicin Kanamycin Cephalosporin (1st generation) Enrofloxacin	Cephalosporins Chloramphenicol
Leptospira	Penicillin G	Doxycycline
Lyme borreliosis	Ampicillin Tetracycline	Doxycycline Cephalexin Chloramphenicol

Malassezia canis	Cuprimyxin
	2% "tame" iodine or
	  25% glyceryl tri-
	  acetate topically
		Itraconazole
		Ketoconazole

Mycobacterium	Isoniazid with rifampin +
	  enrofloxacin or
	  clarithromycin	

Atypical mycobacteria *M. fortuitum* and *M. chelonei*	Aminoglycosides Doxycycline Enrofloxacin Clofazimine Chloramphenicol	

(*continued*)

Organism	Drug(s) of Choice	Alternative Drug(s)
Mycoplasma	Chloramphenicol Erythromycin Tetracycline Enrofloxacin	
Mycoplasma hemofelis (formerly *Hemobartonella felis*)	Tetracyclines	Chloramphenicol
Mycoplasma haemocanis (formerly *Hemobartonella canis*)	Doxycycline Oxytetracycline	Amoxicillin
Mycotic disease *Aspergillus* *Blastomyces* *Candida* *Coccidioides* *Cryptococcus* Sporotrichosis	Amphotericin B ± Itraconazole Clotrimazole (nasal aspergillosis) Sodium or potassium iodide (sporotrichosis)	Flucytosine (*Candida, Cryptococcus*) Ketoconazole Thiabendazole (*Aspergillus*) Fluconazole
Neorickettsia	Chloramphenicol Chlortetracycline Oxytetracycline Penicillin Sulfonamides	Ampicillin with erythromycin
Neospora caninum	Clindamycin	Pyrimethamine + a sulfonamide
Nocardia	Sulfonamides + ampicillin or Trimethoprim-sulfa	Ampicillin + erythromycin Amikacin Minocycline
Pasteurella multocida	Penicillin G	Ampicillin Tetracyclines Trimethoprim-sulfamethoxazole
Pentatrichomonas	Metronidazole	
Proteus mirabilis	Ampicillin Cephalexin Nitrofurantoin (UTI only) Enrofloxacin	Chloramphenicol Trimethoprim-sulfamethoxazole
Pseudomonas	Gentamicin + Ticarcillin or carbenicillin	Chloramphenicol Fluoroquinolones

Organism	Drug(s) of Choice	Alternative Drug(s)
	Ceftazidime Enrofloxacin Tetracycline Tobramycin	Carbenicillin Ticarcillin Trimethoprim-sulfa
Salmonella sp.	Trimethoprim- sulfamethoxazole	Ampicillin Cephalosporin (3rd generation) Chloramphenicol Fluoroquinolones
Staphylococcus aureus	Penicillin G-sensitive Penicillin G	Ampicillin Cephalosporin (1st generation)
	Penicillin G-resistant Cephalosporin (1st generation) Cloxacillin	Cephalosporins Chloramphenicol
Staphylococcus intermedius	Clavamox Trimethoprim-sulfa Ormetoprim-sulfa Chloramphenicol Lincomycin Erythromycin Cephalosporins Enrofloxacin	Aminoglycoside Vancomycin
Streptococcus	Penicillin G Ampicillin Amoxicillin	Ampicillin/amoxicillin Cephalosporins Erythromycin Chloramphenicol Trimethoprim-sulfa
Toxoplasmosis	Clindamycin	Pyrimethamine + sulfonamide
Yersinia enterocolitica	Trimethoprim- sulfamethoxazole	Ampicillin Tetracycline

TABLE 2-2   **Suggested Antimicrobial Treatment Pending Culture**

Condition	Bacteria	Antibiotic Choices
Bacteremia Septicemia	AEROBIC BACTERIA *Staphylococcus*	AEROBIC BACTERIA Aminoglycoside + a penicillin or cephalosporin
Endotoxemia	*Streptococcus* *Escherichia coli (E. coli)* *Klebsiella* *Enterobacter* *Pseudomonas*	
	ANAEROBIC BACTERIA *Clostridium* *Bacteroides*	ANAEROBIC BACTERIA Penicillin Chloramphenicol Clindamycin Metronidazole Cefoxitin Moxalactam
		EMPIRIC CHOICES Cefazolin/Amikacin Cefazolin/Gentamicin Ampicillin/Amikacin Ampicillin/Gentamicin Enrofloxacin/Clindamycin Enrofloxacin/Ampicillin 3rd-generation cephalosporin
Bacterial endocarditis	*Staphylococcus* *E. coli* β-Hemolytic streptococci	Ampicillin + gentamicin, cephalosporins, or fluoroquinolones
Dentistry; in those with preexisting valvular heart disease	*Staphylococcus* *Streptococcus* Facultative bacteria Anaerobes	Ampicillin Amoxicillin Penicillin G Clindamycin
Soft tissue infection	Dogs: *Staphylococcus*	*Staphylococcus:* Cefazolin Cefadroxil Ormetroprim-sulfa
	Cats: *Pasteurella*	*Pasteurella:* Penicillin G Ampicillin

Condition	Bacteria	Antibiotic Choices
		Tetracycline Trimethoprim-sulfa
		Bacteroides: Clavamox
Contaminated wounds, including bite wounds	*Streptococcus* *Pasteurella* Penicillinase-producing staphylococci	Clavamox Oxacillin Dicloxacillin Cephalosporins Tetracyclines Trimethoprim-sulfa Enrofloxacin
		POLYMICROBIAL AEROBIC AND ANAEROBIC INFECTION: Enrofloxacin + metronidazole
Burns	*Pseudomonas* *Staphylococcus* *Proteus* *Klebsiella* *Candida* spp.	Systemic drugs: Aminoglycosides Oxacillin Dicloxacillin Clavamox Fluoroquinolones
		Topical creams: Silver sulfadiazine Polymyxin-neomycin-bacitracin Gentamicin
Gingivitis-stomatitis	Anaerobes	Clindamycin Metronidazole Tetracycline Clavamox
Gastrointestinal tract bacterial overgrowth	Mixed population Anaerobes	Tetracyclines Trimethoprim-sulfa Tylosin and/or metronidazole
Severe gastroenteritis	Aerobic and anaerobic bacteria	Ampicillin or cephalothin ± aminoglycoside Penicillin G (HGE) Metronidazole Fluoroquinolones Trimethoprim-sulfa

(continued)

Condition	Bacteria	Antibiotic Choices
Gastroduodenal surgery	Gram-positive cocci Enteric gram-negative bacilli	Cefazolin Ampicillin
Colorectal surgery	Enteric gram-negative bacilli Anaerobes	Metronidazole + enrofloxacin or ciprofloxacin Oral neomycin + erythromycin
Hepatobiliary infections	*E. coli* *Clostridium* spp. *Staphylococcus* *Pasteurella*	Chloramphenicol Cefoxitin Cephalothin Metronidazole Kanamycin Gentamicin Ampicillin Amoxicillin Tetracyclines (dog)
Upper respiratory infections	Difficult to interpret because of abundant normal flora	Ampicillin Clavamox Cephalosporin Chloramphenicol *Chlamydia:* Tetracycline
Lower respiratory infections	Dog: *E. coli* *Klebsiella* *Pasteurella* *Pseudomonas* *Bordetella* *Strep. zooepidemicus* Cat: *Bordetella* *Pasteurella*	General: Amikacin Ceftizoxime Enrofloxacin Gentamicin Gram-positives: Cephalexin Trimethoprim-sulfa Clavamox Amoxicillin Ampicillin Anaerobes: Ampicillin Clavamox Chloramphenicol Clindamycin Metronidazole

Condition	Bacteria	Antibiotic Choices
		Mycoplasma: Erythromycin Tylosin Chloramphenicol Tetracycline Fluoroquinolones
		Bordetella: Enrofloxacin Chloramphenicol Doxycycline Trimethoprim-sulfa Aminoglycosides Cephalexin Clavamox
		Pyothorax: Ampicillin Cephalothin Chloramphenicol Trimethoprim-sulfa
Urinary tract infection	*E. coli* *Proteus* *Klebsiella* *Pseudomonas* *Enterobacter* *S. aureus* β-Streptococci	Ampicillin Clavamox Cephalosporins Trimethoprim-sulfa Sulfa-ormetoprim Fluoroquinolones
		Recurrent gram-negative infection: Trimethoprim-sulfa Enrofloxacin Cephalexin
		Recurrent gram-positive infection: Ampicillin
		Pyelonephritis: Chloramphenicol Trimethoprim-sulfa Enrofloxacin Norfloxacin
		Fungal and yeast: Fluconazole

(continued)

Condition	Bacteria	Antibiotic Choices
		Itraconazole Amphotericin B
Prostatitis	*E. coli* *Proteus* sp. *Staphylococcus* *Streptococcus*	Gram-positive: Erythromycin Clindamycin Chloramphenicol Fluoroquinolones
		Gram-negative: Trimethoprim-sulfa Chloramphenicol Enrofloxacin Norfloxacin
Vaginitis	*E. coli* *Proteus* *Staphylococcus* *Streptococcus*	Chloramphenicol Amoxicillin Lincomycin
Pyometra and metritis	*E. coli* *Proteus* *Streptococcus*	Chloramphenicol Trimethoprim-sulfa Fluoroquinolones
Intraocular infection	*Chlamydia* *Mycoplasma*	Chloramphenicol
	Gram-positive	Sulfacetamide Neomycin-polymyxin- bacitracin
	Gram-negative	Gentamicin Polymyxin
Central nervous system (CNS) infection		Chloramphenicol Trimethoprim-sulfa Metronidazole Fluoroquinolones Cefotaxime Ceftazidime
		Inflammation allowing entry into CNS by: Minocycline Doxycycline Erythromycin
Dermatologic infections	*Staphylococcus*	Trimethoprim-sulfa Ormetoprim-sulfa Chloramphenicol Dicloxacillin

Condition	Bacteria	Antibiotic Choices
		Oxacillin Clavamox Cephalosporins Erythromycin Lincomycin Fluoroquinolones
Osteomyelitis	*Staphylococcus* *Streptococcus* *E. coli* *Proteus* *Pseudomonas*	Gram-positive: Cephalosporins Clavamox Imipenem
		Gram-negative: Gentamicin Amikacin Fluoroquinolones
		Penicillinase-producing staphylococci: Oxacillin Cloxacillin Clavamox
		Acute infection: Oxacillin + gentamicin
		Anaerobes: Penicillins or 3rd-generation cephalosporins with clindamycin
Orthopedic surgery	*Staphylococcus*	Cefazolin
Mixed or unknown infection	Mixed and/or unknown	Clindamycin + enrofloxacin or imipenem
Neutropenia	Aminoglycoside + 1st-generation cephalosporin Aminoglycoside + ampicillin	Enrofloxacin + 1st-generation cephalosporin Enrofloxacin + ampicillin

TABLE 2-3 **Antiparasitics in Dogs and Cats**

Drug	Ancylostoma spp.	Uncinaria stenocephala	Toxascaris leonina	Toxocara canis	Toxocara cati	Trichuris vulpis	Dipylidium spp.	Taenia spp.	Echinococcus granulosus	Echinococcus multilocularis	Mesocestoides spp.	Dirofilaria immitis	Ctenocephalides spp.	Demodex canis	Otodectes spp.	Sarcoptes scabei	Aedes aegypti (mosquitoes)	Dermacentor variabilis	Rhipicephalus sanguineus	Ixodes scapularis	Amblyomma americanum
Amitraz (Mitaban)														D							
Amitraz (Preventic collar)																D		D	D		
Diethylcarbamazine citrate (Filaribits)			D	D								D									
Diethylcarbamazine citrate/oxibendazole (Filaribits Plus)	D		D	D		D						D									
Epsiprantel (Cestex)							C,D	C,D													
Fenbendazole (Panacur)	D	D	D	D		D		D													
Fipronil (Frontline)													C,D					C,D	C,D	C,D	C,D
Fipronil/methoprene (Frontline Plus)													C,D					C,D	C,D	C,D	C,D

Ticks: Dermacentor variabilis, Rhipicephalus sanguineus, Ixodes scapularis, Amblyomma americanum

Drug (trade name)								
Imidacloprid (Advantage)					C,D		D	D	D D
Imidacloprid/Permethrin (K9 Advantix)					D		D	D	D D
Ivermectin (Heartgard)	C,D				C,D				
Ivermectin/pyrantel (Heartgard Plus)	D	D			D				
Lufenuron (Program)	C	C			C				
Lufenuron/Milbemycin (Sentinel)	C	C			C				
Melarsomine (Immiticide)					D				
Milbemycin (Interceptor)	D	D			C,D		D	D	D D
Moxidectin (ProHeart6)	C,D	D			C,D				
Nitenpyram (Capstar)					C,D				
Nitroscanate (Lopatol)	D	D	D	D	D		D	D	
Permethrin (Defend Exspot, ProTICall)	D						D	D	
Piperazine	C,D	C,D							
Piperazine/Dichlorophene	D	D	C,D	C,D					
Praziquantel (Droncit)	C	C	C	C					
Praziquantel/Pyrantel pamoate (Drontal)	C		D	D	D	D			
Praziquantel/Pyrantel pamoate/Febantel (Drontal Plus)	D	D	D	D	D				
Pyrantel pamoate (Pyr-a-pam)	C,D	D	C,D						
Pyrantel pamoate and oxantel pamoate (Pyr-a-pam Plus)	D	D	D						
Pyrethrins	C,D	C,D	C,D	C,D	C,D	C,D			
Selamectin (Revolution)	C	D	C,D	C,D	D	D	C,D	C,D	D

C = cats; D = dogs.

TABLE 2-4 **Analgesics for Acute Pain in Dogs and Cats**[a]

Drug	Dog Dose	Cat Dose	Duration of Action or Dosing Interval	Relative Potency
Moderate to severe pain				
Morphine (use low end of the dose for moderate pain)	0.3 to 1.0 mg/kg; IM, SC For IV dosing use half the low-end dose, administer over 5 minutes (histamine release)	0.1 to 0.2 mg/kg; IM, SC	2 to 6 hours IM, SC 1 to 4 hours IV	1
Morphine, sustained release (oral)	2 to 5 mg/kg	NA	12 hours	
Oxymorphone	0.05 to 0.2 mg/kg; IV, IM	0.02 to 0.1 mg/kg; IV, IM	2 to 6 hours	10
Hydromorphone (use low end of the dose for moderate pain)	0.08 to 0.3 mg/kg; IV, IM, SC	0.08 to 0.3 mg/kg; IV, IM, SC	2 to 6 hours	10 to 15
Fentanyl (use low end of the dose for moderate pain)	0.001 to 0.01 mg/kg	0.001 to 0.01 mg/kg	0.3 hours	100
Ketamine (use low end of the dose for moderate pain)	1 to 4 mg/kg; IV 2 to 10 mg/kg; PO	1 to 4 mg/kg; IV 2 to 10 mg/kg; PO	As needed (~0.5 hours)	

Mild to moderate pain

Butorphanol	0.1 to 0.4 mg/kg; IV 0.1 to 0.4 mg/kg; IM, SC	0.1 to 0.4 mg/kg; IV 0.4 to 0.8 mg/kg; IM, SC	0.25 to 1.0 hours IV 2 to 4 hours for cat IM 1 to 2(3) hours for dog IM	3 to 5
Butorphanol, oral	0.5 to 2 mg/kg; PO	0.5 to 1 mg/kg; PO	6 to 8 hours	
Buprenorphine	0.005 to 0.02 mg/kg; IV, IM	0.005 to 0.01 mg/kg; IV, IM	4 to 8 hours	25
Meperidine (pethidine)	5 to 10 mg/kg; IM, SC	5 to 10 mg/kg; IM, SC	0.3 to 0.5 hours	0.1

Reprinted with permission from Mathews KA. Pain assessment and general approach to management. Vet Clin North Am [Small Anim Pract]
2000;30:729–755.

NA = Not applicable.

[a]Opioids should be given to effect even beyond dosing and frequency noted.

TABLE 2-5 **Analgesics for Chronic Pain (>5 days) in Dogs and Cats**[a]

Drug	Dog Dose	Duration of Action or Dosing Interval for Dogs	Cat Dose	Duration of Action or Dosing Interval for Cats
Fentanyl patch	≤10 kg: 25 µg/hour 10 to 20 kg: 50 µg/hour 20 to 30 kg: 75 µg/hour >30 kg: 100 µg/hour	As needed up to q 3 days	≤10 kg: 25 µg/hour	As needed up to q 5 days
Meloxicam (Metacam)	≤0.2 mg/kg; PO, then ≤0.1 mg/kg	Once, then q 12 to 24 hours	≤0.2 to 0.3 mg/kg; SC, PO then ≤0.1 mg/kg; PO ≤0.025 mg/kg; PO	Once daily for 3 days, then 2 to 3 times weekly
Carprofen (Rimadyl)	≤2 to 4 mg/kg; PO, then ≤2.2 mg/kg; PO	Once, then q 24 or 12 hours (if needed)	NA	
Etodolac (Etogesic)	≤10 to 15 mg/kg; PO	Once daily	NA	
Tolfenamic acid (Tolfedine)	≤4.0 mg/kg; PO	Every 24 hours for 4 days, then 3 days off and repeat cycle	≤4.0 mg/kg; PO	Every 24 hours for 4 days, then 3 days off, and repeat cycle

	Dogs		Cats	
Morphine syrup	≤0.5 mg/kg; PO	Every 4 to 6 hours	≤0.5 mg/kg; PO	Every 4 to 6 hours
Deracoxib (Deramaxx)	1 to 2 mg/kg; 3 to 4 mg/kg (<7 days)	Once daily; Once daily for ≤7 days	NA	
Tepoxalin (Zubrin)	10 to 20 mg/kg; PO, then 10 mg/kg; PO	Once, then Every 24 hours	NA	
Aspirin	10 mg/kg; PO	Every 8 hours	≤10 mg/kg; PO	Every 72 hours
Corticosteroids	1 to 2 mg/kg; Not in combination with NSAIDs	Every 24 hours with reduced daily dose based on the underlying disease	1 to 2 mg/kg; Not in combination with NSAIDs	Every 24 hours with reduced daily dose based on the underlying disease

Reprinted with permission from Mathews KA. Pain assessment and general approach to management. Vet Clin North Am [Small Anim Pract] 2000;30:729–755.

NA = not applicable.

[a]Manufacturer's recommendations are used for polysulfated glycosaminoglycans, glucosamine chondroitin sulfate, and shark or bovine cartilage.

CHEMOTHERAPY PROTOCOLS FOR DOGS

CANINE LYMPHOSARCOMA
Doxorubicin

Single-agent doxorubicin (Adriamycin) 30 mg/m^2 (or 1 mg/kg for dogs < 10 kg); IV q 21 days for a total of 4 to 6 treatments

Postorino NC, Susaneck SJ, Withrow SJ et al: Single agent therapy with adriamycin for canine lymphosarcoma. J Am Anim Hosp Assoc 1989;25:221–225.

COP Protocols

(**C**ytoxan [cyclophosphamide], **O**ncovin [vincristine], **P**rednisone)

These protocols are generally of two types: frequent low doses or infrequent high-dose blasts, both with the same drugs.

COP (1)

Cyclophosphamide 300 mg/m^2; PO once q 3 weeks (nearest 25 mg on the low side of 300 mg/m^2)

Vincristine 0.75 mg/m^2; IV once weekly for 4 weeks, then once q 3 weeks with cyclophosphamide

Prednisone 1 mg/kg per day; PO for 22 days, then every other day

Week 1:	Vincristine 0.75 mg/m^2; IV
	Cyclophosphamide 300 mg/m^2; PO
	Prednisone 1 mg/kg; PO q 24 hours
Week 2:	Vincristine 0.75 mg/m^2; IV
	Prednisone 1 mg/kg; PO q 24 hours
Week 3:	Vincristine 0.75 mg/m^2; IV
	Prednisone 1 mg/kg; PO q 24 hours
Week 4:	Vincristine 0.75 mg/m^2; IV
	Cyclophosphamide 300 mg/m^2; PO
	Prednisone 1 mg/kg; PO q 48 hours
Week 7:	Vincristine 0.75 mg/m^2; IV
	Cyclophosphamide 300 mg/m^2; PO
	Prednisone 1 mg/kg; PO q 48 hours
Week 10:	Vincristine 0.75 mg/m^2; IV
	Cyclophosphamide 300 mg/m^2; PO
	Prednisone 1 mg/kg; PO q 48 hours

Continue every 3 weeks to week 52, then every 4 weeks for an additional 6 months.

If hemorrhagic cystitis occurs, chlorambucil at a dose of 0.6 mg/kg PO is substituted on the same schedule for cyclophosphamide.

Cotter SM. Treatment of lymphoma and leukaemia with cyclophosphamide, vincristine, and prednisone: I. Treatment of dog. J Am Anim Hosp Assoc 1983;19:159–165.

COP (2)

Vincristine 0.5 mg/m^2; IV once weekly for 8 weeks, then every other week (EOW) for maintenance

Cyclophosphamide 50 mg/m^2; PO for 4 consecutive days or every other day for 8 weeks, then EOW
Prednisone 10 mg/m^2; PO q 12 hours for 1 week, then 10 mg/m^2 daily

Week 1:	Vincristine 0.5 mg/m^2; IV
	Cyclophosphamide 50 mg/m^2; PO for 4 consecutive days
	Prednisone 10 mg/m^2; PO q 12 hours
Week 2:	Vincristine 0.5 mg/m^2; IV
	Cyclophosphamide 50 mg/m^2; PO for 4 consecutive days
	Prednisone 10 mg/m^2; PO q 24 hours
Week 3:	Vincristine 0.5 mg/m^2; IV
	Cyclophosphamide 50 mg/m^2; PO for 4 consecutive days
	Prednisone 10 mg/m^2; PO q 24 hours
Week 4:	Vincristine 0.5 mg/m^2; IV
	Cyclophosphamide 50 mg/m^2; PO for 4 consecutive days
	Prednisone 10 mg/m^2; PO q 24 hours
Week 5:	Vincristine 0.5 mg/m^2; IV
	Cyclophosphamide 50 mg/m^2; PO for 4 consecutive days
	Prednisone 10 mg/m^2; PO q 24 hours
Week 6:	Vincristine 0.5 mg/m^2; IV
	Cyclophosphamide 50 mg/m^2; PO for 4 consecutive days
	Prednisone 10 mg/m^2; PO q 24 hours
Week 7:	Vincristine 0.5 mg/m^2; IV
	Cyclophosphamide 50 mg/m^2; PO for 4 consecutive days
	Prednisone 10 mg/m^2; PO q 24 hours
Week 8:	Vincristine 0.5 mg/m^2; IV
	Cyclophosphamide 50 mg/m^2; PO for 4 consecutive days
	Prednisone 10 mg/m^2; PO q 24 hours

Cycle is repeated every 2 weeks to week 24; then every 3 weeks to week 48; and then every 4 weeks.
Chlorambucil 2 mg/m^2; PO is substituted for cyclophosphamide on the same schedule from week 8.
Madewell BR. Chemotherapy for canine lymphosarcoma. Am J Vet Res 1975;36:1525–1528.

COAP

(**C**ytoxan [cyclophosphamide], **O**ncovin [vincristine], cytosine **A**rabinoside, **P**rednisone)
Vincristine 0.5 mg/m^2; IV once weekly for 8 weeks, then every other week (EOW) for maintenance
Cyclophosphamide 50 mg/m^2; PO every other day for 8 weeks, then EOW
Prednisone 20 mg/m^2; PO q 12 hours for 1 week, then 10 mg/m^2 q 12 hours every other day for 7 weeks
Cytosine arabinoside 100 mg/m^2; IV q 24 hours for first 4 days

Week 1:	Vincristine 0.5 mg/m^2; IV
	Cyclophosphamide 50 mg/m^2; PO q 48 hours

Cytosine arabinoside 100 mg/m²; IV q 24 hours for 4 days
Prednisone 20 mg/m²; PO q 12 hours

Week 2:   Vincristine 0.5 mg/m²; IV
Cyclophosphamide 50 mg/m²; PO q 48 hours
Prednisone 10 mg/m²; PO q 12 hours every other day

Week 3:   Vincristine 0.5 mg/m²; IV
Cyclophosphamide 50 mg/m²; PO q 48 hours
Prednisone 10 mg/m²; PO q 12 hours every other day

Week 4:   Vincristine 0.5 mg/m²; IV
Cyclophosphamide 50 mg/m²; PO q 48 hours
Prednisone 10 mg/m² hours PO q 12 every other day

Week 5:   Vincristine 0.5 mg/m²; IV
Cyclophosphamide 50 mg/m²; PO q 48 hours
Prednisone 10 mg/m²; PO q 12 hours every other day

Week 6:   Vincristine 0.5 mg/m²; IV
Cyclophosphamide 50 mg/m²; PO q 48 hours
Prednisone 10 mg/m²; PO q 12 hours every other day

Week 7:   Vincristine 0.5 mg/m²; IV
Cyclophosphamide 50 mg/m²; PO q 48 hours
Prednisone 10 mg/m²; PO q 12 hours every other day

Week 8:   Vincristine 0.5 mg/m²; IV
Cyclophosphamide 50 mg/m²; PO q 48 hours
Prednisone 10 mg/m²; PO q 12 hours every other day

Cycle is repeated every 2 weeks to week 24; then every 3 weeks to week 48. Treatment is discontinued at week 48.

Chlorambucil 2 mg/m²; PO on days 1 and 4 of each week is substituted for cyclophosphamide starting with week 9.

Theilen GH, Worley M, Benjamini E. Chemoimmunotherapy for canine lymphosarcoma. J Am Vet Med Assoc 1977;170:607–610.

COPA

(**C**ytoxan [cyclophosphamide], **O**ncovin [vincristine], **P**rednisone, **A**driamycin [doxorubicin])

Vincristine 0.75 mg/m²; IV once weekly for 4 weeks, then once every 3 weeks with either cyclophosphamide or doxorubicin

Cyclophosphamide 300 mg/m²; PO once every 3 to 6 weeks (nearest 25 mg on the low side of 300 mg/m²)

Doxorubicin 30 mg/m²; IV in place of every third cyclophosphamide (i.e., every 9 weeks starting at week 7)

Prednisone 1 mg/kg per day PO for 22 days, then every other day

Week 1:   Vincristine 0.75 mg/m²; IV
Cyclophosphamide 300 mg/m²; PO
Prednisone 1 mg/kg; PO q 24 hours

Week 2:   Vincristine 0.75 mg/m²; IV
Prednisone 1 mg/kg; PO q 24 hours

Week 3: Vincristine 0.75 mg/m^2; IV
         Prednisone 1 mg/kg; PO q 24 hours
Week 4: Vincristine 0.75 mg/m^2; IV
         Cyclophosphamide 300 mg/m^2; PO
         Prednisone 1 mg/kg; PO q 48 hours
Week 7: Vincristine 0.75 mg/m^2; IV
         Doxorubicin 30 mg/m^2; IV
         Prednisone 1 mg/kg; PO q 48 hours
Week 10: Vincristine 0.75 mg/m^2; IV
         Cyclophosphamide 300 mg/m^2; PO
         Prednisone 1 mg/kg; PO q 48 hours
Week 13: Vincristine 0.75 mg/m^2; IV
         Cyclophosphamide 300 mg/m^2; PO
         Prednisone 1 mg/kg; PO q 48 hours
Week 16: Vincristine 0.75 mg/m^2; IV
         Doxorubicin 30 mg/m^2; IV
         Prednisone 1 mg/kg; PO q 48 hours

For weeks 19 to 52, treatments are continued every 3 weeks repeating the week 10 to week 16 cycle 4 times. After week 52, treatments are continued every 4 weeks repeating the week 10 to week 16 cycle twice. At week 78, treatment is discontinued.

If hemorrhagic cystitis occurs, chlorambucil at a dose of 0.8 mg/kg; PO is substituted on the same schedule for cyclophosphamide.

Cotter SM, Goldstein MA. Comparison of two protocols for maintenance of remission of dogs in lymphoma. J Am Anim Hosp Assoc 1987;23:495–499.

ACOPA

(L-**A**sparginase, **C**ytoxan [cyclophosphamide], **O**ncovin [vincristine], **P**rednisone, **A**driamycin [doxorubicin])

L-Asparginase 10,000 IU/m^2; IM once weekly for 4 weeks (maximum dose 10,000 IU per administration)

Vincristine 0.75 mg/m^2; IV once weekly for 4 weeks, then once q 3 weeks with cyclophosphamide or doxorubicin

Cyclophosphamide 250 mg/m^2; PO once q 3 to 6 weeks (nearest 25 mg on the low side of 250 mg/m^2) starting at week 7

Doxorubicin 30 mg/m^2; IV q 9 weeks in place of cyclophosphamide starting at week 10

Prednisone 1 mg/kg per day; PO for 22 days, then every other day

Week 1: L-Asparaginase 10,000 IU/m^2; IM
         Vincristine 0.75 mg/m^2; IV
         Prednisone 1 mg/kg; PO q 24 hours
Week 2: L-Asparaginase 10,000 IU/m^2; IM
         Vincristine 0.75 mg/m^2; IV
         Prednisone 1 mg/kg; PO q 24 hours

Week 3:   L-Asparaginase 10,000 IU/m^2; IM
           Vincristine 0.75 mg/m^2; IV
           Prednisone 1 mg/kg; PO q 24 hours
Week 4:   L-Asparaginase 10,000 IU/m^2; IM
           Vincristine 0.75 mg/m^2; IV
           Prednisone 1 mg/kg; PO q 48 hours
Week 7:   Vincristine 0.75 mg/m^2; IV
           Cyclophosphamide 250 mg/m^2; PO
           Prednisone 1 mg/kg; PO q 48 hours
Week 10:   Vincristine 0.75 mg/m^2; IV
           Doxorubicin 30 mg/m^2; IV
           Prednisone 1 mg/kg; PO q 48 hours
Week 13:   Vincristine 0.75 mg/m^2; IV
           Cyclophosphamide 250 mg/m^2; PO
           Prednisone 1 mg/kg; PO q 48 hours
Week 16:   Vincristine 0.75 mg/m^2; IV
           Cyclophosphamide 250 mg/m^2; PO
           Prednisone 1 mg/kg; PO q 48 hours
Week 10:   Vincristine 0.75 mg/m^2; IV
           Doxorubicin 30 mg/m^2; IV
           Prednisone 1 mg/kg; PO q 48 hours
Week 13:   Vincristine 0.75 mg/m^2; IV
           Cyclophosphamide 250 mg/m^2; PO
           Prednisone 1 mg/kg; PO q 48 hours
Week 22:   Vincristine 0.75 mg/m^2; IV
           Doxorubicin 30 mg/m^2; IV
           Prednisone 1 mg/kg; PO q 48 hours
Week 25:   Vincristine 0.75 mg/m^2; IV
           Cyclophosphamide 250 mg/m^2; PO
           Prednisone 1 mg/kg; PO q 48 hours
Week 28:   Vincristine 0.75 mg/m^2; IV
           Doxorubicin 30 mg/m^2; IV
           Prednisone 1 mg/kg; PO q 48 hours

For weeks 31 to 49, treatments are continued every 3 weeks as shown in weeks 13 through 28. For weeks 52 to 68, treatments are continued every 4 weeks as shown in weeks 16 through 28. Week 78 treatment is the same as week 13 treatment, and then therapy is discontinued.

If hemorrhagic cystitis occurs, chlorambucil at a dose of 15 mg/m^2; PO daily for 4 days, is substituted on the same schedule.

Stone MS, Goldstein MA, Cotter SM. Comparison of two protocols for induction of remission in dogs with lymphoma. J Am Anim Hosp Assoc 1991;27:315–321.

AMC Protocol (L-VCMP)

(**L**-Asparginase, **V**incristine, **C**ytoxan [cyclophosphamide], **M**ethotrexate, **P**rednisone)

L-Asparginase 400 IU/kg; IP/IM (maximum dose 10,000 IU per administration)
Vincristine 0.7 mg/m^2; PO every other week
Cyclophosphamide 200 to 250 mg/m^2; IV
Methotrexate 0.6 to 0.8 mg/kg; PO

Week 1:	L-Asparginase 400 IU/kg; IP/IM
	Vincristine 0.7 mg/m^2; IV
	Prednisone 2 mg/kg; PO q 24 hours
Week 2:	Cyclophosphamide 200 to 250 mg/m^2; IV
	Prednisone 1.5 mg/kg; PO q 24 hours
Week 3:	Vincristine 0.7 mg/m^2; IV
	Prednisone 1.0 mg/kg; PO q 24 hours
Week 4:	Methotrexate 0.6 to 0.8 mg/kg; IV
	Prednisone 0.5 mg/kg; PO q 24 hours

Repeat except for L-asparginase on a weekly to biweekly cycle.

After complete response achieved, chlorambucil (1.4 mg/kg; PO) is substituted for cyclophosphamide.

MacEwen EG, Hayes AA, Matus RE, et al. Evaluation of some prognostic factors for advanced multicentric lymphosarcoma in the dog: 147 cases (1978–1981). J Am Vet Med Assoc 1987;190:564–568.

Current Veterinary Therapy (CVT) X Protocol (L-VCAMP)

(**L**-Asparginase, **V**incristine, **C**ytoxan [cyclophosphamide], **A**driamycin [doxorubicin], **M**ethotrexate, **P**rednisone)

Week 1:	Vincristine 0.7 mg/m^2; IV
	L-Asparginase 400 IU/kg; IP (maximum dose 10,000 IU per administration)
	Prednisone 30 mg/m^2; PO q 24 hours
Week 2:	Cyclophosphamide 200 mg/m^2; IV
	Prednisone 20 mg/m^2; PO q 24 hours
Week 3:	Doxorubicin 30 mg/m^2; IV
	Prednisone 10 mg/m^2; PO q 24 hours
Week 4:	Vincristine 0.7 mg/m^2; IV
Week 5:	Cyclophosphamide 200 mg/m^2; IV
Week 6:	Doxorubicin 30 mg/m^2; IV
Week 8:	Vincristine 0.7 mg/m^2; IV
Week 10:	Cyclophosphamide 200 mg/m^2; IV
Week 12:	Vincristine 0.7 mg/m^2; IV
Week 14:	Methotrexate 0.5 mg/kg; IV

Treatment is continued every 2 weeks as above for weeks 8 to 14 for 12 months, then every 3 weeks for 6 months, then monthly for 6 months.

Matus RE. Chemotherapy of lymphoma and leukemia. In Kirk RW (ed): Current Veterinary Therapy X. Philadelphia: WB Saunders, 1989:482–488.

Madison-Wisconsin Protocol (L-VCAMP)

(**L**-Asparginase, **V**incristine, **C**ytoxan [cyclophosphamide], **A**driamycin [doxorubicin], **M**ethotrexate, **P**rednisone)

Week 1:   Vincristine 0.5 to 0.7 mg/m²; IV
          L-Asparginase 400 IU/kg; IM (maximum dose 10,000 IU per administration)
          Prednisone 2 mg/kg; PO q 24 hours
Week 2:   Cyclophosphamide 200 mg/m²; IV
          Prednisone 1.5 mg/kg; PO q 24 hours
Week 3:   Vincristine 0.5 to 0.7 mg/m²; IV
          Prednisone 1.0 mg/kg; PO q 24 hours
Week 4:   Doxorubicin 30 mg/m²; IV
          Prednisone 0.5 mg/kg; PO q 24 hours
Week 6:   Vincristine 0.5 to 0.7 mg/m²; IV
Week 7:   Cyclophosphamide 200 mg/m²; IV
Week 8:   Vincristine 0.5 to 0.7 mg/m²; IV
Week 9:   Doxorubicin 30 mg/m²; IV
Week 11: Vincristine 0.5 to 0.7 mg/m²; IV
Week 13: Chlorambucil 1.4 mg/kg; PO (if in CR), or Cyclophosphamide 200 mg/m²; IV (if not in CR)
Week 15: Vincristine 0.5 to 0.7 mg/m²; IV
Week 17: Methotrexate 0.5 to 0.8 mg/kg; IV
Week 19: Vincristine 0.5 to 0.7 mg/m²; IV
Week 21: Chlorambucil 1.4 mg/kg; PO, or Cyclophosphamide 200 mg/m²; IV (if not in CR)
Week 23: Vincristine 0.5 to 0.7 mg/m²; IV
Week 25: Doxorubicin 30 mg/m²; IV

Treatment is continued as above (Weeks 11 to 25) with 3-week interval between treatments until week 104, then treatment is discontinued if in complete remission.

Maximum dose of doxorubicin is 180 to 200 mg/m². Then, stop doxorubicin and continue methotrexate or substitute actinomycin-D 1.1 mg/m²; IV.

If hemorrhagic cystitis occurs, chlorambucil (1.4 mg/kg; PO) is substituted on the same schedule for cyclophosphamide.

Keller ET, MacEwen EG, Rosenthal RC: Evaluation of prognostic factors and sequential combination of chemotherapy with doxorubicin for canine lymphoma. J Vet Intern Med 1993;7:289–295.

Madison-Wisconsin Short Protocol (L-VCAP-Short)

(**L**-Asparginase, **V**incristine, **C**ytoxan [cyclophosphamide], **A**driamycin [doxorubicin], **P**rednisone)

Intensified Madison-Wisconsin dose protocol with increased cyclophosphamide dose (250 mg/m² compared to 200 mg/m²) and doxorubicin (37.5 mg/m²; IV, compared with 30 mg/m²; IV) with no crossover to chlorambucil or methotrexate; and no maintenance phase

Week 1:   Vincristine 0.7 mg/m^2; IV
          L-Asparginase 400 IU/kg; SC (maximum dose 10,000 IU
          per administration)
          Prednisone 2 mg/kg; PO q 24 hours
Week 2:   Cyclophosphamide 250 mg/m^2; IV
          Prednisone 1.5 mg/kg; PO q 24 hours
Week 3:   Vincristine 0.7 mg/m^2; IV
          Prednisone 1.0 mg/kg; PO q 24 hours
Week 4:   Doxorubicin 37.5 mg/m^2; IV
          Prednisone 0.5 mg/kg; PO q 24 hours
Week 6:   Vincristine 0.7 mg/m^2; IV
Week 7:   Cyclophosphamide 250 mg/m^2; IV
Week 8:   Vincristine 0.7 mg/m^2; IV
Week 9:   Doxorubicin 37.5 mg/m^2; IV
Week 11: Vincristine 0.7 mg/m^2; IV
Week 13: Cyclophosphamide 250 mg/m^2; IV
Week 15: Vincristine 0.7 mg/m^2; IV
Week 17: Doxorubicin 37.5 mg/m^2; IV
Week 19: Vincristine 0.7 mg/m^2; IV
Week 21: Cyclophosphamide 250 mg/m^2; IV
Week 23: Vincristine 0.7 mg/m^2; IV
Week 25: Doxorubicin 37.5 mg/m^2; IV

Treatment is discontinued after week 25 if in complete remission.
If hemorrhagic cystitis occurs, chlorambucil (1.4 mg/kg; PO) is substituted on the same schedule for cyclophosphamide.

Chun R, Garrett LD, Vail DM. Evaluation of a high-dose chemotherapy protocol with no maintenance therapy for dogs with lymphoma. J Vet Intern Med 2000;14:120–124.

VELCAP-L (Long) Protocol

(**V**incristine, **El**spar [L-asparginase], **C**ytoxan [cyclophosphamide],
Adriamycin [doxorubicin], **P**rednisone)

Week 1:   Vincristine 0.75 mg/m^2; IV
          Prednisone 40 mg/m^2; PO q 24 hours
Week 2:   Vincristine 0.75 mg/m^2; IV
          Doxorubicin 25 mg/m^2; IV
          Prednisone 40 mg/m^2; PO q 24 hours
Week 3:   Vincristine 0.75 mg/m^2; IV
          Prednisone 40 mg/m^2; PO q 48 hours
Week 4:   Doxorubicin 25 mg/m^2; IV
          Prednisone 40 mg/m^2; PO q 48 hours
Week 7:   Vincristine 0.75 mg/m^2; IV
          Cyclophosphamide 250 mg/m^2; PO
          L-Asparaginase 10,000 IU/m^2; IM (maximum dose 10,000 IU
          per administration)
          Prednisone 40 mg/m^2; PO q 48 hours

Week 8:   L-Asparaginase 10,000 IU/m²; IM
          Prednisone 40 mg/m²; PO q 48 hours
Week 9:   L-Asparaginase 10,000 IU/m²; IM
          Prednisone 40 mg/m²; PO q 48 hours
Week 12: Vincristine 0.75 mg/m²; IV
          Cyclophosphamide 250 mg/m²; PO
          Prednisone 40 mg/m²; PO q 48 hours
Week 15: Vincristine 0.75 mg/m²; IV
          Cyclophosphamide 250 mg/m²; PO
          Prednisone 40 mg/m²; PO q 48 hours
Week 18: Vincristine 0.75 mg/m²; IV
          Doxorubicin 25 mg/m²; IV
          Prednisone 40 mg/m²; PO q 48 hours
Week 21: Vincristine 0.75 mg/m²; IV
          Cyclophosphamide 250 mg/m²; PO
          Prednisone 40 mg/m²; PO q 48 hours
Week 24: Cyclophosphamide 250 mg/m²; PO
          L-Asparaginase 10,000 IU/m²; IM
          Prednisone 40 mg/m²; PO q 48 hours
Week 25: L-Asparaginase 10,000 IU/m²; IM
          Prednisone 40 mg/m²; PO q 48 hours
Week 27: Vincristine 0.75 mg/m²; IV
          Doxorubicin 25 mg/m²; IV
          Prednisone 40 mg/m²; PO q 48 hours

From week 30, repeat weeks 12 to 18 for 3 times to week 54, then treatments are given every 4 weeks to week 78.

If hemorrhagic cystitis occurs, chlorambucil (15 mg/m²; PO for 4 days) is substituted on the same schedule for cyclophosphamide.

Zemann BI, Moore AS, Rand WM, et al. A combination chemotherapy protocol (VELCAP-L) for dogs with lymphoma. J Vet Intern Med 1998;12:465–470.

VELCAP-S (Short) Protocol

Week 1:   Vincristine 0.75 mg/m²; IV
          Prednisone 40 mg/m²; PO q 24 hours
Week 2:   Vincristine 0.75 mg/m²; IV
          Doxorubicin 25 mg/m²; IV
          Prednisone 40 mg/m²; PO q 48 hours
Week 3:   Vincristine 0.75 mg/m²; IV
          Prednisone 40 mg/m²; PO q 48 hours
Week 4:   Doxorubicin 25 mg/m²; IV
          Prednisone 40 mg/m²; PO q 48 hours
Week 7:   Vincristine 0.75 mg/m²; IV
          Cyclophosphamide 250 mg/m²; PO
          L-Asparaginase 10,000 IU/m²; IM (maximum dose 10,000 IU
          per administration)

Prednisone 40 mg/m^2; PO q 48 hours
Week 8: L-Asparaginase 10,000 IU/m^2; IM
Prednisone 40 mg/m^2; PO q 48 hours
Week 9: L-Asparaginase 10,000 IU/m^2; IM
Prednisone 40 mg/m^2; PO q 48 hours
Week 12: Vincristine 0.75 mg/m^2; IV
Cyclophosphamide 250 mg/m^2; PO
Prednisone 40 mg/m^2; PO q 48 hours

Week 12 to 15 prednisone dose is decreased by half each week. Week 15 treatment is discontinued.

If hemorrhagic cystitis occurs, chlorambucil (15 mg/m^2; PO for 4 days) is substituted on the same schedule for cyclophosphamide.

Moore AS, Cotter SM, Rand WM, et al. Evaluation of a discontinuous treatment protocol (VELCAP-S) for canine lymphoma. J Vet Intern Med 2001;15:348–354.

COPA/LVP

(**C**ytoxan [cyclophosphamide], **O**ncovin [vincristine], **P**rednisone, **A**driamycin [doxorubicin])/**L**eukeran [Chlorambucil], **V**incristine, **P**rednisone)

Vincristine 0.5 mg/m^2; IV once weekly for 11 weeks, omitting weeks 6, 9, and 10; starting at week 13, every 3 weeks for 3 treatments; then every 4 weeks for 4 treatments; then every 6 weeks

Cyclophosphamide 50 mg/m^2; PO every other day for 8 weeks
Prednisone 20 mg/m^2; PO q 24 hours for 1 week, then every other day for 4 weeks, then 10 mg/m^2 every other day for 7 weeks

L-Asparginase 10,000 IU/m^2; SC week 1 and week 2
Doxorubicin 30 mg/m^2; IV on weeks 6, 9, and 12
Chlorambucil 4.0 mg/m^2; PO every other day starting at week 9

Week 1: Vincristine 0.5 mg/m^2; IV
Cyclophosphamide 50 mg/m^2; PO q 48 hours
L-Asparginase 10,000 IU/m^2; SC
Prednisone 20 mg/m^2; PO q 24 hours
Week 2: Vincristine 0.5 mg/m^2; IV
Cyclophosphamide 50 mg/m^2; PO q 48 hours
L-Asparginase 10,000 IU/m^2; SC
Prednisone 20 mg/m^2; PO q 48 hours
Week 3: Vincristine 0.5 mg/m^2; IV
Cyclophosphamide 50 mg/m^2; PO q 48 hours
Prednisone 20 mg/m^2; PO q 48 hours
Week 4: Vincristine 0.5 mg/m^2; IV
Cyclophosphamide 50 mg/m^2; PO q 48 hours
Prednisone 20 mg/m^2; PO q 48 hours
Week 5: Vincristine 0.5 mg/m^2; IV
Cyclophosphamide 50 mg/m^2; PO q 48 hours
Prednisone 20 mg/m^2; PO q 48 hours

Week 6:   Doxorubicin 30 mg/m²; IV
           Cyclophosphamide 50 mg/m²; PO q 48 hours
           Prednisone 10 mg/m²; PO q 48 hours
Week 7:   Vincristine 0.5 mg/m²; IV
           Cyclophosphamide 50 mg/m²; PO q 48 hours
           Prednisone 10 mg/m²; PO q 48 hours
Week 8:   Vincristine 0.5 mg/m²; IV
           Cyclophosphamide 50 mg/m²; PO q 48 hours
           Prednisone 10 mg/m²; PO q 48 hours
Week 9:   Doxorubicin 30 mg/m²; IV
           Chlorambucil 4.0 mg/m²; PO q 48 hours
           Prednisone 10 mg/m²; PO q 48 hours
Week 10:   Chlorambucil 4.0 mg/m²; PO q 48 hours
           Prednisone 10 mg/m²; PO q 48 hours
Week 11:   Vincristine 0.5 mg/m²; IV
           Chlorambucil 4.0 mg/m²; PO q 48 hours
           Prednisone 10 mg/m²; PO q 48 hours
Week 12:   Doxorubicin 30 mg/m²; IV
           Chlorambucil 4.0 mg/m²; PO q 48 hours
           Prednisone 10 mg/m²; PO q 48 hours
Week 13:   Vincristine 0.5 mg/m²; IV
           Chlorambucil 4.0 mg/m²; PO q 48 hours
Week 14:   Chlorambucil 4.0 mg/m²; PO q 48 hours
Week 15:   Chlorambucil 4.0 mg/m²; PO q 48 hours

Chlorambucil is continued every other day. Vincristine is given every 3 weeks from week 16 to 21, then every 4 weeks from week 22 to 38, then every 6 weeks until week 104 (or until dog comes out of remission).

Boyce KL, Kitchell BE. Treatment of canine lymphoma with COPA/LVP. J Am Anim Hosp Assoc 2000;36:395–403.

Ontario Veterinary College Protocol

Similar to intensified Madison-Wisconsin dose protocol with addition of two half-body radiation treatments and substitution of epirubicin (30 mg/m²) for doxorubicin, but with no maintenance phase

Week 1:   Vincristine 0.7 mg/m²; IV
           L-Asparginase 400 IU/kg; IM (maximum dose 10,000 IU per administration)
           Prednisone 30 mg/m²; PO q 24 hours
Week 2:   Cyclophosphamide 250 mg/m²; PO
           Prednisone 20 mg/m²; PO q 24 hours
Week 3:   Epirubicin 30 mg/m²; IV
           Prednisone 10 mg/m²; PO q 24 hours
Week 4:   Vincristine 0.7 mg/m²; IV
Week 5:   Cyclophosphamide 250 mg/m²; PO
Week 6:   Epirubicin 30 mg/m²; IV
Week 8:   Cranial half-body radiation 800 cGy
           Vincristine 0.7 mg/m²; IV

Week 10: Vincristine 0.7 mg/m^2; IV
Week 12: Caudal half-body radiation 800 cGy

Abrams-Ogg ACG, Norris AM, Woods JP, et al. Half-body radiation therapy versus maintenance chemotherapy for the treatment of dogs with multicentric lymphoma in remission. Proc Vet Cancer Soc 1999;19:8.

CANINE OSTEOSARCOMA
Cisplatinum

Adjuvant therapy with cisplatinum is used in dogs without preexisting renal disease (not safe in cats) with pre and post treatment saline diuresis to help protect the kidneys and antemetics.

0.9% saline 18.3 mL/kg per hour for 4 hours pretreatment
Butorphanol 0.4 mg/kg; IM, or metoclopramide 0.5 to 1.0 mg/kg; PO or SC 1/2 hour prior to end of diuresis
Cisplatinum 50 to 70 mg/m^2; IV over 1 to 3 hours
0.9% saline at 18.3 mL/kg per hour for 2 hours posttreatment

Treatment is repeated every 21 to 28 days for 2 to 6 treatments.

Straw RC, Withrow SJ, Richter SL, et al. Amputation and cisplatin for treatment of canine osteosarcoma. J Vet Intern Med 1991;5:205–210.

Ogilvie GK, Krawiec DR, Gelberg HB, et al. Evaluation of a short-term saline diuresis protocol for the administration of cisplatin. Am J Vet Res 1988;49:1076–1078.

Doxorubicin

Adjuvant therapy with doxorubicin 30 mg/m^2; IV q 14 days for a total of 5 treatments

Berg J, Weinstein MJ, Springfield DS, et al. Results of surgery and doxorubicin chemotherapy in dogs with osteosarcoma. J Am Vet Med Assoc 1995;206:1555–1560.

Carboplatinum

Adjuvant therapy with carboplatinum (300 mg/m^2; IV q 21 to 28 days for 4 treatments or more) is used in place of cisplatinum due to less renal toxicity with carboplatinum.

Bergman PJ, MacEwen EG, Kurzman ID, et al. Amputation and carboplatinum for treatment of dogs with osteosarcoma: 48 cases (1991–1993). J Vet Intern Med 1996;10:76–81.

Cisplatinum or Carboplatinum and Doxorubicin

Alternating either cisplatinum or carboplatinum with doxorubicin

Cisplatinum and Doxorubicin

Day 1:   Doxorubicin 30 mg/m^2; IV
Day 21: Cisplatinum 60 mg/m^2; IV with saline diuresis pre and post treatment

Repeat cycle once in 21 days.

Mauldin GN, Matus RE, Withrow SJ, et al. Canine osteosarcoma treatment by amputation versus amputation and adjuvant chemotherapy using doxorubicin and cisplatin. J Vet Intern Med 1988;2:177–180.

or

Day 1:   Doxorubicin 15 to 20 mg/m^2; IV
Day 1:   Cisplatinum 60 mg/m^2; IV with saline diuresis pre and post treatment

Repeat cycle twice every 21 days.

Berg J, Gebhardt MC, Rand WM. Effect of timing of postoperative chemotherapy on survival of dogs with osteosarcoma. Cancer 1997; 79:1343–1350.

or

Day 1:   Cisplatinum 50 mg/m^2; IV with saline diuresis pre and post treatment
Day 2:   Doxorubicin 15 mg/m^2; IV

Repeat cycle up to 3 times every 21 days.

Chun R, Kurzman ID, Couto CG, et al. Cisplatin and doxorubicin combination chemotherapy for the treatment of canine osteosarcoma: a pilot study. J Vet Intern Med 2000;14:495–498.

Carboplatinum and Doxorubicin

Day 1:   Carboplatinum 175 mg/m^2; IV with saline diuresis pre and post treatment
Day 2:   Doxorubicin 15 mg/m^2; IV

Repeat cycle up to 3 times every 21 days.

Bailey D, Erb H, Williams L, et al. Carboplatin and doxorubicin combination chemotherapy for the treatment of appendicular osteosarcoma in the dog. J Vet Intern Med 2003;17:199–205.

CANINE SARCOMAS
Doxorubicin

Doxorubicin 30 mg/m^2 (or 1 mg/kg for dogs < 10 kg); IV q 14 to 21 days for a total of 4 to 6 treatments

Ogilvie GK, Reynolds HA, Richardson RC, et al. Phase II evaluation of doxorubicin for treatment of various canine neoplasms. J Am Vet Med Assoc 1989;195:1580–1587.

Ogilvie GK, Powers BE, Mallinckrodt CH, et al. Surgery and doxorubicin in dogs with hemangiosarcoma. J Vet Intern Med 1996;10:379–384.

Mitoxantrone

Mitoxantrone 5 mg/m^2; IV q 3 weeks

Ogilvie GK, Obradovich JE, Elmslie RE, et al. Efficacy of mitoxantrone against various neoplasms in dogs. J Am Vet Med Assoc 1991; 198:1618–1621.

VAC

(**V**incristine, **A**driamycin [doxorubicin], **C**ytoxan [cyclophosphamide])

Day 1:   Doxorubicin 30 mg/m^2; IV
         Cyclophosphamide 100 to 150 mg/m^2; IV or PO
Day 8:   Vincristine 0.5 to 0.75 mg/m^2; IV
Day 15: Vincristine 0.5 to 0.75 mg/m^2; IV

Repeat cycle day 22 for a total of 4 to 6 cycles.

or

Day 1:   Doxorubicin 30 mg/m^2; IV
         Cyclophosphamide 200 mg/m^2; IV or PO
Day 14: Vincristine 0.7 mg/m^2; IV

Repeat cycle day 21 for a total of 4 to 6 cycles.

Hammer AS, Couto CG, Filippi J, et al. Efficacy and toxicity of VAC chemotherapy (vincristine, doxorubicin and cyclophosphamide) in dogs with hemangiosarcoma. J Vet Intern Med 1991;5:160–166.

AC

(**A**driamycin [doxorubicin], **C**ytoxan [cyclophosphamide])

Day 1:   Doxorubicin 30 mg/m^2; IV
         Cyclophosphamide 100 to 150 mg/m^2; IV or PO

Repeat cycle day 22 for a total of 4 to 6 cycles.

or

Day 1:   Doxorubicin 30 mg/m^2; IV
Days 3 to 6: Cyclophosphamide 50 to 75 mg/m^2; PO

Repeat cycle day 22 for a total of 4 to 6 cycles.

Sorenmo KU, Jeglum KA, Helfand SC. Chemotherapy of canine hemangiosarcoma with doxorubicin and cyclophosphamide. J Vet Intern Med 1993;7:370–376.

CANINE CARCINOMAS
Doxorubicin

Doxorubicin 30 mg/m^2 (or 1 mg/kg for dogs < 10 kg) IV q 14 to 21 days for a total of 4 to 6 treatments

Ogilvie GK, Reynolds HA, Richardson RC, et al. Phase II evaluation of doxorubicin for treatment of various canine neoplasms. J Am Vet Med Assoc 1989;195:1580–1587.

Mitoxantrone

Mitoxantrone 5 mg/m^2; IV q 3 weeks

Ogilvie GK, Obradovich JE, Elmslie RE, et al. Efficacy of mitoxantrone against various neoplasms in dogs. J Am Vet Med Assoc 1991; 198:1618–1621.

Cisplatinum

Adjuvant therapy with cisplatinum is used in dogs without preexisting renal disease (not safe in cats) with pretreatment and posttreatment saline diuresis to help protect the kidneys and antemetics.

0.9% saline 18.3 mL/kg per hour for 4 hours pretreatment

Butorphanol 0.4 mg/kg; IM, or chlorpromazine 0.5 mg/kg; IM, or metoclopramide 0.5 to 1.0 mg/kg; PO or SC 1/2 hour prior to end of diuresis

Cisplatinum 50 to 70 mg/m^2; IV over 1 to 3 hours

0.9% saline at 18.3 mL/kg per hour for 2 hours posttreatment

Treatment is repeated every 21 to 28 days for 2 to 6 treatments.

Shapiro W, Kitchell BE, Fossum TW, et al. Cisplatin for treatment of transitional and squamous cell carcinomas in dogs. J Am Vet Med Assoc 1988;193:1530–1533.

Chun R, Knapp DW, Widmer WR, et al. Cisplatin treatment of transitional cell carcinoma of the urinary bladder in dogs (1983–1993). J Am Vet Med Assoc 1996;209:1588–1591.

Moore AS, Cardona A, Shapiro W, et al. Cisplatin (cisdiamminedichloroplatinum) for treatment of transitional cell carcinoma of the urinary bladder or urethra. J Vet Intern Med 1990;4:148–152.

Piroxicam

0.3 mg/kg; PO q 24 hours

Knapp DW, Richardson RC, Chan TCK, et al. Piroxicam therapy in 34 dogs with transitional cell carcinoma of the urinary bladder. J Vet Intern Med 1994;8:273–278.

AC

(**A**driamycin [doxorubicin], **C**ytoxan [cyclophosphamide])

Day 1:   Doxorubicin 30 mg/m^2; IV
Days 3 to 6: Cyclophosphamide 50 to 100 mg/m^2; PO

Repeat cycle day 22 for a total of 4 to 6 cycles.

Helfand SC, Hamilton TA, Hungerford LL, et al. Comparison of three treatments for transitional cell carcinoma of the bladder in the dog. J Am Anim Hosp Assoc 1994;30:270–275.

CANINE MAST CELL TUMOR
Prednisone

Prednisone 1 mg/kg; PO q 24 hours

McCaw DL, Miller MA, Ogilvie GK, et al. Response of canine mast cell tumors to treatment with oral prednisone. J Vet Intern Med 1994; 8:406–408.

or

Prednisone 40 mg/m^2; PO q 24 hours for 1 week
Then 20 mg/m^2; PO q 24 hours for 3 weeks

Then 20 mg/m²; PO q 48 hours for 3 weeks

Then reduce dose by 50% every 3 weeks to lowest dose that maintains remission or stable disease

O'Keefe DA. Canine mast cell tumors. Vet Clin North Am [Small Anim Pract] 1990;20:1105–1115.

Triamcinolone

Triamcinolone 3 to 6 mg/dog intralesionally once/week

Hess PW, MacEwen EG, McClelland AJ. Chemotherapy of canine and feline tumors. J Am Anim Hosp Assoc 1976;12:350–358.

or

Triamcinolone 1 mg/1 cm (tumor diameter), maximal dose 10 to 40 mg, q 14 days

Tams TR, Macy DW. Canine mast cell tumors. Comp Cont Educ Pract Vet 1981;3:869–878.

CCNU (lomustine)

CCNU (lomustine) 70 to 90 mg/m²; PO q 3 weeks

Rassnick KM, Moore AS, Williams LE, et al. Treatment of canine mast cell tumors with CCNU (lomustine). J Vet Intern Med 1999;13:601–605.

Prednisone/Vinblastine

Prednisone 2 mg/kg; PO q 24 hours

Vinblastine 2 mg/m²; IV q week for 4 weeks followed by 4 treatments q 2 weeks

Week 1:	Vinblastine 2 mg/m²; IV
	Prednisone 2 mg/kg; PO q 24 hours
Week 2:	Vinblastine 2 mg/m²; IV
	Prednisone 2 mg/kg; PO q 24 hours
Week 3:	Vinblastine 2 mg/m²; IV
	Prednisone 2 mg/kg; PO q 24 hours
Week 4:	Vinblastine 2 mg/m²; IV
	Prednisone 2 mg/kg; PO q 24 hours
Week 6:	Vinblastine 2 mg/m²; IV
	Prednisone 2 mg/kg; PO q 24 hours

Continue Vinblastine 2 mg/m²; IV q 2 weeks for as long as appears to have an objective response. Taper and discontinue prednisone over 12 to 26 weeks.

Thamm DH, Mauldin EA, Vail DM. Prednisone and vinblastine chemotherapy for canine mast cell tumor—41 cases (1992–1997). J Vet Intern Med 1999;13:491–497.

CVP

(**C**yclophosphamide/**V**inblastine/**P**rednisone)

Cyclophosphamide 50 mg/m²; PO q 48 hours or for 4 days per week
   Vinblastine 2 mg/m²; IV once a week
   Prednisone 20 to 40 mg/m²; PO q 48 hours
   O'Keefe DA. Canine mast cell tumors. Vet Clin North Am [Small Anim Pract] 1990;20:1105–1115.

or

Day 1:   Vinblastine 2 to 3 mg/m²; IV (start at 2 mg/m² and increase by 10% to 30% with each dose if tolerated)
Days 8,9,10,11: Cyclophosphamide 50 to 75 mg/m²; PO
Daily: Prednisone 1 mg/kg; PO q 24 hours

Repeat cycle at day 21 for 6 months. Prednisone tapering begins at 4 months and is discontinued by 7 months.
   Elmslie R. Combination chemotherapy with and without surgery for dogs with high grade mast cell tumors with regional lymph node metastases. Vet Cancer Soc Newsl 1997;20:6–7.

CANINE MULTIPLE MYELOMA
Melphalan/Prednisone
Melphalan 0.1 mg/kg; PO q 24 hours for 10 days, then 0.05 mg/kg; PO q 24 hours continuously
   Prednisone 0.5 mg/kg; PO q 24 hours for 10 days, then 0.5 mg/kg; PO q 24 to 48 hours

Discontinue prednisone at 60 days.
   Matus RE, Leifer CE, MacEwen EG, et al. Prognostic factors for multiple myeloma in the dog. J Am Vet Med Assoc 1986;188:1288–1292.

or

Melphalan 7 mg/m²; PO days 1 to 5; repeat q 3 weeks
   Prednisone 0.5 mg/kg; PO q 24 hours for 10 days, then 0.5 mg/kg; PO q 24 to 48 hours

Discontinue prednisone at 60 days.
   Vail DM. Plasma cell neoplasms. In: Withrow SJ, MacEwen EG, eds. Small Animal Clinical Oncology, 3rd ed. Philadelphia: WB Saunders, 2001:626–638.

CHEMOTHERAPY PROTOCOLS FOR CATS

FELINE LYMPHOSARCOMA
COP
(**C**ytoxan [cyclophosphamide], **O**ncovin [vincristine], **P**rednisone)
Cyclophosphamide 300 mg/m²; PO once q 3 weeks (nearest 25 mg on the low side of 300 mg/m²)
   Vincristine 0.75 mg/m²; IV once weekly for 4 weeks, then once q 3 weeks with cyclophosphamide

Prednisone 2 mg/kg; PO per day

Week 1:   Vincristine 0.75 mg/m^2; IV
          Cyclophosphamide 300 mg/m^2; PO
          Prednisone 2 mg/kg; PO q 24 hours
Week 2:   Vincristine 0.75 mg/m^2; IV
          Prednisone 2 mg/kg; PO q 24 hours
Week 3:   Vincristine 0.75 mg/m^2; IV
          Prednisone 2 mg/kg; PO q 24 hours
Week 4:   Vincristine 0.75 mg/m^2; IV
          Cyclophosphamide 300 mg/m^2; PO
          Prednisone 2 mg/kg; PO q 24 hours
Week 7:   Vincristine 0.75 mg/m^2; IV
          Cyclophosphamide 300 mg/m^2; PO
          Prednisone 2 mg/kg; PO q 24 hours
Week 10: Vincristine 0.75 mg/m^2; IV
          Cyclophosphamide 300 mg/m^2; PO
          Prednisone 2 mg/kg; PO q 24 hours

Continue every 3 weeks to week 52, then treatment is discontinued. Prednisone is continued for 1 year, then tapered and stopped over a 3 weeks.

Cotter SM. Treatment of lymphoma and leukaemia with cyclophosphamide, vincristine, and prednisone: II. Treatment of cats. J Am Anim Hosp Assoc 1983;19:166–172.

Teske E, van Straten G, van Noort R, et al. Chemotherapy with cyclophosphamide, vincristine and prednisolone (COP) in cats with malignant lymphoma: new results with an old protocol. J Vet Intern Med 2002;16:179–186.

COPA

(**C**ytoxan [cyclophosphamide], **O**ncovin [vincristine], **P**rednisone, **A**driamycin [doxorubicin])

COP used for induction followed by doxorubicin

Cyclophosphamide 300 mg/m^2; PO once q 3 weeks (nearest 25 mg on the low side of 300 mg/m^2)

Vincristine 0.75 mg/m^2; IV once weekly for 4 weeks, then once q 3 weeks with cyclophosphamide

Prednisone 40 mg/m^2; PO per day

Doxorubicin 25 mg/m^2; IV q 3 weeks after induction

Week 1:   Vincristine 0.75 mg/m^2; IV
          Cyclophosphamide 300 mg/m^2; PO
          Prednisone 40 mg/m^2; PO per day
Week 2:   Vincristine 0.75 mg/m^2; IV
          Prednisone 40 mg/m^2; PO per day
Week 3:   Vincristine 0.75 mg/m^2; IV
          Prednisone 40 mg/m^2; PO per day

Week 4:   Vincristine 0.75 mg/m^2; IV
           Cyclophosphamide 300 mg/m^2; PO
           Prednisone 40 mg/m^2; PO per day
Week 7:   Doxorubicin 25 mg/m^2; IV
Week 10:   Doxorubicin 25 mg/m^2; IV
Week 13:   Doxorubicin 25 mg/m^2; IV

Continue every 3 weeks to 6 months, then treatment is discontinued.
Moore SA, Cotter SM, Frimberger AE, et al. A comparison of doxorubicin and COP for maintenance of remission in cats with lymphoma. J Vet Intern Med 1996;10:372–375.

VCM

(**V**incristine, **C**ytoxan [cyclophosphamide], **M**ethotrexate)
    Vincristine 0.025 mg/kg; IV weeks 1 and 3
    Cyclophosphamide 10 mg/kg; IV week 2
    Methotrexate 0.8 mg/kg; PO (IV if GI lymphoma)

Four-week cycle is continued.

Week 1:   Vincristine 0.025 mg/kg; IV
Week 2:   Cyclophosphamide 10 mg/kg; IV
Week 3:   Vincristine 0.025 mg/kg; IV
Week 4:   Methotrexate 0.8 mg/kg; PO (IV if GI lymphoma)

Repeat 4-week cycle for 2 years.
Jeglum KA, Whereat A, Young K. Chemotherapy of lymphoma in 75 cats. J Am Vet Med Assoc 1987;190:174–178.

L-VCMP

(**L**-Asparginase, **V**incristine, **C**ytoxan [cyclophosphamide], **M**ethotrexate, **P**rednisone)
    L-Asparginase 400 IU/kg; IP in week 1
    Vincristine 0.025 mg/kg; IV weeks 1 and 3
    Cyclophosphamide 10 mg/kg; IV week 2
    Methotrexate 0.8 mg/kg; PO
    Prednisone 2 mg/kg; PO q 24 hours

Four-week cycle is repeated except for use of L-asparginase.

Week 1:   L-asparginase 400 IU/kg; IP
           Vincristine 0.025 mg/kg; IV
           Prednisone 2 mg/kg; PO
Week 2:   Cyclophosphamide 10 mg/kg; IV
           Prednisone 2 mg/kg; PO
Week 3:   Vincristine 0.025 mg/kg; IV
           Prednisone 2 mg/kg; PO
Week 4:   Methotrexate 0.8 mg/kg; PO
           Prednisone 2 mg/kg; PO

Repeat 4-week cycle. After 2 months, intervals between treatments are extended to 10 days for another 8 treatments, then intervals between treatments are extended to 2 weeks for next 7 months, then treatment intervals are extended to 3 weeks for second year, to 4 weeks in the third year, 6 weeks in the fourth year, and 8 weeks in the fifth year. In the second year of treatment, the prednisone dose is halved.

Mooney SC, Hayes AA, MacEwen EG, et al. Treatment and prognostic factors in lymphoma in cats: 103 cases (1977–1981). J Am Vet Med Assoc 1989;194:696–699.

Current Veterinary Therapy (CVT) X Protocol (L-VCAMP)

(**L**-Asparginase, **V**incristine, **C**ytoxan [cyclophosphamide], **A**driamycin [doxorubicin], **M**ethotrexate, **P**rednisone)

Week 1:   Vincristine 0.025 mg/kg; IV
          L-Asparginase 400 IU/kg; IP
          Prednisone 5 mg PO q 12 hours
Week 2:   Cyclophosphamide 10 mg/kg; IV
          Prednisone 5 mg PO q 12 hours
Week 3:   Doxorubicin 20 mg/m²; IV
          Prednisone 5 mg PO q 12 hours
Week 4:   Vincristine 0.025 mg/kg; IV
          Prednisone 5 mg PO q 12 hours
Week 5:   Cyclophosphamide 10 mg/kg; IV
          Prednisone 5 mg PO q 12 hours
Week 6:   Doxorubicin 20 mg/m²; IV
          Prednisone 5 mg PO q 12 hours
Week 8:   Vincristine 0.025 mg/kg; IV
          Prednisone 5 mg PO q 12 hours
Week 10: Cyclophosphamide 10 mg/kg; IV
          Prednisone 5 mg PO q 12 hours
Week 12: Vincristine 0.025 mg/kg; IV
          Prednisone 5 mg PO q 12 hours
Week 14: Methotrexate 0.8 mg/kg; IV
          Prednisone 5 mg PO q 12 hours

Treatment is continued every 2 weeks as above for weeks 8 to 14 for 12 months, then every 3 weeks for 6 months, then monthly for 6 months.

Matus RE. Chemotherapy of lymphoma and leukemia. In Kirk RW (ed): Current Veterinary Therapy X. Philadelphia: WB Saunders, 1989:482–488.

L-VCAMP

(**L**-Asparginase, **V**incristine, **C**ytoxan [cyclophosphamide], **A**driamycin [doxorubicin], **M**ethotrexate, **P**rednisone)

Week 1:   Vincristine 0.025 mg/kg; IV
          L-Asparginase 400 IU/kg; SC
          Prednisone 5 mg PO q 12 hours

Week 2:   Cyclophosphamide 10 mg/kg; IV
           Prednisone 5 mg PO q 12 hours
Week 3:   Doxorubicin 1 mg/kg; IV
           Prednisone 5 mg PO q 12 hours
Week 4:   Vincristine 0.025 mg/kg; IV
           Prednisone 5 mg PO q 12 hours
Week 5:   Cyclophosphamide 10 mg/kg; IV
           Prednisone 5 mg PO q 12 hours
Week 6:   Doxorubicin 1 mg/kg; IV
           Prednisone 5 mg PO q 12 hours
Week 8:   Vincristine 0.025 mg/kg; IV
           Prednisone 5 mg PO q 12 hours
Week 10:   Cyclophosphamide 10 mg/kg; IV
           Prednisone 5 mg PO q 12 hours
Week 12:   Vincristine 0.025 mg/kg; IV
           Prednisone 5 mg PO q 12 hours
Week 14:   Methotrexate 0.5 mg/kg; IV
           Prednisone 5 mg PO q 12 hours

Treatment is continued every 2 weeks as above for weeks 8 to 14 for 12 months, then every 3 weeks for 6 months, then monthly for 6 months.

Zwahlen CH, Lucroy MD, Kraegel SA, et al. Results of chemotherapy for cats with alimentary malignant lymphoma: 21 cases (1993–1997). J Am Vet Med Assoc 1998;213:1144–1149.

Madison-Wisconsin Protocol (L-VCAM)

(L-Asparginase, Vincristine, Cytoxan [cyclophosphamide], Adriamycin [doxorubicin]), Methotrexate)

Week 1:   Vincristine 0.025 mg/kg; IV
           L-Asparginase 400 IU/kg; IM
           Prednisone 2 mg/kg; PO q 24 hours
Week 2:   Cyclophosphamide 250 mg/m^2; IV
           Prednisone 2 mg/kg; PO q 24 hours
Week 3:   Vincristine 0.025 mg/kg; IV
           Prednisone 1 mg/kg; PO q 24 hours
Week 4:   Doxorubicin 20 mg/m^2; IV
           Prednisone 1 mg/kg; PO q 24 hours
Week 6:   Vincristine 0.025 mg/kg; IV
           Prednisone 1 mg/kg; PO q 24 hours
Week 7:   Cyclophosphamide 250 mg/m^2; IV
           Prednisone 1 mg/kg; PO q 24 hours
Week 8:   Vincristine 0.025 mg/kg; IV
           Prednisone 1 mg/kg; PO q 24 hours
Week 9:   Doxorubicin 20 mg/m^2; IV
           Prednisone 1 mg/kg; PO q 24 hours

Week 11: Vincristine 0.025 mg/kg; IV
          Prednisone 1 mg/kg; PO q 24 hours
Week 13: Cyclophosphamide 250 mg/m^2; IV
          Prednisone 1 mg/kg; PO q 24 hours
Week 15: Vincristine 0.025 mg/kg; IV
          Prednisone 1 mg/kg; PO q 24 hours
Week 17: Methotrexate 0.8 mg/kg; IV
          Prednisone 1 mg/kg; PO q 24 hours
Week 19: Vincristine 0.025 mg/kg; IV
          Prednisone 1 mg/kg; PO q 24 hours
Week 21: Cyclophosphamide 250 mg/m^2; IV
          Prednisone 1 mg/kg; PO q 24 hours
Week 23: Vincristine 0.025 mg/kg; IV
          Prednisone 1 mg/kg; PO q 24 hours
Week 25: Doxorubicin 20 mg/m^2; IV
          Prednisone 1 mg/kg; PO q 24 hours

Treatment is continued biweekly as above (Weeks 11 to 25) for 12 months; then with 3-week interval between treatments for 6 months; then monthly for 6 months; then treatment is discontinued.

Vail DM, Moore AS, Ogilvie GK. Feline lymphoma (145 cases): proliferation indices, cluster of differentiation 3 immunoreactivity, and their association with prognosis in 90 cats. J Vet Intern Med 1998; 12:349–354.

COPA/LVP

(**C**ytoxan [cyclophosphamide], **O**ncovin [vincristine], **P**rednisone, **A**driamycin [doxorubicin])/**L**eukeran [Chlorambucil], **V**incristine, **P**rednisone)

Vincristine 0.5 mg/m^2; IV once weekly for 11 weeks, omitting weeks 6, 9, and 10; starting at week 13, every 3 weeks for 3 treatments; then every 4 weeks for 4 treatments; then every 6 weeks

Cyclophosphamide 50 mg/m^2; PO q 48 hours (25 mg per cat PO once or twice a week)

Prednisone 20 mg/m^2; PO q 24 hours for 1 week, then every other day for 4 weeks, then 10 mg/m^2 every other day for 7 weeks

L-Asparginase 400 IU/kg; SC week 1 and week 2
Doxorubicin 20 mg/m^2; IV on weeks 6, 9, and 12
Chlorambucil 4.0 mg/m^2; PO every other day starting at week 9

Week 1: Vincristine 0.5 mg/m^2; IV
         Cyclophosphamide 50 mg/m^2; PO q 48 hours
         L-Asparginase 400 IU/kg; SC
         Prednisone 20 mg/m^2; PO q 24 hours
Week 2: Vincristine 0.5 mg/m^2; IV
         Cyclophosphamide 50 mg/m^2; PO q 48 hours
         L-Asparginase 400 IU/kg; SC
         Prednisone 20 mg/m^2; PO q 48 hours

Week 3:   Vincristine 0.5 mg/m^2; IV
          Cyclophosphamide 50 mg/m^2; PO q 48 hours
          Prednisone 20 mg/m^2; PO q 48 hours
Week 4:   Vincristine 0.5 mg/m^2; IV
          Cyclophosphamide 50 mg/m^2; PO q 48 hours
          Prednisone 20 mg/m^2; PO q 48 hours
Week 5:   Vincristine 0.5 mg/m^2; IV
          Cyclophosphamide 50 mg/m^2; PO q 48 hours
          Prednisone 20 mg/m^2; PO q 48 hours
Week 6:   Doxorubicin 20 mg/m^2; IV
          Cyclophosphamide 50 mg/m^2; PO q 48 hours
          Prednisone 10 mg/m^2; PO q 48 hours
Week 7:   Vincristine 0.5 mg/m^2; IV
          Cyclophosphamide 50 mg/m^2; PO q 48 hours
          Prednisone 10 mg/m^2; PO q 48 hours
Week 8:   Vincristine 0.5 mg/m^2; IV
          Cyclophosphamide 50 mg/m^2; PO q 48 hours
          Prednisone 10 mg/m^2; PO q 48 hours
Week 9:   Doxorubicin 20 mg/m^2; IV
          Chlorambucil 4.0 mg/m^2; PO q 48 hours
          Prednisone 10 mg/m^2; PO q 48 hours
Week 10: Chlorambucil 4.0 mg/m^2; PO q 48 hours
          Prednisone 10 mg/m^2; PO q 48 hours
Week 11: Vincristine 0.5 mg/m^2; IV
          Chlorambucil 4.0 mg/m^2; PO q 48 hours
          Prednisone 10 mg/m^2; PO q 48 hours
Week 12: Doxorubicin 20 mg/m^2; IV
          Chlorambucil 4.0 mg/m^2; PO q 48 hours
          Prednisone 10 mg/m^2; PO q 48 hours
Week 13: Vincristine 0.5 mg/m^2; IV
          Chlorambucil 4.0 mg/m^2; PO q 48 hours
Week 14: Chlorambucil 4.0 mg/m^2; PO q 48 hours
Week 15: Chlorambucil 4.0 mg/m^2; PO q 48 hours

Chlorambucil is continued every other day. Vincristine is given every 3 weeks from weeks 16 to 21, then every 4 weeks from week 22 to 38, then every 6 weeks until week 104 (or until cat comes out of remission).

Kitchell BE. Treatment of feline lymphoma with COPA/LVP. (personal communication, 2003).

FELINE SARCOMAS
Doxorubicin

Doxorubicin 1 mg/kg; IV q 21 days for a total of 5 treatments

Chun RA. Feline and canine hemangiosarcoma. Comp Cont Educ Pract Vet 1999;21:622–629.

Bregazzi VS, LaRue SM, McNeil E, et al. Treatment with combination of doxorubicin, surgery, and radiation versus surgery and radiation alone for cats with vaccine-associated sarcomas: 25 cases (1995–2000). J Am Vet Med Assoc 2001;218:547–550.

Mitoxantrone

Mitoxantrone 5 to 6.5 mg/m^2; IV q 3 weeks

Ogilvie GK, Moore AS, Obradovich JE, et al. Toxicoses and efficacy associated with administration of mitoxantrone to cats with malignant tumors. J Am Vet Med Assoc 1993;202:1839–1844.

Carboplatin

Carboplatin 150 to 250 mg/m^2; IV q 3 weeks for 2 to 6 doses

Kobayashi T, Hauck ML, Dodge R, et al. Preoperative radiotherapy for vaccine associated sarcoma in 92 cats. Vet Radiol Ultrasound 2002;43:473–479.

AC

(**A**driamycin [doxorubicin], **C**ytoxan [cyclophosphamide])

Day 1:   Doxorubicin 20 to 30 mg/m^2; IV
Day 3:   Cyclophosphamide 25 mg/cat PO
Day 5:   Cyclophosphamide 25 mg/cat PO

Repeat cycle day 22 for a total of 4 to 6 cycles.

Barber LG, Sorenmo KU, Cronin KL, et al. Combined doxorubicin and cyclophosphamide chemotherapy for nonresectable feline fibrosarcoma. J Am Anim Hosp Assoc 2000;36:416–421.

or

Day 1:   Doxorubicin 20 mg/m^2; IV
             Cyclophosphamide 100 mg/m^2; IV

Repeat every 3 weeks for a total of 4 cycles.

Cohen M, Wright JC, Brawner WR, et al. Use of surgery and electron beam irradiation, with or without chemotherapy, for treatment of vaccine-associated sarcomas in cats: 78 cases (1996–2000). J Am Vet Med Assoc 2001;219:1582–1589.

or

Day 1:   Doxorubicin 25 mg/m^2; IV
Day 3,4,5,6: Cyclophosphamide 50 mg/m^2; PO

Repeat cycle every 21 days for a total of 4 to 6 cycles

Mauldin GN, Matus RE, Patnaik AK, et al. Efficacy and toxicity of doxorubicin and cyclophosphamide used in the treatment of selected malignant tumors in 23 cats. J Vet Intern Med 1988;2:60–65.

FELINE CARCINOMAS
Doxorubicin

Doxorubicin 1 mg/kg; IV q 21 days for a total of 5 to 6 treatments

Slawienski MJ, Mauldin GE, Mauldin GN, et al. Malignant colonic neoplasia in cats: 46 cases (1990–1996). J Am Vet Med Assoc 1997;211:878–881.

Mitoxantrone

Mitoxantrone 5 to 6.5 mg/m^2; IV q 3 weeks

Ogilvie GK, Moore AS, Obradovich JE, et al. Toxicoses and efficacy associated with administration of mitoxantrone to cats with malignant tumors. J Am Vet Med Assoc 1993;202:1839–1844.

Carboplatin

Carboplatin 210 mg/m^2; IV q 3 weeks for 3 doses (as adjuvant to radiation)

Wood CA. Combination coarse fractionation radiation therapy and carboplatin chemotherapy for treatment of feline oral squamous cell carcinoma: an interim analysis. Vet Cancer Soc Newsl 1998;22(4):1–4.

AC

(**A**driamycin [doxorubicin], **C**ytoxan [cyclophosphamide])

Day 1:   Doxorubicin 25 mg/m^2; IV
Day 3,4,5,6: Cyclophosphamide 50 mg/m^2; PO

Repeat cycle every 21 days for a total of 4 to 6 cycles.

Mauldin GN, Matus RE, Patnaik AK, et al. Efficacy and toxicity of doxorubicin and cyclophosphamide used in the treatment of selected malignant tumors in 23 cats. J Vet Intern Med 1988;2:60–65.

or

Day 1:   Doxorubicin 20 to 30 mg/m^2; IV
Day 3,4,5,6: Cyclophosphamide 100 mg/m^2; PO

Repeat cycle every 3 to 5 weeks until death.

Jeglum KA, deGuzman E, Young KM. Chemotherapy of advanced mammary adenocarcinoma in 14 cats. J Am Vet Med Assoc 1985;187: 157–160.

Handbook of Veterinary Drugs, Third Edition, edited by Dana Allen,
Lippincott Williams & Wilkins, Baltimore. © 2005

Section 3

Description of Drugs for Small Animals

ACEMANNAN

INDICATIONS: Acemannan Immunostimulant ★ (Carrasyn ★—human product) enhances macrophage release of interleukin-1, interleukin-6, tumor necrosis factor-α, prostaglandin E_2, and interferon-γ. It increases natural killer cell activity and enhances T-cell function. This agent may be beneficial in dogs and cats with fibrosarcoma when used in conjunction with surgery and radiation treatment. It also has been used in cats with feline leukemia virus (FeLV)-induced diseases. Appetite improved. Hematocrit, hemoglobin, and leukocyte numbers also apparently improved. Finally, this agent (available in the United States as a hydrogel—Carravet Wound Dressing and Carra Sorb M) may enhance wound healing.

ADVERSE AND COMMON SIDE EFFECTS: None reported. Anaphylaxis has been reported after bolus IV administration; this can be eliminated by diluting acemannan in 100 to 150 mL saline and by infusing the IV solution over 15 to 30 minutes. The drug has not been studied in pregnant animals.

DRUG INTERACTIONS: None reported.

SUPPLIED AS VETERINARY PRODUCT:
For injection in 10-mg vials

ACEPROMAZINE

INDICATIONS: Acepromazine [formerly Acetylpromazine] (Atravet ♣, PromAce ★, Aceproject ★, Aceprotabs ★, Acevet ♣) is a pheno-thiazine drug used as a sedative and a preanesthetic agent. Acepro-mazine is used to facilitate restraint of patients. It also has antiemetic, antispasmodic, and hypothermic properties. The drug significantly decreases intraurethral pressures and may be useful in the manage-ment of feline functional urethral obstruction. It also may have a pro-tective effect on barbiturate-, halothane-, and epinephrine-induced cardiac arrhythmias.

ADVERSE AND COMMON SIDE EFFECTS: The following side effects have been noted with the use of acepromazine: constipation, paradoxical aggression, sinus bradycardia, depression of myocardial contractility, hypotension, collapse, and prolongation of pseudocyesis. Acepromazine lowers the seizure threshold and should not be used in animals with the potential for seizure activity, including those patients that have undergone procedures that may precipitate seizure activity, e.g., myelography. In addition, acepromazine should not be given to animals with tetanus.

Prolonged effects of the drug (even at low doses) may be seen in older animals. Giant breeds, as well as greyhounds, appear quite sen-sitive to the clinical effects of the drug, yet terrier breeds appear more resistant. Conversely, boxer dogs are predisposed to the hypotensive and bradycardic effects of the drug. Concurrent administration of atropine often is recommended to counter the bradycardia.

DRUG INTERACTIONS: Acepromazine is contraindicated in animals with strychnine or organophosphate poisoning and should not be given to animals treated with succinylcholine or other cholinesterase inhibitors. Concurrent anesthetic or narcotic preparations may exacer-bate central nervous system (CNS) depression associated with the use of acepromazine. Kaolin-pectin and bismuth subsalicylate compounds and antacids decrease the absorption of oral acepromazine. Concurrent administration of propranolol and acepromazine may lead to serum elevations of both drugs. Phenytoin activity may be decreased if given along with acepromazine, and concurrent use of quinidine may cause additional cardiac depression. Finally, phenothiazines are α-adrenergic blocking agents and, if used with epinephrine, may lead to profound vasodilation and tachycardia. Other CNS depressants enhance hypo-tension and respiratory depression if used concurrently. Atropine and other anticholinergics have additive anticholinergic potential and reduce the antipsychotic effect of phenothiazines. Barbiturate drugs increase the metabolism of phenothiazines and may reduce their effects. Barbiturate anesthetics may increase excitation (tremor, invol-untary muscle movements) and hypotension. Phenothiazines may mask the ototoxic effects of aminoglycoside antibiotics. Phenothiazines inhibit phenytoin metabolism and increase its potential for toxicity. In humans, there is the unexplained possibility of sudden death if phenothiazines are used concurrently with phenylpropanolamine. Tricyclic antidepressants, e.g., amitriptyline, may intensify the sedative and anticholinergic effects of phenothiazines.

SUPPLIED AS VETERINARY PRODUCTS:
Tablets containing 10 and 25 mg
For injection containing 10 mg/mL

OTHER USES
Dogs
AMPHETAMINE TOXICOSIS
0.05 to 1 mg/kg; IM, IV, SC

PREANESTHETIC DOSE
0.1 to 0.2 mg/kg; IV, IM (maximum of 3 mg)

FUNCTIONAL URETHRAL OBSTRUCTION
0.1 mg/kg; IV

Dogs and Cats
ARTERIAL THROMBOEMBOLIC DISEASE

i)   0.05 to 0.11 mg/kg bid to tid; SC (to promote arterial vasodilation)

ii) 0.15 to 0.30 mg/kg bid to tid; IM, SC

ACETAMINOPHEN

INDICATIONS: Acetaminophen (Atasol ♣, Tempra ♣ ★, Tylenol ♣ ★) is an antipyretic, analgesic agent useful for the treatment of mild to moderate pain in dogs. The drug is reported to be as effective as aspirin in the reduction of pain and fever. It is a weak anti-inflammatory agent and is not useful in the management of rheumatoid arthritis.

ADVERSE AND COMMON SIDE EFFECTS: A dosage of 150 to 200 mg/kg in dogs and 50 to 60 mg/kg in cats may cause toxicity, although it has also been reported that a dose as low as 10 mg/kg may cause toxicity in the cat. The incidence of gastric ulceration is less than that reported with aspirin. Vomiting and depression are the most common clinical signs of toxicosis noted in dogs. Anorexia and abdominal pain also are reported. The drug is extremely toxic to cats. Methemoglobinemia, Heinz-body anemia, hepatic necrosis, hematuria, cyanosis, depression, anorexia, vomiting, salivation, edema of the face and paws, and death have been reported in this species. Coma indicates a poor prognosis. Supportive treatment includes parenteral fluids and electrolytes, cimetidine (to reduce acetaminophen hepatic metabolism), and

N-acetylcysteine (loading dose of 140 mg/kg, followed by 70 mg/kg every 6 hours; PO or IV for 7 more treatments). Dogs exhibit similar clinical toxic signs, but centrilobular hepatic necrosis is more common.

DRUG INTERACTIONS: None of significance in small animal medicine.

SUPPLIED AS HUMAN PRODUCTS:
Tablets containing 325 and 500 mg
Syrup containing 80 mg/5 mL solution
Drops containing 80 mg/mL

OTHER USES
Dogs
ANALGESIA
Acetaminophen plus codeine 1 to 2 mg/kg bid to tid; PO (dose based upon amount of codeine)

ACETAZOLAMIDE

INDICATIONS: Acetazolamide (Acetazolam ✤, Diamox ✤ ★) is a carbonic anhydrase inhibitor used in the treatment of glaucoma. The drug promotes renal bicarbonate and potassium excretion accompanied by water. These properties have made it useful as a diuretic and for the management of metabolic alkalosis. Acetazolamide reduces cerebrospinal fluid (CSF) production and may be of use in the management of hydrocephalus.

ADVERSE AND COMMON SIDE EFFECTS: In dogs, carbonic anhydrase inhibitors have been associated with causing drowsiness, behavioral changes, disorientation, vomiting (oral acetazolamide causes vomiting more often than other carbonic anhydrase inhibitors, e.g., methazolamide), diarrhea, hyperventilation, polydipsia (which usually decreases after a few weeks of use), and pruritus of the paws. Other potential adverse effects include bone marrow depression (anemia, leukopenia, thrombocytopenia) and hypercalciuria. Acetazolamide is contraindicated in animals with known hypersensitivity to the sulfonamides and derivatives, e.g., thiazides.

Acetazolamide should not be used in patients with marked renal or hepatic dysfunction, hypoadrenocorticism, hyponatremia, hypokalemia, or hyperchloremic acidosis. Long-term use is contraindicated in patients with hyphema or chronic, noncongestive angle-closure glaucoma. Long-term use may cause metabolic acidosis. Caution is recommended if the drug is used in patients with diabetes mellitus or obstructive pulmonary disease, or for those receiving digitalis.

DRUG INTERACTIONS: Oral use of acetazolamide may inhibit the absorption of primidone. Concurrent use of acetazolamide with primidone or phenytoin may cause osteomalacia. Concurrent use with corticosteroids, amphotericin B, or other diuretics may predispose to hypokalemia.

SUPPLIED AS HUMAN PRODUCTS:
Capsules (extended release) containing 500 mg
Tablets containing 125 and 250 mg
For injection in 500-mg vials

OTHER USES
Dogs
HYDROCEPHALUS
10 mg/kg every 6 to 8 hours

ACETYLCYSTEINE

INDICATIONS: Acetylcysteine (Mucomyst ✤ ★) is used as a mucolytic agent to help liquefy viscous or inspissated mucous secretions of the respiratory tract and eye. The drug also is used as antidotal therapy in the management of acetaminophen toxicity. It is effective if given within 12 hours of acetaminophen ingestion but is still recommended up to 80 hours after ingestion.

ADVERSE AND COMMON SIDE EFFECTS: Nebulization of the drug may cause bronchospasm, especially in patients with asthma. When given orally, nausea and vomiting may occur. Because the drug has a bad taste, stomach intubation may be required for oral administration. Perivascular injection can cause phlebitis, and rapid IV injection can cause hypotension, bronchospasm, and flushing.

DRUG INTERACTIONS: Acetylcysteine is incompatible with (based on the possible formation of a precipitate or a change in the color or clarity): tetracycline, oxytetracycline, chlortetracycline, and hydrogen peroxide.

SUPPLIED AS HUMAN PRODUCT:
For oral inhalation, as an oral solution, or intratracheal instillation containing a 10% or 20% sterile solution

ALBENDAZOLE

INDICATIONS: Albendazole (Valbazen ✤ ★) is an anthelmintic marketed for use in cattle. However, it has been used in small animals in the treatment of filaroidiasis, capillariasis, giardiasis, and paragonimiasis infections. The drug is safer and more effective than metronidazole or quinacrine for the treatment of giardiasis. Efficacy against *Metorchis conjunctus* in cats also is likely.

ADVERSE AND COMMON SIDE EFFECTS: Adverse drug effects have not been seen in dogs at dosages of 25 mg/kg bid, for 2 days, or at dosages of 30 mg/kg once daily for 13 weeks, but dosages of 30 to 60 mg/kg once daily for 26 weeks have resulted in leukopenia, blood dyscrasia, and reduced bone marrow cellularity. Idiosyncratic or dose-dependent pancytopenia has been reported in a dog given the drug at a dosage of 100 mg/kg once daily. The pancytopenia may resolve after drug withdrawal. Anorexia may develop in dogs receiving 50 mg/kg twice daily. In cats, lethargy, depression, and anorexia sometimes develop. Drug dosages of 100 mg/kg once daily for 14 to 21 days have caused leukopenia in cats.

DRUG INTERACTIONS: None reported.

SUPPLIED AS VETERINARY PRODUCT:
Suspension containing 113.6 mg/mL (11.36%)

OTHER USES
Dogs
FILAROIDES HIRTHI
50 mg/kg bid; PO for 5 days, repeat in 21 days
Note: Symptoms may worsen with therapy because of the reaction to dying worms.
FILAROIDES OSLERI
25 mg/kg bid; PO for 5 days, repeat in 2 weeks
CAPILLARIA PLICA
50 mg/kg bid; PO for 10 to 14 days
GIARDIA CANIS
25 mg/kg bid; PO for 2 consecutive days

Cats
PARAGONIMUS KELLICOTTI
25 mg/kg bid; PO for 10 to 21 days
METORCHIS CONJUNCTUS
50 mg/kg divided bid; PO for 10 to 14 days
GIARDIA
25 mg/kg bid; PO for 5 days

ALBUTEROL

INDICATIONS: Albuterol or Salbutamol (Ventolin ✤ ★, Proventil ★) is a synthetic sympathomimetic amine and moderately selective β_2-adrenergic agonist. It has more prominent effects on β_2 receptors—particularly smooth muscles in bronchi, uteri, and vascular supply to skeletal muscles—than on β_1 receptors in the heart. Some peripheral vasodilation may occur. The drug produces bronchodilation and inhibits histamine release. It is used to relieve bronchospasm and alleviate cough.

ADVERSE AND COMMON SIDE EFFECTS: Caution is advised with use of the drug in patients with cardiovascular disease, hypertension, hyperthyroid disease, or diabetes mellitus. In dogs, muscle tremors and nervousness may be noted with initiation of therapy. Side effects disappear within 5 to 7 days of therapy. Additional side effects often include tachycardia, premature ventricular contractions, vomiting, tachypnea and panting, and depression. In humans, other reported side effects have included increased or decreased blood pressure, nausea, paradoxical bronchospasm, difficulty in voiding, muscle cramps, and aggravation of diabetes mellitus. A β-blocking agent such as propranolol or metoprolol may be of benefit in cases of albuterol toxicosis.

DRUG INTERACTIONS: The concurrent use of epinephrine and other sympathomimetic (adrenergic) agents and antihistamines may have additive effects and is not recommended. Monoamine inhibitors, possibly amitraz, may potentiate the action of the drug on the vascular system. Propranolol and other β-adrenergic blocking agents may inhibit the effect of the drug. Theophyllines may potentiate the bronchodilatory effects of albuterol.

SUPPLIED AS HUMAN PRODUCTS:
Tablets containing 2 or 4 mg
Oral liquid containing 0.4 mg/mL

OTHER USES
Cats

ASTHMA
Mild cases 100 mg metered dose inhaler; 1 puff as needed
Moderate or severe cases (clinical signs occurring on a daily basis) 1 to 2 puffs bid to qid

ALLOPURINOL

INDICATIONS: Allopurinol (Zyloprim ✿ ★, Aloprim ★, Purinol ✿) is indicated in the treatment of urate urolithiasis in dogs. It inhibits the enzyme xanthine oxidase and blocks the formation and urinary excretion of uric acid. Urine urate/creatinine ratio decreases with drug administration. Urine urate/creatinine ratio in Dalmatian dogs ranges from 0.5 to 0.6 in one study to 0.6 to 1.5 in another study, versus 0.2 to 0.4 in non-Dalmatian dogs. A 50% reduction in the urine urate/creatinine ratio (reduced to 0.25 to 0.3) is recommended to decrease the recurrence of urate urolithiasis. The drug also has been used to treat leishmaniasis in a dog.

ADVERSE AND COMMON SIDE EFFECTS: Although adverse effects in dogs are uncommon, in humans the drug has been associated with nausea, vomiting, diarrhea, pancreatitis, and a reversible hepatopathy associated with transient increases in serum alkaline phosphatase, alanine aminotransferase, and aspartate aminotransferase. Rare cases of bone marrow suppression with leukopenia and thrombocytopenia also have been documented. The drug should be used with caution in patients with renal disease. In these cases, the dose should be decreased and the patient closely monitored for further deterioration in renal function. It has been reported that chronic use of the drug at doses of 30 mg/kg per day may predispose the patient to xanthine urolith formation. Allopurinol metabolism is not influenced by diet. If long-term use of the drug is required, drug dose probably should be decreased.

DRUG INTERACTIONS: Allopurinol potentiates the effects of cyclophosphamide, increasing the risk for bone marrow suppression. Because azathioprine metabolism depends on xanthine oxidase, concurrent use of this drug with allopurinol may lead to toxic levels of azathioprine. Urinary acidifiers, e.g., methionine and ammonium chloride, may reduce the solubility of uric acid and promote urolithiasis. Thiazides and possibly other diuretics increase the risk of allopurinol toxicity and hypersensitivity, especially in those with impaired renal function. Rarely, when used with trimethoprim/sulfamethoxazole, allopurinol has been associated with thrombocytopenia in humans. Large doses of allopurinol may decrease the metabolism of aminophylline and theophylline and increase their serum levels.

SUPPLIED AS HUMAN PRODUCTS:
Tablets containing 100, 200, and 300 mg
For injection containing 500 mg (★ only)

OTHER USES
Dogs
LEISHMANIA SPP.
11 mg/kg per day for 4 months; PO, dose then was increased to 15 mg/kg per day for an additional 9 months

ALPHA KERI

INDICATIONS: Alpha Keri ❧ ★ is a water-dispersible, antipruritic oil. It contains a dewaxed, oil-soluble, keratin-moisturizing fraction of lanolin, mineral oil, and nonionic emulsifiers. It is indicated for dry, pruritic skin conditions, including seborrhea, to relieve itching and to lubricate and soften the skin.

ADVERSE AND COMMON SIDE EFFECTS: This product should not be used on acutely inflamed skin.

DRUG INTERACTIONS: None.

SUPPLIED AS HUMAN PRODUCTS:
Bath oil available in 200- and 480-mL plastic bottles
Bar soap containing 110 g

ALUMINUM HYDROXIDE

INDICATIONS: Aluminum hydroxide (Amphojel ✤ ★, Nephrox ★) is an antacid, antiflatulent medication useful in the treatment of gastric ulcers and hyperphosphatemia associated with renal failure. The aluminum component is presumed to have a cytoprotective effect on the gastrointestinal tract (GIT) mucosa because of local prostaglandin synthesis, which is in addition to its buffering activity. The drug may have a protective effect on the GIT when administered with poorly tolerated drugs, e.g., aminophylline and nonsteroidal anti-inflammatory agents. Aluminum hydroxide may be combined with magnesium hydroxide. The advantage of combining aluminum with magnesium hydroxide (Amphojel 500 ★, Maalox ✤ ★) is to optimize the extent and rate of acid neutralization. See also ANTACIDS.

ADVERSE AND COMMON SIDE EFFECTS: The drug is contraindicated in animals with alkalosis. It is poorly palatable, and the aluminum component may predispose to constipation. Aluminum-containing antacids may delay gastric emptying and should be used with caution in patients with gastric outlet obstruction. Also, aluminum hydroxide supposedly may lead to phosphate depletion, muscle weakness, bone resorption, and hypercalcemia.

DRUG INTERACTIONS: Antacid products may interfere with the absorption of oral iron preparations, digoxin, phenothiazines, glucocorticoids, captopril, ketoconazole, nitrofurantoin, penicillamine, phenothiazines, phenytoin, ranitidine, cimetidine, and the tetracyclines. Increased absorption and serum levels of the following drugs may be seen if given concurrently with antacid compounds: aspirin, quinidine, and sympathomimetic agents.

SUPPLIED AS HUMAN PRODUCTS:
Liquid containing 320 mg/5 mL [Amphojel]
400 mg/5 mL [Aluminum Hydroxide Gel ★]
600 mg/5 mL [AlternaGEL ★, Aluminum Hydroxide Concentrated ★]
Capsules containing 400 mg [Alu-Cap ★] and 500 mg [Dialume]
Tablets containing 600 mg [Amphojel] [each tablet has an antacid effect = 10 mL of Amphojel liquid (320 mg/5 mL)]

AMIKACIN

INDICATIONS: Amikacin (Amiglyde-V ✿ ★, Amikin ✿ ★, Amiject D ★) is an aminoglycoside antibiotic indicated in the treatment of genitourinary tract infections in the dog caused by susceptible strains of *Escherichia coli* and *Proteus* sp., and skin and soft tissue infections caused by *Pseudomonas* sp., *E. coli*, and *Staphylococcus* sp. Amikacin is especially useful in those infections caused by *E. coli*, *Pseudomonas* sp., *Klebsiella* sp., *Proteus* spp., and *Staphylococcus* spp. resistant to gentamicin, kanamycin, or other aminoglycoside antibiotics. See also AMINOGLYCOSIDE ANTIBIOTICS.

ADVERSE AND COMMON SIDE EFFECTS: The LD_{50} of amikacin is in excess of 250 mg/kg in dogs. Like other aminoglycosides, amikacin has nephrotoxic, neurotoxic, and ototoxic potential, but usually only at exaggerated parenteral doses over a prolonged period of time. Amikacin serum concentrations should be monitored in all patients because of the large inter-animal variation in pharmacokinetics. Peak serum concentrations (determined 1 hour after injection) should be 4 to 5 times the minimum inhibitory concentration (MIC) of the offending organism, but no higher than 25 µg/mL. Trough concentrations (taken just before the next dose) should be less than 5 µg/mL. In cats, amikacin has less ototoxic potential than gentamicin. Transient pain may be noted on injection.

DRUG INTERACTIONS: See AMINOGLYCOSIDE ANTIBIOTICS.

SUPPLIED AS VETERINARY PRODUCT:
For injection containing 50 mg/mL [Amiglyde-V, Amiject D]

SUPPLIED AS HUMAN PRODUCT:
For injection containing 50 and 250 mg/mL [Amikin]

AMINOGLYCOSIDE ANTIBIOTICS

INDICATIONS: The aminoglycoside antibiotics, which include amikacin, dihydrostreptomycin, gentamicin, kanamycin, neomycin, streptomycin, and tobramycin, are indicated in the treatment of certain gram-negative, gram-positive, and mycobacterial infections. They primarily are effective against aerobic gram-negative bacteria such as *E. coli, Klebsiella, Proteus,* and *Enterobacter;* some also are effective against *Pseudomonas* infections. Gentamicin is more effective than kanamycin but less effective than tobramycin against *Pseudomonas aeruginosa*. Amikacin sulfate injection is especially useful against *Pseudomonas* and *Klebsiella* spp. resistant to gentamicin. Steady-state drug levels of gentamicin are established in 6.5 hours in the dog. Serum concentrations are measured 1 to 2 hours after dosing (peak levels) or just before the next dose (trough levels). To establish optimum dosing levels, it is desirable to take samples at peak and trough times.

ADVERSE AND COMMON SIDE EFFECTS: Nephrotoxicity, deafness, vestibular toxicity, respiratory paralysis, and cardiovascular depression have been reported with the use of these drugs, although otic preparations of gentamicin sulfate do not adversely affect vestibular or cochlear function in healthy dogs. Endotoxemia predisposes to cardiovascular-induced depression. These drugs should be avoided in puppies and kittens because they are more likely to develop renal failure. Neomycin is the most nephrotoxic aminoglycoside, followed in decreasing order of nephrotoxicity by gentamicin, tobramycin, kanamycin, amikacin, and streptomycin. Monitoring the urine for the appearance of casts, which in this case is a more sensitive indicator of impending renal dysfunction than serum urea or creatinine, is recommended if blood levels are not measured. Hypokalemia, hypocalcemia, hypomagnesemia, metabolic acidosis, and low-sodium diets may enhance gentamicin nephrotoxicity. Topical administration of gentamicin (i.e., wound lavage) also has caused nephrotoxicity in a cat.

DRUG INTERACTIONS: Aminoglycoside antibiotics can potentiate the action of neuromuscular blocking agents, leading to respiratory depression, apnea, or muscle weakness, especially in animals with renal insufficiency. The neuromuscular blocking activity can be reversed with neostigmine. Furosemide may enhance the ototoxicity and nephrotoxicity of the aminoglycosides. Gentamicin, dihydrostreptomycin, kanamycin, neomycin, and streptomycin may decrease cardiac output and produce hypotension and bradycardia and should be avoided in animals in shock or with serious cardiac insufficiency. Intravenous calcium gluconate should be used to reverse myocardial depression and restore blood pressure. Prolonged high oral doses of neomycin may cause diarrhea and malabsorption because of selective overgrowth of resistant indigenous intestinal flora. Aminoglycosides may cross the placental barrier and produce fetal intoxication and should not be given to pregnant animals. Penicillins should not be mixed with aminoglycosides before injection because inactivation of the aminoglycoside may occur.

SUPPLIED AS: See individual drug.

AMINOPENTAMIDE SULFATE

INDICATIONS: Aminopentamide (Centrine ★) is an antiemetic drug. It has antispasmodic and anticholinergic properties and is recommended for the treatment of acute abdominal visceral spasm, tenesmus, pylorospasm, or hypertrophic gastritis, and associated nausea, vomiting, and/or diarrhea in dogs and cats.

ADVERSE AND COMMON SIDE EFFECTS: Adverse effects may include dry mouth, dry eyes, blurred vision, and urinary hesitancy, the latter of which usually is the result of excessive dosing. The drug is contraindicated in patients with glaucoma, and it should be given cautiously, if at all, to those with pyloric obstruction. Aminopentamide should not be used in animals with a history of sensitivity to anticholinergic drugs, tachycardia, cardiac disease, obstructive gastrointestinal (GI) disease, paralytic ileus, ulcerative colitis, urinary obstruction, or myasthenia gravis. The drug also should not be used in those with GI infections because the antimuscarinic effects decrease GI motility, contributing to retention of the infection within the GIT. In addition, antimuscarinic agents should be used with caution in patients with liver or renal disease, hyperthyroid disease, congestive heart failure, esophageal reflux, or prostatic hypertrophy, and in geriatric or pediatric patients. Although no specific information is given concerning treatment of overdose, therapy for atropine overdose may be applicable here. If oral ingestion is recent, the GIT should be emptied and the patient given activated charcoal and a saline cathartic. The animal then is treated symptomatically. Avoid the use of phenothiazines because they are likely to contribute to the anticholinergic effects. Physostigmine should only be considered in those exhibiting severe supraventricular tachyarrhythmias or extreme agitation to the point of possibly inflicting injury to themselves. The human pediatric dose that may be applicable to small animals is 0.02 mg/kg slowly IV. If clinical response is not seen, the drug is repeated every 10 minutes until anticholinergic or antimuscarinic signs have disappeared. Adverse effects of physostigmine (bronchoconstriction, bradycardia, seizure) are treated with small doses of IV atropine.

DRUG INTERACTIONS: Although none are listed for this product, those drugs that interact with atropine may react similarly with aminopentamide. Antihistamines, procainamide, quinidine, meperidine, benzodiazepines, and phenothiazines may enhance the activity of aminopentamide. The following drugs may potentiate the adverse effects of aminopentamide: primidone, disopyramide, nitrates, and long-term corticosteroid use. Atropine (and possibly aminopentamide) may enhance the activity of nitrofurantoin, the thiazide diuretics, and sympathomimetic agents and they may antagonize the action of metoclopramide.

SUPPLIED AS VETERINARY PRODUCTS:
Tablets containing 0.2 mg
For injection containing 0.5 mg/mL

AMINOPHYLLINE

INDICATIONS: Aminophylline (Phylloconton ✚ ★ and generics) is a bronchodilator principally used for the management of cough due to bronchospasm. It has mild inotropic properties and mild, transient diuretic activity.

ADVERSE AND COMMON SIDE EFFECTS: Side effects may include vomiting, anorexia or polyphagia, diarrhea, polydipsia, polyuria, restlessness, muscle twitching, cardiac arrhythmias, tachycardia, hyperglycemia, and nervousness. The drug should be used with caution in patients with cardiac disease, systemic hypertension, cardiac arrhythmias, GIT ulcers, impaired renal or hepatic function, diabetes mellitus, hyperthyroid disease, and glaucoma. Serum or plasma concentrations of theophylline should be measured after steady-state concentrations have been attained (approximately 30 hours after initiation of therapy in dogs and 40 hours in cats) and just before the next dose. Therapeutic serum concentrations are 10 to 20 µg/mL (55 to 110 µmol/L). See also THEOPHYLLINE.

DRUG INTERACTIONS: Serum levels may be increased by the concurrent use of thiabendazole, cimetidine, allopurinol, clindamycin, and erythromycin. Phenobarbital decreases the therapeutic effect of the drug. Concurrent use of aluminum or magnesium antacid preparations slows the absorption of theophylline. Propranolol has direct antagonistic effects because propranolol is a β-adrenergic blocking agent and aminophylline is a β-adrenergic stimulant. Phenytoin increases theophylline clearance, requiring larger doses of the drug for effect. Aminophylline should not be mixed in a syringe with other drugs. Because aminophylline solutions are alkaline, they are incompatible with epinephrine, isoproterenol, or penicillin G potassium. Aminophylline contains approximately 80% theophylline. Concurrent use of this drug with allopurinol, cimetidine, furosemide, or epinephrine may cause excessive CNS stimulation. See also THEOPHYLLINE.

SUPPLIED AS HUMAN PRODUCTS:
Tablets containing 100 mg aminophylline (78.9 mg theophylline) and 225 mg aminophylline (157.8 mg theophylline)
Theophylline timed-release capsules and tablets are available in 50-, 75-, 100-, 125-, 200-, 250-, 300-, and 350-mg strengths.
For injection containing 25 mg/mL (19.7 mg/mL theophylline) and 50 mg/mL (39.4 mg/mL theophylline)

AMITRAZ

INDICATIONS: Amitraz (Mitaban ♣ ★, Preventic Collar ♣ ★) is indicated for the eradication of demodicosis and sarcoptic mange in dogs. The drug is classified as a monoamine oxidase (MAO) inhibitor (causes a buildup of norepinephrine in the CNS), although the exact mechanism of its action is unknown. It also inhibits prostaglandin synthesis and is an α-adrenergic agonist. Amitraz has stronger and more sustained effects against brown dog tick infestation than fipronil. Amitraz impregnated collars also appear useful for the prevention of borreliosis in dogs. Although not specifically indicated for use in cats, the drug has been used safely as outlined below.

ADVERSE AND COMMON SIDE EFFECTS: The most common side effects of mild toxicosis are ataxia and depression. Other side effects may include transient sedation, mydriasis, hypersalivation, transient pruritus (due to the effect of dead mites), hypothermia or hyperthermia, vomiting, diarrhea, and occasionally bradycardia. Clinical signs of severe toxicosis may include hypotension, hyperglycemia, mydriasis, and hypothermia. Puppies are especially sensitive, and cats may become toxic even when treated aurally. Safe use of the drug in pregnant bitches and puppies less than 4 months of age has not been established and is not recommended.

DRUG INTERACTIONS: Atropine potentiates the pressor effects of amitraz and may cause hypertension and cardiac arrhythmias. It also may potentiate ileus and gastric distention. Yohimbine (0.1 mg/kg; IV) is a safe and effective antidote. The effective half-life of yohimbine is 1.5 to 2 hours. Therefore, it may need to be repeated. Atipamezole (50 μg/kg; IM), a potent $α_2$ antagonist, also is an effective antagonist. Reversal of clinical signs of toxicosis are apparent within 10 minutes after injection. In cases of ingestion, and before the onset of clinical signs of toxicosis, vomiting should be induced.

When drug interactions to MAO inhibitors are reported throughout this text, amitraz is given as a possible example, even though studies directly implicating it may not be available.

SUPPLIED AS VETERINARY PRODUCTS:
Available in 10.6-mL units
Impregnated tick collar for dogs containing 9% amitraz

OTHER USES
Cats

NOTOEDRES CATI
Single application of 0.025% solution applied with a toothbrush to affected skin and repeated in 2 weeks

LOCALIZED DEMODECTIC MANGE
Topical application of 0.025% solution to affected lesions twice weekly for 3 weeks

AMITRIPTYLINE HYDROCHLORIDE

INDICATIONS: Amitriptyline (Apo-Amitriptyline ✤, Elavil ✤ ★, Levate ✤, Endep ★, Novotriptyn ✤) is a tricyclic antidepressant drug with antihistaminic, anticholinergic, and local anesthetic properties. It is recommended for the management of anxiety-related behavioral disorders, including depression, separation anxiety in dogs, narcolepsy, compulsive behaviors and anxiety, urine spraying, and excessive grooming in cats. The drug also may have antipruritic properties in dogs. The drug may also ameliorate clinical signs of lower urinary tract inflammation in cats with recurrent idiopathic cystitis for at least 6 months in some patients, although results from a recent report (Kruger JM, et al. Randomized controlled trial of the efficacy of short-term amitriptyline administration for treatment of acute, nonobstructive, idiopathic lower urinary tract disease in cats. JAVMA 2003;222(6): 749–758) indicated that short-term treatment (7 days) had no benefit in the resolution of pollakiuria and hematuria and use of the drug may be associated with an increased risk of recurrence of clinical signs.

ADVERSE AND COMMON SIDE EFFECTS: Sedation may be marked initially. Anticholinergic effects may include dry mouth, urine retention, constipation, tachycardia, and vomiting. Other side effects may include hallucinations, disorientation, and hyperactivity. Amitriptyline is contraindicated in animals with cardiac disease, urinary retention, or a history of seizure activity because the drug lowers the seizure threshold. Adverse effects noted in small animals may include vomiting, hyperexcitability, ataxia, lethargy, tremors, seizures, and cardiac arrhythmias. Diazepam (2.5 to 5 mg/kg; PO or IV) may be used to control the hyperexcitability. Caution is recommended if the drug is used in patients with diabetes mellitus, hyperthyroid disease, and hepatic or renal disease. After long-term use, withdrawal of the drug should be gradual.

DRUG INTERACTIONS: Amitriptyline should not be given within 14 days of an animal receiving an MAO inhibitor, e.g., amitraz (Mitaban) and selegiline (Anipryl). Tachycardia, hyperpyrexia, seizures, and cardiovascular instability may result. Potentiation of CNS depression may occur if the drug is given with barbiturates or sedatives. Concurrent use of epinephrine or norepinephrine and amitriptyline may cause hypertension and hyperpyrexia. Concurrent use with thyroid drugs may accelerate the onset of therapeutic effects, but also may increase the likelihood of cardiac arrhythmias.

SUPPLIED AS HUMAN PRODUCT:
Tablets containing 10, 25, 50, 75 mg

OTHER USES
Cats
IDIOPATHIC CYSTITIS
10 mg per cat daily; PO (at bedtime)

AMLODIPINE

INDICATIONS: Amlodipine besylate (Norvasc ★ ✿) is a calcium channel blocker used to treat systemic hypertension and congestive heart failure. It also has mild natriuretic and diuretic properties. Amlodipine has a slow onset of action and long-lasting effects. The plasma half-life in dogs is 24 hours. In some patients it may be ineffective when used as a single antihypertensive agent yet a combination of amlodipine and a β blocker, e.g., propranolol, may be more effective. Amlodipine has an antihypertensive effect in cats with coexistent systemic hypertension and renal insufficiency.

ADVERSE AND COMMON SIDE EFFECTS: No adverse effects have been reported in cats. Possible adverse effects may include hypotension, bradycardia, hyperkalemia, hyponatremia, and dehydration.

DRUG INTERACTIONS: In clinical trials in people, amlodipine has been safely administered with thiazide diuretics, β blockers, angiotensin-converting enzyme inhibitors, long-acting nitrates, digoxin, warfarin, nonsteroidal anti-inflammatory drugs (NSAIDs), antibiotics, and oral hypoglycemic drugs.

SUPPLIED AS HUMAN PRODUCT:
Tablets containing 2.5, 5, and 10 mg

AMMONIUM CHLORIDE

INDICATIONS: Ammonium chloride is used in the treatment of metabolic alkalosis and has a mild expectorant action. The drug also is used to acidify urine, as adjunctive therapy in the treatment of urinary tract infection, feline lower urinary tract inflammation, and struvite urolithiasis. Ammonium chloride may enhance the antibacterial properties of penicillin G, nitrofurantoin, methenamine mandelate, chlortetracycline, and oxytetracycline. It also is used to enhance the renal excretion of quinidine and the amphetamines in cases of drug intoxication.

ADVERSE AND COMMON SIDE EFFECTS: Nausea and vomiting may occur with oral use of the drug. Intoxication may follow IV use of the drug, demonstrated by metabolic acidosis, hyperventilation, arrhythmias, depression, stupor, coma, and seizure. Ammonium chloride is contraindicated in animals with severe hepatic disease and in those with renal failure. The drug may cause fetal acidosis and should not be given to pregnant animals.

DRUG INTERACTIONS: Acidification of urine may decrease the efficacy of the aminoglycosides and erythromycin.

SUPPLIED AS HUMAN PRODUCTS (★ Only):
Tablets containing 500 mg
For injection; 26.75% (5 mEq/mL) [dilute 1 or 2 vials (100 to 200 mEq) in 500 or 1,000 mL of sodium chloride 0.9% for injection—do not exceed 5 mL/minute] (adult human)

SUPPLIED AS VETERINARY PRODUCTS:
Uroeze ★
Granules containing 400 or 200 mg/teaspoonful
Tablets containing 200 mg

There are no products containing ammonium chloride alone in Canada. It is available in Canada in combination with atropine, hyoscyamine, scopolamine, and sulfisoxazole as Renazone for treatment of renal bacterial infections and renal spasm in small animals.

OTHER USES: Ammonium chloride sometimes is used in cough mixtures for its expectorant activity.

AMOXICILLIN

INDICATIONS: Amoxicillin (Amoxi-Tabs ★, Amoxi-Drop ★, Amoxi-Inject ★, Amoxil ♣, Moxilean ♣, Robamox-V ★) is indicated for the treatment of genitourinary, GI, respiratory, and skin/soft tissue infections in dogs and cats sensitive to the drug. Amoxicillin has the same antibacterial spectrum as ampicillin but is better absorbed from the GIT and has a more rapid bactericidal activity and a longer duration of action. A combination of amoxicillin, metronidazole, and famotidine has been used to treat clinical signs of *Helicobacter* infection in dogs and cats. For more information, see PENICILLIN ANTIBIOTICS.

ADVERSE AND COMMON SIDE EFFECTS: See PENICILLIN ANTIBIOTICS.

DRUG INTERACTIONS: See PENICILLIN ANTIBIOTICS.

SUPPLIED AS VETERINARY PRODUCTS:
Tablets containing 50, 100, 150, 200, and 400 mg
Oral suspension containing 50 mg/mL [Amoxi-Drop, Moxilean, Robamox-V]
For injection containing 3 g/vial [Amoxi-Inject]

OTHER USES
Dogs
LYME BORRELIOSIS
5 mg/kg bid; PO for 10 to 14 days

AMPHOTERICIN B

INDICATIONS: Amphotericin B (Fungizone ♣ ★, Amphocin ★) is an effective antifungal agent. The drug has been used to treat the following infections: blastomycosis, histoplasmosis, cryptococcosis, coccidioidomycosis, *Sporothrix schenckii, Fusarium* species, and candidiasis. The lipid complex form is less toxic and has been found to be as effective as amphotericin B in the treatment of blastomycosis in dogs. Mucoraceae is variably susceptible, and aspergillosis usually is resistant. Relapse may occur when therapy is discontinued.

ADVERSE AND COMMON SIDE EFFECTS: The most important side effect is renal dysfunction. Serum urea and creatinine levels and urinalysis should be monitored frequently throughout the treatment regimen. Administration of the drug is discontinued, at least temporarily, when the blood urea nitrogen (BUN) exceeds 30 to 40 mg/dL (10.7 to 14.3 mmol/L) or serum creatinine exceeds 3 mg/dL (265 μmol/L). Two regimens have been recommended to decrease the nephrotoxicity of amphotericin B (AMB). Mannitol (12.5 g or 0.5 to 1 g/kg) is given concurrently with AMB by slow infusion. However, this technique may decrease the efficacy of AMB, especially in patients with blastomycosis. With the second method, sodium chloride (0.9%) is administered at a rate of 5 mL/kg, half of which is given before injection of AMB and half after AMB injection. Anorexia, nausea, vomiting, fever, phlebitis, normocytic normochromic anemia, hemolytic anemia, and cardiac arrhythmias also have been documented with use of the drug. Cats appear to be more sensitive to the drug than dogs, and lower doses are recommended by some authors. Potassium loss has not been a problem in dogs and cats as it is in humans treated with the drug.

DRUG INTERACTIONS: The concurrent use of aminoglycosides, polymyxin B, cisplatin, methoxyflurane, or vancomycin may potentiate the nephrotoxicity of AMB. When AMB is combined with minocycline and flucytosine, serum concentrations of AMB needed to inhibit growth of *Candida* or *Cryptococcus neoformans* are reduced. Rifampin enhances the effect of AMB on *Aspergillus, Candida,* and *Histoplasma capsulatum.* Similarly, ketoconazole appears to potentiate the efficacy of AMB against blastomycosis and histoplasmosis.

SUPPLIED AS HUMAN PRODUCT:
For injection containing 50 mg lyophilized AMB per vial

For detailed regimens on the preparation and administration of AMB, the reader is directed to Kirk's Current Veterinary Therapy IX: 1102.

OTHER USES
Dogs

BLASTOMYCOSIS
1 mg/kg; IV every Monday, Wednesday, and Friday, and administered at a rate of 4 mg/kg per hour (cumulative dose of 12 mg/kg; AMB lipid complex)

AMPICILLIN

INDICATIONS: Ampicillin (Omnipen ★, Polyflex ✚ ★) is indicated in the treatment of urinary tract, GI, and respiratory tract infections susceptible to the antibiotic. Ampicillin has increased antibacterial activity against many gram-negative bacteria not affected by the natural penicillins or penicillinase-resistant penicillins, including some strains of *E. coli* and *Klebsiella*. Ampicillin also has activity against anaerobic bacteria, including clostridial organisms. Ampicillin is susceptible to β-lactamase bacteria, e.g., *S. aureus.*

ADVERSE AND COMMON SIDE EFFECTS: See PENICILLIN ANTIBIOTICS.

DRUG INTERACTIONS: Do not administer ampicillin with bacteriostatic drugs, e.g., chloramphenicol, erythromycin, or tetracyclines, because the combination may reduce the bactericidal activity of the ampicillin.

SUPPLIED AS VETERINARY PRODUCT:
For injection in 10- and 25-g vials [Polyflex]

SUPPLIED AS HUMAN PRODUCTS:
Capsules containing 250 and 500 mg
Oral suspension containing 100, 125, 250, and 500 mg/5 mL
For injection containing 125-, 250-, and 500-mg and 1-, 2-, and 10-g vials

AMPROLIUM

INDICATIONS: Amprolium (Amprol ♣, Corid ★) is an antiprotozoal agent (coccidiosis). The drug is a thiamine inhibitor.

ADVERSE AND COMMON SIDE EFFECTS: Vomiting, diarrhea, anorexia, depression, and nervous symptoms may develop. In such cases, the drug should be discontinued and the animal treated with thiamine (1 to 10 mg/day; IM, IV). The drug should not be used for more than 12 days in puppies.

DRUG INTERACTIONS: None reported.

SUPPLIED AS VETERINARY PRODUCTS:
Oral solution containing 96 mg/mL (9.6%) [Amprol, Corid] approved for use in calves
Soluble powder containing 200 mg/mL (20%) [Corid] approved for use in calves

ANABOLIC STEROIDS

INDICATIONS: Anabolic androgenic steroids have been used in the treatment of aplastic anemia, myeloproliferative disease, and lymphoma accompanied by nonregenerative anemia. In addition to increasing erythrocyte mass, androgens stimulate myelopoiesis, and thrombopoiesis to a lesser degree. These drugs stimulate the production of erythropoietin, potentiate its effects, and increase the production of erythrocytes. Because of the lack of an extrarenal source of erythropoietin, dogs with anemia secondary to renal failure are less likely to respond, and the expected response essentially is proportional to the amount of functional renal tissue remaining. Several weeks to months may be required for a positive response to be seen, and reportedly, only one third of dogs and cats show a positive erythropoietic response to these drugs. These agents also are hypothesized to stimulate appetite, promote a positive nitrogen balance, enhance skeletal calcium deposition, and promote intestinal absorption of calcium. In dogs with acute uremia, however, boldenone undecylenate failed to enhance appetite or promote an anabolic effect. Danazol, a modified androgen, also has been used with corticosteroids in the management of autoimmune hemolytic anemia and immune-mediated thrombocytopenia. These agents are classified into two groups: alkylated agents (methyltestosterone, fluoxymesterone, oxymetholone, methandrostenolone, stanozolol, norethandrolone) and nonalkylated agents (testosterone, methenolone, nandrolone).

ADVERSE AND COMMON SIDE EFFECTS: Animals with compromised cardiac or renal function should be monitored closely because of the potential for sodium and water retention. Interference with normal female reproductive cycling, masculinization of fetuses during pregnancy, and a reduction in spermatogenesis may occur. Early closure of bony epiphyses in young animals and pain at injection sites have been reported. Additional adverse effects of androgens may include sodium and water retention, hepatotoxicity, recurrence and exacerbation of perianal adenoma, perineal hernia, and prostatomegaly. The nonalkylating drugs are less hepatotoxic but appear to be less effective in stimulating erythrocyte production. In addition, hepatotoxicity occurs primarily with the oral androgens. Parenteral forms essentially are considered nonhepatotoxic. Anabolic steroids also have been implicated in the etiology of hepatic carcinoma.

DRUG INTERACTIONS: See specific drug.

SUPPLIED AS: See specific drug.

ANTACIDS

INDICATIONS: Orally administered antacids contain aluminum hydroxide (Amphojel, Dialume), calcium carbonate (Titralac, Tums), magnesium compounds (Phillips' Milk of Magnesia), combinations of aluminum and magnesium hydroxide (Amphojel Plus, DiGel, Gelusil, Maalox), or aluminum and magnesium hydroxide with calcium carbonate. The use of sodium bicarbonate (baking soda) is not recommended because this drug can lead to systemic alkalosis with repeated use. These drugs are useful in the management of gastric and duodenal bleeding or ulceration and reflux esophagitis. Aluminum-containing products bind intestinal phosphorus and also are used in the management of hyperphosphatemia associated with renal failure. Antacids reduce the amount of gastric acid and decrease the proteolytic effects of pepsin by inactivating the enzyme when the gastric pH is 6 or higher. They have a cytoprotective function through their ability to stimulate the release of prostaglandins and bind bile salts. Astringent properties enhance gastric mucus production. Onset of action is rapid (less than 30 minutes), but the duration of action is brief. For optimal effect, these drugs should be given every 3 to 4 hours.

ADVERSE AND COMMON SIDE EFFECTS: The use of calcium- and aluminum-containing preparations may be associated with constipation; the use of magnesium-containing preparations may be associated with diarrhea. Calcium-containing preparations also may cause hypercalcemia, stimulation of gastric secretion, and impairment of renal function. Aluminum hydroxide also may lead to phosphate depletion, muscle weakness, bone resorption, and hypercalcemia.

DRUG INTERACTIONS: Antacid products may interfere with the absorption of oral iron preparations, digoxin, phenothiazines, glucocorticoids, captopril, ketoconazole, nitrofurantoin, penicillamine, phenothiazines, phenytoin, ranitidine, cimetidine, and the tetracyclines. Increased absorption and serum levels of the following drugs may be seen if given concurrently with antacid compounds: aspirin, quinidine, and sympathomimetic agents.

SUPPLIED AS: See specific drug.

ANTIHISTAMINES

INDICATIONS: Antihistamines, including chlorpheniramine, clemastine, cyproheptadine, diphenhydramine, hydroxyzine, trimeprazine, and terfenadine, have been used to help alleviate pruritus in dogs. The percentage of dogs with atopic dermatitis that respond favorably to antihistamines is 54%, with 27% of the responses rated as good and 27% as moderate. Response to antihistamines is better in dogs having an onset of clinical signs at a younger age. Diphenhydramine and hydroxyzine were the most frequently effective antihistamines. Chlorpheniramine and clemastine had lower positive response rates. Chlorpheniramine and clemastine have been used successfully to control pruritus in some cats. These drugs are histamine (H_1) antagonists with anticholinergic, local anesthetic properties and with some of those listed, sedative properties. At low doses, they block the release of histamine from mast cells and basophils. At higher doses, they may stimulate histamine release. An animal may respond to one form of an antihistamine drug and not another. It is suggested that if one form of an antihistamine is ineffective in controlling pruritus associated with atopic dermatitis in dogs after a 7- to 14-day period, another should be tried for a 7- to 14-day period. Response is better when antihistamines are used in conjunction with omega-3 and omega-6 fatty acids, topical antipruritic therapy, or H_2-blocking agents. These drugs also have been used as antiemetics (by depressing the chemoreceptor trigger zone and inhibiting input from the vestibular apparatus), although they are less effective than the phenothiazines in this regard. Antihistamines also may relieve neuromuscular blockade associated with organophosphate toxicity. Response to antihistamines and sensitivity to toxic effects vary among individual patients.

ADVERSE AND COMMON SIDE EFFECTS: Antihistamines are divided into first-generation and second (nonsedating)-generation drugs. First-generation drugs are small lipophilic molecules capable of crossing the blood-brain barrier. Second-generation antihistamines are less lipophilic and are thought to lack central nervous system and anticholinergic effects at therapeutic dosages. Sedation may be seen with the use of chlorpheniramine, cyproheptadine, diphenhydramine, and trimeprazine; sedative effects are mild with hydroxyzine and minimal or nonexistent with the use of terfenadine. Generally nausea, vomiting, diarrhea, and an increase in pruritus may occur. With drug overdose, hyperexcitability, seizure, and death may occur. Dogs receiving 100 mg/kg per day of terfenadine developed ataxia, trembling, rigidity or weakness, disorientation, or convulsions. Dosages of 150 mg/kg induced vomiting. These drugs should be avoided in patients with glaucoma, urinary retention, CNS disorders, and gastric and duodenal disorders. Some antihistamines are teratogenic and should be avoided during pregnancy.

DRUG INTERACTIONS: In humans, antihistamines should be discontinued for 4 days before skin testing for allergies. Anxiolytic agents, sedatives, narcotics, and barbiturates may enhance CNS depression, and MAO inhibitors, possibly amitraz and selegiline, may prolong and intensify the anticholinergic (drying) effects of antihistamines. Concurrent use of chlorpheniramine with phenytoin may increase the pharmacologic effects of phenytoin. In humans, normal doses of terfenadine when used in conjunction with ketoconazole or erythromycin, or in patients with severe liver disease, may cause severe and life-threatening cardiac arrhythmias. In addition, conditions that increase the risk of cardiac arrhythmias, e.g., electrolyte imbalance or the use of drugs that prolong the QT interval on an electrocardiogram, also may be associated with increased risk.

SUPPLIED AS: See specific drug.

APOMORPHINE HYDROCHLORIDE

INDICATIONS: Apomorphine ★, Britaject ♣, is a useful and effective centrally acting emetic agent for dogs. Use of the drug in cats is controversial. Xylazine or syrup of ipecac is safer and more effective in this species. Apomorphine produces vomiting by directly stimulating the chemoreceptor trigger zone and possibly by excitation of the vestibular apparatus. Gastric emptying may be induced readily in cases of recent (less than 4 hours) oral intoxication.

ADVERSE AND COMMON SIDE EFFECTS: Respiratory depression, sedation, bradycardia, hypotension, salivation, and protracted vomiting have been reported. These signs may be controlled with the IV use of a narcotic antagonist (e.g., naloxone 0.04 mg/kg, levallorphan 0.02 mg/kg, or nalorphine 0.1 mg/kg). Where indicated, the bradycardia may be treated with atropine. The drug is contraindicated in patients with respiratory or CNS depression. Induction of vomiting is contraindicated in unconscious animals and in those that have ingested strong acids, bases, petroleum products, tranquilizers, or other antiemetics. Local induration has been reported in people at SC sites of injection. Safe use of the drug during pregnancy has not been determined.

DRUG INTERACTIONS: Phenothiazine drugs may counter the emetic effects of apomorphine. The drug is contraindicated in those patients with strychnine poisoning and in those with narcosis due to barbiturate, opiate, or other CNS depressant drug use.

SUPPLIED AS HUMAN PRODUCTS:
Note: Apomorphine is difficult to obtain. In Canada, it only can be obtained on an emergency drug-release basis.
Tablets containing 6 mg ★
Ampules containing 10 mg/mL [Britaject]

ASCORBIC ACID

INDICATIONS: Ascorbic acid or vitamin C (Apo-C ♣, Redoxon ♣) is essential for the synthesis and maintenance of collagen and intercellular ground substance of body tissue cells, blood vessels, bone, cartilage, tendons, and teeth. It also is important in wound healing and resistance to infection. It may influence the immune response. Ascorbic acid is used for the treatment of methemoglobinemia due to acetaminophen toxicosis. However, acetylcysteine is the drug of choice in the treatment of acetaminophen toxicosis. Vitamin C has been recommended as adjunctive therapy in the treatment of copper-induced hepatopathy and as a urinary acidifier. Some authors also have supported its use in cases of hypertrophic osteodystrophy. However, the use of vitamin C in these cases actually may accelerate dystrophic calcification and decrease the rate of bone remodeling.

ADVERSE AND COMMON SIDE EFFECTS: Use of the vitamin is very safe. With high doses, nausea, vomiting, diarrhea, abdominal cramping, dysuria, crystalluria (calcium oxalate, cystine, or urate stones), pain at injection sites, and deep venous thrombosis with IV use have been reported in humans.

DRUG INTERACTIONS: Large doses of ascorbic acid may reduce the hypoprothrombinemic effect of oral anticoagulants in some patients.

SUPPLIED AS HUMAN PRODUCT:
Tablets containing 100, 250, 500, or 1,000 mg

OTHER USES
Dogs
COPPER-INDUCED HEPATOPATHY
500 to 1,000 mg once daily; PO

Vitamin C also is used to prevent and treat cancer. The role of vitamin C in reducing established malignancies remains controversial.

ASPARAGINASE

INDICATIONS: Asparaginase (Elspar ★, Kidrolase ♣) is a chemotherapeutic agent used in the treatment of lymphoma, lymphoblastic leukemia, mast cell tumors, and idiopathic thrombocytopenia. The drug inhibits asparaginase synthetase and depletes asparagine in tumor cells. Despite the drug's limited ability to penetrate the blood-brain barrier, it remains effective in the treatment of central nervous system lymphoma. Asparaginase has also been shown to suppress cell-mediated and humoral immunity, which may give this drug a role in the management of immune-mediated disease.

ADVERSE AND COMMON SIDE EFFECTS: Because this drug is a foreign protein, repeated use can lead to immediate hypersensitivity and urticaria, vomiting, diarrhea, dyspnea, hypotension, pruritus, and collapse. Anaphylaxis was reported in up to 30% of dogs given the drug intraperitoneally. Administration of the drug intramuscularly eliminated the occurrence of anaphylaxis. Prior administration of an antihistamine, e.g., diphenhydramine, may decrease the risk of hypersensitivity. If a hypersensitivity reaction does occur, diphenhydramine (0.2 to 0.5 mg/kg; slowly IV), dexamethasone sodium phosphate (1 to 2 mg/kg; IV), and fluid support is recommended. If the reaction is severe, epinephrine (0.1 to 0.3 mL of a 1:1,000 solution; IV) is suggested. Hemorrhagic pancreatitis also has been observed in the dog. Chronic administration has been associated with a regenerative anemia that resolved when the drug was discontinued. The drug should be used with caution in patients with liver disease, diabetes mellitus, infection, or a history of urate calculi.

DRUG INTERACTIONS: For dogs with multicentric lymphoma receiving doxorubicin, intramuscular treatment with asparaginase is more effective than subcutaneous administration. Asparaginase inhibits the activity of methotrexate. These drugs should not be given concurrently. Asparaginase may reduce the hypoglycemic effect of insulin. In humans, increased toxicity may occur if the drug is used concurrently with or before prednisone or vincristine.

SUPPLIED AS HUMAN PRODUCT:
For injection containing 10,000 IU powder in 10-mL vials

OTHER USES: Asparaginase has been reported to be of some benefit to patients with hypoglycemia associated with islet cell tumors. However, the efficacy remains to be determined.

ASPIRIN

INDICATIONS: Aspirin (ASA) or acetylsalicylic acid (ArthriCare ★, Entrophen ✤, and many others) is an effective analgesic for the management of mild to moderate pain. Therapeutic serum concentrations are in the range of 50 to 100 µg/mL. This agent is not effective for the treatment of visceral pain. ASA is an antipyretic and anti-inflammatory agent. Effective anti-inflammatory serum concentrations range from 150 to 300 µg/mL. Aspirin often is used in the therapy of degenerative joint disease. Its antiplatelet activity makes it useful in the prevention of arterial thromboembolic disease as occurs with feline cardiomyopathy (although many cats still form emboli—warfarin may be more effective), heartworm disease, and membranoproliferative glomerulonephritis. A dose that effectively and consistently inhibits thromboembolic formation in cats with cardiomyopathy or in dogs undergoing adulticide therapy for heartworm disease has not yet been established. A recent study documented that there was no significant difference in survival (median survival for those discharged was 117 days) or recurrence of thromboembolic disease in cats receiving high-dose aspirin (>40 mg/cat q 72 hours) and those receiving a lower and safer dose of aspirin (5 mg/cat q 72 hours).

As a topical agent, salicylic acid (2%) has keratolytic, keratoplastic, mildly antipruritic, and bacteriostatic properties. It often is used in conjunction with captan and sulfur as a shampoo for seborrhea, pyoderma, and dermatophytosis. When combined with sulfur, a synergistic effect occurs, and the keratolytic effect is enhanced.

ADVERSE AND COMMON SIDE EFFECTS: Side effects of ASA are dose dependent. Anorexia, vomiting, gastrointestinal ulceration, seizure, and coma have been reported. The presence of food within the GIT may decrease gastric irritation. Although misoprostol may be effective in decreasing GI hemorrhage when given to dogs treated with aspirin, gastritis still tends to occur. The recommended dose of misoprostol for preventing aspirin-induced gastric injury is 3 µg/kg bid; PO. Chronic high doses of the drug have been associated with an increased incidence of gastric carcinoma in the dog. Buffered aspirin also is associated with gastric irritation, and although enteric-coated aspirin produces fewer gastric side effects, absorption of the drug is less consistent. Hepatotoxicosis has also been reported in dogs. Adverse renal effects are less common and tend to occur in dogs with preexisting renal disease or a concurrent disorder that causes renal hypoperfusion.

Aspirin has a much longer half-life in cats (44.6 hours) than in dogs (7.5 hours). The toxic dose reported in cats is greater than 25 mg/kg per day and is greater than 50 mg/kg 3 times daily in dogs (serum concentrations greater than 500 µg/mL). Consequently, more than 7 mL/kg of Pepto-Bismol contains enough aspirin to cause toxicity. Severe toxicity is characterized by vomiting, fever, metabolic acidosis, increased respiratory rate, GIT ulceration and bleeding, depression, seizure, and coma. In cases of toxicity, vomiting should be induced and activated charcoal given. Serum concentrations are increased in hypoalbuminemia, and drug dosages should be decreased in these animals. Serum salicylate concentrations of 50 to 100 µg/mL are in the analgesic range, and concentrations of 150 to 300 µg/mL are anti-inflammatory. Concentrations greater than 500 µg/mL usually are toxic. Serum samples are taken just before the next dose and after steady-state levels have been attained (40 hours in dogs and 8 days in cats). In cases of toxicity, treatment should include the induction of vomiting or gastric lavage with 3% to 5% sodium bicarbonate to delay salicylate absorption. Activated charcoal (2 g/kg) should be given orally to bind any unabsorbed drug. Alkalinization of the urine with sodium bicarbonate (1 to 4 mEq/kg; IV) will increase urinary excretion of the salicylate, and diuretic use (5 mg/kg IV; furosemide) will further augment urinary excretion.

Aspirin is contraindicated in animals with GIT ulceration, renal insufficiency, von Willebrand's disease, or asthma and should be discontinued approximately 1 week before elective surgery. ASA may exacerbate clinical signs associated with Scotty cramp. The drug should not be used in pregnant animals. Reproductive abnormalities, including fetal resorption and stillbirth, have been reported.

Topically applied solutions containing salicylic acid may be irritating to the skin.

DRUG INTERACTIONS: Aspirin is highly protein-bound and if administered to a patient already receiving warfarin, warfarin will be displaced and severe bleeding may occur. ASA may decrease the vasodilatory activity of captopril and enalapril and decrease the efficacy of spironolactone. Concurrent administration with digoxin may lead to increased serum digoxin levels. Its antiplatelet activity in cats may be impaired when used concurrently with propranolol. Simultaneous administration with acidifying agents, e.g., ammonium chloride, may increase the risk of ASA toxicity. Sodium bicarbonate increases the ionization of ASA in urine, promotes its excretion, and is of potential use in cases of aspirin toxicity. Increased hypoglycemic activity of insulin preparations may be seen if ASA (in moderate to large doses) and insulin preparations are given to the same animal. Concurrent use with carbonic anhydrase inhibitors, e.g., acetazolamide, may induce metabolic acidosis and enhance ASA intoxication. Concurrent use of ASA with glucocorticoids increases the risk of GI ulceration and decreases serum levels of ASA by increasing renal excretion of the drug. ASA may increase toxic methotrexate levels. Salicylates in large doses antagonize spironolactone-induced urinary excretion of sodium. Use in conjunction with diuretics may potentiate nephrotoxicity. Methotrexate competes with ASA for plasma protein binding sites predisposing to methotrexate toxicity.

SUPPLIED AS VETERINARY PRODUCTS:
Tablets containing 273 mg [ArthriCare ★]
Tablets containing 60 gr (3.89 g)
Note: 1 gr = 1 grain = 65 mg

SUPPLIED AS HUMAN PRODUCTS:
Tablets containing 65 mg (1 g) and 81 mg (1.25 g)
Tablets (uncoated) containing 325 mg (5 g) and 500 mg (7.8 g)
Tablets (buffered uncoated) containing 325 mg (5 g) and 500 mg (7.8 g)

OTHER USES
Dogs
DISSEMINATED INTRAVASCULAR COAGULATION
150 to 300 mg/20 kg once daily to once every other day for 10 days; PO

ATENOLOL

INDICATIONS: Atenolol (Novo-Atenol ✿, Tenormin ✿ ★) is a selective β_1-blocking agent equal in potency to propranolol. It is the preferred drug in patients with pulmonary disease, e.g., asthma. Atenolol is useful in the management of supraventricular tachyarrhythmias, ventricular premature contractions, systemic hypertension, and hypertrophic cardiomyopathy in cats.

ADVERSE AND COMMON SIDE EFFECTS: The drug is excreted through the kidneys and should be used with caution in animals with compromised renal function. Nausea, vomiting, and diarrhea are less common in small animals than they are in people. Diarrhea, depression, lethargy, hypoglycemia (in diabetics), bradycardia, impaired atrioventricular conduction, syncope, and congestive heart failure have been documented with the use of β blockers. The acute onset of congestive heart failure should respond to dobutamine (1 to 5 µg/kg per minute; IV), furosemide (1 mg/kg; IM), and oxygen therapy. Glycopyrrolate (0.01 mg/kg; IM) and dopamine hydrochloride (1 to 5 µg/kg per minute; IV) can be used to counter the bradycardia, and 5% dextrose in water can be used to manage the hypoglycemia.

DRUG INTERACTIONS: The simultaneous administration of negative inotropic agents, e.g., calcium channel-blocking drugs such as verapamil and diltiazem, or hypoglycemic agents, e.g., insulin, may exacerbate the adverse effects of β blockers. Atropine and other anticholinergic agents enhance GIT absorption of atenolol. Serum lidocaine levels may be increased, predisposing to lidocaine toxicity if both drugs are used concurrently.

SUPPLIED AS HUMAN PRODUCT:
Tablets containing 50 and 100 mg

ATIPAMEZOLE

INDICATIONS: Atipamezole (Antisedan ✿ ★) is a synthetic α-adrenergic antagonist marketed for the reversal of the sedative and analgesic effects of medetomidine hydrochloride in dogs. Atipamezole is given on a volume-per-volume basis (mL for mL) of medetomidine administered.

ADVERSE AND COMMON SIDE EFFECTS: Occasionally, vomiting is seen. Transient excitement or apprehension may be noted, and hypersalivation, diarrhea, and tremors may occur. The drug can cause a rapid reversal of sedation and analgesia predisposing to apprehension and aggression. Patients should be monitored for persistent hypothermia, bradycardia, and depression of respiration until recovery is complete. Safety of the drug in pregnant or lactating bitches has not been established.

DRUG INTERACTIONS: Unknown.

SUPPLIED AS VETERINARY PRODUCT:
For injection containing 5 mg/mL

ATRACURIUM

INDICATIONS: Atracurium (Tracrium ✿ ★) is a nondepolarizing neuromuscular blocking agent used in conjunction with general anesthesia to produce muscle relaxation during surgery or mechanical ventilation and endotracheal intubation.

ADVERSE AND COMMON SIDE EFFECTS: The drug should not be used in patients with myasthenia gravis. Although rare, it may cause histamine release and should be used with caution in susceptible patients, e.g., asthmatics. Adverse reactions are rare and primarily related to histamine release. Side effects may include allergic reactions, prolonged or inadequate neuromuscular block, hypotension, bradycardia, tachycardia, dyspnea, bronchospasm, laryngospasm, rash, urticaria, and reaction at the site of injection. Reversal of blockade can be achieved by the use of an anticholinesterase, e.g., edrophonium, physostigmine, or neostigmine, in conjunction with an anticholinergic, e.g., atropine or glycopyrrolate. Reversal usually is complete within 8 to 10 minutes.

DRUG INTERACTIONS: Neuromuscular blockade may be potentiated by procainamide, quinidine, verapamil, aminoglycoside antibiotics, lincomycin, clindamycin, bacitracin, polymyxin B, magnesium sulfate, thiazide diuretics, enflurane, isoflurane, and halothane. Furosemide may increase or decrease the efficacy of atracurium. Theophylline and phenytoin may inhibit or reverse the blocking action of atracurium. Succinylcholine may hasten the onset of action and enhance the blockade of atracurium.

SUPPLIED AS HUMAN PRODUCT:
For injection containing 10 mg/mL

ATROPINE

INDICATIONS: Atropine ♣ ★ is an anticholinergic, antispasmodic, and mydriatic drug. It is indicated in the treatment of sinus bradycardia, sinus block or arrest, and incomplete atrioventricular block. It is a parasympatholytic agent that causes relaxation of the GIT, biliary, and genitourinary tract and suppresses salivary, gastric, and respiratory tract secretions (given preoperatively). Atropine is a mydriatic and cycloplegic agent, making it useful in the management of ocular inflammation. It also is used in the treatment of organophosphate and carbamate poisoning.

ADVERSE AND COMMON SIDE EFFECTS: Sinus tachycardia (at higher doses), bradycardia (at low doses or seen with initial injection), and second-degree heart block may occur. Atropine also decreases the threshold at which premature ventricular contractions are likely to occur. Dry mouth, dysphagia, constipation, vomiting, thirst, urinary hesitancy, CNS stimulation, drowsiness, ataxia, seizures, and respiratory depression may occur. With drug overdose, respiratory depression and hypotension are likely to occur. Atropine should not be used in patients with asthma because it will have a drying effect on mucous plugs in bronchi, making them difficult to mobilize. The drug should not be given to patients with glaucoma or paralytic ileus or adhesions between the iris and lens. Use of the drug also has been associated with keratoconjunctivitis sicca. Atropine should be used with caution in those with GIT infections because impaired GIT motility will prolong retention of the offending organism(s). In cases of oral drug overdose, cleanse the stomach by inducing vomiting or performing gastric lavage; follow with installation of activated charcoal. Physostigmine (0.1 to 0.6 mg/kg; slowly IV, repeated every 10 minutes until toxicity reversed) may be used as an antidote and diazepam may be used to control CNS stimulation. Additional supportive care includes oxygen therapy and fluid support.

DRUG INTERACTIONS: Atropine may decrease GIT absorption of oral phenothiazine drugs. Antihistamines, procainamide, quinidine, meperidine, benzodiazepines, and the phenothiazines may enhance the activity of atropine. Primidone, disopyramide, nitrates, and long-term corticosteroid use may potentiate adverse effects of atropine. Atropine may enhance the activity of nitrofurantoin, thiazide diuretics, and sympathomimetic agents. Atropine may antagonize the actions of metoclopramide.

SUPPLIED AS VETERINARY PRODUCT:
For injection containing 0.5 mg/mL, 2 mg/mL, and 15 mg/mL (organophosphate toxicity)

SUPPLIED AS HUMAN PRODUCTS:
Ophthalmic ointment (0.5% and 1% atropine sulfate)
Ophthalmic solution (0.5%, 1%, and 2% atropine sulfate)
For injection containing 0.05 and 0.1 mg/mL (in syringes)
For injection containing 0.3, 0.4, 0.5, 0.6, 1.0, and 1.2 mg/mL
Tablets containing 0.4 mg (regular and soluble) and 0.3, 0.4, and 0.6 mg (soluble)

AURANOFIN

INDICATIONS: Auranofin (Ridaura ♣ ★) is an oral gold salt (triethylphosphine) that has been used in dogs to treat idiopathic polyarthritis and pemphigus foliaceus. Gold compounds stabilize lysosomal membranes, decrease migration and phagocytic activity of macrophages and neutrophils, inhibit prostaglandin synthesis, and suppress immunoglobulin synthesis. Furthermore, oral gold therapy inhibits helper T-cell responses without affecting the suppressor T-cell population. A beneficial response in humans may take 3 to 4 months to be seen.

ADVERSE AND COMMON SIDE EFFECTS: An immune-mediated thrombocytopenia may develop. High doses (2.4 to 3.6 mg/kg per day) result in thrombocytopenia and moderate to severe hemolytic anemia. Rapid reversal of these side effects can be expected after cessation of therapy and the administration of corticosteroids. Dose-dependent diarrhea has been reported in some dogs. It resolves with discontinuation of the drug or lowering of the dose. Proteinuria has been documented in people, the incidence of which is low. A complete blood count, platelet count, serum creatinine, and urinalysis should be completed every 2 weeks for the first month, monthly until the third month, and every 3 to 4 months thereafter. Serum biochemistry should be monitored every 6 months or sooner if warranted. In humans, the drug should be used with caution in inflammatory bowel disease, liver disease, bone marrow suppression, diabetes mellitus, and congestive heart failure. The drug has been shown to be embryotoxic in rats and should not be used during pregnancy.

DRUG INTERACTIONS: None.

SUPPLIED AS HUMAN PRODUCT:
Capsules containing 3 mg

AUROTHIOGLUCOSE

INDICATIONS: Aurothioglucose suspension (Solganal ♣ ★) is used in the treatment of pemphigus foliaceus in cats, feline plasma cell stomatitis, plasma cell pododermatitis, canine bullous pemphigoid and pemphigus complex, and rheumatoid arthritis. Gold compounds stabilize lysosomal membranes, decrease migration and phagocytic activity of macrophages and neutrophils, inhibit prostaglandin synthesis, and suppress immunoglobulin synthesis. Positive clinical response should not be expected before 6 to 12 weeks of therapy. If a positive response is not noted after 16 weeks, the dose can be increased to 1.5 mg/kg per week. Once a positive response is seen, the drug can be given as needed; i.e., every 2 to 8 weeks. Aurothioglucose is the preferred parenteral form of gold therapy.

ADVERSE AND COMMON SIDE EFFECTS: Although rare, oral ulcerations, leukopenia, thrombocytopenia, anemia, nephrotic syndrome, hepatitis, miliary dermatitis, stomatitis, and anaphylaxis have been reported. There also has been a possible relationship between the use of aurothioglucose and death associated with toxic epidermal necrolysis in dogs. A complete blood count, serum biochemistry, and urinalysis should be completed every 2 weeks during the first 2 months of therapy and then monthly to quarterly as the dose is reduced. It is recommended to use a test dose for the first and second weeks (as outlined in Section 1: Common Dosages for Dogs and Cats) to rule out potential idiosyncratic reactions. Gold-containing drugs are contra-indicated in patients with renal or hepatic disease, systemic lupus ery-thematosus, uncontrolled diabetes mellitus, or preexisting hematologic disorders. In humans, overdose is treated with BAL (dimercaprol) [to chelate the gold] at a dose of 3 mg/kg IM every 4 hours for the first 2 days, 4 injections on the third day, and 2 injections daily thereafter for 10 days until complete recovery. In milder cases, the dose may be reduced to 2.5 mg/kg.

DRUG INTERACTIONS: The concurrent use of gold salt compounds and immunosuppressant drugs (other than corticosteroids), penicil-lamine, or phenylbutazone increases the risk of blood dyscrasias.

SUPPLIED AS HUMAN PRODUCT:
For injection containing 50 mg/mL

AZATHIOPRINE

INDICATIONS: Azathioprine (Imuran ♣ ★) is a thiopurine anti-metabolite immunosuppressive agent used primarily in the treatment of autoimmune disease. It suppresses primary and secondary antibody responses and has significant anti-inflammatory activity. More specif-ically, the drug has been used in the treatment of immune-mediated skin disease, autoimmune hemolytic anemia, thrombocytopenia, rheumatoid arthritis, polyarthritis, polymyositis, eosinophilic enter-itis, lymphocytic-plasmacytic enteritis, myasthenia gravis, atrophic gastritis, ulcerative colitis, autoimmune uveitis with dermal depig-mentation, systemic lupus erythematosus, ocular histiocytoma, and chronic active hepatitis. Azathioprine also has been used to prevent organ transplant rejection (although it is not effective in reversing ongoing rejection), and as a last resort, to control pruritus in intractable atopic dogs. The drug often is used in combination with glucocorticoids or cyclophosphamide in the management of these disorders. Accord-ing to some researchers, the onset of action is slow, taking 4 to 6 weeks to produce beneficial clinical effects. However, there is no evidence that azathioprine has a slower onset of action than cyclophosphamide. In fact, it has been shown that T-cell suppression is evident within 1 week of initiation of drug use. Azathioprine is less immunosuppressive than cyclophosphamide, and it has fewer deleterious side effects.

ADVERSE AND COMMON SIDE EFFECTS: Leukopenia, anemia, and thrombocytopenia may occur. Cats are especially sensitive to bone marrow toxicity, and for this reason, it generally is not recommended in this species. If used, it is given at a reduced dose. Leukocyte counts should be monitored biweekly during the first 8 weeks of therapy, then monthly. If leukocyte counts decrease to less than 4,000 per microliter, the drug should be discontinued until the leukopenia has resolved.

Other potential adverse effects associated with azathioprine may include pancreatitis, jaundice, skin eruptions, and poor hair growth. Teratogenicity also is a concern, and the drug should not be used in pregnant animals.

DRUG INTERACTIONS: Azathioprine may potentiate the neuromuscular blockade induced by succinylcholine chloride. It may inhibit the neuromuscular blocking activity of pancuronium and tubocurarine. The concurrent use of azathioprine and allopurinol increases the pharmacologic effects and toxicity of the former drug. In humans, it is recommended that the dose of azathioprine should be reduced by one third to one quarter if the two agents are used together.

SUPPLIED AS HUMAN PRODUCTS:
For injection containing 50 mg
Tablets containing 50 mg

OTHER USES
Dogs
INTRACTABLE PRURITUS
2.2 mg/kg per day until pruritus controlled (usually 2 to 3 weeks); then reduced to lowest effective dose
CHRONIC INFLAMMATORY BOWEL DISEASE
i)   1 to 2 mg/kg every 24 to 48 hours; PO

ii) 2 mg/kg per day for 1 week, then every 48 hours; PO

Cats
CHRONIC INFLAMMATORY BOWEL DISEASE
i)   0.3 to 0.5 mg/kg every 24 to 48 hours; PO

ii) 0.3 mg/kg every 48 hours; PO

AZITHROMYCIN

INDICATIONS: Azithromycin (Zithromax ★ ♦) is a macrolide antibiotic, and like other macrolide antibiotics it inhibits protein synthesis by penetrating the cell wall and binding to ribosomal subunits in susceptible bacteria. It is considered a bacteriostatic antibiotic with activity against gram-positive bacteria such as *Streptococcus* and *Staphylococcus* and gram-negative organisms including *Bordetella* spp., *Borrelia burgdorferi*, *Toxoplasma* spp., and *Mycoplasma pneumoniae*.

ADVERSE AND COMMON SIDE EFFECTS: Experience with the drug is limited in small animals. Vomiting and diarrhea may occur, but gastrointestinal signs are likely less frequent than those associated with erythromycin use. Use with caution in animals with hepatic disease. Local skin irritation may occur with intravenous use.

DRUG INTERACTIONS: Azithromycin may increase serum cyclosporine levels. Oral antacids may reduce the rate of absorption of the drug. Where still available, the drug cisapride should not be given concurrently with azithromycin.

SUPPLIED AS HUMAN PRODUCT:
Capsules containing 250 and 600 mg
Oral suspension containing 100 and 200 mg/5 mL
Injection containing 500 mg/vial

BAL: DIMERCAPROL

INDICATIONS: BAL ✤ ★, or dimercaprol, is a sulfhydryl-containing compound that chelates arsenic. It is used principally for the treatment of arsenical toxicity and occasionally for toxicity caused by lead, mercury, copper, antimony, chromium, zinc, and gold. BAL is not very effective in advanced cases of toxicity. Therefore, it is best to administer the drug shortly after exposure.

ADVERSE AND COMMON SIDE EFFECTS: The drug is contraindicated in patients with hepatic insufficiency unless caused by the offending toxin. It should be used with caution in patients with renal impairment. To offset possible renal toxicosis, the urine should be alkalinized. Intramuscular injection is painful. Administer the drug deep into muscle. Signs of BAL toxicity include vomiting, tremors, ataxia, nystagmus, seizures, coma, and death. Tachycardia and a transient increase in blood pressure sometimes are reported. Toxic effects at therapeutic doses generally are not severe and tend to wear off as the drug is excreted over a 3- to 4-hour period.

DRUG INTERACTIONS: Do not administer dimercaprol within 24 hours of iron or selenium compounds. Dimercaprol can form toxic complexes with iron, selenium, uranium, and cadmium.

SUPPLIED AS HUMAN PRODUCT:
For injection containing 100 mg/mL

BARBITURATES

INDICATIONS: The barbiturate drugs are used for sedation and general anesthesia and for control of seizure disorders. The barbiturates are classified as ultrashort-acting agents, including thiopental, and methohexital, with a rapid onset of action (15 to 30 seconds) and short duration of action (5 to 20 minutes) primarily used as induction agents and as the primary anesthetic for short procedures. The short-acting agents include pentobarbital, hexobarbital, and secobarbital. These drugs have a rapid onset of action (30 to 60 seconds) after IV injection and a duration of action of 1 to 2 hours. Pentobarbital is the principal agent used in veterinary medicine in this group as a sedative and general anesthetic. Barbiturates provide little analgesia, thus necessitating high doses in painful procedures. The long-acting barbiturates include barbital and phenobarbital. These drugs have a slow onset of action after IV administration (12 minutes for phenobarbital, 22 minutes for barbital) and a duration of action of 6 to 12 hours after IV injection. This group of drugs is used mainly as sedatives and hypnotics and to control seizure activity.

ADVERSE AND COMMON SIDE EFFECTS: If given perivascularly, the alkaline pH of barbiturates irritates tissues. Apnea and respiratory depression are common after bolus administration. Other side effects may include myocardial depression, arrhythmogenesis (especially thiopental), hypotension, and hypothermia. At sedative doses, barbiturates have a wide margin of safety with few side effects. These drugs should be used with caution in animals with preexisting arrhythmias, renal or hepatic disease, and hypoalbuminemia or acidosis (increased response and possible toxicity to barbiturates). Lack of body fat can predispose to prolonged recovery because recovery is determined by redistribution from the CNS to other organs, including body fat. Greyhounds and other sight hounds metabolize thiobarbiturates more slowly than methohexital, an oxybarbiturate, making the latter the preferred barbiturate in these breeds. The obese animal is at risk for relative drug overdose. The very young and very old patient also are at increased risk for barbiturate effects because of immature development of hepatic enzyme systems (the young) and impaired liver function (the old), leading to delayed metabolism. Hypothyroidism may predispose to increased sensitivity to anesthetic drugs. Treatment of drug overdose includes doxapram (2% solution: 3 to 5 mg/kg; IV, repeat as necessary), oxygen, and fluid support. See specific drug for more details. Repeated doses of barbiturates can result in excessive anesthetic times and prolonged recovery. Thiobarbiturates may induce anaphylactoid reactions mediated by histamine release via a nonimmunologic mechanism that can occur without prior drug exposure.

DRUG INTERACTIONS: Metabolic acidosis, hypoalbuminemia, renal or hepatic disease, the administration of nonsteroidal anti-inflammatory agents, certain sulfonamides, glucose, and atropine augment the anesthetic effect of barbiturates and potentiate toxicity. Any CNS depressant enhances the response to barbiturates.

SUPPLIED AS: See specific product.

BENAZEPRIL HYDROCHLORIDE

INDICATIONS: Benazepril hydrochloride (Fortekor ✤) is a second-generation angiotensin-converting enzyme (ACE) inhibitor. Like other

ACE inhibitors, captopril and enalapril, it is used to manage patients with congestive heart failure caused by mitral valvular regurgitation or dilated cardiomyopathy. The drug may be an effective treatment to slow the rate of progression of renal failure in cats.

ADVERSE AND COMMON SIDE EFFECTS: Renal failure has no effect on elimination of the drug, and drug dosage does not need to be adjusted in dogs with renal insufficiency. Although overdosage of up to 200 times was not accompanied by deleterious effects, transient reversible hypotension signaled by fatigue and dizziness may occur with overdosage. Benazepril is eliminated by biliary excretion. It is recommended that plasma urea and creatinine be monitored in patients with renal insufficiency. The safety of the drug in breeding or lactating animals has not been studied.

DRUG INTERACTIONS: Benazepril may be used safely in conjunction with digoxin, diuretics, and antiarrhythmic agents.

SUPPLIED AS VETERINARY PRODUCT:
Tablets containing 5 and 20 mg

BENZOYL PEROXIDE

INDICATIONS: Benzoyl peroxide (Oxydex ★, Pyoben ✿ ★) is a degreasing, astringent, keratolytic, keratoplastic, antipruritic, topical anesthetic, wound-healing, follicular-flushing, and anti-inflammatory agent useful in the treatment of Schnauzer comedo syndrome, canine and feline acne, seborrhea, superficial pyoderma, pruritus, crusts, and scales.

ADVERSE AND COMMON SIDE EFFECTS: The 5% solution can be irritating to animals, causing dryness and local irritation. The gel often is too irritating for use in cats. Avoid contact with the eyes and mucous membranes. If irritation develops, discontinue use. Benzoyl peroxide may discolor fabrics.

DRUG INTERACTIONS: None.

SUPPLIED AS VETERINARY PRODUCTS:
Gel 5% [Oxydex]
Shampoo 2.5% [Oxydex]
Shampoo 3% [Pyoben]

BETAMETHASONE

INDICATIONS: Betamethasone (Betasone ★) is a long-acting injectable glucocorticoid used for the control of pruritus in dogs. Betamethasone valerate (Valisone cream) is the cream formulation. For more information on INDICATIONS, ADVERSE AND COMMON SIDE EFFECTS, and DRUG INTERACTIONS, see GLUCOCORTI-COID AGENTS.

ADVERSE AND COMMON SIDE EFFECTS: Betamethasone should be used with caution in dogs with congestive heart failure, diabetes mellitus, and renal disease. Injections of betamethasone have resulted in decreased sperm output, increased percentages of abnormal sperm, and decreased concentrations of serum testosterone. This drug, therefore, should be used with caution in stud dogs. Potent topical corticosteroid agents may be associated with the induction of steroid acne, aggravation of folliculitis, atrophy of epidermal, dermal, and SC tissues, telangiectasia, purpura, poor healing, exacerbation of ulceration, hypopigmentation, hypertrichosis, and aggravation of preexisting disease.

DRUG INTERACTIONS: The concurrent use of barbiturate agents, phenytoin, or rifampin reduces the pharmacologic effects of betamethasone by increasing its metabolism through the induction of liver enzymes. Betamethasone reduces the pharmacologic effects of other corticosteroids and aspirin, requiring higher doses of these drugs if they are given concurrently with betamethasone.

SUPPLIED AS VETERINARY PRODUCT:
For injection containing betamethasone dipropionate equivalent to 5 mg/mL betamethasone and betamethasone sodium phosphate equivalent to 2 mg/mL betamethasone

BETHANECHOL CHLORIDE

INDICATIONS: Bethanechol (Duvoid ✿ ★, Urecholine ✿ ★) is a cholinergic agent used to stimulate muscular contraction of the bladder in cases of detrusor atony. Although the efficacy of the drug has been questioned in humans, in cats unable to urinate because of dysautonomia, bethanechol stimulated urination 30 to 60 minutes after an oral dose of 0.125 or 0.25 mg.

ADVERSE AND COMMON SIDE EFFECTS: Mild vomiting, diarrhea, anorexia, abdominal cramping, bradycardia, increased salivation, and lacrimation may occur with oral doses. Arrhythmias, hypotension, and bronchospasm generally are seen only with overdosage. The drug is contraindicated if urethral obstruction is present. Drugs used to decrease urethral outflow resistance, e.g., diazepam or phenoxybenzamine, may be used concurrently in cases of reflex dyssynergia. The drug is contraindicated in patients with obstructive pulmonary disease, bronchial asthma, hyperthyroidism, cystitis, bacteriuria, peptic ulcer, peritonitis, atrioventricular conduction defects, severe bradycardia, hypotension, hypertension, and epilepsy. Overdosage is treated with atropine. Epinephrine may be used to treat symptoms of bronchospasm.

DRUG INTERACTIONS: Bethanechol should not be used concurrently with neostigmine because additive cholinergic effects and possible toxicity may occur. Procainamide and quinidine may antagonize the cholinergic effects of the drug, and this combination should be used with caution.

SUPPLIED AS HUMAN PRODUCTS:
For injection containing 5 mg/mL
Tablets containing 5, 10, 25, and 50 mg

BISACODYL

INDICATIONS: Bisacodyl (Dulcolax ❦ ★, Correctol ★ ❦) is a laxative used to help alleviate constipation and to help cleanse the colon for colonoscopy. After rehydration to soften feces, it is a useful drug for the treatment of severe impaction. The drug induces contractions by direct stimulation of sensory nerve endings in the colonic wall and expands intestinal fluid volume by increasing epithelial permeability. The drug generally acts within 6 to 12 hours.

ADVERSE AND COMMON SIDE EFFECTS: Rarely, mild cramping, nausea, and diarrhea have been observed in some patients.

DRUG INTERACTIONS: It is advised not to give oral medication within 2 hours of administering a laxative.

SUPPLIED AS HUMAN PRODUCTS:
Microenema containing 10 mg [Dulcolax]
Suppositories containing 5 and 10 mg
Tablets containing 5 mg

BISMUTH SUBSALICYLATE

INDICATIONS: Bismuth subsalicylate (Pepto-Bismol ❦ ★) is used in the treatment of diarrhea. It inhibits the synthesis of prostaglandins responsible for GIT hypermotility and inflammation. The drug also may have antibacterial and antisecretory properties. Bismuth subsalicylate relieves indigestion by forming insoluble complexes with offending noxious agents and by forming a protective coating. This agent has also been reported to be useful in the management of flatulence. It has antibacterial properties and reduces the odor of flatus yet it likely has to be given several times daily, which precludes its long-term use.

ADVERSE AND COMMON SIDE EFFECTS: The drug is contra-indicated in those patients sensitive to salicylate drugs. Cats may be especially sensitive to the salicylate content especially in the presence of an inflamed bowel. Although doses above 7 mL/kg per day are theorized to be potentially toxic, no reports of clinical toxicity have been reported and the salicylate in bismuth subsalicylate does not induce as much GI blood loss as an equivalent dose of aspirin. See also ASPIRIN. Stool color may darken with its use. With high doses, fecal impaction may occur. Bismuth subsalicylate is radiopaque and may interfere with radiographic GIT studies.

DRUG INTERACTIONS: The antimicrobial action of tetracyclines may be reduced if these drugs are used concurrently. It is advised that tetracycline be given at least 2 hours before or after bismuth administration.

SUPPLIED AS HUMAN PRODUCTS:
Suspension containing 17.47 mg/mL
Tablets (chewable) containing 262 mg

BLEOMYCIN

INDICATIONS: Bleomycin (Blenoxane ✤ ★) is an antineoplastic glycopeptide antibiotic. In small animals, it may be useful in the treatment of nonfunctional thyroid tumors, malignant teratoma, lymphoma, and squamous cell carcinoma. Intralesional bleomycin has been used effectively in the management of acanthomatous epulis in dogs.

ADVERSE AND COMMON SIDE EFFECTS: Clinical signs of acute toxicity may include nausea, vomiting, fever, anaphylaxis, and other allergic reactions. Signs of delayed toxicity may include pneumonitis and pulmonary fibrosis, rash, stomatitis, and alopecia.

DRUG INTERACTIONS: Other antineoplastic agents used in conjunction with bleomycin predispose to bleomycin toxicity, including bone marrow suppression. Bleomycin decreases the GIT absorption, and pharmacologic effects of digoxin and phenytoin are reduced if used concurrently.

SUPPLIED AS HUMAN PRODUCT:
For injection containing 15 units/vial

BROMIDE SALTS

INDICATIONS: Bromide salts (potassium, sodium, and ammonium) have been used effectively in the management of seizure disorders in people. Potassium bromide has been used in dogs unresponsive to therapeutic serum concentrations of phenobarbital (as adjunctive therapy with phenobarbital), epileptic patients with suspected anticonvulsant-induced hepatotoxicity, and in epileptics with pre-existing liver dysfunction. It may also be used as the sole anticonvulsant agent in dogs in which phenobarbital is contraindicated because of its potential hepatotoxic effects. The drug penetrates the CNS, raises the seizure threshold, and prevents the spread of epileptic discharge. Steady-state drug levels are achieved after 4 to 6 months in the dog (serum levels are measured 1, and 4 to 6 months after initiation of therapy and are taken before the next dose, preferably in the morning). Reported therapeutic serum concentrations of potassium bromide range from 0.5 to 1.6 mg/mL or 0.7 to 1.9 mg/mL and 0.7 to 2.3 mg/mL and 1 to 3 mg/mL, or 100 to 200 mg/dL and 7 to 17 mmol/L. Toxic levels are in excess of 20 mmol/L. When dogs are treated with bromide and phenobarbital, therapeutic serum bromide concentrations are in the order of 0.81 to 2.4 mg/mL and phenobarbital concentrations are in the range of 9 to 36 μg/mL. When bromide is used alone, therapeutic serum concentrations are in the range of 0.88 to 3.0 mg/mL. Seizure control has been achieved in 80 to 90% of dogs treated with a combination of potassium bromide and phenobarbital. Potassium bromide is also used in cats when phenobarbital alone does not effectively decrease the frequency or severity of seizure activity. Steady state levels in cats may be attained within 2 months. Therapeutic concentrations may be attained within 2 weeks when cats are dosed at 30 mg/kg per day. Although somewhat effective in controlling seizure activity in this species, the incidence of adverse effects may not warrant its routine use. One report documented seizure control in only 6 of 17 cats.

ADVERSE AND COMMON SIDE EFFECTS: Bromide sensitivity may be affected by diets high in chloride content (e.g., Hill's S/D and I/D), dehydration, vomiting, diarrhea, and impaired renal function. High chloride-containing diets decrease bromide levels necessitating an increase in drug dose. In dogs, reported side effects include polydipsia, polyphagia, excessive sedation, ataxia, depression, anisocoria, muscle pain, and stupor. Pancreatitis also has been reported from use of the combination of bromide and phenobarbital (at least 10% of dogs as opposed to only 0.3% on phenobarbital alone). Occasional nausea may be resolved by dividing the daily dose or switching to sodium bromide. Twenty milligrams per kilogram of potassium bromide is equal to 17.3 mg/kg of sodium bromide, i.e., if changing from potassium to sodium bromide, decrease the dose by 15%. Discontinuation of the drug and supportive therapy, including IV isotonic saline, hastens recovery from drug toxicity. Diuretic therapy, e.g., loop diuretics, also may be beneficial. In humans, neonatal bromide intoxication causing growth retardation has been associated with maternal use of the drug during pregnancy. Clinical signs of intoxication also have been reported in human infants nursing from mothers taking the drug. Experience with use of the drug in cats is limited. In cats a persistent cough develops in a number of patients (>40%), which resolves upon discontinuation of the drug and concurrent use of glucocorticoids.

The most common laboratory abnormality noted in dogs given potassium bromide is an artifactual hyperchloremia (DACOS colorimetric methodology). However, flame photometric analysis will correctly determine serum chloride levels.

DRUG INTERACTIONS: Bromide may enhance the effects of other anticonvulsants on the CNS. The use of potassium bromide alone or in combination with primidone and diphenylhydantoin predisposes to hepatotoxicity. The toxicity of bromide may be reduced by a reduction in the drug dose or frequency when it is used in conjunction with other anticonvulsants. Bromide levels increase after halothane anesthesia and remain elevated for days to weeks thereafter, although the increase is reportedly small (40 to 88 mg/L). Loop diuretics (ethacrynic acid, furosemide) may enhance bromide elimination.

SUPPLIED AS HUMAN PRODUCT:
Potassium bromide [Fischer Scientific, Pittsburgh, PA; ICN Biomedicals, Costa Mesa, CA; Sigma Chemical Co., St. Louis, MO; Aldrich, Milwaukee, WI; VWR Scientific, Bridgeport, NJ]

In Canada, the drug is available only through a limited number of pharmacies.

BUDESONIDE

INDICATIONS: Budesonide (Entocort ♣ ★) is a glucocorticoid that may be useful in the management of inflammatory bowel disease. Budesonide has a high topical glucocorticoid activity and a substantial first-pass elimination. The drug is rapidly inactivated in the liver resulting in lower systemic bioavailability and reduced effects on the hypothalamic-pituitary-adrenal axis making iatrogenic hyperadrenocorticism less common. One abstract described superior efficacy with budesonide versus prednisone for dogs and cats with inflammatory bowel disease.

ADVERSE AND COMMON SIDE EFFECTS: Little experience is available in small animals. See GLUCOCORTICOIDS.

DRUG INTERACTIONS: Co-administration of ketoconazole results in an increase in serum levels of budesonide. Since the dissolution of the coating of ENTOCORT EC is pH dependent (dissolves at pH > 5.5), the release properties and uptake of the compound may be altered after treatment with drugs that change the gastrointestinal pH. However, the gastric acid inhibitory drug omeprazole does not affect the absorption or pharmacokinetics of ENTOCORT EC. When an uncoated oral formulation of budesonide is co-administered with a daily dose of cimetidine, a slight increase in the budesonide peak plasma concentration and rate of absorption occurs, resulting in significant cortisol suppression.

A mean delay in time to peak concentration is observed with the intake of a high-fat meal.

SUPPLIED AS HUMAN PRODUCTS:
Capsules containing 3 mg
Enema containing 0.02 mg/mL

BUPRENORPHINE HYDROCHLORIDE

INDICATIONS: Buprenorphine hydrochloride (Buprenex ★) is a partial opiate agonist with analgesic properties. It is used for the management of mild pain. In dogs and cats, analgesia lasts 4 to 8 hours and longer after epidural administration. It is less effective than morphine or oxymorphone for moderate to severe pain.

ADVERSE AND COMMON SIDE EFFECTS: Respiratory depression may occur. In humans, sedation also may be noted. Opiates should be used with caution in animals with hypothyroid disease, severe renal insufficiency, hypoadrenocorticism, debilitated patients, those with head trauma or CNS dysfunction, and geriatrics. The drug is resistant to antagonism by naloxone.

DRUG INTERACTIONS: The concurrent use of other CNS depressants (anesthetics, antihistamines, tranquilizers) may potentiate CNS and respiratory depression. This drug may inhibit the analgesic effects of opiate agonists, e.g., morphine.

SUPPLIED AS HUMAN PRODUCT:
For injection containing 0.324 mg/mL in 1-mL ampules

BUSPIRONE

INDICATIONS: Buspirone (BuSpar ✤ ★) is a nonbenzodiazepine antianxiety drug. It is used to treat various behavioral disorders in dogs and cats, e.g., chronic fears/anxiety, phobias, aggression, and stereotypy-obsessive disease. It does not promote sedation or behavioral dependence. The drug is considered by some to be the drug of choice in the management of urine spraying and inappropriate urination in cats. If after one week the drug is successful in the management of urine spraying in cats, it is continued for 8 weeks and then the dose is gradually reduced. If urine spraying resumes, buspirone is continued for 6 to 12 months, and then the dose is gradually reduced. Cats from multicat households favorably respond more often than cats from single-cat households. Only half of the cats treated with buspirone resumed spraying when the drug was discontinued after 2 months of treatment versus those treated with diazepam in which more than 90% resumed spraying.

ADVERSE AND COMMON SIDE EFFECTS: Rarely sedation may occur. Agitation after administration of the drug is similarly rare. An increase in affection toward owners and aggression toward other cats also is reported. In humans, the drug may cause an increase in liver enzymes [alanine transaminase (ALT), aspartate transaminase (AST)].

DRUG INTERACTIONS: None of significance to small animals.

SUPPLIED AS HUMAN PRODUCT:
Tablets containing 5 and 10 mg

BUSULFAN

INDICATIONS: Busulfan (Myleran ★ ♣, Busulfex ★ ♣) is an alkylating chemotherapeutic agent used most often in combination with other chemotherapeutic agents in the treatment of chronic granulocytic leukemias.

ADVERSE AND COMMON SIDE EFFECTS: The most common adverse effect is myelosuppression. In people, anemia, leukemia, and thrombocytopenia may be noted with the onset of leukemia 10 to 15 days after initiation of treatment and leukocyte nadirs occurring around 11 to 30 days. In humans, other adverse effects reported include stomatitis, pulmonary fibrosis, and uric acid nephropathy.

DRUG INTERACTIONS: Concurrent use with other chemotherapeutic agents may potentiate likelihood of myelosuppression. Use with thioguanine may cause a hepatopathy.

SUPPLIED AS HUMAN PRODUCTS:
Tablets containing 2 mg
For injection containing 6 mg/mL

BUTORPHANOL

INDICATIONS: Butorphanol (Torbugesic ♣ ★, Torbutrol ♣ ★) is a narcotic agonist/antagonist analgesic with potent antitussive activity in dogs. It has minimal cardiovascular effects and causes only slight respiratory depression. Alone, it causes little sedation. Analgesia occurs 30 minutes after IM injection and reaches peak activity in 1 hour. With IV injection, the analgesic effect is immediate, with peak activity in 30 minutes. Pain relief lasts 2 to 3 hours. The drug is 5 times more potent in pain relief than morphine, 15 to 30 times more potent than pentazocine, and 30 to 50 times more potent than meperidine. It provides effective visceral analgesia at low doses for up to 6 hours in cats; however, somatic analgesia is only attained at higher IV doses (0.8 mg/kg) and is only of short duration (1 to 2 hours). Butorphanol tartrate is 15 to 20 times more effective in the management of cough than codeine or dextromethorphan.

ADVERSE AND COMMON SIDE EFFECTS: Although rare, side effects after oral use may include slight sedation, anorexia, nausea, and diarrhea. Because the drug suppresses the cough reflex, it should not be used in dogs with a productive cough. Moderate to marked cardiopulmonary depression has been reported only with IV infusions given at rapid rates (0.2 mg/kg per minute). Panting may occur with doses of 0.4 mg/kg IV. In conscious dogs, the drug produces minimal cardiovascular or respiratory effects. Mydriasis lasting as long as 3 hours after an IV dose of 0.2 mg/kg may be seen in cats. Until further studies are complete, the drug should not be used in pregnant animals or male stud dogs. Butorphanol should not be given to animals with liver disease. The safety of butorphanol use in heartworm-positive dogs has not been established. The drug should not be given with other analgesic agents as the effects are additive. All opiates should be used with caution in debilitated animals and those with head trauma, increased CSF pressure, hypothyroidism, severe renal disease, or adrenocortical insufficiency.

DRUG INTERACTIONS: Butorphanol can be used as an antagonist to narcotic agonists, such as meperidine, morphine, and oxymorphone. As an antagonist, butorphanol is approximately equivalent to nalorphine and 30 times more potent than pentazocine. Marked sedation occurs when butorphanol is combined with acepromazine, more so in medium to large breed dogs. When used with other CNS depressants, such as the barbiturates and phenothiazine tranquilizers, additive respiratory depression may occur. Use these combinations with caution. Concurrent use of pancuronium may lead to conjunctival changes.

SUPPLIED AS VETERINARY PRODUCTS:
Tablets containing 1-, 5-, and 10-mg base activity
For injection containing 0.5 and 10 mg/mL

OTHER USES
Dogs
ANTITUSSIVE
i)   0.05 to 0.12 mg/kg bid to tid; PO
ii) 0.05 to 0.1 mg/kg bid to qid; SC, PO

ANALGESIA
0.2 to 0.4 mg/kg; IM, IV

ANTIEMETIC IN CISPLATIN-INDUCED EMESIS
0.4 mg/kg; IM at the beginning and end of a 3-hour cisplatin infusion

PREANESTHETIC
i)   0.05 mg/kg; IV or 0.4 mg/kg; SC, IM

ii) 0.1 to 0.2 mg/kg; IM

iii) 0.2 to 0.4 mg/kg; IM (with acepromazine 0.02 to 0.04 mg/kg; IM)

NEUROLEPTANALGESIA DOSE
Butorphanol 0.2 mg/kg; IV
Acepromazine 0.05 mg/kg; IV
Atropine 0.02 mg/kg; IV
To make a 20 mL solution mix together the following:
Butorphanol 4 mL of 10 mg/mL = 40 mg
Acetylpromazine 0.5 mL of 10 mg/mL solution = 5 mg
Atropine 8 mL of 0.5 mg/mL solution = 4 mg (atropine may be
replaced by 8 mL glycopyrrolate of a 0.2 mg/mL solution). Make the
mixture up to 20 mL with sterile water. All three agents can be mixed
in one syringe. Sedation can be reversed with naloxone.

PREANESTHETIC DOSE OF THIS MIXTURE:
Dogs 0.05 to 0.1 mL/kg; IM, SC
Cats 0.1 to 0.13 mL/kg; IM, SC

Cats
PREANESTHETIC
i)   0.1 to 0.2 mg/kg; IM

ii) 0.2 to 0.4 mg/kg; IM (with glycopyrrolate 0.01 mg/kg; IM and
     ketamine 4 to 10 mg/kg; IM)

ANALGESIA
i)   0.1 to 0.2 mg/kg; IM, IV

ii) 0.4 mg/kg; SC

CALCITONIN SALMON

INDICATIONS: Calcitonin salmon (Calcimar ✚ ★) may be an effective
adjunct (in addition to fluid therapy, diuretics, and corticosteroids) to
the management of hypercalcemia. The drug inhibits bone resorption.
Efficacy usually is noted 4 to 12 hours after injection.

ADVERSE AND COMMON SIDE EFFECTS: Little data are available
in small animals. In humans, transient nausea, anorexia, and vomiting are encountered most frequently. Local inflammatory reactions at
the injection site develop in a few patients. In a few cases, administration of calcitonin has resulted in allergic reactions, e.g., bronchospasm,

swelling of the tongue, and anaphylactic shock. Some hypercalcemic dogs become refractory to treatment with the drug after several days and hypercalcemia recurs. The drug may result in decreased fetal birth weights and is not advised for use in pregnancy. Calcitonin also inhibits lactation and should not be given to nursing animals.

DRUG INTERACTIONS: None.

SUPPLIED AS HUMAN PRODUCT:
For injection containing 200 IU/mL in 400-IU vials

OTHER USES: In humans, the drug also has been shown to decrease increased serum calcium levels in patients with carcinoma, multiple myeloma, and primary hyperparathyroidism.

CALCITRIOL

INDICATIONS: Calcitriol (Calcijex ✤ ★, Rocaltrol ✤ ★), a vitamin D_3 metabolite, is used in the management of hypocalcemia. It also may be used to prevent or reverse renal secondary hyperparathyroidism in dogs and cats with chronic renal failure. It has a rapid onset of action (1 to 4 days) and a short half-life (4 to 6 hours). Oral calcitriol is administered to patients after initial stabilization with fluid therapy, dietary protein, and phosphorus restriction, the use of intestinal phosphate binders and H_2 blockers as needed. Serum phosphorus should be less than 6 mg/dL (1.9 mmol/L) before initiating calcitriol.

ADVERSE AND COMMON SIDE EFFECTS: Hypercalcemia leading to polyuria, polydipsia, listlessness, depression, anorexia, vomiting, nephrocalcinosis, muscle weakness, and trembling or muscle twitching may occur. If hypercalcemia results from drug overdosage, it generally will resolve within 4 days of discontinuing the drug. Hypercalcemia usually only occurs if calcitriol is used in conjunction with intestinal phosphate binders, especially calcium carbonate. Safety of the use of this product in pregnant or lactating animals has not been established.

DRUG INTERACTIONS: Hypercalcemia may precipitate cardiac arrhythmias in patients on digitalis. Intestinal absorption may be impaired by cholestyramine and by mineral oil (when used as a laxative). Long-term use of phenytoin and the barbiturates may interfere with the action of the drug, necessitating higher doses of calcitriol. Thiazide diuretics may enhance the effects of calcitriol predisposing to hypercalcemia. Calcitriol-induced hypercalcemia may antagonize the antiarrhythmic effects of calcium channel-blocking agents.

SUPPLIED AS HUMAN PRODUCTS:
Capsules containing 0.25 and 0.50 µg
Oral solution containing 1.0 µg/mL
For injection containing 1 and 2 µg/mL

CALCIUM CARBONATE

INDICATIONS: Calcium carbonate (Apo-Cal ✿, Calsan ✿, Os-Cal ✿
★, Calci-Chew ★) is a rapid-acting antacid drug with high neutralizing
properties and relatively prolonged duration of action. It also increases
lower esophageal sphincter tone. The drug also is used for the management of hyperphosphatemia associated with renal failure. Calcium
carbonate is not as potent a phosphorus binder as the aluminum salts.

ADVERSE AND COMMON SIDE EFFECTS: The use of calcium-
containing antacid preparations may be associated with constipation or
diarrhea. Calcium-containing preparations also may cause hypercalcemia, stimulation of gastric secretion, and impairment of renal function. A slight alkalosis may develop with prolonged use of the drug.
Gastric acid rebound may be caused by the release of gastrin triggered
by the action of calcium in the small intestines. Liberation of carbon
dioxide in the stomach causes belching in some patients. The drug is
contraindicated in patients with hypercalcemia, hypercalciuria, severe
renal disease, renal calculi, gastrointestinal hemorrhage or obstruction,
dehydration, hypochloremic alkalosis, ventricular fibrillation, cardiac
disease, and pregnancy. Cautious use of the drug is recommended in
patients with decreased bowel motility, e.g., those receiving anticholinergics, antidiarrheals, or antispasmodics. Also see ANTACIDS.

DRUG INTERACTIONS: Calcium carbonate may decrease oral iron
absorption. The absorption of oral tetracyclines and phenytoin may
be decreased. Administer the tetracycline up to 3 hours before or after
calcium carbonate. Calcium carbonate may antagonize the effects of
calcium channel-blocking agents, e.g., verapamil, diltiazem, nifedipine. Thiazide diuretics used concurrently with large doses of calcium
may cause hypercalcemia.

SUPPLIED AS HUMAN PRODUCTS:
Tablets containing 250, 500, and 750 mg
Capsules containing 500 mg

OTHER USES
Dogs

HYPOCALCEMIA ASSOCIATED WITH HYPOPARATHYROIDISM
100 to 200 mg/kg bid to tid; PO

HYPERPHOSPHATEMIA ASSOCIATED WITH RENAL FAILURE
100 mg/kg per day divided bid or tid; PO

CALCIUM CHLORIDE

INDICATIONS: Calcium chloride ♣ ★ (Calciject ♣) is used in the treatment of cardiac arrest (ventricular asystole and electromechanical dissociation) to stimulate cardiac excitation when epinephrine fails to improve myocardial contractions and hyperkalemic myocardial toxicity. It also may be used in the acute treatment of hypocalcemia.

ADVERSE AND COMMON SIDE EFFECTS: Hypercalcemia may occur. With rapid IV injection, hypotension, bradycardia, syncope, cardiac arrhythmias, and cardiac arrest may occur. Extravascular injection causes inflammation, tissue necrosis, and sloughing. If perivascular injection occurs, recommendations include injection of the area with normal saline, corticosteroids, 1% procaine, and hyaluronidase. In addition, heat should be applied to the affected area and the limb should be kept elevated. Calcium chloride should be used with caution in animals with nephrocalcinosis. The safety of its use during pregnancy has not been established.

DRUG INTERACTIONS: Calcium chloride may increase the risk of digitalis toxicity in patients receiving digitalis drugs. Calcium chloride-induced hypercalcemia may negate the efficacy of calcium channel-blocking agents, e.g., verapamil, diltiazem, and nifedipine. Calcium chloride for injection is incompatible with amphotericin B, bicarbonates, carbonates, cephalothin sodium, chlorpheniramine, phosphates, sulfates, and tartrate admixtures. Thiazide diuretics used concurrently with large doses of calcium may cause hypercalcemia.

SUPPLIED AS HUMAN PRODUCT:
For injection containing 100 mg/mL providing a 10% solution

CALCIUM EDTA

INDICATIONS: Calcium disodium EDTA (Calcium Disodium Versenate ♣ ★) is a favored chelating agent for the treatment of lead toxicity in the dog and cat. Before administration, calcium EDTA is diluted to a 1% solution using 5% dextrose in water.

ADVERSE AND COMMON SIDE EFFECTS: The drug is contraindicated in patients with anuria, and drug dosage should be decreased in those with renal failure. Intravenous administration may cause an increase in CSF pressure and the potential for fatal lead-induced cerebral edema. Therefore, the SC route of administration is recommended. High concentrations can cause pain at the injection site. Lidocaine can be mixed with the solution to prevent pain. Depression, vomiting, and diarrhea may occur but may be alleviated by concurrent zinc supplementation. The most serious potential side effect of calcium EDTA is reversible renal tubular necrosis. Dosages greater than 12 g/kg are fatal in dogs. During the first 72 hours of chelation, blood lead concentrations rapidly decrease and clinical improvement is noted, but then they become constant or even increase during the remainder of the treatment schedule. Therefore, blood lead levels should be submitted only 10 to 14 days after treatment to evaluate the efficacy of therapy.

DRUG INTERACTIONS: Concurrent administration with zinc insulin preparations will decrease the sustained action of the insulin. Renal toxicity of calcium EDTA may be potentiated by the use of corticosteroids. Calcium EDTA should be used with caution with other potentially nephrotoxic agents, e.g., aminoglycosides and amphotericin B.

SUPPLIED AS HUMAN PRODUCT:
For injection containing 200 mg/mL

CALCIUM GLUCONATE

INDICATIONS: Calcium gluconate ✤ ★ is indicated for the treatment of hypocalcemia, ventricular asystole, severe bradycardia, hyperkalemic cardiotoxicity, and eclampsia (puerperal tetany). Although calcium gluconate rapidly corrects hyperkalemic cardiotoxicity, its beneficial effects usually last only 10 to 15 minutes (it does not lower serum potassium levels). The oral form of calcium gluconate also is used to manage hypocalcemia associated with chronic renal failure.

ADVERSE AND COMMON SIDE EFFECTS: The drug is relatively contraindicated in patients with ventricular fibrillation, renal calculi, and hypercalcemia. It should be used with caution in those concurrently receiving digitalis therapy or those with renal or cardiac insufficiency. Intravenous injections must be given slowly to avoid hypercalcemia (vomiting, abdominal pain, ileus, decreased excitability of nerves and muscles, azotemia, acute pancreatitis, and potential cardiotoxicity). If the heart rate decreases significantly, infusion should be discontinued until the rate returns to normal, at which time reinfusion can begin. Extravascular injection causes inflammation, tissue necrosis, and sloughing. Oral preparations predispose to constipation and increased gastric acid secretion. Also see CALCIUM CHLORIDE.

DRUG INTERACTIONS: Calcium gluconate may potentiate the inotropic and toxic effects of digitalis and can precipitate arrhythmias in patients receiving these drugs. Oral calcium complexes with and decreases the effect of oral tetracyclines. Do not administer these drugs within 3 hours of each other. Calcium gluconate-induced hypercalcemia may antagonize the effectiveness of the calcium channel-blocking agents, e.g., verapamil, diltiazem, and nifedipine. Calcium

gluconate reportedly is incompatible with IV fat emulsions, amphotericin B, cefamandole, cephalothin, dobutamine, methylprednisolone
sodium succinate, and metoclopramide. Thiazide diuretics used concurrently with large doses of calcium may cause hypercalcemia.

SUPPLIED AS VETERINARY PRODUCT:
For injection containing 23% w/v as calcium borogluconate

SUPPLIED AS HUMAN PRODUCTS:
1-g tabs contain 90 mg elemental calcium
975-mg tabs contain 87.75 mg elemental calcium
650-mg tabs contain 58.5 mg elemental calcium
500-mg tabs contain 45 mg elemental calcium
For injection as a 10% solution

OTHER USES: Calcium gluconate also has been used to antagonize
aminoglycoside-induced neuromuscular blockade and as a calcium
challenge to diagnose Zollinger-Ellison syndrome (causes increased
plasma gastrin levels in affected dogs).

CALCIUM LACTATE

INDICATIONS: The INDICATIONS, ADVERSE AND COMMON
SIDE EFFECTS, and DRUG INTERACTIONS of calcium lactate ♣ ★
are similar to those of calcium gluconate. Calcium lactate generally
is used to treat mild hypocalcemia and for maintenance calcium
therapy.

SUPPLIED AS HUMAN PRODUCT:
Tablets containing 325 mg (contain 42.25 mg elemental calcium) and
650 mg (contain 84.5 mg elemental calcium)

CAPTOPRIL

INDICATIONS: Captopril (Capoten ♣ ★) is an angiotensin-converting
enzyme (ACE) inhibitor. It significantly increases cardiac output while
reducing systemic vascular resistance, pulmonary capillary wedge
pressure, and right atrial pressure. Heart rate usually is unaffected.
The drug has been shown to be more efficacious in improving cardiac
function in people than prazosin. It is useful in conditions of congestive heart failure and in the management of systemic hypertension.
Angiotensin-converting enzyme inhibitors often improve even mild
cases of congestive heart failure. Experimentally, ACE inhibitors may
slow the progression of renal disease via decreasing glomerular pressures (which contribute to the progression of renal disease) and possibly by limiting the growth/proliferation of glomerular cells, although
clinical improvement has yet to be proven.

ADVERSE AND COMMON SIDE EFFECTS: Hypotension causing lethargy, anorexia, weakness, and difficulty rising—possibly in association with dehydration or azotemia—has been reported. Consequently, low initial doses are recommended, titrating the drug to effect. Anorexia, vomiting, and diarrhea (sometimes with blood) have been observed in some dogs. Discontinuation of the drug results in prompt resolution of these signs, and therapy usually can be resumed at lower doses. Hyperkalemia may occur, especially if the drug is used with potassium-sparing diuretics. Renal insufficiency has been observed in small animals (usually at doses greater than 2 mg/kg tid). Proteinuria may occur in some patients. The drug should be used cautiously in animals with renal disease. Captopril does not require hepatic conversion and consequently is a better choice for patients with liver disease than enalapril. Drug overdose may be treated with a β agonist, e.g., dobutamine (2.5 to 10 µg/kg per minute; IV). Bradyarrhythmias may respond to atropine or glycopyrrolate. A case of pancytopenia in a dog has been reported. The pancytopenia resolved after discontinuation of the drug and the institution of erythropoietin and recombinant human granulocyte colony-stimulating factor (Filgrastim, Neupogen).

DRUG INTERACTIONS: Hypotension may be enhanced if captopril is used in conjunction with other vasodilators, e.g., nitroglycerin. Low-salt diets and accelerated salt loss induced by loop diuretics may predispose to renal insufficiency and azotemia associated with ACE inhibitor use. Treatment includes a reduction of diuretic dose and liberalization of dietary salt intake. The antihypertensive effects of captopril may be decreased when captopril is used in conjunction with aspirin or other nonsteroidal anti-inflammatory drugs (NSAIDs). Hyperkalemia is a concern if captopril is used with potassium-sparing diuretics (e.g., spironolactone) or potassium supplements. Serum digoxin levels may increase if the two drugs are used simultaneously. Absorption from the GIT may be decreased if captopril is given at the same time as antacid preparations. Separate dosing of these drugs by at least 2 hours is recommended.

SUPPLIED AS HUMAN PRODUCT:
Tablets containing 12.5, 25, 50, and 100 mg

OTHER USES: Captopril may be useful in hemorrhagic or endotoxic shock by helping maintain peripheral tissue perfusion.

CARBAMATE INSECTICIDES

INDICATIONS: The carbamate insecticides are cholinesterase inhibitors used to eradicate mites, lice, fleas, and ticks. Included in this group are propoxur (Baygon, Sendran, Vet-Kem), carbaril (Sevin, Vet-Kem), methomyl (Lannate), bendiocarb (Ficam), aldicarb (Temik), and carbofuran (Furadan).

ADVERSE AND COMMON SIDE EFFECTS: Toxicity results in miosis, salivation, frequent urination and defecation, vomiting, bronchoconstriction, ataxia, incoordination, muscle tremors, convulsions, respiratory depression, paralysis, and possibly death. Carbamate products should not be used on puppies or kittens younger than 12 weeks of age or on pregnant or nursing animals. In some animals, skin irritation may develop with use of the collars, especially if the collars are applied too tightly. In case of accidental poisoning, exposed skin should be cleansed. If the drug has been ingested, gastric lavage is indicated. After lavage, activated charcoal should be given by way of stomach intubation. In all cases, atropine (0.2 mg/kg) is given to effect. One fourth of the total dose is given intravenously, and the balance is given intramuscularly or subcutaneously. Diazepam has been used to augment the effects of atropine, hastening recovery. The use of pralidoxime chloride (2-PAM) is discouraged in carbamate toxicity because it may predispose to increased toxicity.

DRUG INTERACTIONS: Phenothiazine tranquilizers may potentiate the adverse effects of carbamate products. Concurrent use of physostigmine, pyridostigmine, neostigmine, morphine, or succinylcholine also should be avoided.

CARBENICILLIN

INDICATIONS: Carbenicillin (Geopen ✤ ★, Geocillin ★, Pyopen ✤) is an extended spectrum, penicillinase-sensitive, semisynthetic penicillin. It is bactericidal against a variety of gram-negative and gram-positive organisms and some anaerobes. Among susceptible bacteria are *Pseudomonas aeruginosa, Proteus,* susceptible strains of *E. coli, Enterobacter,* and *Streptococcus.*

ADVERSE AND COMMON SIDE EFFECTS: See PENICILLIN ANTIBIOTICS.

DRUG INTERACTIONS: A synergistic action occurs when carbenicillin is combined with aminoglycoside antibiotics. If, however, carbenicillin is given concurrently with a tetracycline, the bactericidal activity of the former compound may be reduced.

SUPPLIED AS HUMAN PRODUCTS:
For injection containing 1-, 2-, 5-, 10-, and 30-g vials [Geopen, Pyopen]
Tablets containing 382 mg [Geocillin ★, Geopen Oral ✤]

CARBOPLATIN

INDICATIONS: Carboplatin (Paraplatin ✤ ★) is a second-generation platinum compound that differs from cisplatin because it is less nephrotoxic and does not require saline diuresis. It also may be useful for dogs that cannot receive cisplatin because of preexisting congestive heart failure. The drug has been used in the management of canine osteosarcoma. Treatment with amputation and four doses of the drug given every 21 days resulted in a median survival time of 321 days with 35% of dogs alive at 1 year, which is longer than that reported for amputation alone and similar to that noted with two to four doses of cisplatin. Carboplatin has demonstrated activity against malignant melanomas in dogs and should be considered as an adjunctive treatment for microscopic local or metastatic tumors. It has also been used in the management of feline oral and cutaneous squamous cell carcinoma.

ADVERSE AND COMMON SIDE EFFECTS: The dose-limiting toxicity in dogs is neutropenia and thrombocytopenia. Transient vomiting and elevations in serum urea and creatinine may occur. Dose-limiting neutropenia and thrombocytopenia also have been documented in the cat at dosages of 200 and 250 mg/m^2. The neutrophil nadir is seen on day 17 (at 200 mg/m^2) and lasts from day 14 through 25 after drug administration.

DRUG INTERACTIONS: In people, concomitant use with aminoglycoside antibiotics may predispose to renal and auditory toxicity. Carboplatin should not be used in conjunction with other potentially nephrotoxic drugs.

SUPPLIED AS HUMAN PRODUCTS:
For injection containing 100, 250, and 500 mg
For injection containing 10 mg/mL [Paraplatin-AQ]

CARNITINE

INDICATIONS: Carnitine (Carnitor ★ ✤, VitaCarn ★, L-Carnitine ✤ ★) supplementation may be useful adjunctive therapy in the management of some dogs with dilated cardiomyopathy. It has been reported that myocardial-free carnitine deficiency occurs in approximately 50% to 90% of dogs with dilated cardiomyopathy. It has been concluded that American cocker spaniels with dilated cardiomyopathy are taurine deficient and are responsive to taurine and carnitine supplementation. Although myocardial function did not return to normal, it improved enough to allow discontinuation of cardiovascular drug therapy. Survival of Dobermans with myocardial carnitine deficiency treated with carnitine in addition to conventional pharmacotherapy reportedly has been significantly improved. Although conventional pharmacotherapy for heart failure occasionally can be withdrawn from patients responding to carnitine, it is not considered a reasonable expectation. The drug also may have a protective effect against myocardial infarction and doxorubicin-induced cardiomyopathy. It also has been recommended as adjunct therapy in feline hepatic lipidosis, for which it is believed the drug may facilitate hepatic lipid metabolism, although other investigators suggest that carnitine deficiency has no role in the pathogenesis of this disease.

ADVERSE AND COMMON SIDE EFFECTS: The drug is very safe. Excessive drug doses have not been associated with adverse effects, although mild diarrhea has been reported in one dog. D, L-Carnitine has been associated with a myasthenia-like syndrome. Therefore, it is recommended that the L-isomer (L-carnitine) formulation be used.

DRUG INTERACTIONS: D, L-Carnitine sold in health food stores as vitamin B$_T$ inhibits L-carnitine and may cause a deficiency.

SUPPLIED AS POWDER [L-Carnitine; Ward Robertson Chemicals; Scarborough, Ontario]:
For injection containing 200 mg/mL ❦
Tablets containing 330 mg ★ ❦
Capsules containing 250 mg ★
Oral solution containing 100 mg/mL ★ ❦

OTHER USES
Dogs
AMERICAN COCKER SPANIEL DILATED CARDIOMYOPATHY
500 mg taurine bid to tid; PO with 1 g carnitine bid to tid; PO

CARPROFEN

INDICATIONS: Carprofen (Rimadyl ❦ ★) is a carboxylic acid nonsteroidal anti-inflammatory agent with analgesic, anti-inflammatory and antipyretic properties. Its potency is comparable to that of indomethacin and greater than that of aspirin or phenylbutazone. The drug has been shown to be clinically effective in the management of osteoarthritis in dogs.

ADVERSE AND COMMON SIDE EFFECTS: Clinically significant adverse side effects did not develop in dogs receiving up to 5 times the recommended dosage for 42 days or 10 times the recommended dosage for 14 days. Short-term use of the drug in dogs is unlikely to result in an increased risk of surgical hemorrhage. Use of the drug may be associated with vomiting, diarrhea, melena, changes in appetite, lethargy, constipation, or aggression. In animal studies carprofen has been shown to be approximately 35 times less likely than aspirin to cause gastric ulceration. Acute hepatocellular necrosis and death have also been reported. Clinical signs associated with carprofen-induced hepatic toxicosis include anorexia, vomiting, and jaundice.

Progression of the disease and the extent of clinical signs did not correlate with the dose of drug used, the magnitude of elevation of hepatic enzymes, or histopathologic severity of hepatic lesions. More than one-half of the reported cases were Labrador retrievers. Renal effects may include azotemia, electrolyte and acid-base disturbances, isosthenuria, proteinuria, glucosuria without hyperglycemia, tubular casts, renal tubular necrosis, and acute renal failure. Animals with renal, cardiac, and hepatobiliary disease are at increased risk. Most dogs recover uneventfully after discontinuation of the drug and administration of supportive care. Safe use of the drug in pregnant, breeding, or lactating dogs has not been established.

The drug is not licensed for use in cats in America and should be used with caution because its safety in this species has not been adequately established. There have been anecdotal reports of a possible association between the use of carprofen and a perforated duodenum in cats.

DRUG INTERACTIONS: Carprofen should not be used concurrently with glucocorticoids because the possibility of adverse GI effects may be increased.

SUPPLIED AS VETERINARY PRODUCTS:
Caplets containing 25, 75, and 100 mg
Chewable tablets containing 25, 75, and 100 mg

CARVEDILOL

INDICATIONS: Carvedilol (Coreg ♣ ★) is an α_1- and β-adrenergic blocking agent with arteriolar vasodilating and positive inotrope properties. It is useful in the treatment of congestive heart failure and systemic hypertension. It is 4 times more potent than propranolol. It also possesses antioxidant properties, which may attenuate the progression of doxorubicin-induced myocardial damage. The drug may also be antiarrhythmic.

ADVERSE AND COMMON SIDE EFFECTS: In people, bradycardia, dizziness, edema, hypotension, nausea, and diarrhea are reported. Deterioration of renal function is rarely reported. The drug should be discontinued in patients if liver enzymes increase, and it should not be given to those with preexisting liver disease. Overdose can result in bradycardia and hypotension.

DRUG INTERACTIONS: Carvedilol has proven therapeutic benefit when given as adjunctive therapy with diuretics and ACE inhibitors with or without digoxin. Drugs known to inhibit the cytochrome P450 enzyme system, e.g., diltiazem, itraconazole, ketoconazole, erythromycin, cimetidine, and metoclopramide, may increase serum levels. Drugs known to induce this enzyme system, e.g., phenobarbital and phenytoin, may decrease blood levels of carvedilol. Plasma digoxin levels rise slightly in patients given carvedilol.

SUPPLIED AS HUMAN PRODUCT:
Tablets containing 3.125, 6.25, 12.5, and 25 mg

CEFACLOR

INDICATIONS: Cefaclor (Ceclor ✤ ★, Apo-Cefaclor ✤) is a second-generation cephalosporin antibiotic. It has a similar spectrum of activity as other oral cephalosporins but is more active. For more information, see CEPHALOSPORIN ANTIBIOTICS.

ADVERSE AND COMMON SIDE EFFECTS AND DRUG INTER-ACTIONS: See CEPHALOSPORIN ANTIBIOTICS.

SUPPLIED AS HUMAN PRODUCTS:
Capsules containing 250 and 500 mg
Oral suspension containing 125 mg/5 mL, 250 mg/5 mL, and 375 mg/5 mL

CEFADROXIL

INDICATIONS: Cefadroxil (Cefa-Tabs ✤ ★, Cefa-Drops ✤ ★) is a first-generation cephalosporin. The drug is used in dogs and cats to treat infections caused by susceptible organisms of the skin, soft tissue, and genitourinary tract, including *E. coli, Proteus mirabilis, Pasteurella multocida, Staphylococcus aureus,* and *S. epidermidis,* as well as *Streptococcus* spp. For more information, see CEPHALOSPORIN ANTIBIOTICS.

ADVERSE AND COMMON SIDE EFFECTS: Occasional nausea and vomiting have been reported with the use of Cefa-Tabs. Administration with food appears to decrease nausea. Diarrhea and lethargy also may occur. See also CEPHALOSPORIN ANTIBIOTICS.

DRUG INTERACTIONS: See CEPHALOSPORIN ANTIBIOTICS.

SUPPLIED AS VETERINARY PRODUCTS:
Tablets in 50-mg, 100-mg, 200-mg, and 1-g strengths [Cefa-Tabs]
For oral administration in 750 mg/15-mL bottles and 2,500 mg/50-mL bottles

CEFAMANDOLE

INDICATIONS: Cefamandole (Mandol ★) is a second-generation cephalosporin with wide tissue distribution, including bile and synovia. The drug exerts high activity against *E. coli, Klebsiella, Enterobacter, Proteus, Salmonella, Haemophilus,* and *Shigella* species. For additional information, see CEPHALOSPORIN ANTIBIOTICS.

ADVERSE AND COMMON SIDE EFFECTS AND DRUG INTERACTIONS: See CEPHALOSPORIN ANTIBIOTICS.

SUPPLIED AS HUMAN PRODUCT:
For injection containing 1- and 2-g vials [Mandol]

CEFAZOLIN

INDICATIONS: Cefazolin (Ancef ✿ ★, Kefzol ✿ ★) is a short-acting, first-generation cephalosporin that attains the greatest serum concentration and has the longest half-life. It is more active against *E. coli, Klebsiella,* and *Enterobacter* species. For additional information, see CEPHALOSPORIN ANTIBIOTICS.

ADVERSE AND COMMON SIDE EFFECTS AND DRUG INTERACTIONS: See CEPHALOSPORIN ANTIBIOTICS.

SUPPLIED AS HUMAN PRODUCTS:
For injection as a powder containing 500 mg and 1, 5, 10, and 20 g
For injection (IV infusion) 500 mg and 1 g in vials and in 5% dextrose [in water] (D$_5$W) 50-mL bags

CEFIXIME

INDICATIONS: Cefixime (Suprax ✿ ★) is a third-generation cephalosporin antibiotic. Experience with use of the drug in small animals at this time is limited. As with other third-generation cephalosporins, cefixime has an expanded range of activity against gram-negative bacteria. Its bacteriocidal activity includes *E. coli, Klebsiella, Proteus, Streptococcus,* and *Haemophilus* species. It also has some activity against *Staphylococcus aureus,* but not *Bordetella bronchiseptica* or *Pseudomonas aeruginosa.*

ADVERSE AND COMMON SIDE EFFECTS AND DRUG INTERACTIONS: See CEPHALOSPORIN ANTIBIOTICS.

SUPPLIED AS HUMAN PRODUCTS:
Capsules containing 200 and 400 mg
Oral suspension containing 100 mg/5 mL

CEFOTAXIME

INDICATIONS: Cefotaxime (Claforan ✿ ★) is a third-generation cephalosporin. It readily penetrates into the CSF. Unlike other cephalosporins, the third-generation drugs, including cefotaxime, are somewhat effective against *Pseudomonas aeruginosa*. For more information, see CEPHALOSPORIN ANTIBIOTICS.

ADVERSE AND COMMON SIDE EFFECTS AND DRUG INTERACTIONS: See CEPHALOSPORIN ANTIBIOTICS.

SUPPLIED AS HUMAN PRODUCTS:
For injection as a powder containing 500 mg and 1, 2, or 10 g
For injection in 50 mL, 5% dextrose bags containing 1 and 2 g cefotaxime

CEFOTETAN

INDICATIONS: Cefotetan (Cefotan ✿ ★) is classified as a second- or third-generation cephalosporin similar to cefoxitin but with a longer half-life in dogs. The drug's in vitro spectrum includes *E. coli, Klebsiella, Proteus, Salmonella, Staphylococcus,* and most *Streptococcus* sp. Cefotetan is also efficacious against *Actinomyces, Bacteroides, Clostridium, Peptococcus, Peptostreptococcus,* and *Propionibacterium.* Cefotetan is superior to cefoxitin in activity against *E. coli,* and it should be used at 30 mg/kg IV, tid or SC, bid. For more information, see CEPHALOSPORIN ANTIBIOTICS.

ADVERSE AND COMMON SIDE EFFECTS: Experience with this drug in small animals is limited, but it appears to be well tolerated. For more information, see CEPHALOSPORIN ANTIBIOTICS.

DRUG INTERACTIONS: None of significance to small animals.

SUPPLIED AS HUMAN PRODUCT:
For injection in 1-, 2-, and 10-mg vials

CEFOXITIN

INDICATIONS: Cefoxitin (Mefoxin ✿ ★) is a semisynthetic, broad-spectrum, second-generation cephalosporin antibiotic. For more information, see CEPHALOSPORIN ANTIBIOTICS. Cefoxitin has activity against gram-positive cocci, although less so than first-generation cephalosporins. It does, however, have good activity against many strains of *E. coli, Klebsiella,* and *Proteus* organisms that may be resistant to the first-generation drugs. Cefoxitin is one of the most effective cephalosporins for treating anaerobic infections, including those caused by Enterobacteriaceae and *Bacteroides fragilis.*

ADVERSE AND COMMON SIDE EFFECTS: See CEPHALOSPORIN ANTIBIOTICS.

DRUG INTERACTIONS: An additive or synergistic effect is gained against some organisms when cefoxitin is used in conjunction with the penicillins, chloramphenicol, or the aminoglycoside antibiotics. However, the manufacturer advises that cefoxitin should not be administered with aminoglycoside antibiotics because of possible incompatibility. The concurrent use of cefoxitin and aminoglycosides, vancomycin, polymyxin B, or a diuretic increases the potential for nephrotoxicity, thus dictating close monitoring of renal function. Pain may occur on intramuscular injection.

SUPPLIED AS HUMAN PRODUCTS:
For injection containing 1, 2, and 10 g
For injection containing 1 and 2 g in 5% dextrose (frozen) as 1 g (20 mg/mL) and 2 g (40 mg/mL)

CEFTAZIDIME

INDICATIONS: Ceftazidime (Fortaz ✤ ★, Ceptaz ✤ ★) is a third-generation, broad-spectrum cephalosporin similar to cefotaxime, with activity against gram-negative bacteria but with greater activity against *Pseudomonas aeruginosa*. The drug is used to treat infections of the lower respiratory tract, skin, urinary tract, bones and joints, CNS infections (including meningitis), and bacteremia.

ADVERSE AND COMMON SIDE EFFECTS: The drug is contraindicated in patients with known hypersensitivity to cephalosporins and related β-lactam antibiotics. Drug dose should be decreased in patients with renal impairment. Safe use in pregnancy has not been established. Experience with use of the drug in small animals is limited. The most common adverse effects in humans include local reactions after injection (phlebitis, thrombophlebitis, pain), fever, pruritus, diarrhea, nausea, transient elevations in serum urea and creatinine, and hepatic enzymes. See also CEPHALOSPORIN ANTIBIOTICS.

DRUG INTERACTIONS: Concurrent use with aminoglycosides may cause an additive nephrotoxic effect. Concomitant use of furosemide and ethacrynic acid may increase the risk of renal toxicity. Chloramphenicol is antagonistic in vitro with ceftazidime. Ampicillin may produce antagonism against group B streptococci and *Listeria monocytogenes*. See also CEPHALOSPORIN ANTIBIOTICS.

SUPPLIED AS HUMAN PRODUCTS:
For IM or direct IV injection vials containing 500 mg or 1 g
For IV injection or infusion vials containing 1, 2, or 6 g
For injection containing 1 g in 4.4% dextrose (20 mg/mL) and 2 g in 3.2% dextrose (40 mg/mL)

CEPHALEXIN

INDICATIONS: Cephalexin (Keflex ❦ ★, Keftab ★, Novo-Lexin ❦, Nu-Cephalex ❦) is a broad-spectrum, first-generation cephalosporin. For more information, see CEPHALOSPORIN ANTIBIOTICS.

ADVERSE AND COMMON SIDE EFFECTS: In addition to the side effects noted for the CEPHALOSPORIN ANTIBIOTICS, cephalexin has been reported to cause salivation, tachypnea, and excitability in dogs, and vomiting and fever in cats. See CEPHALOSPORIN ANTIBIOTICS.

DRUG INTERACTIONS: See CEPHALOSPORIN ANTIBIOTICS.

SUPPLIED AS HUMAN PRODUCTS:
Capsules containing 250 and 500 mg
Tablets containing 250 and 500 mg
Oral suspension containing 25 mg/mL and 50 mg/mL

CEPHALOSPORIN ANTIBIOTICS

INDICATIONS: The cephalosporin antibiotics are bactericidal to gram-positive and several gram-negative strains. They are used in the treatment of respiratory, skeletal, genitourinary, skin, and soft tissue infections. In addition, these drugs are recommended for prophylactic use in biliary tract surgery and for treating biliary tract disease. All are effective against anaerobic infections except *Bacteroides fragilis* (with the exception of cefoxitin). Cephalosporins may be more effective than penicillin antibiotics in the treatment of β-lactamase–producing staphylococci. The cephalosporins usually are not effective against resistant strains of *Pseudomonas aeruginosa* (with the exception of ceftazidime). The first- and second-generation cephalosporin antibiotics do not readily cross the blood–brain barrier.

First-generation cephalosporins (cefadroxil, cephalexin, cephradine, cephalothin, cefazolin, cephapirin) are active against gram-positive bacteria, including penicillin-resistant staphylococci, and against some gram-negative bacteria, including *E. coli, Proteus,* and *Klebsiella* spp. First-generation drugs are relatively ineffective against *Bacteroides.* They enter the CSF only in the presence of inflammation. In vitro antimicrobial activity and serum concentrations after oral administration of cephalexin, cefadroxil, and cephradine are similar; however, serum and urine concentrations of cefadroxil are more sustained than those seen with cephalexin. These drugs are less expensive than the second- and third-generation cephalosporins.

Second-generation cephalosporins (cefamandole, cefaclor, cefotetan, cefoxitin) have a broader spectrum of activity and greater efficacy against gram-negative bacteria and anaerobes than the first-generation cephalosporins, but their activity against gram-positive organisms is less than that of the first-generation drugs. Cefoxitin also is effective against *Serratia* and *B. fragilis.* Cefamandole is active against *Salmonella* and *Shigella.*

Third-generation cephalosporins (cefixime, cefotaxime, cefoperazone, ceftazidime, moxalactam) have increased antibacterial activity against gram-negative bacteria and anaerobes, but activity against gram-positive organisms is minimal. The third-generation drugs have increased resistance to β-lactamase–producing bacteria and increased activity against gram-negative bacteria, including *Pseudomonas, Proteus, Enterobacter,* and *Citrobacter* spp. Moxalactam and cefotaxime readily penetrate into the CSF in healthy and inflamed meninges.

A fourth-generation cephalosporin (cefepime) is an injectable drug that has similar gram-negative activity as third-generation agents but maintains good gram-positive activity.

ADVERSE AND COMMON SIDE EFFECTS: As a group, the cephalosporin antibiotics are quite safe. Vomiting and diarrhea may occur with oral administration. Administration with food decreases nausea. Because most cephalosporins are eliminated by the kidney, their concentration is increased and their half-life is extended in cases of renal failure. All parenteral forms may cause phlebitis and myositis after IV or IM injection, respectively. Reversible blood dyscrasias, including anemia, thrombocytopenia, and neutropenia, have been induced with high-dose, long-term use of these drugs in some dogs as a result of a direct bone marrow toxic effect and immune-mediated destruction of blood cells. After withdrawal of the drug, hematologic recovery generally occurs within 1 week. The cephalosporins may cause elevations in serum alkaline phosphatase, alanine transferase, and aspartate transferase, as well as an increase in serum urea nitrogen. False-positive Coombs' test results and false-positive urinary glucose reactions also have been documented. Third-generation cephalosporins can prolong the partial thromboplastin time and the prothrombin time by inhibiting vitamin K activation of clotting factors. Allergic skin reactions have been reported with the use of cephalexin. Cephalothin produces pain and may cause sterile abscess formation on injection. Cross-allergenicity with penicillins may occur. An additive or synergistic effect is gained against some organisms when cefoxitin is used in conjunction with the penicillins, chloramphenicol, or the aminoglycoside antibiotics. For additional information, see the specific cephalosporin.

DRUG INTERACTIONS: The cephalosporins are potentially nephrotoxic, and it is advised that these drugs be used with caution when administered concurrently with other potentially nephrotoxic drugs, e.g., aminoglycosides, amphotericin B, vancomycin, polymyxin B, or a diuretic.

SUPPLIED AS: See specific drug.

CEPHALOTHIN

INDICATIONS: Cephalothin (Keflin ✤, Ceporacin ✤) is a first-generation cephalosporin.

ADVERSE AND COMMON SIDE EFFECTS: In experimental studies, cephalothin impairs platelet aggregation. However, clinical evidence of a bleeding tendency has not been demonstrated. For more information, including DRUG INTERACTIONS, see CEPHALOSPORIN ANTIBIOTICS.

SUPPLIED AS HUMAN PRODUCT:
For injection containing 1 and 2 g in vials

CEPHAPIRIN

INDICATIONS: Cephapirin (Cefadyl ★) is a first-generation cephalosporin. It resists β-lactamase and has been used when a relatively short-acting, injectable, first-generation cephalosporin is indicated. For additional information, see CEPHALOSPORIN ANTIBIOTICS.

ADVERSE AND COMMON SIDE EFFECTS AND DRUG INTERACTIONS: See CEPHALOSPORIN ANTIBIOTICS.

SUPPLIED AS HUMAN PRODUCT:
For injection containing 1g/vial

CEPHRADINE

INDICATIONS: Cephradine (Velosef ★) is a first-generation cephalosporin with a spectrum of activity similar to that of cephalexin. For additional information, see CEPHALOSPORIN ANTIBIOTICS.

ADVERSE AND COMMON SIDE EFFECTS AND DRUG INTERACTIONS: See CEPHALOSPORIN ANTIBIOTICS.

SUPPLIED AS HUMAN PRODUCTS:
Capsules containing 250 and 500 mg
Oral suspension containing 125 mg/5 mL and 250 mg/5 mL

CHARCOAL, ACTIVATED

INDICATIONS: Activated charcoal (Charcodote ✤, Toxiban ★, Liquichar ✤ ★, UAA ★) is an excellent absorbent used in the treatment of accidental poisoning. Repetitive dosing (e.g., every 6 hours for 1 to 2 days) increases clearance of drugs already absorbed into the systemic circulation. It often is used in conjunction with emetics and gastric lavage. Activated charcoal must be of vegetable origin, not mineral or animal. A slurry is made and administered by stomach tube. A cathartic (sodium sulfate) often is given 30 minutes after the administration of charcoal. Activated charcoal is most useful when used for acetaminophen, atropine, digitalis glycosides, phenytoin, mercuric chloride, strychnine, morphine sulfate, atropine, and ethylene glycol poisoning.

ADVERSE AND COMMON SIDE EFFECTS: Vomiting (rapid ingestion of high doses), constipation, and diarrhea may occur with its use.

DRUG INTERACTIONS: Activated charcoal reportedly is not effective in the treatment of poisoning by cyanide, mineral acids, caustic alkalis, organic solvents, ethanol, lead, iron, or methanol. Syrup of ipecac should not be used with activated charcoal because ipecac negates the absorbent activity of the charcoal. If used for the relief of GI upset, other oral drugs should not be given within 2 hours. Stools will be discolored black.

SUPPLIED AS VETERINARY PRODUCTS:
[Toxiban Granules] containing 47.5% charcoal, 10% kaolin in 1-lb bottles and 5-kg pails
[Toxiban Suspension] containing 10.4% charcoal, 6.25% kaolin in 240-mL bottles
[Liquichar] containing 50 g charcoal in 240-mL tubes
[UAA] gel in 8-fl-oz bottle and 60-mL and 300-mL tubes

SUPPLIED AS HUMAN PRODUCTS:
[Charcodote] 200 mg/mL; total 50 g in 250-mL bottles and Pediatric suspension containing 200 mg/mL for a total of 25 g in 125-mL bottles
[Charcodote Aqueous] 200 mg/mL; total 50 g in 250-mL bottle and Pediatric aqueous suspension 200 mg/mL; total 25 g in 125-mL bottle

OTHER USES: Activated charcoal also has been used to absorb intestinal gases in the treatment of dyspepsia, flatulence, and gastric distention.

CHLORAMBUCIL

INDICATIONS: Chlorambucil (Leukeran ✤ ★) is an alkylating chemotherapeutic agent indicated for the treatment of lymphocytic leukemia, polycythemia vera, multiple myeloma, ovarian adenocarcinoma, and macroglobulinemia. The drug also has been used in the treatment of immune-mediated glomerulonephritis, immune-mediated nonerosive arthritis, and immune-mediated skin diseases.

ADVERSE AND COMMON SIDE EFFECTS: Alkylating agents generally cause leukopenia, thrombocytopenia, and anemia with the nadir of leukocyte counts observed 7 to 14 days after treatment and recovery noted in an additional 7 to 14 days. Bone marrow suppression occurs less often with chlorambucil than it does with cyclophosphamide. The complete blood count should be monitored on a regular basis. The drugs busulfan, cyclophosphamide, and chlorambucil also have been associated with the occurrence of bronchopulmonary dysplasia leading to pulmonary fibrosis. Hair regrowth is delayed in shaved areas, and chlorambucil may cause alopecia is some dogs (poodles, Kerry blue terriers). Gastrointestinal side effects are rare, and occasional urticarial reactions have been reported. The drug may affect spermiogenesis and cause embryotoxicity or malformations in the newborn. Seizures, facial twitching, jerking of the muscles of the head and limbs, and myoclonus were reported in one cat under treatment for intestinal lymphosarcoma.

DRUG INTERACTIONS: None of relevance to small-animal medicine.

SUPPLIED AS HUMAN PRODUCT:
Tablets containing 2 mg

CHLORAMPHENICOL

INDICATIONS: Chloramphenicol (Azramycine ✤, Chlor Palm ✤, Chlor Tablets ✤, Chloromycetin ✤ ★, Karomycin Palmitate ✤, and many others) is a bacteriostatic antibiotic with activity against a number of pathogens including *Bacteroides, Staphylococcus, Salmonella, Pasteurella, Bordetella, Haemophilus,* enteric coliforms, most anaerobes, mycoplasmas, chlamydiae, rickettsiae, and some protozoa. It is well absorbed after oral administration, is distributed widely throughout the body—including the prostate, CSF, aqueous and vitreous humor, milk, and amniotic fluid, and is excreted in the bile and urine. It is used commonly in the treatment of eye, skin, urinary, and mucous membrane infections. Serum concentrations are monitored just before the next dose or 6 to 12 hours after the last dose, depending on the regimen, and after steady-state levels have been attained (21 hours in the dog and 26 hours in the cat). The therapeutic serum concentration for dogs and cats is less than or equal to 8 µg/mL (trough). Toxic levels are listed as greater than 20 µg/mL.

ADVERSE AND COMMON SIDE EFFECTS: The most common side effect after oral administration is GI upset manifested by transient depression, anorexia, nausea, vomiting, or diarrhea. Adverse reactions also may include a reversible bone marrow suppression and nonregenerative anemia, thrombocytopenia, and leukopenia. Cats are more sensitive to the adverse effects of the drug. Bone marrow changes may occur after 1 week of therapy at doses of 50 mg/kg bid.

After 3 weeks of therapy, neutropenia, lymphopenia, nonregenerative anemia, and thrombocytopenia may be seen. Resolution of these changes occurs within several days after discontinuation of the drug. Toxic changes are not seen if the drug is given intermittently at a lower dose. Decreased antibody production may be a sequelae of chloramphenicol use. Other clinical signs seen have included ataxia and even death. The drug should not be used in breeding animals and should not be given to pregnant animals because the fetus is unable to metabolize it. The drug should not be used in animals with severe liver impairment or those with severe myocardial dysfunction because of myocardial depression associated with its use. Chloramphenicol should not be used in animals with extensive wounds because it interferes with protein synthesis. Chloramphenicol may cause a false-positive result for glucose in urine when glucose oxidase strips are used.

DRUG INTERACTIONS: Chloramphenicol is a hepatic microsomal enzyme inhibitor. It potentiates the activity of barbiturate drugs, codeine, cyclophosphamide, phenytoin, primidone, warfarin, inhalation anesthetics, digitalis, and aspirin, and yet phenobarbital and other barbiturates actually may reduce the efficacy of chloramphenicol if given concurrently. Its bacteriostatic action inhibits the efficacy of penicillin and cephalosporin antibiotics and the aminoglycosides.

SUPPLIED AS VETERINARY PRODUCTS:
Tablets containing 100, 250, and 500 mg, and 1 g
Oral suspension containing 25 and 50 mg/mL [Azramycine, Chlor Palm, Karomycin Palmitate]

SUPPLIED AS HUMAN PRODUCTS:
Capsules containing 250 mg [Chloromycetin, Kapseals]
Oral suspension containing 25 mg/mL [Chloramphenicol Palmitate]
For injection containing 100 mg/mL (chloramphenicol sodium succinate)

CHLORHEXIDINE

INDICATIONS: Chlorhexidine (ChlorhexiDerm ★, Hibitane ♣, Nolvadent ★, Nolvasan ★, Savlon ♣) is a commonly used antiseptic and disinfectant. It is effective against *Proteus* and *Pseudomonas*. Chlorhexidine can be important adjunct topical therapy in the management of pyoderma and dermatophytosis. It is an effective and nonirritating antiseptic useful for the flushing of wounds. Concentrations of 0.5% chlorhexidine in water or alcohol reduce bacterial contamination of wounds and surgical sites but tend to retard granulation tissue formation and epithelialization. Lower concentrations (0.1%) are less antiseptic, but do not inhibit wound repair. As a disinfectant, it can be used against canine infectious tracheobronchitis virus, canine distemper virus, parainfluenza virus, rabies virus, and feline respiratory viruses. Flushing dental surfaces once daily with 0.1% to 0.2% chlorhexidine may delay the accumulation of tartar.

ADVERSE AND COMMON SIDE EFFECTS: Chlorhexidine has a low order of toxicity after oral ingestion. It is poorly absorbed from the GIT or the skin. It is, however, absorbed across serous membranes, the uterus, and bladder. Sufficient quantities can be absorbed to cause intravascular hemolysis with hemoglobinemia and hemoglobinuria because of a direct effect on the erythrocyte membrane. If these signs occur, diuresis should be promoted to prevent renal damage. Deafness may occur if the product comes in contact with the middle ear.

CHLORINATED HYDROCARBONS

INDICATIONS: Included in this group are chlorpyrifos (Duratrol), cythioate (Proban), diazinon (various generic products), dichlorvos (Vapona), fenthion (Spotton, Pro-Spot), malathion (various generic products), and phosmet (Louse Kill, Vet-Kem Paramite Flea, and Tick Dip). These agents have been used in the eradication of mites, fleas, lice, mosquitoes, and some ticks in dogs.

ADVERSE AND COMMON SIDE EFFECTS: Muscarinic effects include salivation, lacrimation, miosis, pallor, cyanosis, dyspnea, vomiting, and diarrhea. Nicotinic effects include twitching of the facial and tongue muscles, progressing to all musculature and followed by paralysis. Central nervous system effects include depression and tonic–clonic seizures. Respiratory muscle paralysis, bronchoconstriction, excessive pulmonary secretions, and pulmonary edema lead to dyspnea and death.

Treatment includes removal of unabsorbed drug by cleansing the affected area of skin or inducing vomiting, followed by oral administration of activated charcoal to prevent further absorption of insecticide remaining in the GIT. This is followed by the use of atropine (0.2 mg/kg; one fourth given intravenously and the remainder given intramuscularly or subcutaneously as needed to control clinical signs) and pralidoxime chloride (20 mg/kg bid to tid; IM or slow IV; most efficacious if given within the first 12 to 18 hours—of little benefit after 24 hours). Diazepam can be used to control seizures. In addition, diphenhydramine (4 mg/kg tid; PO) has been shown to block the effects of nicotine stimulation and prevent the receptor paralysis associated with organophosphate-induced myasthenia-like syndrome. Maintenance of fluid balance will help hasten recovery. Where indicated, ventilatory support is used. Respiratory failure is the most common cause of death.

DRUG INTERACTIONS: Other drugs that inhibit cholinesterase, e.g., physostigmine, morphine, succinylcholine, phenothiazine, pyridostigmine, and neostigmine, should be avoided.

CHLOROTHIAZIDE

INDICATIONS: Chlorothiazide (Diuril ★) is a thiazide diuretic used in the management of congestive heart failure, pulmonary edema, and systemic hypertension. Thiazide diuretics inhibit sodium and chloride absorption in the distal tubules. Potassium secretion is promoted, and loss is comparable to that seen with furosemide. The onset of action occurs within 1 hour and peaks in 4 hours. Because thiazide diuretics work in a different part of the kidney than other diuretics, the thiazides and other diuretics often are used concurrently.

ADVERSE AND COMMON SIDE EFFECTS: Hypokalemia and excessive extravascular volume depletion are the most notable concerns associated with the use of these drugs, although hypokalemia rarely is severe enough to cause clinical signs. Other possible adverse effects include vomiting, diarrhea, hematologic toxicity, hyperglycemia, hyperlipidemia, polyuria, and hypersensitivity dermal reactions.

DRUG INTERACTIONS: When used with amphotericin B or the corticosteroids, there may be enhancement of the hypokalemic effect of chlorothiazide. When chlorothiazide is used with insulin preparations, the hypoglycemic effects of the insulin may be antagonized by the hyperglycemic effect of the thiazide. Hypokalemia may predispose to digitalis toxicity when these drugs are used concurrently. The half-life of quinidine may be prolonged by thiazides. Hypercalcemia may be exacerbated if thiazides are used with vitamin D or calcium salts.

SUPPLIED AS HUMAN PRODUCTS:
Tablets containing 250 and 500 mg
Oral suspension containing 50 mg/mL
For injection in 500-mg vial

OTHER USES
Dogs
CONGENITAL NEPHROGENIC DIABETES INSIPIDUS
20 to 40 mg/kg bid (in conjunction with a salt-restricted diet)

CHLORPHENIRAMINE MALEATE

INDICATIONS: Chlorpheniramine (Chlor-Trimeton ★, Chlor-Tripolon ♣) may be useful in the management of pruritus in dogs and cats. It also may be of some benefit in treating feline miliary dermatitis and excessive grooming in cats. For additional information see ANTIHISTAMINES.

ADVERSE AND COMMON SIDE EFFECTS: The most common adverse effects are lethargy and somnolence. Anorexia, vomiting,

and diarrhea also may occur. For additional information, see ANTI-
HISTAMINES.

DRUG INTERACTIONS: Concurrent use with phenytoin may lead
to increased pharmacological effects of phenytoin. Also see ANTI-
HISTAMINES.

SUPPLIED AS HUMAN PRODUCTS:
Tablets containing 4 mg
Tablets containing 8 and 12 mg (timed-release)
Oral syrup containing 1 and 2 mg/5 mL

CHLORPROMAZINE

INDICATIONS: Chlorpromazine (Largactil ✦, Thorazine ★) is a
phenothiazine derivative. It primarily is used as an antiemetic agent.
The drug also has been used to sedate and reduce activity. It has pharmacological properties similar to acepromazine but is less potent and
has a longer duration of activity.

ADVERSE AND COMMON SIDE EFFECTS: Constipation, paradoxical aggression, hypotension, collapse, and the initiation of seizure
activity in animals with epilepsy have been reported. The drug should
not be used in animals with tetanus. In cats, the drug may cause extrapyramidal signs at high doses, e.g., tremors, shivering, muscle rigidity, and the patient's inability to right itself. Lethargy, diarrhea, and
loss of anal sphincter tone also may be seen. For additional information see ACEPROMAZINE.

DRUG INTERACTIONS: Chlorpromazine should not be used with
organophosphates or strychnine toxicity. Phenothiazines should not
be given within 1 month of worming with organophosphate medications because their effects may be potentiated. If used concurrently
with dipyrone, serious hypothermia may result. Physostigmine toxicity may be enhanced by chlorpromazine. Other CNS depressants
enhance chlorpromazine-induced hypotension and respiratory depression if used concurrently. The concurrent use of quinidine may cause
additive cardiac depression. Antacids and antidiarrheal compounds
decrease absorption of oral phenothiazines. Space concurrent drug
administration by at least 2 hours. Atropine and other anticholinergics have additive anticholinergic potential and reduce the antipsychotic effect of phenothiazines. Barbiturate drugs increase the
metabolism of phenothiazines and may reduce their effects. Barbiturate anesthetics may increase excitation (tremor, involuntary muscle
movements) and hypotension. Propranolol may have additive hypotensive effects. Phenothiazines may mask the ototoxic effects of aminoglycoside antibiotics. Chlorpromazine inhibits phenytoin metabolism

and increases its potential for toxicity. In humans, there is the unexplained possibility of sudden death if chlorpromazine is used concurrently with phenylpropanolamine. Tricyclic antidepressants, e.g., amitriptyline, may intensify the sedative and anticholinergic effects of chlorpromazine. Also see ACEPROMAZINE.

SUPPLIED AS HUMAN PRODUCTS:
Tablets containing 10, 25, 50, 100, and 200 mg [Thorazine]
Capsules (extended-release) containing 30, 75, 150 mg [Thorazine Spanule]
Oral solutions available as 2, 30 mg/mL
For injection containing 25 mg/mL
Rectal suppositories in 25- and 100-mg strengths

OTHER USES: Chlorpromazine raises the threshold for ventricular ectopia and may be used to protect the heart from arrhythmias. The drug also has been used as adjunct therapy in the management of pulmonary edema by its effect in decreasing venous return. In addition, chlorpromazine has been used in the treatment of feline infectious anemia (*Hemobartonella felis*), where it is believed that the drug affects erythrocyte permeability and facilitates detachment of *H. felis* from the erythrocyte membrane.

CHLORPROPAMIDE

INDICATIONS: Chlorpropamide (Diabinese ★, Novo-Propamide ❧) is an oral hypoglycemic agent used in humans in the management of diabetes mellitus. In small animals, it has been used in the treatment of partial diabetes insipidus, where it potentiates the effect of antidiuretic hormone at the renal tubules and reduces polyuria. The efficacy in canine diabetes insipidus has been variable, with a 20% to 50% reduction in urine output reported by some and no reduction in output reported by others. The drug has been used successfully in a cat with central diabetes insipidus to control urine output. A positive response may require several consecutive days of therapy.

ADVERSE AND COMMON SIDE EFFECTS: Hypoglycemia is the most common expected side effect. Other side effects are not well documented in small animals. In humans, anorexia, drowsiness, weakness, diarrhea, and jaundice have been reported, as have anemia, leukopenia, and thrombocytopenia.

DRUG INTERACTIONS: Chloramphenicol, phenylbutazone, the salicylates, sulfonamides, and ammonium chloride may potentiate the hypoglycemic effects of chlorpropamide if given concurrently. Thiazide diuretics, sodium bicarbonate, and β-blocking agents (propranolol, atenolol) may decrease the hypoglycemic effects of chlorpropamide. The hyperglycemic actions of diazoxide may be antagonized by the concurrent use of chlorpropamide.

SUPPLIED AS HUMAN PRODUCT:
Tablets containing 100 and 250 mg

CIMETIDINE

INDICATIONS: Cimetidine (Tagamet ✤ ★, Novo-Cimetine ✤), a histamine (H_2)-blocking agent, reduces gastric acid secretion and is useful in the management of gastric and duodenal ulceration associated with renal failure, liver disease, mast cell tumor, and gastrinoma. It is less effective than antacids in the treatment of acute gastrointestinal bleeding because it impairs the secretory capacity of the gastric mucosa and decreases bicarbonate concentrations. However, some researchers state that the drug also may increase luminal bicarbonate secretion, increase mucus production, and increase mucosal blood flow. Histamine (H_2) antagonists are not effective in preventing NSAID-induced gastric ulceration. The drug has been recommended to help prevent gastrointestinal side effects of corticosteroids. Cimetidine may be beneficial in cases of esophagitis and gastroesophageal reflux, where it increases caudal esophageal sphincter tone and promotes gastric emptying. In uremic dogs, cimetidine decreases the secretion of parathyroid hormone, decreases bone resorption and serum phosphate levels, and increases serum calcium levels.

ADVERSE AND COMMON SIDE EFFECTS: Adverse effects in small animals appear rare. In humans, confusion, headache, gynecomastia, and, rarely, agranulocytosis may occur. Pain at the injection site may occur. The drug should not be used in animals with significantly impaired renal or hepatic function. Histamine enhances cardiac automaticity; cimetidine blocks histamine and may cause bradycardia, hypotension, and cardiac arrest. Cimetidine has been implicated as a cause of infertility in men (decreased sperm counts, loss of libido, decreased plasma testosterone).

DRUG INTERACTIONS: By interfering with hepatic microenzyme systems, cimetidine decreases the metabolism of many drugs, including warfarin-type anticoagulants, phenytoin, theophylline, digitoxin, and diazepam, resulting in delayed excretion. Ketoconazole concentrations are decreased if the drugs are used concurrently because ketoconazole requires adequate stomach acidity for maximal oral absorption. Propranolol, lidocaine, and morphine plasma concentrations are increased, associated with decreased metabolism caused by cimetidine-induced decreased hepatic blood flow. Tetracycline, erythromycin, penicillin G, and procainamide plasma concentrations also are increased because of better oral absorption in a stomach with lower acidity (tetracycline, erythromycin, penicillin G) and because of competitive inhibition of renal tubular secretion (procainamide). Antacids may reduce GI absorption of cimetidine and, if used, should be given no less than 1 hour before or after cimetidine. Because sucralfate can absorb drugs, it is recommended that cimetidine be given parenterally or that dosage times be staggered by approximately 2 hours. Cardiac toxicity is increased with the infusion of lidocaine. Cimetidine may affect the oral absorption of cyclosporine in dogs and monitoring of blood concentrations of cyclosporine during treatment is advised.

SUPPLIED AS HUMAN PRODUCTS:
Tablets containing 200, 300, 400, 600, and 800 mg
Oral solution containing 60 mg/mL
For injection containing 150 mg/mL or premixed bag containing 300 mg cimetidine in 50 mL 0.9% saline

OTHER USES
Dogs
IMMUNOMODULATOR
10 to 25 mg bid; PO

It enhances cell-mediated immunity and suppresses T suppressor cell function and has been used in conjunction with antibiotics in dogs with chronic pyoderma and other recurrent infectious dermatoses.

PANCREATIC EXOCRINE INSUFFICIENCY
5 to 10 mg/kg tid to qid; PO 30 minutes preprandially to reduce gastric acid destruction of pancreatic enzyme preparations

RENAL FAILURE/VOMITING
5 to 10 mg/kg bid to qid; IV, PO

CIPROFLOXACIN

INDICATIONS: Ciprofloxacin (Cipro ♣ ★) is a fluoroquinolone antibiotic with activity against *E. coli, Klebsiella, Proteus, Pseudomonas, Staphylococcus, Salmonella, Shigella, Yersinia, Campylobacter,* and *Vibrio* species. It has little activity against anaerobic cocci or clostridia or *Bacteroides* organisms. The fluoroquinolone antibiotics are indicated in the treatment of genitourinary tract infections, including prostatitis, severe bacterial gastroenteritis, and infections of the respiratory tract and external auditory canal. In humans, ciprofloxacin is a preferred drug in the treatment of prostatitis. See also FLUOROQUINOLONE ANTIBIOTICS.

ADVERSE AND COMMON SIDE EFFECTS: See FLUOROQUINO-LONE ANTIBIOTICS.

DRUG INTERACTIONS: Absorption is hindered by antacid preparations. The concomitant use of theophylline and ciprofloxacin increases the plasma concentration of theophylline. See FLUOROQUINOLONE ANTIBIOTICS.

SUPPLIED AS HUMAN PRODUCTS:
Tablets containing 250, 500, and 750 mg
For injection containing 200 mg/20 mL, 400 mg/40 mL, and 1,200 mg/120 mL in dextrose and vials of 20 and 40 mL containing 10 mg ciprofloxacin
Note: For IV use, dilute to concentration of 1 to 2 mg/mL.

CISAPRIDE

INDICATIONS: Cisapride has been associated with serious and sometimes fatal arrhythmias in people and has consequently been removed from the North American market. It may still be available from selected veterinary pharmacies. In people, suggested alternatives to cisapride for the management of gastroparesis include erythromycin, metoclopramide or domperidone, for gastroesophageal reflux consider an H_2-receptor antagonist or proton pump inhibitor. Cisapride is chemically related to metoclopramide and may be useful in small animals in cases of gastroesophageal reflux and to stimulate GI motility in cases of primary motility disorders. It stimulates GI motility by increasing acetylcholine release. The drug increases lower esophageal pressure and lower esophageal peristalsis (in those species in which the distal esophageal muscularis is composed of smooth muscle, e.g., cat; the dog esophagus is composed entirely of striated muscle and would not be expected to respond to the drug at this level), accelerates gastric emptying, and enhances small intestinal and colonic activity. In small animals, the drug may be useful in the management of regurgitation associated with idiopathic megaesophagus, gastroparesis, idiopathic megacolon in cats (along with a stool softener and a fiber-augmented diet), gastroesophageal reflux, and postoperative ileus. It has only weak antiemetic properties. The drug generally is given 15 minutes before a meal.

ADVERSE AND COMMON SIDE EFFECTS: A single oral dose of 640 mg/kg is lethal to dogs. Signs of acute toxicosis include diarrhea, dyspnea, ptosis, tremors, loss of righting reflex, hypotonia, catalepsy, and convulsions. Use of the drug is contraindicated in those with GI hemorrhage, obstruction, or perforation.

DRUG INTERACTIONS: Because cisapride increases gastric emptying, absorption of drugs from the stomach may be decreased whereas absorption from the small bowel may be increased. Coagulation times of anticoagulant drugs may be increased if cisapride is used concurrently. The sedative effects of benzodiazepines may be enhanced. Concurrent use of cimetidine or ranitidine increases the bioavailability of cisapride. Concurrent use of anticholinergic agents, e.g., atropine, aminopentamide, and isopropamide, antagonize the beneficial effects of cisapride on the GIT.

SUPPLIED AS HUMAN PRODUCT:
Tablets containing 10 and 20 mg
Oral suspension containing 1 mg/mL

OTHER USES
Dogs
DELAYED GASTRIC EMPTYING
0.5 to 1.0 mg/kg

Cats
IDIOPATHIC CONSTIPATION
2.5 mg bid to tid; PO

CISPLATIN

INDICATIONS: Cisplatin (Platinol ★ and generics ♣) is a chemotherapeutic agent that as a single agent has modest efficacy in the treatment of some adenocarcinomas, squamous cell carcinomas, and osteosarcomas. It is a reasonable choice for palliation in patients with nonresectable carcinoma or metastatic osteosarcoma and has been used in the treatment of transitional cell carcinoma of the bladder. However, in the case of transitional cell carcinoma and even at higher dosages (60 mg/m²), none of the dogs treated achieved complete remission, suggesting that a more effective approach should be sought. Recent reports suggest that dogs treated with cisplatin alone after amputation for osteosarcoma have increased survival times. Intracavitary cisplatin chemotherapy has been used in dogs with pleural or abdominal effusion associated with neoplasia of the thoracic cavity (mesotheliomas and carcinomatosis of unknown origin). Its use resulted in rapid resolution of the effusion in five of six dogs treated. Finally the drug has been used with some success following surgical resection in a limited number of male dogs with testicular tumor (Sertoli cell tumor, seminoma).

ADVERSE AND COMMON SIDE EFFECTS: The principal side effects of cisplatin are gastrointestinal upset, nephrotoxicity, bone marrow suppression, and ototoxicity. Transient vomiting is the most common side effect reported in dogs. Dogs that receive butorphanol (0.4 mg/kg; IM) immediately after cisplatin therapy are much less likely to vomit. Anorexia and diarrhea also may occur, and seizure activity has been reported. Mild granulocytopenia and thrombocytopenia have been documented. Saline (0.9%) diuresis (18.3 mL/kg per hour over a 4-hour period) before and after (same rate for 2 hours) use of the drug is recommended to decrease the incidence of renal pathology. Several protocols involving the use of saline diuresis have been proposed, the most effective of which has not been determined. Concurrent administration of methimazole (40 mg/kg; IV over 1 minute) has been found to decrease the incidence of renal toxicity of cisplatin. Intravenous sodium thiosulfate delivered during and after intracavitary cisplatin administration has been recommended in humans to protect against renal toxicosis. The incidence of cisplatin-induced renal toxicosis is decreased if the drug is administered in the latter part of the afternoon as opposed to the morning. The concurrent use of mannitol appears to do little to further limit renal toxicity and does not appear to be required. Carboplatin, a second-generation platinum compound, is less nephrotoxic and does not require saline diuresis. Intracavitary cisplatin (50 mg/m^2 every 4 weeks), however, was not associated with toxicity in the dog. Cisplatin is quite toxic to cats. Its use has led to dose-related pulmonary edema, dyspnea, and death in this species. The drug should not be used in patients with renal disease or myelosuppression. Complete blood counts should be monitored on a weekly basis when the low-dose regimen is used and before therapy if the monthly high-dose regimen is chosen. Reduction of dosage is recommended if the leukocyte count or platelet count significantly decreases or if serum creatinine or urea nitrogen increases. Use of the drug is discontinued if the leukocyte count decreases to less than 3,200/μL, if the platelet count decreases to less than 100,000/μL, or if endogenous creatinine clearance decreases to less than 1.4 mL/minute per kg.

DRUG INTERACTIONS: Concurrent use with aminoglycoside antibiotics, amphotericin B, or furosemide increases the risk of ototoxicity and nephrotoxicity. Serum phenytoin levels are decreased by cisplatin.

SUPPLIED AS HUMAN PRODUCT:
For injection containing 10 mg and 50 mg/vial and 1 mg/mL [Platinol AQ 1 mg]

CLAVAMOX

INDICATIONS: Clavamox ♣ ★ (amoxicillin/clavulanate) is an amoxicillin and clavulanic acid combination. This combination increases efficacy against *E. coli, Klebsiella,* and *Proteus. Pseudomonas* usually is resistant. The drug is indicated in the treatment of skin and soft tissue infections caused by susceptible organisms, including β-lactamase–producing and non-β-lactamase–producing *Staphylococcus aureus* and *Staphylococcus* spp. and *E. coli.* It is useful in the treatment of cystitis, and in cats, the drug combination also is effective against *Pasteurella* spp. and *Chlamydia psittaci*. Amoxicillin penetrates most body tissues with the exception of the brain and spinal fluid, where entry occurs only if the meninges are inflamed. For additional information, see PENICILLIN ANTIBIOTICS.

ADVERSE AND COMMON SIDE EFFECTS: The drug combination is contraindicated in animals with sensitivity to the penicillins or the cephalosporin antibiotics. Also see PENICILLIN ANTIBIOTICS.

DRUG INTERACTIONS: See PENICILLIN ANTIBIOTICS.

SUPPLIED AS VETERINARY PRODUCTS:
Tablets containing 50, 100, 200, and 300 mg amoxicillin and 12.5, 25, 50, and 75 mg clavulanic acid, respectively for a total of 62.5, 125, 250, and 375 mg of Clavamox
Oral suspension containing amoxicillin 50 mg/mL and clavulanic acid 12.5 mg/mL

CLEMASTINE

INDICATIONS: Clemastine (Tavist ♣ ★), an antihistamine, has been used in dogs and cats to control chronic pruritus. The drug effectively controlled pruritus in 26% to 30% of dogs and in 50% of cats.

ADVERSE AND COMMON SIDE EFFECTS: In people, it is suggested that if a patient has any of the following medical problems a lower dose of the drug may be indicated. These medical problems include glaucoma, stomach ulcer, enlarged prostate, difficulty urinating, hypertension or heart disease, or asthma.

Clemastine passes into breast milk. Newborns are especially sensitive to the effects of antihistamines, and serious side effects could occur.

DRUG INTERACTIONS: In people, it is suggested not to take clemastine if you have taken an MAO inhibitor, which in veterinary medicine may include amitraz or selegiline in the last 14 days. A very dangerous drug interaction could occur, leading to serious side effects.

SUPPLIED AS HUMAN PRODUCTS:
Tablets containing 1 and 2 mg
Syrup containing 5,000 µg/5 mL

CLINDAMYCIN

INDICATIONS: Clindamycin (Antirobe ♣ ★, Clindrops ★) is a lincosamide antibiotic with activity against gram-positive cocci (staphylococci and streptococci). It often is effective against gram-positive organisms that are resistant to penicillin and the cephalosporins. The drug also may be effective against *Salmonella, Pseudomonas, Pasteurella, Actinomyces, Nocardia, Mycoplasma,* and *Toxoplasma* organisms, *Neospora caninum,* and anaerobic bacteria (*Bacteroides fragilis,* fusobacteria, *Propionibacterium, Eubacterium, Actinomyces* species, peptostreptococci, *Clostridium perfringens*) and possibly *Babesia canis* infections. It has greater activity than lincomycin but is more expensive. The drug is distributed extensively in most body tissues, and it appears that clindamycin may penetrate the CSF and ocular tissue if inflammation is present.

ADVERSE AND COMMON SIDE EFFECTS: Adverse effects may include vomiting and diarrhea (sometimes hemorrhagic) after oral use of the drug. Intramuscular injection may cause local pain. Clindamycin dosage should be reduced or the drug avoided in animals with hepatic insufficiency or cholestasis. The drug also should be used with caution in animals with renal impairment. The drug in cats induces transient vomiting occasionally during the first few days of therapy. Vomiting is controlled by stopping the drug for 24 hours, and then reintroducing it at a lower dosage, gradually increasing it to 25 mg/kg. Small bowel diarrhea occurs in some cats. It tends to resolve within 1 week after therapy. Caution is advised by the manufacturer if the drug is used in atopic animals. The safety of its use in pregnant and breeding animals has not been established.

DRUG INTERACTIONS: Clindamycin may potentiate the effects of neuromuscular-blocking agents (e.g., atracurium, tubocurarine, pancuronium) during anesthesia. Mutual antagonism is expected if erythromycin or chloramphenicol are used with clindamycin. Diphenoxylate [Lomotil] and the opiates, e.g., paregoric, may reduce the rate (not the extent of absorption) of clindamycin and prolong diarrhea if present.

SUPPLIED AS VETERINARY PRODUCTS:
Capsules containing 25, 75, and 150 mg
Oral solution containing 25 mg/mL

OTHER USES
Dogs
NEOSPORA CANINUM
13.5 mg/kg tid; PO

BABESIA CANIS
10 mg/kg tid; PO for 2 weeks with imidocarb dipropionate at 5 mg/kg; IM

CLOFAZIMINE

INDICATIONS: Clofazimine (Lamprene ★) is an antimicrobial agent used in the treatment of feline leprosy, and localized *Mycobacterium avium* in conjunction with doxycycline. Clofazimine is bacteriocidal to *Mycobacterium leprae.*

ADVERSE AND COMMON SIDE EFFECTS: Adverse effects may include a reddish-orange discoloration of skin and mucous membranes.

DRUG INTERACTIONS: Clofazimine is often used safely with other drugs in combination therapy. Clofazimine's anti-inflammatory effects may be inhibited if the drug is used concurrently with dapsone. If inflammatory reactions associated with leprosy are observed while these drugs are used concurrently, it is still advisable to continue with the treatment combination.

SUPPLIED AS HUMAN PRODUCT:
Capsules containing 50 and 100 mg

CLOMIPRAMINE

INDICATIONS: Clomipramine (Clomicalm ✿ ★) is a tricyclic anti-depressant drug that works by inhibiting serotonin reuptake in the brain. It is used as part of a behavioral management program for the treatment of separation anxiety in dogs greater than 6 months of age and for inappropriate barking, destructive behavior, tail chasing, canine acral lick dermatitis, noise phobia, psychogenic alopecia in cats, and inappropriate elimination. The drug should not be used to treat aggression.

ADVERSE AND COMMON SIDE EFFECTS: Vomiting, diarrhea, lethargy, thirst, decreased appetite, aggression, and seizure activity may occur. The drug should not be used in dogs with a history of sensitivity to tricyclic antidepressant drugs or to dogs with a history of seizure activity. Use with caution in patients with cardiovascular disease. Because of its anticholinergic effects, it should not be used in dogs with ocular disease, e.g., glaucoma, urinary retention, or reduced gastrointestinal motility. In cats drowsiness, pupillary dilation, and urinary retention were most often noted.

Clomipramine use in dogs may cause a significant decrease in serum T_4 and FT_4 concentrations leading to a misdiagnosis of hypothyroid disease.

DRUG INTERACTIONS: Clomipramine should not be given to dogs with drugs that may lower the seizure threshold. It should not be given concurrently or within 14 days of a monoamine oxidase (MOA) inhibitor, e.g., amitraz or selegiline. The drug should not be given to breeding male dogs. It should be used with caution if used concurrently with anticholinergic agents, sympathomimetic drugs, or other CNS-active drugs including general anesthetics and neuroleptics. Co-administration with phenobarbital increases plasma concentrations of phenobarbital.

Plasma levels of several closely related tricyclic antidepressants have been reported to be increased by the concomitant administration of methylphenidate or hepatic enzyme inhibitors (e.g., cimetidine, fluoxetine) and decreased by the concomitant administration of hepatic enzyme inducers (e.g., barbiturates, phenytoin), and such an effect may be anticipated as well. Administration of clomipramine has been reported to increase the plasma levels of phenobarbital, if given concomitantly. Because clomipramine is highly bound to serum protein, the administration of clomipramine to patients taking other drugs that are highly bound to protein (e.g., warfarin, digoxin) may cause an increase in plasma concentrations of these drugs, potentially resulting in adverse effects.

SUPPLIED AS VETERINARY PRODUCT:
Tablets containing 20, 40, and 80 mg

CLONAZEPAM

INDICATIONS: Clonazepam (Klonopin ★, Rivotril ✤) is a benzodiazepine drug that is potentially useful in the management of status epilepticus. It should not, however, be considered a major anticonvulsant in the dog. Clonazepam may be used in conjunction with phenobarbital in the management of intractable epilepsy. Peak serum concentrations are reached within 3 hours.

ADVERSE AND COMMON SIDE EFFECTS: Ataxia and sedation occur at higher doses. Vomiting and pronounced ataxia were noted in dogs at doses of 0.2 mg/kg; IV. Other side effects noted in humans include bradycardia, dry mouth, anorexia, nausea, increased appetite, constipation, diarrhea, dysuria, urinary retention, dyspnea, hepatomegaly, leukopenia, anemia, and thrombocytopenia. Tolerance develops after a 3- to 9-month period.

DRUG INTERACTIONS: Cimetidine may increase the pharmacological effects of clonazepam.

SUPPLIED AS HUMAN PRODUCTS:
Tablets containing 500 µg and 2 mg [Rivotril]
Tablets containing 0.5, 1, and 2 mg [Klonopin]

CLORAZEPATE

INDICATIONS: Clorazepate (Tranxene ♣ ★) is an anxiolytic, sedative benzodiazepine that has been used in the management of behavioral problems in dogs, e.g., anxiety and noise phobia. It also may prove useful as a secondary anticonvulsant in the management of refractory canine epilepsy in conjunction with phenobarbital.

ADVERSE AND COMMON SIDE EFFECTS: The drug is contraindicated in myasthenia gravis. In one study in dogs, mild and transient sedation and ataxia were noted only infrequently and did not recur on additional dosing. In humans, drowsiness, ataxia, paradoxical excitement, GI disturbances, hypotension, and blood dyscrasias have been reported. Safe use during pregnancy has not been established.

DRUG INTERACTIONS: Antacids delay absorption of the drug. Cimetidine may increase the pharmacological effects of clonazepam.

SUPPLIED AS HUMAN PRODUCT:
Capsules containing 3.75, 7.5, and 15 mg

CLOTRIMAZOLE

INDICATIONS: Clotrimazole (Canesten ♣, Lotrimin ★, Mycelex ★) is a topical imidazole useful in the treatment of localized dermatophytosis and candidal stomatitis in small animals. A 1% solution has been used successfully in the topical treatment of nasal aspergillosis in dogs where the drug is infused into the nasal cavities. Therapeutic success approaches 80% to 100%. For detailed information concerning its use for the treatment of nasal aspergillosis, the reader is referred to Smith SA, Andrews G, Biller DS. Management of nasal aspergillosis in a dog with a single, noninvasive intranasal infusion of clotrimazole. J Am Anim Hosp Assoc 1998;34:487; and Mathews KG, et al. Comparison of topical administration of clotrimazole through surgically placed versus non-surgically placed catheters for treatment of nasal aspergillosis in dogs: 60 cases (1990 to 1996). JAVMA 1998;213:501. The drug has also been infused in the bladder to treat cystitis caused by *Candida* spp. in a cat.

ADVERSE AND COMMON SIDE EFFECTS: Local irritation may occur in some patients. Mild subcutaneous emphysema and inflammation associated with placement of the infusion tubes occurs in some dogs.

DRUG INTERACTIONS: None.

SUPPLIED AS HUMAN PRODUCTS:
Topical cream containing 10 mg/g (1%) [Canesten, Lotrimin, Mycelex]
Topical solution containing 10 mg/mL [Canesten, Lotrimin, Mycelex]
Topical lotion containing 10 mg/g (1%) [Lotrimin]
Powder containing 2% [Lotrimin]

OTHER USES

Cats

CANDIDIASIS (BLADDER)
50 mL of 1% clotrimazole instilled into the bladder; cat rotated through 360° over 15 to 90 minutes; evacuated voluntarily; repeated once weekly over 3 weeks

CLOXACILLIN

INDICATIONS: Cloxacillin (Cloxapen ★, Orbenin ❤) is a penicillin antibiotic used primarily against gram-positive, β-lactamase–producing bacteria, especially staphylococcal spp. For further information, see PENICILLIN ANTIBIOTICS.

ADVERSE AND COMMON SIDE EFFECTS AND DRUG INTERACTIONS: See PENICILLIN ANTIBIOTICS.

SUPPLIED AS HUMAN PRODUCTS:
Capsules containing 250 and 500 mg [Cloxapen]
Oral suspension containing 125 mg/5 mL

COAL TAR

INDICATIONS: Coal tar shampoos are keratolytic and keratoplastic. They are used in the treatment of seborrhea, to relieve pruritus, and to remove crusts and scales. Coal tar is found alone or in combination with other agents in the following products: MicroPearls Coal Tar ★, Lytar ★, and Allerseb T ❤ ★.

ADVERSE AND COMMON SIDE EFFECTS: Coal tar shampoos may be irritating and may cause excessive drying, photosensitization, and superficial necrolytic dermatitis. Reduce frequency of use or discontinue if this occurs. These products may be toxic to cats and should not be used in this species.

DRUG INTERACTIONS: None.

SUPPLIED AS: See specific product.

CODEINE

INDICATIONS: Codeine (Tylenol No. 1 ❤) often is used in the management of mild to moderate pain. It is only 10% as potent an analgesic as morphine sulfate. It also is useful as an antidiarrheal agent and as an antitussive.

ADVERSE AND COMMON SIDE EFFECTS: Drowsiness, nausea, ileus, vomiting, and constipation may occur with its use. Its use is contraindicated in liver disease, intestinal obstruction, and invasive or toxigenic bowel disease. Spasm of the biliary and pancreatic ducts can occur. The respiratory depressant effects and the capacity to increase CSF pressure may be exacerbated in cases of head injury. Use of the drug is cautioned in patients with a history of seizure or cardiac arrhythmias. In cats, opiate agonists may cause CNS excitation with hyperexcitability, tremors, and seizure activity.

DRUG INTERACTIONS: The concurrent use of barbiturates, phenothiazines, and other CNS depressants potentiate CNS depression.

SUPPLIED AS HUMAN PRODUCTS:
For injection containing 30 and 60 mg codeine phosphate
Caplets containing 8 mg (#1), 15 mg (#2), 30 mg (#3), and 60 mg (#4) codeine with acetaminophen and caffeine [Tylenol with codeine]
Elixir containing 8 mg/5 mL codeine with acetaminophen [Tylenol with codeine elixir]
Tablets containing 15, 30, and 60 mg codeine phosphate

COLCHICINE

INDICATIONS: Colchicine (generic products ✤ ★) has been recommended in the treatment of chronic hepatic fibrosis in the dog. The drug works by decreasing collagen formation and promoting its breakdown. Its anti-inflammatory properties are mediated by the drug's inhibition of mononuclear cell and neutrophil migration. Colchicine also may have hepatoprotective effects by stabilizing hepatocyte plasma membranes and restoring hepatic enzyme activities. It also has been used in the treatment of amyloidosis. In this condition, the drug impairs the release of serum amyloid A (SAA) from hepatocytes, prevents the production of amyloid-enhancing factor, and delays tissue deposition of amyloid. Because of the advanced state in which veterinary patients present, colchicine is unlikely to benefit those with amyloidosis.

ADVERSE AND COMMON SIDE EFFECTS: Reports of its use in dogs are scant; however, no toxicity was observed in a dog treated with the drug over a 7-month period at a dose of 0.03 mg/kg per day. In humans, nausea, vomiting, and diarrhea are most common. Muscular weakness, hematuria, oliguria, agranulocytosis, and anemia also have been reported with chronic use. Use of the drug is contraindicated in patients with serious GIT, renal, or cardiac disease. It is not recommended for use in breeding or pregnant animals.

DRUG INTERACTIONS: Colchicine action is inhibited by acidifying agents and potentiated by alkalinizing agents.

SUPPLIED AS HUMAN PRODUCT:
Tablets containing 0.5, 0.6, and 1 mg colchicine

CYCLOPHOSPHAMIDE

INDICATIONS: Cyclophosphamide (Cytoxan ❧ ★, Procytox ❧) is an alkylating agent with potent immunosuppressive properties and has been used in small animals in the treatment of lymphosarcoma, hemangiosarcoma, mammary gland carcinoma, mastocytoma, transmissible venereal tumor, bladder carcinoma, macroglobulinemia, multiple myeloma, and autoimmune diseases not responsive to other immunosuppressive agents, including autoimmune skin diseases, immune-mediated arthritis, lymphocytic-plasmacytic enteritis, autoimmune anemia, thrombocytopenia, and polymyositis. The drug impairs B- and T-cell responses and suppresses macrophage function and thus, inflammation. However, short-term use (1 week) of the drug does not affect the humoral or cell-mediated immune response. A beneficial clinical response may take 1 to 4 weeks.

ADVERSE AND COMMON SIDE EFFECTS: Bone marrow depression, hemorrhagic cystitis (especially if therapy exceeds 2 months), and an association with the induction of transitional cell carcinoma of the bladder have been documented. Measures aimed at decreasing the frequency or severity of cystitis have included administering the drug in the morning, encouraging diuresis (promoting increased water intake and the concurrent use of furosemide), administering prednisone on the same day, and intravesicular administration of 50% dimethyl sulfoxide (DMSO), 1% formalin, or acetylcysteine. Chlorambucil may be substituted should adverse effects necessitate discontinuation of the drug. Alkylating agents generally cause leukopenia, thrombocytopenia, and anemia, with the nadir of the leukocyte counts observed 7 to 14 days after treatment and recovery noted in an additional 7 to 14 days. The complete blood count should be monitored weekly for the first 2 months and monthly thereafter. If the segmented neutrophil count falls below 1000 to 1500 cells/µl, prophylactic oral antibiotic therapy may be warranted (trimethoprim-sulfadiazine 15 mg/kg bid). Other side effects include GI inflammation causing vomiting, diarrhea, anorexia, depression, infertility, teratogenicity, alopecia (especially in poodles, old English sheepdogs), and altered wound healing. The drug should not be used for more than 4 to 5 months.

DRUG INTERACTIONS: The pharmacological activity of digoxin may be reduced if the two drugs are used concurrently. Cyclophosphamide inhibits the metabolism of succinylcholine, potentially leading to prolonged neuromuscular-blocking activity. Barbiturate drugs including phenobarbital may increase the rate of cyclophosphamide metabolism via hepatic microsomal enzyme induction. Allopurinol and the thiazide diuretics may potentiate the myelosuppression associated with cyclophosphamide. Cyclophosphamide should be used with caution in patients receiving doxorubicin because potentiation of cardiotoxicity may occur.

SUPPLIED AS HUMAN PRODUCTS:
Tablets containing 25 or 50 mg
For injection containing either 500-, 1,000-, and 2,000-mg base lyophilized in mannitol or 100 and 200 mg nonlyophilized with sodium chloride

CYCLOSPORINE

INDICATIONS: Cyclosporine (Atopica ★, Sandimmune ✤ ★, Optimmune ✤ ★) is an effective immunosuppressant agent. It inhibits B- and T-lymphocyte activation. It exerts its major effect on helper T cells by blocking the release of interleukin-2. Cyclosporine may be useful in the management of autoimmune disease, in perianal fistulae, to control pruritus associated with atopic dermatitis in dogs, and to block rejection of organ and tissue transplants. Cyclosporine may be used in conjunction with ketoconazole in the treatment of perianal fistulas. A recent study failed to demonstrate beneficial effects of the drug in dogs with glomerulonephritis. Susceptibility to infection appears to be less common than that observed with common immunosuppressive agents. A 0.2% solution (Optimmune ✤ ★) is quite effective in the treatment of dogs with keratoconjunctivitis sicca. Causes varied, but tear production improved and corneal pigmentation decreased. The drug appears to inhibit T cells within the lacrimal gland from secreting inflammatory mediators that damage lacrimal acini. Lacrimation increases, and superficial pigmentation, vascularization, and granulation decrease. Days to weeks may be required before ocular improvement is noted.

ADVERSE AND COMMON SIDE EFFECTS: In dogs, vomiting, diarrhea, anorexia, gingival hyperplasia, pyoderma, predisposition to infection, and papillomatosis have been reported. These adverse effects tend to abate when the dosage of the drug is decreased. Dogs treated with the microemulsified preparation may develop a dose-dependent, antibiotic-responsive psoriasiform-lichenoid-like dermatosis that may represent an atypical staphylococcal infection. The incidence of nephrotoxicity and hepatotoxicity in dogs appears to be less than that observed in humans and has not been demonstrated in cats. Many cats find the oral solution unpalatable, resulting in ptyalism and head shaking. Intravenous administration causes acute anaphylactoid reactions in a high percentage of dogs. Use of the ophthalmic preparation may be associated with local irritation with periocular redness, blepharospasm, and excessive rubbing. Expense and systemic toxicity may limit the use of the systemic drug in veterinary medicine.

DRUG INTERACTIONS: Gentamicin, amphotericin B, and melphalan may potentiate cyclosporine nephrotoxicity. Ketoconazole, erythromycin, and cimetidine depress hepatic metabolism of cyclosporine. Phenobarbital and phenytoin increase hepatic metabolism of cyclosporine and result in lower than anticipated blood levels. Cimetidine may affect absorption of orally administered cyclosporine but does not affect the pharmacokinetics of the drug. Monitoring of blood concentrations is recommended. Ketoconazole slows the clearance of cyclosporine, reduces the amount of cyclosporine required, and lowers the cost of treatment. Concurrent administration of D-α-tocopheryl polyethylene glycol 1,000 succinate (10 IU vitamin E TPGS) increases the bioavailability of cyclosporine (Sandimmune, not Neoral), allowing the oral dose of the Sandimmune product to be reduced significantly.

SUPPLIED AS HUMAN PRODUCTS:
Capsules containing 25, 50, and 100 mg
Oral solution containing 100 mg/mL
Solutions for IV injection are NOT recommended

SUPPLIED AS VETERINARY PRODUCTS:
Atopica as capsules containing 10, 25, 50, or 100 mg
Optimmune as an ointment

OTHER USES
Dogs
KERATOCONJUNCTIVITIS SICCA
Applied topically; bid
PERIANAL FISTULAE
i) 3 to 5 mg/kg bid; PO continued for 2 weeks beyond clinical remission (not less than 8 weeks; average treatment duration 16 weeks)
ii) Cyclosporine 2.5 mg/kg bid; PO OR 4 mg/kg once daily; PO with goal to attain trough concentration of 400 to 600 ng/mL PLUS ketoconazole at 8 mg/kg; PO
ATOPIC DERMATITIS
5 mg/kg once daily PO

CYPROHEPTADINE

INDICATIONS: Cyproheptadine (Periactin ♣ ★) is an antihistamine-antiserotonin, and acetylcholine antagonist. The drug has been used to stimulate appetite in cats (it may not be effective in dogs). Cyproheptadine may be useful in the management of bronchospasm associated with allergic airway disease in cats. It also has been used with limited success in the treatment of pituitary-dependent hyperadrenocorticism in dogs. It is ineffective in the management of allergic pruritus.

ADVERSE AND COMMON SIDE EFFECTS: Excitability and aggressive behavior have been documented in some cats. Other adverse effects sometimes noted in people include nausea, vomiting, jaundice, and drowsiness. The drug is contraindicated in patients with glaucoma, pyloric or duodenal obstruction, urinary retention, and acute asthma.

DRUG INTERACTIONS: Monoamine oxidase inhibitors, possibly amitraz and selegiline, prolong and intensify the anticholinergic effects of the drug. Central nervous system depressant drugs may have an additive effect if used concurrently with cyproheptadine.

SUPPLIED AS HUMAN PRODUCTS:
Tablets containing 4 mg
Syrup containing 2 mg/5 mL

OTHER USES
Dogs
PITUITARY-DEPENDENT HYPERADRENOCORTICISM
0.3 to 3.0 mg/kg daily for 4 to 27 weeks (8 of 10 dogs failed to improve)

CYTARABINE

INDICATIONS: Cytarabine (Cytosar ♣, Cytosar-U ★) is a chemo-therapeutic agent that has been used in the treatment of lympho-reticular neoplasms, mastocytoma, and myeloproliferative disease. It also has been injected intrathecally in the treatment of lymphoma involving the CNS.

ADVERSE AND COMMON SIDE EFFECTS: Nausea, vomiting, diarrhea, and, rarely, anaphylaxis have been reported. Bone marrow suppression (nadir at 5 to 7 days, recovery at 7 to 14 days), oral ulcer-ation, hepatotoxicity, and fever also may occur. The drug is poten-tially teratogenic and embryotoxic.

DRUG INTERACTIONS: Cytarabine may decrease the amount of orally administered digoxin, an effect that may persist for several days after discontinuation of cytarabine. Cytarabine may decrease the efficacy of gentamicin and flucytosine.

SUPPLIED AS HUMAN PRODUCT:
For injection containing 100-, 200-, and 500-mg and 1- and 2-g vials

DACARBAZINE

INDICATIONS: Dacarbazine (DTIC ♣ ★) is a chemotherapeutic agent with alkylating and antimetabolite properties. It has been used pri-marily in the treatment of lymphosarcoma and malignant histiocytosis.

ADVERSE AND COMMON SIDE EFFECTS: Nausea, anorexia, vomiting, diarrhea, and cytopenia have been reported. A burning sensation may occur when injected intravenously, and extravascular injection may cause tissue damage and severe pain. Anaphylaxis has been reported in some patients. Delayed toxicity may cause alopecia, photosensitivity, and renal and hepatic impairment.

DRUG INTERACTIONS: None reported.

SUPPLIED AS HUMAN PRODUCT:
For injection in vials containing 100 and 200 mg

DACTINOMYCIN

INDICATIONS: Dactinomycin, or actinomycin-D (Cosmegen ✤ ★), is a potent antibiotic used in the treatment of bone and soft tissue sarcomas, anal sac adenocarcinoma, perianal adenocarcinoma, squamous cell carcinoma, thyroid carcinoma, transitional cell carcinoma, lymphoma, and malignant melanomas. It has been recommended as a rescue drug for dogs with lymphoma after traditional combination chemotherapy studies have failed to demonstrate a beneficial effect.

ADVERSE AND COMMON SIDE EFFECTS: In dogs, GI (anorexia, vomiting, diarrhea) and hematologic (thrombocytopenia, neutropenia) toxicity are reported. At this point, no toxicity has been documented in the limited number of cats on which the drug has been used. Dactinomycin is contraindicated in patients with viral infections, and use is cautioned in patients that have had radiation therapy within the past 3 to 6 weeks, bone marrow suppression, infections, obesity, and renal or hepatic impairment.

DRUG INTERACTIONS: Dactinomycin may cause elevations in uric acid levels if used concurrently with allopurinol. Potentiation of myelosuppression may occur if the drug is used concurrently with other myelosuppressive agents. Radiation may potentiate the effects of dactinomycin and vice versa. Dactinomycin decreases vitamin K effects, leading to prolonged clotting time and potential hemorrhage.

SUPPLIED AS HUMAN PRODUCT:
For injection containing 500 μg/vial

DANAZOL

INDICATIONS: Danazol (Danocrine ★, Cyclomen ✤) is a modified androgen. It has been shown to be effective in the treatment of canine immune-mediated thrombocytopenia and anemia in conjunction with prednisolone or prednisone. When combined with corticosteroids, the immunomodulating effects are synergistic. Response to danazol reduces the need for other therapies and may replace them when remission is achieved. A clinically significant response may not be apparent for 2 to 3 months. A recent study in dogs with autoimmune hemolytic anemia given prednisone and azathioprine failed to show additional benefit when danazol was added to the regimen. Danazol decreases immunoglobulin G production, cell-bound immunoglobulin, and complement. It also modulates the balance between T suppressor and helper cells. The therapeutic effects reportedly are slow. In cases of autoimmune hemolytic anemia (AIHA), elevations in packed cell volume may not be apparent for 1 to 3 weeks. Also see ANABOLIC STEROIDS.

ADVERSE AND COMMON SIDE EFFECTS: In humans, side effects are rare but may include virilization and hepatic dysfunction. Hepatopathy also has been documented in dogs.

DRUG INTERACTIONS: None reported.

SUPPLIED AS HUMAN PRODUCT:
Capsules containing 50, 100, and 200 mg

DANTROLENE

INDICATIONS: Dantrolene (Dantrium ✽ ★) is a skeletal muscle relaxant that may be useful in reducing external urethral sphincter tone in cases of urinary incontinence associated with urethral hypertonia. Dantrolene also is used in the prevention and treatment of malignant hyperthermia.

ADVERSE AND COMMON SIDE EFFECTS: Sedation, nausea, vomiting, constipation, and, possibly, hypotension occur. Drug overdose may cause generalized muscle weakness. Hepatotoxicity has been documented in humans after long-term drug therapy.

DRUG INTERACTIONS: Concurrent use of other CNS depressants may cause additive CNS depression. Use of calcium channel-blocking agents, e.g., verapamil, diltiazem, may predispose to ventricular fibrillation.

SUPPLIED AS HUMAN PRODUCTS:
Capsules containing 25, 50, and 100 mg
For injection containing 20 mg

OTHER USES
Dogs
FUNCTIONAL URETHRAL OBSTRUCTION
i)   1 to 5 mg/kg tid; PO

ii) 3 to 15 mg/kg divided bid to tid; PO

ADJUNCTIVE THERAPY FOR BLACK WIDOW SPIDER BITES
1 mg/kg; IV; followed by 1 mg/kg every 4 hours; PO

Cats
FUNCTIONAL URETHRAL OBSTRUCTION
i)   0.5 to 2 mg/kg tid; PO

ii) 1 mg/kg; PO in conjunction with prazosin (0.03 mg/kg; IV)

DAPSONE

INDICATIONS: Dapsone (Avlosulfon ♣ and generic products ★) is an anti-inflammatory, antibacterial agent that has been used in the dog for treatment of pemphigus foliaceus, dermatitis herpetiformis, subcorneal pustular dermatosis, leprosy, and leukocytoclastic vasculitis.

ADVERSE AND COMMON SIDE EFFECTS: In dogs, hepatotoxicity, mild anemia and neutropenia, severe thrombocytopenia, GI signs, and skin reactions may occur. Gastrointestinal signs usually can be reduced or eliminated by giving the drug with food. A complete blood count and serum biochemistry should be performed every other week during the first 6 weeks of therapy and reduced in frequency after the dose is reduced.

DRUG INTERACTIONS: Pyrimethamine increases the risk of adverse dapsone-induced hematologic effects. Rifampin lowers dapsone blood levels by increasing plasma clearance. Higher doses of dapsone may be required.

SUPPLIED AS HUMAN PRODUCT:
Tablets containing 25 and 100 mg

DEHYDROCHOLIC ACID

INDICATIONS: Dehydrocholic acid (Atrocholin ★, Dycholium ♣, Decholin ★) is a bile acid that may stimulate flow of watery bile and help alleviate cholestasis. The drug only should be used once a positive diagnosis of biliary sludge or precipitation has been established. Dehydrocholic acid is used until urine is negative for bilirubin. Dehydrocholic acid in conjunction with fluid therapy may improve biliary flow, although it does not hasten the clearance of jaundice. Because biliary sludging and precipitation may be associated with infection, the drug always should be used in conjunction with fluid therapy and antibiotics. There is little evidence that this drug is of benefit in cats with cholestatic disorders. Ursodeoxycholic acid may be more effective.

ADVERSE AND COMMON SIDE EFFECTS: The drug is not to be used in the presence of jaundice, hepatic insufficiency, or cholelithiasis, or in complete mechanical obstruction of the common bile duct. Nausea, vomiting, diarrhea, abdominal discomfort, and dizziness are observed in people.

DRUG INTERACTIONS: None reported.

SUPPLIED AS HUMAN PRODUCTS:
Tablets containing 300 mg [Dycholium]
Tablets containing 130 mg [Atrocholin]
Tablets containing 250 mg [Decholin]

DEMECLOCYCLINE

INDICATIONS: Demeclocycline (Declomycin ✤ ★) is an intermediate-acting tetracycline antibiotic. For more information, see TETRACYCLINE ANTIBIOTICS.

ADVERSE AND COMMON SIDE EFFECTS: Demeclocycline has been shown to induce a reversible nephrogenic diabetes insipidus in humans. Experience with the drug in small animals is limited.

DRUG INTERACTIONS: See TETRACYCLINE ANTIBIOTICS.

SUPPLIED AS HUMAN PRODUCT:
Tablets containing 150 and 300 mg

DERACOXIB

INDICATIONS: Deracoxib (Deramaxx ★) is an NSAID for the relief of postoperative pain in dogs, especially with fracture repair and cruciate rupture, and for osteoarthritic pain. Deracoxib acts by inhibiting COX-2 prostaglandins responsible for pain and inflammation, but does not inhibit COX-1, important in maintaining kidney perfusion and protection of the stomach lining. It is generally given several hours before surgery and continued for up to 7 days.

ADVERSE AND COMMON SIDE EFFECTS: The most commonly reported side effects include anorexia, vomiting, diarrhea, and leakage from the surgery site. Melena may be observed at dosages above 25 mg/kg. Deracoxib may cause renal damage at high doses or after prolonged administration. Deracoxib should not be used in animals with known hypersensitivity or allergy to the drug. It should be used with caution in animals with renal, cardiac, or hepatic disease. The drug is not recommended for puppies less than 4 months of age or dogs weighing less than 4 pounds (2 kg). Deracoxib is contraindicated in cats.

DRUG INTERACTIONS: Concurrent use of other NSAIDs or cortico-steroids increases the risk of NSAID-related disorders such as bleeding ulcers or renal damage.

SUPPLIED AS VETERINARY PRODUCT:
Chewable tablets containing 25 or 100 mg

DERM CAPS

INDICATIONS: Derm caps ♣ ★ are a fatty acid nutritional supplement containing eicosapentaenoic, linoleic, and gamma-linolenic acid. It may be of benefit in lessening or eliminating pruritus associated with atopic disease in some dogs. The anti-inflammatory action is likely the result of the decreased production of inflammatory eicosanoids. The drug also has been used to treat idiopathic seborrhea in dogs and may be effective in controlling seborrhea and pruritus in cats. Pruritus was eliminated in 40% of cats with nonlesional pruritus or miliary dermatitis, and approximately 67% of cats with eosinophilic granuloma complex responded favorably to the drug.

ADVERSE AND COMMON SIDE EFFECTS: Side effects are rare. Vomiting, lethargy, diarrhea, urticaria, and increased pruritus have been reported in a few dogs. Although not well documented, these agents may induce pancreatitis in animals predisposed to the disease.

DRUG INTERACTIONS: None reported.

SUPPLIED AS VETERINARY PRODUCTS:
DERM CAPS capsules for small and medium breeds
DERM CAPS ES capsules for medium and large breeds
DERM CAPS ES liquid for medium and large breeds
DERM CAPS liquid for small and medium breeds

OTHER USES
Cats
NONLESIONAL PRURITUS OR MILIARY DERMATITIS AND EOSINOPHILIC GRANULOMA COMPLEX
1 mL per 9.1 kg daily; PO for 14 days

DESMOPRESSIN

INDICATIONS: Desmopressin acetate (DDAVP ♣ ★) is a vasopressin analog used in the management of central diabetes insipidus and type I von Willebrand's disease [quantitative deficiency of von Willebrand factor (vWF)]. DDAVP exerts its maximal effect in diabetes insipidus in 2 to 8 hours, and the duration of activity lasts from 8 to 24 hours. It causes an increase in factor VIII:C and vWF by stimulating the release of preformed factor VIII from storage sites. Maximal levels are attained within 30 minutes, but the duration of effect of DDAVP in von Willebrand's disease is only 2 to 4 hours. Multiple doses of DDAVP are not effective because release of preformed vWF depletes its storage pool, decreasing subsequent responses. Because not all dogs with von Willebrand's disease respond to DDAVP, a response test should be performed in dogs. Buccal mucosal bleeding time and plasma vWF are measured before and after administration of DDAVP and before surgical procedures or possible future hemorrhagic events. DDAVP is not effective in the management of hemophilia A.

ADVERSE AND COMMON SIDE EFFECTS: Side effects in small animals are rare; however, hypersensitivity reactions and fluid retention leading to hyponatremia are a possibility. At the doses required for hemostasis, adverse effects may include a decrease in blood pressure, peripheral vasodilation, and tachycardia. German short-haired pointers (GSHPs) typically have type II von Willebrand's disease, a qualitative vWF disorder, and if this breed reacts as humans with type II disease do, GSHPs may respond to DDAVP with platelet aggregation and thrombocytopenia.

DRUG INTERACTIONS: The use of demeclocycline, lithium, or epinephrine may decrease the antidiuretic response. Carbamazepine, chlorpropamide, and clofibrate may prolong the antidiuretic effect of desmopressin.

SUPPLIED AS HUMAN PRODUCTS:
For injection in ampules containing 4 µg/mL
For intranasal use containing 10 µg/0.1 mL metered spray and 100 µg/mL as drops
Tablets containing 0.1 and 0.2 mg

OTHER USES:
Dogs
MODIFIED WATER DEPRIVATION TEST
After the failure to concentrate urine after water deprivation, 2 µg of DDAVP is given subcutaneously or intravenously, or 20 µg (approximately 4 drops of the 100 µg/mL intranasal solution) is given intranasally or conjunctivally. Urine-specific gravity or osmolality are monitored every 2 hours for a total of 6 to 10 hours. Further increases in urine osmolality greater than 10% are supportive of central diabetes insipidus (DI) or partial nephrogenic DI. Increases less than 10% are suggestive of complete nephrogenic DI or psychogenic polydipsia.

DESOXYCORTICOSTERONE

INDICATIONS: Desoxycorticosterone acetate [DOCA (Percorten-V)] and desoxycorticosterone pivalate [DOCP (Percorten pivalate)] are mineralocorticoid preparations that have been used in the management of hypoadrenocorticism. DOCA (where available) is used in the management of the acute crisis of the disease, and DOCP is used for maintenance therapy.

ADVERSE AND COMMON SIDE EFFECTS: DOCP is well tolerated even at higher than recommended dosages. Depression, polyuria, polydipsia, anorexia, skin and coat changes, vomiting, diarrhea, weakness, weight loss, incontinence, pain on injection, and injection site abscess may occur. Hypokalemia, hypernatremia, and hypertension have also been reported in some patients. Do not use in pregnant dogs or dogs with congestive heart failure, severe renal disease or edema.

DRUG INTERACTIONS: None reported.

SUPPLIED AS VETERINARY PRODUCT:
For injection containing 25 mg/mL in 4-mL vials

DEXAMETHASONE

INDICATIONS: Dexamethasone (Azium ♣ ★, Azium SP ♣ ★, Dex-5 ♣) is a glucocorticoid used in the treatment of nonspecific dermatosis and inflammatory conditions involving the joints (in the absence of structural damage). It also is used in the management of hydrocephalus in toy breeds, in the reduction of intracerebral pressure and edema, as adjunctive therapy of fibrocartilaginous embolic myopathy, for the treatment of shock, for the management of acute hypoadrenocortical insufficiency, for treatment of acquired thrombocytopenia, and as adjunctive therapy in endotoxemia secondary to gastric dilation-volvulus, and cholecalciferol toxicity. There is however little support for the use of this drug in the treatment of acute spinal cord injury, and in light of the frequency of associated adverse gastrointestinal effects, its use in this condition is discouraged. Dexamethasone decreases the frequency of vomiting in cats caused by xylazine. Dexamethasone sodium phosphate is used in the diagnosis of hyperadrenocorticism. For further information, see GLUCOCORTICOID AGENTS.

ADVERSE AND COMMON SIDE EFFECTS AND DRUG INTERACTIONS: See GLUCOCORTICOID AGENTS.

SUPPLIED AS VETERINARY PRODUCTS:
For injection containing 2 mg/mL dexamethasone [Azium solution]
For injection containing dexamethasone 21-isonicotinate 1 mg/mL [Voren ★]

For injection containing 4 mg/mL [Azium-SP], 2 mg/mL [Dex-2], and 5 mg/mL [Dex-5] as dexamethasone sodium phosphate
Tablets containing 0.25 mg [Azium, Dextab ♣]

OTHER USES
Cats
VOMITING ASSOCIATED WITH XYLAZINE USE
4 or 8 mg/kg IM

DEXTRANS

INDICATIONS: Dextran 70 (Gentran 70 ♣) and dextran 40 (Gentran 40 ♣) are polysaccharide solutions of high molecular weight that are used for plasma volume expansion and the treatment of hypovolemic shock (dextran 70). Dextran 40, with its smaller molecular size, has a greater osmotic effect per gram. Dextran 70 has a particle size similar to that of albumin. The half-life of dextran 40 is 2.5 hours and that of dextran 70 is 25 hours. Infusion of 1 L of dextran 70 expands plasma volume by 800 mL. Less than 30% of the product is retained within the vascular compartment, leading to a rapid (4 to 6 hours) dissipation of its initial volume-expanding effect. Infusion of 1 L of 10% dextran 40 in normal saline increases plasma volume by 1,000 mL for approximately 2 to 6 hours. The smaller molecular weight of dextran 40 compared with that of dextran 70 accounts for its shorter duration of vascular volume expansion and its rapid removal from the intravascular compartment.

ADVERSE AND COMMON SIDE EFFECTS: Hypervolemia, hyperviscosity, hemorrhagic diathesis (abnormal platelet function, precipitation of coagulation factors, increased fibrinolytic activity, decrease in vWF), and anaphylaxis are reported. Dextran 70 may exacerbate intravascular erythrocyte sludging. These effects are rare in dogs and usually are the result of too rapid or excessive administration. Dextrans should be used with caution in cases with cardiac decompensation, and with oliguric or anuric renal failure. Dextran 40 has been associated more often with renal failure. Large volumes of dextran may cause a dilutional lowering of plasma protein levels. Dextrans may interfere with cross-matching of blood and cause artifactual increases in serum glucose. Colloid administration may lower hematocrit concentrations, lower serum potassium, and cause dilution of plasma proteins. Colloids can exacerbate pulmonary edema in cases with increased microvascular permeability and interstitial edema, and alveolar flooding may occur if the alveolar epithelium is also damaged.

DRUG INTERACTIONS: None reported.

SUPPLIED AS HUMAN PRODUCTS:
Dextran 70:
For injection containing 6 g dextran 70 and 900 mg sodium chloride per 100 mL
For injection containing 6 g dextran 70 and 5 g dextrose per 100 mL
Dextran 40:
For injection containing 10 g dextran 40 and 900 mg saline per 100 mL
For injection containing 10 g dextran 40 and 5 g dextrose per 100 mL

OTHER USES
Dogs

SHOCK
7% saline in 6% dextran 70 at a dosage of 5 mL/kg, given slowly over a 5-minute period; IV, followed by lactated Ringer's solution at a dosage of 20 mL/kg per hour

DEXTROAMPHETAMINE

INDICATIONS: Dextroamphetamine (Dexedrine ♣ ★) is an isomer of amphetamine. In dogs, the drug has been used in the treatment of hyperkinesis and narcolepsy.

ADVERSE AND COMMON SIDE EFFECTS: Amphetamines are potent stimulators of the CNS and the cardiovascular system. The drug is contraindicated in glaucoma, hyperthyroid disease, significant heart disease, or hypertension, or within 14 days of having used an MAO inhibitor, possibly amitraz and selegiline. Side effects may include hyperexcitability, hyperesthesia, tachycardia, hypertension, hyperthermia, panting, mydriasis, vomiting, diarrhea, trembling, and seizures. Amphetamines also have been implicated as a potential cause of thrombocytopenia. Treatment of drug overdose may include diazepam (2.5 to 20 mg; IV, as needed).

DRUG INTERACTIONS: Ammonium chloride and other urinary acidifiers may reduce the pharmacological effect of the drug by enhancing urinary excretion. Phenothiazines are mutually antagonistic with amphetamines. Furazolidone increases the risk of dextroamphetamine toxicity from an additive pressor response.

SUPPLIED AS HUMAN PRODUCTS:
Capsules containing 5, 10, and 15 mg
Tablets containing 5 and 10 mg

DEXTROMETHORPHAN

INDICATIONS: Dextromethorphan (Broncho-Grippol-DM ♣, Balminil DM ♣, Benylin DM ♣ ★) is a nonnarcotic opiate with antitussive activity equal to that of codeine but is 15 to 20 times less potent than butorphanol.

ADVERSE AND COMMON SIDE EFFECTS: In humans, nausea and drowsiness are infrequent complaints. With large doses, confusion, nervousness, irritability, and excitability may occur.

DRUG INTERACTIONS: Other CNS depressants may potentiate CNS depression.

SUPPLIED AS HUMAN PRODUCT:
Syrup containing 15 mg/5 mL

DIAZEPAM

INDICATIONS: Diazepam (Valium ❖ ★, Valrelease ★) is an effective anticonvulsant for the control of seizure in status epilepticus. For cats with more long-term use of the drug, the recommended therapeutic range for benzodiazepine concentration, measured 2 weeks after the initiation of treatment, is 500 to 700 ng/mL. Because of the development of tolerance, the oral form is less useful as an anticonvulsant except in cats where tolerance is rarely seen. It also is useful in the management of toxicity associated with metaldehyde and methylxanthine (chocolate and caffeine), nicotine, amphetamine, strychnine, chlorinated hydrocarbon, and salicylate poisoning. Diazepam has been used in functional urethral obstruction and in canine and feline behavioral problems, including noise phobias, fear-induced and defensive aggression, destructive behavior, excessive grooming, anxiety, and urine spraying. The drug is useful as adjunctive therapy to promote relaxation in cases with tetanus. The drug also is used as a preanesthetic. Diazepam is used to stimulate appetite. It is more effective in cats than dogs for this purpose, but oxazepam (Serax) actually is even more effective than diazepam in stimulating appetite. Flurazepam (Dalmane) also is an effective appetite stimulant, and it has a longer duration of action. The use of benzodiazepines to stimulate appetite in cats with hepatic disease should be viewed with caution. These drugs require hepatic biotransformation for elimination and may promote sedation in addition to appetite stimulation, and, finally, a benzodiazepine receptor has been characterized as one of the causal factors in the development of hepatic encephalopathy.

ADVERSE AND COMMON SIDE EFFECTS: The benzodiazepines generally are safe drugs. They have minimal cardiopulmonary effects and are short-acting. Dose-related sedation, ataxia, excitement, and sometimes paradoxical aggression may occur. The benzodiazepines should not be used for more than 2 days to stimulate appetite. Acute fulminant hepatic necrosis has been associated with the ingestion of 1.25 to 2 mg once or twice daily in cats. Many cats became lethargic, ataxic, anorectic, and jaundiced within 96 hours of administration. Death may ensue. An idiosyncratic drug reaction is suspected. The authors recommend baseline serum ALT and AST be completed before and within 5 days of initiation of diazepam treatment.

DRUG INTERACTIONS: Metabolism may be decreased and excessive sedation may occur if diazepam is given with cimetidine, erythromycin, ketoconazole, or propranolol. Additive CNS effects may be anticipated if diazepam is given with barbiturates, narcotics, or anesthetics. Antacids may slow the rate of drug absorption. The pharmacological effects of digoxin may be potentiated. Rifampin may induce hepatic microsomal enzyme activity and decrease the efficacy of diazepam. An increase in the duration and intensity of respiratory depression may occur if diazepam is used with pancuronium or succinylcholine.

SUPPLIED AS HUMAN PRODUCTS:
Tablets containing 2, 5, and 10 mg
Timed-release tablets containing 15 mg [Valrelease]
Oral solution containing 1 mg/mL in 500-mL containers [PMS-Diazepam ♣] and unit dose (5 and 10 mg) 5 mg/mL in 30-mL dropper bottles [Diazepam Intensol ★]
For injection containing 5 mg/mL

OTHER USES
Dogs
SCOTTY CRAMP
0.5 to 2 mg/kg to effect; IV, or tid; PO

It decreases the clinical signs associated with the disease and its recurrence.

WHITE DOG SHAKER SYNDROME
0.25 mg/kg tid to qid; PO
It is used to reduce tremors associated with this syndrome.

Cats
URINE SPRAYING
1 to 2 mg bid; PO for an initial 2-week period. If therapy is successful, then this dose is continued for 6 to 8 weeks. After the treatment period, diazepam is reduced gradually, and if spraying does not recur, further treatment is not given. Recurrences are treated at the previous effective dose. If spraying does not subside, the dose is increased to 2 to 3 mg bid; PO for an additional 2-week trial period. For cats that respond to the increased dose, treatment is continued for 6 to 8 weeks. If cats still spray urine at this dose, diazepam is decreased gradually over the next 2 weeks and then discontinued. It is reported that a better response can be expected from female cats with diazepam (approximately 50% of cats respond) than with progestins (approximately 20% of cats respond), whereas the response of male cats is approximately the same for both drugs (approximately 50% of cats respond).

DIAZOXIDE

INDICATIONS: Diazoxide (Proglycem ✤ ★) is an antihypertensive agent. In dogs, it has been used for the management of hypoglycemia associated with islet cell tumors (insulinomas). It inhibits pancreatic insulin secretion, enhances epinephrine-induced glycogenolysis, and inhibits peripheral glucose use.

ADVERSE AND COMMON SIDE EFFECTS: Side effects primarily are anorexia, vomiting, and diarrhea. Other possible side effects include diabetes mellitus, anemia, agranulocytosis, thrombocytopenia, sodium and fluid retention, and cardiac arrhythmias.

DRUG INTERACTIONS: Diazoxide in conjunction with frequent small meals and prednisone (1 mg/kg per day divided) transiently controls hypoglycemia in most dogs with islet cell neoplasia. Hydrochlorothiazide (2 to 4 mg/kg per day) may potentiate the hyperglycemic effects of diazoxide if diazoxide alone is not effective. Phenothiazines may enhance the hyperglycemic effects. Diazoxide may increase the metabolism or decrease the protein binding of phenytoin, and the risk of hyperglycemia may be increased when these two drugs are used concurrently. Diazoxide may potentiate the hypotensive effects of other hypotensive agents, e.g., hydralazine and prazosin.

SUPPLIED AS HUMAN PRODUCTS:
Capsules containing 50 and 100 mg
Oral suspension containing 50 mg/mL

DICHLORPHENAMIDE

INDICATIONS: Dichlorphenamide (Daranide ★) is a carbonic anhydrase inhibitor used in the management of glaucoma.

ADVERSE AND COMMON SIDE EFFECTS: The drug is contraindicated in significant liver disease, obstructive pulmonary disease, renal or adrenocortical insufficiency, hyponatremia, hypokalemia, and hyperchloremic acidosis. Long-term use of the drug is contraindicated in chronic, noncongestive angle-closure glaucoma because the drug may mask the severity of the disease by lowering intraocular pressure.

Adverse effects may include GI upset, sedation, depression, excitement, bone marrow depression, dysuria, polyuria, crystalluria, hypokalemia, hyponatremia, hyperglycemia, hepatic insufficiency, skin rash, and hypersensitivity.

DRUG INTERACTIONS: The drug may inhibit primidone absorption from the GIT. Primidone or phenytoin used concurrently with dichlorphenamide may cause osteomalacia. Concurrent use of corticosteroids, amphotericin B, or diuretics may enhance potassium depletion. This may be especially important to patients receiving digitalis compounds. Carbonic anhydrase preparations may interfere with the efficacy of insulin.

SUPPLIED AS HUMAN PRODUCT:
Tablets containing 50 mg

DICHLORVOS

INDICATIONS: Dichlorvos (Task ★) is a cholinesterase inhibitor anthelmintic used for the elimination of *Toxocara canis, Toxascaris leonina, Ancylostoma caninum, Uncinaria stenocephalia,* and *Trichuris vulpis.*

ADVERSE AND COMMON SIDE EFFECTS AND DRUG INTER-ACTIONS: See ORGANOPHOSPHATES.

SUPPLIED AS VETERINARY PRODUCT:
Capsules containing 68, 136, and 204 mg

DICLOXACILLIN

INDICATIONS: Dicloxacillin (Dynapen ★) is a β-lactamase–resistant penicillin antibiotic with activity against gram-positive bacteria. Also see CLOXACILLIN.

ADVERSE AND COMMON SIDE EFFECTS: See PENICILLIN ANTIBIOTICS.

DRUG INTERACTIONS: Tetracyclines and other bacteriostatic anti-biotics may interfere with the antibacterial activity of penicillin antibiotics.

SUPPLIED AS HUMAN PRODUCTS:
Oral suspension containing 62.5 mg/5 mL
Capsules containing 500 mg

DIETHYLCARBAMAZINE

INDICATIONS: Diethylcarbamazine; DEC (Filaribits ★, Decacide ♣, Nemacide ★) is recommended for the prevention of heartworm dis-ease and as an aid in the treatment of ascarid infection in dogs and cats. Filaribits Plus combines DEC and oxibendazole and is used for the elimination of heartworms (*Dirofilaria immitis*), roundworms

(*Toxocara canis*), hookworms (*Ancylostoma caninum*), and whipworms (*Trichuris vulpis*) in dogs.

ADVERSE AND COMMON SIDE EFFECTS: Vomiting and diarrhea occasionally are noted. Administration with food reduces this problem. Low sperm counts have been reported in dogs receiving the drug. If given to dogs with microfilaremia, hypersensitivity or anaphylaxis and death may occur. The use of Filaribits Plus has been associated with a hepatopathy that is potentially fatal. The drug should not be given to dogs with a history of liver disease.

DRUG INTERACTIONS: Levamisole and pyrantel may enhance the toxic effects of DEC, and vice versa.

SUPPLIED AS VETERINARY PRODUCTS:
Oral liquid containing 60 mg/mL [Nemacide]
Tablets containing 50, 100, 200, 300, and 400 mg [Decacide, Nemacide Tablets]
Tablets containing 60, 120, and 180 mg DEC [Filaribits]

DIETHYLSTILBESTROL

INDICATIONS: Diethylstilbestrol; DES (Stilboestrol ✤) is used in the management of estrogen-responsive urinary incontinence, vaginitis, perianal gland adenoma, and benign prostatic gland hyperplasia. It is not effective when used alone to prevent pregnancy.

ADVERSE AND COMMON SIDE EFFECTS: Thrombocytopenia may be observed approximately 2 weeks after the initiation of treatment with estrogens. Leukocytosis with a left shift may develop at approximately 16 to 20 days, and anemia may become gradually apparent. Leukopenia may follow at approximately 22 to 25 days. Bone marrow suppression is unlikely at doses recommended to control urinary incontinence. There is considerable variation in sensitivity to the adverse effects of DES. Feminization or the induction of estrus also is possible. Estrogens induce squamous metaplasia and fibromuscular proliferation of the prostate gland, which predisposes to fluid stasis and infection.

DRUG INTERACTIONS: Estrogen activity may be decreased if the drug is used concurrently with rifampin, phenytoin, or barbiturate drugs. Estrogens may enhance glucocorticoid activity, necessitating adjustment of the glucocorticoid dose.

SUPPLIED AS VETERINARY PRODUCT:
Tablets containing 1 mg

SUPPLIED AS HUMAN PRODUCTS:
Tablets containing 1 and 5 mg ★
Tablets (enteric-coated) containing 0.1, 0.5, 1, and 5 mg

OTHER USES
Dogs
PERIANAL GLAND ADENOMA AND PROSTATIC HYPERPLASIA
0.1 to 1 mg every 24 to 48 hours; PO

DIGITOXIN

INDICATIONS: Digitoxin (Crystodigin ★, Digitaline ✤) is a cardiac glycoside used in the treatment of supraventricular tachyarrhythmias (atrial flutter or fibrillation), premature atrial contractions, and tachycardia. Because the drug has less parasympathetic activity than digoxin, it is less effective in the management of supraventricular arrhythmias. However, it is preferred to digoxin in patients with renal dysfunction. Measurements of serum concentrations are taken after steady-state levels are attained (after approximately 5 days of therapy). Normal serum values are 15 to 35 ng/mL, 6 to 8 hours after treatment. Toxicity generally is noted when serum levels exceed 40 ng/mL.

ADVERSE AND COMMON SIDE EFFECTS: Anorexia, vomiting, diarrhea, depression, atrioventricular block, ectopia, and junctional tachycardia have been documented. Patients with hypokalemia, hypernatremia, and hypercalcemia are predisposed to toxicity. Because of the exceedingly long half-life in the cat (greater than 100 hours), it is not recommended in this species.

DRUG INTERACTIONS: See DIGOXIN.

SUPPLIED AS HUMAN PRODUCTS:
Tablets containing 0.05 and 0.1 mg digitoxin [Crystodigin]
Tablets containing 0.1 and 0.2 mg [Digitaline]

DIGOXIN

INDICATIONS: Digoxin (Lanoxin ★, Cardoxin ✤ ★) decreases sympathetic nerve activity and is a positive inotropic and negative chronotropic agent. Its chronotropic properties make it a popular choice in the management of supraventricular tachyarrhythmias, e.g., atrial flutter and fibrillation and sinus tachycardia associated with congestive heart failure. Its inotropic value is questionable. However, digoxin is used in an effort to improve cardiac output in conditions of congestive heart failure and cardiomyopathy. Samples for the determination of serum blood concentration should be taken after steady-state levels have been attained (greater than 7 days in dogs and cats). Blood samples are taken just before the next dose or at least 8 hours after the previous dose. Normal serum concentrations are between 0.9 and 3 ng/mL in dogs and between 0.9 and 2 ng/mL in cats. Concurrent measurement of serum electrolytes helps interpret the digoxin concentration and its effect on the patient.

ADVERSE AND COMMON SIDE EFFECTS: Toxic serum levels are in excess of 3 ng/mL in dogs and in excess of 2.4 ng/mL in cats. Vomiting, diarrhea, anorexia, lethargy, ataxia, arrhythmias, and conduction abnormalities may occur. Toxicity is enhanced by hypokalemia, hypercalcemia, decreased glomerular filtration, and hyperthyroid states. It does not appear necessary to adjust drug doses in hypothyroid dogs. Doberman pinschers with dilated cardiomyopathy appear to be more sensitive to digitalis intoxication. Acute increases in serum digoxin levels are better tolerated than prolonged high concentrations.

Intoxication can be managed by preventing further digoxin absorption from the GIT with activated charcoal that binds digoxin, correction of electrolyte imbalances and acid–base status, and management of arrhythmias. Lidocaine and phenytoin are effective in managing digitalis-induced arrhythmias.

DRUG INTERACTIONS: Furosemide, quinidine, and verapamil may potentiate digoxin toxicity. Serum digoxin levels also may increase with the concurrent use of spironolactone, diltiazem, triamterene, erythromycin, and prazosin. Antacid preparations, cimetidine, metoclopramide, oral neomycin, cyclophosphamide, doxorubicin, vinca alkaloids, and cytarabine decrease GIT digoxin absorption. Drugs that inhibit hepatic microsomal activity, e.g., chloramphenicol, quinidine, and tetracycline, decrease digoxin excretion and should be used with caution if given concurrently. Drugs that predispose to hypokalemia, e.g., amphotericin B, glucocorticoids, laxatives, sodium polystyrene sulfonate, and high-dose dextrose solutions, may potentiate digoxin toxicity.

SUPPLIED AS VETERINARY PRODUCT:
Elixir containing 0.05 and 0.15 mg/mL [Cardoxin]

SUPPLIED AS HUMAN PRODUCTS:
Capsules containing 0.05, 0.1, and 0.2 mg [Lanoxicaps ★]
Tablets containing 0.125, 0.25, and 0.5 mg [Lanoxin]
Elixir containing 0.05 mg/mL [Lanoxin]
For injection containing 0.1, 0.25, and 0.5 mg/mL [Lanoxin]

DIHYDROSTREPTOMYCIN

INDICATIONS: Dihydrostreptomycin (Ethamycin ♣) is an aminoglycoside antibiotic used for the treatment of leptospirosis. For information on INDICATIONS, ADVERSE AND COMMON SIDE EFFECTS, and DRUG INTERACTIONS, see AMINOGLYCOSIDE ANTIBIOTICS.

SUPPLIED AS VETERINARY PRODUCT:
For injection containing 500 mg/mL

DIHYDROTACHYSTEROL

INDICATIONS: Dihydrotachysterol (DHT ★, Hytakerol ✚ ★) is used in the treatment of hypocalcemia. The time required for the drug to exert its maximal effect may not be attained for 2 to 4 weeks, and the duration of effect after cessation of therapy may be as long as 1 week.

ADVERSE AND COMMON SIDE EFFECTS: Hypercalcemia leading to polyuria, polydipsia, listlessness, depression, anorexia, vomiting, nephrocalcinosis, muscle weakness, and trembling or muscle twitching may occur. Serum calcium levels should be monitored every 2 weeks.

DRUG INTERACTIONS: None established.

SUPPLIED AS HUMAN PRODUCTS:
Tablets containing 0.125, 0.2, and 0.4 mg [DHT]
Capsules containing 0.125 mg [Hytakerol]
Oral concentrate containing 0.2 mg/mL [DHT Intensol]

DILTIAZEM

INDICATIONS: Diltiazem (Cardizem ✚ ★), like nifedipine and verapamil, is a calcium channel-blocking agent. Calcium channel-blocking agents decrease heart rate, myocardial contractility, and oxygen demand, decrease systolic pressure gradients, improve myocardial relaxation, and dilate coronary blood vessels. Diltiazem decreases afterload, prolongs atrioventricular conduction (although not as much as verapamil), and is a less potent negative inotrope than verapamil or nifedipine. The drug appears to be useful in the treatment of supraventricular tachycardia, e.g., atrial fibrillation and hypertrophic cardiomyopathy. Diltiazem causes less peripheral arterial vasodilation and reflex tachycardia than verapamil or nifedipine. The drug also may be useful in the management of congestive cardiomyopathy because it decreases ventricular response to atrial fibrillation, decreases peripheral resistance and afterload, and has minimal cardiodepressant effects. Because they inhibit angiotensin II and α-adrenergic–mediated vasoconstriction, calcium channel-blocking agents have renoprotective effects, the extent and clinical utility of which in veterinary medicine have yet to be determined.

ADVERSE AND COMMON SIDE EFFECTS: Bradycardia appears to be the most common side effect in dogs. Diltiazem also can cause depression and hypotension and can contribute to heart failure. Acute toxicity can be managed with 10% calcium gluconate infusion (1 mL/ 10 kg; IV) or the administration of a positive inotrope, e.g., dopamine. The drug has been used at standard doses without side effects in most cats.

DRUG INTERACTIONS: Diltiazem is reported to increase serum digoxin levels in humans and to attenuate the positive inotropic effects of the cardiac glycosides. Diltiazem and verapamil inhibit hepatic microsomal enzyme, affecting the clearance of propranolol, theophylline, and quinidine. Cimetidine increases serum levels. Prolongation of atrioventricular conduction is potentiated by the concurrent use of β blockers, e.g., propranolol and atenolol, or digoxin. Propranolol has been shown to reduce the clearance of orally administered diltiazem and vice versa.

SUPPLIED AS HUMAN PRODUCTS:
Tablets containing 30, 60, 90, and 120 mg
Capsules (sustained-release) containing 60, 90, and 120 mg
Capsules (controlled-delivery) containing 120, 180, 240, 300, and 360 mg
For injection containing 5 mg/mL

DIMETHYL SULFOXIDE

INDICATIONS: Dimethyl sulfoxide; DMSO (Domoso ♣ ★) is reported to have a number of beneficial properties, yet little scientific evidence is available to support these claims. The drug often is used to help transport drugs across the skin into the general circulation. It has anti-inflammatory activity and is a potent diuretic, local analgesic, muscle relaxant, vasodilator, and inotropic agent. Dimethyl sulfoxide inhibits platelet aggregation, decreases fibroplasia, and is bacteriostatic and antifungal. The drug is recommended for topical treatment in dogs with acute and chronic musculoskeletal disease, otitis externa, and ophthalmic disease. It also has been recommended in the treatment of trauma to the head and spine and in renal amyloidosis, where the beneficial effects are attributed to its anti-inflammatory activity.

ADVERSE AND COMMON SIDE EFFECTS: Topical application can lead to erythema, edema, pruritus, vesiculation, and pain. Dryness of the skin and oyster-like breath odor also may be noted. Toxicity after IV injection may include sedation, hematuria, seizure, coma, dyspnea, and pulmonary edema. Intravascular injection of concentrations greater than 20% leads to severe hemolysis. Side effects of repeated administration of DMSO in dogs may include perivascular inflammation and local thrombosis (if used in undiluted form), reversible hemolytic anemia (when given repeatedly intravenously), and reduced lucency of the lens cortex (which resolves with discontinuation of the drug). The drug is potentially teratogenic during the first trimester of pregnancy.

Dimethyl sulfoxide should not be given to animals with ocular, renal, or liver disease, or those with a history of allergy, and it should not be used in animals weighing less than 4.5 kg.

DRUG INTERACTIONS: None established.

SUPPLIED AS VETERINARY PRODUCTS:
Gel 90% in 60- and 120-g tubes and 425-g jars
Topical solution 90% in 4-oz (± spray bottle), 16-oz, and 1-gal bottle
Otic preparation containing DMSO 60% [Synotic ✣ ★]

OTHER USES
Dogs
CYCLOPHOSPHAMIDE-INDUCED HEMORRHAGIC CYSTITIS
10 mL of 50% DMSO solution diluted in equal volume of sterile saline instilled in urinary bladder for 20 minutes; repeat in 1 week
RENAL AMYLOIDOSIS
80 mg/kg 3 times weekly; SC

DIPHENHYDRAMINE

INDICATIONS: Diphenhydramine (Benadryl ✣ ★) is an antihistamine used as an antiemetic and to help alleviate urticaria and angioedema, canine atopy, canine pruritus, and to guard against the effects of histamine release from mast cell tumors. Diphenhydramine also is used to prevent allergic reactions in animals receiving doxorubicin. This drug also has been used to manage a number of behavioral problems, e.g., compulsive scratching, self-trauma, and waking at night. It has mild sedative properties. Diphenhydramine also may be useful in the treatment of organophosphate and carbamate poisoning, where nicotinic signs predominate, e.g., muscular twitching. For further information, refer to ANTIHISTAMINES.

SUPPLIED AS HUMAN PRODUCTS:
Capsules containing 25 and 50 mg
Tablets containing 25 and 50 mg
Elixir and syrup containing 12.5 mg/5 mL
For injection containing 10 and 50 mg/mL
Solution and cream containing 1% and 2% w/v diphenhydramine

OTHER USES
Dogs
PREMEDICATION FOR DOGS RECEIVING DOXORUBICIN
10 mg before doxorubicin; IV (dogs = 9 kg)
20 mg before doxorubicin; IV (dogs 9 to 27 kg)
30 mg before doxorubicin; IV (dogs > 27 kg)

PREOPERATIVE THERAPY FOR SPLENIC MAST CELL TUMOR
2.2 mg/kg bid; IM (with cimetidine 5 mg/kg tid to qid; PO, IV)
ANTIPRURITIC
25 to 50 mg bid to tid; PO

ANTIEMETIC
2 to 4 mg/kg tid; PO

BEHAVIORAL DISORDERS
2 to 4 mg/kg bid to tid; PO

Cats
ANTIEMETIC
2 to 4 mg/kg tid; PO

BEHAVIORAL DISORDERS
2 to 4 mg/kg bid to tid; PO

DIPHENOXYLATE

INDICATIONS: Diphenoxylate (Lomotil ♣ ★) is indicated for the management of diarrhea. The drug increases intestinal segmentation, decreases the frequency of bowel movements, decreases abdominal pain and tenesmus, and possibly inhibits fluid secretion.

ADVERSE AND COMMON SIDE EFFECTS: Constipation, bloating, and sedation may occur. It should only be used for a 36- to 48-hour period and should not be used in cases with infectious enteritis. In cats, the use of opiate antidiarrheal preparations may cause excitement.

DRUG INTERACTIONS: Diphenoxylate may potentiate the action of barbiturates, phenothiazines, antihistamines, and anesthetic agents.

SUPPLIED AS HUMAN PRODUCTS:
Tablets containing 2.5 mg diphenoxylate with atropine (0.025 mg)
Oral liquid containing 2.5 mg/5 mL diphenoxylate with atropine (0.025 mg)

DIPYRONE

INDICATIONS: Dipyrone (generic products ♣) is an anti-inflammatory, antipyretic, antispasmodic, and analgesic agent. It is prescribed for the relief of pain, reducing fever, and relaxing smooth muscle.

ADVERSE AND COMMON SIDE EFFECTS: Sedation is common. Subcutaneous injection may cause irritation and is not recommended. At high doses or with prolonged therapy, agranulocytosis and leukopenia may develop. Nausea, vomiting, skin rashes, pain at the injection site, hemolytic anemia, tremors, GI hemorrhage, and prolongation of bleeding times also may occur. Novolate may discolor urine red. The drug should not be used in animals with a history of blood dyscrasias.

DRUG INTERACTIONS: Phenothiazines may predispose to hypothermia in patients given dipyrone. The drug should not be used in animals receiving phenylbutazone or barbiturates because of drug interaction involving hepatic microsomal systems.

SUPPLIED AS VETERINARY PRODUCT:
For injection containing 500 mg/mL

DISOPYRAMIDE PHOSPHATE

INDICATIONS: Disopyramide (Norpace ♣ ★) is an antiarrhythmic drug used for the management of ventricular tachyarrhythmias. It has anticholinergic effects and is a potent negative inotrope. Although disopyramide has been of benefit in humans with supraventricular tachycardia, e.g., atrial fibrillation, it does not appear to be as effective for this use in the dog.

ADVERSE AND COMMON SIDE EFFECTS: Disopyramide should be avoided in patients in congestive heart failure or shock because of its negative inotropic effects. Dry mouth, vomiting, urinary retention, glaucoma, depression, atrioventricular block, sinus node depression, and multiform ventricular tachycardia also may occur. Hyperkalemia potentiates its myocardial depressant effects, and hypokalemia reduces its therapeutic effects.

DRUG INTERACTIONS: Dilantin and other drugs that induce hepatic microsomal enzymes may increase the metabolism of disopyramide.

SUPPLIED AS HUMAN PRODUCTS:
Capsules containing 100 and 150 mg
Tablets (controlled-release) containing 100 and 150 mg

DOBUTAMINE

INDICATIONS: Dobutamine (Dobutrex ♣ ★) is a rapid-acting synthetic catecholamine that predominantly stimulates β_1 receptors and is useful for short-term increases in cardiac output in conditions of shock, congestive heart failure, and cardiomyopathy.

ADVERSE AND COMMON SIDE EFFECTS: Generally the drug has little effect on heart rate and blood pressure, except at higher doses. Sinus tachycardia and ventricular arrhythmias may occur. An increase in atrioventricular conduction may occur. Animals with atrial fibrillation should be pretreated with a cardiac glycoside or calcium channel-blocking agent, e.g., diltiazem. The drug is contraindicated in animals with aortic stenosis. Vomiting and seizure activity have been reported in some cats.

DRUG INTERACTIONS: Propranolol, atenolol, and metoprolol may negate the effects of dobutamine. Halothane may increase the likelihood of arrhythmias. Insulin requirements may increase in diabetic patients.

SUPPLIED AS HUMAN PRODUCT:
For injection containing 12.5 mg/mL in 20-mL vials

DOCUSATE CALCIUM

INDICATIONS: Docusate calcium (Surfak ♣ ★) is an anionic surface-active agent with emulsifying and wetting properties. Detergent action lowers surface tension, permitting water and fats to penetrate and soften stools. It is used for the prevention and treatment of constipation. The drug acts at the small and large bowel and generally takes 12 to 72 hours to work effectively.

ADVERSE AND COMMON SIDE EFFECTS: Mild, transient cramping may occur. A bitter taste, nausea, vomiting, and diarrhea also are reported. The drug should not be administered with mineral oil because increased absorption of the oil may occur, resulting in tumor-like deposits. Liquid preparations may cause throat irritation.

DRUG INTERACTIONS: None established.

SUPPLIED AS HUMAN PRODUCT:
Capsules containing 240 mg

DOCUSATE SODIUM

INDICATIONS: Docusate sodium (Colace ♣ ★). For INDICATIONS, ADVERSE AND COMMON SIDE EFFECTS, and DRUG INTERACTIONS, see DOCUSATE CALCIUM.

SUPPLIED AS VETERINARY PRODUCTS:
Liquids available in gallon formulations containing 50 mg/mL (refer to Part II, Section 6, Large Animal Preparations, for further discussion)
Enema containing 250 mg in 12 mL glycerin [Docu-Soft Enema ★]

SUPPLIED AS HUMAN PRODUCTS:
Capsules containing 50 and 100 mg
Syrup containing 60 mg/15 mL

Solution containing 10 mg/mL
Tablets containing 50 and 100 mg

DOMPERIDONE

INDICATIONS: Domperidone (Motilium ✤) is a gastrointestinal motility modifier similar in action to metoclopramide, but unlike metoclopramide it apparently does not cross the blood–brain barrier and therefore does not have adverse CNS effects. The drug is a dopamine antagonist. It may be useful as a prokinetic or antiemetic agent.

ADVERSE AND COMMON SIDE EFFECTS: Galactorrhea and gynecomastia may occur and are a reflection of increases in serum prolactin levels caused by the drug.

DRUG INTERACTIONS: Antacids or H_2-blocking agents, e.g., ranitidine, may reduce absorption of the drug. Domperidone should not be used concurrently with dopamine or dobutamine.

SUPPLIED AS HUMAN PRODUCT:
Tablets containing 10 mg

DOPAMINE

INDICATIONS: Dopamine (Intropin ✤, generic products ★) is an endogenous precursor of norepinephrine that stimulates β_1 receptors and dopaminergic receptors. Dopaminergic receptors are located predominantly in renal, mesenteric, coronary, and cerebral arterioles. Intermediate dosages (3 to 10 μg/kg per minute) increase cardiac output with little change in heart rate or blood pressure. High infusion rates (10 to 20 μg/kg per minute) stimulate α- and β-adrenergic receptors and lead to an increase in cardiac contractility, heart rate, and blood pressure. It is indicated in cases of acute or chronic congestive heart failure and shock unresponsive to other methods. The drug also is used as adjunctive therapy in oliguric and anuric renal failure to promote renal vasodilation and an improvement in glomerular filtration. The drug also has been used experimentally to protect against hemorrhagic pancreatitis in cats when it was given up to 12 hours after initiation of the insult.

ADVERSE AND COMMON SIDE EFFECTS: Nausea, vomiting, hypotension or hypertension, and dyspnea may occur. Overdose may cause tachycardia, increases in blood pressure, and ventricular ectopia. Extravascular injection may cause tissue necrosis and sloughing. Should perivascular injection occur, the site should be infiltrated with phentolamine (5 to 10 mg) in 10 to 15 mL of saline. The drug is contraindicated in patients with ventricular arrhythmias.

DRUG INTERACTIONS: Phenytoin may decrease the effects of dopamine, leading to hypotension and bradycardia.

SUPPLIED AS HUMAN PRODUCTS:
For injection containing 40, 80, and 160 mg/mL in 5-mL vials or additive syringes
For infusion containing 0.8, 1.6, and 3.2 mg/mL in D_5W in 250- and 500-mL bags

OTHER USES
OLIGURIC RENAL FAILURE
1 to 3 µg/kg per minute

Cats
HEMORRHAGIC PANCREATITIS
5 µg/kg per minute; IV, continued for 6 hours

DOXAPRAM

INDICATIONS: Doxapram (Dopram-V ♣ ★) is used to stimulate respiration in patients with postanesthetic respiratory depression or apnea and to encourage the return of laryngopharyngeal reflexes in patients with mild to moderate respiratory and CNS depression due to anesthetic overdose. In the neonate, doxapram may be used to stimulate respiration after dystocia or Cesarean-section birth.

ADVERSE AND COMMON SIDE EFFECTS: Cough, dyspnea, and laryngospasm may occur. Overdose may cause tremor, lacrimation, excessive salivation, occasional vomiting, diarrhea, and stiffness of the extremities. Excessive doses may initiate hyperventilation and respiratory alkalosis. Arrhythmias and urinary retention may occur, and seizure activity may be provoked in epileptic patients.

DRUG INTERACTIONS: Do not mix with alkaline solutions. The concomitant use with sympathomimetic agents or MAO inhibitors (possibly amitraz and selegiline) may lead to serious increases in blood pressure and arrhythmias. Halothane and enflurane may precipitate arrhythmias. It is recommended that doxapram use be delayed approximately 10 minutes after discontinuation of these anesthetic agents.

SUPPLIED AS VETERINARY PRODUCT:
For injection containing 20 mg/mL

DOXORUBICIN

INDICATIONS: Doxorubicin (Adriamycin ♣ ★, Rubex ★) is a chemotherapeutic agent used in the treatment of lymphoma, osteosarcoma

(30 mg/m² every 2 weeks; IV), thyroid carcinomas, mammary gland adenocarcinoma (in one case at a dose of 30 mg/m² every 3 weeks; IV), and as an adjuvant to surgery in cases of canine hemangiosarcoma (1 mg/kg every 3 weeks for 5 treatments). It has been suggested that six treatments of doxorubicin (30 mg/m²) may be more advantageous in maintaining longer remission length than three treatments for cases of canine lymphoma. Preliminary results in cats have shown response with lymphoma, mammary adenocarcinoma, and fibrosarcoma.

ADVERSE AND COMMON SIDE EFFECTS: A study in 1994 suggested that dose based on body weight, as opposed to body surface area, results in more uniform therapeutic and predictable toxic responses in the dog. In the dog, doxorubicin toxicity can be classified as acute, short-term, and chronic. Acute toxicity occurs during or immediately after treatment and includes head-shaking, pruritus, erythema, and occasionally acute collapse. Diphenhydramine (Benadryl) given at a dose of 2.2 mg/kg intramuscularly 20 minutes before doxorubicin use has been recommended to prevent anaphylactic reactions. The efficacy of this precaution is unknown. Severe local tissue damage occurs if the drug is injected extravascularly. If this occurs the affected area should be infiltrated with hyaluronidase (300 units diluted with 6 mL of saline administered circumferentially by SC injections and repeated in 7 to 14 days). The drug may discolor urine orange or red for 1 to 2 days after treatment.

Short-term toxicity occurs 5 to 10 days after treatment and includes myelosuppression, anorexia, vomiting, diarrhea, and weight loss. Bone marrow suppression peaks 10 to 14 days after the initiation of treatment, followed by recovery in 21 days. Complete blood counts should be monitored 10 days after initiation of therapy and before each dose. If neutrophil counts decrease to less than 2,000/μL or platelet numbers decrease to less than 50,000/μL, the drug should be discontinued until counts return to normal. Alopecia also may occur within a few weeks of therapy and most commonly occurs in curly-coated breeds. Dose-dependent congestive cardiomyopathy is reported, and dose-independent cardiac arrhythmias occur with chronic toxicity. Do not exceed a cumulative dose of 250 mg/m². Prolongation of infusion time to greater than 6 hours or using a low-dose weekly schedule may be helpful in reducing cardiotoxicity by decreasing peak plasma concentrations. In addition, it has been suggested that carnitine supplementation also may reduce the cardiac toxicity of chronic doxorubicin therapy, although the efficacy of this recommendation has yet to be established. Dexrazoxane (Zinecard, Cardioxane), a cyclic derivative of EDTA, has been shown to reduce the cardiotoxic effects of the anthracyclines. It prevents cardiotoxicity. The recommended dose ratio of dexrazoxane to doxorubicin is 10:1. The reconstituted solution is administered over a 15 minute period with a 30 minute fixed interval from completion of dexrazoxane infusion to the start of doxorubicin therapy.

In cats, short-term toxicities include neutropenia (nadir 8 to 11 days) and poikilocytosis. Neutrophil counts return to normal within 14 days in the cat. Thrombocytopenia is uncommon and mild when it does occur. A complete blood count and platelet numbers should be completed on days 1 and 8 of each treatment cycle. Anorexia, vomiting, diarrhea, and weight loss also have been reported in some cats. No clinical evidence of cardiotoxicity has been seen. Mild azotemia also has been reported. Other uncommon adverse effects have included whisker loss and testicular atrophy.

DRUG INTERACTIONS: Barbiturates may decrease pharmacological effects by increasing hepatic metabolism. Streptozocin may prolong doxorubicin half-life, necessitating a decrease in dose.

SUPPLIED AS HUMAN PRODUCTS:
For injection containing 10, 20, 50, 100, and 150 mg
For injection containing 2 mg/mL in 5-, 10-, and 25-mL vials

DOXYCYCLINE

INDICATIONS: Doxycycline (Vibramycin ♣ ★) is a second-generation, long-acting, lipid-soluble tetracycline antibiotic used in the treatment of actinomycosis, ehrlichiosis, *Chlamydia,* leptospirosis, borreliosis, Rocky Mountain spotted fever, toxoplasmosis, and *Hemobartonella* infections. Doxycyline and minocycline have greater activity against anaerobes and facultative intracellular bacteria such as *Brucella canis* than other tetracyclines. It is a useful tetracycline in patients with renal failure. For more information, see TETRACYCLINE ANTIBIOTICS.

ADVERSE AND COMMON SIDE EFFECTS: The most common side effects of oral tetracycline use in small animals are vomiting and diarrhea. Mixing the drug with food decreases the incidence of these reactions. See also TETRACYCLINE ANTIBIOTICS.

DRUG INTERACTIONS: Barbiturate drugs and carbamazepine decrease the serum half-life of doxycycline. Antacid preparations containing aluminum, calcium, iron, or magnesium, antidiarrheal compounds containing kaolin and pectin or bismuth, and laxatives reduce GIT absorption of doxycycline. Sodium bicarbonate interferes with gastric absorption of oral tetracyclines. Schedule doxycycline 1 to 2 hours before use of these preparations.

SUPPLIED AS HUMAN PRODUCTS:
Tablets and capsules containing 50 and 100 mg
Oral suspension containing 5 mg/mL after reconstitution
Oral syrup containing 10 mg/mL
For injection in 100-mg vials

ECADOTRIL—*INVESTIGATIONAL*

INDICATIONS: Ecadotril is a neutral endopeptidase inhibitor. Studies in dogs indicate that the drug may be effective in alleviating clinical signs in patients with left-sided heart failure and may be particularly effective in those refractory to traditional diuretic therapy.

ADVERSE AND COMMON SIDE EFFECTS: Dogs that received 300 mg/kg per day for 3 months developed pronounced anemia, bone marrow suppression, and some evidence of hepatic impairment. Reversibility of toxic effects was evident. Dogs that received less than or equal to 100 mg/kg per day for 3 or 12 months did not demonstrate evidence of toxicity.

DRUG INTERACTIONS: Unknown.

EDROPHONIUM CHLORIDE

INDICATIONS: Edrophonium chloride (Tensilon ♣ ★, Enlon ★) is a cholinesterase inhibitor. It is used in the diagnosis of myasthenia gravis and in the treatment of curare poisoning and unresponsive atrial tachycardia.

ADVERSE AND COMMON SIDE EFFECTS: Cholinergic reactions, including bradycardia, pupillary constriction, laryngospasm, bronchiolar constriction, nausea, vomiting, diarrhea, and muscle weakness, may occur. In the case of accidental overdose, atropine should be administered. The drug should be used with caution in patients with asthma or cardiac arrhythmias.

DRUG INTERACTIONS: The anticholinergic properties of procainamide and quinidine may antagonize the cholinergic effects of edrophonium.

SUPPLIED AS HUMAN PRODUCT:
For injection containing 10 mg/mL in 10-mL vials

EFA-CAPS ♣, EFA CAPS HP ♣, EFA-Z PLUS ♣, EFAVITE CAPSULES ♣, AND EFAVITE HP CAPSULES ♣

INDICATIONS: These products are dietary multivitamin and mineral supplements containing fatty acids derived from primrose and fish oil. They have useful anti-inflammatory properties and may be used in the management of seborrhea and pruritus in dogs and cats. Potential ben-

eficial effects of omega-3 fatty acid supplementation include the alleviation of pain, control of pruritus, suppression of inflammation and
autoimmune disease, decrease in serum triglyceride levels, decreased
formation of thrombi, anti-arrhythmogenesis, and inhibition of tumori-
genesis. Supplementation of diets with linoleic acid increases glomerular filtration rate and decreases proteinuria. Omega-3 fatty acid supplementation may be renoprotective and may also decrease intestinal
inflammation. Diets containing fish oil can decrease blood pressure.
However, clinical relevance of these claims remains to be established.

ADVERSE AND COMMON SIDE EFFECTS: Although rare, use of
these products may be associated with GIT disorders (softening of the
stools and diarrhea), increased pruritus, and urticaria. Although the
cutaneous bleeding time may be slightly prolonged, the risk of bleeding is low. Although not well documented, these agents may induce
pancreatitis in animals predisposed to the disease.

DRUG INTERACTIONS: None.

SUPPLIED AS VETERINARY PRODUCTS:
These products are available in liquid formulations and as capsules.

ENALAPRIL

INDICATIONS: Enalapril (Enacard ✤ ★, Vasotec ✤ ★) is an ACE
inhibitor. Peak concentrations occur 4 to 6 hours after oral administration. It has a longer duration of action than captopril. ACE inhibitors
are used for their vasodilatory properties in the treatment of congestive heart failure, systemic hypertension, renal disease, and shock. ACE
inhibitors may significantly improve even mild cases of congestive
heart failure, although long-term treatment with enalapril does not
delay the onset of heart failure in dogs with mitral valvular disease.
Enalapril appears to be ineffective in managing hypertension in most
cats. Experimentally, ACE inhibitors actually may slow the progression of renal disease via decreasing glomerular pressures (which contribute to the progression of renal disease) and possibly by limiting the
growth/proliferation of glomerular cells.

ADVERSE AND COMMON SIDE EFFECTS: Hypotension causing
lethargy, anorexia, weakness, and difficulty rising, possibly in association with dehydration or azotemia, is rare. In one report administration of the drug for up to 2 years in dogs with severe, compensated
mitral regurgitation did not have any demonstrable adverse effects on
renal function. Vomiting, diarrhea, sinus tachycardia, and hyperkalemia also have been documented. In addition, in people, pruritus,
proteinuria, bone marrow-induced neutropenia, anemia, vasculitis,

and deterioration of renal function have been noted with the use of ACE inhibitors. Doses should be reduced in patients with renal disease or severe congestive heart failure. Renal function should be determined before use of the drug is initiated, rechecked after 5 to 7 days, and reevaluated every 2 months thereafter. Drug overdose may be treated with a β agonist, e.g., dobutamine. Bradyarrhythmias may respond to atropine or glycopyrrolate. Unlike captopril, enalapril requires hepatic hydrolysis to become activated. Therefore, captopril or lisinopril are better choices in patients with liver disease. Use of the drug in pregnant bitches is not recommended.

DRUG INTERACTIONS: Indomethacin may decrease the antihypertensive activity of the drug. Potassium-sparing diuretics, e.g., spironolactone, may potentiate the hyperkalemia associated with enalapril use. Vomiting may occur in patients given digoxin in combination with enalapril. Low-salt diets and accelerated salt loss induced by loop diuretics may predispose to renal insufficiency associated with ACE inhibitor use. Drugs that cause volume depletion, e.g., diuretics, may predispose to azotemia. If clinical signs of hypotension or azotemia develop, the dose of the diuretic should be reduced first. If signs persist, it may be necessary to further decrease the dose of the diuretic, or discontinue it altogether. Persistence of clinical signs necessitates reduction of the dosing frequency or discontinuation of enalapril.

SUPPLIED AS VETERINARY PRODUCT:
Tablets containing 1, 2.5, 5, 10, and 20 mg [Enacard]

SUPPLIED AS HUMAN PRODUCT:
Tablets containing 2.5, 5, 10, and 20 mg [Vasotec]

ENILCONAZOLE

INDICATIONS: Enilconazole (Imaverol ♣) is a topical imidazole antifungal agent successfully used intranasally in the dog for the treatment of nasal aspergillosis. Nasal discharge resolved in approximately 80% of affected dogs when the drug was administered topically twice daily for 7 to 14 days. It also has activity against *Penicillium* and is recommended for the treatment of dermatophyte infections.

ADVERSE AND COMMON SIDE EFFECTS: Side effects are rare. Sneezing and salivation and inappetence occur with intranasal use. Because of extensive destruction caused by the fungus, some animals may continue to have a mucopurulent nasal discharge, even with successful elimination of the fungus. Secondary bacterial infection may respond to appropriate antibiotic therapy. Slight weight loss may occur. Anorexia may occur at higher doses.

DRUG INTERACTIONS: Unknown.

SUPPLIED AS VETERINARY PRODUCT:
Solution containing 100 mg/mL

ENROFLOXACIN

INDICATIONS: Enrofloxacin (Baytril ✤ ★) is a fluoroquinolone antibiotic with activity against *E. coli, Klebsiella pneumoniae, Salmonella* spp., *Staphylococcus aureus* and *epidermidis, Actinobacillus, Brucella, Leptospira, Pasteurella multocida,* and *Proteus mirabilis,* as well as *Mycoplasma* spp., *Rickettsia rickettsii, Ehrlichia,* and atypical mycobacteria. The fluoroquinolone antibiotics are indicated in the treatment of genitourinary tract infections including prostatitis, dermal infections, and infections of the respiratory tract in the dog. Enrofloxacin has limited activity against anaerobes, although it is reported to have activity against some obligate anaerobic bacteria. Increasing the dose (up to 20 mg/kg) increases the potential for antibacterial efficacy and may be indicated for *Pseudomonas aeruginosa* infections.

ADVERSE AND COMMON SIDE EFFECTS: Isolated incidents of vomiting and anorexia occur at higher than recommended (e.g., 10 times) doses. Oral treatment of 15- to 28-week-old puppies at doses of 25 mg/kg (recommended dose is 2.5 mg/kg bid) induced abnormal carriage of the carpal joints and weakness in the hindquarters. Significant improvement followed drug withdrawal. Cartilage damage occurred after treatment for 30 days at 5, 15, and 25 mg/kg in this age group. Cartilaginous lesions did not occur in puppies 29- to 34-weeks-old after treatment at 25 mg/kg for a 30-day period. The drug is contraindicated in small and medium breeds of dogs during the rapid growth phase (between 2 and 8 months). Large breed dogs may be in the rapid growth phase for as long as 1 year and giant breeds for up to 18 months. Because of the risk of induction of cartilage defects, the drug is not recommended for use in pregnant animals. Other side effects may include GI upset, polydipsia, and CNS dysfunction, i.e., seizures. In cats, dosages in excess of 5 mg/kg per day may result in mild to severe retinal and/or visual changes including blindness. Splitting the dose, i.e., 2.5 mg/kg bid; PO and avoiding rapid IV infusion may help reduce the risk. Doses of 50 mg/kg have been reported to cause CNS dysfunction. See also FLUOROQUINOLONE ANTIBIOTICS.

DRUG INTERACTIONS: Absorption is hindered by antacid preparations and sucralfate. Nitrofurantoin may antagonize the effects of enrofloxacin. Fluoroquinolone antibiotics may potentiate the nephrotoxicity of cyclosporine. In humans, concurrent use of NSAID drugs may promote CNS-related side effects. See FLUOROQUINOLONE ANTIBIOTICS.

SUPPLIED AS VETERINARY PRODUCTS:
Tablets containing 22.7, 68, and 136 mg ★
Tablets containing 15, 50, and 150 mg ♣
For injection containing 22.7 and 50 mg/mL

OTHER USES
Dogs and Cats
ATYPICAL MYCOBACTERIA
5 to 15 mg/kg bid; PO for 3 to 4 weeks

Dogs
PSEUDOMONAS AERUGINOSA
5.5 mg/kg bid; PO is effective, although 11 mg/kg bid; PO may be more efficacious

EPHEDRINE

INDICATIONS: Ephedrine sulfate is an α-receptor stimulant. It is useful in the management of urinary incontinence, as a bronchodilator, as a nasal decongestant, and in the management of hypotension.

ADVERSE AND COMMON SIDE EFFECTS: Tachycardia, hypertension, tremors, restlessness, anxiety, hyperexcitability, and urine retention may occur. The drug is minimally arrhythmogenic.

DRUG INTERACTIONS: Sodium bicarbonate may increase the pharmacological effects of ephedrine with excessive CNS stimulation and cardiovascular effects. Use with amitriptyline may potentiate α-adrenergic effects, leading to hypertension and fever.

SUPPLIED AS HUMAN PRODUCTS:
Capsules containing 25 and 50 mg (generic products ★)
For injection containing 50 mg/mL (generic products ♣ ★)
Tablets containing 8, 15, 25, and 30 mg (generic products ♣)

OTHER USES
Dogs and Cats
NASAL DECONGESTANT
1 drop per nostril tid to qid (0.5% solution)

Dogs
NASAL DECONGESTANT
5 to 15 mg tid to qid; PO

Cats
NASAL DECONGESTANT
2 to 5 mg tid to qid; PO

EPINEPHRINE

INDICATIONS: Epinephrine is indicated for the treatment of cardiac arrest associated with ventricular standstill. It accelerates atrial and ventricular rates. A topical solution (2%) is used to treat glaucoma.

ADVERSE AND COMMON SIDE EFFECTS: Fear, anxiety, excitability, vomiting, hypertension, and arrhythmias are reported. The topical preparations are locally irritating, resulting in conjunctival hyperemia, chemosis, and blepharospasm.

DRUG INTERACTIONS: The use of other sympathomimetic agents, e.g., isoproterenol, may have additive and potentially toxic effects. The antihistamines diphenhydramine and chlorpheniramine and l-thyroxine also may potentiate the effects of epinephrine. Epinephrine potentiates halothane-induced arrhythmias, especially with the concurrent use of barbiturate or xylazine anesthesia. Acepromazine given 20 minutes before anesthesia may decrease the incidence of epinephrine-induced arrhythmias. Propranolol, metoprolol, and atenolol may potentiate hypertension and antagonize the effect of epinephrine on the heart and bronchi. Nitrates, α-blocking agents, and diuretics may mitigate the pressor effects of the drug.

SUPPLIED AS VETERINARY AND HUMAN PRODUCTS (✿ ★): For injection containing 0.1 mg/mL (1:10,000) and 1.0 mg/mL (1:1,000) epinephrine

OTHER USES
Dogs
BRONCHODILATION AND ANAPHYLAXIS
0.02 mg/kg; IV, SC, IM

Cats
ASTHMA AND ANAPHYLAXIS
0.1 mg every 4 to 6 hours; SC or 0.2 mg in 100 mL D_5W bid to tid PRN; IV

EPSIPRANTEL

INDICATIONS: Epsiprantel (Cestex ✿ ★) is an anthelmintic used for the eradication of *Dipylidium caninum* and *Taenia pisiformis* in dogs and *Dipylidium caninum* and *Taenia taeniaeformis* in cats.

ADVERSE AND COMMON SIDE EFFECTS: The drug should not be given to puppies and kittens less than 7 weeks of age. Significant side effects at recommended doses are unreported.

DRUG INTERACTIONS: None reported.

SUPPLIED AS VETERINARY PRODUCT:
Tablets containing 12.5, 25, 50, and 100 mg

ERYTHROMYCIN

INDICATIONS: Erythromycin (Erythro-100 ★) is a macrolide anti-biotic with primary activity against gram-positive bacteria. It is effective against streptococci, staphylococci, *Erysipelothrix, Clostridium, Bacteroides, Borrelia, Fusobacterium, Pasteurella,* and *Bordetella.* The drug also has activity against *Campylobacter fetus,* mycoplasmas, chlamydiae, rickettsiae, spirochetes, some atypical mycobacteria, *Leptospira,* and amoebae. At lower dosages, the drug may be used to treat gastroesophageal reflux and reflux esophagitis in cats and perhaps dogs, to promote gastric emptying, and to stimulate small intestinal motility, but not colonic motility.

ADVERSE AND COMMON SIDE EFFECTS: Adverse effects are rare, but nausea, vomiting, abdominal pain, anorexia, and diarrhea may occur with oral use of the drug. Liver dysfunction and/or abnormal liver function tests may be noted. Erythromycin estolate and ethylsuccinate have been associated with an increased risk of cholestasis and hepatotoxicity. Allergic reactions, including urticaria, mild skin eruptions, and anaphylaxis, have been reported. All parenteral preparations are irritating at the site of injection.

DRUG INTERACTIONS: Kaolin, pectin, and bismuth decrease GI absorption of the drug. Because of competitive protein binding, erythromycin should not be used in patients given chloramphenicol, lincomycin, or clindamycin. At low doses, erythromycin may antagonize the antimicrobial action of the penicillins. Increased serum levels leading to toxicity may occur in those concurrently receiving theophylline. The occurrence in small animals is unknown. Erythromycin may cause prolongation of bleeding times in those receiving warfarin therapy. Methylprednisolone metabolism may be inhibited by erythromycin. Concurrent use of erythromycin with terfenadine (Seldane) may predispose to severe and life-threatening cardiac arrhythmias in humans.

SUPPLIED AS VETERINARY PRODUCT:
For injection containing 100 mg/mL [Gallimycin 100 ★] and 200 mg/mL [Erythro-200 ♣, Gallimycin ★] for use in large animals

SUPPLIED AS HUMAN PRODUCTS:
Tablets (enteric-coated) containing 250 and 333 mg as erythromycin base [E-Mycin ★]
Tablets (film-coated) containing 250 and 500 mg as erythromycin stearate

Capsules containing 250 mg as erythromycin base [Eryc ✤ ★]
Oral drops containing 125 mg/5 mL

Note: There are several other human preparations available.

OTHER USES
Dogs and Cats
GASTROINTESTINAL STIMULANT
0.5 to 1 mg/kg tid; PO

ERYTHROPOIETIN

INDICATIONS: Human recombinant erythropoietin (Epogen ★, Eprex ✤) is used to stimulate the production of erythrocytes in patients with anemia due to renal failure. The product also has been used successfully in dogs and cats. Improved appetite (may precede increases in hematocrit), increased activity levels, weight gain, reduced sleep requirements, and improved grooming behavior also have been reported in cats.

ADVERSE AND COMMON SIDE EFFECTS: Although rare, skin rash at the injection site, fever, arthralgia, and mucocutaneous ulcers have been reported. Autoantibodies may develop in 20% of dogs and 30% of cats, leading to a progressive decline in the hematocrit. In humans, additional adverse effects may include systemic hypertension, hyperkalemia, iron deficiency, and seizures. In cats, polycythemia, systemic hypertension, iron depletion, mucocutaneous reactions, and seizures have been reported. Seizures have been reported in cats with severe azotemia or hypertension.

DRUG INTERACTIONS: None reported.

SUPPLIED AS HUMAN PRODUCT:
For injection in vials containing 1,000, 2,000, 3,000, 4,000, 6,000, 8,000, 10,000, and 20,000 units

ESMOLOL

INDICATIONS: Esmolol (Brevibloc ★ ✤) is an ultra-short-acting selective β_1-receptor–blocking agent indicated for the short-term management of supraventricular arrhythmias, e.g., atrial flutter or fibrillation, sinus tachycardia and ventricular arrhythmias associated with increases in sympathetic tone, or arrhythmias caused by drugs that sensitize the myocardium to arrhythmias, e.g., halothane, thiobarbiturates.

ADVERSE AND COMMON SIDE EFFECTS: At recommended dosages adverse effects are uncommon. Hypotension and bradycardia may be noted, which are mild and generally transient. This drug should be avoided in patients with evidence of heart failure or volume depletion, heart block, or sinus bradycardia. Extravasation from venous injection can cause skin irritation.

DRUG INTERACTIONS: Concurrent use with a calcium channel-blocking agent, e.g., diltiazem, may potentiate the occurrence of significant bradycardia. Esmolol may increase serum digoxin levels. Morphine may increase esmolol serum concentrations. Neuromuscular blockade effects of succinylcholine may be prolonged if used concurrently with esmolol. Mutual inhibition of effects of drugs may occur if esmolol is used with aminophylline or theophylline. Hypertension may occur if esmolol is used concurrently with MAO, e.g., amitraz or selegiline.

SUPPLIED AS HUMAN PRODUCT:
For injection containing 10 mg/mL, 20 mg/mL, 250 mg/mL

ESTRADIOL CYPIONATE

INDICATIONS: Estradiol cypionate (ECP ♣ ★) has been used for the prevention of pregnancy. It likely causes expulsion of the ova into the uterus or delays transport of the ova through the oviduct, predisposing to its degeneration. This agent also has been used in the treatment of urinary incontinence in spayed female dogs and for palliation of benign anal tumors in aged male dogs.

ADVERSE AND COMMON SIDE EFFECTS: Feminization or the induction or prolongation of estrus may occur. Estrogens predispose to the development of cystic endometrial hyperplasia and pyometra. Thrombocytopenia may be observed approximately 2 weeks after the initiation of treatment with estrogens. Leukocytosis with a left shift may develop at approximately 16 to 20 days, and anemia may become gradually apparent. Leukopenia may follow at approximately 22 to 25 days. There is considerable variation in sensitivity to the adverse effects of estrogens. In some dogs, severe and fatal myelotoxicosis develops, whereas others may have only mild to moderate reversible marrow damage. Bone marrow hypoplasia appears more likely to occur after repeated use or high doses of long-acting preparations such as ECP. Estrogens induce squamous metaplasia and fibromuscular proliferation of the prostate gland, which predisposes to fluid stasis and infection.

DRUG INTERACTIONS: Estrogen activity may be decreased if the drug is used concurrently with rifampin, phenytoin, or barbiturate drugs. Estrogens may enhance glucocorticoid activity, necessitating adjustment of the glucocorticoid dose.

SUPPLIED AS:
For injection containing 1 (♣) and 2 (★) mg/mL

OTHER USES
Dogs
MISMATING
i)   0.02 mg/kg; IM within 72 hours of mating
ii) 0.044 mg/kg; IM once during 3 to 5 days of standing heat or within
     72 hours of mating

Cats
MISMATING
0.125 to 0.25 mg; IM within 40 hours of mating

ETIDRONATE

INDICATIONS: Etidronate (Didronel ♣ ★) is potentially useful in
the management of refractory hypercalcemia.

ADVERSE AND COMMON SIDE EFFECTS: In humans, nausea,
diarrhea, and loose stools may occur. With drug overdose, hypocalcemia may occur. Absorption is decreased by food and dairy
products.

DRUG INTERACTIONS: None.

SUPPLIED AS HUMAN PRODUCTS:
Tablets containing 200 and 400 mg
For injection containing 50 mg/mL ♣ ★

ETODOLAC

INDICATIONS: Etodolac (Etogesic ★) is an NSAID used to manage
pain and inflammation associated with osteoarthritis in dogs. The
drug preferentially inhibits cyclooxygenase (COX-2), and prostaglandin
E_2. Tolerance to the drug may develop. The half-life of the drug is
between 9.7 and 14.4 hours.

ADVERSE AND COMMON SIDE EFFECTS: Etodolac causes fewer
gastrointestinal reactions than aspirin. The following adverse reactions, however, may be observed and include vomiting, diarrhea,
regurgitation, lethargy, hypoproteinemia, urticaria, behavioral
change, and anorexia. As a class of drugs, NSAIDs may be associated
with gastrointestinal and renal toxicity. Because COX-2 is expressed
constitutively in the kidney, use of selective COX-2 inhibitors may
cause renal damage. Those at greatest risk are dogs with preexisting
renal disease, those that are dehydrated, on diuretic therapy, and those

with concurrent cardiovascular and/or hepatic disease. In rodent studies, selective COX-2 inhibitors delay healing of acute-stage ulcers. Safety in breeding, pregnant, or lactating dogs has not been established or in dogs under 12 months of age.

DRUG INTERACTIONS: Concurrent use with other NSAIDs or glucocorticoids should be avoided. Etodolac increases serum levels of cyclosporine, lithium, methotrexate, and digoxin, putting patients at risk for toxicity related to these drugs.

SUPPLIED AS VETERINARY PRODUCT:
Tablets containing 150 and 300 mg

FAMOTIDINE

INDICATIONS: Famotidine (Pepcid ✿ ★) is a histamine (H_2)-receptor antagonist. Although it is more potent than cimetidine, studies have not indicated that it actually is more efficacious than cimetidine or ranitidine in the management of gastric hyperacidity and gastrointestinal ulcers. It is indicated in the treatment or prophylaxis of gastric and duodenal ulcers, uremic gastritis, stress-related and drug induced erosive gastritis, esophagitis, duodenal gastric reflux, and esophageal reflux. It is not effective in preventing ulcers when glucocorticoids or nonsteroidal anti-inflammatory agents are used concurrently with famotidine.

ADVERSE AND COMMON SIDE EFFECTS: In humans, depression, anxiety, insomnia, cardiac arrhythmias, conjunctival injection, nausea, vomiting, anorexia, dry mouth, diarrhea, arthralgia, bronchospasm, pruritus, fever, and thrombocytopenia have been reported. There is little experience with use of the drug in small animals.

DRUG INTERACTIONS: Food enhances the bioavailability of famotidine while antacids decrease the amount of drug available. Administration of antacids should be given 2 hours before or after famotidine. Drugs affected by an increase in pH, e.g., metoclopramide, digoxin, ketoconazole, should be administered 2 to 4 hours before or after famotidine.

SUPPLIED AS HUMAN PRODUCTS:
Tablets containing 20 and 40 mg
For injection containing 10 mg/mL

FELBAMATE

INDICATIONS: Felbamate (Felbatol ★) is an anticonvulsant drug used in dogs refractory to other anticonvulsant agents. It is believed the drug works by inhibiting excitatory neurotransmission.

ADVERSE AND COMMON SIDE EFFECTS: Little information regarding its use in dogs is available. Sedation, nausea, and vomiting have been reported in dogs. In people adverse effects may include tremor, limb rigidity, salivation, and restlessness/anxiety. In people, aplastic anemia and hepatic necrosis have been documented.

DRUG INTERACTIONS: Felbamate may increase serum phenobarbital levels. The same increase in drug levels may occur if felbamate is used concurrently with phenytoin or valproic acid.

SUPPLIED AS HUMAN PRODUCTS:
Tablets containing 400 and 600 mg
Oral liquid containing 120 mg/mL

FENBENDAZOLE

INDICATIONS: Fenbendazole (Panacur ✿ ★) is an anthelmintic recommended for the elimination of roundworms (*Toxocara canis, Toxascaris leonina*), hookworms (*Ancylostoma caninum, Uncinaria stenocephala*), whipworms (*Trichuris vulpis*), and tapeworms (*Taenia pisiformis*) as well as *Physaloptera* infections. The drug also has been shown to reduce the burden of *Ancylostoma caninum* and *Toxocara canis* in newborn pups when the bitch is treated during the last trimester of pregnancy. Fenbendazole is effective and safe for treating *Giardia* and *Heterobilharzia americana* in dogs. The drug also may have some efficacy against crenosomiasis. It also has been used to treat the fluke *Eurytrema procyonis* in cats.

ADVERSE AND COMMON SIDE EFFECTS: Although the drug generally does not have side effects, vomiting and diarrhea may occur. Fenbendazole appears safe for use in cats.

DRUG INTERACTIONS: None in small animals.

SUPPLIED AS VETERINARY PRODUCT:
Granules (222 mg fenbendazole/g) to be mixed with food

OTHER USES
Dogs
CAPILLARIA AEROPHILA
25 to 50 mg/kg bid for 10 to 14 days; PO

CAPILLARIA PLICA
i)   50 mg/kg once daily for 3 days; PO, repeat in 3 weeks
ii) 50 mg/kg once daily for 3 to 10 days; PO

CRENOSOMA VULPIS
50 mg/kg once daily; PO for 3 days

FILAROIDES HIRTHI
50 mg/kg once daily for 14 days; PO
Note: Clinical signs may worsen during therapy, ostensibly because of reaction to dying worms.

PARAGONIMUS KELLICOTTI
50 to 100 mg/kg divided bid for 10 to 14 days; PO

TRICHURIS VULPIS COLITIS
50 mg/kg once daily for 3 days; repeat in 2 to 3 weeks and again in 2 months

GIARDIA CANIS
50 mg/kg once daily; PO for 3 doses

Cats

ASCARIDS, HOOKWORMS, STRONGYLOIDES,
AND TAPEWORMS (Taenia spp.)
50 mg/kg for 5 days; PO

AELUROSTRONGYLUS ABSTRUSUS
i)   20 mg/kg once daily for 5 days; repeat 5 days later

ii) 25 to 50 mg/kg bid for 10 to 14 days; PO

CAPILLARIA AEROPHILA
50 mg/kg for 10 days; PO

CAPILLARIA FELISCATI
25 mg/kg bid for 10 days; PO

PARAGONIMUS KELLICOTTI
50 mg/kg daily for 10 days; PO

EURYTREMA PROCYONIS
30 mg/kg daily for 6 days

FENTANYL

INDICATIONS: Fentanyl (Duragesic ♣ ★, Sublimaze ★) is a synthetic narcotic with an analgesic potency approximately 100 times that of morphine and 500 times that of meperidine. Its onset of action is rapid. The drug induces profound analgesia, sedation, and respiratory depression within 6 to 8 minutes after injection. It has a short duration of action; peak effects last approximately 30 to 60 minutes. Narcotic antagonists can reverse fentanyl.

Its use in the form of a transdermal slow-release formulation also has been described in the dog and cat. Plasma concentrations of 1 to 2 ng/mL are considered analgesic in dogs. There may be a wide range of variation in analgesic effect because of differences in absorption of the product. For management of postoperative pain, the patch should be placed 12 to 24 hours before surgery in dogs and 6 to 12 hours before surgery in cats to attain effective concentrations at the time of surgery. The patch is designed to release the drug at a constant rate for at least 72 hours. After removal of the patch plasma opioid concentrations fall rapidly in dogs (half-life of 1.4 hours).

ADVERSE AND COMMON SIDE EFFECTS: Respiratory depression, constipation, and decreased appetite may occur. Fentanyl is eliminated by hepatic biotransformation, and most of its metabolites are excreted in the urine. Its use in patients with compromised hepatic or renal function may be contraindicated. It should not be used in patients with compromised respiratory function, increased intracranial pressure, brain tumors, or altered consciousness. It should be used with caution in those patients with bradyarrhythmias. In humans, side effects may include sedation, respiratory depression, bronchoconstriction, constipation, muscle rigidity, miosis, suppression of the cough reflex, bradycardia, and mood changes. Tolerance to the drug may occur. Concurrent administration of atropine prevents bradycardia. In cats given the transdermal patches, no adverse effects have been noted.

DRUG INTERACTIONS: Barbiturates, other narcotics, and general anesthetics potentiate cerebral and respiratory depression associated with its use.

SUPPLIED AS HUMAN PRODUCTS:
Patches delivering 25, 50, 75, and 100 µg/hour as fentanyl (Duragesic ❦ ★)

For injection containing 50 µg as fentanyl citrate (Sublimaze ★, generic products ❦)

FENTANYL-DROPERIDOL

See INNOVAR-VET.

FERROUS SULFATE

INDICATIONS: Ferrous sulfate (Fer-In-Sol, Slow-Fe, and others, as listed below) is used for the treatment and prevention of iron-deficiency anemia.

ADVERSE AND COMMON SIDE EFFECTS: Mild GIT upset may occur after oral administration. The drug is contraindicated in patients with GIT ulcers, enteritis, colitis, and hemolytic anemia.

DRUG INTERACTIONS: Oral iron supplements may interfere with the absorption of tetracycline antibiotics. Antacids decrease iron absorption from the GIT. Chloramphenicol and cimetidine may delay the hematologic response to iron. Iron may decrease the efficacy of penicillamine by decreasing its absorption.

SUPPLIED AS HUMAN PRODUCTS:
Tablets (20% elemental iron) containing 195 mg (39 mg iron), 300 mg (60 mg iron), and 325 mg (65 mg iron) as ferrous sulfate
Tablets containing 195 mg [Mol-Iron ★]
Tablets containing 300 mg ferrous sulfate [Apo-Ferrous ✤], 525 mg (105 mg elemental iron) in timed-release form
[Fero-Grad ✤, Film tabs], 160 mg (50 mg elemental iron)
[Slow-Fe ✤]
Capsules (timed-release) containing 150 mg (30 mg iron) and 250 mg (50 mg iron) [Ferospace ★ for (American drug), Ferra-TD ★]
Syrup containing 18 mg/mL (3.6 mg iron/mL) [Fer-In-Sol ★]
Elixir containing 44 mg/mL (8.8 mg iron/mL) [Feosol ★ for]
Drops containing 125 mg/mL (25 mg iron/mL) [Fer-Iron Drops ★]

FINASTERIDE

INDICATIONS: Finasteride (Proscar ✤ ★) is a 5α-reductase enzyme inhibitor that blocks the production of dihydrotestosterone from testosterone. It is used to reduce prostatic size in patients with benign prostatic hyperplasia (BPH) without affecting semen quality or libido at the dosages suggested here. It is estimated that more than 80% of intact male dogs have gross or microscopic evidence of BPH.

ADVERSE AND COMMON SIDE EFFECTS: In humans adverse effects may include decreased libido, impotence, and decreased ejaculation volume. No adverse effects have been reported in dogs.

DRUG INTERACTIONS: No drug interactions of clinical importance have been identified.

SUPPLIED AS HUMAN PRODUCT:
Tablets containing 5 mg

FLORFENICOL

INDICATIONS: Florfenicol (Nuflor ✤ ★) is a chloramphenicol derivative with a wide spectrum of antibacterial activity and has been used when chloramphenicol is not available.

ADVERSE AND COMMON SIDE EFFECTS: Experience with the drug in small animals is limited; however, like chloramphenicol, the drug may be associated with dose-dependent bone marrow suppression.

DRUG INTERACTIONS: None reported. Also see CHLORAM-PHENICOL.

**SUPPLIED AS VETERINARY PRODUCT
(Approved for Use in Cattle Only):**
For injection containing 300 mg/mL

FLUCONAZOLE

INDICATIONS: Fluconazole (Diflucan ✝ ★) is an azole derivative that has been used to treat canine nasal aspergillosis and penicilliosis infections. It has demonstrated efficacy against *Blastomyces, Candida, Coccidioides, Cryptococcus,* and *Histoplasma* infections. Fluconazole has greater water solubility, better oral bioavailability, higher plasma extravascular levels, and a longer plasma half-life than ketoconazole and penetrates the CSF and brain tissue. Overall, fluconazole is successful in approximately half the dogs treated, which is similar to what can be expected with thiabendazole or ketoconazole treatment of the same condition. Therefore, fluconazole is recommended only if topical treatment (i.e., enilconazole or clotrimazole) is not feasible. The drug also has been used to treat systemic cryptococcosis in the cat.

ADVERSE AND COMMON SIDE EFFECTS: Although experience with the drug in small animals is limited, no adverse effects were noted in dogs during therapy. In subacute toxicity studies in dogs, a dose of 30 mg/kg caused slight increases in plasma transaminase activity. In humans, adverse effects may include nausea, vomiting, diarrhea, abdominal pain, skin rash, and elevations in serum ALT, alkaline phosphatase, and AST.

DRUG INTERACTIONS: High doses of fluconazole may increase serum cyclosporine levels. Fluconazole also increases serum phenobarbital and phenytoin levels. Prothrombin time may increase if used concurrently with warfarin. Hydrochlorothiazide increases fluconazole plasma levels. Rifampin decreases serum levels of fluconazole, necessitating an increase in fluconazole drug dosages. Fluconazole decreases the elimination of oral sulfonylurea drugs, e.g., glipizide, predisposing to hypoglycemia.

SUPPLIED AS HUMAN PRODUCTS:
For injection containing 2 mg/mL
Tablets containing 50, 100, 150, and 200 mg
Oral suspension containing 10 and 40 mg/mL

FLUCYTOSINE

INDICATIONS: Flucytosine (Ancobon ★) has been recommended for the treatment of cryptococcosis and candidiasis. It also has been used in combination with amphotericin B and ketoconazole in the treatment of cryptococcosis. *Aspergillus* spp. has an intermediate sensitivity to the drug. It is deaminated to 5-fluorouracil in fungal cells.

ADVERSE AND COMMON SIDE EFFECTS: Leukopenia and thrombocytopenia (which may occur within days of onset of treatment), hepatotoxicity, cutaneous eruption, rash, nausea, diarrhea, and abdominal pain have been reported. The drug is teratogenic and should not be given to pregnant animals. Resistance to the drug develops rapidly, especially when low doses are used.

DRUG INTERACTIONS: An additive or synergistic response may be expected when used with amphotericin B; however, toxicity of flucytosine may be increased with this combination because of decreased renal clearance. Combination therapy with flucytosine and ketoconazole in cats is especially toxic.

SUPPLIED AS HUMAN PRODUCT:
Capsules containing 250 and 500 mg [Ancobon]

OTHER USES
Dogs
URINARY TRACT CANDIDIASIS
200 mg/kg per day divided tid to qid; PO. The drug is continued at least 2 to 3 weeks beyond clinical resolution of the disease.

FLUDROCORTISONE

INDICATIONS: Fludrocortisone (Florinef ✤ ★) is a long-acting steroid with potent mineralocorticoid and moderate glucocorticoid activity. It is indicated in the treatment of hypoadrenocorticism, where it promotes sodium retention and urinary potassium excretion. In larger doses, it inhibits endogenous cortisol secretion.

ADVERSE AND COMMON SIDE EFFECTS: Adverse effects are rare but with overdose may include sodium retention causing edema and hypertension, hypokalemia, and muscle weakness. At higher drug dosages clinical signs of glucocorticoid excess may become apparent, e.g., polyuria, polydipsia, or urinary incontinence. To help resolve these problems, switch the patient to DOCP and then gradually taper the dog off fludrocortisone over a 4 to 5 day period.

DRUG INTERACTIONS: The likelihood of hypokalemia is increased with the concurrent use of amphotericin B, thiazide diuretics, and furosemide. The drug may increase insulin requirements of diabetic patients.

SUPPLIED AS HUMAN PRODUCT:
Tablets containing 0.1 mg

OTHER USES
Dogs
HYPERKALEMIA
0.1 to 1 mg/dog per day (as adjunctive therapy)

FLUMAZENIL

INDICATIONS: Flumazenil (Romazicon ★, Anexate ♣) is a benzodiazepine receptor antagonist that can be used to reverse the sedative effects of diazepam or midazolam. The drug has also been used in people to treat clinical signs of hepatic encephalopathy, the efficacy of which is unknown in small animals.

ADVERSE AND COMMON SIDE EFFECTS: Flumazenil has a wide margin of safety and few adverse effects. The drug should be used with caution in dogs with CNS disease as seizures may occur.

DRUG INTERACTIONS: None of significance have been reported at this time. Clinical effects of long-acting benzodiazepines may recur after flumazenil's effects have abated.

SUPPLIED AS HUMAN PRODUCT:
For injection containing 0.1 mg/mL

FLUMETHASONE

INDICATIONS: Flumethasone (Flucort ♣ ★) is a long-acting glucocorticoid recommended for use in dogs and cats for inflammatory musculoskeletal conditions, acute and chronic dermatoses to help control pruritus, irritation and inflammation associated with these disorders, in allergic states, in shock, and in cats for appetite stimulation along with B-complex vitamins. For further information on INDICATIONS, ADVERSE AND COMMON SIDE EFFECTS, and DRUG INTERACTIONS, see GLUCOCORTICOID AGENTS.

SUPPLIED AS VETERINARY PRODUCT:
For injection containing 0.5 mg/mL in 100-mL vials

FLUNIXIN MEGLUMINE

INDICATIONS: Flunixin meglumine (Banamine ✤ ★) is a potent antiprostaglandin with anti-inflammatory and antipyretic properties that make it useful in the treatment of inflammation and pain associated with musculoskeletal disease. Its analgesic properties are considered superior to those of aspirin, meperidine, pentazocine, codeine phosphate, and phenylbutazone. The drug also has been recommended as adjunctive therapy in the treatment of shock in the dog. In addition, flunixin has been used for the short-term relief of ocular inflammation, e.g., conjunctivitis, corneal trauma, uveitis, chorioretinitis, and panophthalmitis.

ADVERSE AND COMMON SIDE EFFECTS: Increased serum concentrations of ALT, nephrotoxicity, and gastric ulceration may be noted. Gastric ulceration may be exacerbated by the concurrent use of prednisone. At higher doses, salivation, panting, vomiting, and tremors have been reported. Kidney necrosis may occur in patients with preexisting kidney disease. Intramuscular injection can be irritating.

DRUG INTERACTIONS: None established. Concurrent use of methoxyflurane may predispose to acute renal tubular necrosis.

SUPPLIED AS VETERINARY PRODUCTS:
Granules containing 25 mg/g
Paste containing 50 mg/g
For injection containing 50 mg/mL

FLUOROQUINOLONE ANTIBIOTICS

INDICATIONS: Norfloxacin (Noroxin ✤ ★), enrofloxacin (Baytril ✤ ★), ciprofloxacin (Cipro ✤ ★), marbofloxacin (Zeniquin ★ ✤), and orbifloxacin (Orbax ✤ ★) constitute the fluoroquinolone group. These antibiotics have activity against *E. coli, Enterobacter, Klebsiella, Proteus, Pseudomonas,* some *Staphylococcus, Salmonella, Shigella, Vibrio, Yersinia,* and *Campylobacter* organisms. They have little activity against anaerobic cocci, *Bacteroides,* or clostridial organisms. Resistance does occur, especially with *Pseudomonas, Klebsiella, Acinetobacter,* and Enterococcus organisms. Ciprofloxacin has more activity than other quinolones against *Pseudomonas* and *Acinetobacter.* Streptococci (particularly enterococci) generally are resistant, which may limit the use of fluoroquinolone antibiotics in the treatment of respiratory infections, where streptococci often are present. Orbifloxacin appears more effective than enrofloxacin in the treatment of urinary tract infection and equally as effective as enrofloxacin in the treatment of skin wounds and abscesses in dogs. Fluoroquinolone antibiotics may be effective against atypical mycobacteria (*M. fortuitum* and *M. chelonei*), although higher dosages may be needed. The fluoroquinolone antibiotics are effective in the treatment of respiratory tract infections, bronchopneumonia, enteric infections, bacterial prostatitis, bacterial meningoencephalitis, osteomyelitis, and skin and soft tissue infections.

ADVERSE AND COMMON SIDE EFFECTS: Side effects are rare but may include vomiting and diarrhea. Rapid IV injection in anesthetized dogs or cats may cause hypotension related to histamine release. At high doses, renal toxicity may develop from crystalluria and crystal deposition in renal tubules. Drug dose should be decreased in patients with renal disease. Fluoroquinolone antibiotics also may cause erosion of cartilage and a permanent lameness in young animals, and they are not recommended between 2 and 8 months of age in small and medium-sized breeds of dogs, before 1 year of age in large breeds, and before 18 months of age in giant breed dogs. These drugs should not be given to lactating bitches. The drugs are potentially teratogenic and should not be given to pregnant animals. Seizure activity may be precipitated with the concurrent use of NSAIDs. Dogs given high doses have had subcapsular cataract formation of the lens and associated inflammatory response after treatment for 8 to 12 months. Cats given high doses of ciprofloxacin developed erythema of the pinnae, vomiting, and clonic muscle spasm. Retinal degeneration leading to partial, temporary, or total blindness has been reported in some cats given enrofloxacin. The reported incidence is 0.0008%. This adverse effect may be seen with other fluroquinolones. Dosing on an exact body weight using split dosing (2.5 mg/kg bid; PO) and avoiding rapid IV infusions, and drug interactions may reduce the risk of retinal degeneration.

DRUG INTERACTIONS: Food impairs the absorption of these drugs. Absorption also is hindered by antacid preparations, multivitamin compounds and sucralfate, and agents containing divalent and trivalent cations, e.g., iron, aluminum, calcium, magnesium, and zinc. Nitrofurantoin may impair pharmacological efficacy. Enrofloxacin and ciprofloxacin may increase plasma theophylline levels. Fluoroquinolones may exacerbate the nephrotoxic potential of cyclosporine. Antibiotic synergism may occur if these agents are used with aminoglycosides, third-generation cephalosporins, and extended-spectrum penicillins.

SUPPLIED AS: See specific product.

FLUOROURACIL

INDICATIONS: Fluorouracil (Adrucil ✤ ★) is an antimetabolite chemotherapeutic agent that has been used in the treatment of various canine carcinomas and sarcomas.

ADVERSE AND COMMON SIDE EFFECTS: Nausea, vomiting, and diarrhea may occur. Oral and GI ulceration, leukopenia, thrombocytopenia, anemia, cerebellar ataxia, and alopecia also have been reported. The drug is extremely neurotoxic to cats and should not be used in this species.

DRUG INTERACTIONS: The concurrent use of other myelosuppressive agents or radiation therapy may require adjustment of fluorouracil dose.

SUPPLIED AS HUMAN PRODUCT:
For injection containing 50 mg/mL

FLUOXETINE

INDICATIONS: Fluoxetine (Prozac ✤ ★) is a selective serotonin reuptake inhibitor used in dogs and cats in the management of behavioral disorders, e.g., canine aggression and compulsive disorders. A beneficial clinical response may not be noted for 1 to 4 weeks. A 15% (w/v) pluronic lecithin organogel (PLO gel) can be absorbed through the skin, but the relative bioavailability is only 10% of that of an oral dose.

ADVERSE AND COMMON SIDE EFFECTS: The drug may cause lethargy, anxiety, irritability, insomnia or hyperactivity, panting, and gastrointestinal effects. Transient anorexia is common in dogs.

DRUG INTERACTIONS: Fluoxetine is highly protein bound and could displace similarly bound drugs, e.g., warfarin, phenylbutazone, digitoxin. Fluoxetine may potentiate the effects of diazepam, lithium, buspirone, and the tricyclic antidepressants. The concurrent use with MAO inhibitors, e.g., amitraz and selegiline, may be associated with significant morbidity.

SUPPLIED AS HUMAN PRODUCTS:
Tablets containing 10 mg
Tablets or capsules containing 10, 20, and 40 mg
Liquid formulations containing 20 mg/5 mL

FOLIC ACID

INDICATIONS: Folic acid (Folvite ★ and generic products ✤ ★) is a member of the vitamin B complex group and is essential for the maintenance of normal erythropoiesis. Folic acid deficiency may occur with blood loss, prolonged malabsorption, or sulfonamide administration. It may be indicated in cases in which pyrimethamine is used on a long-term basis.

ADVERSE AND COMMON SIDE EFFECTS: The drug is reportedly nontoxic.

DRUG INTERACTIONS: Chloramphenicol may antagonize the hematologic response.

SUPPLIED AS HUMAN PRODUCTS:
Tablets containing 100, 400, 800 µg and 1 and 5 mg
For injection containing 5 and 10 mg/mL

FOMEPIZOLE

INDICATIONS: Fomepizole (Antizol-Vet ★) is a synthetic alcohol dehydrogenase inhibitor used in the treatment of ethylene glycol (antifreeze) toxicity in dogs. Its chemical name is 4-methylpyrazole, and it is a more potent inhibitor of alcohol dehydrogenase than ethanol. Once inhibition of alcohol dehydrogenase has been effected, the remaining unmetabolized ethylene glycol and its metabolites are excreted in the urine. This agent is only effective if it is administered before complete metabolism of ethylene glycol has occurred. Efficacy of the product can be determined before the initiation of therapy by measuring serum creatinine and BUN after clinical dehydration has been corrected. Blood urea nitrogen levels in excess of 40 mg/dL (14.28 mmol/L) and serum creatinine levels greater than 1.8 mg/dL (159.12 µmol/L) imply that ethylene glycol has been metabolized completely and that significant renal impairment probably has occurred. However, if urine output can be maintained, treatment with fomepizole still may be beneficial. Experimental studies with 4-methylpyrazole have indicated that most dogs survive if treatment is begun within 8 hours of ingestion of ethylene glycol. In another study, all dogs treated within 5 hours of antifreeze ingestion survived. 4-Methylpyrazole does not appear to be as effective as ethanol in the treatment of ethylene glycol toxicity in cats.

ADVERSE AND COMMON SIDE EFFECTS: At higher-than-recommended dosages, fomepizole can cause CNS depression. Dosages of 25 mg/kg resulted in decreased food consumption, weight loss, and a sweet breath. At 30 mg/kg, the drug caused hypoactivity. At 50 mg/kg, ataxia, hypoactivity, hypothermia, tremors and/or prostration, injected sclera, ptosis, protruding tongues, and decreased defecation were noted. Anaphylaxis, as documented by tachypnea, gagging, excessive salivation, and trembling, is rare. Safe use of the drug in pregnant or breeding dogs has not been established.

DRUG INTERACTIONS: There are no specific drug interactions documented to date. Supportive care, in the form of maintaining adequate hydration status, and normal acid–base and electrolyte balance are vital to successful outcome.

SUPPLIED AS VETERINARY PRODUCT:
For injection containing 1.5 g Kit (after addition of 30 mL saline resultant solution contains 50 mg/mL) [Antizol-Vet]

SUPPLIED AS HUMAN PRODUCT:
For injection containing 1 g/mL [Antizol]

FUCIDIC ACID

INDICATIONS: Fucidic acid (Fucithalmic Vet ✤) is an ophthalmic antibiotic preparation that exerts its activity by interfering with bacterial protein synthesis. The drug is active against a number of gram-positive and gram-negative cocci, e.g., *Staphylococcus* including penicillinase-producing strains and in particular *S. intermedium* and *aureus*, which are responsible for the majority of external eye infections in dogs. The slow release formulation results in prolonged retention within the conjunctival sac allowing once daily application. One of the main actions of Fucithalmic Vet may be the carbomer that lubricates the eye and stops the ocular pruritus.

ADVERSE AND COMMON SIDE EFFECTS: The drug should be discontinued if hypersensitivity occurs. It should not be used to treat *Pseudomonas* infections. If a clinical response is not apparent within 5 days the diagnosis should be reevaluated.

DRUG INTERACTIONS: None reported.

SUPPLIED AS VETERINARY PRODUCT:
Tubes containing 3 grams

FUROSEMIDE

INDICATIONS: Furosemide (Lasix ✤ ★) is a potent loop diuretic effective in reducing preload and pulmonary edema in patients with congestive heart failure. The drug also may be used after adequate rehydration to promote diuresis in patients with oliguria. It promotes significant sodium and water excretion by inhibiting chloride resorption in the ascending loop of Henle. It also redistributes blood flow from the juxtamedullary region of the kidney to the cortex and may act as a venous vasodilator by increasing systemic and venous capacitance. The drug is beneficial in the management of systemic hypertension. Activity is noted 5 minutes after IV injection and 1 hour after oral use. Peak activity occurs 30 minutes after IV injection and 1 to 2 hours after oral dosing. Duration of activity is 2 hours after IV injection and 6 hours after oral administration.

ADVERSE AND COMMON SIDE EFFECTS: Dehydration, hypokalemia, hyponatremia, and hypochloremic alkalosis may occur. The drug should not be used in patients with anuria or with progressive renal disease in the face of increasing azotemia. Ototoxicity may occur in cats, especially with high IV doses. Other side effects may include GI upset, anemia, leukopenia, weakness, and restlessness.

DRUG INTERACTIONS: Furosemide-induced hypokalemia may enhance the toxic potential of digitalis. The likelihood of hypokalemia may be increased if used with amphotericin B or the glucocorticoids. Pharmacological effects of theophylline may be increased with furosemide. Ototoxicity and nephrotoxicity of the aminoglycosides may be potentiated. Competition for renal excretory sites may require adjustment of aspirin doses. Furosemide may inhibit muscle relaxation produced by tubocurarine, but it may enhance the effects of succinylcholine. Adjustments in insulin requirements also may need to be addressed. With continuous use, the loss of water-soluble vitamins may occur, and it may be advisable to supplement these patients with B-complex vitamins.

SUPPLIED AS VETERINARY PRODUCTS:
Tablets containing 20 and 40 mg ❧
Tablets containing 12.5 and 50 mg ★
Oral solution containing 10 mg/mL ❧
For injection containing 50 mg/mL ❧ ★

GENTAMICIN

INDICATIONS: Gentamicin (Gentocin ❧ ★, Gentasul ❧, Garagen ★) is an aminoglycoside antibiotic. For information on ADVERSE AND COMMON SIDE EFFECTS and DRUG INTERACTIONS, see AMINOGLYCOSIDE ANTIBIOTICS.

SUPPLIED AS VETERINARY PRODUCTS:
Ophthalmic preparation containing 3 mg/mL [Gentocin ❧ ★]
Ophthalmic preparation containing 3 mg/mL that includes betamethasone [Gentocin Durafilm ❧ ★]
Otic preparation containing 3 mg/mL gentamicin as well as betamethasone [Garagen ★, Gentocin Otic ❧ ★]
For injection containing 50 mg/mL and 100 mg/mL gentamicin

GLIPIZIDE

INDICATIONS: Glipizide (Glucotrol ★) is an oral sulfonylurea hypoglycemic agent. It stimulates functioning pancreatic β cells to secrete insulin within 10 minutes of oral administration. Indirectly, glipizide leads to increased insulin binding at receptor sites, and it causes inhibition of hepatic glucose production and a reduction in serum glucagon levels. The drug has been used successfully in some cats with type II (non–insulin-dependent) diabetes mellitus. Approximately 35% of cats may be responsive to oral hypoglycemic agents when used in conjunction with dietary therapy and correction of obesity. Response often is not apparent during the first 2 to 6 weeks of therapy. If response does occur, it usually is apparent by week 8 of treatment, although some cats require up to 12 weeks of therapy before clinical response occurs. Which cats will respond cannot be predicted. Initial response to glipizide does not rule out the possible need for exogenous insulin in the future. Glipizide loses its effectiveness in 5% to 10% of patients and is related to the progressive loss of β cells and insulin secretory capacity. The drug also has been used in some cases of type II and type III canine diabetes, but most dogs tend to be type I (insulin-dependent) diabetics, undermining the effect of the drug. In addition, some type II and type III diabetic animals have insulin antagonism as a result of hyperadrenocorticism or excessive growth hormone secretion. The cause of the diabetes should be determined before therapy is instituted.

ADVERSE AND COMMON SIDE EFFECTS: The drug is contra-indicated in diabetic ketoacidosis. Caution is advised in patients with impaired renal or hepatic function and those with adrenal or pituitary insufficiency. Experience with the drug in small animals is limited; however, adverse reactions in cats have included anorexia, vomiting, hypoglycemia, icterus, and increased serum alanine aminotransferase levels. Icterus is reported to have resolved within 5 days of cessation of drug administration. Hypoglycemia has been noted in 12% to 15% of cats. Chronic treatment may result in decreased insulin content in β cells and decreased nutrient-stimulated insulin secretion. The drug should be discontinued and insulin treatment initiated if clinical signs of the disease worsen, if the cat becomes ill or develops ketoacidosis or neuropathy, if blood glucose levels remain greater than 350 mg/dL (19.4 mmol/L), or if owners become dissatisfied with the treatment. If cats suffer from side effects of the drug but the owners wish to try the drug again, these cats may be started at a lower dose, e.g., 2.5 mg every other day or once daily, slowly increasing the dose on a weekly basis. In humans, other side effects may include nausea, diarrhea, constipation, cholestatic jaundice, leukopenia, thrombocytopenia, hemolytic anemia, agranulocytosis, and pruritus.

DRUG INTERACTIONS: Oral anticoagulants, cimetidine, chloramphenicol, phenylbutazone, salicylates, and sulfonamides may potentiate the hypoglycemic action of the drug. β-Adrenergic–blocking agents may increase the frequency and severity of hypoglycemia, and if these drugs must be used, a selective β_1-blocking agent, e.g., atenolol or metoprolol, is recommended. Cimetidine may potentiate the hypoglycemic effects of glipizide. Diazoxide and the thiazide diuretics may antagonize the action of glipizide, decreasing its hypoglycemic effect.

SUPPLIED AS HUMAN PRODUCT:
Tablets containing 5 and 10 mg

GLUCOCORTICOID AGENTS

INDICATIONS: Glucocorticoid agents are recommended for the treatment of allergic and immune-mediated diseases, pruritus, cardiogenic and septic shock, and trauma and edema of the CNS and spinal cord. The benefit of steroid use in traumatic shock has not been proven to decrease morbidity or mortality. Corticosteroids are absorbed by cells wherein they affect the formation of new mRNA and initiate new protein synthesis. The newly formed proteins mediate the effects of these drugs. Beneficial effects include stabilization of lysosomal and capillary membranes; decrease in activation of the complement and clotting cascades; binding of endotoxin; positive inotropic effect; prevention of GI mucosal ischemia associated with shock; increase in glucogenesis; inhibition of the formation of vasoactive substances (kinins, prostaglandins); decreased chemotaxis, phagocytosis, and bactericidal activity; depressed T-cell responses and interleukin-2 production; decrease in collagen and scar formation; and decrease in the accumulation of phagocytes at areas of inflammation. In autoimmune disease, glucocorticoids have a rapid onset of action. They interfere with the F_c receptors of immunoglobulin G and C_{3b} receptors on macrophages and decrease immunoglobulin affinity for erythrocytes in cases of autoimmune hemolytic anemia. In large doses, they decrease antibody production. They do not decrease the concentration of antibody already present. Analgesic activity is only related to prostaglandin inhibition. These agents do not possess direct analgesic activity.

The glucocorticoids are classified according to their duration of action. As biologic half-life increases, anti-inflammatory potency increases and mineralocorticoid potency decreases. Short-acting drugs (less than 12 hours) include hydrocortisone and cortisone acetate. Intermediate-acting drugs (12 to 36 hours) include prednisone, prednisolone, methylprednisolone, and triamcinolone. The long-acting steroids (more than 48 hours) include paramethasone, flumethasone, betamethasone, and dexamethasone. Topical corticosteroids are used for their local anti-inflammatory, antipruritic, and vasoconstrictive effects.

ADVERSE AND COMMON SIDE EFFECTS: Polyuria, polydipsia, polyphagia, panting, lethargy, weakness, and bilateral symmetrical alopecia are the most common clinical signs of glucocorticoid excess. Changing to a corticosteroid with little or no mineralocorticoid activity (methylprednisolone, dexamethasone, triamcinolone, DOCP) can reduce or eliminate excessive polyuria-polydipsia. Weight loss, anorexia, and diarrhea may follow use of these drugs. Hemorrhagic gastroenteritis, pancreatitis, glomerulonephritis, and hepatopathy have been reported with the use of corticosteroids. Corticosteroid administration is only considered a predisposing cause of gastrointestinal ulcer if multiple doses of short-acting preparations are given or if single or multiple doses are given concurrently with NSAIDs. In one study, although daily doses of prednisone (4 mg/kg; PO or IM) caused an increase in serum lipase values (and a decrease in serum amylase), the drug did not induce pancreatitis. Urine protein to creatinine ratios may increase (generally values less than 3) in dogs treated with large doses of prednisone over long-term use. Laboratory changes noted with these drugs may include elevations in serum alanine transferase, alkaline phosphatase, gamma-glutamyl transpeptidase, hyperglycemia, hypokalemia, hypocalcemia, a stress leukogram, increases in red blood cell numbers, a decrease in serum total T_4 and free T_4, but did not affect endogenous thyroid-stimulating hormone (TSH). Alternate day treatment did not prevent suppression. Glucocorticoid drugs suppress inflammation, reduce fever, and increase protein catabolism and their conversion to carbohydrates leading to a negative nitrogen balance, promote sodium retention and potassium diuresis, retard wound healing, lower resistance to infection, and cause a reduction in the number of circulating lymphocytes. Only prolonged or high-dose therapy started before surgery actually delays wound healing, an effect potentiated by starvation or protein depletion. Once the inflammatory phase is established, usually within 1 to 3 days of injury, glucocorticoid therapy has little effect on subsequent healing. If preoperative corticosteroid use is necessary, vitamin A or zinc supplementation may help counter the effects of the steroids on collagen production and metabolism. An increase in the incidence of osteoporosis may be noted, especially in older dogs, with prolonged use of these drugs. Their use during the healing phase of bone fractures is not recommended. Iatrogenic hyperadrenocorticism may follow prolonged use of parenteral as well as topical glucocorticoid agents. Glucocorticoids are contraindicated in animals with acute or chronic bacterial infections unless therapeutic doses of an effective bactericidal agent are used concurrently. Corticosteroids may mask signs of infection, such as elevation in body temperature. These drugs should be used with caution in animals with congestive heart failure, diabetes mellitus, and renal disease. These drugs may retard growth if given to young growing animals. Corticosteroids have been associated with an increased incidence of cleft palate and other congenital malformations. In addition, their use may be associated with the induction of the first stage of parturition when administered during the last trimester of pregnancy, and may precipitate premature parturition followed by dystocia, fetal death, retained placenta, and metritis.

Iatrogenic hyperadrenocorticism can be induced by topical, parenteral, or oral administration of glucocorticoids. Even alternate day administration of 1 mg/kg prednisolone in dogs significantly suppresses plasma ACTH concentration for 18 to 24 hours. The most common adverse effects noted in dogs with iatrogenic hyperadrenocorticism were polydipsia, polyuria, polyphagia, skin lesions, lethargy, increases in alkaline phosphatase and alanine transferase, and hypercholesterolemia. Baseline cortisol levels were at the lower end of the reference range and affected dogs exhibited a suppressed or absent response to adrenocorticotropic hormone (ACTH) stimulation. Observable clinical signs were noted only in dogs medicated orally or parenterally, not topically. The mean time for initial clinical signs of hyperadrenocorticism to develop was about 9 months, although they may develop in as little as 1 month. The mean time for each dog to show initial improvement following glucocorticoid withdrawal was 6 weeks, with an additional mean time of 12 weeks for complete remission. Cessation of polyuria, polydipsia, and polyphagia were the first signs of clinical recovery. All dogs recovered without progressing into secondary hypoadrenocorticism and without glucocorticoid support.

DRUG INTERACTIONS: Glucocorticoids may decrease the efficacy of bacteriostatic antibiotics by decreasing the inflammatory response and diminishing the phagocytic activity of leukocytes. Amphotericin B, furosemide, and the thiazide diuretics may potentiate hypokalemia. Hypokalemia may predispose to digitalis toxicity. Glucocorticoids may reduce serum salicylate levels. Phenytoin, phenobarbital, and rifampin may increase the metabolism of glucocorticoids, and insulin requirements of diabetic patients may increase. Hepatic metabolism of methylprednisolone may be inhibited by erythromycin. The concomitant use of glucocorticoids and cyclosporine may lead to increases in serum levels of both drugs. The dose of steroids used in animals receiving mitotane may have to be increased. Live attenuated-virus vaccines generally should not be given to animals receiving glucocorticoid drugs. Concurrent use of NSAIDs may increase the potential for GIT ulceration. Estrogens may potentiate the effects of hydrocortisone and other glucocorticoids.

SUPPLIED AS: See specific product.

GLYBURIDE

INDICATIONS: Glyburide (Diaβeta ✤ ★, Micronase ★) is an oral sulfonylurea hypoglycemic drug with indications similar to those of glipizide. The drug has a longer duration of effect (24 hours) in people than glipizide (10 to 16 hours). The practitioner is advised that experience with use of this specific agent is limited in small animals. Also see GLIPIZIDE.

ADVERSE AND COMMON SIDE EFFECTS: Experience with use of this oral sulfonylurea hypoglycemic agent is limited. See GLIPIZIDE.

DRUG INTERACTIONS: Glyburide is less likely to be displaced or cause the displacement of highly protein-bound drugs than glipizide.

Phenylbutazone may potentiate the hypoglycemic effects of the drug. Thiazide diuretics may exacerbate diabetes mellitus, increasing the dosage requirement of the sulfonylurea drugs. Nonselective β-blocking agents may potentiate the hypoglycemic effects of these drugs. These effects may be mitigated by the use of selective β_1-blocking agents. Monoamine oxidase inhibitors (possibly amitraz and selegiline) may enhance the hypoglycemic effect of sulfonylurea agents. Drugs that may decrease the hypoglycemic effect include furosemide, corticosteroids, phenothiazines, estrogens, thyroid agents, phenytoin, calcium channel-blocking drugs, rifampin, and sympathomimetic agents.

SUPPLIED AS HUMAN PRODUCT:
Tablets containing 1.25, 2.5, and 5 mg

GLYCOPYRROLATE

INDICATIONS: Glycopyrrolate (Robinul-V ★, Robinul ❀ ★) is an anticholinergic agent used in preanesthetic regimens to reduce salivary, tracheobronchial, and pharyngeal secretions, to reduce the volume and acidity of gastric secretion, and to inhibit cardiac vagal inhibitory reflexes during anesthetic induction and intubation.

ADVERSE AND COMMON SIDE EFFECTS: Mydriasis and xerostomia may be noted with its use. Excretion of the drug may be prolonged in animals with impaired renal or gastrointestinal function. It should not be given to pregnant animals. Refer also to ADVERSE AND COMMON SIDE EFFECTS of ATROPINE, which are similar.

DRUG INTERACTIONS: As for atropine, interactions include enhancement of activity if used with antihistamines, procainamide, quinidine, meperidine, benzodiazepines, and phenothiazines. Adverse effects may be potentiated by primidone, disopyramide, nitrates, and long-term corticosteroid use (via increasing intraocular pressure). Glycopyrrolate may enhance the actions of nitrofurantoin, thiazide diuretics, and sympathomimetic agents. The drug may antagonize the activity of metoclopramide.

SUPPLIED AS VETERINARY PRODUCT:
For injection containing 0.2 mg/mL ★

SUPPLIED AS HUMAN PRODUCT:
Tablets containing 1 and 2 mg

OTHER USES
Dogs
REDUCE SECRETIONS
0.01 mg/kg PRN; SC, IM, IV

PREANESTHETIC
0.01 to 0.02 mg/kg; SC, IM

Cats
PREANESTHETIC
0.011 mg/kg; IM (15 minutes before anesthetic)

GONADORELIN

INDICATIONS: Gonadorelin (Cystorelin ❋ ★), also known as gonadotropin-releasing hormone (GnRH), has been used experimentally in dogs to diagnose reproductive failure and to identify intact animals from neutered ones by maximally stimulating follicle-stimulating hormone (FSH) and luteinizing hormone (LH) production. This agent also has been used experimentally via pulse-dosing to induce estrus in dogs. The drug has been used to induce estrus in cats with prolonged anestrus.

ADVERSE AND COMMON SIDE EFFECTS: None reported.

DRUG INTERACTIONS: In humans, it has been noted that response may be blunted by phenothiazines and dopamine antagonists, which cause a rise in prolactin.

SUPPLIED AS VETERINARY PRODUCT:
For injection in 50 µg/mL [Cystorelin]

SUPPLIED AS HUMAN PRODUCT:
For injection in 800 µg/vial [Lutrepulse ❋]

GRANULOCYTE COLONY-STIMULATING FACTOR

INDICATIONS: Filgrastim (Neupogen ❋ ★) is a human granulocyte colony-stimulating factor that has been used to manage dogs and cats with chemotherapy-induced neutropenia. More specifically, it is indicated in animals with febrile neutropenia (counts less than 1,000/µL), prolonged (more than 72 hours) severe neutropenia (counts less than 500/µL), or a history of febrile neutropenia associated with previous dosages of chemotherapy. Canine recombinant granulocyte colony-stimulating factor, although not commercially available at this time, is effective in dogs.

ADVERSE AND COMMON SIDE EFFECTS: Neutrophilia accompanied by a left shift, Dohle bodies, vacuolation, and toxic granulation of leukocytes are to be expected with use of the product and do not necessarily indicate sepsis. Increases in alkaline phosphatase activity also have been reported in people receiving this therapy. Initially, a significant and rapid (within 12 hours and steadily rising over a 2-week period) increase in neutrophil numbers is to be expected. In healthy dogs and cats, the increase in neutrophil numbers is followed by a decrease in neutrophil numbers (after 23 days in dogs and as early as day 14 and after 17 to 21 days in cats), which in the case of healthy dogs is due to the formation of antibodies directed against the product. Antibody formation apparently does not occur in dogs with cancer that are receiving the drug. It is suggested that the drug only be used as aforementioned, for short courses only, and that it be discontinued 2 days after segmented neutrophil numbers exceed 3,000/μL. The most common adverse effect reported in people is medullary bone pain, which in most cases is readily controlled with nonopioid analgesics. Other less common adverse effects in people include exacerbation of skin disease (psoriasis, cutaneous vasculitis), hematuria, proteinuria, and thrombocytopenia. Long-term (up to 4.5 years) adverse effects in people include osteoporosis. No systemic toxicity has been noted in cats. There is the possibility that filgrastim may potentiate the growth of certain tumor types, particularly myeloid malignancies.

DRUG INTERACTIONS: Because of the potential sensitivity of rapidly dividing myeloid cells to cytotoxic chemotherapy, filgrastim should not be given 24 hours before or after cytotoxic chemotherapy is administered. The efficacy of this agent in patients receiving nitrosourea compounds or with myelosuppressive dosages of 5-fluorouracil or cytosine arabinoside has not been established. Nor has filgrastim's safety and efficacy been established in those patients undergoing concurrent radiation therapy.

SUPPLIED AS HUMAN PRODUCTS:
For injection containing 300 μg/mL
In a syrup containing 600 μg/mL

GRISEOFULVIN

INDICATIONS: Griseofulvin (Fulvicin U/F ♣ ★) is used for the treatment of dermatophyte infections. The drug is detectable in the skin within 4 to 8 hours of oral administration. High dietary fat facilitates absorption.

ADVERSE AND COMMON SIDE EFFECTS: Nausea, vomiting, and diarrhea are the most common side effects. Hepatotoxicity and photosensitization also have been reported but are rare. Cats, especially kittens, are more sensitive to the adverse effects of the drug. Anemia and panleukopenia also have been documented. Seropositive cats with FIV are at increased risk for griseofulvin-associated neutropenia. Anorexia, dehydration, edema of the skin and mucosae, pruritus, and ataxia also have been reported in cats. The drug may inhibit spermatogenesis and is potentially teratogenic and mutagenic in a number of species and may cause cleft palate, skeletal, and brain malformations in kittens if administered during the first trimester of pregnancy.

DRUG INTERACTIONS: Phenobarbital decreases absorption of the drug. Coumarin anticoagulant activity may be reduced by griseofulvin. Vaccination or viral infection induce interferon synthesis, which in turn inhibits hepatic enzyme systems and may prolong the elimination of griseofulvin.

SUPPLIED AS VETERINARY PRODUCT:
Tablets (microsize) containing 250 and 500 mg ★

SUPPLIED AS HUMAN PRODUCT:
Tablets (microsize) containing 125, 250, 330, and 500 mg ✤ ★

GUAIFENESIN

INDICATIONS: Guaifenesin (Guiatuss ★, Organidin NR ★, Robitussin ✤ ★, Benylin ✤ ★, Anti-Tuss ★, Breonesin ★, Fenesin ★, Glytuss ★, Humibid ★), formerly glyceryl guaiacolate, is used as an adjunct to anesthesia to induce muscle relaxation and restraint for short procedures. In humans, the drug is used as an expectorant in the management of dry, unproductive cough. It stimulates gastric receptors that initiate a reflex secretion of bronchial glands, thereby increasing the volume and decreasing the viscosity of bronchial secretions. Its efficacy in improving mucociliary clearance, however, is questionable.

ADVERSE AND COMMON SIDE EFFECTS: A mild decrease in blood pressure and an increase in heart rate may occur. Thrombophlebitis has been reported, and perivascular injection may cause tissue reaction. Hemolysis may occur if solutions greater than 5% concentration are used. If overdose occurs, apneustic breathing, nystagmus, hypotension, and paradoxical muscle rigidity have been noted. With oral preparations, nausea, gastric upset, and drowsiness are reported in people. The drug may prolong activated clotting time and impair platelet function. It should be avoided in animals with bleeding tendencies. Because it is a creosote derivative, it should probably not be given to cats.

DRUG INTERACTIONS: Physostigmine and other cholinesterase agents, e.g., neostigmine, pyridostigmine, and edrophonium, are contraindicated with its use.

SUPPLIED AS HUMAN PRODUCTS:
Capsules containing 200 mg
Extended release capsules containing 300 mg

Liquid containing 100 mg/5 mL and 200 mg/5 mL
Syrup containing 50 mg/5 mL and 100 mg/5 mL
Tablets containing 100 mg and 200 mg
Extended release tablets containing 575 mg, 600 mg, 800 mg, 1000 mg, and 1200 mg

HALOTHANE

INDICATIONS: Halothane (Fluothane ✤ ★, Halothane ✤ ★) is an inhalant anesthetic agent. It is a fast, potent anesthetic that allows for smooth induction without excitement and a quick uneventful recovery.

ADVERSE AND COMMON SIDE EFFECTS: Dose-dependent hypotension has been documented. Hepatic necrosis, although rare, may occur with the use of halothane, the incidence of which increases with each use of this agent. Should unexplained fever, jaundice, or other signs of liver dysfunction occur after use of the drug, its subsequent use in that animal is contraindicated. High doses of halothane may cause uterine atony and postpartum bleeding, and generally, it is not recommended for obstetric procedures unless uterine relaxation is required.

DRUG INTERACTIONS: The drug is potentially arrhythmogenic, especially in the presence of epinephrine and the thiobarbiturates. D-Tubocurare causes a marked decrease in blood pressure when used with halothane.

SUPPLIED AS VETERINARY AND HUMAN PRODUCTS:
Halothane is supplied in 250-mL bottles

HEPARIN

INDICATIONS: Heparin may be indicated in cases of aortic and venous thrombosis, pulmonary thromboembolic disease, and disseminated intravascular coagulation (DIC). It inactivates thrombin, blocks the conversion of fibrinogen to fibrin, and—in combination with antithrombin III—inactivates factors IX, X, XI, and XII and prevents the formation of a stable fibrin clot via the inactivation of factor XIII. Heparin does not lyse clots. The drug promotes resolution of thromboemboli by preventing deposition of fibrin and platelets on the thrombin surface, inhibiting thrombus formation and allowing natural thrombolytic mechanisms to decrease the size of the thrombus. In the case of burn victims, heparin has been used to increase the effectiveness of repair mechanisms, decrease thrombosis and the development of gangrene, and protect against the development of DIC. Heparin not only has anticoagulant and antithromboembolic properties, it also has antiallergic, antiviral, antiendotoxic, and antiinflammatory properties as well.

Low-molecular weight heparin [Enoxaparin] has superior bioavailability at low dosages and more predictable anticoagulant response. It may be useful in the management of inflammatory bowel disease.

ADVERSE AND COMMON SIDE EFFECTS: Bleeding and thrombocytopenia are the most common adverse effects of the drug, leading to prolonged activated partial thromboplastin time (APTT). Protamine zinc may be used to reverse the adverse effects of bleeding. Intramuscular injection can result in hematoma formation. Other side effects reported have included osteoporosis with long-term use, diminished renal function after long-term use, high-dose therapy, rebound hyperlipidemia, hyperkalemia, alopecia, suppressed aldosterone synthesis, and priapism. Standard screening tests, e.g., thrombin time, APTT, are not useful for monitoring the anticoagulant efficacy of low-molecular weight heparin.

DRUG INTERACTIONS: Heparin may antagonize the action of corticosteroids, insulin, and ACTH and increase serum levels of diazepam. Antihistamines, IV nitroglycerin, digoxin, and tetracyclines may antagonize the effects of heparin. Heparin should be used with caution with other drugs that may adversely affect coagulation, e.g., aspirin, phenylbutazone, dipyridamole, or warfarin.

SUPPLIED AS HUMAN PRODUCTS:
For injection containing 1,000, 5,000, 10,000, 20,000, and 40,000 U/mL ★
For injection containing 100, 1,000, 10,000, and 25,000 U/mL [Heparin Leo ✚]

OTHER USES
Dogs
HEARTWORM DISEASE
300 U/kg tid; SC (prevention of pulmonary thromboembolism associated with adulticide therapy)

HEPARIN STIMULATION TEST
100 U/kg; IV to stimulate lipoprotein lipase
A lack of increase in lipolytic activity is suggestive of lipoprotein lipase inactivity.

DISSEMINATED INTRAVASCULAR COAGULATION
i)   5 to 10 U/kg per hour by continuous intravenous infusion
ii) 75 U/kg tid; SC

Monitoring of APTT at these dosages is not necessary because the risk of bleeding is minimal.

PULMONARY THROMBOEMBOLISM
200 U/kg; IV followed by 100 to 200 U/kg qid; SC or 15 to 20 U/kg per hour IV infusion adjusted to prolong APTT by 1.5 to 2.0 times baseline

values. Warfarin is recommended if anticoagulant therapy is required for longer periods. Warfarin requires 2 to 7 days to become effective. A dose of 0.2 mg/kg; PO is used initially, followed by 0.05 to 0.10 mg/kg per day to maintain prothrombin time (PT) 1.5 to 2 times baseline values. Heparin therapy is tapered gradually and discontinued when desired PT is achieved.

Cats

ACUTE ARTERIAL EMBOLIZATION
100 U/kg tid; SC

AORTIC THROMBOEMBOLISM
Heparin 100 U/kg; tid; SC in conjunction with warfarin 0.5 mg/day; PO. Discontinue heparin after 3 to 4 days. Adjust warfarin dose to maintain international normalized ratio (INR) PT, which is the patient's PT divided by control PT, to 2 to 3.

HETASTARCH

INDICATIONS: Hetastarch or hydroxyethyl starch (Hespan ★) is a colloidal plasma volume expander used in cases requiring intravascular volume expansion, e.g., shock. It also has been used successfully to manage patients with hypoalbuminemia with or without accompanying peripheral edema or body cavity transudates. The product is eliminated primarily by the kidneys. Hetastarch has a half-life of 25 hours in plasma. Intravenous infusion of 1 L of hetastarch expands plasma volume by approximately 700 mL, with 40% of the resultant increase in plasma volume persisting approximately 24 to 36 hours. A recent study in dogs with hypoalbuminemia, however, demonstrated that a single dose of hetastarch raised colloid oncotic pressure for less than 12 hours, indicating that multiple doses may be required to prolong the beneficial effects.

ADVERSE AND COMMON SIDE EFFECTS: Large volumes may adversely affect coagulation and cause a decrease in platelet numbers and a prolongation of prothrombin time, partial thromboplastin time, and clotting times. Large volumes may decrease the hematocrit, lower serum potassium, and cause dilution of plasma proteins. In people, serum amylase levels may be increased with administration of the product as a result of drug binding and reduced excretion. Hypervolemia may occur, and patients with congestive heart failure or anuric renal failure are at increased risk. Because the product is eliminated via the kidneys, caution is advised if it is used in patients with renal insufficiency. Other adverse effects reported in people include vomiting, pruritus, chills, elevated body temperature, muscle pain, edema of the extremities, and anaphylaxis. Colloids can exacerbate pulmonary edema in cases with increased microvascular permeability, and interstitial edema and alveolar flooding may occur if the alveolar epithelium is also damaged.

DRUG INTERACTIONS: None established.

SUPPLIED AS HUMAN PRODUCT:
For injection containing 6% hetastarch in 0.9% sodium chloride

OTHER USES
Dogs
HYPOALBUMINEMIA
25 to 30 mL/kg over 6 to 8 hours; IV. A second dose may be given immediately after the first without concurrent crystalloid fluid administration in cases of severe hypoalbuminemia combined with intravascular volume depletion and moderate to marked peripheral edema or body cavity effusions. In less severe cases, give concurrent crystalloids at approximately two thirds of the daily dosing requirements. Most dogs require at least 2 doses of hetastarch given 12 to 24 hours apart.

HYDRALAZINE

INDICATIONS: Hydralazine (Apresoline ♣ ★) is an arterial vasodilator. It facilitates increased cardiac output and decreases mitral regurgitation and left atrial size. It helps alleviate the cough associated with compression of the left principal bronchus from enlargement of the left atrium secondary to mitral valvular regurgitation. The drug also is used to manage systemic hypertension, often in conjunction with a diuretic and a β blocker.

ADVERSE AND COMMON SIDE EFFECTS: Hypotension, increases in heart rate, sodium and water retention, vomiting, diarrhea, and tolerance to the drug have been described. Initial weakness and lethargy, which generally resolve in 3 to 4 days, may be noted.

DRUG INTERACTIONS: Phenylpropanolamine may exacerbate the tachycardia associated with use of hydralazine. Hydralazine may increase the absorption of propranolol and other β blockers; in addition, the concurrent use of β blockers or diazoxide may predispose to hypotension. The pressor response to epinephrine may be mitigated by hydralazine.

SUPPLIED AS HUMAN PRODUCTS:
Tablets containing 10, 25, 50, and 100 mg
For injection containing 20 mg/mL

HYDROCHLOROTHIAZIDE

INDICATIONS: Hydrochlorothiazide (HydroDiuril ★, Apo-Hydro ♣) is a diuretic used to decrease pulmonary edema in patients with congestive heart failure and cardiomyopathy. It is a less potent diuretic than furosemide. The drug (2 mg/kg bid; PO) also may be beneficial in reducing the recurrence of calcium oxalate urolithiasis, especially when used concurrently with Hill's Prescription Diet U/D.

ADVERSE AND COMMON SIDE EFFECTS: Hypokalemia, hypochloremic alkalosis, dilutional hyponatremia, and loss of water-soluble vitamins may occur with chronic use. Other side effects may include vomiting, diarrhea, polyuria, hyperglycemia, hyperlipidemia, hypotension, and hypersensitivity/dermatologic reactions.

DRUG INTERACTIONS: Concurrent use with corticosteroids or amphotericin B may predispose to hypokalemia. Thiazide hypokalemia predisposes to digitalis toxicity, and hydrochlorothiazide may prolong the half-life of quinidine. Sulfonamides may potentiate the action of hydrochlorothiazide. Hydrochlorothiazide may increase the activity of tubocurarine. The concurrent use of diazoxide may predispose to hyperglycemia, hypotension, and hyperuricemia. This drug also may alter the requirements of insulin.

SUPPLIED AS HUMAN PRODUCT:
Tablets containing 25, 50, and 100 mg

OTHER USES
Dogs
NEPHROGENIC DIABETES INSIPIDUS
i)   0.5 to 1 mg/kg bid; PO

ii) 2.5 to 5 mg/kg bid; PO

SYSTEMIC HYPERTENSION
2 to 4 mg/kg once to twice daily; PO (along with dietary salt restriction)

HYPOGLYCEMIA
2 to 4 mg/kg bid; PO (along with diazoxide)

HYDROCHLOROTHIAZIDE-SPIRONOLACTONE

INDICATIONS: Hydrochlorothiazide-spironolactone (Aldactazide ★, Spirozide ★, Novo-Spirozine ♣) acts at Henle's loop and the proximal and distal convoluted tubules, exerting a synergistic diuretic effect. The principal advantage of this combination is its potassium-sparing effect. The onset of action is slower, and its effect is longer lasting. In humans, this drug combination is recommended in patients with congestive heart failure unresponsive or poorly tolerant to other diuretics, diuretic-induced hypokalemia in those requiring diuretic therapy, cirrhosis of the liver accompanied by edema and/or ascites, essential hypertension, and nephrotic syndrome unresponsive to glucocorticoids or other diuretics.

ADVERSE AND COMMON SIDE EFFECTS: Aldactazide should not be used in patients with anuria, acute renal insufficiency, or hyperkalemia, or those sensitive to spironolactone or thiazide agents. In humans, adverse effects may include nausea, anorexia, vomiting, cramping, diarrhea or constipation, jaundice, acute pancreatitis, leukopenia, thrombocytopenia, agranulocytosis, aplastic anemia, impotence, abnormal sperm motility or counts, and irregularities of the menstrual cycle.

DRUG INTERACTIONS: Spironolactone has been shown to increase the half-life of digoxin and may result in digitalis toxicity. The drug may alter insulin requirements in diabetic patients.

SUPPLIED AS HUMAN PRODUCT:
Tablets containing 25 and 50 mg

HYDROCODONE

INDICATIONS: Hydrocodone (Hycodan ♣ ★) is a narcotic antitussive that is especially useful in the control of cough not responsive to other agents. The drug also has been used to treat compulsive, behaviorally related skin disorders.

ADVERSE AND COMMON SIDE EFFECTS: Sedation, vomiting, and constipation with chronic use may occur. In cats, opiate agonists may cause CNS excitation with hyperexcitability, tremors, and seizure activity.

DRUG INTERACTIONS: Antihistamines, phenothiazines, barbiturates, and other CNS depressants may potentiate CNS depression.

SUPPLIED AS HUMAN PRODUCTS:
Tablets containing 5 mg
Syrup containing 1 mg/mL

OTHER USES
Dogs
BEHAVIORAL DISORDERS
0.22 mg/kg bid to tid; PO

Cats
BEHAVIORAL DISORDERS
0.25 to 1 mg/kg bid to tid; PO

HYDROCORTISONE SODIUM SUCCINATE

INDICATIONS: Hydrocortisone sodium succinate (Solu-Cortef ❦ ★) is a glucocorticoid used primarily in cases of shock, feline asthma, and animals in acute hypoadrenocortical crisis. For information concerning ADVERSE AND COMMON SIDE EFFECTS and DRUG INTERACTIONS, see GLUCOCORTICOID AGENTS.

SUPPLIED AS HUMAN PRODUCT:
For injection containing 100, 250, 500, and 1,000 mg/vial

HYDROXYUREA

INDICATIONS: Hydroxyurea (Hydrea ❦ ★) is a chemotherapeutic agent used in the treatment of leukemia, mastocytoma, primary polycythemia (polycythemia vera), polycythemia secondary to right to left shunting patent ductus arteriosus, and essential thrombocythemia.

ADVERSE AND COMMON SIDE EFFECTS: In the dog, anorexia, vomiting, arrest of spermatogenesis, bone marrow hypoplasia, and sloughing of the nails have been reported. A complete blood count and platelet count should be done every 7 to 14 days until the hematocrit has normalized and repeated every 3 to 4 months thereafter. If leukopenia, thrombocytopenia, or anemia develop, the drug should be discontinued until blood counts return to normal. The drug should then be resumed at a lower dose. Other side effects may include transient hair loss, skin pigment changes, stomatitis, and dysuria.

DRUG INTERACTIONS: None established.

SUPPLIED AS HUMAN PRODUCT:
Capsules containing 500 mg

OTHER USES
Dogs
PRIMARY POLYCYTHEMIA
30 mg/kg daily for 5 to 7 days, then 15 mg/kg daily; PO
*POLYCYTHEMIA SECONDARY TO RIGHT
TO LEFT SHUNTING PDA*
40 to 50 mg/kg every 48 hours; PO
ESSENTIAL THROMBOCYTHEMIA

Dogs

25 to 50 mg/kg per day; PO for 10 days or until platelet counts return to normal at which time dose is reduced to 15 mg/kg per day

Cats

125 mg/cat every 24 to 48 hours; PO

HYDROXYZINE

INDICATIONS: Hydroxyzine (Atarax ❧ ★) is an anxiolytic, antihistaminic agent. It has been used to manage some behavioral disorders, e.g., compulsive scratching and self-trauma, and to provide mild sedation. The drug also has anticholinergic, antiemetic, and bronchodilator effects. It has been used in small animals primarily for its antihistaminic properties. For more information concerning ADVERSE AND COMMON SIDE EFFECTS and DRUG INTERACTIONS, see ANTIHISTAMINES.

ADVERSE AND COMMON SIDE EFFECTS: Transitory drowsiness is the most common side effect. Other adverse effects may include fine rapid tremors, seizures, xerostomia, hypotension, diarrhea, and decreased appetite.

DRUG INTERACTIONS: Barbiturates and other sedatives may potentiate CNS depression.

SUPPLIED AS HUMAN PRODUCTS:
Capsules containing 10, 25, and 50 mg
Syrup containing 10 mg/5 mL
For injection containing 50 mg/mL

IBUPROFEN

INDICATIONS: Ibuprofen (Advil ❧ ★, Motrin ❧ ★) is a nonsteroidal anti-inflammatory agent with antipyretic and analgesic properties that make it useful in the management of joint pain secondary to degenerative joint disease. However, the drug is not routinely recommended because of its GI side effects and the availability of other safer NSAIDs, e.g., aspirin, meloxicam.

ADVERSE AND COMMON SIDE EFFECTS: The drug appears to cause gastric irritation and ulceration more frequently in dogs than it does in people. Toxicity develops in dogs at a dosage of 50 to 125 mg/kg and may include vomiting, depression, diarrhea, anorexia, ataxia and incoordination, and melena. Polyuria-polydipsia may occur. Hemorrhagic gastroenteritis can be severe and lead to perforation. Less often, ataxia and stupor have been reported. Cats appear less prone to gastro-enteritis, but are more apt to show tachypnea.

DRUG INTERACTIONS: Use of heparin and other anticoagulants may augment ibuprofen's inhibition of platelet aggregation, predisposing to bleeding. The pharmacological activity of lithium may be increased if both drugs are used concurrently.

SUPPLIED AS HUMAN PRODUCT:
Tablets containing 200, 300, 400, and 600 mg

IMIPENEM-CILASTATIN

INDICATIONS: Imipenem-cilastatin (Primaxin ❖ ★) is a fixed combination of a β-lactam antibiotic and cilastatin, an inhibitor of the dipeptidase that inactivates imipenem. This drug combination has the widest antibacterial spectrum of any β-lactam antibiotic, surpassing even that of the third-generation cephalosporins. The spectrum of activity includes gram-positive, gram-negative, anaerobic bacteria, *Acinetobacter baumannii*, and *Pseudomonas aeruginosa*. Infections resistant to cephalosporins, penicillins, and aminoglycosides often respond favorably to this combination.

ADVERSE AND COMMON SIDE EFFECTS: The drug combination is contraindicated in patients with hypersensitivity to penicillins or cephalosporins. Cautious use is recommended in patients with a history of seizures, brain lesions, recent head injury, or renal impairment. Drug dosage should be reduced in cases of renal failure. Nausea, salivation, vomiting, diarrhea, pain upon injection, phlebitis at the infusion site, fever, pruritus, tachycardia, hypotension, and seizure activity have been reported. Safe use during pregnancy has not been established.

DRUG INTERACTIONS: The antibacterial effect of imipenem and aminoglycosides is additive or synergistic against some gram-positive bacteria. Imipenem antagonizes the antibacterial activity of other β-lactam antibiotics, including most cephalosporins and extended spectrum penicillins against *P. aeruginosa* and some strains of *Enterobacter* and *Klebsiella*. Chloramphenicol may antagonize the bactericidal activity of imipenem.

SUPPLIED AS HUMAN PRODUCT:
For injection containing 250 and 500 mg

IMIPRAMINE

INDICATIONS: Imipramine (Tofranil ❖ ★) is a tricyclic antidepressant, structurally related to phenothiazines and used in dogs for the treatment of canine narcolepsy/cataplexy, separation anxiety, and lick granuloma. The drug also has been used to manage cases of urinary sphincter incontinence.

ADVERSE AND COMMON SIDE EFFECTS: In humans, hypotension, tachycardia, arrhythmias, anxiety, ataxia, seizure, constipation, mydriasis, urinary retention, pruritus, anorexia, vomiting, diarrhea, jaundice, and bone marrow suppression leading to granulocytopenia and thrombocytopenia have been documented. Experience with the drug in small animals is limited.

DRUG INTERACTIONS: Barbiturates potentiate the adverse effects but decrease serum levels of imipramine. Cimetidine increases serum levels. Phenothiazines may enhance the drug's effects. Thyroid medication may potentiate tachycardia and arrhythmias when used concurrently with imipramine.

SUPPLIED AS HUMAN PRODUCT:
Tablets containing 10, 25, 50, and 75 mg

OTHER USES
Dogs
URINARY SPHINCTER INCONTINENCE
5 to 15 mg bid; PO

BEHAVIORAL PROBLEMS
2.2 to 4.4 mg/kg once to twice daily; PO

Cats
URINARY SPHINCTER INCONTINENCE
2.5 to 5 mg bid; PO

BEHAVIORAL PROBLEMS
1 to 2 mg/kg bid to tid; PO

IMMUNOGLOBULIN

INDICATIONS: Pooled human immunoglobulin, primarily IgG (Iveegam ♣ ★, Gamimune ♣ ★), has been used in the treatment of autoimmune hemolytic anemia and immune-mediated thrombocytopenia. It blocks the F_c receptor on macrophages, enhances C_8 function, causes suppression of polyclonal B biosynthesis, inhibits inflammation, and blocks the uptake of antibody-coated cells in the spleen. In one study, the drug improved short-term survival of dogs with autoimmune hemolytic anemia, but it did not improve long-term survival, i.e., survival longer than 1 year. In another study, an 85% response rate was observed in dogs unresponsive to conventional immunosuppressive therapy alone.

ADVERSE AND COMMON SIDE EFFECTS: Experience with use of the drug in small animals is limited; however, no adverse effects have been documented with its use in dogs thus far. In humans, IV use has been associated with nausea, chills, wheezing, skeletal pain, abdominal cramps, and anaphylaxis.

DRUG INTERACTIONS: Antibodies in immunoglobulin may interfere with response to live virus vaccines. In humans, it is recommended that live virus vaccines be given 14 days before or 3 months after use of this agent.

SUPPLIED AS HUMAN PRODUCT:
For injection containing 4.5% to 5.5% protein containing approximately 50 mg/mL protein

INAMRINONE (FORMERLY AMRINONE)

INDICATIONS: Inamrinone (Inocor ★) is a positive inotropic agent with mild arteriolar dilating properties. It is of potential benefit in increasing cardiac output and decreasing pulmonary capillary pressure in animals with congestive heart failure and cardiomyopathy.

ADVERSE AND COMMON SIDE EFFECTS: Although side effects are rare, anorexia, nausea, vomiting, diarrhea, tachycardia, arrhythmias, and hypotension may be seen. The drug should be used with caution in patients with compromised renal or hepatic function or aortic stenosis.

DRUG INTERACTIONS: If used with disopyramide, excessive hypotension may occur.

SUPPLIED AS HUMAN PRODUCT:
For injection containing 5 mg/mL

INDOMETHACIN

INDICATIONS: Indomethacin (Indocid ✤ ★, Indocin ★) is a nonsteroidal anti-inflammatory agent recommended by some clinicians for the management of joint pain secondary to degenerative joint disease. Use of the drug, however, has been associated with hepatotoxicity in dogs and cats and fatal GI hemorrhage in dogs, and because of the availability of other suitable NSAID agents, it is not recommended by this author for use in small animals.

INNOVAR-VET

INDICATIONS: Innovar-Vet ✤ ★ is a combination of droperidol and fentanyl citrate. The drug has tranquilizing and analgesic properties and is used as a preanesthetic sedative or as an anesthetic induction agent. Given intramuscularly, it provides 30 to 40 minutes of analgesia.

ADVERSE AND COMMON SIDE EFFECTS: Respiratory depression and centrally mediated vagal bradycardia occur. A standard dose of atropine may be used to reverse or prevent the bradycardia. Naloxone (0.4 mg; IM, IV, SC) counters the respiratory depression of 0.4 mg fentanyl. Intramuscular injection may be associated with local pain, nystagmus, flatulence, and defecation. Salivation and bradycardia may occur, especially in those not pretreated with atropine. Innovar-Vet may cause panting. Some patients still may respond to loud noises and mechanical stimulation. Analgesia and tranquility may not be obtained in some dogs with this drug combination, especially Australian terriers. Behavioral changes, including aggression, have been reported in some dogs after its use. The drug should not be used in animals with significant renal or hepatic disease or in those in which respiration is depressed. Perivascular injection is irritating to surrounding tissues. Overdose may cause tonic-clonic convulsions and long-lasting extension and rigidity of the neck, which may be antagonized by small IV doses (6.6 mg/kg) of sodium pentobarbital. The drug causes CNS excitation in cats and is not recommended in this species.

DRUG INTERACTIONS: Tranquilizers, antitussives, or analgesics must not be given in conjunction with or for at least 8 hours after use of Innovar-Vet. Sodium pentobarbital has an additive effect and should not be used for 4 hours after use of Innovar-Vet.

SUPPLIED AS VETERINARY PRODUCT:
For injection containing 0.628 mg/mL fentanyl citrate and 20 mg/mL droperidol

INSULIN

INDICATIONS: Insulin preparations ✤ ★ are used in the management of diabetes mellitus. Although the clinical significance of insulin resistance due to insulin antibodies in small animals is unknown, dog insulin and pork insulin are identical in structure, and pork insulin may be expected to be less antigenic than beef insulin. In the cat, beef insulin is more similar to cat insulin. Protamine zinc insulin is the only insulin available as a beef formulation (Blue Ridge Pharmaceuticals Inc, Greensboro, NC).

Regular insulin has the fastest onset of action and the shortest duration. Semilente insulin also is classified as a short-acting insulin but is only available as a component of Lente insulin.

Intermediate-acting insulins include isophane insulin suspension (NPH) and insulin zinc suspension (Lente insulin). Lente is a mixture of Semilente (3 parts) and Ultralente insulin (7 parts). Lente insulin is the insulin of choice for the dog with uncomplicated diabetes. If the duration of effect of NPH or Lente or Ultralente insulin is 10 to 14 hours, administer it twice daily. If the duration of NPH or Lente insulin is less than 10 hours, switch to Ultralente insulin given once or twice daily. If NPH or Lente insulin has a duration of effect of 16 to 20 hours and clinical signs of hyperglycemia are present, consider changing to Ultralente insulin.

Long-acting insulin formulations include Ultralente insulin. Human insulin preparations (Humulin and Novolin) appear better absorbed than beef/pork insulin in cats. The dosage of Ultralente Humulin insulin is approximately 1 to 4 units per cat. Ultralente is the insulin of choice for the uncomplicated diabetic cat. If Ultralente insulin has a duration of effect of 16 to 20 hours in the dog and clinical signs of hyperglycemia are present, consider a supplemental dose of regular insulin administered in the late evening. Otherwise, discontinue the Ultralente insulin and replace it with Lente or NPH administered twice daily.

Peak effect and duration of activity, as listed below, serve as guidelines only and will vary according to individual response and the effects of diet, exercise, and concurrent illness. Caninsulin is a product specifically designed for use in dogs and cats. It is a purified porcine insulin consisting of 30% amorphous and 70% crystalline zinc insulin. The amorphous fraction reaches its maximum effect approximately 3 hours after SC injection, and the total duration of effect lasts about 8 hours. The crystalline zinc portion has an onset of action of 7 to 12 hours and a total duration of activity of approximately 24 hours.

Insulin mixtures of rapid-acting and intermediate-acting insulins also are available. Some authors have used insulin mixtures in diabetic dogs that required twice daily NPH insulin. In these patients, a mixture of 1 part regular insulin and 3 parts Ultralente was effective. Early peak activity was noted within 2 to 4 hours, a second peak occurred 10 to 12 hours later, and total duration of activity was 20 to 24 hours. When mixing insulins in the same syringe, the short-acting insulin should be drawn up first. Feeding several small meals is preferable to feeding one large meal. For diabetics receiving one injection per day, a suitable feeding schedule would consist of three equally sized meals fed at 6-hour intervals. Dogs receiving two injections of insulin per day would benefit best from four equally sized meals: immediately after each insulin injection, at mid-afternoon, and at late evening.

ADVERSE AND COMMON SIDE EFFECTS: Overdose may cause hypoglycemia, leading to disorientation, weakness, hunger, seizure, coma, and death. If overdose occurs, the animal should be fed sugar with water or food. If seizures occur, dextrose solutions should be given intravenously until seizure activity stops. If poor SC absorption is present, changing the type of insulin to a more potent form may be useful. Insulins in increasing order of potency include Ultralente, Lente, NPH, Semilente, and regular crystalline insulin.

DRUG INTERACTIONS: Anabolic steroids, including stanozolol, β-blocking agents, including propranolol and metoprolol, phenylbutazone, tetracycline, aspirin, and other salicylates may potentiate hypoglycemia induced by insulin. Glucocorticoids, dobutamine, epinephrine, estrogens, progesterones, furosemide, and thiazide diuretics may antagonize the hypoglycemic effects of insulin. Similarly, thyroid preparations may increase blood glucose levels in diabetic patients when thyroid preparations are first initiated. Insulin preparations may alter serum potassium levels, which is of importance in those receiving digitalis, especially if the patient is also receiving a diuretic.

SUPPLIED AS HUMAN PRODUCTS:
ELI LILLY
Humulin 100 units/mL—regular, NPH, Lente, Ultralente
Humalog 100 units/mL—Insulin Lispro (rapid acting, short duration)

NOVO-NORDISK
Novolin ge 100 units/mL—regular, NPH, Lente, Ultralente plus premixes

SUPPLIED AS VETERINARY PRODUCTS:
Caninsulin ♣ containing 40 U/mL (pork source). See manufacturer's instructions for dosage and use of the product.

BLUE RIDGE PHARMACEUTICALS
PZI Insulin (beef/pork) 40 units/mL

OTHER USES
Dogs
ADJUNCTIVE TREATMENT OF HYPERKALEMIA
5 U/kg per hour regular insulin; IV with 2 g glucose/unit of insulin given

Cats
ADJUNCTIVE TREATMENT OF HYPERKALEMIA
0.5 U/kg regular insulin; IV with 2 g of glucose/unit of insulin

INTERFERON

INDICATIONS: Interferon (Roferon A ♣ ★) has immunomodulating and antiproliferative capabilities and antiviral activity. It has been used in the treatment of FeLV infection. In one study, treated cats improved clinically, and hematocrit values returned to normal. In a second study, cats improved clinically (increased appetite, weight gain, increased physical activity, loss of fever), peripheral blood values improved, and recovery from secondary bacterial infections improved when antibiotics were used. Despite treatment, 95% of cats remained persistently viremic. However, because adequate controls were not included in these studies, definitive conclusions concerning the efficacy of this agent in this disease cannot be made. A more recent study failed to demonstrate any beneficial effects in clinically ill FeLV-infected cats. Experimentally, the drug also has been used alone or in combination with *Propionibacterium acnes* in cats with feline infectious peritonitis, where the combination apparently suppressed clinical signs of the disease and prolonged survival. The drug combination did not prevent death.

ADVERSE AND COMMON SIDE EFFECTS: None were observed in the cats in the studies noted here. In humans, however, hypersensitivity may develop, and nausea, anorexia, vomiting, diarrhea, fever, somnolence, depression, seizure, and coma have been reported.

DRUG INTERACTIONS: Interferon-α-2a may affect CNS function, and interaction with other centrally acting drugs is possible.

SUPPLIED AS HUMAN PRODUCT:
Solution containing 3, 6, or 9 million IU/mL

Note: Dilute the 3 million IU into 1 L of sterile saline, which then can be divided into aliquots of 1 to 10 mL and frozen. The original stock solution (3 million IU) can be frozen for years without losing activity. Once reconstituted, it can be stored in a refrigerator (4°C) for several months without losing activity. The activity of the diluted solution after frozen storage is unknown.

IPECAC

INDICATIONS: Syrup of ipecac ♣ ★ is a useful emetic agent. It acts via gastric irritation and stimulation of the medullary chemoreceptor trigger zone. Only half of the patients that the formulation is given to will vomit.

ADVERSE AND COMMON SIDE EFFECTS: At regular doses, side effects are rare but may include lacrimation, salivation, and an increase in bronchial secretions. In humans, diarrhea and lethargy also may occur. With drug overdose, syrup of ipecac is potentially cardiotoxic, leading to arrhythmias, hypotension, and fatal myocarditis. The total dose should not exceed 15 mL (1 tablespoon).

DRUG INTERACTIONS: Syrup of ipecac should not be used with activated charcoal because the charcoal will decrease the activity of ipecac. Vomiting may be induced initially with syrup of ipecac and then followed by activated charcoal.

SUPPLIED AS HUMAN PRODUCT:
Oral syrup available in 15- and 30-mL and pint and gallon bottles

IRON DEXTRAN

INDICATIONS: Iron dextran is indicated for the treatment of iron deficiency anemia.

ADVERSE AND COMMON SIDE EFFECTS: Intramuscular injection can be irritating. Allergic reactions and anaphylaxis occasionally have been reported in humans.

DRUG INTERACTIONS: Clinical response may be delayed in patients concurrently receiving chloramphenicol.

SUPPLIED AS VETERINARY PRODUCT:
For injection containing 100 and 200 mg elemental iron/mL [Ferrodex ★, Ironol-100 ♣, and generic products]

ISOFLURANE

INDICATIONS: Isoflurane (Forane ♣ ★, Isoflo ♣ ★) is an inhalant anesthetic agent that is especially useful for short surgical procedures. It is well tolerated in debilitated patients and those with hepatic or renal impairment. Induction and recovery times are more rapid with isoflurane than with halothane. Cardiovascular status is better maintained with isoflurane, and isoflurane does not sensitize the heart to epinephrine-induced cardiac arrhythmias as does halothane.

ADVERSE AND COMMON SIDE EFFECTS: Dose-dependent cardiac and respiratory depression occurs. Hypotension, respiratory depression, arrhythmias, nausea, vomiting, and postoperative ileus have been reported.

DRUG INTERACTIONS: Isoflurane potentiates the effects of muscle relaxants.

SUPPLIED AS VETERINARY AND HUMAN PRODUCTS:
Supplied in 100- and 250-mL bottles

ISOPROTERENOL

INDICATIONS: Isoproterenol ♣ ★ is a β-adrenergic agent used for the short-term management of incomplete heart block, sinus bradycardia, and sick sinus syndrome. The drug increases atrioventricular conduction and ventricular excitability. It also causes peripheral vascular dilation and bronchial smooth muscle relaxation and is used to promote bronchodilation.

ADVERSE AND COMMON SIDE EFFECTS: Vomiting, nervous excitation, weakness, tachycardia, and ectopic beat formation are reported. The drug is considered more arrhythmogenic than dopamine or dobutamine, so it rarely is used in the treatment of heart failure or shock.

DRUG INTERACTIONS: Digitalis and amitriptyline may have additive effects and lead to arrhythmias if used with isoproterenol. The use of β blockers, e.g., propranolol or metoprolol, may antagonize the β-adrenergic effects of isoproterenol. If used with theophylline, there is a possibility of increased cardiotoxic effects.

SUPPLIED AS HUMAN PRODUCT:
For injection containing 0.2 mg/mL (1:5,000)

OTHER USES
Dogs and Cats
BRONCHODILATION
0.1 to 0.2 mg qid; IM, SC

ISOTRETINOIN

INDICATIONS: Isotretinoin (Accutane ♣ ★) appears to be useful in the treatment of disorders of keratinization, abnormalities in follicular keratinization, and quantitative or qualitative disorders of sebaceous gland secretion, e.g., seborrhea. It appears to cause a reduction in sebum production, has an anti-inflammatory effect, an effect on the microflora population, and an antikeratinizing effect. It has been used successfully to treat sebaceous adenitis in standard poodles, canine lamellar ichthyosis, Schnauzer comedo syndrome, intracutaneous cornifying epitheliomas, multiple epidermal inclusion cysts, idiopathic seborrheic disorders, and cutaneous T-cell lymphoma (mycosis fungoides).

ADVERSE AND COMMON SIDE EFFECTS: The incidence of adverse effects appears to be low. Lethargy, anorexia, vomiting, conjunctivitis, pruritus, polydipsia, erythema of mucocutaneous junctions and feet, hyperactivity, abdominal distention, collapse, and a swollen tongue have been reported. All side effects were reversible on discontinuation of the drug. Occasional laboratory changes include increases in serum triglyceride and cholesterol levels, accompanied by corneal lipid deposits, increases in alanine aminotransferase levels, and thrombocytosis. A higher incidence of side effects has been noted in cats. Erythema, periocular crusting, epiphora, blepharospasm, and diarrhea have been reported. The drug is potentially teratogenic and may inhibit spermatogenesis and should not be used in breeding animals.

DRUG INTERACTIONS: In humans, minocycline and tetracycline may increase the risk of papilledema and cerebral edema.

SUPPLIED AS HUMAN PRODUCT:
Capsules containing 10 and 40 mg

OTHER USES
Dogs
SEBACEOUS ADENITIS
1 mg/kg once daily; PO (Vizslas)

CUTANEOUS LYMPHOMA
3 to 4 mg/kg once daily

INTRACUTANEOUS CORNIFYING EPITHELIOMA
1 to 2 mg/kg daily

ITRACONAZOLE

INDICATIONS: Itraconazole (Sporanox ✤ ★) is active against histoplasmosis, blastomycosis, coccidioidomycosis, and cryptococcosis. It is more effective than amphotericin B or ketoconazole in the treatment of canine nasal aspergillosis and is as effective as a combination of amphotericin B and ketoconazole in the treatment of blastomycosis. The drug also is active against *Microsporum, Trichophyton, Sporothrix, Pythium, Candida, Leishmania,* and *Trypanosoma cruzi.* Unlike ketoconazole, itraconazole may reach adequate levels in the CNS at therapeutic doses. Itraconazole is best absorbed when given with a fatty meal. Treatment should be continued for 1 to 2 months beyond clinical remission.

ADVERSE AND COMMON SIDE EFFECTS: Minimal toxicity has been seen in dogs. Anorexia secondary to hepatotoxicity and vasculitis characterized by ulcerative dermatitis and increases in blood urea nitrogen have been reported. If adverse effects occur, the drug should be discontinued until the appetite returns. Treatment then can be reinstituted at half the original dose. It appears that adequate serum concentrations can be maintained at this decreased dose level. Anorexia and hepatotoxicity, with a concurrent mild to moderate increase in serum alanine aminotransferase activity, are the most frequently observed adverse effects reported in cats. Teratogenic effects have been documented in rat studies. The potential risk versus the benefit must be ascertained in pregnant animals before the drug is used.

DRUG INTERACTIONS: Concurrent use with terfenadine is contraindicated. Rare cases of ventricular tachycardia and death have been reported in people. Itraconazole will cause elevations in plasma levels of calcium channel-blocking agents (amlodipine, verapamil, diltiazem), as well as digoxin, midazolam, quinidine, cyclosporine, and warfarin.

Rifampin and H₂ antagonists given concurrently will lower serum itraconazole levels.

SUPPLIED AS HUMAN PRODUCTS:
Capsules containing 100 mg
Liquid containing 10 mg/mL

OTHER USES
Cats
MICROSPORUM CANIS
i)   10 mg/kg daily; PO

ii)   20 mg/kg every other day; PO

iii) 10 mg/kg per day for 28 days then on alternate weeks (treatment stopped when 2 consecutive negative fungal cultures obtained)

HISTOPLASMOSIS
5 mg/kg bid; PO for 60 or more days

IVERMECTIN

INDICATIONS: Ivermectin (Heartgard ♣ ★, Ivomec ♣ ★, Eqvalan ♣ ★) is used for the eradication of demodectic, sarcoptic, otodectic, and *Cheyletiella* mites in dogs. It also has been used in the treatment of *Capillaria aerophila* and is marketed for the prevention of canine heartworm [Heartgard]. The drug has been used as a microfilaricide in heartworm disease. In fact, ivermectin has been shown to be effective against heartworm infection when 1 year of monthly prophylactic dosing is started as late as 4 months after infection. In cats, the drug has been used for the prevention of heartworm and in the treatment of ear mites, *Cheyletiella blakei, Physaloptera preputialis, Demodex,* and fleas.

ADVERSE AND COMMON SIDE EFFECTS: Ivermectin has a wide margin of safety. In dogs, mydriasis and tremors were noted at doses of 5,000 μg/kg, and more pronounced tremors and ataxia were reported at doses of 10,000 μg/kg. Some collies and related breeds have a variable sensitivity to the drug. The prevalence of sensitivity to the drug in collies ranges from 30% to 40%. Collies suffering from ivermectin toxicity can have a severe and prolonged adverse clinical course with up to 3 weeks for clinical recovery. Clinical improvement is generally noted by day 6 after ivermectin administration.

In approximately 5% of dogs with microfilaremia, vomiting, trembling, tachypnea, and collapse develop within 1 to 4 hours of use of the drug. Fatalities are rare. The drug is not recommended for use in puppies younger than 6 weeks of age. It is apparently safe to use in cats.

DRUG INTERACTIONS: None.

SUPPLIED AS VETERINARY PRODUCTS:

For injection Ivomec 1% (10 mg/mL) (for use in cattle, sheep, and swine)

Oral paste 1.87% (for equine use)

Ivermectin liquid 1% (10 mg/mL) [Eqvalan] (for equine use)

Tablets containing 68, 136, and 272 µg [Heartgard]

Otic suspension containing 0.01% ivermectin [ACAREXX]

OTHER USES

Dogs

OTODECTES CYNOTIS AND SARCOPTES SCABEI

Single dose 200 µg/kg; SC, PO, repeat in 14 days

SARCOPTES SCABEI

i) 0.2 to 0.3 mg/kg; PO, SC given twice 2 weeks apart

ii) 50 µg/kg; PO on day 1, 100 µg/kg on day 2, 150 µg/kg on day 3, 200 µg/kg day 4 to a final dose of 300 µg/kg on day 5, which is continued 4 times at 7-day intervals

DIROFILARIA IMMITIS

i) 50 µg/kg 3 to 4 weeks after adulticide therapy (microfilaricide)

ii) 50 to 200 µg/kg as a single oral dose

iii) 6 µg/kg once monthly; PO (preventative dose)

CHEYLETIELLA YASGURI

300 µg/kg once; SC, repeat in 3 weeks if required

GENERALIZED DEMODICOSIS

i) 400 µg/kg weekly; SC (total of 8 treatments)—efficacy questionable

ii) 0.6 mg/kg daily; PO (median duration of treatment was 10 weeks)

iii) 50 µg/kg; PO on day 1; 100 µg/kg on day 2; 150 µg/kg on day 3; 200 µg/kg day 4 to a final dose of 300 µg/kg on day 5, which is continued daily until resolution

CAPILLARIA SPP.

0.2 mg/kg once; PO

ROUNDWORMS, HOOKWORMS, AND WHIPWORMS

Single dose 200 µg/kg; PO

PNEUMONYSSUS CANINUM

i) 200 µg/kg; SC, repeat in 3 weeks

ii) 200 to 400 µg/kg; SC, PO

STRONGYLOIDES STERCORALIS

200 µg/kg; PO. A second treatment at the same dose may be required.

Cats

ANCYLOSTOMA BRAZILIENSE AND TUBAEFORME

24 µg/kg; PO

OTODECTES CYNOTIS
i)   Single dose 200 μg/kg; SC

ii) Otic solution (0.01%) applied once in ears

NOTOEDRES CATI AND CHEYLETIELLA MITES
Single dose 400 μg/kg; SC

CHEYLETIELLA BLAKEI
300 μg/kg twice at 5 week intervals; SC

DEMODEX
300 μg/kg; SC, 2 weeks apart with concurrent use of 2.5% lime sulfur

PHYSALOPTERA PREPUTIALIS
Single dose 200 μg/kg; SC

HEARTWORM PROPHYLAXIS
24 μg/kg per month; PO

KANAMYCIN

INDICATIONS: Kanamycin (Kantrim ★) is an aminoglycoside anti-biotic with activity against *Staphylococcus aureus* and *albus, Klebsiella pneumonia, Salmonella, Pasteurella, Corynebacterium, Bacillus anthracis, Proteus, E. coli,* and *A. aerobacter.* It penetrates most body fluids other than spinal fluid. Also see AMINOGLYCOSIDES.

ADVERSE AND COMMON SIDE EFFECTS: Impairment of vestibu-lar function or irreversible hearing loss may occur if dosage is exces-sive or use prolonged. Nephrotoxicity may occur, especially in toxic, poorly hydrated patients. At higher doses, local irritation at the injec-tion site may occur. The drug also has been shown to decrease cardiac output and produce hypotension and bradycardia. Cardiac arrest has been reported in humans receiving overdoses of the drug. Also see AMINOGLYCOSIDES.

DRUG INTERACTIONS: The potential for ototoxicity increases if kanamycin is used with other aminoglycosides. Furosemide potentiates ototoxicity. Amphotericin B, cisplatin, methoxyflurane, vancomycin, and succinylcholine may have an additive neuromuscular blocking effect. Calcium gluconate can be given intravenously to reverse aminoglycoside-induced neuromuscular blockade or myocardial depression and to restore blood pressure. Penicillins and aminoglyco-sides should not be mixed in the same syringe because inactivation of the aminoglycoside may result. Also see AMINOGLYCOSIDES.

SUPPLIED AS VETERINARY PRODUCT:
For injection containing 200 mg/mL

KAOLIN-PECTIN

INDICATIONS: Kaolin-pectin (Kaopectate ❧ ★, others) is a GI protectant used in the management of diarrhea. It coats the surface of the gut and exerts a mild demulcent and absorbent effect. It actually is relatively ineffective in absorbing toxins produced by enteropathogenic bacteria. It appears to act by adding particulate matter to the feces, which serves to improve consistency until the disease spontaneously resolves. Kaolin is a potent coagulation activator and may be of some benefit in treating diarrhea associated with mucosal disruption and hemorrhage.

ADVERSE AND COMMON SIDE EFFECTS: Kaolin-pectin may cause constipation, especially in poorly hydrated patients.

DRUG INTERACTIONS: The absorption of lincomycin is decreased if given concurrently with kaolin-pectin. Administer kaolin-pectin 2 hours before or 3 to 4 hours after lincomycin. Absorption of digoxin also may be hindered by kaolin-pectin.

SUPPLIED AS VETERINARY PRODUCT:
Oral suspension containing:
Kaolin 197 mg and pectin 4.33 mg per mL (large animal preparation)
[Kaopectate ❧, Kaopectolin ★]

KETAMINE

INDICATIONS: Ketamine (Ketaset ❧ ★, Vetalar ❧ ★) is a nonbarbiturate anesthetic used in cats. It generally is used for chemical restraint or anesthesia of short duration. Supplemental doses can be given, providing anesthesia for 6 hours or more. The drug is characterized by a rapid onset of action, profound analgesia, maintenance of normal muscle tone and laryngeal reflex, mild cardiac stimulation, and respiratory depression. Recovery generally is smooth and uneventful, especially if animals are not stimulated by sound or handling during recovery. At lower doses, recovery is complete within 4 to 5 hours. At high doses, complete recovery may take as long as 24 hours or more, especially if the patient is in poor condition or suffering from renal impairment. In cats, ketamine often is combined with acepromazine or midazolam. The combination provides dependable chemical restraint with minimal cardiovascular effects. In addition, ketamine may be combined with atropine to decrease respiratory and salivary secretions. Somatic analgesia is moderate and only of short duration; it provides little to no visceral analgesia.

ADVERSE AND COMMON SIDE EFFECTS: Pain on IM injection may occur. The use of ketamine is associated with increased muscle tone and should not be used as the sole anesthetic for procedures requiring muscle relaxation. Used alone, ketamine may induce seizure activity in dogs and in up to 20% of cats. In fact, the drug should not be used in dogs or cats with a history of seizure disorders. The incidence of seizure can be reduced if ketamine is combined with diazepam or midazolam. Dose-dependent respiratory depression and hypotension may occur with larger doses. The drug is eliminated via the kidney and should be used with caution in patients with renal impairment. The drug may cause elevations in CSF pressure and should not be used in cases with suspect increases in CSF or trauma to the head. Ketamine should not be used in animals with increased intraocular pressure or trauma to the globe, or for procedures involving the pharynx, larynx, and trachea. Eyes remain open after ketamine induction and should be protected from drying with an ophthalmic lubricant.

At high doses, respiratory depression, vomiting, vocalization, erratic and prolonged recovery, dyspnea, spastic jerking movements, convulsions, muscular tremors, hypertonicity, opisthotonos, and cardiac arrest may occur. In the cat, the myoclonic jerking and clonic-tonic convulsions can be controlled by ultrashort-acting barbitutes or acepromazine given slowly intravenously and to effect.

DRUG INTERACTIONS: Concurrent barbiturate, narcotic, or diazepine use may prolong recovery time after ketamine use. Ketamine may potentiate the neuromuscular blocking action of tubocurarine. Concomitant use of halothane can cause cardiac depression. Chloramphenicol may prolong the anesthetic actions of ketamine. Marked hypertension and tachycardia after induction with ketamine has been documented in people if the drug is used concurrently with thyroid medications.

SUPPLIED AS VETERINARY PRODUCT:
For injection containing 100 mg/mL

OTHER USES
SHORT, PAINFUL SURGICAL PROCEDURES
1 to 2 mg/kg; IV

KETOCONAZOLE

INDICATIONS: Ketoconazole (Nizoral ✤ ★) has been used in the treatment of *Trichophyton mentagrophytes* and *Microsporum canis* infections, candidiasis, coccidioidomycosis, cryptococcosis, blastomycosis, histoplasmosis, and canine nasal aspergillosis. The drug also has been used effectively in the treatment of Malassezia infection in dogs and cats. Therapeutic concentrations are achieved in all body fluids except the skin, bone, bile, brain, testes, and eye. The drug also has been used in the treatment of canine hyperadrenocorticism. Ketoconazole effectively blocks cortisol synthesis in dogs with pituitary-dependent hyperadrenocorticism and those with adrenocortical tumor. Long-term administration of the drug does not suppress plasma cortisol concentrations in clinically normal cats.

ADVERSE AND COMMON SIDE EFFECTS: Nausea, anorexia, vomiting, diarrhea, lightening of the hair coat, transient elevations in liver enzymes, and jaundice have been reported. Gastrointestinal side effects may be prevented by administering the drug with food (which also may serve to increase its absorption) and by dividing the daily dose and administering the drug 2 to 4 times daily. In the management of hyperadrenocorticism, overdose of the drug could result in hypo-cortisolism and resultant vomiting, diarrhea, anorexia, weakness, and depression. The drug should not be given to pregnant animals because its use has been associated with stillbirths and mummified fetuses. In addition, decreased libido and impotence occur in humans and may occur in dogs.

DRUG INTERACTIONS: Antacids, cimetidine, and ranitidine decrease the absorption of ketoconazole. Phenytoin may antagonize the actions of ketoconazole. Rifampin and isoniazid reduce the antifungal effects of ketoconazole. Mitotane and ketoconazole should not be used concurrently in the treatment of hyperadrenocorticism because the adrenolytic effects of mitotane may be inhibited by ketoconazole's inhibition of cytochrome P-450 enzymes. Ketoconazole may increase the anticoagulant effects of warfarin. The duration of activity of methylprednisolone is prolonged with ketoconazole. Ketoconazole may decrease serum concentrations of theophylline in some patients. Cyclosporine levels may be increased by ketoconazole. Concurrent use of ketoconazole and terfenadine (Seldane) or astemizole (Hismanal) may predispose to severe and life-threatening cardiac arrhythmias in humans.

SUPPLIED AS HUMAN PRODUCTS:
Tablets containing 200 mg
Shampoo containing 20 mg/mL
Cream containing 20 mg/mL

OTHER USES
Dogs
ASPERGILLOSIS
Ketoconazole 20 mg/kg for at least 6 weeks; long-term maintenance may be required

BLASTOMYCOSIS
i) Ketoconazole 10 mg/kg bid; PO (15 to 20 mg/kg bid; PO if CNS involvement) for at least 3 months with amphotericin B, initially at 0.25 to 0.5 mg/kg every other day; IV. If tolerated, increase dose

of amphotericin B to 1 mg/kg until a cumulative dose of 4 to 5 mg/kg is attained.

ii) Ketoconazole 20 mg/day; once daily or divided bid PO; 40 mg/kg divided bid for ocular or CNS involvement (for at least 2 to 3 months or until remission, then start maintenance) with amphotericin B 0.15 to 0.5 mg/kg; IV 3 times a week. When the total dose of amphotericin reaches 4 to 6 mg/kg, start maintenance dose of amphotericin at 0.15 to 0.25 mg/kg; IV, once a month, or use ketoconazole at 10 mg/kg once daily or divided bid; PO or ketoconazole at 2.5 to 5 mg/kg once daily; PO. If there is ocular or CNS involvement, use ketoconazole at 20 to 40 mg/kg divided bid; PO.

CANDIDAL STOMATITIS
10 mg/kg tid; PO until lesions resolve

COCCIDIOIDOMYCOSIS
i)   5 to 10 mg/kg bid; PO (systemic disease)

ii) 15 to 20 mg/kg bid; PO (CNS disease)

Continue treatment for 3 to 6 months. Those with bony lesions or relapses may require lifelong treatment at 5 mg/kg every other day; PO.

CRYPTOCOCCOSIS
Amphotericin B 0.15 to 0.4 mg/kg 3 times a week; IV with flucytosine at 150 to 175 mg/kg divided tid to qid; PO. When total dose of amphotericin B reaches 4 to 6 mg/kg, start maintenance dose of amphotericin B at 0.15 to 0.25 mg/kg once monthly; IV or with ketoconazole at 10 mg/kg once daily or divided bid; PO.

HISTOPLASMOSIS
i)   10 mg/kg once daily or bid; PO for at least 3 months. Continue treatment for at least 30 days beyond complete remission. If relapse occurs, retreat as indicated and put on maintenance of 5 mg/kg every other day indefinitely.

ii) Ketoconazole 10 to 20 mg/kg once daily; PO or divided bid (for at least 2 to 3 months or until remission, then start maintenance) with amphotericin B at 0.15 to 0.5 mg/kg; IV 3 times weekly. When a total dose of amphotericin B reaches 2 to 4 mg/kg, start maintenance dose of amphotericin B at 0.15 to 0.25 mg/kg once a month; IV, or use ketoconazole at 10 mg/kg once daily or divided bid; PO or at 2.5 to 5 mg/kg once daily; PO.

MALASSEZIA
5 to 10 mg/kg bid; PO for 30 to 45 days

HYPERADRENOCORTICISM
i)   30 mg/kg once daily or divided bid; PO

ii) Initially at 10 mg/kg bid; PO for 7 to 10 days. Discontinue drug for 24 to 48 hours if adverse reactions occur. Reevaluate ACTH stimulation at end of 7- to 10-day period. If response is inadequate, increase dose to 15 mg/kg bid; PO, and reevaluate again in 7 to 10 days. Once controlled, continue on that dose long term.

iii) Initially at 5 mg/kg bid; PO for 7 days to evaluate for side effects. If none occur, increase dose to 10 mg/kg bid; PO for an additional 14 days. Perform ACTH stimulation 1 to 3 hours after last dose. If no improvement noted, increase dose again to 15 mg/kg bid; PO and reevaluate in 14 days.

Cats

ASPERGILLOSIS
20 mg/kg; PO for at least 6 weeks; long-term maintenance therapy may be required

BLASTOMYCOSIS
i) Ketoconazole at 10 mg/kg bid; PO (15 to 20 mg/kg bid if CNS involvement) for at least 3 months with amphotericin B, initially at 0.25 to 0.5 mg/kg every other day; IV. If tolerated, increase dose to 1 mg/kg until a total dose of 4 to 5 mg/kg is attained.

ii) Ketoconazole at 10 mg/kg bid; PO (for at least 2 months) with amphotericin B at 0.25 mg/kg in 30 mL D5W IV over 15 minutes every 48 hours. Continue amphotericin until total dose of 4 mg/kg is attained or until BUN is greater than 50 mg/dL (18 mmol/L). If renal toxicity does not occur, increase amphotericin dose to 0.5 mg/kg.

iii) Ketoconazole at 10 mg/kg once daily; PO or divided bid (for at least 2 to 3 months or until clinical remission, then start maintenance) with amphotericin B at 0.15 to 0.5 mg/kg 3 times a week; IV. When total amphotericin B dose reaches 4 to 6 mg/kg, start maintenance dose of 0.15 to 0.25 mg/kg once monthly; IV, or use ketoconazole at 10 mg/kg once daily; PO or divided bid or ketoconazole at 2.5 to 5 mg/kg once daily; PO. For ocular or CNS disease, use ketoconazole at 20 to 40 mg/kg divided bid; PO.

COCCIDIOIDOMYCOSIS
i) 5 to 10 mg/kg bid; PO (systemic disease) and 15 to 20 mg/kg bid; PO (CNS disease)

Continue treatment for 3 to 6 months. Those with relapses or with bony lesions may require lifelong therapy at 5 mg/kg every other day; PO.

ii) 10 mg/kg once or twice daily; PO for at least 6 months

iii) 50 mg/day; PO (in several cases treatment periods continued 28 to 43 months)

CRYPTOCOCCOSIS
i) 10 mg/kg once or twice daily; PO for 3 months or for at least 30 days beyond clinical remission

ii) 10 to 20 mg/kg divided bid; PO (20 to 30 mg/kg per day if CNS involvement). Continue for at least 3 to 4 weeks beyond clinical remission.

iii) Amphotericin B at 0.15 to 0.4 mg/kg 3 times a week; IV with flucytosine at 125 to 250 mg/kg divided tid to qid; PO. Start maintenance dose of amphotericin of 0.15 to 0.25 mg/kg once a month; IV after a total dose of 4 to 6 mg/kg has been reached along with flucytosine at the dose indicated or with ketoconazole at 10 mg/kg once daily or divided bid; PO.

HISTOPLASMOSIS

i) 10 mg/kg once or twice daily; PO for at least 3 months. Continue for at least 30 days after clinical remission. If relapse occurs, retreat as indicated and maintain on 5 mg/kg every other day; PO indefinitely.

ii) Ketoconazole at 10 mg/kg bid; PO with amphotericin at 0.25 mg in 30 mL of D_5W; IV given over 15 minutes every 48 hours. Continue amphotericin for 4 to 8 weeks or until BUN is greater than 50 mg/dL (18 mmol/L). If BUN increases to greater than 50 mg/dL (18 mmol/L), continue ketoconazole alone for at least 6 months.

iii) Ketoconazole at 10 mg/kg once daily or divided bid; PO (for at least 2 to 3 months or until clinical remission is apparent, then start maintenance dose) with amphotericin B at 0.15 to 0.5 mg/kg 3 times a week; IV. When total amphotericin B dose reaches 2 to 4 mg/kg, start maintenance dose of 0.15 to 0.25 mg/kg once a month; IV, or use ketoconazole at 10 mg/kg once daily or divided bid or at 2.5 to 5 mg/kg once daily; PO.

MALASSEZIA
5 mg/kg every 24 to 48 hours; PO for a minimum of 30 days

Dogs and Cats
DERMATOPHYTOSIS
10 mg/kg once to twice daily; PO with food
Continue treatment until lesions have resolved and fungal cultures yield no growth (median duration of treatment 6 weeks).

Note: Griseofulvin may be more effective than ketoconazole for the treatment of dermatophytosis.

KETOPROFEN

INDICATIONS: Ketoprofen (Anafen ♣) is an NSAID with potent analgesic and antipyretic properties. The drug inhibits the cyclooxygenase and lipoxygenase inflammatory pathways. Most NSAIDs only inhibit the cyclooxygenase pathway. Ketoprofen is used in the management of fever and acute, subacute, and chronic pain associated with musculoskeletal disease. Onset of activity of the drug occurs within

30 minutes of parenteral administration and 1 hour after oral use. The terminal half-life in cats and dogs is 2 to 3 hours. Duration of action is approximately 12 hours. It reportedly can be used for several months for the management of chronic pain in dogs and cats. The drug is 50 to 100 times more potent than phenylbutazone as an analgesic. Ketoprofen is more effective and longer lasting than oxymorphone or butorphanol in the management of postoperative orthopedic pain.

ADVERSE AND COMMON SIDE EFFECTS: Ketoprofen has a wide margin of safety. In dogs, mild and self-limiting cases of vomiting, diarrhea, anorexia, melena, increased thirst, and weight loss have been documented with drug overdose. In cats occasional vomiting may occur. The drug should not be given to animals with GI ulceration, or impaired renal or hepatic function, or those with coagulation disorders. Preoperative administration inhibited platelet aggregation but did not alter bleeding time and can safely be given before surgery in healthy dogs. It may be inadvisable to use the drug before surgical procedures in which noncompressible hemorrhage may be a problem (e.g., laparotomy, laminectomy, rhinotomy). The effects of ketoprofen on breeding animals are not known.

DRUG INTERACTIONS: Concomitant use of ketoprofen and high-dose methotrexate may cause prolonged excretion and increased serum levels predisposing to methotrexate toxicity. Ketoprofen may impair platelet aggregation and prolong bleeding times. Concurrent use of aspirin decreased ketoprofen protein binding and increased plasma clearance. Patients taking diuretic agents are at greater risk of developing renal failure because of prostaglandin production. Ketoprofen is highly protein bound and may compete with sulfonamides, warfarin, phenylbutazone, oral hypoglycemic agents, and phenytoin for binding sites.

SUPPLIED AS VETERINARY PRODUCTS:
For injection containing 10 and 100 mg/mL
Tablets containing 5, 10, and 20 mg

KETOROLAC

INDICATIONS: Ketorolac tromethamine (Toradol ✤ ★) is a nonsteroidal anti-inflammatory analgesic with antipyretic properties. It is used in the management of moderate to severe pain. Its principal mode of action is via prostaglandin inhibition. The analgesic properties of the drug are estimated to be approximately 180 to 350 times greater than those of aspirin. In humans and apparently in dogs, the onset of analgesia after IM injection is apparent within 10 minutes and peaks within 75 to 150 minutes, and analgesia may be maintained for 8 to 12 hours. The duration of analgesia is greater than that observed with morphine or meperidine. For the management of anticipated postsurgical pain, the drug is best given at least 30 minutes before extubation.

ADVERSE AND COMMON SIDE EFFECTS: Like other NSAIDs, ketorolac has the potential to adversely affect renal function, inhibit platelet aggregation, and cause gastric mucosal damage, which may result in ulceration and bleeding. However, the incidence of these side effects is less common than that observed with other NSAIDs. Drug dose should be cut in half in patients with renal impairment, and the drug should only be used when the apparent benefits outweigh the risks of the drug. Patients have been reported to recover from renal injury after discontinuation of the drug. The drug should be used with caution in dehydrated/hypovolemic or hypotensive patients. Fluid retention and edema have been reported in humans with congestive heart failure.

DRUG INTERACTIONS: Ketorolac may be used concurrently with morphine or meperidine in the management of moderate to severe pain. The combined use results in reduced opiate analgesic requirements. Diuretic use increases the risk of renal injury. Ketorolac may decrease the diuretic response to furosemide. Ketorolac may increase serum lithium concentrations. It also may increase serum methotrexate concentrations, predisposing to toxicity by decreasing its clearance.

SUPPLIED AS HUMAN PRODUCTS:
For injection containing 10, 15, and 30 mg/mL
Tablets containing 10 mg

LACTULOSE

INDICATIONS: Lactulose (Cephulac ✤ ★, Chronulac ✤ ★) is a synthetic nonabsorbable disaccharide. It acts as a mild osmotic laxative, increases the rate of passage of ingesta, and leads to the reduction of bacterial production of ammonia, making it useful in the management of hepatic encephalopathy. Enteric bacteria ferment lactulose to acidic by-products, decrease intraluminal pH, and favor the formation of ammonium ions, which are poorly absorbed.

ADVERSE AND COMMON SIDE EFFECTS: Transient gastric distention, flatulence, and abdominal cramping may occur. With excessive doses, diarrhea may occur. The preparation is distasteful to cats and may be difficult to administer.

DRUG INTERACTIONS: Antacids decrease the efficacy of the drug. Neomycin and other oral antibiotics may inhibit lactulose activity by reduction or removal of resident colonic bacteria. However, clinical experience suggests that combined therapy in hepatic encephalopathy actually may be synergistic.

SUPPLIED AS HUMAN PRODUCT:
Syrup containing 10 g/15 mL

LEVAMISOLE

INDICATIONS: Levamisole (Levasole ✤ ★, Tramisol ✤ ★) is an anthelmintic licensed for use in large animals. It also has been used for the elimination of *Dirofilaria immitis* microfilaria and for the treatment of *Filaroides osleri*, *Crenosoma vulpis*, and *Capillaria* infection in dogs and *Aelurostrongylus abstrusus*, *Capillaria aerophila,* and *Ollulanus tricuspis* infection in cats. Levamisole may help restore immune function by increasing the number and function of T lymphocytes and macrophages. It also has been reported to stimulate antibody production, increase macrophage phagocytosis, inhibit tumor growth, and stimulate suppressor cell activity.

ADVERSE AND COMMON SIDE EFFECTS: Vomiting, diarrhea, anorexia, salivation, agranulocytosis, depression, panting, head shaking, muscular tremors, and agitation are reported in dogs. In cats, hypersalivation, excitement, mydriasis, and vomiting are reported. Atropine is only partially effective as an antidote. If toxicity progresses to flaccid paralysis, respiratory assistance should be given until recovery has occurred.

DRUG INTERACTIONS: The concurrent use of chloramphenicol has led to death in some cases. Pyrantel, diethylcarbamazine, and organophosphate drugs may enhance the toxic effects of levamisole.

**SUPPLIED AS VETERINARY PRODUCTS
(For Large Animals):**
For injection containing 136.5 mg/mL
Soluble drench powder containing 11.7 g/packet [Levasole]
Soluble drench containing 46.8 and 93.6 g/packet [Tramisol, Levasole]
Oral tablets/boluses containing 184 mg and 2.19 g bolus

OTHER USES
Dogs
AS AN IMMUNOSTIMULANT
i)   For recurrent skin infections, use 2.2 mg/kg every other day; PO along with appropriate antibiotic therapy.
ii) As adjunctive therapy for chronic pyoderma, give 0.5 to 1.5 mg/kg 2 to 3 times weekly; PO.

MICROFILARICIDE
11 mg/kg for 6 to 12 days; PO
Examine blood on day 6 and discontinue therapy when microfilaria are negative. Retching and vomiting are common. Discontinue if ataxia or abnormal behavior occurs.

CRENOSOMA VULPIS
8 mg/kg once; PO

CAPILLARIA
7 to 12 mg/kg once daily for 3 to 7 days; PO

FILAROIDES OSLERI
7 to 12 mg/kg once daily for 20 to 45 days; PO

Cats

LUNGWORMS
Aelurostrongylus abstrusus: 100 mg daily every other day for 5 treatments; PO; give atropine (0.5 mg; SC, 15 minutes before levamisole) or 15 mg/kg every other day for 3 treatments, then 3 days later, 30 mg/kg; PO, then 2 days later, 60 mg/kg; PO

CAPILLARIA AEROPHILA
4.4 mg/kg; SC for 2 days, then 8.8 mg/kg once 2 weeks later; or 5 mg/kg once daily for 5 days, followed by 9 days without therapy; repeat twice

OLLULANUS TRICUSPIS
5 mg/kg; SC

MICROFILARICIDE
10 mg/kg for 7 days; PO

EOSINOPHILIC GRANULOMA
5 mg/kg 3 times weekly; PO

LEVOTHYROXINE

INDICATIONS: Levothyroxine (Eltroxin ♣ ★, Synthroid ♣ ★, Levotec ♣, Soloxine ♣ ★, Thyro-Tab ♣ ★) is a synthetic form of T_4 used in the treatment of hypothyroid disease. Peak serum concentrations are reached in 4 to 12 hours. Some animals require the drug twice daily. Serum levels can be measured after steady-state levels have been attained (as early as 5 to 10 days, but preferably 1 month because the increased metabolism induced by the drug may change the rate of T_4 catabolism). For those on once-daily treatment, serum samples for T_4 levels are taken 24 hours after the last dose. Timing is not as important for those on twice-daily dosing. Individual response to recommended starting dosages is quite variable and should be evaluated. Levothyroxine also has been used (at standard doses) in the management of dogs with von Willebrand's disease, and problems of platelet dysfunction. The drug causes an increase in vWF antigen (vWF:Ag) and platelet adhesiveness and platelet production and release, corresponding to a correction in bleeding times. However, other reports have not demonstrated efficacy in hypothyroid patients with von Willebrand's disease.

ADVERSE AND COMMON SIDE EFFECTS: Thyroid replacement should be undertaken with caution in animals with hypoadrenocorticism, diabetes mellitus, or congestive heart failure. The increase in metabolism may place undue stress on the heart. Increased metabolism of adrenal hormones may precipitate a hypoadrenocortical crisis, and increased metabolism may enhance ketone production and potentiate ketoacidosis in animals with diabetes mellitus. Clinical signs consistent with drug overdose include polyuria, polydipsia, polyphagia, weight loss, panting, vomiting, diarrhea, abnormal pupillary light reflexes, nervousness, and tachycardia. Clinical signs resolve 1 to 3 days after discontinuation of the drug. After this time, levothyroxine can be reinstituted at a lower dose and serum levels reevaluated in 2 to 4 weeks. Levothyroxine overdose in recently exposed dogs, without clinical signs of toxicity, can be managed by the induction of vomiting followed by the administration of activated charcoal (1 to 2 g/kg; PO) and a saline cathartic (e.g., 250 mg/kg; PO of magnesium sulfate or sodium sulfate). Repeated administration of activated charcoal (every 4 to 8 hours at a reduced dose of 0.5 to 1 g/kg) may further reduce the reabsorption of thyroxine by interfering with enterohepatic recirculation. A saline cathartic may be used with the second dose of activated charcoal at one half the initial dose. Further cathartic use is not recommended. Propranolol may be useful in the management of significant tachycardia.

DRUG INTERACTIONS: The activity of epinephrine and norepinephrine increases with the use of levothyroxine. Insulin requirements may increase, and the therapeutic effects of digitalis products may decrease. With the use of thyroid medications, marked hypertension and tachycardia after induction with ketamine have been documented in humans.

SUPPLIED AS VETERINARY PRODUCTS:
Tablets containing 0.1, 0.2, 0.3, 0.4, 0.5, 0.6, 0.7, and 0.8 mg [Soloxine, Thyro-Tabs]
Tablets (chewable) containing 0.2, 0.5, and 0.8 mg [Thyro-Form ★]

SUPPLIED AS HUMAN PRODUCTS:
Tablets containing 25, 50, 75, 88, 100, 112, 125, 150, 175, 200, and 300 µg [Eltroxin, Synthroid]
For injection containing 200- and 500-µg vials [Synthroid]

OTHER USES
Dogs
HEMOSTATIC DEFECTS, INCLUDING
VON WILLEBRAND'S DISEASE
22 µg/kg bid; PO

LIDOCAINE

INDICATIONS: Lidocaine ♣ ★ is licensed as a local anesthetic in small animals. It also is the drug of choice for the management of ventricular premature contractions or tachycardia in dogs. Serum concentrations are measured after steady-state levels have been attained (5 hours in the dog). Therapeutic serum concentrations in dogs range from 2 to 6 µg/mL. Toxic levels are in excess of 8 µg/mL. Topical administration of a liposome-encapsulated preparation [ELA-Max] appears safe for use in healthy cats.

ADVERSE AND COMMON SIDE EFFECTS: With drug overdose, drowsiness, vomiting, tremors, nystagmus, seizure (especially in cats), excitation, hypotension, and increased atrioventricular conduction with atrial flutter and fibrillation have been reported. The neurologic signs can be controlled with diazepam. Hypokalemia reduces anti-arrhythmic effects.

DRUG INTERACTIONS: Cimetidine, propranolol, metoprolol, and quinidine increase the activity of lidocaine. Barbiturates decrease lidocaine action via enzyme induction. Phenytoin increases the cardiac depressant effect of lidocaine. Procainamide may have additive neurologic and cardiac effects.

SUPPLIED AS VETERINARY PRODUCT:
For injection containing 20 mg/mL (2%)
To prepare IV infusion (without epinephrine) using 2% veterinary solution, add 1 g (50 mL) of 2% solution to 1 L of D₅W, thus providing 1 mg/mL (1,000 µg/mL).
With a minidrop (60 drops/mL) IV set, each drop will contain approximately 17 µg.

SUPPLIED AS HUMAN PRODUCTS:
For injection containing 0.2%, 0.4%, or 0.8% in 5% dextrose and 2% in disposable syringes
Topical 5% cream containing 25 mg lidocaine and 25 mg prilocaine [Emla ♣ ★]
Patch containing 1 g of emulsion [Emla patch ♣ ★]

OTHER USES
Dogs
SYSTEMIC ANALGESIA
40 to 70 µg/kg per minute; constant rate IV infusion (without epinephrine)

LINCOMYCIN

INDICATIONS: Lincomycin (Lincocin ♣ ★) is a lincosamide antibiotic with activity against gram-positive cocci, particularly *Streptococcus* spp. and *Staphylococcus* spp. It also is active against *Clostridium tetani* and *perfringens, Mycoplasma* spp., *Leptospira pomona,* and *Erysipelothrix insidiosa.* In dogs, the drug is indicated in the treatment of upper respiratory infections and skin infections, nephritis, and metritis. In cats, lincomycin is indicated in the treatment of localized infections, such as abscesses. Lincomycin is effective against penicillinase-producing staphylococci. Significant concentrations of the drug are achieved in most tissues of the body other than CSF. The drug is excreted in the bile and urine.

ADVERSE AND COMMON SIDE EFFECTS: Vomiting and loose stools may occur. Hemorrhagic diarrhea infrequently occurs in dogs. Pain at the injection site has been reported.

DRUG INTERACTIONS: Kaolin, pectin, and bismuth subsalicylate decrease GI absorption. Chloramphenicol and erythromycin may be mutually antagonistic with lincomycin. Lincomycin has intrinsic neuromuscular blocking properties and should be used with caution with other neuromuscular blocking agents.

SUPPLIED AS VETERINARY PRODUCTS:
Tablets containing 100, 200, and 500 mg
Drops containing 50 mg/mL [Lincocin Aquadrops ★]
For injection containing 100 mg/mL [Lincocin ★] [Lincomix ♣ (approved for use in swine only)]

LIOTHYROXINE

INDICATIONS: Liothyroxine or liothyronine (Cytomel ♣ ★) is a synthetic form of T_3 that has been used in the treatment of some forms of hypothyroid disease. Specifically it is indicated in animals with an inability to convert thyroxine (T_4) to triiodothyronine (T_3), e.g., animals on corticosteroid therapy, and in those with impaired absorption of thyroxine from the GIT. Conversion abnormalities in small animals are rare, if they occur at all. Peak serum concentrations occur 2 to 5 hours after oral administration. Serum T_3 levels are measured just before and 2 to 4 hours after administration (T_4 levels will be low to undetectable because of negative feedback suppression on the remaining functional thyroid tissue).

ADVERSE AND COMMON SIDE EFFECTS: As for LEVOTHY-ROXINE. Clinical signs of drug overdose resolve within 1 to 2 days after discontinuation of the drug. After this time, liothyronine can be reinstituted at a lower dose.

DRUG INTERACTIONS: As for LEVOTHYROXINE.

SUPPLIED AS HUMAN PRODUCT:
Tablets containing 5, 25, and 50 µg [Cytomel]

LISINOPRIL

INDICATIONS: Lisinopril (Prinivil ♣ ★, Zestril ♣ ★) is an ACE inhibitor. It is better tolerated than captopril in dogs. It is a longer acting lysine analog of enalapril that does not require hepatic activation. Experience with the drug in small animals is limited.

ADVERSE AND COMMON SIDE EFFECTS: See CAPTOPRIL and ENALAPRIL.

DRUG INTERACTIONS: The following information is data obtained from human medicine. Patients on diuretics and especially those in which diuretic therapy was recently instituted may occasionally experience an excessive reduction of blood pressure after initiation of therapy with lisinopril. The possibility of hypotensive effects with lisinopril can be minimized by either discontinuing the diuretic or increasing the salt intake prior to initiation of treatment with lisinopril. When a diuretic is added to the therapy of a patient receiving lisinopril, an additional antihypertensive effect is usually observed. Studies with ACE inhibitors in combination with diuretics indicate that the dose of the ACE inhibitor can be reduced when it is given with a diuretic. Lisinopril has been used concomitantly with nitrates and/or digoxin without evidence of clinically significant adverse interactions. No clinically important pharmacokinetic interactions occurred when lisinopril was used concomitantly with propranolol or hydrochlorothiazide. Lisinopril attenuates potassium loss caused by thiazide-type diuretics. Use of lisinopril with potassium-sparing diuretics (e.g., spironolactone, triamterene), potassium supplements, or potassium-containing salt substitutes may lead to significant increases in serum potassium. Potassium sparing agents should generally not be used in patients with heart failure who are receiving lisinopril.

SUPPLIED AS HUMAN PRODUCT:
Tablets containing 2.5, 5, 10, 20, and 40 mg

LITHIUM CARBONATE

INDICATIONS: Lithium carbonate (Lithotabs ★, Carbolith ♣) is used to stimulate granulopoiesis and increase neutrophil numbers in patients following cancer therapy and bone marrow suppression subsequent to estrogen therapy. In humans, it is also used to treat depression.

ADVERSE AND COMMON SIDE EFFECTS: In one report lithium treated cats became ill and exhibited anorexia, vomiting, diarrhea, changes in behavior, muscular tremors, and a decrease in neutrophils. The authors of this paper did not recommend its use in this species.

DRUG INTERACTIONS: Nonsteroidal anti-inflammatory agents including indomethacin and piroxicam increase plasma lithium levels. Angiotensin-converting enzyme inhibitors including enalapril and captopril also may increase serum lithium concentrations. Concurrent use of metronidazole and lithium may potentiate lithium toxicity due to decreased renal clearance, and concurrent use of calcium channel-blocking agents in people have been noted to increase the risk of neurotoxicity resulting in ataxia, tremors, nausea, vomiting, and diarrhea. Sodium bicarbonate and xanthine preparations may lower serum lithium levels. Drug interactions have also been reported with diuretics and SSRI antidepressants.

SUPPLIED AS HUMAN PRODUCTS:
Capsules containing 150, 300, and 600 mg
Tablets containing 300 mg
Syrup containing 300 mg/6 mL

LOMUSTINE

INDICATIONS: Lomustine, CCNU (CeeNU ♣ ★) is an alkylating nitrosourea compound that has been used as a rescue agent in the management of lymphoma in dogs (median response duration 86 days). Complete response rate was only 7% and overall response (complete and partial) was 28%, which is similar to most rescue protocols. It has also been used to treat mast cell tumors (37% had partial response with a median and mean duration of 77 and 109 days respectively, and 32% had stable disease for a median and a mean duration of 78 and 122 days) and brain tumors in dogs. Because of its lipophilic nature, this drug has the ability to cross the blood–brain barrier. All dogs with gliomas had partial remissions with survival times comparable to that expected with radiation therapy (mean survival 10.25 months). The drug has also been effective in some cats with lymphoma and mast cell tumors.

ADVERSE AND COMMON SIDE EFFECTS: Use of the drug is contraindicated with immunization of live virus vaccines or active viral infections. It should be used with caution in those with decreased numbers of circulating platelets, red or white blood cells, or in patients with renal or hepatic impairment, infection, or previous cytotoxic or radiation therapy. The drug is potentially embryotoxic, teratogenic, and carcinogenic. In dogs the most significant side effect is bone marrow suppression (neutrophil nadir occurs 1 week after initiation of treatment and platelet counts reach nadir 1 to 3 weeks after treatment). The drug should be discontinued if platelet counts fall lower than 200,000/μL. Occasional vomiting is reported but is mild and does not require treatment. CCNU may cause a chronic, possibly cumulative, hepatotoxicity in dogs. Discontinuation of the drug at an early stage of recognition of liver dysfunction may prevent progression to advanced liver disease. Renal toxicity has been reported in some dogs.

DRUG INTERACTIONS: None reported.

SUPPLIED AS HUMAN PRODUCT:
Capsules containing 10, 40, and 100 mg

LOPERAMIDE

INDICATIONS: Loperamide (Imodium ♣ ★) is a narcotic analgesic useful for the management of diarrhea in dogs. It also has been used in the treatment of acute colitis and malabsorption/maldigestion.

ADVERSE AND COMMON SIDE EFFECTS: The drug is relatively safe. Sedation, constipation, and ileus may occur. Dose-dependent vomiting (doses greater than 0.63 mg/kg) is reported. With chronic use, soft stools, bloody diarrhea, vomiting, and weight loss also have been reported. Collie dogs may be predisposed to toxicity, and additional toxic signs may include mydriasis, prostration, excitation, and coma. Severe cased may be treated with reloxone. The drug should not be used to treat cases of suspect invasive bacterial enteritis such as *Salmonella,* because decreased intestinal transit can delay clearance of the pathogen. Loperamide also is contraindicated in patients with liver disease, obstructive GI disease, glaucoma, and obstructive uropathy. The drug should be discontinued if diarrhea has not been controlled within 48 hours. Use of opiate antidiarrheal products in cats may be associated with CNS excitation.

DRUG INTERACTIONS: None established.

SUPPLIED AS HUMAN PRODUCTS:
Capsules containing 2 mg
Oral liquid containing 0.2 mg/mL

MAGNESIUM HYDROXIDE

INDICATIONS: Magnesium hydroxide (Phillips' Milk of Magnesia ♣ ★) acts as an antacid at low doses and as a mild laxative at higher doses. For more information on ADVERSE AND COMMON SIDE EFFECTS and DRUG INTERACTIONS, see ANTACIDS.

SUPPLIED AS VETERINARY PRODUCTS (Large Animal Preparations):
Oral powder containing 310 g of magnesium hydroxide/lb of powder [Magnalax ★]
Oral powder containing 361 g of magnesium hydroxide/lb of powder [Carmilax ★]
Oral boluses containing 27 g [Carmilax ★, Magnalax ★]
Oral powder containing 400 mg of magnesium hydroxide/teaspoon of powder [Milk of Magnesia (for dogs and horses) ♣]

SUPPLIED AS HUMAN PRODUCTS:
Oral suspension containing 408 mg/5 mL
Tablets containing 310 mg

MAGNESIUM SULFATE

INDICATIONS: Magnesium maintains the electrolyte balance across all membranes. Magnesium deficiency may occur with decreased intake and increased loss through gastrointestinal and renal disease, endocrine disease, and other miscellaneous causes in people (allergic rhinitis, asthma, immunosuppression, malignancy). Magnesium-deficient states predispose to ventricular arrhythmias. Magnesium slows the rate of sinoatrial node impulse formation and prolongs conduction time. Clinical signs of hypomagnesemia may include muscle weakness. Hypokalemia and hyponatremia may be seen in association with hypomagnesemia. Animals at greater risk for the development of hypomagnesemia include critically ill animals on peritoneal dialysis, dogs with congestive heart failure being treated with furosemide and, low serum albumin, potassium, blood urea nitrogen and total CO_2 concentrations.

ADVERSE AND COMMON SIDE EFFECTS: Cumulative infusion dosage of 0.1 to 0.2 mEq/kg may be given without affecting hemodynamic properties. At higher cumulative infusion dosages acceleration in heart rate occurs. Dangerous arrhythmias occur at total dosages exceeding 3.9 mEq/kg. Clinical signs of drug overdose include depression, weakness, hypotension, loss of deep tendon reflexes, and prolongation of PR and QRS intervals on electrocardiograms. At toxic levels, respiratory depression and coma may be observed. Treatment of hypermagnesemia includes IV calcium (antagonizes magnesium) and fluid therapy with concurrent use of furosemide to enhance excretion.

DRUG INTERACTIONS: Magnesium sulfate can be diluted in normal saline, 2.5% dextrose in 0.45% saline, or 5% dextrose in water. Concurrent administration of CNS depressants (barbiturates, opiates, general anesthetics) may augment CNS depression. Magnesium sulfate may enhance the neuromuscular blockade of agents used to induce neuromuscular blockade. Cautious use of the drug is recommended in patients on digitalis therapy.

SUPPLIED AS HUMAN PRODUCT:
For injection at various concentrations, e.g., 10%, 12.5%, 20%, and 50% (magnesium sulfate) and 20% (magnesium chloride)

MANNITOL

INDICATIONS: Mannitol (Osmitrol ♣ ★) is a potent osmotic diuretic agent. It is used in the prevention and treatment of oliguria and acute glaucoma and in the management of acute cerebral edema. The use of the drug in animals with intracranial injury is controversial. These patients may have a damaged blood–brain barrier that allows the drug to leak into the brain and cause the area to swell further. This effect is most notable with longer contact times. Because of this constant rate, infusion of mannitol is not recommended and intermittent intravenous boluses are used instead. The drug also has been used to enhance the renal elimination of toxins, such as aspirin, ethylene glycol, some barbiturates, and bromides.

ADVERSE AND COMMON SIDE EFFECTS: Volume overload and pulmonary edema may occur, especially in patients with compromised renal or cardiac function. With drug overdose, hyponatremia and seizures have been reported. Other side effects may include nausea, vomiting, and dizziness.

DRUG INTERACTIONS: Mannitol may increase the renal elimination of lithium.

SUPPLIED AS VETERINARY PRODUCTS:
For injection containing 20% (20 g/100 mL) [Am-Vet Mannitol Injection] and 180 mg/mL [Manniject]

SUPPLIED AS HUMAN PRODUCT:
For injection containing 5%, 10%, 15%, 20%, and 25%

OTHER USES
Dogs and Cats
ACUTE GLAUCOMA
1 to 2 g/kg over a 15- to 20-minute period; IV (withhold water for 30 to 60 minutes after administration)

ACUTE CEREBRAL EDEMA
i)   Mannitol (20%) 2 g/kg once; slowly IV
ii) 0.5 to 1 g/kg bid to qid; slowly (over 20 minutes) IV

OLIGURIC RENAL FAILURE
Mannitol (20% to 25%) 0.5 g/kg; slowly IV after adequate rehydration; repeat dose at 15-minute intervals up to 1.5 g/kg total dose.

MARBOFLOXACIN

INDICATIONS: Marbofloxacin (Zeniquin ✤ ★) is a fluoroquinolone antibiotic, the spectrum of activity of which includes some strains of *Pseudomonas aeruginosa, Klebsiella* spp., *E. coli, Enterobacter, Campylobacter, Shigella, Salmonella, Aeromonas, Proteus, Yersinia, Serratia,* and *Vibrio* spp. *Brucella* sp., *Chlamydia trachomatis,* staphylococcus, *Mycoplasma,* and *Mycobacterium* are generally susceptible as well.

ADVERSE AND COMMON SIDE EFFECTS: As for other fluoroquinolone agents this drug is not recommended for dogs between 2 and 8 months of age (small and medium-sized breeds), before 1 year of age (large breeds), and before 18 months of age (giant breeds). It may cause nausea and vomiting, lethargy, and diarrhea. Marbofloxacin may cause CNS stimulation and should be used with caution in animals with a history of seizure activity.

DRUG INTERACTIONS: Antacids and sucralfate may bind to and prevent absorption of the drug. Separate drug dosing by at least 2 hours. Nitrofurantoin may antagonize the bacteriocidal effect of marbofloxacin. Drug synergism may occur against some bacteria (*Pseudomonas aeruginosa,* other *Enterobacteriaceae*) if used in conjunction with aminoglycosides, third-generation cephalosporins, and extended spectrum penicillins.

SUPPLIED AS VETERINARY PRODUCT:
Tablets containing 25, 50, 100, and 200 mg

MEBENDAZOLE

INDICATIONS: Mebendazole (Telmin ✤) is an anthelmintic used for the elimination of *Toxocara canis, Ancylostoma caninum, Uncinaria stenocephala, Trichuris vulpis,* and *Taenia pisiformis* in dogs.

ADVERSE AND COMMON SIDE EFFECTS: Although rare, vomiting and diarrhea are the most common side effects. Hepatotoxicity is rare. The drug is contraindicated in dogs with a history of hepatic disease.

DRUG INTERACTIONS: None established.

SUPPLIED AS VETERINARY PRODUCT:
Paste containing 200 mg mebendazole (for horses)

SUPPLIED AS HUMAN PRODUCT:
Tablets (chewable) containing 100 mg [Vermox ♣ ★]

MECLOFENAMIC ACID

INDICATIONS: Meclofenamic acid (Arquel ♣ ★) is a nonsteroidal anti-inflammatory agent with analgesic and antipyretic properties. The drug may act by inhibiting the migration of monocytes from inflamed blood vessels, their phagocytic activity, and the release of prostaglandins. Centrally, meclofenamic acid may raise the pain threshold. It has been used to treat inflammatory conditions of the musculoskeletal system in dogs.

ADVERSE AND COMMON SIDE EFFECTS: Anorexia, vomiting, diarrhea with or without blood, small intestinal ulcers, anemia, and leukocytosis may occur. Drug dosage should not exceed 1.1 mg/kg. The drug should not be used in animals with GI, hepatic or renal disease, or in those with asthma. The drug may delay parturition and should be avoided in the last stages of pregnancy.

DRUG INTERACTIONS: The drug is highly protein bound and may displace other agents, e.g., phenytoin, salicylates, sulfonamides, and oral anticoagulants, resulting in increased serum levels of these drugs. Aspirin may decrease plasma levels of meclofenamic acid and increase the likelihood of adverse GIT effects.

SUPPLIED AS VETERINARY PRODUCTS:
Granules containing 50 mg/g [Arquel] (for use in the horse)
Tablets containing 10 and 20 mg [Arquel ★] (for use in the dog)

MEDETOMIDINE

INDICATIONS: Medetomidine (Domitor ♣ ★) is an α_2 agonist pre-anesthetic agent with sedative and analgesic properties. When used with barbiturates, ketamine, or inhalation anesthetics, it produces safe and reliable sedation (1 to 2 hours), muscle relaxation, and analgesia. The drug should not be used alone. Medetomidine should only be used in young healthy animals undergoing routine or diagnostic procedures not requiring muscle relaxation or tracheal intubation.

ADVERSE AND COMMON SIDE EFFECTS: Paradoxical excitation, prolonged sedation, bradycardia, cyanosis, vomiting, apnea, death from circulatory failure, and recurrence of sedation have been reported. Urination during recovery is common, and adrenergic-induced hyperglycemia is seen. The drug should not be used in animals with cardiac, respiratory, renal, or liver disease, dogs in shock, debilitated patients, or dogs stressed due to extremes in heat, cold, or fatigue. Acutely stressed dogs may not respond to medetomidine and if they should not, repeat dosing is discouraged. Bradycardia, second-degree heart block, marked sinus arrhythmia, decreased respiratory rate, pain on injection, muscle jerking, and vomiting have been reported. Atipamezole, an α_2-adrenergic antagonist, shortens the recovery times of medetomidine in dogs.

DRUG INTERACTIONS: Medetomidine should be used with caution with other analgesic or sedative agents since clinical effects may be enhanced. Atropine and glycopyrrolate given at the same time as or after medetomidine may induce bradycardia, heart block, premature ventricular contractions, and sinus tachycardia. In cats medetomidine in combination with isoflurance may promote severe vasoconstriction and sustained increases in left ventricular preload and afterload and should be avoided.

SUPPLIED AS VETERINARY PRODUCT:
For injection containing 1 mg/mL

MEDIUM CHAIN TRIGLYCERIDE (MCT) OIL

INDICATIONS: MCT oil ✤ ★ is used in the management of patients that cannot efficiently digest and absorb long chain food fats, e.g., animals with lymphangiectasia. Medium chain triglycerides are absorbed directly into mucosal cells and transported to the liver by the portal system. The clinical use of MCTs are as a substitute for normal dietary fat, which is composed of almost entirely long-chain fatty acids. Its use has been advocated in patients with diseases of lipid transport including chylothorax and lymphangiectasia. In one study, however, the oil appeared to be directly absorbed through intestinal lymphatic vessels and not into the portal venous system as was previously held, and provided little benefit for dogs with chylothorax.

ADVERSE AND COMMON SIDE EFFECTS: The oil is distasteful and should be mixed with small amounts of food. It may lead to signs of hepatic encephalopathy in patients with advanced cirrhosis or portacaval shunts and should not be used in these patients. The hyperosmolality may worsen diarrhea, so it is best introduced gradually. The product is contraindicated in cats because of the concern for predisposition to hepatic encephalopathy and fatty liver.

DRUG INTERACTIONS: None established.

SUPPLIED AS HUMAN PRODUCT:
Oil in 500-mL bottles

MEDROXYPROGESTERONE ACETATE

INDICATIONS: Medroxyprogesterone (Depo-Provera ❦ ★, Provera ❦ ★) is a synthetic prolonged-action progestational compound that suppresses secretion of FSH and LH, thus arresting the development of Graafian follicles and corpora lutea within the ovary. The drug has been used to treat benign prostatic hyperplasia in the dog. It also has been used to treat feline endocrine alopecia, eosinophilic granuloma complex, psychogenic alopecia and dermatitis, miliary dermatitis, stud tail, intermale aggression, and urine spraying by male cats.

ADVERSE AND COMMON SIDE EFFECTS: Overdose or prolonged treatment may cause cystic endometritis. Transient or permanent diabetes mellitus, acromegaly, mammary hyperplasia or adenocarcinoma, adrenocortical suppression, polydipsia, polyphagia, depression, immunosuppression, suppression of fibroblast function (which may delay healing), inhibition of spermatogenesis, and pyometra in intact females also are reported. Injection may cause temporary local alopecia, cutaneous atrophy, and pigmentary changes. Use the inguinal area for injection. Medroxyprogesterone acetate also has been associated with causing calcinosis circumscripta in two poodle bitches at the site of injection. The lesions were successfully removed surgically.

DRUG INTERACTIONS: None established.

SUPPLIED AS HUMAN PRODUCTS:
Tablets containing 2.5, 5, 10, and 100 mg [Provera]
For injection containing 50, 150, and 400 mg/mL [Depo-Provera]

OTHER USES
Dogs
ADJUNCTIVE THERAPY TO AGGRESSIVE BEHAVIOR
10 mg/kg; IM, SC as indicated (not to exceed 3 injections per year)
BENIGN PROSTATIC HYPERPLASIA
3 mg/kg; SC, repeat in 4 to 6 weeks if needed or if relapse occurs

Cats
RECURRENT ABORTION
1 to 2 mg once weekly; IM. Stop treatment 7 to 10 days before parturition.
TO ALLEVIATE SIGNS OF ESTRUS AND MATING ACTIVITY
i)   5 mg once daily; PO for up to 5 days; alleviates signs in 24 hours

ii) 25 mg injected every 6 months to postpone estrus

LONG-TERM REPRODUCTIVE CONTROL
2.5 to 5 mg once weekly; PO

BEHAVIORAL DISORDERS
Male cats: 100 mg; IM initially, then reduce dose by 1/3 to 1/2 and repeat every 30 days
Female cats: 50 mg; IM initially, then reduce dose by 1/3 to 1/2 and repeat every 30 days

PSYCHOGENIC ALOPECIA
75 to 150 mg; IM, SC, repeat PRN, but not more often than every 2 to 3 months

URINE SPRAYING
100 mg; SC for male cats
50 mg; SC for female cats

MEGESTROL ACETATE

INDICATIONS: Megestrol acetate (Ovaban ♣ ★) is a progestational compound marketed for the postponement of estrus and the alleviation of false pregnancy in bitches. The drug also is used to treat acral lick dermatitis and dominance aggression in dogs. In cats, the drug has been used to treat neurodermatitis (psychogenic alopecia), eosinophilic granuloma complex, eosinophilic keratitis, miliary dermatitis, pemphigus foliaceous, endocrine alopecia, hyperesthesia, urine spraying, intermale aggression, and aggression toward people. It also has been used in cats to prevent or postpone estrus.

ADVERSE AND COMMON SIDE EFFECTS: The drug should not be given to bitches with reproductive problems, pregnant bitches, or bitches with mammary tumors. Polyphagia, polydipsia, weight gain, and a change in behavior are common side effects. Overdose or prolonged use may result in cystic endometritis. Transient or permanent diabetes mellitus, mammary hyperplasia or adenocarcinoma, adrenocortical suppression (especially in cats), immunosuppression, suppression of fibroblast function (which may delay healing), and pyometra are other possible side effects. Rare reports of jaundice and hepatotoxicity in cats have been documented.

DRUG INTERACTIONS: None established.

SUPPLIED AS VETERINARY PRODUCT:
Tablets containing 5 and 20 mg

OTHER USES
Dogs
UNACCEPTABLE MASCULINE BEHAVIOR
1.1 to 2.2 mg/kg once daily; PO for 2 weeks, then 0.5 to 1.1 mg/kg once daily for 2 weeks (used in conjunction with behavior modification)

Cats

EOSINOPHILIC KERATITIS
0.5 mg/kg per day; PO until a response is seen, then maintain on
1.25 mg 2 to 3 times weekly to prevent recurrence

EOSINOPHILIC ULCERS
5 to 10 mg every other day for 10 to 14 treatments, then every 2 weeks;
PO (alone or with methylprednisolone acetate)

*URETHRITIS: FELINE LOWER URINARY
TRACT INFLAMMATION*
2.5 to 5 mg once daily to every other day; PO

IMMUNE SKIN DISEASE
2.5 to 5 mg once daily for 10 days, then every other day; PO

URINE SPRAYING, ANXIETY, INTRASPECIES AGGRESSION
5 mg once daily for 5 to 7 days, then once weekly; PO

MELARSOMINE

INDICATIONS: Melarsomine (Immiticide ★) is indicated in the treatment of heartworm disease caused by immature (4-month-old, stage
L₅) to mature adult infections of *Dirofilaria immitis* in dogs. The drug
causes greater worm mortality than thiacetarsamide and is associated
with fewer complications.

ADVERSE AND COMMON SIDE EFFECTS: Melarsomine has a low
margin of safety. Three times the recommended dosage may cause
pulmonary inflammation, edema, and death. Pain and irritation at the
injection site accompanied by swelling, tenderness, and reluctance to
move occurs in up to 30% of dogs. Recovery from signs of pain occurs
over 1 week to 1 month. Firm nodules may persist indefinitely. Other
adverse effects may include coughing, gagging, depression, lethargy,
anorexia, fever, lung congestion, and vomiting. Hypersalivation and
panting are infrequent. Various degrees of neurologic impairment
have been identified and may include unilateral lameness, proprioceptive deficits, paresis that may be bilateral, marked paraparesis to
paralysis of the hind legs, dementia, coma, and death. Some dogs may
partially recover. Safety for use in pregnant bitches or lactating or
breeding animals has not been established.

DRUG INTERACTIONS: None reported.

SUPPLIED AS VETERINARY PRODUCT:
For injection containing 25 mg/mL

MELOXICAM

INDICATIONS: Meloxicam (Metacam ✤) is a nonsteroidal anti-
inflammatory agent with analgesic and antipyretic properties. It is
indicated for the relief of inflammation and pain in acute and chronic

musculoskeletal disease. Clinical benefit is generally noted within 3 to 4 days. Preoperative administration of meloxicam is a safe and effective method of controlling postoperative pain for 20 hours in dogs undergoing abdominal surgery. The analgesic effects are comparable to those of ketoprofen and superior to those of butorphanol. The drug inhibits prostaglandin synthesis and is primarily a COX-2 inhibitor. It is 12 times more effective in inhibiting COX-2 activity than COX-1 activity.

ADVERSE AND COMMON SIDE EFFECTS: Vomiting, diarrhea, loss of appetite, apathy, and hematochezia may occur. Side effects are generally transient and disappear following cessation of drug use. Avoid use of the drug during lactation or during the last third of pregnancy, if gastrointestinal bleeding is suspect, if there is evidence of cardiac, hepatic, or renal disease, or if there is a coagulation disorder.

DRUG INTERACTIONS: Do not administer the drug concurrently or within 24 hours of other steroidal or nonsteroidal anti-inflammatory products, aminoglycoside antibiotics, or other anticoagulation products.

SUPPLIED AS VETERINARY PRODUCTS:
Plastic squeeze dropper bottles containing 1.5 mg/mL in 10-, 32-, or 100-mL bottles
For injection containing 5 mg/mL

MELPHALAN

INDICATIONS: Melphalan (Alkeran ✤ ★) is an alkylating chemotherapeutic agent indicated in the treatment of lymphoreticular neoplasms, osteosarcoma, mammary and lung tumors, ovarian adenocarcinoma, and multiple myeloma.

ADVERSE AND COMMON SIDE EFFECTS: Nausea, anorexia, and vomiting have been reported. Leukopenia, thrombocytopenia, and anemia also may occur. The complete blood count should be monitored on a regular basis. Pulmonary infiltrates and fibrosis are reported.

DRUG INTERACTIONS: In humans, the concomitant use of melphalan and cyclosporine has resulted in nephrotoxicity.

SUPPLIED AS HUMAN PRODUCTS:
Tablets containing 2 mg
For injection containing 50 mg/vial

MEPERIDINE

INDICATIONS: Meperidine (Demerol ✤ ★) is a short-acting narcotic analgesic used for the relief of moderate to severe pain or as a preanesthetic. It has minimal sedative effects and is only approximately one eighth as potent as morphine in providing pain relief. It has a more rapid onset of action and shorter duration than morphine, causes less depression of the cough reflex, and is spasmolytic for some smooth muscle-containing tissues. Given orally, the onset of action occurs within 15 minutes with a peak effect within 1 hour. The analgesic effect is only approximately one half as effective when given orally as opposed to that given parenterally. Given parenterally, the onset of analgesia occurs within 10 minutes, and the duration of effect is 2 to 4 hours. In cats, its duration of action is short (60 minutes). Meperidine is the only narcotic with depressant effects on the heart, and it also may cause histamine release.

ADVERSE AND COMMON SIDE EFFECTS: Nausea, vomiting, and decreased peristalsis are reported. With drug overdose, respiratory depression, cardiovascular collapse, hypothermia, skeletal muscle hypotonia, and seizure are possible side effects. Naloxone should be used to reverse the respiratory depression. Bronchoconstriction after IV use in dogs has been reported. The drug is quite irritating given subcutaneously. Meperidine should not be given to animals with head trauma because it may increase intracranial pressure. It should be used with caution in animals with adrenocortical insufficiency, hypothyroid disease, and renal disease, in geriatrics, in those with respiratory disease, and in debilitated patients. Meperidine may potentiate the toxicity of venom of the scorpion *Centruroides sculpturatus*. In cats, the drug may cause CNS excitation with hyperexcitability, tremors, and seizure activity at doses greater than 20 mg/kg.

DRUG INTERACTIONS: Central nervous system depression or stimulation induced by meperidine may be potentiated by amphetamines, barbiturates, or cimetidine. Phenytoin may increase meperidine toxicity and decrease its analgesic effects.

SUPPLIED AS HUMAN PRODUCTS:
Tablets containing 50 and 100 mg
Syrup containing 10 and 25 mg/mL
For injection containing 50-, 75-, and 100-mg/mL single- or multiple-dose units and 25-, 75-, and 100-mg single-dose ampules

MERCAPTOPURINE

INDICATIONS: Mercaptopurine (Purinethol ✤ ★) is an antimetabolite chemotherapeutic agent used in the treatment of lymphosarcoma, acute lymphocytic and granulocytic leukemia, and rheumatoid arthritis. In humans, the drug also has been used to treat granulomatous and ulcerative colitis unresponsive to corticosteroids or sulfasalazine.

ADVERSE AND COMMON SIDE EFFECTS: Nausea, anorexia, vomiting, and diarrhea have been reported. Bone marrow suppression and hepatotoxicity may occur. Leukopenia is rare. In addition, cholestasis, oral and intestinal ulcers, and pancreatitis have been documented in humans.

DRUG INTERACTIONS: Allopurinol delays the metabolism of mercaptopurine and enhances its antineoplastic effect and toxicity. Mercaptopurine may reverse the neuromuscular blocking effect of tubocurarine.

SUPPLIED AS HUMAN PRODUCT:
Tablets containing 50 mg

MEROPENEM

INDICATIONS: Meropenem (Merrem ✤ ★) is a carbapenems β-lactam antibiotic similar in spectrum of activity as imipenem. This antibiotic has increased activity against gram-negative organisms; it has a 2- to 4-fold greater activity against *Pseudomonas aeruginosa* and a 2- to 32-fold increased activity against Enterobacteriaceae than imipenem in vitro. See also IMIPENEM-CILASTATIN.

ADVERSE AND COMMON SIDE EFFECTS: Compared to imipenem, meropenem causes minimal nausea and vomiting and is not nephrotoxic or neurotoxic. Seizure activity is less common than that associated with imipenem. In people, systemic adverse events reported also include diarrhea, vomiting, and headache.

DRUG INTERACTIONS: Experience with use of this drug in small animals is limited. In people, probenecid (agent used in people to increase the excretion of uric acid in chronic gout and gouty arthritis) has been found to inhibit the renal excretion of meropenem, leading to statistically significant increases in the elimination half-life and extent of systemic exposure. See also IMIPENEM-CILASTATIN.

SUPPLIED AS HUMAN PRODUCT:
For injection in 20-mL vials containing 500 mg or 30-mL vials containing 1 g

METAMUCIL

INDICATIONS: Metamucil ✤ ★ is a psyllium hydrophilic mucilloid used for the management of constipation and colitis. It may require 12 to 24 hours to be effective.

ADVERSE AND COMMON SIDE EFFECTS: Side effects are minimal. Temporary cramping, flatulence, and bloating may occur. It should not be used in patients with abdominal pain, vomiting, nausea, or fecal impaction.

DRUG INTERACTIONS: None established.

SUPPLIED AS HUMAN PRODUCT:
Powder containing 3.4 to 3.6 g psyllium hydrophilic mucilloid/ packet and 3.4 g psyllium hydrophilic mucilloid per rounded teaspoonful

METHENAMINE MANDELATE

INDICATIONS: Methenamine mandelate (Mandelamine ❖ ★, Rena-Tone ❖) is a urinary antibacterial agent. It is used in the management of urinary tract infection. In the presence of acidic urine (pH less than 6), the drug is hydrolyzed to formaldehyde. Concurrent use of a urinary acidifier is common. It also is effective against fungal urinary tract infections.

ADVERSE AND COMMON SIDE EFFECTS: The drug may cause GI upset and dysuria (due to urinary tract irritation). It should not be given to patients with renal insufficiency.

DRUG INTERACTIONS: Methenamine should not be given to patients receiving sulfamethizole because formaldehyde and sulfamethizole form insoluble precipitates in acid urine. Drugs that increase urine pH, e.g., acetazolamide and sodium bicarbonate, prevent hydrolysis of methenamine and decrease its antimicrobial efficacy.

SUPPLIED AS VETERINARY PRODUCT:
Liquid containing 100 g

SUPPLIED AS HUMAN PRODUCTS:
Tablet containing 500 mg and 1 g
Oral suspension containing 0.5 g/5 mL

METHIMAZOLE

INDICATIONS: Methimazole (Tapazole ❖ ★) is the drug of choice for the medical management of feline hyperthyroid disease. It is safer and more potent than propylthiouracil in blocking thyroid hormone synthesis. Use of the drug generally will bring serum T_4 into normal ranges within 2 to 3 weeks in 87% of cases. In those cats that remain hyperthyroid after this time, increasing the dose to 15 to 20 mg/day generally is successful. A small number of cats are methimazole resistant. The drug also is used to decrease renal toxicity of cisplatin in dogs. Its efficacy in this regard is probably related to its antioxidant properties.

ADVERSE AND COMMON SIDE EFFECTS: Adverse effects have been observed in approximately 15% of cats and generally are transient. Anorexia, vomiting, and transient lethargy have been reported. Serum antinuclear antibodies develop in many cats with long-term use of the drug. A glucocorticoid-responsive pruritus involving the face, ears, and neck may occur. Hepatopathy, icterus, and bleeding tendencies (epistaxis, oral hemorrhage, excessive bleeding during surgery) may occur. Methimazole interferes with the activation of vitamin K-dependent coagulation factors. In less than 2% of cases, thrombocytopenia and agranulocytosis have been reported in cats treated with the drug. Withdrawal of the drug and provision of care for thrombocytopenia or agranulocytosis generally results in resolution of the drug reaction. Transient eosinophilia, lymphocytosis, and leukopenia have also been noted in a small number of cases. Myasthenia gravis has been reported in cats after treatment with methimazole. Cats with hyperthyroidism have increased glomerular filtration rates (GFR). Treatment with methimazole results in a decreased GFR and may be associated with increased serum urea concentrations. Cats on chronic methimazole therapy should be rechecked every 3 to 6 months to assay serum T_4 levels and to check for signs of drug toxicity.

DRUG INTERACTIONS: The activity of anticoagulants may be potentiated by methimazole.

SUPPLIED AS HUMAN PRODUCT:
Tablets containing 5 and 10 mg

METHIONINE

INDICATIONS: Methionine (Methio-Tabs ♣, Methigel ♣ ★, Methio-Form ♣ ★) is a urinary acidifying agent used in the treatment and prevention of struvite urolithiasis and to control urine odor. Urine acidification also may be effective adjunctive therapy to optimize the efficacy of certain antibiotics, e.g., penicillin, ampicillin, carbenicillin, tetracycline, and nitrofurantoin, in the treatment of urinary tract infections.

ADVERSE AND COMMON SIDE EFFECTS: The drug is contraindicated in patients with renal failure or pancreatic disease. The drug has no place in the treatment of hepatic lipidosis unless it is caused by choline deficiency, as with pancreatic exocrine insufficiency. It may potentiate clinical signs of hepatic encephalopathy by leading to the increased production of mercaptan-like compounds. The drug is not recommended for use in kittens.

DRUG INTERACTIONS: Methionine may increase the renal excretion of quinidine. The antibacterial efficacy of the aminoglycosides and erythromycin may be decreased in the presence of an acid urine produced by methionine.

SUPPLIED AS VETERINARY PRODUCTS:
Tablets containing 200 and 500 mg
Chewable tablets containing 500 mg
Gel containing 400 mg/5 g [Methigel]

METHOCARBAMOL

INDICATIONS: Methocarbamol (Robaxin-V ★, Robaxin ♣ ★) is a central-acting muscle relaxant that may be used as adjunct therapy to rest and physical therapy in the treatment of musculoskeletal injury. It also has been used to reduce muscular spasm associated with tetanus and metaldehyde or strychnine poisoning.

ADVERSE AND COMMON SIDE EFFECTS: Excessive salivation, sedation, vomiting, muscular weakness, and ataxia have been reported. Extravascular injection may cause tissue necrosis. The drug should not be given to animals with renal dysfunction, nor should it be used in pregnant animals.

DRUG INTERACTIONS: Other CNS depressants may potentiate CNS depressive effects of methocarbamol.

SUPPLIED AS VETERINARY PRODUCTS (★ Only):
Tablets containing 500 mg
For injection containing 100 mg/mL

SUPPLIED AS HUMAN PRODUCTS (♣ ★):
Tablets containing 500 and 750 mg
For injection containing 100 mg/mL

METHOHEXITAL

INDICATIONS: Methohexital (Brevital ★) is an ultra-short-acting barbiturate anesthetic. It is approximately 2 to 3 times more potent than pentothal but with a shorter duration of action. Also see BARBITURATES.

ADVERSE AND COMMON SIDE EFFECTS: This agent may cause profound respiratory depression. The lethal dose is only 2 to 3 times that of the anesthetic dose. To limit the likelihood of muscle tremors and seizure activity upon recovery, premedication is recommended. If seizures do occur they can be managed with diazepam. Too rapid an injection may cause apnea and hypotension. Also see BARBITURATES.

DRUG INTERACTIONS: Methohexital may augment CNS depression if used with drugs associated with a similar response.

SUPPLIED AS HUMAN PRODUCT:
For injection in vials containing 0.5, 2.5, and 5 gm

METHOTREXATE

INDICATIONS: Methotrexate ♣ ★ is an antimetabolite chemotherapeutic agent that has been recommended in the treatment of lymphoreticular neoplasms, myeloproliferative disease, osteosarcoma, transmissible venereal tumor, and Sertoli cell tumor.

ADVERSE AND COMMON SIDE EFFECTS: Vomiting, nausea, diarrhea, leukopenia, thrombocytopenia, and anemia are reported. Delayed toxicity may be associated with oral and GI ulceration, renal tubular necrosis, hepatic necrosis, alopecia, pulmonary infiltrates and fibrosis, encephalopathy, and anaphylactoid reactions with high doses. Leucovorin calcium, a reduced folate, given at 3 mg/m^2 within 3 hours of methotrexate administration, helps ameliorate these effects. Methotrexate may adversely affect spermiogenesis and may cause embryotoxicity or congenital malformations.

DRUG INTERACTIONS: Chloramphenicol, salicylates, sulfonamides, phenylbutazone, phenytoin, tetracyclines, and p-aminobenzoic acid (PABA) displace methotrexate from plasma proteins, causing increased toxicity. Oral aminoglycoside antibiotics may reduce GIT absorption. Penicillin and probenecid increase methotrexate plasma levels predisposing to toxicity.

SUPPLIED AS HUMAN PRODUCTS:
Tablets containing 2.5 mg
For injection (parenteral solution) containing equivalent of 2.5, 10, and 25 mg/mL methotrexate
Lyophilized powder equivalent to 25 and 1000 mg/vial

METHOXYFLURANE

INDICATIONS: Methoxyflurane (Metafane ♣) is used for induction and maintenance of general anesthesia. Because induction time for methoxyflurane alone is slow (5 to 10 minutes), an ultrashort-acting IV anesthetic generally is used for induction.

ADVERSE AND COMMON SIDE EFFECTS: The drug should be used cautiously in animals with liver disease. Minimal hepatic damage may occur with drug overdose. Hypoxia at deep levels of anesthesia predisposes to hepatic damage. The drug is potentially nephrotoxic.

Nephrotoxicity is enhanced by dehydration and the concurrent use of other potentially nephrotoxic drugs, e.g., flunixin meglumine.

DRUG INTERACTIONS: Large doses of epinephrine may produce atrioventricular block and arrhythmias. Vomiting is infrequent and mild when it does occur. The drug will cross the placental barrier and depress the fetus. If depression of a newborn does occur, administration of oxygen usually brings about prompt recovery.

SUPPLIED AS VETERINARY PRODUCT:
Available in 118-mL bottles

METHYLENE BLUE

INDICATIONS: Methylene blue ✦ ★ is used in the treatment of methemoglobinemia. The drug reduces ferric^{+3} iron to the ferrous^{+2} state thus improving oxygen carrying capacity. It also has been used for the intraoperative identification of parathyroid and pancreatic islet cell tumors in dogs.

ADVERSE AND COMMON SIDE EFFECTS: The drug is contraindicated in patients with renal insufficiency. Methylene blue may cause Heinz body hemolytic anemia and possibly acute renal failure. Cats are especially sensitive to Heinz body formation.

In people, additional side effects may include bladder irritation, nausea, vomiting, diarrhea, and abdominal pain. With large IV doses, fever, cardiovascular abnormalities, methemoglobinemia, and profuse sweating have been recorded in humans.

DRUG INTERACTIONS: None reported.

SUPPLIED AS HUMAN PRODUCT:
For injection containing 10 mg/mL

OTHER USES
Dogs
TO STAIN ISLET CELL TUMORS
3 mg/kg in 250 mL saline over 30 to 40 minutes intraoperatively; IV. Tumors appear reddish-violet against a dusky blue background.
TO STAIN PARATHYROID TUMORS
Dose as aforementioned; tumor staining becomes evident starting 15 minutes after infusion. Tumors appear dark blue.

METHYLPHENIDATE

INDICATIONS: Methylphenidate (Ritalin ✦ ★) is used in dogs in the management of narcolepsy (as a supplement to imipramine) and hyperkinesis.

ADVERSE AND COMMON SIDE EFFECTS: In humans, nervousness, anorexia, and tachycardia are reported. Overdose may cause vomiting, tremors, muscle twitching, convulsions, arrhythmias, mydriasis, and dryness of the mucous membranes. The drug tends to lose its effect over time. Experience with the drug in small animals is limited. Signs of toxicosis reported in a cat included muscle tremors, mydriasis, agitation, and tachycardia. In severe toxicosis, supportive treatment, anxiolytic drugs, e.g., diazepam, and the use of an adrenergic blocking agent, e.g., propranolol, may be required.

DRUG INTERACTIONS: Combination with MAO inhibitors, e.g., possibly amitraz and selegiline, may cause hypertension.

SUPPLIED AS HUMAN PRODUCTS:
Tablets (sustained-release) containing 20 mg
Tablets containing 5, 10, and 20 mg

METHYLPREDNISOLONE

INDICATIONS: Methylprednisolone (Medrol ✤ ★, Depo-Medrol ✤ ★) is an intermediate-acting glucocorticoid used for its anti-inflammatory properties, to control autoimmune skin diseases in dogs, as adjunctive therapy in spinal cord trauma, and in the treatment of shock. In cats, it also is used to treat eosinophilic ulcers, plasma cell gingivitis-pharyngitis, and for the adjunctive treatment of asthma.

ADVERSE AND COMMON SIDE EFFECTS AND DRUG INTERACTIONS: See GLUCOCORTICOID AGENTS.

SUPPLIED AS VETERINARY PRODUCTS:
Tablets containing 4 mg [Medrol]
For injection containing 20 and 40 mg/mL methylprednisolone acetate [Depo-Medrol]

SUPPLIED AS HUMAN PRODUCTS:
Tablets containing 2, 4, 8, 16, 24, and 32 mg [Medrol ✤ ★]
For injection containing 40 mg/mL, 125 mg/2 mL, 500 mg/8 mL, 1,000 mg/16 mL, and 2,000 mg/32 mL methylprednisolone sodium succinate [Solu-Medrol ✤ ★]

OTHER USES
Dogs
ANTI-INFLAMMATORY DOSE
i) 1 mg/kg tid; PO methylprednisolone
ii) 1.1 mg/kg; SC, IM methylprednisolone acetate (lasts 1 to 3 weeks in skin conditions)

AUTOIMMUNE SKIN DISEASE "PULSE THERAPY"
Methylprednisolone sodium succinate 11 mg/kg in 250 mL D₅W infused over 1 hour for 3 consecutive days. Maintenance therapy includes oral prednisone at 1.1 mg/kg every 1 to 2 days and azathioprine (2.2 mg/kg daily for 2 weeks, then every 48 hours). Cimetidine may be given concurrently to reduce the incidence of GIT ulcerations.

Cats

ANTI-INFLAMMATORY AGENT
Methylprednisolone acetate 5.5 mg/kg; IM or SC (effects for skin conditions may last from 1 week to 6 months)

EOSINOPHILIC ULCER
Methylprednisolone acetate 20 mg; SC every 2 weeks for 2 to 3 doses

PLASMA CELL GINGIVITIS/PHARYNGITIS
Methylprednisolone acetate 10 to 20 mg PRN; SC

INFLAMMATORY BOWEL DISEASE
i)   Methylprednisolone acetate 20 mg; SC, IM, repeated at 1- to 2-week intervals for 2 to 3 doses, then given every 2 to 4 weeks PRN

ii)   20 mg; IM every 2 to 4 weeks

FELINE ASTHMA
Methylprednisolone acetate 1 to 2 mg/kg; IM

METOCLOPRAMIDE

INDICATIONS: Metoclopramide (Reglan ★, generics ♣ ★) is an antiemetic agent with central (chemoreceptor trigger zone) and peripheral activity. It stimulates and coordinates esophageal, gastric, pyloric, and duodenal motor activity, contributes to lower esophageal sphincter competence, and promotes gastric emptying. It is useful in the management of vomiting, gastroesophageal reflux, and gastric motility disorders. It has no effect on colon motility. The drug has also been used to stimulate detrusor contractions in dogs.

ADVERSE AND COMMON SIDE EFFECTS: Metoclopramide should not be used in patients with gastric outlet obstruction or those with a history of epilepsy. Renal disease may increase blood levels of the drug. Central nervous system reactions include increased frequency of seizure activity, vertigo, hyperactivity, depression, and disorientation. Clinical signs of overdose also include dyspnea, lacrimation, ataxia, miosis, tachycardia, tremors, and tonic seizures. Diphenhydramine may be useful in controlling extraparamidal effects of the drug.

DRUG INTERACTIONS: Phenothiazine drugs may potentiate CNS effects. Digoxin, cimetidine, tetracycline, narcotic agents, and sedatives enhance CNS effects. Digoxin absorption also may be decreased, whereas acetaminophen, aspirin, diazepam, and tetracycline absorption may be accelerated. Atropine will block the effects of the drug on GIT motility.

SUPPLIED AS HUMAN PRODUCTS:
Tablets containing 5 and 10 mg
Syrup containing 1 mg/mL and 5 mg/mL
For injection containing 5 mg/mL

OTHER USES
Dogs
DISORDERS OF GASTRIC MOTILITY
0.2 to 0.4 mg/kg tid; PO, SC given 30 minutes before meals

ESOPHAGEAL REFLUX
i)   0.5 mg/kg tid; PO

ii) 0.2 to 0.5 mg/kg tid; PO, SC given 30 minutes before meals and at bedtime

Cats
GASTRIC MOTILITY DISORDERS AND ESOPHAGEAL REFLUX
0.2 to 0.4 mg/kg tid to qid; PO

METOPROLOL

INDICATIONS: Metoprolol (Lopressor ♣ ★) is a selective β_1-blocking agent equal in potency to propranolol. It is a preferred β-blocker in patients with pulmonary disease such as asthma. The drug also is useful in the management of supraventricular tachyarrhythmias, ventricular premature contractions, and hypertrophic cardiomyopathy.

ADVERSE AND COMMON SIDE EFFECTS: Depression, lethargy, bradycardia, impaired atrioventricular conduction, and congestive heart failure have been reported with the use of β-blocking drugs. Glycopyrrolate and dopamine may be used to counter bradycardia. The drug should be used with caution in patients with renal insufficiency.

DRUG INTERACTIONS: Barbiturates and rifampin may decrease the pharmacological effects of metoprolol. Cimetidine, methimazole, and propylthiouracil may increase the pharmacological effects of metoprolol. Digitalis may potentiate bradycardia associated with metoprolol. The pharmacological effects of hydralazine and metoprolol may be increased if both drugs are used concurrently. Indomethacin may cause a decrease in the antihypertensive effects of the drug.

SUPPLIED AS HUMAN PRODUCTS:
Tablets containing 50 and 100 mg
Tablets (slow-release) containing 100 and 200 mg
For injection containing 1 mg/mL

METRONIDAZOLE

INDICATIONS: Metronidazole (Flagyl ✿ ★) is a synthetic antibacterial, antiprotozoal agent that has been used in the treatment of giardiasis, trichomoniasis, amoebiasis, balantidiasis, and trypanosomiasis. It is as effective and is better tolerated than quinacrine for the treatment of giardiasis, but it is not as safe or as efficacious as albendazole. It is bactericidal to many anaerobic bacteria, including *Bacteroides* spp., *Fusobacterium, Clostridium* spp., *Veillonella, Peptococcus,* and *Peptostreptococcus.* It has been recommended in conjunction with amoxicillin and famotidine for the management of *Helicobacter* spp. infection. Metronidazole has been used in the treatment of septicemia, meningitis, peritonitis, biliary infections, inflammatory bowel disease including colitis, and gingivostomatitis in which anaerobic bacteria are involved. The drug also may have immunosuppressive or immunostimulatory properties. It inhibits cell-mediated immunity.

ADVERSE AND COMMON SIDE EFFECTS: Clinical signs generally begin 7 to 12 days after initiation of therapy. Nausea, anorexia, vomiting, diarrhea, hepatotoxicity, hematuria, neutropenia, lethargy, weakness, bradycardia, and dose-dependent neurologic signs (ataxia, nystagmus, blindness, hypermetria, hyperesthesia, tremors, proprioceptive deficits, seizure, head tilt, rigidity, and stiffness) have been reported. Recovery times range from 1 to 2 weeks. Faster recovery times may be promoted by the administration of diazepam (initial IV bolus of 0.43 mg/kg followed by an oral dose of 0.43 mg/kg tid for 3 days). Metronidazole toxicity with ataxia, alterations in mentation, and seizures has been reported in cats. Neutropenia and hematuria also have been seen in some dogs. It is potentially hepatotoxic. The tablets have a bitter taste and should not be crushed before use. The drug also may be mutagenic and should not be given to pregnant animals.

DRUG INTERACTIONS: Blood levels may be decreased by concurrent use of phenobarbital or phenytoin, and blood levels may be increased by cimetidine use.

SUPPLIED AS HUMAN PRODUCTS:
Tablets containing 250 and 500 mg
Capsules containing 375 mg
For injection containing 500 mg/vial and 500 mg in 100 mL of isotonic saline

OTHER USES
Dogs

LYMPHOCYTIC/PLASMOCYTIC ENTERITIS-COLITIS
i) 30 to 60 mg/kg once daily; PO
ii) 10 to 30 mg/kg 1 to 3 times daily for 2 to 4 weeks; PO (refractory cases)

ANAEROBIC INFECTIONS
i)   30 mg/kg per day divided tid to qid; PO

ii) 25 to 50 mg/kg bid; PO (bacterial meningitis)

GIT BACTERIAL OVERGROWTH
20 to 40 mg/kg once daily; PO (in food)

AMOEBIASIS, BALANTIDIASIS
60 mg/kg once daily; PO for 5 days

ADJUNCTIVE THERAPY IN HEPATIC ENCEPHALOPATHY
i)   20 mg/kg tid; PO

ii) 7.5 mg/kg tid for 2 to 4 weeks; PO

CHOLANGITIS
i)   7.5 mg/kg tid; PO

ii) 25 to 30 mg/kg bid; PO (may be used with chloramphenicol); 4 to
6 weeks of therapy may be required

STOMATITIS
15 mg/kg tid; PO

Cats

ANAEROBIC INFECTION
i)   10 mg/kg once daily; PO (adjunctive therapy of plasmacytic/
lymphocytic enteritis)

ii) 25 to 30 mg/kg bid; PO for 2 to 3 weeks (adjunctive therapy of hepatic lipidosis—efficacy unknown)

PLASMA CELL GINGIVITIS/PHARYNGITIS
50 mg/kg once daily; PO for 5 days (antibacterial effects)

INFLAMMATORY BOWEL DISEASE
10 to 20 mg/kg bid to tid; PO with prednisone 2 mg/kg per day; PO
(refractory cases)

BALANTIDIUM
10 to 25 mg/kg once to twice daily; PO for 5 days

MEXILETINE

INDICATIONS: Mexiletine (Mexitil ★, generic brands ❧) is an analog of lidocaine with electrophysiologic properties similar to those of
tocainide. The drug has been used in dogs to treat ventricular arrhythmias, including premature contractions and runs of tachycardia.

ADVERSE AND COMMON SIDE EFFECTS: Side effects are uncommon but may include vomiting. In humans, gastric irritation, anorexia,
and tremor are reported infrequently and resolve upon cessation of
therapy.

DRUG INTERACTIONS: Mexiletine may be used in combination with quinidine (6.6 to 22 mg/kg) in those cases refractory to either drug alone. Enhanced activity and a reduction in toxicity are noted when these drugs are used concurrently. Antacids, cimetidine, and narcotic analgesics may slow GI absorption. Hepatic enzyme inducers, e.g., phenobarbital, phenytoin, and rifampin, may increase drug clearance. Mexiletine may increase theophylline levels because of decreased hepatic metabolism of theophylline.

SUPPLIED AS HUMAN PRODUCT:
Capsules containing 100, 150, and 200 mg

MIBOLERONE

INDICATIONS: Mibolerone (Cheque Drops ★) is an androgenic, anabolic, antigonadotropic agent used for the prevention of estrus in adult female dogs.

ADVERSE AND COMMON SIDE EFFECTS: Mibolerone is contraindicated in female dogs with perianal adenoma, perianal adenocarcinoma, and liver and renal disease. The drug also is not recommended for use in Bedlington terriers. The drug should not be given to pregnant bitches because it will cause masculinization of the female fetus. In prepuberal females, the drug may cause premature closure of epiphyses, clitoral enlargement, and vaginitis. In the adult bitch, adverse effects may include mild clitoral enlargement, vulvovaginitis, and abnormal behavior, including riding behavior, urinary incontinence, exacerbation of seborrhea oleosa, and epiphora. Significant hepatic disease is rare, and renal changes generally are not pathologic. With the exception of mild residual clitoral enlargement, all changes resolve after discontinuation of the drug.

In the cat, dosages of 60 µg/day induced hepatic dysfunction, and dosages of 120 µg/day caused death. Other adverse effects noted in cats include clitoral enlargement, thyroid dysfunction, cervical dermis thickening, and pancreatic dysfunction. Although not approved for use in cats, the drug has been used to prevent estrus at doses of 50 µg/day. The potential for adverse side effects, however, is great. The drug may incite seizure activity in dogs predisposed to seizures.

DRUG INTERACTIONS: Mibolerone should not be used in conjunction with estrogen or progestin products.

SUPPLIED AS VETERINARY PRODUCT:
Oral drops containing 100 µg/mL

OTHER USES
Dogs
PSEUDOCYESIS
16 µg/kg once daily for 5 days; PO

GALACTORRHEA
8 to 18 µg/kg once daily for 5 days; PO (once discontinued galactorrhea may resume because of effects of prolactin)

MIDAZOLAM

INDICATIONS: Midazolam (Versed ❈ ★) is a short-acting parenteral benzodiazepine, CNS depressant with sedative-hypnotic, anxiolytic, muscle-relaxing, and anticonvulsant properties useful in small animals as a preanesthetic agent. The drug is 2 to 3 times more potent than diazepam and has a shorter half-life.

ADVERSE AND COMMON SIDE EFFECTS: No significant cardiovascular effects are noted. Respiratory depression and dose-dependent sedation occur.

DRUG INTERACTIONS: Barbiturates prolong respiratory depression predisposing to apnea and underventilation. Fentanyl and droperidol (Innovar-Vet) increase the hypnotic effect. Hypotension has been reported with the concurrent use of meperidine.

SUPPLIED AS HUMAN PRODUCTS:
For injection containing 1 and 5 mg/mL
In a syrup containing 2 mg/mL

MILBEMYCIN

INDICATIONS: Milbemycin oxime (Interceptor ❈ ★, Sentinel ❈ ★) is an anthelmintic used in dogs for the prevention of heartworm caused by *Dirofilaria immitis,* as a microfilaricide, and for the control of hookworm (*Ancylostoma caninum*) and roundworm (*Toxocara canis*) infections. It also may be effective against *Trichuris vulpis* infections. It has been used for the eradication of the nasal mite (*Pneumonyssoides caninum*) in dogs. The drug also prevents the development of infection in cats by larvae of *Dirofilaria immitis* and has been used in the treatment of generalized demodicosis in adult dogs.

ADVERSE AND COMMON SIDE EFFECTS: At therapeutic doses no adverse effects are seen. With drug overdose (5 times recommended dose), the only adverse effects seen were transient ataxia and trembling in 8-week-old puppies. If milbemycin is administered to heartworm-infected dogs, a mild shock-like reaction may occur.

DRUG INTERACTIONS: None reported.

SUPPLIED AS VETERINARY PRODUCTS:
Tablets containing 2.3, 5.75, 11.5, and 23 mg [Interceptor]
Tablets containing 2.3, 5.75, 11.5, and 23 mg with lufenuron [Sentinel]

OTHER USES
Dogs
JUVENILE GENERALIZED DEMODICOSIS
11.5 mg/22.7 kg once daily. Treat until no mites are detected and then for an additional 30 days thereafter. If mite counts are still high after 90 days, double the dose. Resolution has been reported in 83% of previously untreated cases, and cure is reported in 60% of cases.

ADULT CHRONIC GENERALIZED DEMODICOSIS
i) 0.52 to 3.8 mg/kg once daily; PO for 30 days after mites are no longer detected on skin scraping

NB: relapse may occur

ii) 1 mg/kg per day; PO until 30 days after skin scraping fails to detect mites. If the mite count has not decreased by 25%, increase the drug dose to 2 mg/kg per day.

DIROFILARIA IMMITIS
500 µg/kg 3 to 4 weeks after adulticide therapy (microfilaricide)

PNEUMONYSSOIDES CANINUM
0.5 to 1.0 mg/kg once weekly for 3 consecutive weeks; PO

Cats
DIROFILARIA IMMITIS
0.5 to 0.9 mg/kg 60 and 90 days after inoculation with infective larvae prevents development of infection

MINERAL OIL

INDICATIONS: Mineral oil ♣ ★ is used for the relief of constipation. It softens stools by coating the feces and preventing the colonic absorption of water. The agent works at the level of the colon and may take 6 to 12 hours to work effectively. It also has been used to retard the absorption of lipid-soluble toxins (kerosene, metaldehyde).

ADVERSE AND COMMON SIDE EFFECTS: Mineral oil is contra-indicated in patients with nausea, vomiting, abdominal pain, intestinal obstruction, or dysphagia. A small amount of oil is absorbed, but it generally is of no clinical significance. Because of the lack of taste, accidental aspiration and subsequent pneumonia may occur. Occasionally, pruritus ani may occur. Interference with postoperative anorectal wound healing may occur. Prolonged use may cause anorexia and vomiting.

DRUG INTERACTIONS: Increased absorption may occur if mineral oil is given concurrently with docusate sodium or docusate calcium. Mineral oil may interfere with the absorption of fat-soluble vitamins and should only be given between meals. Mineral oil may interfere with action of nonabsorbable sulfonamides.

SUPPLIED AS VETERINARY PRODUCTS:
Several products are available, including generic mineral oil as well
as petrolatum preparations, Hairball Preparations ✤ ★, Tonic-Lax ✤,
and many others.

MINOCYCLINE

INDICATIONS: Minocycline (Minocin ✤ ★) is a second-generation,
long-acting, lipid-soluble tetracycline. It is more active against anaerobes and several facultative intracellular bacteria, such as *Brucella canis*,
than other tetracyclines except for doxycycline. It is more active against
Nocardia and staphylococcus than other tetracyclines. The drug has
been used in the treatment of actinomycosis, canine ehrlichiosis, nocar-
diosis, and Rocky Mountain spotted fever. Minocycline does not reach
high enough concentrations in the urine to be effective in treating urinary tract infection. Also see TETRACYCLINE ANTIBIOTICS.

ADVERSE AND COMMON SIDE EFFECTS: Hypotension, shock,
and urticaria developed in dogs given rapid doses of minocycline.
Doses of 10 to 20 mg/kg per day caused the erythrocyte count to
decrease and alanine transferase (ALT) activity to increase in dogs.
Daily IV doses of 40 mg/kg caused decreased appetite and weight loss.
None of these side effects were noted at similar oral doses.

DRUG INTERACTIONS: Minocycline and doxycycline are less affected by the presence of food. In fact, these two agents often are given
with food to decrease GIT irritation.

SUPPLIED AS HUMAN PRODUCTS:
Capsule containing 50 and 100 mg
Oral syrup containing 10 mg/mL

MISOPROSTOL

INDICATIONS: Misoprostol (Cytotec ✤ ★) is a synthetic prostaglandin E_1 analog used to prevent gastric ulceration. It mitigates nonsteroidal anti-inflammatory drug-induced gastroduodenal injury.
Although partial protection is provided, gastritis still may occur and
contribute to vomiting. The drug decreases gastric acid secretion,
increases bicarbonate and mucus secretion, increases epithelial cell
turnover, and increases mucosal blood flow. The drug did not prevent
gastric hemorrhage in dogs treated with methylprednisolone and is
not effective in the healing or prevention of gastric mucosal lesions in
dogs with acute degenerative disc disease treated with corticosteroids.
Less common reported uses include intravaginal administration in
conjunction with prostaglandin $F_{2\alpha}$ for pregnancy termination in the
mid to late stages of gestation. Misoprostol is reported to be effective

in the treatment of canine atopic dermatitis, reducing pruritus and the severity of skin lesions in patients with uncomplicated nonseasonal chronic atopic dermatitis.

ADVERSE AND COMMON SIDE EFFECTS: Vomiting, diarrhea, flatulence, and abdominal pain are reported. The incidence of diarrhea can be minimized by adjusting the dose, by administering the drug after food, and by avoiding the administration of misoprostol with magnesium-containing antacids. The drug may induce abortion in pregnant animals. Experience with the drug in small animals is limited.

DRUG INTERACTIONS: No clinically significant drug interactions have been reported.

SUPPLIED AS HUMAN PRODUCT:
Tablets containing 100 and 200 µg

MITOTANE

INDICATIONS: Mitotane or o,p′-DDD (Lysodren ✤ ★) is indicated in the treatment of pituitary-dependent hyperadrenocorticism in dogs. It causes selective necrosis of the zona fasciculata and reticularis in the adrenal gland. Damage to the zona glomerulosa is slight. The drug also is used to manage primary adrenal hyperadrenocorticism, but patients with adrenal tumors causing hyperadrenocorticism appear more resistant and require higher drug doses. Target serum cortisol levels after ACTH stimulation are between 2 and 4 µg/dL (less than ~112 nmol/L). Hyperadrenocorticism in cats, although rare, can also be treated with mitotane. The drug is fat soluble and should be given with food.

ADVERSE AND COMMON SIDE EFFECTS: Mitotane is effective and relatively safe for treatment of canine pituitary-dependent hyperadrenocorticism. More than 80% of dogs are reported to have a good to excellent response. Lethargy, vomiting, weakness, anorexia, and diarrhea are reported. Dividing the dose, increasing the time interval, or both and, administering the drug with food will help reduce the gastrointestinal side effects. In approximately 5% of dogs, adrenal insufficiency develops. Although cats appear more sensitive to the chlorinated hydrocarbons, the drug has been used in this species. It is well tolerated by 75% of cats and results in adrenocortical suppression in half.

DRUG INTERACTIONS: Spironolactone may decrease pharmacological effects of the drug. Mitotane may induce hepatic microsomal enzymes and increase the metabolism of barbiturates and warfarin. Insulin requirements in diabetic patients may be decreased as the hyperadrenocortical situation is brought under control. Additive depression may occur if the drug is used concurrently with CNS depressants. Phenobarbital may decrease serum concentrations of the drug.

SUPPLIED AS HUMAN PRODUCT:
Tablets containing 500 mg

OTHER USES
Dogs
ADRENAL TUMORS CAUSING HYPERADRENOCORTICISM
50 to 75 mg/kg per day for 10 to 14 days (induction) with prednisone at 0.2 mg/kg per day; PO; maintenance regimen is 75 to 100 mg/kg per week

MITOXANTRONE

INDICATIONS: Mitoxantrone (Novantrone ♣ ★) is a chemothera-peutic agent related to doxorubicin. It has been used in dogs to treat various malignancies, including lymphoma, fibrosarcoma, thyroid car-cinomas, transitional cell carcinoma, hemangiopericytoma, and renal adenocarcinoma. The drug also has been used in cats with malignant tumors.

ADVERSE AND COMMON SIDE EFFECTS: The drug is considered safe and effective. The most common signs of toxicosis noted in dogs include depression, vomiting, diarrhea, anorexia, and sepsis secondary to myelosuppression. Use of the drug has not been associated with car-diotoxicity, as noted with doxorubicin. Toxicity is not dose dependent in dogs. Neutropenia may occur (nadir on day 10). The use of recom-binant canine granulocyte colony-stimulating factor (Amgen, Thou-sand Oaks, CA) at a dosage of 5 μg/kg per day SC for 20 days after infusion of mitoxantrone reduces the severity and duration of myelo-suppression and neutropenia. Also see GRANULOCYTE COLONY-STIMULATING FACTOR (Neupogen).

The most common adverse effects in cats include vomiting, anorexia, diarrhea, lethargy, sepsis secondary to myelosuppression, and seizures. The drug may even cause death in some cats.

DRUG INTERACTIONS: Mitoxantrone should not be mixed with heparin because precipitates may form.

SUPPLIED AS HUMAN PRODUCT:
For injection containing 2 mg/mL

MORPHINE

INDICATIONS: Morphine (Astramorph ★, Duramorph ★, Roxanol ★, M.S. Contin ♣ ★, M.O.S. ♣ ★, Morphitec ♣, Statex ♣) is a very effec-tive analgesic narcotic agent. It is used for the management of acute pain and as a preanesthetic agent. Analgesia lasts 4 to 6 hours after IM injection. In addition to analgesia, morphine produces CNS depression with sedation or sleep. It increases cardiac output and decreases pulmonary edema associated with congestive heart failure and cardiomyopathy. The drug also has been administered via epidural injection to relieve somatic or visceral pain, especially of the hind limbs, but as far forward as the neck. It is particularly useful after hind limb, fore limb, and pelvic orthopedic surgery. The onset of action is 30 to 60 minutes, and the duration of analgesia is 6 to 24 hours.

ADVERSE AND COMMON SIDE EFFECTS: In dogs morphine may produce initial excitement, restlessness, panting, salivation, nausea, vomiting, urination, defecation, and hypotension. Subsequently, CNS depression, constipation, urinary retention, bradycardia, respiratory depression, hypothermia, and miosis occur. Morphine should be used with caution in animals with biliary tract disease because it will increase bile duct luminal pressure. In cats, analgesia and CNS depression occur at lower doses (0.1 mg/kg qid). At doses of 1 mg/kg, hyperexcitability, tonic spasms, seizure activity, ataxia, aggression, vomiting, and even death may occur. The depressive effects of the drug are antagonized by naloxone (0.1 mg/kg; IV). The drug should not be used in animals with renal failure or a history of seizures or in those in hypovolemic shock. Pruritus may occur after epidural injection.

DRUG INTERACTIONS: Phenothiazines, amitriptyline, antihistamines, fentanyl, and parenteral magnesium sulfate may potentiate the depressant effects of morphine.

SUPPLIED AS HUMAN PRODUCTS:
For injection containing 0.5, 1, 2, 4, 5, 8, 10, 15, 25, and 50 mg/mL
Tablets containing 5, 10, 15, 20, 25, 30, and 50 mg
Tablets (slow-release) containing 15, 30, 60, 100, and 200 mg
Syrup containing 1, 5, and 10 mg/mL
Oral solution containing 2, 4, 20, and 50 mg/mL

OTHER USES
Dogs
POSTOPERATIVE ANALGESIC
0.25 to 1 mg/kg PRN; IM, IV

EPIDURAL ANALGESIA
0.1 mg/kg diluted in 0.2 mL/kg of sterile saline injected into the lumbosacral space

PREANESTHETIC
0.1 to 0.2 mg/kg; SC

SUPRAVENTRICULAR PREMATURE BEATS
0.2 mg/kg; IM, SC

MOXIDECTIN

INDICATIONS: Moxidectin (ProHeart 6 ♣ ★, Guardian ♣) is an injectable heartworm preventative that provides protection for a full season for dogs six months and older. The drug is effective in preventing heartworm and is also indicated for the treatment of canine hookworms *Ancylostoma caninum* and *Uncinaria stenocephala*.

ADVERSE AND COMMON SIDE EFFECTS: Moxidectin is considered to have a wider safety margin than ivermectin or milbemycin in ivermectin-sensitive collies. The manufacturer claims that in extensive studies the drug has been found to be safe in dogs with existing heartworm infections, safe in collies with known sensitivity to ivermectin, safe in breeding animals and pregnant animals, and safe at up to 20 times the recommended dose. Lethargy, vomiting, ataxia, anorexia, diarrhea, nervousness, weakness, polydipsia, and pruritus may occur.

DRUG INTERACTIONS: ProHeart 6 was safely used in conjunction with a variety of veterinary products commonly used in dogs (vaccines, antibiotics, anesthetics, and others).

SUPPLIED AS VETERINARY PRODUCT:
For injection containing 3.4 µg/mL after mixing [ProHeart]
Tablets containing 30, 68, or 136 µg

NAFCILLIN

INDICATIONS: Nafcillin (Unipen ★) is a β-lactamase–resistant parenterally administered penicillin effective against gram-positive bacteria, especially staphylococcal bacteria. For information see PENICILLIN ANTIBIOTICS.

ADVERSE AND COMMON SIDE EFFECTS: Nausea, vomiting, and diarrhea are reported in humans. Rash, pruritus, urticaria, and thrombophlebitis with IV injection also are reported. Intraoperative use of the drug may be associated with the development of acute azotemia in dogs. Experience with the drug in small animals is limited. Also see PENICILLIN ANTIBIOTICS.

DRUG INTERACTIONS: Also see PENICILLIN ANTIBIOTICS.

SUPPLIED AS HUMAN PRODUCT:
For injection containing 1, 2, and 10 g powder

NALOXONE

INDICATIONS: Naloxone ♣ ★ is a narcotic antagonist. It is the preferred agent for reversal of narcotic-induced depression, including respiratory depression induced by morphine, oxymorphone, meperidine, or fentanyl. Survival times have been shown to increase and mortality rates decrease in animals in endotoxic shock given naloxone. Naloxone increases cardiac output and arterial blood pressure, decreases hemoconcentration and metabolic acidosis, and helps prevent hypoglycemia.

ADVERSE AND COMMON SIDE EFFECTS: At recommended doses, the drug is relatively free of adverse effects. At high doses, seizure activity has been reported. The duration of its action may be less than that of the opioid it is antagonizing; consequently, animals should be monitored for signs of returning narcosis. The safety of the drug in pregnant animals has not been established, although reproductive studies in rats did not reveal any adverse effects.

DRUG INTERACTIONS: Naloxone also reverses the effects of butorphanol and pentazocine. One milliliter (0.4 mg) of P/M Naloxone counteracts the following narcotic dosages: 1.5 mg oxymorphone, 15 mg morphine sulfate, 100 mg meperidine, and 0.4 mg fentanyl.

SUPPLIED AS HUMAN PRODUCT:
For injection containing 0.02, 0.4, and 1 mg/mL

NALTREXONE

INDICATIONS: Naltrexone (Trexan ★, ReVia ♣ ★) is an opiate antagonist similar to naloxone other that it is longer-acting and is administered orally. It has been used in small animals to treat stereotypic compulsive behavioral disorders, e.g., licking, chewing, scratching, and tail chasing.

ADVERSE AND COMMON SIDE EFFECTS: The only reported adverse effect reported in dogs was drowsiness. In people the drug may cause nausea, cramping, vomiting, nervousness, insomnia, joint and muscle pain, skin rash, and pruritus. Dose dependent hepatotoxicity has also been reported in people.

DRUG INTERACTIONS: Naltrexone will block the effects of pure opiate agonists, e.g., morphine, meperidine, codeine, oxymorphone, as well as the opioid agonist/antagonist agents, e.g., butorphanol, pentazocine.

SUPPLIED AS HUMAN PRODUCT:
Tablets containing 50 mg

NANDROLONE

INDICATIONS: Nandrolone decanoate (Deca-Durabolin ♣ ★) is an anabolic steroid that has been recommended for the treatment of nonresponsive anemia. The efficacy of anabolic steroids in promoting a positive nitrogen balance, in stimulating appetite, and in stimulating an increase in erythrocyte mass is questionable. The positive nitrogen balance that has been linked with their use is a reflection of an increase in appetite rather than an alteration in the patient's metabolism. Also see ANABOLIC STEROIDS.

ADVERSE AND COMMON SIDE EFFECTS: Prolonged use of anabolic steroids may result in hepatotoxicity. Also see ANABOLIC STEROIDS.

DRUG INTERACTIONS: None of clinical importance.

SUPPLIED AS HUMAN PRODUCT:
For injection containing 100 mg/mL

OTHER USES
Dogs
APPETITE STIMULANT
5 mg/kg weekly; IM (maximum of 200 mg/week)

NEOMYCIN

INDICATIONS: Neomycin (Biosol-M ♣ ★), an aminoglycoside antibiotic, generally is less effective against many bacteria than amikacin or gentamicin. It is used most often as a topical antibiotic and orally for its local antibiotic effects. Systemic use of the drug is very toxigenic.

ADVERSE AND COMMON SIDE EFFECTS: Neomycin is the most nephrotoxic aminoglycoside. The drug also is potentially toxic to the vestibular and auditory nerves. Ototoxicity is especially a concern if the drug is instilled into external ear canals with ruptured tympanic membranes. It also may cause a contact hypersensitivity and otitis externa. Neomycin may decrease cardiac output and produce hypotension.

DRUG INTERACTIONS: Orally administered, neomycin may decrease the absorption of digitalis, methotrexate, penicillin VK, and vitamin K.

SUPPLIED AS VETERINARY PRODUCT:
Oral liquid containing 140 mg/mL [Biosol]

SUPPLIED AS HUMAN PRODUCT:
Tablets containing 500 mg

OTHER USES
Dogs
HEPATIC ENCEPHALOPATHY
i)   22 mg/kg tid to qid; PO
ii) After evacuation enema, instill 10 to 20 mg/kg neomycin sulfate diluted in water as an enema for emergency treatment of hepatic encephalopathy.

Cats
HEPATIC ENCEPHALOPATHY
10 to 20 mg/kg bid; PO

NEOSTIGMINE

INDICATIONS: Neostigmine methylsulfate (Prostigmin ✽ ★) is a cholinesterase inhibitor used in the diagnosis and treatment of myasthenia gravis. There is marked clinical variability in response to dose.

ADVERSE AND COMMON SIDE EFFECTS: Salivation, urination, and diarrhea may occur if the drug dose is too high. With severe overdose, generalized weakness similar in appearance to that which occurs with myasthenia gravis occurs. A test dose of edrophonium will differentiate between the two. A cholinergic crisis should be treated with atropine.

DRUG INTERACTIONS: Corticosteroids and magnesium administration may decrease the anticholinesterase activity of neostigmine. Aminoglycosides, which have some neuromuscular blocking activity, may decrease the efficacy of neostigmine in the diagnosis and treatment of myasthenia gravis. Neostigmine antagonizes the action of pancuronium and tubocurarine. Atropine antagonizes the muscarinic effects of neostigmine and often is used to treat adverse effects of the drug.

SUPPLIED AS HUMAN PRODUCTS:
Tablets containing 15 mg neostigmine bromide
For injection containing 0.25, 0.5, 1, and 2.5 mg/mL neostigmine methylsulfate

NITROFURANTOIN

INDICATIONS: Nitrofurantoin (Apo-Nitrofurantoin ✽, Equifur ✽, Furadantin ★, Macrodantin ✽ ★, Novofuran ✽) is bacteriostatic or bactericidal, depending on susceptibility of the organisms and the concentration of the drug at the site of infection. It is active against *E. coli, Klebsiella, Enterobacter, Enterococci, Staphylococcus aureus* and *epidermidis, Citrobacter, Salmonella, Shigella,* and *Corynebacterium.* The drug is used in the treatment of canine tracheobronchitis (kennel cough) and urinary tract infections.

ADVERSE AND COMMON SIDE EFFECTS: The drug is contraindicated in patients with significant renal impairment, including anuria and oliguria. Cautious use is advised if the drug is to be given to patients with a history of asthma, anemia, diabetes, or electrolyte imbalance. Nausea, vomiting, hypersensitivity reactions, peripheral nervous system toxicity (weakness, numbness), polymyositis, and hepatopathy have been reported. The drug can cause yellow discoloration of permanent teeth if given before tooth eruption.

DRUG INTERACTIONS: Drugs that tend to alkalinize urine (acetazolamide, thiazides) may decrease the effect of nitrofurantoin. Antacids may delay absorption of nitrofurantoin. Magnesium-containing drugs may decrease the antimicrobial efficacy of the drug. Concomitant administration of probenecid or sulfinpyrazone may increase serum nitrofurantoin concentrations predisposing to toxicity. Nitrofurantoin may interfere with the action of fluoroquinolone antibiotics, and it may antagonize the effects of nalidixic acid. Food and anticholinergic drugs may increase bioavailability of the drug.

SUPPLIED AS VETERINARY PRODUCT (♣):
Oral suspension containing 15 mg/mL [Equifur]

SUPPLIED AS HUMAN PRODUCTS:
Tablets and capsules containing 50 and 100 mg [Furadantin, Novofuran]
Capsules (macrocrystals) containing 25, 50, and 100 mg [Macrodantin]
Oral suspension containing 5 mg/mL [Furadanin, Novofuran]

NITROGLYCERIN

INDICATIONS: Nitroglycerin (Nitro-Bid ★, Nitrol ♣ ★) is a venous vasodilator used to treat cases of congestive heart failure, especially those with pulmonary edema.

ADVERSE AND COMMON SIDE EFFECTS: Rash and hypotension are reported.

DRUG INTERACTIONS: Use of calcium channel-blocking agents, e.g., verapamil and diltiazem; β-blocking agents, e.g., propranolol, atenolol, or metoprolol; and phenothiazine drugs may potentiate hypotension.

SUPPLIED AS HUMAN PRODUCT:
Topical ointment containing 2% nitroglycerin

NITROPRUSSIDE

INDICATIONS: Nitroprusside sodium (Nitropress ★, Nipride ✣) is a potent arterial and venous vasodilator used in refractory cases of heart failure and life-threatening mitral valve regurgitation caused by rupture of the chordae tendineae.

ADVERSE AND COMMON SIDE EFFECTS: The drug should be used with caution in patients with hepatic insufficiency, renal impairment, hypothyroid disease, and hyponatremia. Hypotension is the most serious side effect, but it is reversed readily within 10 minutes of discontinuation of the drug. The drug may be irritating if injected extravascularly.

In humans, prolonged use may result in cyanide toxicity. Monitoring of serum thiocyanate levels is recommended. Levels greater than 100 µg/mL are considered toxic. The administration of hydroxocobalamin (vitamin B_{12}) prevents cyanide toxicity.

DRUG INTERACTIONS: Hypotensive effects are potentiated by the use of β-blockers, e.g., propranolol; ACE inhibitors, e.g., captopril and enalapril; and general anesthetics, e.g., halothane or enflurane.

SUPPLIED AS HUMAN PRODUCT:
For injection containing 50 mg/vial

NITROSCANATE

INDICATIONS: Nitroscanate (Lopatol ✣) is an anthelmintic agent used for the eradication of *Toxocara canis, Toxascaris leonina, Ancylostoma caninum, Uncinaria stenocephala, Taenia* spp., and *Dipylidium caninum* in dogs. It also has been used to eliminate *Echinococcus* and *Trichuris* in dogs and *Ancylostoma* and *T. cati* in cats.

ADVERSE AND COMMON SIDE EFFECTS: The drug is considered to be safe. Vomiting may occur. To help limit the occurrence of vomiting, food should be given 15 minutes before administration of the drug. With drug overdose, depression and anorexia may occur. The drug should not be given to severely debilitated animals. The drug is safe in breeding and pregnant dogs. Some cats given in excess of 400 mg/kg developed a reversible hind-limb paralysis.

DRUG INTERACTIONS: Nitroscanate should not be administered concurrently with other anthelmintics.

SUPPLIED AS VETERINARY PRODUCT:
Tablets containing 100 and 500 mg

NIZATIDINE

INDICATIONS: Nizatidine (Axid ♣ ★) is an H_2-blocking agent similar to cimetidine but up to 10 times more potent. It is primarily used however as a prokinetic agent. The drug stimulates gastric emptying and colonic motility via anticholinesterase activity.

ADVERSE AND COMMON SIDE EFFECTS: The drug is well tolerated. In humans anemia, headache, dizziness, rash, and pruritus have been rarely reported.

DRUG INTERACTIONS: Nizatidine may increase serum salicylate levels in patients on high-dose aspirin. Atropine and propantheline may antagonize the prokinetic effects of the drug.

SUPPLIED AS HUMAN PRODUCT:
Capsules containing 75, 150, and 300 mg

NORFLOXACIN

INDICATIONS: Norfloxacin (Noroxin ♣ ★) is a fluoroquinolone antibiotic. It has been recommended for the treatment of urinary tract infections and bacteremia. Also see FLUOROQUINOLONE ANTIBIOTICS.

ADVERSE AND COMMON SIDE EFFECTS: See FLUOROQUINOLONE ANTIBIOTICS.

DRUG INTERACTIONS: Absorption is impaired by magnesium- and aluminum-containing antacids and sucralfate. Nitrofurantoin may decrease the antibacterial effects of norfloxacin in the urinary tract. Also see FLUOROQUINOLONE ANTIBIOTICS.

SUPPLIED AS HUMAN PRODUCT:
Tablet containing 400 mg

NOVOBIOCIN

INDICATIONS: Novobiocin is active against gram-positive cocci, including staphylococci and some streptococci. Variable effectiveness has been found against *Proteus, Pseudomonas,* and *Pasteurella multocida.* It is marketed for small animals in combination with tetracycline (Albaplex ★) and with tetracycline and prednisolone (Delta-Albaplex ♣ ★).

ADVERSE AND COMMON SIDE EFFECTS: Nausea, vomiting, diarrhea, rashes, and blood dyscrasias are reported.

DRUG INTERACTIONS: Novobiocin may decrease the elimination of penicillin drugs and the cephalosporins.

SUPPLIED AS VETERINARY PRODUCTS:
Tablets containing 60 mg novobiocin with 60 mg tetracycline [Albaplex]
Tablets containing 60 mg novobiocin, 60 mg tetracycline, and 1.5 mg prednisolone [Delta-Albaplex]
Tablets containing 180 mg novobiocin, 180 mg tetracycline, and 4.5 mg prednisolone [Delta-Albaplex 3X ★]

NYSTATIN

INDICATIONS: Nystatin (Mycostatin ♣ ★, Nilstat ♣ ★) is used for the treatment of candidal infections of the skin, mucous membranes, and intestinal tract. The drug also has been recommended for the treatment of *Malassezia pachydermatitis* and otitis externa caused by *Microsporum canis*. It is only partially effective against *Aspergillus* infections.

ADVERSE AND COMMON SIDE EFFECTS: Rarely, topical application causes contact dermatitis. In humans, large oral doses have been associated with diarrhea, nausea, and vomiting. The drug is too toxic for parenteral use in small animals.

DRUG INTERACTIONS: None of clinical significance in small animals.

SUPPLIED AS HUMAN PRODUCTS:
Oral suspension containing 100,000 U/mL
Tablets containing 500,000 U
Cream containing 100,000 U/g
Powder containing 100,000 U/g

OLSALAZINE

INDICATIONS: Olsalazine (Dipentum ♣ ★) is an anti-inflammatory agent consisting of two molecules of aminosalicylic acid joined by an azo bond. It is used to treat colitis.

ADVERSE AND COMMON SIDE EFFECTS: Unlike sulfasalazine, keratoconjunctivitis sicca (KCS) has not been reported in dogs using this product. Diarrhea has been reported in dogs.

DRUG INTERACTIONS: Concurrent use with warfarin may increase prothrombin times.

SUPPLIED AS HUMAN PRODUCT:
Tablets containing 250 mg

OMEPRAZOLE

INDICATIONS: Omeprazole (Prilosec ★, Losec ✿) is a proton pump-inhibitor used for the treatment of esophagitis, erosive gastritis, and gastric ulcers. The drug is 5 to 10 times more potent than cimetidine in inhibiting gastric acid secretion and has a long duration of action (24 hours or more). The drug is more effective than cimetidine in controlling aspirin-induced gastritis but has no effect on ulcer healing. It has cytoprotective (by enhancing mucosal cell prostaglandin production) and acid-reducing properties and may be useful in decreasing gastric hyperacidity. Omeprazole is not effective in the healing or prevention of gastric mucosal lesions in dogs with acute degenerative disc disease treated with corticosteroids.

ADVERSE AND COMMON SIDE EFFECTS: In humans, nausea, vomiting, flatulence, and diarrhea are reported. Long-term, high-dose administration does not cause clinical, hematologic, or biochemical abnormalities in dogs. However, it can result in reversible gastric mucosal hypertrophy as a result of sustained hypergastrinemia, which occurs with prolonged gastric acid suppression. No adverse reactions were noted in cats at doses of 0.7 mg/kg per day.

DRUG INTERACTIONS: The elimination time of diazepam, phenytoin, and warfarin is increased with chronic administration of omeprazole.

SUPPLIED AS HUMAN PRODUCT:
Capsules containing 10, 20, and 40 mg

ONDANSETRON

INDICATIONS: Ondansetron (Zofran ✿ ★) is a potent antiemetic agent. It has been used in human medicine for the control of vomiting in patients undergoing chemotherapy with cisplatin, a drug that frequently causes nausea and vomiting. Ondansetron blocks selective serotonin S_3 receptors (mediators of the vomiting reflex) on neurons located in either the peripheral or central nervous systems. This drug is not effective in preventing motion-induced nausea and vomiting in people.

ADVERSE AND COMMON SIDE EFFECTS: Adverse effects in dogs are uncommon but may include sedation, lip licking, and head shaking. The drug dose should be reduced in patients with reduced liver function.

DRUG INTERACTIONS: Unknown.

SUPPLIED AS HUMAN PRODUCTS:
For injection containing 2 mg/mL
Tablets containing 4, 8, and 24 mg
Oral solution containing 0.8 mg/mL

OTHER USES
Dogs

CISPLATIN CHEMOTHERAPY
0.5 to 1 mg/kg; PO 30 minutes before and 90 minutes after commencing cisplatin

ORBIFLOXACIN

INDICATIONS: Orbifloxacin (Orbax ✤ ★) is a synthetic broad-spectrum bactericidal antibiotic with activity against many gram-positive and gram-negative organisms, including *Staphylococcus intermedius,* coagulase-positive staphylococci, *Pasteurella multocida, E. coli, Pseudomonas aeruginosa, Proteus mirabilis,* and *hemolytic* (group G) *Streptococcus.*

ADVERSE AND COMMON SIDE EFFECTS: Adverse effects in dogs at standard recommended dosages are not seen. Dosages greater than 5 times the recommended maximum daily dose did not produce any treatment-related adverse effects. As with other fluoroquinolone antibiotics, orbifloxacin should not be given to young growing dogs, i.e., between 2 and 8 months of age in small and medium-sized breeds and up to 18 months of age in large and giant breed dogs. These drugs are known to cause arthropathy in immature dogs. Fluoroquinolone antibiotics may predispose to seizure activity and should be used with caution in dogs with CNS pathology. Safe use of the drug in pregnant or breeding animals has not been established.

DRUG INTERACTIONS: Absorption of the drug is hindered by sucralfate, antacids, multivitamin compounds, and agents containing divalent and trivalent cations, e.g., calcium, iron, aluminum, magnesium, and zinc.

SUPPLIED AS VETERINARY PRODUCT:
Tablets containing 5.7, 22.7, and 68 mg

ORGANOPHOSPHATES

INDICATIONS: Organophosphate agents include chlorpyrifos, cythioate, diazinon, dichlorvos, fenthion, malathion, parathion, phosmet, ronnel, safrotin, and tetrachlorvinphos. Some have been used in the treatment of *Cheyletiella* and sarcoptic mange, fleas, ticks, and lice. Not all drugs listed are recommended for use in small animals. All, however, have been associated with toxicity in dogs and cats.

ADVERSE AND COMMON SIDE EFFECTS: These agents, other than malathion, are not approved for use in cats. Cats are especially sensitive to toxicity from organophosphate compounds. In dogs, the greyhound appears more sensitive to the adverse effects of these drugs. Signs of intoxication are due to cholinesterase inhibition resulting in overstimulation of the parasympathetic nervous system and include bradycardia, salivation, vomiting, diarrhea, muscle tremors, convulsions, pupillary constriction, bronchoconstriction, respiratory depression, and paralysis. Death may occur. Some organophosphates are associated with a delayed neurotoxicity characterized by muscular weakness and ataxia that progresses to flaccid paralysis of the hind limbs and occasionally all four limbs 8 to 21 days after administration.

If topical application has resulted in toxicity, the skin should be cleansed. If the drug was ingested within the last 2 hours and the patient is not exhibiting clinical signs of toxicosis, vomiting should be induced with 3% hydrogen peroxide (2 mL/kg; maximum of 45 mL). Otherwise, gastric lavage followed by the oral administration of activated charcoal (2 g/kg) is indicated. In all cases, atropine should be given (0.2 mg/kg). One fourth of the total dose is given intravenously, and the balance is given intramuscularly or subcutaneously. In addition, pralidoxime chloride may be useful (20 mg/kg; IM or IV, repeat every 12 hours as indicated). In addition, the antihistamine diphenhydramine (Benadryl) (4 mg/kg tid; PO) may effectively block the effects of nicotine-receptor stimulation. Although diazepam has been used to augment the effects of atropine and reportedly has aided recovery, some authors suggest that diazepam actually may potentiate toxic signs and should *not* be used.

DRUG INTERACTIONS: Drugs that inhibit cholinesterase, including morphine, neostigmine, physostigmine, pyridostigmine, phenothiazines, and succinylcholine, should be avoided.

SUPPLIED AS: See specific product.

OXACILLIN

INDICATIONS: Oxacillin (Bactocill ★, Prostaphlin ★) is a penicillin antibiotic used in the treatment of gram-positive infections, including staphylococcal infections and infections caused by β-lactamase–producing bacteria. The drug has been used in the treatment of pyoderma, bacterial endocarditis, and blepharitis. Also see PENICILLIN ANTIBIOTICS.

For information concerning ADVERSE AND COMMON SIDE EFFECTS and DRUG INTERACTIONS, see PENICILLIN ANTIBIOTICS.

SUPPLIED AS HUMAN PRODUCTS:
Capsules containing 250 and 500 mg
For injection in 250- and 500-mg and 1-, 2-, 4-, and 10-g vials

OXAZEPAM

INDICATIONS: Oxazepam (Serax ★) is an anxiolytic-sedative benzodiazepine drug that is used to stimulate appetite. Feeding usually commences within 20 minutes. Also see DIAZEPAM.

ADVERSE AND COMMON SIDE EFFECTS: Mild sedation and ataxia may be seen. These drugs are metabolized in the liver and should be used cautiously in animals with liver or renal dysfunction. Oxazepam occasionally may exacerbate grand mal seizures. Abrupt withdrawal in these patients should be avoided. Also see DIAZEPAM.

DRUG INTERACTIONS: Phenothiazines and barbiturates may potentiate the action of oxazepam. Also see DIAZEPAM.

SUPPLIED AS HUMAN PRODUCT:
Tablets containing 10, 15, and 30 mg

OXTRIPHYLLINE

INDICATIONS: Oxtriphylline (Choledyl ✤ ★) contains 64% theophylline, which accounts for its pharmacological effects. The drug is a bronchodilator used in the management of chronic cough.

ADVERSE AND COMMON SIDE EFFECTS: Anorexia, vomiting, restlessness, tachypnea, arrhythmias, and, rarely, seizures are reported.

DRUG INTERACTIONS: Serum levels are increased by cimetidine and erythromycin. Oxtriphylline potentiates the action of thiazide diuretics and the cardiac effects of digitalis. Synergism with ephedrine has been documented. Theophylline antagonizes the effect of propranolol. The concomitant use of morphine or curare may antagonize the effect of theophylline, and because this drug stimulates the release of histamine, bronchoconstriction may result. Acidifying agents increase the urinary excretion and inhibit the action of theophylline. Alkalinizing agents potentiate its effects.

SUPPLIED AS HUMAN PRODUCTS:
Tablets containing 100, 200, and 300 mg
Tablets containing 400 and 600 mg [Choledyl SA]

Elixir containing 100 mg/5 mL [Choledyl]
Syrup containing 50 mg/5 mL

OXYBUTYNIN

INDICATIONS: Oxybutynin (Ditropan ✤ ★) is an anticholinergic agent with direct antispasmodic activity and antimuscarinic activity on smooth muscle. In addition, the drug exerts an analgesic and local anesthetic effect. It is useful in the management of detrusor hyperreflexia.

ADVERSE AND COMMON SIDE EFFECTS: Dry mouth, urinary hesitancy, retention of urine, pupillary dilation, tachycardia, syncope, weakness, nausea, vomiting, anorexia, and constipation may occur. In small animals, diarrhea and sedation are the most common side effects reported. In the case of drug overdose, the stomach should be emptied of any remaining drug, and physostigmine should be given.

Oxybutynin is contraindicated in patients with hyperthyroidism, prostatic disease, glaucoma, myasthenia gravis, partial or complete GIT obstruction, ileus, megacolon, severe colitis, or unstable cardiovascular status.

DRUG INTERACTIONS: None of clinical significance to small animals.

SUPPLIED AS HUMAN PRODUCTS:
Tablets containing 5, 10, and 15 mg
Syrup containing 5 mg/5 mL

OXYGLOBIN

INDICATIONS: Oxyglobin (Oxyglobin ★) is a bovine-derived polymerized hemoglobin solution used as an oxygen carrying fluid in dogs in cases of acute, reversible anemia. The terminal elimination half-life of the drug in dogs is estimated to range between 18 and 43 hours for dosages of 10 to 30 mL/kg. The increase in half-life with dose suggests a saturable elimination process. Depending on the dose, greater than 95% of the administered dose is expected to be eliminated from the body at 4 to 9 days after infusion. Although it has been reported that bovine hemoglobin is more potent than autologous red blood cells in restoring muscular tissue oxygenation after profound isovolemic hemodilution in dogs, it has also been reported that colloids or fresh frozen plasma is as effective as whole blood or hemoglobin in maintaining survival until about 70% of blood volume is removed. The effect of hemoglobin solutions becomes important when the hematocrit falls below 10%. A recent paper suggested that dogs with immune mediated hemolytic anemia treated with a combination of cyclophosphamide and bovine hemoglobin were at increased risk of death. More studies are needed before specific recommendations concerning the efficacy and safety of this product can be made. A recent study concluded that although administration of a hemoglobin-based oxygen carrying solution may provide temporary support to anemic cats, the development of pulmonary edema or pleural effusion potentially associated with rapid infusion rate and large volumes of the solution should be investigated further before recommendations concerning its use in cats is made.

ADVERSE AND COMMON SIDE EFFECTS: The manufacturer states that accidental overdosage or an excessive rate of administration (i.e., >10 mL/kg per hour) could result in immediate cardiopulmonary effects, in which case infusion of Oxyglobin should be discontinued immediately until signs abate. Signs of circulatory overload such as pulmonary edema, pleural effusion, increased central venous pressure, dyspnea, or coughing may occur. Treatment of circulatory overload may be necessary.

Transient hemoglobinuria may be noted. Rapid administration may compromise pulmonary function. The safety and efficacy of repeat administration of Oxyglobin have not been demonstrated in dogs. The safety of Oxyglobin for use in breeding dogs and pregnant or lactating bitches has not been determined. Teratogenic effects were observed in preliminary reproductive toxicity studies in rats using a related polymerized bovine hemoglobin product. The safety and efficacy of Oxyglobin have not been evaluated in dogs with disseminated intravascular coagulopathy, thrombocytopenia with active bleeding, hemoglobinemia and hemoglobinuria, or autoagglutination. If an immediate hypersensitivity reaction occurs, infusion of Oxyglobin should be immediately discontinued and appropriate treatment administered. If a delayed type of hypersensitivity reaction occurs, immunosuppressant therapy is recommended.

Treatment with Oxyglobin at a dosage of 30 mL/kg results in a mild decrease in hematocrit immediately following infusion. Due to the dilutional effects of Oxyglobin at that dose, the hematocrit and red cell counts are not accurate measures of the degree of anemia for 24 hours following administration. Dilutional effects are not seen at a dosage of 15 mL/kg.

The animal should be adequately hydrated (but not overhydrated) prior to administration. Due to the plasma expanding properties of Oxyglobin, the possibility of circulatory overload should be considered especially when administering adjunctive intravenous fluids, particularly colloidal solutions. If concurrent fluid therapy is administered, it should be temporarily discontinued during infusion of Oxyglobin. The patient should be carefully monitored for signs of circulatory overload. Vomiting, diarrhea, anorexia, and purple skin discoloration have been reported.

Adverse effects in cats have included pulmonary edema, pleural effusion, mucous membrane discoloration, pigmenturia, vomiting, and neurologic abnormalities.

DRUG INTERACTIONS: Do not administer this agent with other fluids or drugs via the same IV line.

SUPPLIED AS VETERINARY PRODUCT:
Available as 13 g/dL polymerized bovine hemoglobin in 125 mL dose bags

OXYMETHOLONE

INDICATIONS: Oxymetholone (Anadrol 50 ★) is an anabolic steroid used to stimulate erythrocyte production in cases of nonresponsive anemia. For more discussion on the use of these agents, including ADVERSE AND COMMON SIDE EFFECTS and DRUG INTERACTIONS, see ANABOLIC STEROIDS.

SUPPLIED AS HUMAN PRODUCT:
Tablets containing 50 mg

OXYMORPHONE

INDICATIONS: Oxymorphone (Numorphan ♣ ★) is a narcotic agent used for sedation, preanesthesia, and the management of pain in the dog. Pain relief lasts 2 to 4 hours after IM or IV injection. It is approximately 10 times more potent an analgesic than morphine, causes less sedation, and does not suppress the cough reflex.

ADVERSE AND COMMON SIDE EFFECTS: Respiratory depression and bradycardia are reported. Cats are more sensitive to the drug and may exhibit dose-dependent excitement. The drug should not be used in animals with head trauma because it may increase CSF pressure; it should be used with caution in patients with hypothyroid disease, hepatic impairment, significant respiratory disease, adrenocortical insufficiency, and renal disease, and in the severely debilitated or geriatric animal. Oxymorphone should not be given to animals with diarrhea caused by a toxic agent.

With overdose, profound respiratory and/or CNS depression may occur, as may cardiovascular collapse, hypothermia, and skeletal muscle hypotonia. Adverse effects of the drug can be reversed with naloxone. In cats, use of the drug may be associated with ataxia, hyperesthesia, and behavioral changes. If used at higher doses in this species, it is recommended that it be given with a tranquilizing agent.

DRUG INTERACTIONS: Antihistamines, phenothiazines, barbiturates, and anesthetic agents may potentiate CNS or respiratory depression of the drug. In cats, the drug may be used concurrently with diazepam (0.1 to 0.2 mg/kg; IV, IM) to offset adverse effects of excitement and hyperalgesia.

SUPPLIED AS HUMAN PRODUCT:
For injection containing 1.0 and 1.5 mg/mL (Numorphan)

OTHER USES
Dogs
ANALGESIA
Postoperative dose: 0.05 to 0.1 mg/kg; IM, IV

PREANESTHESIA
0.1 to 0.2 mg/kg; IM, IV (with acepromazine and atropine or glycopyrrolate)

Cats
RESTRAINT/SEDATION
0.02 to 0.03 mg/kg; IM, IV

ANALGESIA/PREANESTHESIA
0.1 to 0.4 mg/kg; IV

POSTOPERATIVE ANALGESIA
0.05 to 0.15 mg/kg; IM, IV (with acepromazine)

OXYTETRACYCLINE

INDICATIONS: Oxytetracycline (Liquamycin ✤ ★, Terramycin ✤ ★) is a short-acting, water-soluble tetracycline. The drug reaches high concentrations in the lung, liver, kidney, and mononuclear phagocyte system. For more information, see TETRACYCLINE ANTIBIOTICS.

ADVERSE AND COMMON SIDE EFFECTS: Oxytetracycline may cause discoloration of the teeth in young animals. High doses or prolonged use may cause delayed bone growth and healing. Tetracyclines cause nausea, anorexia, vomiting, and diarrhea in small animals. In addition, in cats, toxicity may present as fever, colic, hair loss, and depression.

DRUG INTERACTIONS: Antidiarrheal preparations, including kaolin and pectin or bismuth, reduce absorption of tetracyclines. Medications containing aluminum, calcium, iron, magnesium, or zinc, such as antacids, laxatives, mineral supplements, and iron preparations, reduce absorption of oral tetracycline drugs. Methoxyflurane may potentiate the nephrotoxicity of tetracyclines. Sodium bicarbonate may interfere with gastric absorption by increasing gastric pH. Tetracyclines may interfere with the bactericidal activity of the penicillins, cephalosporins, and aminoglycosides. Tetracyclines may increase the bioavailability of digoxin and predispose to digitalis toxicity. Gastrointestinal tract side effects may be increased if the drug is administered concurrently with theophylline. Tetracyclines reportedly have reduced insulin requirements in diabetic patients.

SUPPLIED AS VETERINARY PRODUCTS (For Large Animals):
For injection containing 50 and 100 mg/mL [generic products ✤ ★]
For injection containing long-acting formula 200 mg/mL [Liquamycin-LA]

OXYTOCIN

INDICATIONS: Oxytocin (Pitocin ★, Syntocinon ✤ ★) is a hormone of the posterior pituitary gland and is used for the induction of parturition, for uterine prolapse in dogs and cats, and to stimulate milk letdown in bitches.

ADVERSE AND COMMON SIDE EFFECTS: The drug is contraindicated in animals with dystocia due to abnormal presentation of the fetus or in those with a closed cervix. Full relaxation of the cervix should be accomplished naturally or with the use of estrogen before oxytocin use. Overdose may precipitate intense labor, uterine rupture, fetal injury, or death. Water intoxication may occur if large doses are infused, especially in the presence of electrolyte-free fluid therapy. Intoxication may be manifested by listlessness, depression, seizures, coma, and death. Severe intoxication may be treated with mannitol or dextrose, with or without furosemide.

DRUG INTERACTIONS: Concurrent use of ephedrine or other vasopressors may result in postpartum hypertension.

SUPPLIED AS VETERINARY PRODUCT:
For injection containing 20 IU/mL (products are listed generically)

SUPPLIED AS HUMAN PRODUCT:
For injection containing 10 IU/mL [Pitocin, Syntocinon]

PANCREATIC ENZYME REPLACEMENT

INDICATIONS: Pancreatic enzyme replacement therapies (Pancrease-V ✤, Pancrezyme ★) are mixtures containing porcine pancreatic enzymes, especially lipase and amylase. Other products also may include protease, esterase, peptidase, nuclease, and elastase enzyme supplements. These products are used for the management of pancreatic exocrine insufficiency.

ADVERSE AND COMMON SIDE EFFECTS: Overdose can cause nausea, cramping, and diarrhea. Oral bleeding has been noted and is dose dependent. A reduction in dose will lead to resolution of the bleeding without recurrence or a loss of product efficacy.

DRUG INTERACTIONS: Antacids (magnesium hydroxide, calcium carbonate) may diminish efficacy. Concurrent use of cimetidine may improve efficacy.

SUPPLIED AS VETERINARY PRODUCTS:
Available in tablets and as a powder

PANCURONIUM BROMIDE

INDICATIONS: Pancuronium (Pavulon ★, generics ✲) is a synthetic nondepolarizing neuromuscular blocking agent. It is used as an adjunct to general anesthesia to promote muscle relaxation during surgery and to facilitate mechanical ventilation and endotracheal intubation.

ADVERSE AND COMMON SIDE EFFECTS: The drug should be used with caution in patients with compromised renal function and in those in whom tachycardia may be hazardous. Lower doses are recommended in patients with hepatobiliary disease. It should be used with caution in those with myasthenia gravis. Adverse effects may include tachycardia, increases in blood pressure, hypersalivation in those not pretreated with an anticholinergic, and profound muscle weakness and respiratory depression. Drug toxicity may be treated with mechanical support of ventilation and the use of atropine (0.02 mg/kg; IV) followed by neostigmine (0.06 mg/kg; IV).

DRUG INTERACTIONS: Neuromuscular blockade may be potentiated by aminoglycoside antibiotics (amikacin, gentamicin, kanamycin, neomycin, streptomycin, tobramycin), bacitracin, clindamycin, enflurane, halothane, isoflurane, lincomycin, magnesium sulfate, polymyxin B, and quinidine. Succinylcholine may hasten the onset of action of pancuronium and potentiate neuromuscular blockade. The action of pancuronium is antagonized by acetylcholine, anticholinesterases, and potassium ions. Theophylline may inhibit or reverse the neuromuscular blocking effect of pancuronium and precipitate arrhythmias. Azathioprine may reverse the neuromuscular blocking effect of the drug.

SUPPLIED AS HUMAN PRODUCT:
For injection containing 1 and 2 mg/mL

PANTOPRAZOLE

INDICATIONS: Pantoprazole (Pantoloc ✲, Protonix ★) is a proton pump inhibitor that achieves maximum acid inhibition of 86% within one hour in people. The drug is indicated in patients in whom rapid reduction of gastric acid secretion is warranted, e.g., reflux esophagitis, and in those who cannot take oral medication.

ADVERSE AND COMMON SIDE EFFECTS: No adverse effects have been reported in toxicologic studies completed in beagles. The drug should not be given to patients with liver impairment. If liver enzymes increase during the course of therapy, the drug should be discontinued. Use of the drug in pregnant animals is not advised as safety studies have not been completed. Oral dosages above 15 mg/kg caused pulmonary edema and death in some dogs.

DRUG INTERACTIONS: None.

SUPPLIED AS HUMAN PRODUCTS:
Tablets containing 20 and 40 mg
For injection in 40-mg vials

PAROXETINE

INDICATIONS: Paroxetine (Paxil ★ ✿) is an SSRI similar in action to that of fluoxetine (Prozac) and is used in the management of compulsive disorders and aggression.

ADVERSE AND COMMON SIDE EFFECTS: Experience with the drug is limited, but adverse effects may include lethargy, anxiety, irritability, insomnia, panting, and gastrointestinal effects. Anorexia may be persistent in some dogs. Aggressive behavior may be noted in dogs not demonstrating this type of behavior beforehand. In cats, fluoxetine, another SSRI, may cause anxiety, irritability, anorexia, sleep disturbances, and changes in elimination behavior. The drug should be used with caution in patients with liver, renal or cardiac disease, and those with a history of seizure activity.

DRUG INTERACTIONS: Paroxetine is highly protein bound and may displace other highly bound drugs, e.g., digitoxin, phenylbutazone, warfarin. Paroxetine may augment the CNS effects of diazepam, lithium and buspirone. Increased levels of paroxetine may be noted with drugs that inhibit or compete with the cytochrome P-450 enzyme system, e.g., tricyclic antidepressant agents, cimetidine, some phenothiazines. Significant morbidity may be noted if paroxetine is used concurrently with MAO inhibitors, e.g., amitraz, selegiline.

SUPPLIED AS HUMAN PRODUCTS:
Tablets containing 10, 20, 30, and 40 mg
Oral suspension containing 2 mg/mL

PENICILLAMINE

INDICATIONS: Penicillamine (Cuprimine ✿ ★, Depen ✿ ★) is a thiol compound that chelates cystine, lead, and copper and promotes their excretion in the urine. It is used in the management of cystine urolithiasis, lead poisoning, and hepatitis associated with progressive copper accumulation. The very slow rate of copper dispersion makes use of this drug ineffective in advanced cases of hepatic copper storage disease and in cirrhosis. Trientine is recommended if vomiting remains a problem for animals given penicillamine. Although no more effective than penicillamine, it does have fewer side effects. A dose of 15 to 30 mg/kg bid, PO, given 1 hour before meals has been recommended in dogs. Penicillamine also has been recommended for the treatment of hepatic cirrhosis, where it may work by lessening the formation of collagen and promoting its breakdown.

ADVERSE AND COMMON SIDE EFFECTS: Lethargy, vomiting, oral lesions, anorexia, proteinuria, and thrombocytopenia have been reported. The drug decreases the strength of skin wound closure by its effect on collagen and should only be used after wound healing is complete. Finally, the drug has been used experimentally in the treatment of renal amyloidosis.

DRUG INTERACTIONS: Gold therapy and phenylbutazone may potentiate hematologic and renal toxicity of the drug. Oral iron may inhibit absorption of the drug.

SUPPLIED AS HUMAN PRODUCTS:
Tablets containing 250 mg [Depen]
Capsules containing 125 and 250 mg [Cuprimine]

OTHER USES
Dogs
BEDLINGTON COPPER STORAGE DISEASE
125 mg bid; PO given 30 minutes before eating

PENICILLIN ANTIBIOTICS

INDICATIONS: Penicillin antibiotics, including penicillin G and V, ampicillin, amoxicillin, cloxacillin, carbenicillin, ticarcillin, hetacillin, and nafcillin, are effective bactericidal antibiotics used for the treatment of gram-positive and gram-negative infections. Penicillin drugs are distributed extensively throughout the body to most body fluids and bone except the brain and CSF unless inflamed. Penicillin G is effective against most gram-positive organisms. Penicillin V has the same spectrum but is more reliably absorbed from the GIT. Ampicillin has an extended activity against *E. coli, Shigella,* and *Proteus.* Hetacillin is hydrolyzed to ampicillin in most body fluids. Amoxicillin is similar to ampicillin but is absorbed from the GIT more readily and persists for a longer period of time within the body. It also is available in combination with clavulanate potassium (Clavamox), which protects the drug from β-lactamase–producing staphylococci, and *Chlamydia psittaci* in cats. Cloxacillin is penicillinase-resistant and is useful in the treatment of staphylococcal infections. Carbenicillin is also active against *Pseudomonas* and *Proteus.* Ticarcillin is more effective than carbenicillin against *Pseudomonas* and can be given at a lower dose. Piperacillin and azlocillin are also active against *Pseudomonas.*

ADVERSE AND COMMON SIDE EFFECTS: Toxicity is rare in dogs and cats. Rapid IV injection may cause neurologic signs and seizures. Hypersensitivity reactions, including hives, fever, joint pain, and anaphylaxis, have been reported in dogs and cats. Sensitivity to one penicillin confers sensitivity to all penicillins. Penicillin and its derivatives may exacerbate clinical signs associated with Scotty cramp.

DRUG INTERACTIONS: Food and antacids decrease the absorption of orally administered penicillins. The drug should be given 1 hour before or 2 hours after feeding. Neomycin blocks the absorption of oral penicillins. The bacteriostatic action of chloramphenicol, erythromycin, and the tetracyclines may antagonize the bactericidal activity of the penicillins. Aspirin, indomethacin, and phenylbutazone may increase serum levels of the penicillins by displacing them from plasma protein-binding sites. Penicillins and other β-lactam antibiotics may inactivate aminoglycosides in vitro and should not be mixed together in the same syringe.

PENTASTARCH

INDICATIONS: Pentastarch (Pentaspan ✤ ★) is a colloid used for plasma volume expansion. It has an average molecular weight of 200,000 to 300,000. Volume expansion persists for approximately 18 to 24 hours in people and is expected to improve hemodynamic status for 12 to 18 hours. Infusion of 500 mL results in a 700-mL (140%) increase in plasma volume within 30 minutes. Comparatively, the amount of volume expansion appears greatest with 10% pentastarch followed by 6% dextran 70, 6% hetastarch, and 5% albumin. Pentastarch is especially useful in the management of shock. It was developed to provide a colloidal solution with fewer adverse effects and greater osmotic properties.

ADVERSE AND COMMON SIDE EFFECTS: This agent is contraindicated in patients with bleeding disorders or with congestive heart failure in which volume overload is a potential problem. Large volumes of the drug also may predispose to coagulopathy, although this should not be expected at recommended dosages. The drug should not be used in oliguric or anuric renal failure not related to hypovolemia. Administration of large volumes of pentastarch will decrease hemoglobin concentrations and dilute plasma proteins. Hypersensitivity (wheezing and urticaria) also has been reported in humans. This agent should not be used in pregnant small animals unless the benefit outweighs the risk because it has been demonstrated to be embryocidal at large doses in experimental studies using rabbits and mice. Elevation in serum amylase levels in humans has been noted, but it has not been associated with pancreatitis.

DRUG INTERACTIONS: None established.

SUPPLIED AS HUMAN PRODUCT:
For injection containing 10% pentastarch in 0.9% sodium chloride [Pentaspan]

PENTAZOCINE

INDICATIONS: Pentazocine (Talwin ♣ ★) is a narcotic agonist used in the management of moderate to severe pain in dogs. Its analgesic properties are approximately one fourth as potent as those of morphine and are equivalent to those of meperidine. Onset of action is rapid, and duration of analgesia is at least 3 hours in most patients. In cats, an IV dose of 0.75 mg/kg provides visceral analgesia of approximately 22 minutes. The duration of analgesia is increased at doses of 1.5 mg/kg, but mydriasis and apprehension are noted. The drug does not depress respiration and produces little or no sedation at therapeutic doses.

ADVERSE AND COMMON SIDE EFFECTS: In dogs, the most common side effect is profuse salivation. Other side effects may include tremors, vomiting, and swelling at the injection site. At high doses (6 mg/kg), ataxia, tremors, and seizures have been reported in dogs. In cats, the drug appears to cause dysphoria and is not recommended by some clinicians for use in this species. Others believe that the drug can be used safely in cats. Side effects can be reversed with naloxone. Use of the drug is contraindicated in patients with head injury or increased intracranial pressure. Cautious use is recommended in animals with impaired renal or hepatic function, adrenocortical insufficiency, hypothyroid disease, and respiratory depression, and in severely debilitated animals, geriatrics, and those with nausea or vomiting.

DRUG INTERACTIONS: Do not mix pentazocine with soluble barbiturates because precipitation will occur.

SUPPLIED AS HUMAN PRODUCT:
Tablets containing 50 mg

PENTOBARBITAL

INDICATIONS: Pentobarbital (Somnotol ✦, generic products ★) is a short-acting barbiturate used for promoting sedation and general anesthesia. Anesthesia is induced in 3 to 5 minutes and lasts 45 to 90 minutes, with the animal remaining quiet for several hours afterward. It is used to control intractable seizures in dogs and cats, other than those seizures induced by lidocaine intoxication. For more information on this class of drug, see BARBITURATES.

ADVERSE AND COMMON SIDE EFFECTS: Respiratory depression is the most common concern with the use of the drug. It also may cause excitement in the dog during recovery from anesthetic doses. The use of sodium bicarbonate to increase renal excretion of the drug is not effective with pentobarbital.

DRUG INTERACTIONS: Antihistamines, phenothiazines, narcotic agents, and chloramphenicol may potentiate the effects of the drug. Pentobarbital may decrease the effects of corticosteroids, β blockers (e.g., propranolol, metoprolol), quinidine, metronidazole, and theophylline. Barbiturates may interfere with the metabolism of phenytoin, thus altering its serum levels. Unexplained death has occurred when dogs intoxicated with lidocaine were treated with pentobarbital.

SUPPLIED AS VETERINARY PRODUCT:
For injection containing 65 mg/mL

OTHER USES
Dogs
STATUS EPILEPTICUS
5 to 15 mg/kg to effect; IV

Cats
ANESTHETIC
25 mg/kg; IV; an additional 10 mg/kg may be given if initial dose is inadequate
STATUS EPILEPTICUS
5 to 15 mg/kg to effect; IV

PENTOXIFYLLINE

INDICATIONS: Pentoxifylline (Trental ✦ ★) belongs to the methylxanthine class and is a derivative of theobromine. The drug reduces blood viscosity; the mechanism of which is believed to be related to improved red blood cell deformability. It also inhibits microvascular constriction and red blood cell and platelet aggregation. Pentoxifylline inhibits interleukin-1, -6, and tumor necrosis factor as well as B- and T-cell activation. It has also been of benefit in the treatment of hyper-coagulable states and wound healing. In veterinary medicine the drug has been used in the management of contact dermatitis, atopy, der-matomyositis, systemic lupus erythematosus, erythema multiforme, cutaneous and renal vasculitis of greyhounds, ear margin seborrhea, and acral lick granuloma. Pentoxifylline has been used in dogs to pro-mote healing and reduce inflammation caused by ulcerative der-matosis in Shelties and Collies where improved circulation may be beneficial. Any necrotizing cutaneous lesion may benefit from the increased oxygen delivery. In humans beneficial clinical effects may not be noted for 2 to 4 weeks.

ADVERSE AND COMMON SIDE EFFECTS: Adverse effects reported in dogs include bone marrow suppression, flushing, vomiting, and diarrhea. The drug should be used with caution in patients with hepatic or renal impairment and in those at risk for hemorrhage. Although risk to pregnant dogs and cats has not been studied, pregnant rats and rab-bits did not demonstrate teratogenicity. Experience with the drug in veterinary medicine is limited. In people, vomiting, anorexia, and dizzi-ness have been noted. Overdosage in people has resulted in seizures, hypotension, fever, somnolence, and GI distress.

DRUG INTERACTIONS: In humans, there have been reports of bleed-ing and/or prolonged prothrombin time in patients treated with Trental with and without anticoagulants or platelet aggregation inhibitors. Concomitant administration of Trental and theophylline-containing drugs leads to increased theophylline levels and theophyl-line toxicity in some individuals. Small decreases in blood pressure have been observed in some patients treated with Trental. Periodic sys-temic blood pressure monitoring is recommended for patients receiv-ing concomitant antihypertensive therapy. If indicated, dosage of the antihypertensive agents should be reduced. Concurrent use of NSAIDs is controversial. Ciprofloxacin and cimetidine may increase serum pen-toxifylline levels, increasing the potential for adverse effects. Increased risk of bleeding may occur if the drug is used along with warfarin or other anticoagulants.

SUPPLIED AS HUMAN PRODUCT:
Tablets containing 400 mg

OTHER USES
Dogs

ULCERATIVE DERMATOSIS OF SHELTIES & COLLIES
400 mg once daily; PO or every other day if vomiting occurs

DERMATOMYOSITIS
i) 10 mg/kg once daily to every other day (give with food); clinical improvement may take 2 to 3 months

ii) 25 mg/kg bid; PO to start (median response time 6 weeks)

EAR MARGIN SEBORRHEA
400 mg once daily; PO or 200 mg once daily (dogs < 10 kg)

PHENOBARBITAL

INDICATIONS: Phenobarbital ❦ ★ is one of the most useful drugs for the control of seizure activity in small animals. It is effective in controlling seizures in most dogs (60% to 80%) when adequate serum concentrations are maintained. Other authors indicate that 10% to 50% of epileptic dogs are refractory to phenobarbital alone. Tolerance to the drug may develop over time. The addition of potassium bromide markedly improves (80% to 90%) seizure control. Phenobarbital decreases seizure activity by enhancing responsiveness to the inhibitory postsynaptic effects of gamma-aminobutyric acid (GABA) neurotransmitters. It also inhibits glutamate activity and likely decreases calcium fluxes across the cell membrane. Peak plasma concentrations occur only 4 to 6 hours after administration. Serum levels should be monitored after steady-state levels have been reached (14 days in the dog, 9 days in the cat). Serum samples are collected just before the next dose. Effective serum levels in the dog are in the range of 65 to 170 μmol/L (14 to 45 μg/mL). In cats a level of 23.2 to 30.2 μg/mL should be attained. The drug also is used for its sedative properties. Also see BARBITURATES.

ADVERSE AND COMMON SIDE EFFECTS: Initially, sedation and ataxia may be noted, especially at higher doses. These effects tend to resolve with continued treatment. Respiratory depression may occur with toxicity and should be treated with doxapram and artificial respiration where indicated. Polyuria, polydipsia, and polyphagia are reported. Phenobarbital is a hepatic enzyme inducer. Phenobarbital has been implicated as causing hepatotoxicity, especially with chronic use. Serum alkaline phosphatase (ALP), ALT, and cholesterol increase after prolonged use, but the increase does not necessarily correlate with liver disease. The increases in ALP and ALT may reflect enzyme induction rather than hepatic injury. Continued elevation of hepatic enzymes 6 to 8 weeks after discontinuation of the drug may indicate hepatic disease. Serum AST, fasted bile acids and bilirubin, and hepatic ultrasound evaluation are not affected. Hepatotoxicity has not been documented in cats, but cutaneous hypersensitivity and bone marrow suppression have been documented. Total T_4 and free T_4 concentrations may be reduced and endogenous TSH increased with chronic use of the drug. There is no effect by phenobarbital on the pituitary adrenal axis. Neutropenia, thrombocytopenia, and anemia may develop after prolonged use. Values return to within reference ranges 7 to 21 days after discontinuation of the drug. Chronic administration of the drug (median deveation of therapy was 6 years) may be a risk factor for the development of superficial necrolytic dermatitis. Activated charcoal is given in cases of drug overdose, even when it has been administered parenterally. In addition, sodium bicarbonate increases the renal excretion of the drug and is potentially useful in cases of drug overdose.

DRUG INTERACTIONS: Diet may affect serum concentrations. High fiber may impair absorption. A low-protein, low-fat diet may also be associated with lower serum concentrations. Antihistamines, phenothiazines, narcotic agents, and chloramphenicol may potentiate the effects of the drug. Phenobarbital increases the activity of hepatic microsomal enzymes and may decrease the effects of doxycycline, chloramphenicol, corticosteroids, β blockers (e.g., propranolol, metoprolol), estrogens, androgens, adrenocortical and progestational steroids, thyroid hormone, quinidine, metronidazole, theophylline, cimetidine, chloramphenicol, diltiazem, cyclosporine, digitoxin, doxycycline, itraconazole, phenylbutazone, selegiline, theophylline, felbamate, warfarin, and shortens the anesthetic time of xylazine. Once induced by phenobarbital, it may take up to 7 months for microsomal enzyme systems to return to their baseline state. Phenobarbital may decrease the absorption of griseofulvin. Barbiturates may interfere with the metabolism of phenytoin, thus altering its serum levels.

SUPPLIED AS HUMAN PRODUCTS:

IN THE UNITED STATES
Tablets containing 15, 16, 30, 32, 60, 65, and 100 mg
Capsules containing 16 mg
Elixir containing 20 mg/5 mL
For injection containing 30, 60, 65, and 130 mg/mL
Powder for injection containing 130 mg/amp

IN CANADA
Tablets containing 15, 30, 60, and 100 mg
For injection containing 30 and 120 mg/mL
Elixir containing 4 and 5 mg/mL

OTHER USES

Dogs
SEDATION
2.2 to 6.6 mg/kg bid; PO

Cats
IDIOPATHIC EPILEPSY
i)   8 to 15 mg once to twice daily; PO
ii) 2.2 to 4.4 mg/kg per day divided bid or tid; PO

PHENOXYBENZAMINE

INDICATIONS: Phenoxybenzamine (Dibenzyline ★) is a long-acting α-adrenergic blocking agent. The drug may be of use in reducing urethral sphincter tone, thus facilitating urine flow. Several days of treatment may be required for a desirable effect.

ADVERSE AND COMMON SIDE EFFECTS: Hypotension, reflex tachycardia, weakness, miosis, increased intraocular pressure, nausea, and vomiting are reported.

DRUG INTERACTIONS: Phenoxybenzamine will antagonize the effects of α-adrenergic agonists, e.g., phenylephrine.

SUPPLIED AS HUMAN PRODUCT:
Capsules containing 10 mg

OTHER USES
Dogs
PHEOCHROMOCYTOMA
Presurgical stabilization of blood pressure
0.2 to 1.5 mg/kg bid; PO for 10 to 14 days before surgery

PHENYLBUTAZONE

INDICATIONS: Phenylbutazone (Butazone ♣, Phenylbutazone ♣ ★) has analgesic, antipyretic, and anti-inflammatory properties that make it useful in the treatment of osteoarthritis, rheumatism, and inflammation of the skin and soft tissue. The drug also has been used for the short-term management of corneal injury, acute uveitis, chorioretinitis, endophthalmitis, and trauma to the globe.

ADVERSE AND COMMON SIDE EFFECTS: Gastric irritation with vomiting and GI ulceration may occur. Misoprostol may be effective in the prevention and treatment of the adverse GI side effects of the drug. Thrombocytopenia, neutropenia, and nonregenerative anemia also are reported. Adverse effects are unpredictable and unrelated to dose. Intramuscular or SC injection is irritating and should be avoided. Use of phenylbutazone may exacerbate clinical signs of Scotty cramp. The drug is toxic to cats and is not recommended in this species.

DRUG INTERACTIONS: Phenylbutazone is a hepatic enzyme inducer and may increase the metabolism of digitoxin and phenytoin. Conversely, barbiturates, corticosteroids, chlorpheniramine, and diphenhydramine may decrease the plasma half-life of phenylbutazone. Metabolism of phenylbutazone may be accelerated by hepatic enzyme inducers such as phenobarbital, griseofulvin, and phenytoin. Phenylbutazone may increase the plasma half-life of penicillin G and lithium. The drug also may antagonize the effects of furosemide. Concurrent use with other NSAIDs increases the potential for drug toxicity.

SUPPLIED AS VETERINARY PRODUCTS:
For injection containing 200 mg/mL ♣ ★
Tablets containing 100 mg ♣ ★
Tablets containing 1 g (horses only) ♣ ★

SUPPLIED AS HUMAN PRODUCT:
Tablets containing 100 mg

OTHER USES
Dogs
OPHTHALMIC DISEASE
40 mg/kg tid; PO

Cats
OPHTHALMIC DISEASE
10 to 14 mg/kg bid; PO

PHENYLPROPANOLAMINE

INDICATIONS: In November 2000, the Food and Drug Administration (FDA) issued a public health warning regarding phenylpropanolamine (PPA) due to the risk of hemorrhagic stroke. The FDA, requested that manufacturers voluntarily discontinue marketing products that contain PPA. Whether animals are at risk is unknown, but to the author's knowledge there have been no reports of such toxicity in small animals. Phenylpropanolamine (Propalin ♣) is an α-adrenergic stimulant. The drug is useful in the treatment of urinary incontinence in the dog. Excellent results are reported in 73% to 90% of dogs. Dogs older at the onset of clinical signs (median 5 years) and those with a longer period from the time of ovariohysterectomy to the onset of urinary incontinence (median 2.5 years) respond best. It is preferred to ephedrine because side effects are less severe; ephedrine has greater cardiovascular side effects, and it tends to lose effectiveness over time. Phenylpropanolamine also may be useful in the management of nasal congestion.

ADVERSE AND COMMON SIDE EFFECTS: Anorexia, restlessness, irritability, tremors, tachycardia, cardiac arrhythmias, hypertension, and urine retention are reported. With drug overdose, nausea, anorexia, vomiting, tachycardia, disorientation, and mydriasis may occur.

DRUG INTERACTIONS: Phenylpropanolamine enhances the pressor effects of tricyclic antidepressants, e.g., amitriptyline; NSAIDs, including aspirin and indomethacin, also increase the potential for hypertension. Arrhythmias are more likely in those administered halogenated anesthetic agents. Ephedrine may potentiate sympathetic nervous system stimulation, causing toxicity. An unexplained mechanism leading to the possibility of death is reported in humans taking chlorpromazine with phenylpropanolamine.

SUPPLIED AS VETERINARY PRODUCT:
As an oral liquid containing 50 mg/mL

PHENYTOIN

INDICATIONS: Phenytoin, or diphenylhydantoin (Dilantin ✤ ★), is an anticonvulsant. Phenytoin stops the propagation and spread of neural excitation. Because of undesirable pharmacological activity of the drug in small animals, it has lost favor as a single agent for long-term control of seizure activity. It is used as an alternative or adjunctive drug in dogs that have not responded to or that have developed adverse reactions to phenobarbital or primidone. Serum concentrations are measured just before the next dose and after steady-state levels have been attained (22 hours in the dog). Effective serum concentration levels are in the range of 39.6 to 79.2 μmol/L (10 to 20 μg/mL or, according to another source, 10 to 30 μg/mL). The drug also is useful in the management of digitalis-induced tachyarrhythmias and atrioventricular block. The drug may be used with other antiarrhythmic agents to control difficult ventricular arrhythmias or in the place of lidocaine or procainamide for refractory ventricular arrhythmias.

ADVERSE AND COMMON SIDE EFFECTS: Vomiting, ataxia, tremors, depression, hypotension, and atrioventricular block are reported. Gingival hyperplasia is an uncommon side effect. The drug is toxic to cats and is not recommended in this species.

DRUG INTERACTIONS: Antacids (aluminum, calcium, and magnesium compounds), antihistamines, cisplatin, vinblastine, bleomycin, barbiturates, calcium gluconate, carbamazepine, folic acid, oxacillin, and rifampin decrease serum levels of phenytoin. Serum levels are increased (and the potential for toxicity and loss of seizure control) by chloramphenicol, cimetidine, allopurinol, theophylline, anticoagulants, benzodiazepines, dexamethasone, estrogens, methylphenidate, nitrofurantoin, pyridoxine, phenothiazines, sulfonamides, salicylates, and phenylbutazone. Phenytoin may decrease the activity of corticosteroids, disopyramide, doxycycline, estrogens, quinidine, dopamine, and furosemide. The analgesic properties of meperidine may be decreased and its toxicity enhanced by phenytoin. Additive hepatotoxicity may occur if phenytoin is used in conjunction with primidone or phenobarbital. Pyridoxine (vitamin B_6) may decrease serum phenytoin levels. Lidocaine and propranolol may have additive cardiac depressant effects. Valproic acid may increase or decrease serum concentrations.

SUPPLIED AS HUMAN PRODUCTS (✤ ★):
Capsules (extended) containing 30 and 100 mg ★
Oral suspension containing 6 and 25 mg/mL ✤ ★
Tablets containing 50 mg ✤ ★
For injection containing 50 mg/mL ✤ ★

PHOSPHATE ENEMAS

INDICATIONS: Phosphate-containing enemas (Fleet ✤ ★) are used for the relief of constipation in the dog. Osmotic action draws water into the intestinal lumen.

ADVERSE AND COMMON SIDE EFFECTS: These agents should not be used in the presence of dehydration, abdominal pain, nausea, vomiting, cardiac disease, or severe debility. Their use is contraindicated in cats, small dogs, and those with significant renal disease. Clinical signs of toxicity occur within 1 hour of use and include depression, ataxia, tetany, seizure, vomiting, hemorrhagic diarrhea, tachycardia, pallor, and stupor. Associated biochemical abnormalities may include hyperphosphatemia, hypernatremia, hypocalcemia, hyperglycemia, hyperosmolality, and metabolic acidosis with a high anion gap (increased lactic acid). Death has been reported with the use of these agents in cats.

DRUG INTERACTIONS: None reported.

SUPPLIED AS HUMAN PRODUCT:
For rectal use containing 16 g sodium phosphate and 6 g dibasic sodium phosphate per 100 mL sodium, 8.09 mmol (186 mg)/5 mL

PIMOBENDAN

INDICATIONS: While pimobendan [Vetmedin ✤] does have some phosphodiesterase inhibition activity, it is unique because it is primarily a calcium-sensitizing agent and does not substantially increase intracellular calcium or cyclic AMP. The cardiac myofilaments become more sensitive to intracellular calcium and by this mechanism contractility of the heart is improved. This is in contrast to other inotropic agents including digoxin that improve contractility by increasing intracellular calcium. In humans with heart failure, exercise capacity and quality of life improved significantly. Pimobendan is used in the management of congestive heart failure. In Doberman pinschers, mean survival time was increased from a reported time of 79 days to 280 days in those treated with this drug. The drug did not appear to have an impact upon life expectancy in cocker spaniels with congestive heart failure associated with dilated cardiomyopathy. In both breeds a significant improvement in quality of life was noted. Affected dogs also received standard doses of digoxin, furosemide, and enalapril.

ADVERSE AND COMMON SIDE EFFECTS: The drug is metabolized by the liver. In people, ventricular arrhythmia and sudden death have been reported. Other adverse effects include headache, dizziness, weight gain, and skin rash. In the dogs reported above, no significant side effects were reported.

DRUG INTERACTIONS: Hypotension may occur with concurrent use of ACE inhibitors.

SUPPLIED AS:
Capsules containing 1.25, 2.5, and 5 mg

PIPERAZINE

INDICATIONS: Piperazine (Hartz Once a Month ★, Once a Month Roundworm Treatment ♦, Pipa-Tabs ★, Purina Liquid Wormer ★) is an anthelmintic used for the eradication of roundworms.

ADVERSE AND COMMON SIDE EFFECTS: The most common clinical signs of toxicity, in decreasing order of frequency, are tremors, ataxia, seizures, vomiting, and weakness. For recent ingestion, activated charcoal and a saline or osmotic cathartic are recommended. The drug should not be given to animals with chronic liver or renal disease.

DRUG INTERACTIONS: Piperazine and chlorpromazine may precipitate seizure activity if used at the same time. Piperazine may exaggerate the extrapyramidal effects of phenothiazines. Pyrantel/morantel antagonize the efficacy of piperazine. The concurrent use of laxatives is not recommended because these agents may cause elimination of the drug before it has had an opportunity to work effectively.

SUPPLIED AS VETERINARY PRODUCTS:
Tablets equivalent to 50 mg or 250 mg base [Pipa-Tabs] or
80 and 125 mg base [Once a Month Treatment] or
80 and 303 mg base [Hartz Once a Month]

PIROXICAM

INDICATIONS: Piroxicam (Feldene ❦ ★) is a nonsteroidal anti-inflammatory agent with analgesic, antipyretic, and anti-inflammatory properties. Piroxicam has been used in dogs for the management of pain associated with degenerative joint disease. In humans, it appears equivalent in efficacy to aspirin in the treatment of osteoarthritis and rheumatoid arthritis. The drug also has been used successfully in dogs for the management of transitional cell carcinoma of the bladder (median survival in dogs 181 days in 1 report) and for inducing partial remission of squamous cell carcinoma in dogs (median and mean times for failure were 180 and 223 days respectively).

ADVERSE AND COMMON SIDE EFFECTS: Piroxicam is contraindicated in hemophilia and GI ulceration or bleeding. Caution is advised in patients with renal or cardiac dysfunction, predisposition to fluid retention, hypertension, or coagulation disorders. Standard dosages may cause anorexia, melena, vomiting, anemia, mild to moderate leukocytosis, and a mild increase in serum urea nitrogen in dogs. Use of the drug in dogs at doses of 1 mg/kg has been associated with GI ulceration, peritonitis, and renal papillary necrosis.

DRUG INTERACTIONS: Concurrent use of aspirin may cause a slight reduction in piroxicam plasma levels. Anticoagulants may cause a slight increase in hypoprothrombinemic response. Diazepam, propranolol, and phenylbutazone may be displaced by piroxicam, leading to increased therapeutic and possibly toxic serum levels.

SUPPLIED AS HUMAN PRODUCT:
Capsules containing 10 and 20 mg

OTHER USES
Dogs
*TRANSITIONAL CELL CARCINOMA OF THE BLADDER
AND ORAL SQUAMOUS CELL CARCINOMA IN DOGS*
0.3 mg/kg per day; PO

PLICAMYCIN

INDICATIONS: Plicamycin, formerly known as mithramycin, (Mithracin ★), has been used in dogs to treat hypercalcemia of malignancy and hypercalcemia secondary to vitamin D toxicosis. Clinical effectiveness peaks 1 to 2 days after a single IV dose of 25 µg/kg. The drug has antitumor activity independent of its calcium-lowering effect. Although the drug has minimal immunosuppressive activity, its high toxicity and low therapeutic index have limited its clinical use in human medicine.

ADVERSE AND COMMON SIDE EFFECTS: No significant side effects were documented at a dose of 25 µg/kg. A dose of 100 µg/kg induced severe hepatic necrosis and death. Prolonged daily administration of the drug has been associated with hypocalcemia, hypokalemia, azotemia, and increased liver enzyme activities. These side effects are reversible on discontinuation of the drug. At an IV dose of 0.1 mg/kg (in 250 mL saline), dogs may exhibit shivering and mild pain in the injected leg. In humans, other adverse effects worth noting include thrombocytopenia and bleeding diathesis, anorexia, nausea, vomiting, diarrhea, and stomatitis.

DRUG INTERACTIONS: Concurrent administration of vitamin D may enhance hypercalcemia.

SUPPLIED AS HUMAN PRODUCT:
For injection containing 2.5 mg

POLYSULFATED GLYCOSAMINOGLYCANS

INDICATIONS: Polysulfated glycosaminoglycans may be beneficial in the treatment of osteoarthritis. Administration of the compound to growing pups susceptible to hip dysplasia resulted in better coxofemoral congruity and fewer pathologic changes. The drug stimulates the synthesis of glycosaminoglycans, inhibits collagen and proteoglycan catabolism, and inhibits neutrophil migration into synovial fluid. These agents also inhibit potentially destructive enzymes including cathepsin, collagenase, hyaluronidase, and stromelysin. They have fibrinolytic activity and stimulate hyaluronic acid synthesis. Circulation to subchondral bone and perivascular tissue may improve. To maximize therapeutic benefit treatment should begin soon after the inciting traumatic event.

ADVERSE AND COMMON SIDE EFFECTS: Some studies have reported a potentiation of antithrombin III activity leading to a dose-dependent prolongation of activated partial thromboplastin time, prothrombin time, and activated coagulation time. Recent studies of the product Cosequin in dogs, however, failed to demonstrate clinically significant adverse changes in hematologic, hemostatic, or biochemical parameters under investigation. Adequan should be used with caution in animals with renal and/or hepatic dysfunction. It should not be used in breeding animals because the effects on fertility and reproductive function have not been determined.

DRUG INTERACTIONS: The concurrent use of glucocorticoids or NSAIDs may mask clinical signs of joint sepsis. Use with caution in dogs on long-term NSAIDs.

SUPPLIED AS VETERINARY PRODUCTS:
For injection containing 100 mg/mL [Adequan ♣ ★]
Available in capsules for cats and chewable tablets for dogs [Cosequin from Nutramax Laboratories]

POTASSIUM CHLORIDE

INDICATIONS: Potassium chloride ♣ ★ is indicated in the treatment of hypokalemia in the dog and cat.

ADVERSE AND COMMON SIDE EFFECTS: Infusion of potassium-containing fluids, especially those containing glucose, may initially decrease serum potassium levels further as a result of dilution, increased distal renal tubular flow, and cellular uptake of potassium. To minimize the likelihood of this complication, begin oral potassium supplementation 12 to 24 hours before fluid therapy, use a fluid that does not contain glucose, and administer fluids at an appropriate rate. Infusion of potassium fluid concentrations in excess of 40 mEq/L may be associated with pain and sclerosis of peripheral veins.

Hyperkalemia and cardiac arrest may occur, and patients with impaired ability to excrete potassium, e.g., renal impairment, are at increased risk. Potassium may exacerbate heart block. The drug is contraindicated in patients with renal failure and oliguria, adrenal insufficiency, acute dehydration, and hyperkalemia of any cause. In patients on a low-salt diet, hypokalemic hypochloremic alkalosis may occur that may require calcium supplementation in addition to potassium. Potassium chloride is acidifying and may exacerbate preexisting metabolic acidosis. Clinical signs of hyperkalemia may include muscular weakness, bradycardia, vomiting, and diarrhea.

DRUG INTERACTIONS: The concurrent use of potassium-sparing diuretics, e.g., spironolactone and triamterene, may predispose to severe hyperkalemia, as may the concurrent use of penicillin G potassium.

SUPPLIED AS HUMAN PRODUCTS:
Tablets containing 750 mg potassium chloride equivalent to 10 mEq potassium and tablets containing 1,500 mg equivalent to 20 mEq
Capsules containing 600 mg potassium chloride equivalent to 8 mEq and 750 mg equivalent to 10 mEq potassium
For injection containing 2 mEq/mL in 10-mL (20 mEq) and 20-mL (40 mEq) vials
For injection containing 10, 20, 30, 40, 60, and 90 mEq
Each 7.8 g dose contains 1.85 g [25 mmol (mEq)] potassium and 25 mmol (mEq) chloride [K-Lyte/Cl ♣]

Guidelines for Routine Intravenous Supplementation of Potassium in Dogs and Cats

Serum Potassium (mEq/L)	mEq KCl to Add to 250 mL Fluid	mEq KCl to Add to 1 L Fluid	Maximal Fluid Rate (mL/kg per Hour)
<2.0	20	80	6
2.1 to 2.5	15	60	8
2.6 to 3.0	10	40	12
3.1 to 3.5	7	28	18
3.6 to 5.0	5	20	25

Reprinted with permission from DiBartola SP. Fluid Therapy in Small Animal Practice. 2nd ed. Philadelphia: WB Saunders, 2000:96.

POTASSIUM CITRATE

INDICATIONS: Potassium citrate (Urocit-K ★, K-Lyte ♣) is used for the prevention of calcium oxalate urolithiasis. The citrate complexes with calcium and decreases the urinary concentration of calcium oxalate. Potassium citrate also alkalinizes the urine and increases the solubility of calcium oxalate.

ADVERSE AND COMMON SIDE EFFECTS: Studies in dogs have failed to demonstrate serious side effects with use of the drug. In humans, the drug may be associated with mild GI upset, e.g., abdominal discomfort, nausea, vomiting, diarrhea, and loose stools. Reducing the dose or administering the drug with food may alleviate these complaints. If there is evidence of GI upset, the drug should be discontinued. Hyperkalemia may occur and serum electrolytes should be monitored regularly. The drug is contraindicated in animals with hyperkalemia or renal failure. It also is contraindicated in patients with urinary tract infections because the alkaline urinary pH associated with its use may promote further bacterial growth.

DRUG INTERACTIONS: Drugs that decrease GI transit, e.g., anticholinergics, may predispose to gastric irritation induced by potassium citrate. The concurrent use of potassium-sparing agents, e.g., spironolactone and triamterene, predispose to hyperkalemia and should be avoided.

SUPPLIED AS HUMAN PRODUCTS:
Tablets containing 5 mEq (540 mg) and 10 mEq (1,080 mg)
Tablets containing 2.5 g or 25 mmol (mEq) elemental potassium [K-Lyte]

POTASSIUM GLUCONATE

INDICATIONS: Potassium gluconate (Kaon ♣ ★, Tumil-K ★) is indicated in the treatment of hypokalemia in the dog and cat. Potassium gluconate elixir is more palatable and easier to dose for cats than potassium chloride.

ADVERSE AND COMMON SIDE EFFECTS: As for POTASSIUM CHLORIDE, except that potassium gluconate is nonacidifying.

DRUG INTERACTIONS: As for POTASSIUM CHLORIDE.

SUPPLIED AS VETERINARY PRODUCTS:
Powder containing 468 mg (2 mEq) per 1/4 teaspoon (0.65 g) [Tumil-K]
Tablets containing 468 mg (2 mEq) [Tumil-K]
Gel containing 468 mg (2 mEq) per 1/2 teaspoon (2.34 g) [Tumil-K]

SUPPLIED AS HUMAN PRODUCTS:
Elixir containing 20 mEq per 15 mL [Kaon ♣ ★]
Tablets containing 2, 2.3, 2.5, and 5 mEq [generic products ★] and 10 mEq [Kaon ★]

POTASSIUM IODIDE

INDICATIONS: Supersaturated potassium iodide (SSKI ★) has been used for the treatment of sporotrichosis in dogs and cats. Potassium iodide also is used in cats with hyperthyroidism scheduled for thyroidectomy that do not tolerate methimazole well. Iodine decreases the rate of thyroid hormone synthesis and causes a reduction in the size and vascularity of the adenomatous thyroid gland, although the effects are inconsistent and serum T_3 and T_4 may not normalize. In addition, the antithyroid effect may be short-lived, and escape from inhibition generally occurs. This medication should not be used as the sole therapy for cats with hyperthyroid disease but may be used in conjunction with a β-blocking drug or another antithyroid agent.

ADVERSE AND COMMON SIDE EFFECTS: Cats are especially sensitive to iodides. Toxic signs include anorexia, excessive salivation, vomiting, depression, muscle twitching, hypothermia, cardiomyopathy, cardiovascular collapse, and death. Caution is advised in patients with renal impairment, cardiac disease, or hypoadrenocorticism. Safe use during pregnancy and in lactating mothers has not been established.

DRUG INTERACTIONS: Lithium may potentiate the hypothyroid and goitrogenic effects of potassium iodide. The concurrent use of potassium-sparing diuretics or potassium-containing drugs increases the risk of hyperkalemia, cardiac arrhythmias, and cardiac arrest.

SUPPLIED AS HUMAN PRODUCTS:
Oral solution containing 1 g/mL [SSKI ★, Potassium Iodide Saturated Solution ★]
Lugol's solution (5 g iodine with 10 g potassium iodide per 100 mL; solution yields 6.3 mg iodine/drop)

OTHER USES
Cats
HYPERTHYROID DISEASE
30 to 100 mg/day; PO for 1 to 2 weeks prethyroidectomy; combine with a β-blocker, e.g., propranolol (2.5 to 5 mg tid; PO)

POTASSIUM PHOSPHATE

INDICATIONS: Potassium phosphate ❖ ★ is indicated in the treatment of hypophosphatemia. In dogs and cats, the most common cause of hypophosphatemia is diabetic ketoacidosis. It also has been documented in a cat with hepatic lipidosis.

ADVERSE AND COMMON SIDE EFFECTS: Potassium phosphate is contraindicated in conditions in which high potassium or phosphate or low calcium are expected. To avoid potassium or phosphate intoxication, infuse slowly. Infusing high concentrations of phosphate may cause hypocalcemia. In patients with severe renal or adrenal insufficiency, infusion of the drug may cause hyperkalemia. High serum potassium concentrations may cause weakness, bradycardia, heart block, hypotension, and cardiac arrest.

DRUG INTERACTIONS: Potassium-containing products should be used with caution in patients receiving digitalis agents and are contraindicated in these same patients with evidence of heart block. Captopril and enalapril and potassium-sparing diuretics, e.g., spironolactone and triamterene, may predispose to hyperkalemia with the concurrent use of potassium phosphate.

SUPPLIED AS HUMAN PRODUCT:
For injection providing 3 mmol (285 mg) phosphate and 4.4 mEq (170 mg) potassium per mL

PRAZIQUANTEL

INDICATIONS: Praziquantel (Droncit ❖ ★, Prazarid ❖) is an anthelmintic used in dogs and cats to eliminate tapeworms, including *Taenia* spp., *Dipylidium caninum, Echinococcus granulosus,* and *Mesocestoides* *corti.* The drug also is effective against *Paragonimus* infections in dogs. After use of the drug, the parasite loses its ability to resist digestion by the host, and because of this, it is common to see only disintegrated and partially digested pieces of tapeworm in the stool. Increased dosages have been used to eliminate *Spirometra* in dogs and cats and schistosomiasis (*Heterobilharzia americana*) infestations in dogs. Finally, praziquantel has been used to treat *Amphimerus pseudofelineus,* a liver fluke in cats.

ADVERSE AND COMMON SIDE EFFECTS: The drug is very safe but should not be used in puppies or kittens younger than 4 weeks of age. Administration of the drug at dosages of 5 times the recommended level did not cause signs of toxicity in the dog or cat. Drug overdose may be associated with anorexia, vomiting, salivation, diarrhea, and depression.

DRUG INTERACTIONS: None reported.

SUPPLIED AS VETERINARY PRODUCTS:
For injection containing 56.8 mg/mL
Tablets containing 34 mg (canine formulation) and 23 mg (feline formulation)
Tablets containing 50 mg

OTHER USES
Dogs and Cats
PARAGONIMIASIS
25 mg/kg bid; PO for 2 consecutive days

SPIROMETRA
7.5 mg/kg for 2 consecutive days

SCHISTOSOMIASIS
25 mg/kg bid to tid; PO for 2 to 3 days

Cats
AMPHIMERUS PSEUDOFELINEUS
40 mg/kg once daily for 3 days
SPIROMETRA
25 mg/kg for 2 consecutive days

PRAZOSIN

INDICATIONS: Prazosin (Minipress ♣ ★) is a selective α-adrenergic blocking agent. It causes arterial and venous vasodilation without changes in heart rate or cardiac output and is used to decrease blood pressure in patients with systemic hypertension and decrease pulmonary edema in cases of congestive heart failure. The drug has also been used to manage dogs with functional urethral obstruction. Good long-term results were noted in 41% of cases.

ADVERSE AND COMMON SIDE EFFECTS: Hypotension and syncope may occur and are most common after administration of the first dose. These problems usually are transient, and repeated doses rarely cause them again. Nausea, vomiting, diarrhea, and constipation also have been reported. Tolerance to the drug has been documented, but temporarily discontinuing the drug, adjusting the dose, or adding an aldosterone antagonist, e.g., spironolactone, to the regimen may alleviate this problem.

DRUG INTERACTIONS: Increased frequency of hypotension may occur with the concurrent use of diuretics and β-adrenergic blocking agents, e.g., propranolol. Highly protein-bound drugs, e.g., phenobarbital and phenytoin, may potentiate prazosin side effects. Similarly, prazosin may displace or be displaced by the sulfonamides, phenylbutazone, or warfarin.

SUPPLIED AS HUMAN PRODUCTS:
Capsules containing 1, 2, and 5 mg ★
Tablets containing 1, 2, and 5 mg ❧

PREDNISOLONE

PREDNISOLONE SODIUM SUCCINATE

PREDNISONE

INDICATIONS: Prednisolone (Delta-Cortef ★, PrednisTab ★), and prednisone (Deltasone ❧) are intermediate-acting glucocorticoid agents. Prednisone is converted to prednisolone by the liver. Except for cases of liver failure, the drugs essentially can be used interchangeably. Prednisolone also is available in combination with other agents, e.g., salicylate (Pred-C ❧) or antihistamine (Predniderm ❧). Prednisolone is indicated for the treatment of inflammatory conditions of the skin and joints and for supportive care during periods of stress. Prednisolone sodium succinate (Solu-Delta-Cortef ❧ ★) also is beneficial for the treatment of acute hypersensitivity reactions, atopic and contact dermatitis, summer eczema, and conjunctivitis. This drug also is used in animals with severe overwhelming infections with toxicity (in combination with appropriate antibiotic therapy) and for the prevention and treatment of adrenal insufficiency and shock (in conjunction with fluid support). For further information concerning ADVERSE AND COMMON SIDE EFFECTS and DRUG INTERACTIONS, see GLUCOCORTICOID AGENTS.

SUPPLIED AS VETERINARY PRODUCTS:

PREDNISOLONE
For injection containing 10 and 50 mg/mL as prednisolone acetate ✣
Tablets containing 5 or 20 mg [PrednisTab ★]
For injection containing 10 and 50 mg/mL as prednisolone sodium succinate [Solu-Delta-Cortef ✣ ★]

HUMAN PRODUCTS:
Oral syrup containing 5 mg/5 mL or 15 mg/5 mL [Prelone ★]
Tablets containing 5 mg [generic products ✣ ★]
For injection containing 20 mg/mL as prednisolone sodium phosphate [generic products ✣]

PREDNISONE
VETERINARY PRODUCT:
Tablets containing 5 mg

HUMAN PRODUCTS:
Oral syrup containing 5 mg/mL [Liquid pred ★]
Tablets containing 1, 2.5, 5, 10, 20, 25, and 50 mg ✣ ★

OTHER USES
Dogs
IATROGENIC SECONDARY HYPOADRENOCORTICISM
Administer prednisone or prednisolone at 0.50 mg/kg per day every other morning
Taper dose gradually and discontinue after 1 month
During periods of severe stress, reinstitute prednisone or prednisolone at 1 to 2 mg/kg per day

IATROGENIC HYPERADRENOCORTICISM
Replace current glucocorticoid with prednisone or prednisolone at equivalent doses
Taper dose of prednisone or prednisolone to 0.25 mg/kg per day over 1 to 2 months
If the original condition for steroid use recurs before attaining the 0.25 mg/kg per day dose, double the last effective dose and administer on alternate days.
If the 0.25 mg/kg per day dose is reached without recurrence of the original indication for steroid use, maintain on this dose for 1 month and then treat for adrenocortical atrophy as outlined above.

PRIMIDONE

INDICATIONS: Primidone (Mysoline ✣ ★) is an anticonvulsant agent. In the liver, the drug is metabolized to phenobarbital (contributes approximately 85% of the anticonvulsant activity) and phenylethylmalonamide (which contributes approximately 15% of the anticonvulsant activity). Primidone works by raising the seizure threshold.

Serum concentrations are measured just before the next dose and after steady-state levels have been reached (16 days in the dog). Effective serum concentrations are based on levels of phenobarbital and are in the range of 65 to 170 μmol/L (approximately 14 to 45 μg/mL). The use of primidone for the control of seizures has been discouraged because the drug must be administered 3 times daily to be effective, absorption is poor, clinically it is no more effective than phenobarbital, and finally, primidone is associated with a greater incidence of hepatotoxicity than other anticonvulsant drugs. The drug is not approved for use in cats.

ADVERSE AND COMMON SIDE EFFECTS: Polyuria, polydipsia, and polyphagia are noted during the first few weeks of therapy or when the dose is increased. Sedation and ataxia may occur but tend to resolve with continued treatment. When initiating therapy, transient anxiety and agitation may be observed. Increase in serum liver enzymes and hepatotoxicity is reported, especially with chronic use, e.g., 2 to 3 years. Neutropenia, thrombocytopenia and anemia have also been documented. Hematologic values return to within reference range within 7 to 21 days after discontinuation of the drug.

DRUG INTERACTIONS: Acetazolamide may decrease the absorption of primidone. The combination of primidone and phenytoin potentiates hepatotoxicity. Phenytoin may increase phenobarbital levels by stimulating the conversion of primidone to phenobarbital. The effects of primidone may be enhanced if the drug is used in conjunction with narcotics, phenothiazines, antihistamines, or chloramphenicol. The effects of corticosteroids, β-blockers, quinidine, theophylline, and metronidazole may be decreased if used in conjunction with primidone. Primidone may decrease the absorption of griseofulvin. Patients are predisposed to postural hypotension if the drug is used with furosemide.

SUPPLIED AS VETERINARY PRODUCT:
Tablets containing 250 mg [Neurosyn ★, Mysoline ♣]

SUPPLIED AS HUMAN PRODUCTS:
Tablets containing 50, 125, and 250 mg [Mysoline]
Oral suspension containing 50 mg/mL [Mysoline ★]

PROCAINAMIDE

INDICATIONS: Procainamide (Pronestyl ♣ ★, Procan SR ♣ ★) is an antiarrhythmic drug. It is used for the management of ventricular premature contractions and tachycardia and supraventricular tachycardia associated with Wolff-Parkinson-White syndrome with wide QRS complexes. Serum drug concentrations are measured after steady-state levels have been attained (12 hours in the dog) and before the next dose is administered.

ADVERSE AND COMMON SIDE EFFECTS: Weakness, hypotension, decreased myocardial contractility, and vagolytic effects are reported. Procainamide should be avoided in patients with second- or third-degree heart block unless the patient is supported by cardiac pacing. Electrocardiographic changes may include widened QRS complexes and QT intervals, atrioventricular block, and multiform ventricular tachycardia. In addition, anorexia, vomiting, diarrhea, and agranulocytosis have been reported. The drug is contraindicated in patients with myasthenia gravis and in humans with systemic lupus erythematosus (SLE). Procainamide has been associated with causing an SLE syndrome in humans. The drug should be used with caution in patients with significant renal or hepatic dysfunction or those with congestive heart failure.

DRUG INTERACTIONS: Antiarrhythmic effects are increased if procainamide is used with other antiarrhythmic agents. Concurrent use with digoxin should be avoided. Serum levels are increased with cimetidine. Acetazolamide increases the effect of procainamide. Anticholinergic effects are enhanced if procainamide is used with anticholinergic drugs. Procainamide may antagonize the effects of pyridostigmine or neostigmine in patients with myasthenia gravis. The incidence of hypotension is increased if the drug is used with antihypertensive agents. Procainamide may potentiate or prolong the neuromuscular blocking activity of succinylcholine or other drugs, e.g., aminoglycosides.

SUPPLIED AS HUMAN PRODUCTS:
For injection containing 100 and 500 mg/mL
Tablets and capsules containing 250, 375, and 500 mg
Tablets (sustained-release) containing 250, 500, 750, and 1,000 mg

PROCHLORPERAZINE

INDICATIONS: Prochlorperazine (Stemetil ♥, Compazine ★) is a phenothiazine derivative used principally for its antiemetic properties. The drug depresses the chemoreceptor trigger zone.

ADVERSE AND COMMON SIDE EFFECTS: The drug is contraindicated in glaucoma, pyloric obstruction or stenosis, and prostatic hypertrophy.

DRUG INTERACTIONS: Prochlorperazine may prolong the effects of general anesthetics. Phenothiazines should not be given within 1 month of worming with organophosphate medications because their effects may be potentiated. Other CNS depressants enhance hypotension and respiratory depression if used concurrently. The concurrent use of quinidine may cause additive cardiac depression. Antacids and antidiarrheal compounds decrease absorption of oral phenothiazines. Space administration by at least 2 hours. Atropine and other anticholinergics have additive anticholinergic potential and reduce the antipsychotic effect of phenothiazines. Barbiturate drugs increase the metabolism of phenothiazines and may reduce their effects. Barbiturate anesthetics may increase excitation (tremor, involuntary muscle movements) and hypotension. Propranolol may have additive hypotensive effects. Phenothiazines may mask the ototoxic effects of aminoglycoside antibiotics. Phenothiazines inhibit phenytoin metabolism and increase its potential for toxicity. Tricyclic antidepressants, e.g., amitriptyline, may intensify the sedative and anticholinergic effects of phenothiazines.

SUPPLIED AS HUMAN PRODUCTS:
Capsules containing 10 and 15 mg (sustained-release) [Compazine]
Tablets containing 5 and 10 mg [Stemetil, Compazine]
Oral syrup containing 1 mg/mL [Compazine, Stemetil]
For injection containing 5 mg/mL [Compazine, Stemetil]

OTHER USES
Dogs
ANTIEMETIC
i)   0.5 mg/kg tid to qid; IM (prochlorperazine)
ii) 0.14 to 0.22 mg/kg bid; SC [Darbazine]

Cats
ANTIEMETIC
i)   0.1 mg/kg qid; IM (prochlorperazine)
ii) 0.5 to 0.8 mg/kg; IM or, bid; SC [Darbazine]

PROPANTHELINE

INDICATIONS: Propantheline bromide (Pro-Banthine ♣ ★) is an anticholinergic agent. It is used in the management of diarrhea, detrusor hyperreflexia, sinus bradycardia, atrioventricular block, and sick sinus syndrome.

ADVERSE AND COMMON SIDE EFFECTS: Tachycardia, weakness, nausea, vomiting, constipation, pupillary dilation, and dryness of the mucous membranes may occur. Signs of drug overdose include urinary retention, excitement, hypotension, respiratory failure, paralysis, and coma.

DRUG INTERACTIONS: Antihistamines, procainamide, quinidine, meperidine, benzodiazepines, and the phenothiazines may enhance the activity of propantheline, and primidone, disopyramide, nitrates, and long-term corticosteroid use may potentiate the adverse effects of the drug. Propantheline may enhance the activity of nitrofurantoin, thiazide diuretics, and sympathomimetic drugs. Propantheline delays the absorption of, but increases serum levels of, ranitidine, and it may decrease the absorption of cimetidine.

SUPPLIED AS HUMAN PRODUCT:
Tablets containing 7.5 and 15 mg

OTHER USES
Dogs
DETRUSOR HYPERREFLEXIA
i)   0.2 mg/kg tid to qid; PO, titrate dose to effect

ii) 5 to 30 mg tid; PO

DIARRHEA/COLITIS/IRRITABLE BOWEL SYNDROME AND ANTIEMETIC
0.25 mg/kg tid; PO for no longer than 72 hours (diarrhea)

SINUS BRADYCARDIA AND HEART BLOCK
0.5 to 1 mg/kg tid; PO

Cats
DETRUSOR HYPERREFLEXIA
i)   7.5 mg once daily to once every third day; PO, titrate dose to effect

ii) 5 to 7.5 mg tid; PO

DIARRHEA AND ANTIEMETIC
0.25 mg/kg tid; PO

CHRONIC COLITIS
0.5 mg/kg bid to tid; PO

SINUS BRADYCARDIA AND HEART BLOCK
i)   0.8 to 1.6 mg/kg tid; PO (the drug generally is ineffective in this instance)

ii) 3.75 to 15 mg bid to tid; PO

PROPIONIBACTERIUM ACNES

INDICATIONS: *Propionibacterium acnes* (Immunoregulin ★) has non-specific immunostimulatory properties. It induces macrophage activation and lymphokine production, enhances cell-mediated immunity, and increases natural killer cell activity that may intensify antineoplastic, antiviral, and antibacterial activity and stimulate hemopoiesis. This agent is marketed as adjunct therapy to antibiotic treatment for dogs with chronic pyoderma. In uncontrolled studies, it has been shown to increase survival times in dogs with oral melanoma and mastocytoma and has been used to treat immunosuppressed cats with rhinotracheitis. *P. acnes* also has been used to treat cats with clinical signs of FeLV-induced disease. Almost half the cats improved clinically, and peripheral blood results also improved. Cats may even seroconvert to an FeLV-seronegative status. Lack of adequate control groups in this study, however, makes conclusions difficult to confirm.

ADVERSE AND COMMON SIDE EFFECTS: Occasionally, fever, chills, anorexia, and lethargy are reported shortly after its use. Anaphylaxis may occur, and when it does, the animal should be treated with epinephrine. Extravascular injection may cause tissue inflammation. Safety of the drug has not been evaluated in pregnant animals.

DRUG INTERACTIONS: The beneficial effects of the drug may be negated by the concurrent use of corticosteroids or other immunosuppressive agents. Corticosteroids should be discontinued 1 week before the use of this product.

SUPPLIED AS VETERINARY PRODUCT:
For injection containing 0.4 mg/mL nonviable *Propionibacterium acnes* in 5-mL vials

PROPOFOL

INDICATIONS: Propofol (Rapinovet ❋ ★, Diprivan ❋ ★) is a sedative/hypnotic IV anesthetic agent used for the induction and maintenance of general anesthesia. It is indicated to provide general anesthesia for procedures lasting less than 5 minutes and for induction and maintenance of general anesthesia using incremental doses to effect. It is particularly useful for cases in which a short recovery is desired. Induction, maintenance, and recovery are smooth after single or incremental doses and after IV infusion. Recovery is rapid and occurs partly by redistribution. In unsedated mixed-breed dogs, the recovery time is approximately 15 minutes, and for greyhounds, it is approximately 22 minutes. The drug is rapidly metabolized and noncumulative. It also has been used successfully in young dogs (3 months) and cats (8 months).

ADVERSE AND COMMON SIDE EFFECTS: In dogs, apnea, cyanosis, and pain on injection have been reported. Induction may be associated with a slight bradycardia. Serious cardiac arrhythmias have not been a feature of propofol anesthesia in dogs. Administration (6 mg/kg over 30 seconds) to hypovolemic dogs may cause a profound decrease in arterial blood pressure. Twitching and paddling of the front legs occurs infrequently. Recovery tends to be rapid, smooth and excitement-free but vomiting, retching, and/or salivation may be noted. With drug overdose, transient apnea and dose-related hypotension or hypertension is reported in cats. Hypotension is minimized by slow administration and the prior administration of fluids. Repeated injections may lead to prolonged recovery, and Heinz body anemia, malaise, anorexia, and diarrhea have been documented after sequential daily use in cats.

Propofol should not be administered through the same IV catheter with blood or plasma. The drug should be used with caution in patients with a history of epilepsy and disorders of lipid metabolism, e.g., pancreatitis. The drug is supplied in sterile glass ampules and contains no preservatives. Because of the risk of contamination, any unused drug should be discarded.

DRUG INTERACTIONS: Propofol is compatible with a wide range of inhalation anesthetics and premedicant drugs, although dosage requirements are reduced if used concurrently. Propofol enhances the arrhythmogenic effect of epinephrine.

SUPPLIED AS VETERINARY [Rapinovet] AND HUMAN [Diprivan] PRODUCTS:
For injection containing 10 mg/mL

OTHER USES
Dogs
BALANCED ANESTHESIA
Premedicate with medetomidine (30 µg/kg; IM) and atropine (0.044 mg/kg; IM); follow with loading dose of propofol (2 mg/kg; IV) and continue with IV infusion at 165 µg/kg per minute

PROPRANOLOL

INDICATIONS: Propranolol (Inderal ♣ ★) is a nonselective β_1- and β_2-blocking agent. It is indicated alone or in conjunction with digoxin in the management of atrial fibrillation. The drug may be of benefit in the treatment of ventricular premature contractions and arrhythmias caused by digitalis toxicity and in the management of systemic hypertension. Propranolol also is useful in the treatment of hypertrophic cardiomyopathy, especially that associated with hyperthyroid disease. Diltiazem may be more effective than propranolol in the treatment of idiopathic hypertrophic cardiomyopathy. Propranolol appears to be ineffective in managing hypertension in most cats. The drug also has been recommended for the management of mild fears and anxiety.

ADVERSE AND COMMON SIDE EFFECTS: Drug dosages should be reduced in cats with hyperthyroid disease. Monitoring heart rate is an appropriate method of determining adequate dosage. Propranolol is contraindicated in patients with congestive heart failure unless it is secondary to a tachyrhythmia responsive to β-blockade. The drug also is contraindicated in those with second- or third-degree heart block and sinus bradycardia and those with bronchoconstrictive lung disease, e.g., asthma. Propranolol should not be given to animals with evidence of thromboembolic disease. The drug may cause hypoglycemia and should be used with caution in diabetics. Side effects of propranolol include bronchoconstriction, hypoglycemia, decreased cardiac contractility, hypotension, bradycardia, peripheral vasoconstriction, and diarrhea. Bronchoconstriction can be managed with terbutaline (2 to 5 mg bid; PO) or oxtriphylline (4 to 8 mg tid; PO). Drug-induced congestive heart failure can be treated with dobutamine, furosemide, and oxygen therapy. Dextrose can be used to manage the hypoglycemia.

Propranolol should be withdrawn gradually in patients on long-term therapy because of the possibility of sensitizing these animals to the endogenous release of norepinephrine and epinephrine, which may result in tachycardia, arrhythmias, and hypertension.

DRUG INTERACTIONS: Antacids delay GI absorption of propranolol. Antiarrhythmic effects of quinidine, procainamide, and lidocaine are enhanced by propranolol, but toxic effects may be additive. Serum levels of propranolol are increased by cimetidine. The hypotensive effects of propranolol are enhanced by chlorpromazine, cimetidine, furosemide, phenothiazines, and hydralazine. Propranolol increases the serum levels of lidocaine. It also increases the effects of tubocurarine and succinylcholine. The action of terbutaline, epinephrine, and phenylpropanolamine may be antagonized by propranolol. Concurrent use of digitalis may potentiate bradycardia. Concurrent use of salicylates may inhibit the antihypertensive effects of propranolol. The effect of propranolol may be decreased by the concurrent use of thyroid hormone supplementation, and the dose of propranolol may need to be decreased in animals receiving methimazole. The bronchodilatory effects of theophylline may be antagonized by propranolol.

SUPPLIED AS HUMAN PRODUCTS:
Tablets containing 10, 20, 40, 60, 80, 90, and 120 mg
Capsules (extended-release) containing 60, 80, 120, and 160 mg
Oral solution containing 4, 8, and 80 mg/mL
For injection containing 1 mg/mL

OTHER USES
Dogs
HYPERTROPHIC CARDIOMYOPATHY
0.3 to 1 mg/kg tid; PO (maximum of 120 mg/day)

MILD FEARS AND ANXIETY
0.5 to 3 mg/kg bid or PRN; PO

Cats

HYPERTROPHIC CARDIOMYOPATHY
4.5 kg or less; 2.5 mg bid to tid; PO
5 kg or more; 5 mg bid to tid; PO

MILD FEARS AND ANXIETY
0.2 to 1 mg/kg tid; PO

PROSTAGLANDIN F$_{2\alpha}$

INDICATIONS: Prostaglandin F$_{2\alpha}$ (Lutalyse ✤ ★) is used in the treatment of pyometra in the dog and cat. The drug causes contraction of the myometrium and relaxation of the cervix. Reduction in uterine size and improvement in clinical signs are not evident for at least 48 hours after the start of therapy. It also has been used alone as an abortifacient in small animals and in combination with intravaginal misoprostol. The latter combination is more expedient (abortion mean—5 days) than PGF$_{2\alpha}$ alone (abortion mean—7 days). PGF$_{2\alpha}$ has also been combined with bromocriptine, a dopamine agonist and prolactin inhibitor, for the termination of unwanted pregnancy.

ADVERSE AND COMMON SIDE EFFECTS: Restlessness, vomiting, salivation, diarrhea, tachycardia, fever, pupillary dilation followed by pupillary constriction, and panting occur within the first minute after injection and last approximately 20 to 30 minutes. Walking dogs for 20 to 40 minutes after use of the drug tends to diminish these clinical signs. These signs tend to become less pronounced with subsequent doses and usually are absent by the fifth dose. Death has been reported with use of this product. Additional side effects in cats may include vocalization, restlessness, grooming, tenesmus, salivation, kneading, mydriasis, urination, and lordosis. Reactions in cats may begin as early as 30 seconds after injection and last as long as 1 hour. Normal estrus cycles and normal litters can be expected in most animals after successful therapy. Prostaglandin F$_{2\alpha}$ should be used with caution in animals with closed-cervix pyometra because of the poor therapeutic response, the risk of peritonitis (through retrograde flow of uterine contents via the fallopian tubes), and the risk of uterine rupture (from contraction against a closed cervix).

DRUG INTERACTIONS: The concurrent use of estrogens is not recommended because estrogens enhance the effects of the drug on the uterus.

SUPPLIED AS VETERINARY PRODUCT:
For injection containing 5 mg/mL [Lutalyse] (licensed for use in large animals only)

OTHER USES

Dogs
INDUCTION OF ABORTION

i) After day 25 of gestation, give 60 µg/kg divided bid or tid; IM for 3 to 6 days (abortion usually occurs in 3 to 7 days).

ii) In healthy bitches from midgestation to term, give 25 to 250 µg/kg bid; IM; radiography or ultrasound is completed every 3 to 5 days to determine whether abortion is complete.

iii) 30 to 35 days after an unplanned breeding, give 0.1 mg/kg tid; SC, until abortion is complete.

iv) Treatment initiated between days 30 and 43 of gestation; intra-vaginal misoprostol (1 to 3 µg/kg) once daily given in conjunction with PGF2a (0.1 mg/kg tid for 48 hours, then 0.2 mg/kg tid to effect; SC).

v) Increasing dose of bromocriptine (15 to 30 µg/kg bid; PO) and dinoprost tromethamine, a PGF2a, (0.1 to 0.2 mg/kg per day; SC)—days of treatment required for pregnancy termination ~ 5 days

Cats
INDUCTION OF ABORTION
After day 40 of gestation, give 0.5 to 1 mg/kg; SC, and again in 24 hours (abortion usually occurs in 8 to 24 hours)

PROTAMINE SULFATE

INDICATIONS: Protamine sulfate ♣ is used as an antidote for heparin intoxication.

ADVERSE AND COMMON SIDE EFFECTS: The drug should be used with caution in patients with a history of cardiovascular disease or a history of allergy to fish. An abrupt decrease in blood pressure, bradycardia, dyspnea, nausea, vomiting, and lassitude are reported. These effects are minimized if the drug is injected slowly (over a 3-minute period). Hypersensitivity also is reported. A rebound effect leading to prolonged bleeding may occur several hours after heparin apparently has been neutralized because of the release of heparin from the heparin–protamine complex or release of additional heparin from extravascular spaces.

DRUG INTERACTIONS: None reported.

SUPPLIED AS HUMAN PRODUCT:
For injection containing 10 mg/mL

PSEUDOEPHEDRINE

INDICATIONS: Pseudoephedrine (Eltor ✤, Sudafed ✤ ★) is a sympathomimetic amine used in dogs in the management of urinary incontinence caused by sphincter incompetence. It has less CNS-stimulating and pressor effects than ephedrine. Patients are started at the lower end of the dose range, with an increase in dose if there is no clinical response. The drug is used in humans for its bronchodilatory and nasal decongestant properties.

ADVERSE AND COMMON SIDE EFFECTS: The drug should not be used within 14 days of the use of MAO inhibitors, e.g., possibly amitraz and selegiline. It is contraindicated in patients with hypertension, glaucoma, and hyperthyroid disease and should be used with caution in those with congestive heart disease and urinary retention. Tachycardia, arrhythmias, nervousness, insomnia, anorexia, nausea, vomiting, and dry mouth are reported.

DRUG INTERACTIONS: The drug should not be used in conjunction with other sympathetic amines because an additive effect and potential toxicity may occur. The activity of β-blocking drugs, e.g., propranolol, may be antagonized by pseudoephedrine.

SUPPLIED AS HUMAN PRODUCTS:
Capsules containing 120 mg
Tablets containing 30 and 60 mg
Oral drops containing 9.4 mg/mL

PYRANTEL PAMOATE

INDICATIONS: Pyrantel pamoate (Pyr-A-Pam ✤, Pyran ✤, Nemex ★) is an anthelmintic used to eradicate hookworm (*Ancylostoma caninum, Uncinaria stenocephala*) and roundworm (*Toxocara canis, Toxascaris leonina*) infections in dogs and hookworm (*Ancylostoma* spp.) and roundworm (*Toxocara cati*) infestations in cats. Pyrantel also may be useful in the elimination of *Physaloptera* spp. in dogs and cats. Nemex is only licensed for use in dogs. Pyrantel is a cholinesterase inhibitor.

ADVERSE AND COMMON SIDE EFFECTS: Cautious use of the drug is advised in patients with liver dysfunction, malnutrition, dehydration, and anemia. Although the drug is considered safe, vomiting may occur.

DRUG INTERACTIONS: The drug should not be used concurrently with levamisole because of similar mechanisms of action and potential toxicity. Adverse effects may be potentiated by the concurrent use of organophosphates or diethylcarbamazine. Piperazine and pyrantel have antagonistic actions and should not be used together.

SUPPLIED AS VETERINARY PRODUCTS:
Tablets containing 35 and 125 mg [Pyr-A-Pam, Pyran]
Tablets containing 22.7 mg (of base) [Nemex]
Oral suspension containing 4.54 mg (of base) per mL of suspension [Nemex]

OTHER USES
Dogs and Cats
PHYSALOPTERA
5 mg/kg; PO once, repeat in 2 or 3 weeks

PYRETHRIN-CONTAINING PRODUCTS:

INDICATIONS: Pyrethrin-containing products (Ovitrol ♣, Mycodex ★, and many others) are naturally occurring insecticides derived from the plant *Chrysanthemum cinerariae-folium*, and commonly are used for flea control. These drugs are GABA agonists that stimulate the insect's central nervous system, causing muscular excitation, convulsions, and paralysis. Insect mortality is enhanced when these products are combined with piperonyl butoxide, e.g., Sectrol and Ovitrol. Piperonyl butoxide inhibits pyrethrin metabolism.

ADVERSE AND COMMON SIDE EFFECTS: These products are relatively nontoxic to mammals, and moderate amounts can be ingested without toxic effects. Pyrethrins should not be used in dogs or cats younger than 6 weeks of age. Ingestion of toxic amounts of pyrethrins in mammals causes depression, nausea, vomiting, diarrhea, muscle tremors, convulsions, stupor, pallor, conjunctivitis, respiratory arrest, and death. Hypersalivation is common. Additionally, cats may display ear flicking, paw shaking, and repeated contractions of the superficial cutaneous muscles. Treatment of toxic patients includes cleaning exposed areas of the skin. If ingestion has taken place within the past hour, the induction of emesis (e.g., 1 to 2 mL/kg of 3% hydrogen peroxide) is indicated. If ingestion has taken place within 3 to 4 hours, gastric lavage and activated charcoal (2 g/kg) then magnesium sulfate or sodium sulfate (0.5 g/kg as a 10% solution) are indicated to limit further absorption. Additionally, fluid therapy, methocarbamol (55 to 220 mg/kg; IV) to control muscle tremors, and phenobarbital (6 mg/kg; IV) or pentobarbital (4 to 20 mg/kg; IV) to control seizures may be indicated.

DRUG INTERACTIONS: Because pyrethrins cause extrapyramidal stimulation, phenothiazines are contraindicated. Piperonyl butoxide, sesame oil, and isosafrole act synergistically with pyrethrins and commonly are combined with them.

SUPPLIED AS VETERINARY PRODUCTS:
See specific product.

PYRIDOSTIGMINE

INDICATIONS: Pyridostigmine (Mestinon ♣ ★) is the anticholinesterase agent most often used in the management of myasthenia gravis because of its long duration of activity and fewer GI side effects. Anticholinesterase drugs are effective in controlling clinical signs in some dogs but not others. These agents are often not effective as long-term single agents for acquired myasthenia, and immunosuppressive drugs may be required to control the underlying disease, e.g., azathioprine. Pyridostigmine is more effective in treating acquired myasthenia than the congenital form. The clinical efficacy in improving esophageal function in dogs with megaesophagus is less than that observed on appendicular muscles.

ADVERSE AND COMMON SIDE EFFECTS: The drug is contraindicated in patients with mechanical obstruction of the GIT or urinary tract, bradycardia, and hypotension. The drug should be used with caution in those with asthma, epilepsy, hyperthyroidism, peptic ulcer disease, and cardiac arrhythmias. Intravenous injection may cause thrombophlebitis. With drug overdose, nausea, vomiting, diarrhea, miosis, excessive salivation and bronchial secretion, bronchoconstriction, bradycardia, weakness, fasciculation, and hypotension may occur. The drug does not cross the blood–brain barrier at moderate dosages, but it may do so at excessive dosages causing CNS depression, respiratory depression, paralysis, and death. Treatment for acute toxicity includes cessation of pyridostigmine use, respiratory support, and the intravenous administration of atropine (1 to 4 mg/kg repeated every 5 to 30 minutes as required).

DRUG INTERACTIONS: The aminoglycosides may have some neuromuscular blocking effects that may necessitate increased dosage of pyridostigmine. The concurrent use of the following drugs with pyridostigmine may alter neuromuscular transmission and should be avoided: barbiturates, succinylcholine, quinidine, procainamide, phenothiazine, methoxyflurane, potassium-depleting diuretics, and magnesium sulfate. Atropine antagonizes the muscarinic effects of the drug but should be used with caution because atropine may mask the early symptoms of a cholinergic crisis. The drug should be administered before feeding to facilitate absorption. Corticosteroids may decrease the effect of the drug by initially worsening the disease.

SUPPLIED AS HUMAN PRODUCTS:
Tablets containing 60 mg
Tablets (sustained-release) containing 180 mg
Oral syrup containing 60 mg/5 mL

PYRIMETHAMINE

INDICATIONS: Pyrimethamine (Daraprim ✤ ★) is used in combination with the sulfonamides, i.e., sulfadiazine, in the treatment of *Toxoplasma* infections. Pyrimethamine inhibits folic acid metabolism in the parasite and appears to increase the activity of the sulfonamide against toxoplasmosis.

ADVERSE AND COMMON SIDE EFFECTS: Depression, anorexia, vomiting, and reversible bone marrow suppression (anemia, leukopenia, and thrombocytopenia) may occur within 4 to 6 days of initiation of therapy with the pyrimethamine-sulfonamide combination. Cats are especially sensitive to these side effects, and anemia, leukopenia, and thrombocytopenia may develop rapidly. Bone marrow suppression may be mitigated by the addition of folic acid (50 mg/day), baker's yeast (100 mg/kg per day), or folinic acid (1 mg/kg per day) to the diet.

DRUG INTERACTIONS: Pyrimethamine is synergistic with the sulfonamides. The efficacy of pyrimethamine against toxoplasmosis is decreased by folic acid and *p*-aminobenzoic acid.

SUPPLIED AS HUMAN PRODUCT:
Tablets containing 25 mg

QUINACRINE

INDICATIONS: Quinacrine ★ is used for the eradication of giardiasis and trichomoniasis. In cats, the drug controlled clinical signs of *Giardia* infection but did not stop cyst shedding.

ADVERSE AND COMMON SIDE EFFECTS: Yellowing of the skin, darkening of urine, anorexia, vomiting, nausea, diarrhea, fever, pruritus, and behavioral changes (excessive barking, fly biting) have been reported. The drug should not be given to pregnant animals because it readily crosses the placenta. In humans, hepatotoxicity, agranulocytosis, anemia, and hypersensitivity reactions also have been reported.

DRUG INTERACTIONS: None of significance in small animals.

SUPPLIED AS HUMAN PRODUCT:
Tablets containing 100 mg

QUINIDINE

INDICATIONS: Quinidine gluconate (Quinaglute ♣ ★) and sulfate are used most commonly in the management of ventricular arrhythmias. They also have been used in the treatment of atrial fibrillation. Serum concentrations are measured just before the next dose and after steady-state levels have been attained (28 hours in the dog, 10 hours in the cat). The therapeutic range in dogs is 2.5 to 5 µg/mL.

ADVERSE AND COMMON SIDE EFFECTS: Quinidine is contraindicated in patients with myasthenia gravis, digitalis intoxication, heart block, and escape beats. Anorexia, vomiting, diarrhea, vagolytic response, urine retention, weakness, hypotension, and decreased cardiac contractility are reported. Sinus node suppression, ventricular tachycardia, atrioventricular block, and prolongation of the PR, QRS, and QT intervals also are reported. A paradoxical acceleration in ventricular rate may occur, especially when the drug is used to treat patients with atrial flutter or fibrillation. In these cases, quinidine often is used after patients have first been given a digitalis glycoside. Drug dose should be decreased in cases with liver disease, congestive heart failure, hyperkalemia, or hypoalbuminemia.

DRUG INTERACTIONS: Quinidine increases serum digoxin levels. Cimetidine increases serum quinidine levels. Phenothiazines potentiate the cardiac depressive effects of quinidine. Quinidine potentiates the neuromuscular blocking effects of curariform and depolarizing blocking agents and those induced by neomycin and kanamycin. Anticholinergic drugs have additive vagolytic effects. Phenobarbital and phenytoin decrease the half-life of quinidine, necessitating a readjustment of drug dose. Sodium bicarbonate, antacids, and thiazide diuretics prolong the half-life of quinidine, predisposing to toxicity. Verapamil potentiates hypotension. Nifedipine decreases quinidine serum concentrations predisposing to breakthrough ventricular tachycardia. Quinidine may enhance the hypotensive effects of β-blocking agents and vasodilators.

SUPPLIED AS HUMAN PRODUCTS:
Tablets and capsules containing 200 mg quinidine sulfate
Tablets (sustained-release) containing 300 mg quinidine sulfate
For injection containing 190 mg/mL quinidine sulfate
Tablets containing 325 mg quinidine gluconate
Tablets (sustained-release) containing 324 mg quinidine gluconate

OTHER USES
Dogs and Cats

ATRIAL FIBRILLATION
6 to 8 mg/kg qid; IM

RANITIDINE

INDICATIONS: Ranitidine (Zantac ✿ ★) is a histamine (H_2) antagonist that is used for the treatment of GI ulceration. It is more potent (5 to 12 times) in inhibiting gastric acid secretion than cimetidine, but it clinically is no more effective. The drug also has been used to treat gastric hypersecretion associated with gastrinomas and systemic mastocytosis. H_2 antagonists do not prevent NSAID-induced gastric ulcers, although ranitidine may prevent NSAID-induced duodenal ulceration. Ranitidine also does not appear to protect the stomach from prednisone-induced gastric hemorrhage. Unlike cimetidine, ranitidine increases the passage of ingesta through the gut by stimulating gastric, small intestinal, and colonic motility; it may stimulate pancreatic exocrine secretion, and while it has less affinity for hepatic cytochrome P-450 enzyme systems, it still interferes with the metabolism of drugs removed by this system.

ADVERSE AND COMMON SIDE EFFECTS: Adverse effects in small animals appear rare. Dogs given dosages greater than 225 mg/kg per day exhibited muscle tremors, vomiting, and rapid respiration. In humans, nausea and bradycardia with IV injection are reported. Pain at the injection site with IM use may occur.

DRUG INTERACTIONS: Propantheline delays absorption and increases peak concentration, thus increasing its bioavailability. Theophylline absorption from controlled-release formulations is decreased by ranitidine-induced achlorhydria. Antacids decrease GI absorption, and concurrent use should be spaced by at least 2 hours. Ranitidine may delay the renal clearance of procainamide, the clinical significance of which remains unclear. The drug also decreases renal clearance of cisplatin in dogs.

SUPPLIED AS HUMAN PRODUCTS:
Tablets containing 75, 150, and 300 mg
Oral syrup containing 15 mg/mL
For injection containing 25 mg/mL

RIFAMPIN

INDICATIONS: Rifampin (Rifadin ✿ ★, Rimactane ★, Rofact ✿) is an antibiotic used alone or in combination with other agents in the treatment of actinomycosis, *Coxiella burnetii* (Q Fever), feline leprosy, listeriosis, Rocky Mountain spotted fever, and tuberculosis. It is active against staphylococcus and other intracellular organisms, e.g., *Chlamydia*. The drug also may be useful in the treatment of chronic staphylococcal infection, e.g., severe pyoderma and chronic osteomyelitis, but it always should be used with another antibiotic because resistance develops rapidly.

ADVERSE AND COMMON SIDE EFFECTS: Hepatopathy and discoloration of the urine are reported. Although rare, anorexia, vomiting, diarrhea, thrombocytopenia, hemolytic anemia, and death have been reported in humans.

DRUG INTERACTIONS: Rifampin induces hepatic microsomal enzyme activity, which may contribute to decreased serum levels of barbiturate drugs, benzodiazepines, chloramphenicol, corticosteroid drugs, dapsone, digitoxin, metoprolol, propranolol, and quinidine. Serum levels of ketoconazole also may be reduced if the drugs are used concurrently.

SUPPLIED AS HUMAN PRODUCT:
Capsules containing 150 and 300 mg

OTHER USES
Dogs
ASPERGILLOSIS AND HISTOPLASMOSIS
10 to 20 mg/kg tid; PO with amphotericin and flucytosine
ACTINOMYCOSIS
10 to 20 mg/kg bid; PO

Cats
ASPERGILLOSIS AND HISTOPLASMOSIS
10 to 20 mg/kg tid; PO with amphotericin and flucytosine

S-ADENOSYLMETHIONINE

INDICATIONS: S-adenosyl-L-methionine (SAMe; Denosyl SD4 ★) is the pure and stabilized 1,4-butanedisulfonate salt of SAMe. Supplementation with SAMe increases levels of glutathione and should only be used in cats with liver damage. S-adenosylmethionine is an essential part of three major biochemical pathways: transmethylation, transsulfuration, and aminopropylation. As part of these pathways, SAMe is essential to all cells and is particularly important in hepatocytes because of their central role in metabolism. Deficiency of SAMe has been associated with a spectrum of cellular derangements that have profound effects on hepatocytes, and a deficiency of SAMe may initiate or contribute to abnormalities of cellular structure and function in many body tissues, including the liver. Denosyl SD4 has been shown to increase hepatic glutathione levels in cats and dogs. Glutathione is a potent antioxidant that protects hepatic cells from toxins and death. A recent analysis of 31 dogs and cats with various severe liver problems showed that 45% of these animals had low hepatic glutathione levels. Denosyl SD4 is recommended to improve hepatic glutathione levels to help maintain and protect liver function. Denosyl SD4 may also be used in other conditions of tissue oxidant injury and red blood cell fragility caused by certain toxins or drugs, which are related to reduced glutathione concentrations, e.g., acetaminophen toxicity.

ADVERSE AND COMMON SIDE EFFECTS: Acute and chronic high-dose administration of the identical stabilized salt of SAMe found in Denosyl SD4 demonstrated a wide margin of safety. Clinically healthy cats administered Denosyl SD4 at more than 4 times the recommended daily dose for 118 days remained healthy with no demonstrable adverse changes in complete blood counts, serum chemistries, or liver histology. In acute toxicity trials, even large amounts (100 mg/kg) of SAMe administered by IV bolus to anesthetized dogs and cats did not cause harmful effects. Extremely high, clinically irrelevant doses caused a transient drop in blood pressure and reduced smooth muscle tone of the bladder and uterus in cats. Studies using Denosyl SD4 in dogs substantiate the safety of administration in these species.

DRUG INTERACTIONS: There are no known drug interactions with Denosyl SD4, and research indicates that supplementation with the product to animals receiving large doses of glucocorticoids can result in beneficial effects on glutathione levels, improved hepatic handling of organic anions, and slowed alkaline phosphatase induction. Tablets should be given on an empty stomach, at least one hour before feeding, as the presence of food decreases the absorption of SAMe.

SUPPLIED AS VETERINARY PRODUCT:
Tablets containing 90 and 225 mg

OTHER USES
Dogs
ACETAMINOPHEN TOXICITY
Loading dose of 40 mg/kg; PO followed by a maintenance dose of 20 mg/kg once daily for 7 days

SELAMECTIN

INDICATIONS: Selamectin (Revolution ♣ ★) is a topical parasiticide indicated for the eradication of fleas in dogs and cats. It kills adult fleas and prevents flea eggs from hatching for 1 month. It is also indicated for the prevention of heartworm, and the treatment and control of ear mites (*Otodectes cynotis*) in dogs and cats, and for the treatment and control of sarcoptic mange in dogs. This agent has also been found to be effective in the eradication of nasal mites (*Pneumonyssoides caninum*) in dogs. In cats, it also eliminates hookworm (*Ancylostoma tubaeforme*) and roundworm (*Toxocara cati*) infections.

ADVERSE AND COMMON SIDE EFFECTS: The drug should not be used in animals less than 6 weeks of age. Side effects appear minimal. Less than 1% of cats had hair loss where the medication was applied and less than 1% experienced vomiting and diarrhea. Caution should be used in sick or underweight animals.

DRUG INTERACTIONS: None reported.

SUPPLIED AS VETERINARY PRODUCT:
Each milliliter contains 60 or 120 mg of selamectin

SELEGILINE

INDICATIONS: Selegiline or l-deprenyl (Anipryl ♣ ★, Eldepryl ♣ ★) is a selective, irreversible MAO inhibitor (predominantly type B). It is marketed for the treatment of uncomplicated pituitary-dependent hyperadrenocorticism in dogs. Pituitary-dependent hyperadrenocorticism in dogs may be related to a deficiency of dopamine. In healthy dogs, dopamine serves to inhibit ACTH secretion from the pituitary gland. Anipryl helps restore brain dopamine, facilitates its transmission, increases its synthesis, and inhibits its reuptake. The drug is started at an oral dose of 1 mg/kg per day and continued for a period of 2 months, during which time response is evaluated on the basis of history and physical examination. If a beneficial response is not seen during this time, the dose is increased to a maximum of 2 mg/kg per day. Beneficial effects generally are noted within the first 2 months of therapy. The drug is however clinically effective in dogs in only 20% of cases. Standard tests used to assess success of therapy (urinary cortisol:creatinine, ACTH stimulation, and abdominal ultrasound) are not useful with use of this drug. Finally normalization of the low-dose dexamethasone suppression test was not consistently accompanied by an improvement in clinical signs. It also may be used to manage cognitive dysfunction disorders in dogs recognized as various geriatric-onset–related behavioral disorders, e.g., geriatric-onset inappropriate urination. In addition to its effects on dopamine, the drug is known to decrease the production of and increase the clearance of free radicals and exert a protective effect on damaged neurons.

ADVERSE AND COMMON SIDE EFFECTS: Vomiting and diarrhea are the most common reported adverse effects. Other adverse effects reported include hyperactivity, agitation, restlessness, and insomnia. In dogs, at doses of 2 mg/kg per day, no untoward clinical effects or laboratory abnormalities were seen over a course of 2 months.

DRUG INTERACTIONS: The concurrent use of meperidine or other opiates should be avoided. Stupor, muscle rigidity, agitation, and increased body temperature have been reported in humans. Fourteen days should be allotted between the discontinuation of Anipryl and the initiation of a tricyclic antidepressant, e.g., amitriptyline or imipramine, and the drug should not be given to animals concurrently receiving MAO inhibitors, e.g., possibly amitraz.

SUPPLIED AS HUMAN PRODUCT (ELDEPRYL):
Tablets containing 5 mg

SUPPLIED AS VETERINARY PRODUCT (ANIPRYL):
Tablets containing 2, 5, 10, 15, and 30 mg

SEVOFLURANE

INDICATIONS: Sevoflurane (Sevoflurane ✿, Ultane ★) is a nonflammable, halogenated inhalation anesthetic agent for induction and maintenance of general anesthesia. Recovery time is faster than that for halothane and isoflurane and time for anesthetic induction is quicker. The higher MAC value means that sevoflurane is less potent than isoflurane and will require a higher inspired concentration to maintain anesthesia. One of the major benefits of this agent is the depth of anesthesia can be changed rapidly enabling more precise control.

ADVERSE AND COMMON SIDE EFFECTS: The half-life of the drug may be increased in patients with impaired renal or hepatic function. The drug should not be administered to patients sensitive to other halogenated agents or to those with malignant hyperthermia. The most common side effects noted in dogs are hypotension, tachypnea, and apnea. Dose dependent decreases in blood pressure and respiratory depression are reported. Heart rate may increase.

DRUG INTERACTIONS: None of clinical importance. In studies where epinephrine was administered submucosally in people, the drug was associated with ventricular premature contractions at the same frequency as that associated with isoflurane.

SUPPLIED AS HUMAN PRODUCT:
Bottles containing 100 and 250 mL

SODIUM BICARBONATE

INDICATIONS: Sodium bicarbonate is indicated for the treatment of metabolic acidosis and the management of hyperkalemia and hypercalcemia.

ADVERSE AND COMMON SIDE EFFECTS: The agent is contraindicated in cases with alkalosis, significant chloride loss associated with vomiting, or with hypocalcemia where infusion of this agent will predispose to hypocalcemic tetany. Sodium bicarbonate should be used with caution in those with potential volume overload, e.g., congestive heart failure and renal disease. Hypercapnia predisposing to ventricular fibrillation may occur in patients during cardiopulmonary resuscitation if adequate ventilatory support is not given.

The use of this drug may cause metabolic alkalosis, hypokalemia, hypocalcemia, hypernatremia, volume overload, and paradoxical CSF acidosis leading to respiratory arrest. Myocardial depression and peripheral vasodilation leading to hypotension, hyperosmolality, CSF acidosis, increased intracranial pressure, and intracranial hemorrhage have been reported. Caution should be used when administering this agent to cats at doses greater than 2 mEq/kg because of the potential for serious acid–base and electrolyte changes.

DRUG INTERACTIONS: If sodium bicarbonate is mixed with calcium-containing fluids, insoluble complexes may form. The action of epinephrine is impaired if it is mixed with sodium bicarbonate. Oral sodium bicarbonate may reduce the absorption of anticholinergic agents, cimetidine, ranitidine, iron products, ketoconazole, and tetracycline antibiotics and reduce the efficacy of sucralfate. Orally administered drugs are best given 2 hours before or after sodium bicarbonate. The alkalinization of urine decreases the urinary excretion of quinidine and ephedrine, whereas the excretion of weakly acidic drugs, e.g., salicylates, is increased.

SUPPLIED AS VETERINARY PRODUCTS:
For injection containing 8.4% (1 mEq/mL) ★
For injection containing 7.5% (0.89 mEq/mL) ♣

SUPPLIED AS HUMAN PRODUCTS:
Tablets containing 325 mg (5 gr) and 650 mg (10 gr) ★
Tablets containing 300, 500, or 600 mg ♣
For injection containing 4.2% (0.5 mEq/mL), 7.5% (0.9 mEq/mL), and 8.4% (1 mEq/mL) ♣ ★

SODIUM CHLORIDE

INDICATIONS: Sodium chloride ♣ ★ is recommended for the treatment of hyponatremia and metabolic alkalosis, the restoration of normovolemia, and the promotion of urinary calcium excretion. It is not recommended for maintenance fluid requirements because of its supraphysiologic levels of sodium and chloride in solution. Hypertonic sodium chloride (3% to 5%) has been used in cases of sodium depletion associated with a relative increase in body water (syndrome of inappropriate antidiuretic hormone secretion). Isotonic sodium chloride (0.9%) remains in the extracellular space (two thirds in the interstitial space, one third in the intravascular space) after IV injection. Half-strength saline (0.45%) is directed into the intracellular space (one third) and extracellular space (two thirds) after IV administration. Hypertonic saline (7.5%) has been used successfully to reverse the pathologic effects of hemorrhagic/hypovolemic shock in the dog. The effect is almost immediate and of short duration. Plasma volume expansion is negligible in 30 to 60 minutes. Hypertonic saline in conjunction with 6% dextran 70 (5 mL/kg; IV over 5 minutes) is more effective than hypertonic saline used alone in the treatment of hypovolemic shock.

ADVERSE AND COMMON SIDE EFFECTS: Excessive volumes of 0.9% saline may cause hyperchloremic metabolic acidosis and hypokalemia, especially in patients with diarrhea in whom sodium loss is greater than chloride and in those patients in whom the kidney cannot excrete the excess chloride load. Volume overload and pulmonary edema are potential concerns in animals with cardiac or renal insufficiency. Hypernatremia also may occur and lead to irritability, lethargy, weakness, ataxia, stupor, coma, and seizure.

Adverse effects noted with hypertonic saline may include cardiovascular collapse if the product is administered too rapidly, increase in sodium and chloride concentrations, and in osmolality, a decrease in potassium and bicarbonate concentrations, bradyarrhythmias, bronchoconstriction, hemolysis, hemoglobinuria, and signs of pain if the solution is injected into small peripheral veins.

DRUG INTERACTIONS: Glucocorticoids and corticotrophin may predispose to sodium retention and volume overload, especially in patients with congestive heart failure.

SUPPLIED AS HUMAN AND VETERINARY PRODUCTS:
For injection containing 0.45% (77 mEq/L) sodium and chloride
For injection containing 0.9% (154 mEq/L) sodium and chloride
For injection containing 5% and 7.2% [Hypertoninc Saline ✚, ★]

OTHER USES
Dogs
SHOCK
i)   7.5% saline: 4 to 5 mL/kg slowly over 8 to 10 minutes or longer; IV

ii) 7.5% saline in hydroxyethyl starch (Hespan) at 4 mL/kg; IV push, then give additional Hespan at 20 mL/kg; IV push; follow with Plasmalyte, Normosol R, or lactated Ringer's solution; IV to effect

iii) 7% saline in 6% dextran 70 at a dosage of 5 mL/kg given slowly over a 5-minute period; IV, followed by lactated Ringer's solution at a dosage of 20 mL/kg per hour

Cats
SHOCK
7.5% saline alone or in combination with 6% dextran 70; slowly IV at a dose of 3 to 5 mL/kg

Note: Hypertonic saline provokes a rapid improvement in cardiovascular function in cats with hypovolemia; the duration of effect lasts only 15 to 60 minutes. Hypertonic saline combined with dextrose provides a more prolonged effect.

SODIUM IODIDE

INDICATIONS: Sodium iodide ✲ ★ is an antifungal agent used in the treatment of the cutaneous and lymphocutaneous forms of sporotrichosis in small animals.

ADVERSE AND COMMON SIDE EFFECTS: Adverse effects include vomiting, anorexia, lacrimation, depression, cardiomegaly, and cutaneous reactions that generally are reversible when the drug dose is decreased. Nausea can be lessened by mixing the drug with milk before administration. Cats are especially sensitive to iodide toxicosis, necessitating a reduction in drug dosage. Toxicity in cats is manifested by hypothermia, muscle spasms, depression, vomiting, and diarrhea.

DRUG INTERACTIONS: None reported.

SUPPLIED AS VETERINARY PRODUCT:
For injection containing 200 mg/mL [20%] (large animal product)

SODIUM POLYSTYRENE SULFONATE

INDICATIONS: Sodium polystyrene sulfonate (Kayexalate ✲ ★) is a sulfonic cation-exchange resin. The drug is used to lower serum potassium levels in patients with hyperkalemia by the exchange of sodium for potassium.

ADVERSE AND COMMON SIDE EFFECTS: The drug should be used with caution in patients with renal failure or those who cannot tolerate an increase in serum sodium levels, e.g., patients with congestive heart failure, severe hypertension, or marked edema. Hypokalemia, hypocalcemia, anorexia, nausea, vomiting, diarrhea, and/or constipation have been reported.

DRUG INTERACTIONS: Digitalis toxicity may be potentiated. The efficacy may be reduced by the concurrent use of antacids or laxatives containing magnesium or calcium.

SUPPLIED AS HUMAN PRODUCT:
Oral suspension: 15 g/60 mL (sodium 1.5 g, 65 mEq) in 120, 480 mL, and UD 60 mL; 15 g/60 mL in 60, 120, 200, and 500 mL; SPS (Carolina Medical Products Co)

Powder for suspension (for rectal or oral use): sodium content is approximately 100 mg (4.1 mEq) per g; in 1 lb jars Kayexalate

SOTALOL

INDICATIONS: Sotalol (Betapace ★) is a β₁- and β₂-blocking agent similar in action to propranolol (1/3 potency) used in the treatment of heart failure and tachyarrhythmias. Its efficacy may also be related to its antiarrhythmic properties. The drug also possesses some Class III (potassium channel-blocking) activity.

ADVERSE AND COMMON SIDE EFFECTS: β-Adrenergic antagonists are contraindicated in uncontrolled heart failure, bradyarrhythmias, and atrioventricular blocks. These drugs should not be used in cats with feline asthma because of the potential to cause bronchospasm. Adverse effects may include hypotension, bradycardia, depression, nausea, vomiting, and diarrhea.

DRUG INTERACTIONS: Absorption from the gut is delayed by meals containing calcium and elimination is prolonged in those with renal disease.

SUPPLIED AS HUMAN PRODUCT:
Tablets containing 80, 120, 160, and 240 mg

SPIRONOLACTONE

INDICATIONS: Spironolactone (Aldactone ♣ ★) is a potassium-sparing diuretic agent used alone or in combination with other diuretics in the management of edema unresponsive to other diuretics. The drug inhibits the action of aldosterone in the distal renal tubules. It is indicated when hypokalemia is a concern and diuresis is indicated. Desired clinical response generally takes 2 to 3 days, and clinical effects persist for an additional 2 to 3 days after cessation of drug use.

ADVERSE AND COMMON SIDE EFFECTS: The drug is contraindicated in patients with hyperkalemia, anuria, or renal failure. Hyperkalemia and dehydration may occur. Vomiting, anorexia, lethargy, and ataxia also may occur. Safe use of the drug during pregnancy has not been established, and spironolactone inhibits the synthesis of testosterone.

DRUG INTERACTIONS: Spironolactone increases the half-life of digoxin and may increase or decrease the half-life of digitoxin, necessitating monitoring of serum digitalis levels. Spironolactone may decrease the effects of mitotane. The combination of spironolactone and ammonium chloride may produce systemic acidosis. The diuretic action of spironolactone may be antagonized by aspirin and other sa-licylates. The concurrent use of other potassium-sparing diuretics, e.g., triamterene, may predispose to hyperkalemia as may the concurrent use of indomethacin, captopril, and enalapril.

SUPPLIED AS HUMAN PRODUCT:
Tablets containing 25, 50, and 100 mg

STANOZOLOL

INDICATIONS: Stanozolol (Winstrol-V ✽ ★) is an anabolic steroid with strong anabolic and weak androgenic activity. It is potentially useful as an adjunct to the management of catabolic disease states. The drug has been used to stimulate erythropoiesis, arouse appetite, promote weight gain, and increase strength and vitality. The efficacy of promoting these positive changes is questionable, and prolonged treatment (3 to 6 months) may be required before a response in the erythron is seen. The drug may be of benefit in animals with chronic renal failure by stimulating appetite, promoting muscle protein syn-thesis, reversing catabolism, and enhancing general well-being. It has been demonstrated to have positive effects on nitrogen balance and lean body mass in dogs with mild to moderate chronic renal failure. Also see ANABOLIC STEROIDS.

ADVERSE AND COMMON SIDE EFFECTS: The drug should be used with caution in animals with cardiac or renal insufficiency and in those with hypercalcemia. It may promote sodium and water retention and exacerbate azotemia, and it also may promote hypercalcemia, hyperphosphatemia, and hyperkalemia. It should not be used in patients with neoplastic disease. The drug is potentially hepatotoxic even when given at recommended dosages. Changes in grooming, appetite, and activity were apparent within 7 days of initiation of drug use at a dose of 4 mg/day. A more delayed hepatotoxic response (2 to 3 months) may be seen at lower dosage levels (1 mg/day). The earliest indication of hepatotoxicity in cats is an increase in serum ALT. Most cats recover following discontinuation of the drug. Cats with severe cholestatic liver disease may require additional support includ-ing plasma transfusions, vitamin K_1, and nutritional support. Stanozolol should not be used in pregnant animals because of possible masculinization of the fetus.

DRUG INTERACTIONS: Anabolic agents may potentiate the effect of anticoagulants. Anabolic agents may decrease blood glucose and decrease insulin requirements of diabetic patients, and these drugs may potentiate water retention associated with the use of ACTH or adrenal steroids.

SUPPLIED AS VETERINARY PRODUCTS:
Tablets containing 2 mg
For injection containing 50 mg/mL

OTHER USES
Dogs
ANEMIA SECONDARY TO CHRONIC RENAL FAILURE
i)   1 to 4 mg once daily; PO

ii) 2 to 10 mg bid; PO

ANABOLIC/APPETITE STIMULANT
i)   1 to 4 mg bid; PO

ii) 25 to 50 mg weekly; IM

Cats
ANEMIA SECONDARY TO CHRONIC RENAL FAILURE
1 to 4 mg once daily; PO

SUCCIMER

INDICATIONS: Succimer (Chemet ★) is a chelating agent used in the treatment of lead, mercury, and arsenic toxicity.

ADVERSE AND COMMON SIDE EFFECTS: No known adverse effects have been reported in small animals but people may exhibit vomiting, diarrhea, fatigue, and body aching. Increases in liver enzymes and skin rashes have also been reported.

DRUG INTERACTIONS: Concurrent use with other chelating agents, e.g., CaEDTA, dimercaprol, penicillamine, trientine, is advised against.

SUPPLIED AS HUMAN PRODUCT:
Capsules containing 100 mg

SUCRALFATE

INDICATIONS: Sucralfate (Carafate ★, Sulcrate ❦) accelerates the healing of oral, esophageal, gastric, and duodenal ulcers. It forms a complex with proteinaceous exudates that adhere to the ulcer, providing a protective barrier to the penetration of gastric acid. Sucralfate stimulates prostaglandin production, increases mucus production and mucosal turnover, inactivates pepsin, and absorbs bile acids. Sucralfate may be useful for the prevention of NSAID-induced ulceration. It does not protect dogs undergoing spinal surgery having been given corticosteroids from gastrointestinal bleeding. Sucralfate normalizes serum phosphorus levels, which makes it of potential benefit in cases of secondary hyperparathyroidism associated with renal failure.

ADVERSE AND COMMON SIDE EFFECTS: Side effects are rare. Constipation is the only significant problem reported in small animals.

DRUG INTERACTIONS: Antacids and H_2-blocking agents decrease gastric pH and reduce the efficacy of sucralfate and should be spaced apart by at least 1/2 hour. Sucralfate decreases the bioavailability of digoxin, cimetidine, phenytoin, and tetracycline antibiotics. Concurrent oral drug administration should be separated by 2 hours.

SUPPLIED AS HUMAN PRODUCTS:
Tablets containing 1 g
Suspension containing 1 g per 10 mL

SUFENTANIL

INDICATIONS: Sufentanil (Sufenta ♣ ★) is an opioid agonist that is 5 to 7 times more potent than fentanyl. It is reported that 13 to 20 µg of sufentanil produces analgesia equal to 10 mg of morphine.

ADVERSE AND COMMON SIDE EFFECTS: Similar to those of other opiates. See also MORPHINE.

DRUG INTERACTIONS: Sufentanil is metabolized mainly via the cytochrome P-450 enzyme, and although clinical data are lacking, in vitro data suggest that other potent cytochrome P-450 enzyme inhibitors, e.g., ketoconazole and itraconazole, may inhibit the metabolism of sufentanil which could increase the risk of prolonged or delayed respiratory depression. The concomitant use of such drugs requires special patient care and observation; in particular, it may be necessary to lower the dose of sufentanil. An additive effect with sufentanil may be exhibited in patients receiving barbiturates, tranquilizers, opioids, general anesthetics, or other CNS depressants. In such cases of combined treatment, the dose of sufentanil and/or these agents should be reduced. It is recommended that MAO inhibitors, e.g., amitraz and selegiline, be discontinued at least 2 weeks prior to use of sufentanil. A decrease in heart rate and/or blood pressure may be seen when sufentanil is administered to patients receiving β-blocking agents. Sufentanil should be administered with caution to patients with liver or kidney dysfunction, due to the importance of these organs in its metabolism and excretion of the drug.

SUPPLIED AS HUMAN PRODUCT:
For injection containing 50 µg/mL

SULFADIMETHOXINE

INDICATIONS: Sulfadimethoxine (Albon ★, SULFA 125 and 250 ♣) is a sulfonamide drug used in small animals for the treatment of respiratory, genitourinary, enteric, and soft tissue infections caused by susceptible organisms, including streptococci, staphylococci, *Escherichia*, *Salmonella*, *Klebsiella*, *Proteus*, and *Shigella*. It also is used for the eradication of coccidiosis in dogs, although it is not licensed for this purpose.

ADVERSE AND COMMON SIDE EFFECTS: See SULFONAMIDE ANTIBIOTICS.

DRUG INTERACTIONS: Intramuscular injection is associated with pain and poor blood drug levels and is not recommended. See SULFONAMIDE ANTIBIOTICS.

SUPPLIED AS VETERINARY PRODUCTS:
Tablets containing 125, 250, and 500 mg [Albon, SULFA 125 and 250]
Oral suspension containing 50 mg/mL [Albon]
For injection containing 400 mg/mL [Albon]

SULFASALAZINE

INDICATIONS: Sulfasalazine (Azulfidine ★, Salazopyrin ♣) is used in the management of inflammatory bowel disease in the dog and cat. In the colon, bacteria degrade the drug to release aminosalicylic acid and sulfapyridine. The aminosalicylic acid exerts an anti-inflammatory effect by inhibiting prostaglandin synthesis. It also may inhibit the lipoxygenase pathway, and hydroxyeicosatetraenoic and leukotriene synthesis. Sulfasalazine may have immunosuppressive properties, especially on B lymphocytes. Other actions include antibacterial effects, scavenging of reactive oxygen, and inhibition of fibrinolysis.

ADVERSE AND COMMON SIDE EFFECTS: The drug should not be used in animals with sensitivity to salicylates or sulfonamides. It should be used with caution in animals with liver, renal, or hematologic disease. Other newer aminosalicylic drugs without some of the adverse effects of sulfasalazine are available, e.g., olsalazine (10 to 20 mg/kg tid; PO in dogs) and mesalamine (10 mg/kg tid; PO in dogs). Vomiting, cholestasis, exacerbation of colitis, fever, oligospermia, anemia, leukopenia, allergic dermatitis, and keratoconjunctivitis sicca also have been reported. A baseline Schirmer's tear test is advised before initiation of therapy, and monthly monitoring is recommended. Vomiting and anorexia may develop in cats. The use of enteric-coated tablets may alleviate these signs.

DRUG INTERACTIONS: Antibiotics may alter metabolism of sulfasalazine by altering intestinal flora. Sulfasalazine may displace highly protein-bound drugs, such as methotrexate, phenytoin, phenylbuta-zone, salicylates, thiazide diuretics, and warfarin. Phenobarbital may decrease the urinary excretion of sulfasalazine. Sulfasalazine may decrease the bioavailability of folic acid and digoxin.

SUPPLIED AS HUMAN PRODUCTS:
Tablets containing 500 mg
Tablets (enteric-coated) containing 500 mg

SULFONAMIDE ANTIBIOTICS

INDICATIONS: The sulfonamide antibiotics are bacteriostatic drugs that are effective against streptococci, *Bacillus, Corynebacterium, Nocardia, Brucella, Campylobacter, Pasteurella,* and *Chlamydia. Pseudomonas, Serratia,* and *Klebsiella* generally are resistant. The sulfonamides readily enter the CSF and are effective in treating meningeal infections. These drugs are ineffective in the presence of pus and necrotic tissue. The combination of a sulfonamide with trimethoprim or pyrimethamine "potentiated sulfonamides," such as trimethoprim-sulfadiazine (Tribrissen ♣), greatly enhances antimicrobial activity. The enhanced spectrum includes *E. coli, Proteus, Salmonella, Staphylococcus, Klebsiella,* and *Streptococcus.* Another example of a potentiated sulfa is the sulfadimethoxine-ormetoprim combination (Primor ★). This agent is indicated in the treatment of skin and soft tissue infections caused by *Staphylococcus aureus* and *E. coli.*

Sulfonamides are classified according to their duration of effect. Short-acting sulfonamides require dosing at 8-hour intervals and include sulfadiazine, sulfamerazine, sulfamethazine, and sulfamethoxazole, and generally are indicated in the treatment of systemic and urinary tract infections; intermediate-acting sulfonamides require dosing every 12 to 24 hours and include sulfisoxazole and sulfadimethoxine, which primarily are indicated in the treatment of urinary tract infections; and long-acting sulfonamides require dosing every few days and include sulfadoxine, which has been used primarily in humans for the treatment of chronic bronchitis and urinary tract infections.

ADVERSE AND COMMON SIDE EFFECTS: Precipitation and crystalluria generally are not a problem in small animals, but sulfonamides should be used with caution in patients with preexisting renal disease, especially if complicated by dehydration or metabolic acidosis. In dogs given high doses of sulfonamides, sulfonamide cystic urolithiasis can develop. Azotemia and renal failure may develop in cats during sulfonamide or trimethoprim-sulfonamide therapy.

Potentially irreversible KCS has been the most common problem with long-term use of these drugs (sulfadiazine, sulfasalazine). Generally, long-term use (3 to 4 months) of sulfadiazine is necessary before KCS occurs. Pruritus and photosensitization have been reported, and alopecia may occur with long-term use. Other reported conditions associated with the use of these drugs include polyarthritis, urticaria, facial swelling, fever, hemolytic anemia, polydipsia, polyuria, hepatitis, vomiting, diarrhea, anorexia, and seizure. Hypersensitivity, including anaphylaxis, although rare, also has been documented. Dogs with hypersensitivity reactions to potentiated sulfonamides, Samoyeds and miniature Schnauzers especially, may demonstrate thrombocytopenia, fever, hepatopathy, neutropenia, KCS, hemolytic anemia, arthropathy, uveitis, skin and mucocutaneous lesions, proteinuria, facial palsy, pancreatitis, facial edema, hypothyroidism, or pneumonitis. Onset of adverse effects ranged from 5 to 36 days after administration of the drug, and 77% of dogs recovered.

Sulfadimethoxine-ormetoprim should not be given to dogs with liver damage or blood dyscrasias, or those with a history of sulfonamide sensitivity. This drug combination should be used with caution in those with thyroid disease. Safety has not been established in pregnant animals. Long-term therapy at recommended doses resulted in elevation in serum cholesterol, increases in thyroid and liver weights, and enlarged basophilic cells in the pituitary. Potentiated sulfonamides may cause iatrogenic hypothyroidism, as noted by low serum thyroxine levels. Changes in thyroid function may be detected as early as 7 days after initiation of sulfonamide use and may last as long as 8 to 12 weeks after discontinuation of the drug.

DRUG INTERACTIONS: Antacids decrease the absorption of sulfonamides. Methenamine and other acidifying agents increase the risk of sulfonamide crystallization in the urine. *p*-Aminobenzoic acid and local anesthetics may antagonize sulfonamide action. Phenothiazines may increase the toxic effects of sulfonamides.

SUPPLIED AS VETERINARY PRODUCTS:
Tablets containing 100 mg sulfadimethoxine and 20 mg ormetoprim [Primor]
Tablets containing 200 mg sulfadimethoxine and 40 mg ormetoprim [Primor]
Tablets containing 500 mg sulfadimethoxine and 100 mg ormetoprim [Primor]
Tablets containing 1,000 mg sulfadimethoxine and 200 mg ormetoprim [Primor]
For other drugs, see individual product.

OTHER USES
Cats
TOXOPLASMOSIS
15 mg/kg qid; PO (sulfadiazine or sulfamerazine) for at least 2 weeks, along with pyrimethamine at 0.5 to 1 mg/kg daily; PO

SULFUR-CONTAINING SHAMPOOS

INDICATIONS: Sulfur as a topical dermatologic agent is keratolytic, keratoplastic, antibacterial, antifungal, and antiparasitic, and a mild follicular flushing agent. It may be combined with salicylic acid and coal tar (Allerseb T ✤ ★) or with sodium salicylate (Sebolux ✤). The shampoo is indicated for the treatment of mites, lice, chiggers, some fleas, dermatophytosis, seborrhea, pyoderma, pruritus, crusts, and scales. When salicylic acid is combined with sulfur, a synergistic effect occurs, and the keratolytic effect is enhanced.

ADVERSE AND COMMON SIDE EFFECTS: Sulfur may cause scalding if the product is applied to the skin at concentrations greater than 2%. Coal tar may be especially irritating or even toxic to cats.

DRUG INTERACTIONS: None reported.

TACROLIMUS

INDICATIONS: Tacrolimus (Prograf ✤ ★) is a macrolide compound with potent immunosuppressant properties. In dogs it has been used in the management of perianal fistulas and may be useful in the management of other immune-mediated diseases. Dogs with perianal fistulas were treated with topical tacrolimus ointment once to twice daily for 16 weeks. Full healing of the fistulas occurred in 50% and was noticeably improved in 90% of dogs.

ADVERSE AND COMMON SIDE EFFECTS: In people side effects may include tremor, headache, hypertension, nausea, diarrhea, constipation, insomnia, and abdominal pain.

DRUG INTERACTIONS: Drug interaction trials have not been conducted. Due to the potential for impairment of renal function, care should be taken when administering the drug with other drugs known to affect renal function. Tacrolimus is metabolized by cytochrome P-450 enzyme systems. Drugs known to inhibit this system, e.g., diltiazem, itraconazole, ketoconazole, erythromycin, cimetidine, metoclopramide, may increase serum levels. Drugs known to induce this enzyme system, e.g., phenobarbital and phenytoin, may decrease blood levels of tacrolimus.

SUPPLIED AS HUMAN PRODUCT:
The ointment must be prepared by a pharmacist and formulated into a 0.1% w/w preparation with petrolatum (the contents of a 1 mg capsule mixed with 100 g hydrophilic petrolatum). The ointment is applied to the skin twice daily.

TAR-CONTAINING SHAMPOOS

INDICATIONS: Crude coal tars are used in the management of seborrhea, especially the greasy form of the disease. Tars are keratolytic, keratoplastic, antipruritic, and vasoconstrictive. Tar is available in combination with salicylic acid (Allerseb T ✤ ★).

ADVERSE AND COMMON SIDE EFFECTS: Tar shampoos may be drying and irritating to the skin. Photosensitization and superficial necrolytic dermatitis have been reported. Tar is not approved for use in cats because it tends to be very irritating in this species.

DRUG INTERACTIONS: None reported.

TAURINE

INDICATIONS: Taurine plays a role in antioxidation, retinal photoreceptor activity, stabilization of neural membranes, development of the nervous system, reduction in platelet aggregation, reproduction, the regulation of calcium fluxes across membranes, and the conjugation of bile acids. It is used in conjunction with appropriate supportive therapy in the management of feline-dilated cardiomyopathy. Taurine may contribute to the inotropic, metabolic, and osmotic function of the myocardium. It has been concluded that American cocker spaniels with dilated cardiomyopathy are taurine deficient and are responsive to taurine and carnitine supplementation. Although myocardial function did not return to normal, it improved sufficiently enough to allow discontinuation of cardiovascular drug therapy. Taurine deficiency also has been associated with feline central retinal degeneration and reproductive problems characterized by poor growth, survival, and abnormalities of kittens born to taurine-deficient queens. Deficiency has also been linked to dogs with urate and cystine urolithiasis. One investigator has used taurine in conjunction with vitamin B_6 in cats with recurrent seizures. In cases of hepatic lipidosis, supplemental taurine (250 to 500 mg/day; PO) and L-carnitine (250 mg/day; PO) may be given for the first several weeks, with strict attention to caloric intake.

ADVERSE AND COMMON SIDE EFFECTS: No long-term side effects have been reported.

DRUG INTERACTIONS: None reported.

SUPPLIED AS VETERINARY PRODUCT:
Tablets containing 250 mg [Taurine Tablets ♣, Formula V Taurine Tablets ★]

OTHER USES
Cats
SEIZURES
500 mg bid; PO together with vitamin B_6

Dogs
AMERICAN COCKER SPANIEL DILATED CARDIOMYOPATHY
500 mg taurine bid to tid; PO with 1 g carnitine bid to tid; PO

TEPOXALIN

INDICATIONS: Tepoxalin (Zubrin ★) is a nonsteroidal anti-inflammatory agent that inhibits COX-1 and COX-2 as well as 5-lipoxygenase pathways. The drug has anti-inflammatory, analgesic, and antipyretic properties and is indicated for the control of pain and inflammation associated with osteoarthritis in the dog. The tablet rapidly disintegrates in the mouth within seconds after placement on the tongue allowing it to be swallowed with ease.

ADVERSE AND COMMON SIDE EFFECTS: The drug is considered quite safe. The selective nature of the tissue distribution and the inhibition of the lipoxygenase pathway provide for better gastrointestinal safety, but as for other NSAID drugs, vomiting, diarrhea, anorexia, lethargy, and gastrointestinal ulceration may occur. If these clinical signs do appear, the drug should be immediately discontinued. Zubrin should be given with food or within 2 hours after eating. There are no reports of renal or hepatotoxic effects.

DRUG INTERACTIONS: To minimize the possibility of adverse GI effects Zubrin should not be administered concurrently with other NSAIDs or glucocorticoid agents. The safety of the drug has not been established in pregnant, lactating, or breeding dogs or in dogs younger than 6 months.

SUPPLIED AS VETERINARY PRODUCT
Tablets containing 30, 50, 100, and 200 mg

TERBUTALINE

INDICATIONS: Terbutaline (Bricanyl ♣ ★) is a synthetic adrenergic stimulant with selective β_2- and negligible β_1-agonist activity. It is useful as a bronchodilator. In cats a heart rate that approaches 240 beats/minute suggests the drug has been absorbed. A respiratory rate or effort that drops by 50% or more implies a beneficial effect. The drug also has been used in the management of some cases of first- and second-degree heart block.

ADVERSE AND COMMON SIDE EFFECTS: The drug should not be given to patients with tachycardia associated with digitalis intoxication or glaucoma, nor should it be used within 14 days of the use of an MAO inhibitor, e.g., possibly amitraz and selegiline. The drug should be used with caution in patients with hypertension, diabetes mellitus, thyrotoxicosis, a history of seizure disorders, cardiac arrhythmias, and renal or hepatic dysfunction. Side effects may include tachycardia, hypotension or hypertension, nausea, vomiting, tremor, fatigue, or seizure activity. Treatment of terbutaline toxicosis may include volume expansion to mitigate hypotension and β-blocking agents, e.g., propranolol (dogs: 5 to 40 mg tid; PO or 0.1 to 0.3 mg/kg; IV).

DRUG INTERACTIONS: Propranolol antagonizes the bronchodilatory effect of terbutaline. Concurrent use of MAO inhibitors may cause severe hypertension. Use with other sympathetic agents may potentiate the risk of arrhythmias.

SUPPLIED AS HUMAN PRODUCTS:
Tablets containing 2.5 and 5 mg
Aerosol containing 200 µg/metered spray ★ and 500 µg/metered spray ♣

OTHER USES
Dogs
FIRST- AND SECOND-DEGREE HEART BLOCK
2.5 to 5 mg bid to tid; PO

TESTOSTERONE

INDICATIONS: Testosterone is an androgenic steroid used principally in small animals for the management of hormone-responsive urinary incontinence in the neutered male. Veto-Test is marketed in Canada for use in animals with impotence, testicular deficiency, cryptorchidism (in the absence of anatomic defects), and as an aid in the treatment of mammary tumors in bitches. Also see ANABOLIC STEROIDS.

ADVERSE AND COMMON SIDE EFFECTS: The drug is contraindicated in patients with prostatic carcinoma. It should be used with caution in those with renal, hepatic, or cardiac disease. Prostatic enlargement and recurrence or exacerbation of perianal adenoma or perianal hernia, as well as behavioral problems, are occasionally reported. Chronic use or high doses may result in oligospermia or infertility in intact males.

DRUG INTERACTIONS: Testosterone may decrease blood glucose concentrations and decrease the requirement for insulin in diabetic patients. The drug may enhance bleeding tendencies in patients taking oral anticoagulants. Androgens may potentiate edema associated with ACTH or adrenal steroid therapy, the significance of which in small animals is unknown.

SUPPLIED AS VETERINARY PRODUCT:
For injection containing 100 mg/mL testosterone [Veto-Test ♣]

SUPPLIED AS HUMAN PRODUCTS:

For injection containing 100 and 200 mg/mL testosterone cypionate in oil [Depo-Testosterone ✸ ★]

For injection containing 100 and 200 mg/mL testosterone enanthate in oil

For injection containing 25, 50, and 100 mg/mL testosterone propionate in oil

TETRACYCLINE ANTIBIOTICS

INDICATIONS: The tetracycline antibiotics exert a bacteriostatic effect against many aerobic and anaerobic gram-positive and gram-negative bacteria, spirochetes, mycoplasma, and rickettsiae organisms. These drugs are classified as short-acting/water soluble (tetracycline, oxytetracycline, chlortetracycline), intermediate-acting (demeclocycline), and long-acting/lipid soluble (minocycline, doxycycline). Tetracycline antibiotics are especially useful against *Leptospira, Chlamydia, Brucella, Mycoplasma, Pseudomonas, Rickettsia,* and *Actinomyces* organisms. They also are used in the treatment of protozoan infections. Minocycline is the most effective of this group against *Nocardia* and *Staphylococcus.* Tetracycline and doxycycline are effective in the treatment of feline ehrlichiosis. Doxycycline is also used in the treatment of actinomycosis, ehrlichiosis, chlamydia, leptospirosis, borreliosis, Rocky Mountain spotted fever, toxoplasmosis, and *Hemobartonella* infections. Minocycline and doxycycline are second-generation lipid-soluble tetracyclines and are more effective against anaerobes and intracellular bacteria such as *Brucella canis.* These two agents readily diffuse into the eye, brain, CSF, and prostate gland. However, they do not reach sufficient concentrations in the urine to be effective in the treatment of urinary tract infections.

ADVERSE AND COMMON SIDE EFFECTS: Tetracyclines, with the exception of doxycycline, should be avoided in patients with renal failure because of delayed excretion. Tetracyclines, especially chlortetracycline, inhibit protein synthesis. Nausea, vomiting, diarrhea, dose-related renal tubular damage, and metabolic acidosis have been reported. Discoloration of the teeth may occur if these drugs (especially dimethyl chlortetracycline and tetracycline) are given to pregnant bitches in the last 2 to 3 weeks of pregnancy or to puppies in the first 4 weeks after birth. Anaphylaxis associated with the use of parenteral tetracyclines occasionally has been noted in dogs and cats. Hypotension, shock, and urticaria developed in dogs given rapid IV doses of minocycline. Thrombophlebitis frequently occurs after IV injection of tetracycline and is seen more frequently with lipid-soluble tetracyclines. Intramuscular injection is painful and irritating. Intravascular injection of minocycline (10 to 20 mg/kg daily for 1 month) in dogs has been associated with decreased erythrocyte counts, hemoglobin concentration, and hematocrit and elevations in serum ALT activity. Cats are especially sensitive to these drugs. Fever, vomiting, diarrhea, colic, depression, ptyalism, anorexia, and increased serum ALT activity are reported in this species.

DRUG INTERACTIONS: Absorption is decreased by the concurrent use of antacids, antidiarrheal compounds, laxatives, iron, aluminum, or calcium-containing products, including kaolin and pectin or bismuth, and dairy products. Sodium bicarbonate may interfere with absorption of oral tetracyclines by increasing gastric pH. Doxycycline and minocycline are less affected by food or oral products and often are given with food to reduce GI irritation. Tetracyclines potentiate the catabolic effects of glucocorticoids and may contribute to cachexia. In addition, concurrent use of corticosteroids may allow the emergence of resistant organisms during prolonged therapy and may mask clinical signs of infection. Bacteriostatic drugs such as tetracyclines may decrease the bactericidal activity of penicillin, cephalosporin, and aminoglycoside antibiotics. Tetracyclines may increase the bioavailability of digoxin, predisposing to toxicity in a small number of patients; the effects of which can persist for months after discontinuation of the tetracycline. Tetracyclines may potentiate the anticoagulant activity of warfarin, decreasing the dose of the anticoagulant required. Gastrointestinal side effects may be potentiated by theophylline. Tetracyclines may reduce insulin requirements in diabetic patients. Methoxyflurane may contribute to the possibility of nephrotoxicity. Tetracyclines inhibit hepatic microsomal enzymes and may delay the elimination of drugs metabolized by the liver.

SUPPLIED AS: See specific product.

OTHER USES
Dogs
GASTROINTESTINAL BACTERIAL OVERGROWTH
Tetracycline at 10 to 20 mg/kg bid; PO for 1 month
LYME BORRELIOSIS
Tetracycline at 5 mg/kg tid; PO for 10 to 14 days

THEOPHYLLINE

INDICATIONS: Theophylline (Theo-Dur ❧ ★, Theolair ★, Quibron-T/SR ❧ ★, Slo-Bid ❧ ★) is a bronchodilator indicated for the management of cough due to bronchospasm. It has mild inotropic properties and a mild, transient diuretic activity. Serum levels are measured after steady-state serum levels have been attained (29 hours in the dog, 40 hours in the cat) and just before the next dose. The therapeutic range is 10 to 20 µg/mL (55 to 110 µmol/L). Toxic blood levels are in excess of 25 µg/mL.

ADVERSE AND COMMON SIDE EFFECTS: The drug should be used with caution in patients with cardiac disease, systemic hypertension, cardiac arrhythmias, GI ulcers, impaired renal or hepatic function, diabetes mellitus, hyperthyroid disease, and glaucoma. Side effects may include nausea, vomiting, anorexia or polyphagia, diarrhea, polydipsia, polyuria, restlessness, muscle twitching, cardiac arrhythmias, tachycardia, hyperglycemia, and nervousness. Seizure activity may occur with marked drug overdose.

DRUG INTERACTIONS: Serum levels may be increased by the concurrent use of thiabendazole, cimetidine, allopurinol, clindamycin, lincomycin, and erythromycin. Phenobarbital and phenytoin decrease the therapeutic effect of the drug. Concurrent use of aluminum or magnesium antacid preparations slows the absorption of theophylline. Propranolol has direct antagonistic effects because propranolol is a β-adrenergic blocking agent and theophylline is a β-adrenergic stimulant. Phenytoin increases theophylline clearance, requiring larger doses of the drug for a clinically beneficial effect. Halothane may increase the incidence of cardiac arrhythmias. Ketamine may cause an increase incidence of seizure activity.

Concurrent use of this drug with allopurinol, cimetidine, furosemide, or epinephrine may cause excessive CNS stimulation.

SUPPLIED AS HUMAN PRODUCTS:
Tablets [Theo-Dur] and capsules [Slo-Bid] (timed-release) containing 50, 100, 200, 300, and 450 mg and additional strengths
Oral liquid containing 80 mg/15 mL [Theolair]
For injection in 5% dextrose containing 0.8, 1.6, and 4 mg/mL

OTHER USES
Cats
SINUS BRADYCARDIA
25 mg/kg once daily in the evening; PO (sustained-release formulation)

THIABENDAZOLE

INDICATIONS: Thiabendazole (Equizole ★, Mintezol ★, Thibenzole ★) is used in the treatment of nasal aspergillosis (approximately 50% success rate), and penicilliosis and for the elimination of *Toxocara canis, Toxascaris leonina, Strongyloides stercoralis,* and *Filaroides* infections in dogs. The drug also has been used in the treatment of *Oslerus osleri* infestation in a dog.

ADVERSE AND COMMON SIDE EFFECTS: Initially, anorexia, vomiting, and diarrhea may be noted. If these occur, it is best to discontinue medication for several days and reinstitute the drug at half the dose for 1 week, then gradually increase the dose to the recommended level. The drug should be given with food to enhance absorption and to decrease anorexia. Hair loss also has been reported. Dachshunds may be especially sensitive to the drug.

DRUG INTERACTIONS: Thiabendazole may compete with theophylline and aminophylline for metabolism in the liver, resulting in increased serum levels of the latter two drugs.

SUPPLIED AS HUMAN PRODUCT:
Oral suspension containing 500 mg per 5 mL [Mintezol]

OTHER USES
Dogs
STRONGYLOIDES STERCORALIS
50 to 60 mg/kg; PO

FILAROIDES INFECTIONS
i)   30 to 70 mg/kg divided bid; PO in food for 20 to 45 days

ii) 70 mg/kg bid; PO for 2 days then 35 mg/kg bid; PO for 20 days

ASPERGILLOSIS/PENICILLIOSIS
i)   30 to 70 mg/kg divided bid; PO for 20 to 45 days

ii) 20 mg/kg once daily or divided bid; PO for 6 to 8 weeks

OSLERUS OSLERI
35 mg/kg bid; PO for 5 days, followed by 70 mg/kg bid; PO for 21 days

THIAMINE (B_1)

INDICATIONS: Thiamine (vitamin B_1 ✤ ★) is used in the treatment of thiamine deficiency and occasionally as adjunctive therapy in cases of ethylene glycol toxicity and lead poisoning.

ADVERSE AND COMMON SIDE EFFECTS: The vitamin itself is nontoxic, but IM injection may cause muscle soreness. Deficiency of the vitamin is rare. Cats fed commercial diets or raw fish are predisposed. Clinical signs of vitamin B_1 deficiency may include anorexia, vomiting, weight loss, dehydration, paralysis, gallop heart rhythms in the presence of congestive heart failure, muscle weakness, prostration, abnormal reflexes, convulsions, ventral flexion of the neck, and dilated pupils. Laboratory abnormalities may include mild anemia, hypoproteinemia, hyperglycemia, and increased blood and urine concentrations of pyruvate and lactate.

DRUG INTERACTIONS: Thiamine may potentiate the neuromuscular blocking effect of neuromuscular blocking agents.

SUPPLIED AS VETERINARY PRODUCT:
For injection containing 100, 200, and 500 mg/mL

SUPPLIED AS HUMAN PRODUCTS:
Tablets containing 5, 10, 25, 50, 100, 250, and 500 mg
For injection containing 100 mg/mL

OTHER USES
Dogs

ETHYLENE GLYCOL TOXICITY
100 mg/day; PO

THIOGUANINE

INDICATIONS: Thioguanine (Lanvis ✤, Thioguanine ★) is a purine analog chemotherapeutic agent often used in combination with other such agents in the treatment of lymphocytic or granulocytic leukemias in dogs and cats.

ADVERSE AND COMMON SIDE EFFECTS: Nausea, anorexia, vomiting, and diarrhea may occur. Bone marrow suppression, hepatotoxicity, pancreatitis, gastrointestinal ulceration, and skin lesions are also possible.

DRUG INTERACTIONS: In people, it has been shown that there is usually complete cross-resistance between mercaptopurine and thioguanine. In one study, 12 of approximately 330 patients receiving continuous busulfan and thioguanine were found to have esophageal varices associated with abnormal liver function tests. Liver biopsies showed nodular regenerative hyperplasia. The significance of these observations to small animals is unknown but the concurrent use of thioguanine with other agents known to be potentially hepatotoxic should be carried out cautiously, e.g., halothane, ketoconazole, phenobarbital, primidone. Caution should also be exercised if this agent is used concurrently with drugs known to be potentially myelosuppressive (chloramphenicol, flucytosine, amphotericin B) or immunosuppressive.

SUPPLIED AS HUMAN PRODUCT:
Tablets containing 40 mg

THIOPENTAL SODIUM

INDICATIONS: Thiopental sodium (Veterinary Pentothal kit ★, Pentothal ✤ ★) is an ultrashort-acting thiobarbiturate used for procedures requiring general anesthesia of short duration. Its characteristics include short action, smooth recovery, rapid elimination, and minimal side effects. Also see BARBITURATES.

For additional information concerning ADVERSE AND COMMON SIDE EFFECTS and DRUG INTERACTIONS, see BARBITURATES.

SUPPLIED AS VETERINARY PRODUCT:
For injection containing 5 g in 200 mL (reconstituted concentration 2.5% solution) and in 100 mL (reconstituted concentration 5% solution)

SUPPLIED AS HUMAN PRODUCT:
For injection containing 250, 400, and 500 mg and 1, 2.5, 5, and 10 g thiopental base [Pentothal ✤ ★]

TICARCILLIN

INDICATIONS: Ticarcillin (Ticar ★) is an extended spectrum parenteral penicillin antibiotic with activity similar to, but more potent than, carbenicillin. In humans, the drug is active against gram-negative bacteria, including *Klebsiella pneumoniae, Proteus mirabilis* and *vulgaris, E. coli, Enterobacter aerogenes, Serratia marcescens, Pseudomonas aeruginosa,* and *Bacteroides fragilis,* and gram-positive organisms, including *Staphylococcus aureus,* coagulase-positive staphylococci, enterococci, and streptococcal organisms. Bacterial susceptibility is similar in veterinary medicine. The antibiotic is available in combination with clavulanic acid (Timentin ✤ ★) that is effective against many penicillinase-producing strains of bacteria.

ADVERSE AND COMMON SIDE EFFECTS: Use is contraindicated in animals with hypersensitivity to penicillins or the cephalosporins. Intramuscular injection may cause pain. Also see PENICILLIN ANTIBIOTICS.

DRUG INTERACTIONS: Ticarcillin is physically and/or chemically incompatible with aminoglycosides and can inactivate the drug in vitro. Also see PENICILLIN ANTIBIOTICS.

SUPPLIED AS HUMAN PRODUCTS:
For injection containing 1-, 3-, 20-, and 30-g vials
For injection containing 3 g with 100 mg clavulanic acid [Timentin ✤ ★]

TILETAMINE ZOLAZEPAM

INDICATIONS: Tiletamine zolazepam (Telazol ★) is a mixture of a dissociative drug tiletamine and the benzodiazepine zolazepam that may be used for sedation and restraint and anesthetic induction or anesthesia of short duration (30 minutes) requiring mild to moderate analgesia. Tiletamine produces immobilization, but muscle rigidity and occasional seizure-like activity may occur. Zolazepam reduces the incidence of these side effects. Recumbency is generally observed within 5 to 10 minutes following intramuscular injection of 3 to 15 mg/kg. Prolonged sedation and/or residual ataxia may last 2 to 4 hours after dosages of greater than 5 to 7.5 mg/kg are used. The drug combination has no analgesic properties at sedative dosages.

ADVERSE AND COMMON SIDE EFFECTS: Excitation may occur during induction and recovery. Xylazine or acepromazine is recommended to prevent possible self-trauma and hyperthermia. Concurrent use of anticholinergics is recommended because salivation induced by the drug combination may interfere with visualization of the larynx. The drug is contraindicated in animals with pancreatic disease and those with significant cardiac, pulmonary, hepatic, or renal disease. Rapid IM injection is painful. Respiratory depression may occur at higher doses. Other side effects may include salivation, increased bronchial and tracheal secretions (if atropine is not given before its use), increased heart rate and blood pressure, increased cardiac output and myocardial oxygen consumption, and hypertension or hypotension. Vomiting may occur on recovery, and vocalization, hypertonia, muscular twitching, muscle rigidity, erratic and/or prolonged recovery, cyanosis, cardiac arrest, and pulmonary edema also have been reported. The drug should not be used in pregnant animals.

DRUG INTERACTIONS: In cats, anesthesia is prolonged by chloramphenicol by approximately 30 minutes. This does not occur in dogs. Phenothiazines may enhance the cardiac and respiratory depression of the drug. The dose of barbiturate or volatile anesthetic used may need to be reduced. Chemical restraint with this agent will not adversely affect the performance of intradermal skin testing in atopic dogs.

SUPPLIED AS VETERINARY PRODUCT:
For injection containing 250 mg each of tiletamine and zolazepam, each producing a concentration of 50 mg/mL when reconstituted

TOBRAMYCIN

INDICATIONS: Tobramycin (Nebcin ✤ ★) is an aminoglycoside antibiotic. It is closely related to gentamicin in spectrum, activity, and pharmacological properties, but it is more active against some strains of *Pseudomonas* that are resistant to gentamicin, and it is less nephrotoxic. Also see AMINOGLYCOSIDE ANTIBIOTICS.

ADVERSE AND COMMON SIDE EFFECTS: See AMINOGLYCOSIDE ANTIBIOTICS.

DRUG INTERACTIONS: Tobramycin should not be mixed with other drugs. Also see AMINOGLYCOSIDE ANTIBIOTICS.

SUPPLIED AS HUMAN PRODUCT:
For injection containing 10 and 40 mg/mL and in disposable syringes containing 60 mg/1.5 mL and 80 mg/2 mL

TOCAINIDE

INDICATIONS: Tocainide (Tonocard ✤ ★) is an antiarrhythmic agent and analog of lidocaine with similar electrophysiologic and hemodynamic properties. The drug is effective orally. It is used to suppress ventricular premature contractions. Therapeutic plasma levels are quoted as 4 to 10 µg/mL. A positive response to lidocaine appears to be a good predictor of response to tocainide.

ADVERSE AND COMMON SIDE EFFECTS: Adverse effects are common (40%) with use of this drug. Arrhythmias are reported. Tocainide should not be used in patients with second- or third-degree heart block, hypokalemia, myasthenia gravis, and pregnancy. Cautious use is recommended in those with renal or hepatic disease. The drug dose should be reduced or the interval between doses increased in animals with renal disease. Reported adverse effects in dogs include anorexia, vomiting, head trembling, weakness, ataxia, nervousness, and anxiety. Long-term use (greater than 6 months) of the drug appears to predispose to corneal endothelial dystrophy and possibly renal dysfunction. Giving the drug with food decreases side effects.

DRUG INTERACTIONS: Tocainide may be combined with other antiarrhythmic agents, e.g., propranolol, quinidine, or disopyramide, to increase effectiveness. Allopurinol increases the serum concentration of tocainide. Metoprolol has additive effects on wedge pressure and cardiac index. In people, the concurrent use of propranolol may lead to paranoia.

SUPPLIED AS HUMAN PRODUCT:
Tablets containing 400 and 600 mg

TRIAMCINOLONE

INDICATIONS: Triamcinolone (Vetalog ★) is a glucocorticoid. The drug is indicated for the treatment of arthritic disorders and for the treatment of allergic and dermatologic conditions responsive to corticosteroids. Also see GLUCOCORTICOID AGENTS.

ADVERSE AND COMMON SIDE EFFECTS: Subconjunctival injection may be associated with granuloma formation requiring surgical excision. Also see GLUCOCORTICOID AGENTS.

DRUG INTERACTIONS: See GLUCOCORTICOID AGENTS.

SUPPLIED AS VETERINARY PRODUCTS:
Tablets containing 0.5 and 1.5 mg ★
For injection containing 2 and 6 mg/mL

SUPPLIED AS HUMAN PRODUCTS:
Tablets containing 4 mg [Aristocort ♣ ★]
Syrup containing 2 mg/5 mL [Aristocort ♣ ★]

OTHER USES
Dogs and Cats
INFLAMMATORY AND ALLERGIC CONDITIONS
0.11 to 0.22 mg/kg once; IM, SC (remission generally lasts 7 to 15 days; if signs recur, the dose may be repeated or oral corticosteroid treatment begun)

Cats
PLASMACYTIC PHARYNGITIS
2 to 4 mg once daily to once every 48 hours; PO
POLYMYOPATHY
0.5 to 1 mg/kg once daily; PO

TRIAMTERENE

INDICATIONS: Triamterene (Dyrenium ★), like spironolactone, has weak diuretic action and a potassium-sparing effect. Unlike spironolactone, triamterene blocks potassium secretion by a direct action on distal renal tubules rather than by inhibiting aldosterone. It may be used in conjunction with other diuretics to promote diuresis in patients refractory to other diuretics.

ADVERSE AND COMMON SIDE EFFECTS: The drug is contraindicated in severe or progressive renal disease, anuria, severe hepatic dysfunction, or elevated serum potassium concentrations. Cautious use is advised in diabetes mellitus or impaired renal or hepatic function. In humans, adverse effects may include diarrhea, nausea, vomiting, dry mouth, pruritus, weakness, hypotension, muscle cramps, hyperkalemia, elevated serum urea and uric acid, hyperchloremic acidosis, granulocytopenia, eosinophilia, and megaloblastic anemia. There is limited information concerning use of the drug in small animals.

DRUG INTERACTIONS: Digitalis effects may be decreased by triamterene. Antihypertensive agents may have an additive hypotensive effect. Lithium clearance is decreased, predisposing to toxicity. Nonsteroidal anti-inflammatory agents can cause a marked decrease in creatinine clearance.

SUPPLIED AS HUMAN PRODUCT:
Capsules containing 50 and 100 mg ★

TRIIODOTHYRONINE

See LIOTHYROXINE (Cytobin, Cytomel).

TRILOSTANE

INDICATIONS: Trilostane (Modrenal [Great Briain] not commercially available in the United States or Canada at present) is a competitive inhibitor of 3β-hydroxysteroid dehydrogenase, an enzyme that mediates the conversion of pregnenolone to progesterone in the adrenal glands, from which cortisol, aldosterone, and androstenedione are produced. Trilostane inhibits the production of progesterone and its end products. It has been successfully used for the treatment of pituitary-dependent hyperadrenocorticism in dogs. The time required for response to therapy is similar to that of mitotane. Response to therapy can be monitored with the ACTH stimulation test. Target serum cortisol levels after ACTH stimulation are between 1.0 and 2.5 µg/dL.

ADVERSE AND COMMON SIDE EFFECTS: Adverse effects appear rare but may include lethargy and vomiting. Some dogs may have a transient exacerbation of skin lesions before clinical improvement is apparent. Hypoadrenocorticism may also be observed with use of the drug. In people flushing, tingling and swelling of mouth, rhinorrhea, nausea, vomiting, diarrhea, and rashes are reported and rarely, granulocytopenia.

DRUG INTERACTIONS: The concurrent use of potassium-sparing diuretics predisposes to hyperkalemia.

SUPPLIED AS HUMAN PRODUCT:
Capsules containing 60 mg

TRIMEPRAZINE

INDICATIONS: Trimeprazine (Temaril-P ★, Vanectyl-P ❄) is a phenothiazine antihistamine/corticosteroid used for the relief of pruritus caused by allergy. It is also recommended by the manufacturer as an antitussive agent in dogs.

ADVERSE AND COMMON SIDE EFFECTS: Side effects for trimeprazine include sedation, depression, hypotension, rigidity, tremors, weakness, and restlessness. If the combined veterinary product is used, additional side effects may include polyuria, polydipsia, vomiting, diarrhea, weight loss, elevation in liver enzymes, and iatrogenic Cushing's syndrome. Other side effects may include sodium retention, potassium loss, delayed wound healing, osteoporosis, increased susceptibility to infection, and blood dyscrasias.

DRUG INTERACTIONS: Intensification and prolongation of the action of sedatives, analgesics, and anesthetics may be noted, as well as possible potentiation of organophosphate toxicity and procaine hydrochloride activity. Augmented CNS depression may occur with concomitant use of narcotics, barbiturates, and anesthetics. Quinidine may cause additive cardiac depression. Antacids and antidiarrheal compounds may decrease GI absorption. Concurrent use of propranolol may cause increased serum elevation of both drugs. Phenytoin metabolism may be decreased. Phenothiazines are α-adrenergic blocking agents, and if epinephrine is given, unopposed, β-adrenergic activity leading to vasodilation and an increased heart rate may result. Products containing prednisolone, e.g., Temaril-P, may cause hypokalemia if used concurrently with amphotericin B, furosemide, or the thiazide diuretics. In addition, insulin requirements may increase and serum salicylate levels may decrease. Phenytoin and phenobarbital may increase the metabolism of prednisolone.

SUPPLIED AS VETERINARY PRODUCT:
Tablets containing 5 mg trimeprazine and 2 mg prednisolone [Temaril-P and Vanectyl-P]

TRIMETHOPRIM-SULFADIAZINE

INDICATIONS: Trimethoprim-sulfadiazine (or sulphadiazine) (Tribrissen ❀ ★) is a bactericidal antibiotic combination recommended for the treatment of alimentary, respiratory, and urinary tract infections and skin and soft tissue infections caused by susceptible organisms, including *E. coli, Enterobacter, Klebsiella, Streptococcus, Staphylococcus, Pasteurella, Clostridia, Salmonella, Shigella, Brucella* spp., *Actinomyces, Corynebacterium* spp., *Bordetella* spp., *Neisseria* spp., *Vibrio* spp., and *Proteus* organisms. It is especially useful for long-term, low-dose treatment of chronic bacterial urinary tract infections. This drug combination also may be used for the eradication of coccidiosis in dogs and cats.

ADVERSE AND COMMON SIDE EFFECTS: The drug should not be used in animals with marked liver disease or blood dyscrasias or in those with sulfonamide sensitivity. A rare idiosyncratic drug reaction leading to fatal hepatic necrosis has been reported. Prolonged use can result in clinical signs of hypothyroid disease indistinguishable by thyroid gland function testing from endogenous hypothyroid disease. Recovery of thyroid gland function may require several months.

Anemia, leukopenia, thrombocytopenia, hyperkalemia, anorexia, and ataxia have been noted at higher doses. Dietary supplementation with folinic acid (leucovorin calcium at 0.5 to 1 mg/day) may protect the patient against the anemia and leukopenia that accompany the interference of folic acid metabolism. This drug combination has been associated with fever and polyarthritis (Doberman pinschers may be predisposed), cutaneous eruptions, hepatitis, cholestasis, vomiting, anorexia, diarrhea, urticaria, facial swelling, polydipsia, polyuria, keratoconjunctivitis sicca, glomerulonephropathy, and polymyositis. Signs of polyarthritis and fever typically occur 8 to 20 days after the initiation of therapy. Complete recovery of clinical signs is apparent within 1 week after withdrawal of the drug. Skin changes resolve within 3 weeks.

The drug should not be used for more than 14 days in the cat. Excessive salivation may occur in cats given uncoated tablets. In addition, Tribrissen may cause anemia, leukopenia, and anorexia and interfere with thyroid function in cats.

DRUG INTERACTIONS: Antacids may decrease the bioavailability of trimethoprim-sulfadiazine if administered concurrently. Trimethoprim-sulfadiazine may prolong clotting times in patients receiving warfarin and decrease the effect of cyclosporine while increasing the risk of nephrotoxicity of the drug. Sulfonamides may increase the effects of methotrexate, phenylbutazone, phenytoin, salicylates, thiazide diuretics, and probenecid.

SUPPLIED AS VETERINARY PRODUCTS:
For injection containing 40 mg/mL trimethoprim and 200 mg/mL sulfadiazine [Tribrissen 24% ♣ ★]
Tablets containing 5 mg trimethoprim and 25 mg sulfadiazine ♣ ★
Tablets containing 20 mg trimethoprim and 100 mg sulfadiazine ♣ ★
Tablets containing 80 mg trimethoprim and 400 mg sulfadiazine ♣ ★
Tablets containing 160 mg trimethoprim and 800 mg sulfadiazine ★
Oral suspension containing 10 mg trimethoprim and 50 mg sulfadiazine ★

OTHER USES
Dogs
ANTIBIOTIC-RESPONSIVE DIARRHEA (FORMERLY SMALL INTESTINAL BACTERIAL OVERGROWTH)
15 mg/kg bid; PO for 1 month

Dogs and Cats
COCCIDIOSIS/TOXOPLASMOSIS
15 to 30 mg/kg bid; PO, SC [Tribrissen]

TYLOSIN

INDICATIONS: Tylosin (Tylan ♣ ★, Tylocine ♣, Tylosin ♣ ★) is a macrolide antibiotic. It has activity against gram-negative and gram-positive bacteria, spirochetes, chlamydiae, and mycoplasma organisms. The drug is effective in the treatment of bronchitis, tracheobronchitis, laryngitis, tonsillitis, pneumonia, rhinitis, sinusitis, cellulitis, otitis externa, cystitis, metritis, endometritis, and pyogenic dermatitis caused by susceptible organisms. It also has been used to manage canine and feline inflammatory bowel disease, the mechanism of action for which is unknown.

ADVERSE AND COMMON SIDE EFFECTS: Clinical side effects are rare, but anorexia, diarrhea, and local pain with IM injection are reported.

DRUG INTERACTIONS: Tylosin may increase serum digitalis levels.

SUPPLIED AS VETERINARY PRODUCT:
For injection containing 50 and 200 mg/mL ♣ ★ (for swine and cattle)

OTHER USES
Dogs
CHRONIC COLITIS
40 to 80 mg/kg per day in 2 to 3 divided doses; mixed with food or as a bolus with water for 2 weeks, then taper. Some require long-term therapy. May be alternated with sulfasalazine for long-term maintenance.

Note: Tylan Plus Vitamins is no longer marketed. Tylan Soluble Powder contains 3,000 mg/teaspoon (may require dilution for accurate dosing).

CHRONIC INFLAMMATORY BOWEL DISEASE
20 to 40 mg/kg bid; PO

SUSCEPTIBLE INFECTIONS
6.6 to 11 mg/kg once to twice daily; IM

Cats
CHRONIC COLITIS
10 to 20 mg/kg per day in 2 divided doses mixed with food or as a bolus with water. May be alternated with sulfasalazine for long-term maintenance.

CHRONIC INFLAMMATORY BOWEL DISEASE
10 to 20 mg/kg bid; PO

SUSCEPTIBLE INFECTIONS
i)   6.6 to 11 mg/kg once to twice daily; IM
ii) 10 mg/kg bid; IM

URSODIOL

INDICATIONS: Ursodiol, or ursodeoxycholic acid; UDCA (Urso ♣, Actigall ★), is a chloretic agent used to treat chronic inflammatory cholestatic liver disease, bile sludging, dissolution of radiolucent non-calcified gallstones smaller than 20 mm in diameter, primary biliary cirrhosis, chronic persistent hepatitis, cirrhosis, and biliary atresia. The drug promotes biliary flow and has anti-inflammatory properties. Total endogenous bile acids are reduced. It will not dissolve calcified cholesterol or bile pigment gallstones.

ADVERSE AND COMMON SIDE EFFECTS: None have been reported in dogs or cats. In humans, adverse effects may include diarrhea, vomiting, constipation, stomatitis, abdominal pain, and flatulence. Mean preprandial and postprandial serum bile acid concentrations increased with treatment attributable to the increased UDCA concentration. Thus, serum bile acid concentration may not be an accurate indication of liver function in animals receiving the drug. The drug is contraindicated in patients with extrahepatic biliary obstruction.

DRUG INTERACTIONS: Estrogens and clofibrate may increase hepatic cholesterol secretion and predispose to cholesterol gallstone formation. Aluminum-based antacids absorb bile acids and interfere with ursodiol by decreasing its absorption. Cholestyramine also tends to decrease ursodiol's absorption.

SUPPLIED AS HUMAN PRODUCTS:
Capsules containing 250 mg [Urso]
Capsules containing 300 mg [Actigall]

VALPROIC ACID

INDICATIONS: Valproic acid (Depakene ✽ ★, Depakote ★, Epival ✽) is an anticonvulsant drug. It is costly, has a short half-life (2.8 hours) in the dog, and is potentially hepatotoxic; however, some clinicians use the drug in combination with phenobarbital in patients not responsive to phenobarbital alone. In humans, target serum concentrations are approximately 50 to 150 µg/mL.

ADVERSE AND COMMON SIDE EFFECTS: The drug is contraindicated in patients with significant hepatic disease. It should be used with caution in those with thrombocytopenia or impaired platelet function. The drug is potentially teratogenic and should only be used in pregnant bitches when the benefits appear to outweigh the risks. Side effects may include anorexia, vomiting, and diarrhea. In humans, hepatotoxicity and elevation in liver enzymes occur; this may be of concern in dogs. Other potential side effects may include sedation, ataxia, behavioral changes, leukopenia, anemia, pancreatitis, and edema.

DRUG INTERACTIONS: Valproic acid may increase the serum levels and potentiate the effect of phenobarbital and primidone. Valproic acid may increase or decrease phenytoin levels, predisposing to seizure activity. Concurrent use of tricyclic antidepressants, e.g., amitriptyline, or MAO inhibitors, e.g., possibly amitraz and selegiline, may potentiate CNS depression. Salicylates may increase serum valproic acid levels. The sedative effects of clonazepam may be increased, but the anticonvulsant activity of both drugs decreased when used concurrently.

SUPPLIED AS HUMAN PRODUCTS:
Capsules containing 250 mg [Depakene]
Tablets containing 125, 250, and 500 mg [Depakote, Epival]
Oral syrup containing 50 mg/mL [Depakene]

VASOPRESSIN

INDICATIONS: Vasopressin (Pitressin ★, generics ♣) is a synthetic form of vasopressin or antidiuretic hormone. It has been used in the diagnosis and management of diabetes insipidus.

ADVERSE AND COMMON SIDE EFFECTS: Abdominal pain, nausea, vomiting, bronchial constriction, fluid retention, hyponatremia, pain at the site of injection, and the formation of sterile abscesses have been reported. The drug is contraindicated in patients with cardiorenal disease with hypertension, epilepsy, or hypersensitivity to the drug. The drug should be used with caution in patients with asthma or heart failure.

DRUG INTERACTIONS: Large doses of epinephrine, heparin, and demeclocycline may antagonize the effects of Pitressin. Chlorpropamide, carbamazepine, and fludrocortisone may potentiate the action of Pitressin.

SUPPLIED AS HUMAN PRODUCT:
For injection containing 20 pressor units/mL

VEDAPROFEN

INDICATIONS: Vedaprofen (Quadrisol ♣★) is an NSAID used for reduction of inflammation and relief of pain associated with musculoskeletal disorders and trauma in dogs.

ADVERSE AND COMMON SIDE EFFECTS: Vedaprofen has shown to have potential side effects similar to other NSAIDs, including vomiting, soft feces or diarrhea, bloody stool, gastritis, erosions, reduced appetite, and lethargy. Vedaprofen should be avoided in dehydrated, hypovolemic, or hypotensive animals due to an increased risk of renal toxicity. Vedaprofen is contraindicated in animals with alimentary tract disorders, hemorrhagic diathesis, or impaired renal, hepatic, or cardiac function. Vedaprofen should not be used at the time of parturition, and should not be given to dogs under 12 weeks of age. The safety of use in lactating bitches has not been established.

DRUG INTERACTIONS: Other NSAIDs, diuretics, anticoagulants, and highly protein bound substances may compete for binding and exacerbate toxic effects. Do not give in conjunction with other NSAIDs or glucocorticoids.

SUPPLIED AS VETERINARY PRODUCT:
Oral gel containing 5 mg/mL in 15 and 30 mL "dial a dose" syringes

VERAPAMIL

INDICATIONS: Verapamil (Isoptin ✤ ★) is a calcium channel-blocking agent. The drug may be useful in the management of atrial flutter, atrial fibrillation, and atrial tachycardia. It is a potent arterial vasodilator and is a more potent negative inotropic agent than nifedipine or diltiazem.

ADVERSE AND COMMON SIDE EFFECTS: The drug is contraindicated in sick sinus syndrome, atrioventricular block and myocardial failure (unless tachycardia is contributing to the failure), shock, hypotension, or digitalis-intoxicated patients. The drug should be used with caution in those with hepatic or renal impairment and is contraindicated in Wolff-Parkinson-White syndrome, myocardial failure, and digitalis toxicity.

Adverse effects may include nausea, constipation, fatigue, dizziness, bradycardia, tachycardia, hypotension, exacerbation of congestive heart failure, pulmonary edema, and atrioventricular block. The potential for serious adverse effects and short duration of action have largely caused verapamil to be replaced by diltiazem.

DRUG INTERACTIONS: Verapamil may increase serum digitalis and theophylline levels. Epinephrine, isoproterenol, and theophylline may oppose the calcium-blocking action of verapamil. Propranolol and metoprolol may augment the cardiodepressant effect of verapamil. Calcium salts, vitamin D, and rifampin may decrease the pharmacological effects of verapamil. Cimetidine may increase the pharmacological effects of calcium channel-blocking agents by increasing bioavailability. Highly protein-bound drugs, e.g., oral anticoagulants, salicylates, and sulfonamides, may displace or be displaced by verapamil, predisposing to toxicity. Prazosin and other antihypertensive agents as well as quinidine may cause an acute hypotensive effect.

SUPPLIED AS HUMAN PRODUCTS:
Tablets containing 80 and 120 mg
Tablets (sustained-release) containing 120, 180, and 240 mg
For injection containing 2.5 mg/mL

VINBLASTINE

INDICATIONS: Vinblastine (Velbe ✤, generics ✤) has been used in the treatment of lymphomas, carcinomas, mast cell tumors, and splenic tumors.

ADVERSE AND COMMON SIDE EFFECTS: Vinblastine is contraindicated in patients with leukopenia, granulocytopenia, or bacterial infection. Side effects of vinblastine may include nausea, vomiting, and myelosuppression. Granulocytic depression occurs within 4 to 9 days of administration, with recovery occurring 7 to 14 days later. Additional side effects may include constipation, stomatitis, ileus, jaw and muscle pain, inappropriate antidiuretic hormone (ADH) secretion, and loss of deep tendon reflexes. Perivascular injection causes severe tissue irritation and necrosis. If this occurs, aspiration of the drug should be attempted and the area infiltrated with sodium bicarbonate (8.4%), dexamethasone or hyaluronidase (150 µg/mL), or topical DMSO. In addition, warm compresses should be applied to the area.

DRUG INTERACTIONS: None of significance in small animals.

SUPPLIED AS HUMAN PRODUCT:
For injection containing 1 mg/mL

VINCRISTINE

INDICATIONS: Vincristine (Oncovin ★, generics ✤) is a chemotherapeutic agent used in the management of lymphoid and hematopoietic neoplasms, mammary neoplasms in cats, some sarcomas, transmissible venereal tumors in dogs, and immune-mediated thrombocytopenia (IMT). Administration of vincristine along with prednisone is associated with a more rapid increase in platelet numbers and shortened duration of hospitalization. The drug often is used in conjunction with other chemotherapeutic agents.

ADVERSE AND COMMON SIDE EFFECTS: The drug should be used with caution in those with liver disease, leukopenia, bacterial infection, or preexisting neuromuscular disease.
  Vincristine inhibits platelet aggregation in vitro in dogs with lymphosarcoma, which may be of concern for dogs with concurrent IMT. Vincristine is less myelosuppressive than vinblastine, causing a mild leukopenia, but it has greater potential to cause peripheral neuropathy

(proprioceptive deficits, hyporeflexia, and paralytic ileus and constipation). Perivascular injection causes severe tissue irritation and necrosis. If this occurs, aspiration of the drug should be attempted and the
area infiltrated with sodium bicarbonate (8.4%), dexamethasone or
hyaluronidase (150 µg/mL, or 300 units diluted in 6 mL saline–
repeated in 7 to 14 days), or topical DMSO. In addition, warm compresses should be applied to the area.

Other side effects may include increases in serum liver enzymes,
inappropriate ADH secretion, jaw pain, alopecia, stomatitis, and seizure
activity.

DRUG INTERACTIONS: Concurrent use of asparaginase may contribute to neurotoxicity, the incidence of which is less common if
asparaginase is administered after vincristine.

SUPPLIED AS HUMAN PRODUCT:
For injection containing 1 mg/mL

OTHER USES
Dogs
TRANSMISSIBLE VENEREAL TUMOR
0.025 mg/kg once weekly; IV (maximum 1 mg); usually requires 3 to
6 weeks of therapy
IMMUNE-MEDIATED THROMBOCYTOPENIA
i)   0.01 to 0.025 mg/kg; IV at 7- to 10-day intervals (used alone or in
     combination with corticosteroids)
ii) Vincristine (0.02 mg/kg once; IV) with prednisone (1.5 to 2 mg/kg
     bid; PO or SC)

VITAMIN E

INDICATIONS: Vitamin E (Aquasol E ✤ ★) is a fat-soluble vitamin.
It has been used in the treatment of Scotty cramp and as an anti-
inflammatory agent in discoid lupus, pemphigus erythematosus,
demodicosis, and acanthosis nigricans. The drug may have a steroid-
sparing effect. As an antipruritic agent, it is of limited value and has
not been proven efficacious in the treatment of dermatomyositis. In
cats, it has been used in the treatment of steatitis. The efficacy of the
use of vitamin E in these diseases is unknown.

ADVERSE AND COMMON SIDE EFFECTS: Changes in the hair
coat color have been documented in a tricolored collie. Anorexia also
may occur. In humans, excessive doses may cause muscle weakness,
fatigue, nausea, diarrhea, intestinal cramping, increases in serum
cholesterol and triglyceride levels, and decreases in serum thyroxine
levels.

DRUG INTERACTIONS: The drug should be given 2 hours before a meal because the inorganic iron present in most commercial diets interferes with its absorption. Concomitant administration of vitamin E may enhance oral anticoagulant activity. Vitamin A absorption, use, and storage may be enhanced by vitamin E. Large doses of vitamin E may delay the hematologic response to iron therapy in those with iron deficiency anemia. Mineral oil may reduce the absorption of oral vitamin E.

SUPPLIED AS HUMAN PRODUCTS:
Capsules containing 100, 200, 400, 500, 600, 800, and 1,000 IU
Drops containing 50 IU/mL

OTHER USES
Dogs
SCOTTY CRAMP
70 IU/kg intermittently; IM (it may reduce the likelihood of recurrences but does not alter severity of an episode)
DISCOID LUPUS
i) 400 IU bid; PO or as a topical ointment may be beneficial
ii) 200 to 800 IU bid; PO with prednisone 1 to 1.5 mg/kg per day; PO eventually tapered to every alternate day
VITAMIN E-DEFICIENT MYOPATHY
400 IU once daily; PO

Cats
STEATITIS
10 to 20 IU/kg bid; PO until clinical signs have resolved

VITAMIN K₁

INDICATIONS: Vitamin K_1 or phytonadione (Aqua-Mephyton ★, Mephyton ★, Veta-K1 ✤ ★) is used to treat coagulopathy caused by fat-soluble vitamin malabsorption and vitamin K antagonism caused by salicylates, coumarins, and indanediones. It does not correct hypoprothrombinemia due to hepatic disease. Treatment is continued for 5 to 7 days with first-generation toxicants (warfarin, pindone, fumarin, tomarin, isovaleryl indanedione) and for 4 to 6 weeks for second-generation toxicants (brodifacoum, volak, diphacinone, chlorphacinone, bromadiolone). Oral absorption is enhanced when the drug is given with a fatty meal. With appropriate treatment most dogs can be expected to survive. A lag time of 3 to 12 hours is expected before new clotting factors are synthesized and 12 to 48 hours may elapse before coagulation times normalize. Vitamin K_3 is less expensive but also is less effective. Cats with hepatic lipidosis, severe cholangiohep-

atitis and severe inflammatory bowel disease may develop coagulopathies responsive to vitamin K administration.

ADVERSE AND COMMON SIDE EFFECTS: The drug is contraindicated in patients with severe liver disease. Transient hypotension, dyspnea, and cyanosis are reported rarely. Anaphylaxis has been reported
after IV injection of the drug. Intramuscular injection has been associated with acute bleeding from the site of injection during the initial
stages of therapy (small-gauge needles are recommended).

DRUG INTERACTIONS: Oral, broad-spectrum antibiotics given
long-term potentiate hypoprothrombinemia by suppressing vitamin
K-producing intestinal bacteria. Vitamin K antagonizes the effects of
anticoagulants. Mineral oil decreases GI absorption of vitamin K.
Phenylbutazone, aspirin, chloramphenicol, sulfonamides, diazoxide,
allopurinol, cimetidine, metronidazole, anabolic steroids, erythromycin, ketoconazole, propranolol, and thyroid drugs may antagonize
the therapeutic effects of phytonadione.

SUPPLIED AS VETERINARY PRODUCTS:
Capsules containing 25 mg [Veta-K1 ★]
For injection containing 10 mg/mL [Veta-K1 ♣ ★]

SUPPLIED AS HUMAN PRODUCTS:
For injection containing 2 mg/mL ♣ ★ and 10 mg/mL ♣ ★
Tablets containing 5 mg [Mephyton]

Note: The injectable formulation can be given orally at the same dose
(mg/kg basis) when tablets or capsules are not available.

WARFARIN

INDICATIONS: Warfarin (Coumadin ♣ ★) is an anticoagulant. It
interferes with clotting by depressing hepatic synthesis of vitamin K-
dependent coagulation factors II, VII, IX, and X and anticoagulant proteins C and S. It has no effect on already formed circulating coagulation
factors or on circulating thrombi, but it may prevent extension of existing thrombi and prevent new clots from forming. It augments thrombin inactivation and prevents the conversion of fibrinogen to fibrin.
Warfarin may be more effective prophylaxis for thromboembolic disease than aspirin in cats with cardiomyopathy.

ADVERSE AND COMMON SIDE EFFECTS: A transient hypercoag-
ulable state occurs when warfarin is introduced. The actual antithrom-
botic effects are caused by the decrease in factors IX and X, which does
not occur for 4 to 6 days after the start of therapy in humans. Therefore,
for the first 3 to 4 days when anticoagulant protein C levels are low,
heparin is used in conjunction with warfarin. The drug is contraindi-

cated in patients with preexisting bleeding tendencies or GI ulceration, or those undergoing surgery. It is embryotoxic and is contraindicated in pregnancy. Clinical signs are due to dose-related hemorrhage and include pale mucous membranes, weakness, dyspnea, prostration, and occasionally hematomas, ecchymosis, epistaxis, hematemesis, hematuria, hematochezia, and death. A single toxic dose is listed as 5 to 50 mg/kg for dogs and cats.

DRUG INTERACTIONS: Drugs that may enhance the anticoagulant effect of warfarin include acetaminophen, allopurinol, alkylating agents, aminoglycosides, amiodarone, anabolic steroids, antimetabolites, aspirin, asparaginase, chloramphenicol, chlorpropamide, cimetidine, danazol, dextran, diazoxide, erythromycin, ethacrynic acid, MAO inhibitors, e.g., possibly amitraz and selegiline, metronidazole, mineral oil, miconazole, nalidixic acid, neomycin, NSAIDs, potassium products, propylthiouracil, quinidine, sulfonamides, tetracyclines, thiazide diuretics, tolbutamide, tricyclic antidepressants, e.g., amitriptyline, thyroid drugs, and vitamin E. Concurrent use with itraconazole may cause elevation in serum warfarin levels.

Drugs that may decrease the anticoagulant response include barbiturates, corticosteroids, diuretics, griseofulvin, laxatives, mercaptopurine, rifampin, spironolactone, vitamin C, and dietary vitamin K.

SUPPLIED AS HUMAN PRODUCTS:
Tablets containing 1, 2, 2.5, 3, 4, 5, 6, 7.5, and 10 mg ❦ ★
For injection containing 5.4 mg/vial ❦

XYLAZINE

INDICATIONS: Xylazine (Anased ❦ ★, Rompun ❦ ★) is an anesthetic agent characterized by a rapid onset, good-to-excellent sedation, excellent analgesia of 15 to 30 minutes duration, and a smooth recovery. Its sedative effects last longer (90 to 120 minutes) than its analgesic effects. The drug also is used as a diagnostic aid in cases of pituitary hypofunction, e.g., pituitary dwarfism.

ADVERSE AND COMMON SIDE EFFECTS: Use of the drug is contraindicated in animals receiving epinephrine or those with ventricular arrhythmias. It should be used with caution in animals with heart disease, hypotension, shock, respiratory dysfunction, severe hepatic or renal disease, or a history of seizure activity, or those that are severely debilitated. Vomiting may occur 1 to 5 minutes after administration (especially in cats). Dexamethasone (4 to 8 mg/kg; IM) decreases the frequency of vomiting without compromising the sedative effects in cats and may be used prophylactically. In addition hypotension, bradycardia, second-degree heart block, polyuria, mild respiratory depression, hyperglycemia, glycosuria, and aggression are reported. Dogs may bloat from aerophagia. In cats, apnea and seizures also have been reported. Bradycardia may be prevented by the administration of atropine or glycopyrrolate. The drug may precipitate early parturition if used in the last trimester of pregnancy.

DRUG INTERACTIONS: Xylazine sensitizes the heart to epinephrine-induced arrhythmias, especially in the face of halothane anesthesia. Other CNS depressants, including barbiturates, narcotics, and phenothiazines, may potentiate CNS depression. Yohimbine (dogs 0.1 mg/kg; IV, cats 0.5 mg/kg; IV) can be used to antagonize the effects of xylazine, shorten recovery times, and reduce anesthetic-related complications.

SUPPLIED AS VETERINARY PRODUCT:
For injection containing 20 and 100 mg/mL

OTHER USES
Dogs
GROWTH HORMONE RESPONSE TEST FOR HYPOPITUITARISM
300 µg/kg; IV; collect plasma at time 0 and 15, 30, 45, 60, and 90 minutes
Pituitary dwarfs demonstrate little or no response to xylazine stimulation.

Cats
AS AN EMETIC
0.44 mg/kg IM

ZIDOVUDINE (AZT)

INDICATIONS: Zidovudine (AZT) (Retrovir ✤ ★) inhibits viral enzyme, reverse transcriptase, which prevents the conversion of viral RNA into DNA. It has been used in the treatment of FeLV and FIV infections in cats. Clinical improvement has been noted even though the long-term prognosis is still poor. These reports are not based upon strong statistical science and a firm recommendation can therefore not be given.

ADVERSE AND COMMON SIDE EFFECTS: In cats, decreases in red blood cell counts and hemoglobin are reported. It may also be associated with hepatotoxicity.

DRUG INTERACTIONS: Acetaminophen may decrease blood levels of AZT. The co-administration with doxorubicin, flucytosine, vincristine, or vinblastine may potentiate hematologic toxicity. Fluconazole, trimethoprim, and interferon may increase AZT blood levels.

SUPPLIED AS HUMAN PRODUCTS:
For injection containing 10 mg/mL
Syrup containing 10 mg/mL
Capsule containing 100 mg
Tablet containing 300 mg

ZINC ACETATE

INDICATIONS: Zinc acetate ★ has been used in dogs in the treatment and prophylaxis of hepatic copper toxicosis. The suggested plasma therapeutic concentration is 200 to 500 µg/dL. It appears to take 100 mg of zinc administered twice daily approximately 3 to 6 months to obtain therapeutic serum levels. Zinc cannot be expected to reverse cirrhotic liver changes. Zinc acetate has also been recommended to decrease fecal hydrogen sulfide concentrations in dogs prone to flatulence.

ADVERSE AND COMMON SIDE EFFECTS: Zinc acetate appears to be well tolerated by dogs. Vomiting may occur and may be controlled by giving the drug with a small piece of meat. Note, however, that this drug should not normally be given with food.

DRUG INTERACTIONS: To be effective, zinc must be given separately from food by at least 1 hour.

SUPPLIED AS HUMAN PRODUCT:
Capsules containing 25 and 50 mg [Lemmon Co., Sellersville, PA]

ZINC SULFATE

INDICATIONS: Zinc sulfate (PMS-Egozinc ✿, Orazinc ★) has been used in dogs for the treatment of zinc-responsive dermatoses (especially Siberian huskies and Alaskan malamutes) and as a copper-chelating agent, which has been shown in humans to prevent copper reaccumulation in those whose livers already had been depleted of copper with appropriate chelating agents. Therefore, it may have a more important role in preventive copper-associated liver therapy.

ADVERSE AND COMMON SIDE EFFECTS: The product is contraindicated in patients sensitive to zinc. The most common side effects associated with zinc therapy include nausea, anorexia, and vomiting, which can be controlled by dividing the daily dose into two equal portions and administering the drug with food. Zinc gluconate (3 mg/kg per day divided tid; PO) has been suggested as an alternative because it causes less gastric irritation. Toxic zinc levels may result in iron deficiency and hemolytic anemia.

DRUG INTERACTIONS: Excessive zinc will inhibit iron absorption.

SUPPLIED AS HUMAN PRODUCTS:
Capsules and tablets containing 220 mg zinc sulfate (50 mg zinc)
Tablets containing 66 mg (15 mg zinc), 110 mg (25 mg zinc), and 200 mg
(45 mg zinc) [Orazinc]

OTHER USES
Dogs
ZINC-RESPONSIVE DERMATOSIS
1 mg/kg per day; PO of elemental zinc; continue treatment for
1 month. If clinical condition does not improve, increase dose by 50%.

Part II

Large Animals

Handbook of Veterinary Drugs, Third Edition, edited by Dana Allen,
Lippincott Williams & Wilkins, Baltimore. © 2005

Section 4

Common Dosages for Large Animals

To protect the health and welfare of large animals, veterinarians must
legitimately use therapeutic medications. While drugs are commonly
and appropriately used to treat various disease conditions of horses,
ruminants, and swine, many of them have the ability to affect athletic
performance and/or leave residues in edible tissues. For performance
horses, drug rules exist to ensure fair competition and to protect the
welfare of the horses and riders. For food animals, approved drugs
have label withdrawal times to guide veterinarians as to when meat,
milk, and eggs are safe for human consumption. When medications are
administered to performance animals or to food animals in an extralabel manner, it is the responsibility of the veterinarian to ensure that
violative drug residues do not occur. When using drugs in an extralabel manner in food animals in the United States and Canada or in the
event of animal exposure to pesticides, herbicides, and other toxic
chemicals, veterinarians should contact their global Food Animal
Residue Avoidance Databank (gFARAD) for withdrawal recommendations. In the United States, veterinarians may call 1-888-
USFARAD (1-888-873-2723), send email to FARAD@ncsu.edu, or go to
www.farad.org. In Canada, veterinarians may call 1-866-CGFARAD
(1-866-243-2723), send email to cgfarad@umontreal.ca or go to
www.cgfarad.usask.ca. When contacting a gFARAD center, the veterinarian should be prepared to provide information regarding the
brand name and generic name of the drug, the dose, the type and number of animals treated, and the disease condition prompting treatment.
The gFARAD personnel are veterinary pharmacologists and toxicolo-
gists trained to analyse pharmacokinetic data to provide withdrawal
interval guidelines. This global, science-based system minimizes the

risk of contaminated products entering the human food supply. The service is currently free of charge to veterinarians in each country.

When administering drugs to performance horses, veterinarians need to be familiar with the drug regulations for the treated animal's sport. A local or discipline-specific group, state or provincial agency, national federation or agency, or international federation may regulate equine competitions. Drug rules vary enormously between sport organizations. The current sensitivity of drug testing allows for laboratory detection of very small quantities of drugs, which may even be pharmacologically insignificant. The drug detection laboratories do not reveal the drugs that they test for or their limits of detection. Some information on detection limits can be found in the Schedule of Drugs (2002) from the Canadian Pari-Mutuel Agency (www.cpma-acpm.gc.ca/english/cpma.htm), and guides from the Australian Equine Veterinary Association and the American Association of Equine Practitioners. Most of the detection limits in these guides were determined using small numbers of horses, so this information should be used only as a general guide for determining when it is safe to enter a treated horse in a competition. There is extreme variation in some of the reported drug detection limits. This is mainly due to test methods varying between testing laboratories. The recommended Canadian drug withdrawal times are shorter than most others because the Canadian Pari-Mutuel Agency has made a deliberate effort to limit the sensitivity of their test methods to levels of drug that are performance altering. The Canadian detection times may not be valid for testing done in the United States or other countries, especially if extremely sensitive testing methodology, such as ELISA testing, is used. A veterinarian should consider the published detection times and the sport organization's rules as well as his/her knowledge of the particular horse's physiology to advise a competitor on an appropriate drug withdrawal period prior to a competition.

Drug	Horses (and Miniature Pig Doses, Where Indicated)	Ruminants (Cattle, Sheep, and Goats)
Acepromazine	0.44 to 0.88 mg/kg; IV, IM, SC 0.02 to 0.05 mg/kg IV (preanesthetic) *Miniature pigs:* 0.03 to 0.1 mg/kg; IM (catheter placement), 0.1 to 0.2 mg/kg; IM (calm nursing sow), 0.05 to 0.5 mg/kg; IM (sedation, premedication)	0.01 to 0.02 mg/kg; IV 0.05 to 0.1 mg/kg; IM or SC
Acetazolamide	2.2 mg/kg bid to tid; PO	
Acetic acid (5% w/v solution)	250 mL/450 kg; PO daily (enterolith prevention)	2 to 6 L; PO via rumenal intubation, followed with 20 L cold water; PO (cattle), 0.5 to 1 L; PO via rumenal intubation, followed with 2 to 8 L cold water; PO (sheep and goats) for nonprotein nitrogen-induced ammonia toxicosis
Acetylcysteine (10% w/v solution, in Canada 20% w/v available)	2 to 5 mL/50 kg bid to tid as an aerosol As an enema for meconium impaction of a 4% solution: give 120 to 240 mL per rectum via Foley catheter; hold in place for 4 to 5 minutes; repeat if necessary in 1 hour	
Albendazole		10 mg/kg; PO (cattle) 3 mg/kg per day; PO for 35 days (sheep,

(continued)

Drug	Horses (and Miniature Pig Doses, Where Indicated)	Ruminants (Cattle, Sheep, and Goats)
		prophylaxis against infective metacercariae of *Fasciola hepatica*)
Albuterol	2 to 3 μg/kg via metered dose inhaler	
Altrenogest	0.044 mg/kg once daily; PO (1 mL/50 kg) for 15 days (estrus synchronization); follow with luteolytic dose of prostaglandin $F_{2\alpha}$ 0.044 mg/kg daily; PO to maintain pregnancy in mares with deficient progesterone concentrations	
Aluminum hydroxide: See Antacids	60 mg/kg tid to qid; PO	60 mg/kg tid to qid; PO
Amikacin	2 g IU infusion daily for 3 days 10 mg/kg q 24 hours; IV, IM, SC 20 to 25 mg/kg q 24 hours; IV, IM, SC (neonates)	Use not recommended due to prolonged withdrawal times
Aminophylline	2 to 7 mg/kg IV (for pulmonary edema; dilute in 100 mL of saline and administer over 30 minutes) 11 mg/kg bid to tid; PO	
Ammonium chloride	60 to 250 mg/kg per day; PO (urolithiasis) 132 mg/kg; PO (strychnine intoxication)	0.5% w/w in ration (urolithiasis) 132 mg/kg; PO (strychnine intoxication) 100 g/day; PO administer for 21 days prior to calving (prevention of parturient paresis)

Drug	Horses (and Miniature Pig Doses, Where Indicated)	Ruminants (Cattle, Sheep, and Goats)
Amoxicillin sodium	15 mg/kg qid; IV, IM	62.5 mg/quarter q 24 hours; IM
Amoxicillin trihydrate	20 mg/kg bid; IM	11 mg/kg q 24 hours; IM
Amphoteracin B	0.3 mg/kg IV day 1; 0.4 mg/kg IV day 2; 0.5 mg/kg IV day 3; no treatment days 4 to 7, then q 48 hours until a cumulative dose of 6.75 mg/kg has been administered	
Ampicillin sodium	10 to 50 mg/kg tid to qid; IV, IM *Miniature pigs:* 4 to 10 mg/kg; IM, IV	
Ampicillin sulbactam	6.6 mg/kg of ampicillin daily for 3 days; IM	6.6 mg/kg of ampicillin daily for 3 days; IM
Ampicillin trihydrate	11 to 22 mg/kg bid to tid; IM *Miniature pigs:* 10 to 20 mg/kg tid to qid; IM	22 mg/kg bid; IM
Amprolium	*Miniature pigs:* 100 mg/kg in food or water daily	Mix in drinking water at 0.012% w/v amprolium for 5 days to provide 10 mg/kg per day at normal water consumption 50 to 100 mg/kg daily; PO (prophylaxis against clinical sarcocystosis in lambs)
Antacids	See product labels for dosage	See product labels for dosage

(*continued*)

Drug	Horses (and Miniature Pig Doses, Where Indicated)	Ruminants (Cattle, Sheep, and Goats)
Apramycin	*Miniature pigs:* 12.5 mg/kg per day in water for 7 days	
Aspirin	15 to 100 mg/kg bid to tid; PO *Miniature pigs:* 10 to 20 mg/kg bid to qid; PO	Two to four 240 grain boluses; PO
Atracurium	0.04 to 0.7 mg/kg; IV (foals)	
Atropine	0.1 to 0.4 mg/kg; IV, IM, or SC 5 to 7 mg; IV (test dose for recurrent airway obstruction) *Miniature pigs:* 0.04 mg/kg; IM	0.1 to 0.4 mg/kg; IV, IM, or SC
Azaperone	*Miniature pigs:* 0.25 to 0.5 mg/kg; IM (sedation without ataxia); 2.2 mg/kg; IM (calm nursing sow); 2 to 8 mg/kg; IM (sedation, immobilization)	
Azithromycin	10 mg/kg q 24 hours for 5 days, then q 48 hours; PO	
Bacitracin, neomycin, polymixin B sulfate (and with hydrocortisone)	Apply topically to the cornea qid for ocular infections	Apply topically to the cornea qid for ocular infections
BAL (Dimercaprol) (10% w/v solution in oil)	2.5 to 5 mg/kg qid; IM for 2 days, then bid for the next 10 days or until recovery	2.5 to 5 mg/kg q 4 hours; IM for 2 days, then bid for the next 10 days or until recovery
Beclomethasone	3.75 mg bid via metered dose inhaler	
Betamethasone	0.02 to 0.1 mg/kg; IM 12.5 to 25 mg; IA	5 to 25 mg; IA

Drug	Horses (and Miniature Pig Doses, Where Indicated)	Ruminants (Cattle, Sheep, and Goats)
Bethanechol	0.025 to 0.075 mg/kg tid to qid; SC 0.3 to 0.75 mg/kg tid to qid; PO	
Bismuth subsalicylate	8.75 to 17.5 mg/kg q 4 to 6 hours; PO (foals) 1 to 2 L/450 kg bid; PO (adults) of oral liquid containing 17.5 mg/mL bismuth subsalicylate	3.25 to 5.25 g q 2 to 3 hours; PO (adult cattle) 1 to 2 g q 2 to 3 hours; PO (calves) For bolus products: Generally, one bolus/70 kg calf bid; PO for 2 or 3 days Scour bolus: 1 bolus/45 kg bid; PO for 2 days Read directions on individual products
Boldenone undecylenate	0.28 to 1.1 mg/kg; IM repeated at 2- or 3-week intervals	
Botulinum antitoxin	200 mL; IV, IM (foals) 500 mL; IV, IM (adults)	
Bupivicaine hydrochloride	Local infiltration for nerve blocks	Local infiltration for nerve blocks and epidural anesthesia in sheep
Butorphanol tartrate	0.1 mg/kg; IV, IM 0.01 to 0.02 mg/kg in combination with xylazine, detomidine, or romifidine *Miniature pigs:* 0.1 to 0.3 mg/kg bid to tid; IM, IV 0.05 to 0.2 mg/kg q 3 to 4 hours; SC, IV	0.01 to 0.1 mg/kg; IV, IM
Calcium borogluconate (23% w/v solution)	250 to 500 mL; IV, SC, IP	250 to 500 mL; IV, SC, IP 25 mL; IV, SC, IP (sheep)

(continued)

Drug	Horses (and Miniature Pig Doses, Where Indicated)	Ruminants (Cattle, Sheep, and Goats)
Calcium chloride	1 to 2 g/450 kg; slowly IV to effect	
Calcium disodium edetate	70 to 100 mg/kg divided into 2 to 3 doses daily for 3 days	70 to 100 mg/kg divided into 2 to 3 doses daily for 3 days
Carbachol	2 to 4 mg; SC (adults) 0.5 to 1 mg; SC (yearlings) 0.25 to 0.5 mg; SC (foals) Repeat at intervals no shorter than 30 to 60 minutes, as required	2 to 4 mg; SC (mature cattle) 0.5 to 2 mg; SC (calves)
Carbaryl	Dust entire animal with not more than 500 g dust per head; repeat at 14- to 18-day intervals for louse control Apply spray directly to horse's coat not more than twice per week	Dust top line, sides, and legs; do not apply to underline or udder; repeat not more than twice per week (dairy cattle) Mix 1 kg/100 L of water; spray 5 L of the mixture per head of livestock; repeat if necessary
Cefazolin: See Cephalosporins	15 mg/kg bid to tid; IV, IM 50 mg subconjunctivally	250 mg; IV regional perfusion (for local treatment of septic arthritis/ tenosynovitis)
Cefepime: See Cephalosporins	11 mg/kg tid; IV	
Cefotaxime: See Cephalosporins	40 mg/kg qid; IV	
Cefoxitin: See Cephalosporins	20 mg/kg tid; IV, IM	
Ceftazidime: See Cephalosporins	25 to 50 mg/kg bid; IV, IM	

Drug	Horses (and Miniature Pig Doses, Where Indicated)	Ruminants (Cattle, Sheep, and Goats)
Ceftiofur: See Cephalosporins	2 to 4 mg/kg once daily; IM 5 to 10 mg/kg bid; IV *Miniature pigs:* 3 to 10 mg/kg once daily; IM 1.1 to 2.2 mg/kg once daily; IM for 7 days (rhinitis)	1 to 2 mg/kg once daily; IM (cattle) 2 mg/kg once daily; IM (sheep and goats)
Ceftizoxime: See Cephalosporins	25 to 50 mg/kg bid to tid; IV, IM	
Ceftriaxone: See Cephalosporins	25 to 50 mg/kg bid; IV, IM	
Cefuroxime axetil: See Cephalosporins	25 to 50 mg/kg tid; IV, IM 250 to 500 mg/kg bid; PO	
Cephalothin: See Cephalosporins	20 to 40 mg/kg tid to qid; IV, IM	
Cephapirin: See Cephalosporins		For intramammary infusion; see specific product label
Charcoal, activated	Toxiban: 0.75 to 2 g/kg or 10 to 20 mL/kg; PO 1 to 3 g/kg; PO in a slurry (1 g/5 mL water), repeat in 8 to 12 hours if needed	Toxiban: 0.75 to 2 g/kg or 10 to 20 mL/kg; PO 2 to 9 g/kg; PO in a slurry, repeat as needed
Chloral hydrate	40 to 100 mg/kg; PO (sedation) 60 to 200 mg/kg; IV (foal restraint)	50 to 70 mg/kg; IV (sedation) 10 g/45 kg; PO (acetonemia)
Chloramphenicol	25 mg/kg tid to qid; IV, IM [succinate] 4 to 10 mg/kg tid to qid; PO (foals) 25 to 50 mg/kg tid to qid; PO (adult horses) [palmitate]	Banned from use in food animals

(continued)

Drug	Horses (and Miniature Pig Doses, Where Indicated)	Ruminants (Cattle, Sheep, and Goats)
Chlorhexidine	See product labels	See product labels
Chlorpromazine hydrochloride	Not recommended due to adverse reactions	0.22 to 1 mg/kg; IV 1 to 4.4 mg/kg; IM
Chlortetracycline		22 mg/kg; PO (beef and dairy cattle) 55 mg/kg; PO (calves) 22 mg/kg; PO (lambs)
Chorionic gonadotro-pin (HCG)	1,000 U; IV on the first or second day of estrus, breed 24 or 48 hours later (mares) 1,000 to 2,000 U weekly for 8 injections; IM (stallions) 1,000 U twice weekly for 4 to 6 weeks; IM (cryptorchid foals)	1,000 to 2,500 U; IV 10,000 U; IM, repeat in 21 days if necessary (cystic ovaries in cattle) 500 U; IV on days 19 and 20 of the cycle (hasten ovulation) 400 to 800 U; IV, IM (sheep) 3,000 U; IV (goats)
Cimetidine	4 mg/kg bid; IV 18 mg/kg bid; PO	
Ciprofloxacin	Apply 3 mg/mL solution topically to corneas	
Cisplatin	Inject intralesionally (sarcoids, skin tumors) every 2 weeks	
Clenbuterol	0.8 to 3.2 µg/kg bid; IV (Canada), PO 200 µg; IV (for uterine relaxation) (Canada)	Banned for use in food animals
Cloprostenol: See Prostaglandin F$_{2\alpha}$	100 µg; IM, on day 7 or 8 post estrus (abortifacient)	500 µg; IM 62.5 to 125 µg; IM at 144 days of gesta-tion to induce par-turition in goats
Clorsulon		7 mg/kg; PO (cattle, sheep, llamas)
Cloxacillin		See intramammary product label for directions

Drug	Horses (and Miniature Pig Doses, Where Indicated)	Ruminants (Cattle, Sheep, and Goats)
Cobalt		Top dress the soil with 100 to 150 g cobalt sulfate/acre, alternatively, mixed with mineral or salt blocks (endemic deficiency areas) See acetonemia products
Chondroitin sulfate	13.4 mg/kg daily; PO	
Copper, injectable	See individual product labels	See individual product labels
Copper naphthenate		External use only; remove necrotic tissues, cleanse area, and apply; not to be used on the teats of lactating dairy cattle
Copper sulfate	Apply the powder freely to wounds twice daily; repeat as indicated	Apply the powder freely to wounds twice daily; repeat as indicated 5% w/v solution for footbaths 2 to 4 L as a 0.4% w/v solution; PO (phosphorus toxicity) 1 g/adult cow daily; PO, (copper deficiency) 35 mg/head per day; PO, (swayback prevention in lambs)
Corticotropin (ACTH)	200 IU; IM, SC, repeat every 3 to 7 days as required (adult horse)	200 IU; IM daily (mature cow)

(continued)

Drug	Horses (and Miniature Pig Doses, Where Indicated)	Ruminants (Cattle, Sheep, and Goats)
Coumaphos	1% w/w dust topically 3% w/v spray (KRS) topically or according to labeled instructions for concentrated products	1% w/w dust topically, 55 g/head 3% w/v spray (KRS) topically or according to labeled instructions for concentrated products; directions may vary for lactating and non-lactating cattle
Cromolyn sodium	80 to 300 mg; via inhalation	
Cyproheptadine	0.5 mg/kg bid; PO	
Danofloxacin: See Fluoroquinolones		6 mg/kg, repeat in 48 hours; SC (Fluoroquinolones are banned from extralabel use in food-producing animals in the United States)
Dantrolene	9 mg/kg; PO presurgically (postanesthetic myopathy prevention) 2 mg/kg; slowly IV in saline (acute myopathy) *Miniature pigs:* 2 to 5 mg/kg tid; PO, IV (malignant hyperthermia)	
Decoquinate		0.5 mg/kg body weight per day. Mix according to label directions.
Dembrexine	0.33 mg/kg bid; PO for 10 days	
Deslorelin	Place one implant SC in the neck of an estrous mare that has	

Drug	Horses (and Miniature Pig Doses, Where Indicated)	Ruminants (Cattle, Sheep, and Goats)
	an ovarian follicle greater than 30 mm in diameter. The mare should then be bred or inseminated prior to ovulation within the next 48 hours.	
Detomidine	0.02 to 0.04 mg/kg; IV, IM 0.01 to 0.02 mg/kg; IV followed by butor-phanol (0.044 to 0.066 mg/kg; IV), or ketamine (2.2 mg/kg; IV)	
Dexamethasone	2 to 5 mg; IV, IM 5 to 10 mg; PO daily 0.02 to 0.2 mg/kg; IV, IM, PO 0.5 to 2 mg/kg; IV (shock) 0.1% w/v suspension every 3 to 8 hours applied topically to corneas	5 to 20 mg; IM, IV 5 to 10 mg; PO (anti-inflammatory for adult cattle) 20 mg; IM (parturition induction in cattle) 8 to 16 mg; IM (parturition induction in sheep past 138 days of gestation) 10 mg; IM (parturition induction in goats past 135 days of gestation) 20 mg; IM combined with luteolytic dose of prosta-glandin $F_{2\alpha}$ (for abortion in cattle after 150 days of gestation)
Dextran 70	8 g/kg of 6% w/v dex-tran 70 solution once daily for up to 3 days; slow IV	

(continued)

Drug	Horses (and Miniature Pig Doses, Where Indicated)	Ruminants (Cattle, Sheep, and Goats)
	500 mL of 32% w/v dextran 70 into abdominal cavity during surgery (intestinal adhesion prevention)	
Diazepam	0.03 to 0.5 mg/kg; slowly IV, repeat in 30 minutes if needed *Miniature pigs:* 0.5 to 3 mg/kg; IM (tranquilization), 5.5 mg/kg; IM (sedation)	0.5 to 1.5 mg/kg; IV, IM
Dichlorvos	*Miniature pigs:* 20 mg/kg; PO	See label directions.
Diethylcarbamazine	1 mg/kg once daily; PO for 21 days (onchocerciasis) 50 mg/kg; PO for 10 days (verminous myelitis)	
Digoxin	11 µg/kg: slowly IV (loading dose) 44 µg/kg; PO (loading dose) 11 µg/kg bid; PO (maintenance dose)	
Dihydrostreptomycin		12.5 mg/kg bid for 3 to 5 days; IM
Dimethyl glycine	1 to 1.6 mg/kg daily; PO	
Dimethyl sulfoxide (DMSO)	Gel: topical use 2 to 3 times daily Solution: topical use 2 to 3 times daily; not to exceed 100 g or 100 mL per day 1 g/kg bid; IV, PO (via nasogastric tube) IV solution should be diluted to 10% w/v concentration in saline, LRS, or D_5W	1 g/kg bid; IV, PO (via nasogastric tube) IV solution should be diluted to 10% w/v concentration in saline, LRS, or D_5W

Drug	Horses (and Miniature Pig Doses, Where Indicated)	Ruminants (Cattle, Sheep, and Goats)
Dioctyl sodium sulfosuccinate (docusate sodium)	Orally: 12 g/gal water Enema: 6 to 9 g/gal water 17 to 66 mg/kg q 48 hours; PO (intestinal impaction) 10 mL per rectum in warm water (meconium impaction)	300 mL; PO (adult cattle) 50 mL; PO (sheep and goats), repeat as required (frothy bloat) 50 mg/kg per day; PO (abomasal impaction)
Diphenhydramine	0.25 to 1 mg/kg; IV or IM (anaphylaxis) 2 mg/kg; IV (to reverse CNS effects of metoclopramide or phenothiazine tranquilizers)	0.25 to 1 mg/kg; IV or IM (anaphylaxis)
Dipyrone	Banned for sale in the United States 44 to 66 mg/kg bid to tid; IV, IM, SC. IM injections are highly irritating.	Banned for sale in the United States
Dobutamine	1 to 10 µg/kg per minute; IV (250 mg in 500 mL saline infused at 0.45 mL/kg per hour)	
Domperidone	1.1 mg/kg daily; PO	
Dopamine	2 to 10 µg/kg per minute; IV	2 to 10 µg/kg per minute; IV
Doramectin	*Miniature pigs:* 0.3 mg/kg; IM	0.2 mg/kg; SC or IM in the neck 0.5 mg/kg; topically (pour-on formulation)
Doxapram	0.44 to 0.55 mg/kg; IV 0.5 to 1 mg/kg q 5 minutes; IV, 0.02 to 0.05 mg/kg per minute; IV	5 to 10 mg/kg; IV

(continued)

Drug	Horses (and Miniature Pig Doses, Where Indicated)	Ruminants (Cattle, Sheep, and Goats)
Doxycycline: See Tetracyclines	(resuscitation in neonatal foals); do not exceed 2 mg/kg in foals 10 mg/kg bid; PO (IV administration may cause fatal cardiac arrhythmias)	
Enilconazole	Apply topically for dermatophytosis Flush 60 mL of 33.3 mg/mL solution once daily through endoscope (gutteral pouch mycosis)	
Enrofloxacin	5 to 10 mg/kg once daily; IV, IM, PO *Miniature pigs:* 2.5 to 5 mg/kg once daily; IM	2.5 to 5 mg/kg once daily for 3 days or 7.5 to 12.5 mg/kg once; SC (Fluoroquinolones are banned from extralabel use in food-producing animals in the US.)
Epinephrine	20 µg/kg; IM (anaphylaxis) 2 to 10 µg/kg; IV, intratracheal (cardiopulmonary arrest)	20 µg/kg; IM (anaphylaxis) 2 to 10 µg/kg; IV, intratracheal (cardiopulmonary arrest)
Eprinomectin		0.5 mg/kg applied topically (pour-on formulation)
Ergonovine	1 to 4 mg; IM, IV (mare)	1 to 4 mg; IM, IV (cow) 0.4 to 1 mg; IM, IV (ewe and doe)
Erythromycin	2.5 to 5 mg/kg tid to qid; IV [lactobionate] 25 mg/kg tid to qid; PO [base or estolate] combined with rifam-	2.2 to 4.4 mg/kg once daily; IM (cattle) 11 mg/kg once daily; IM (lambs > 4.5 kg)

Drug	Horses (and Miniature Pig Doses, Where Indicated)	Ruminants (Cattle, Sheep, and Goats)
	pin at 10 mg/kg bid; PO (*R. equi* pneumonia); therapy must often be prolonged (4 to 20 weeks) 0.5 to 1 mg/kg; IV [lactobionate] (postoperative ileus)	2.2 mg/kg; IM (older sheep) 300 mg per quarter (mastitis × 3 treatments) 600 mg/quarter (dry cow treatment)
Estradiol	5 to 10 mg; IM (anestrus) 0.004 to 0.008 mg/kg q 2 days; IM (urinary incontinence)	3 to 5 mg; IM (anestrus in cows) 10 mg; IM (pyometra, retained placenta, mummified fetus; cows) 4 mg; IM (persistent corpus luteum, cow) 3 mg; IM (anestrus, heifers) 0.05 mg/kg; IM with 0.125 mg/kg progesterone bid; IM for 7 days (lactation induction in cattle)
Ethylenediamine dihydroiodide	7.5 to 15 g bid; PO for 7 days	7.5 to 15 g bid; PO for 7 days
Famotidine	0.35 mg/kg bid; IV 2.8 mg/kg bid; PO	
Fenbendazole	5 mg/kg; PO (strongyles, pinworms) 10 mg/kg; PO (ascarids) 50 mg/kg; PO (*S. westeri*) *Miniature pigs:* 10 mg/kg once daily; PO for 3 days (whipworms)	5 mg/kg; PO **OR** 10 mg/kg; PO for *Moniezia benedeni* and arrested 4th stage larvae of *Ostertagia ostertagi* 5 to 15 mg/kg; PO (sheep, goats, llamas)

(*continued*)

Drug	Horses (and Miniature Pig Doses, Where Indicated)	Ruminants (Cattle, Sheep, and Goats)
Fenoterol	2 to 4 µg/kg via metered dose inhaler as needed	
Fenprostalene: See Prostaglandin $F_{2\alpha}$	0.5 mg; SC	1 mg; SC
Fenthion		See label directions.
Florfenicol		20 mg/kg; IM; repeat in 48 hours 40 mg/kg once; SC
Flumethasone	1.25 to 2.5 mg once daily; IV, IM, IA	1.25 to 5 mg once daily; IV, IM, IA
Flunixin meglumine	1.1 mg/kg once daily to tid; PO, IM, IV 0.25 mg/kg tid; IV (endotoxemia) *Miniature pigs:* 0.5 to 1 mg/kg once to twice daily; SC, IV	1.1 to 2.2 mg/kg once daily or divided and given bid for up to 3 days; IV
Flurbiprofen (0.03% solution)	Apply topically to corneas tid to qid	
Fluticasone	2,000 µg bid; via metered dose inhaler	
Folic acid	75 mg; IM (foal) 75 mg; IM every 3 days (during antiprotozoal therapy for equine protozoal encephalomyelitis)	
Follicle-stimulating hormone (FSH)	10 to 50 mg/450 kg; IV, IM, SC	10 to 50; IV, IM, SC
Furosemide	0.5 to 3 mg/kg bid; IV, IM	500 mg once daily or 250 mg bid; IM, IV 2 grams once daily; PO
Gentamicin	4.4 to 6.6 mg/kg q 24 hours; IV, IM, SC (adults) 10 to 14 mg/kg q 24 hours; IV, IM, SC (neonates)	Use not recommended due to prolonged withdrawal times

Drug	Horses (and Miniature Pig Doses, Where Indicated)	Ruminants (Cattle, Sheep, and Goats)
	150 mg (buffered); IA 10 to 40 mg; sub-conjunctivally	
Glycerol	1 g/kg; PO (CNS trauma) 5% w/v as an aerosol (respiratory therapy)	
Glycopyrrolate	5 to 10 µg/kg; IV (bradyarrhythmias) 2 to 3 mg bid to tid; IM (bronchodilation) *Miniature pigs:* 0.01 mg/kg; IM (preanesthetic)	
Gonadorelin (GnRH)	See Deslorelin	100 µg; IM or IV
Griseofulvin	2.5 g/450 kg; PO once daily for 10 days to 3 weeks 10 g/450 kg once daily; PO for 2 weeks, then 5 g/450 kg once daily; PO for 7 weeks	Avoid in food animals due to persistent residues
Guaifenesin (glyceryl guaiacolate)	110 mg/kg; slowly IV to effect (anesthetic induction) 0.1 to 0.2 g/50 kg qid; PO (expectorant)	110 mg/kg; slowly IV to effect (anesthetic induction)
Halothane	Induction: 3% to 5% Maintenance: 1% to 3%	Induction: 3% to 5% Maintenance: 1% to 3%
Heparin	25 to 100 IU/kg bid to qid; SC (acute laminitis, DIC, adhesion prevention)	
Hyaluronate	40 mg; IV 10 to 100 mg; IA	
Hydralazine	0.5 mg/kg; IV 0.5 to 1.5 mg/kg bid; PO	
Hydrochlorothiazide	0.5 mg/kg bid; PO	125 to 250 mg/cow once or twice daily; IV, IM

(continued)

Drug	Horses (and Miniature Pig Doses, Where Indicated)	Ruminants (Cattle, Sheep, and Goats)
Hydrocortisone sodium succinate	1 to 4 mg/kg; IV drip	1 to 4 mg/kg; IV drip
Hydroxyzine	0.5 to 1 mg/kg tid; IM, PO	0.5 to 1 mg/kg tid; IM, PO
Imipramine	100 to 600 mg/450 kg bid; PO for 2 weeks (improve ejaculation) 0.55 mg/kg tid; IM, IV **OR** 1.5 mg/kg tid; PO (narcolepsy)	
Insulin	0.15 U/kg PZI insulin bid; IM, SC 0.1 to 0.2 U regular insulin/kg; SC, IV with simultaneous D₅W at 0.1 to 0.2 mL/kg per minute; IV (hyperkalemia)	200 U ultralente insulin/450 kg bid; SC along with IV glucose drip (hepatic lipidosis, ketosis)
Ipratropium bromide	2 to 3 µg/kg qid; via metered dose inhaler	
Iron dextran	400 to 600 mg/450 kg; IM (split dose in 2 sites) *Miniature pigs* 50 mg/ animal; IM, repeat in 2 to 3 weeks	
Isoflupredone	5 to 20 mg/450 kg as needed; IM, IA 0.02 to 0.03 mg/kg once daily for 5 days then taper for 10 to 20 days; IM (recurrent airway obstruction)	10 to 20 mg/cow once daily to bid; IM, IA (multiple doses may cause hypokalemia)
Isoflurane	Induction: 3% to 5% Maintenance: 1.5% to 1.8%	Induction: 3% to 5% Maintenance: 1.5% to 1.8%
Isoniazid	5 to 15 mg/kg bid; PO	10 mg/kg per day; PO for 1 month (actinomycosis)

Drug	Horses (and Miniature Pig Doses, Where Indicated)	Ruminants (Cattle, Sheep, and Goats)
Isoproterenol	0.4 µg/kg; dilute in saline and administer by slow infusion IV (discontinue when heart rate doubles) 0.05 to 1 µg/kg; IV (foal resuscitation)	
Isoxsuprine	0.6 to 1.8 mg/kg bid; PO	
Itraconazole	5 mg/kg bid; PO	
Ivermectin	0.2 mg/kg; PO *Miniature pigs:* 0.3 mg/kg; PO, SC, IM (repeat in 14 days for sarcoptic mange)	0.2 mg/kg; SC 0.5 mg/kg; topically (pour-on) One sustained-release bolus (1.72 g) per calf weighing at least 100 kg and not more than 300 kg Not for use in lactating cattle 0.2 mg/kg; PO (sheep) 0.2 mg/kg; SC (American bison, reindeer for warbles)
Kaolin-pectin	15 to 30 mL/45 kg; PO q 2 to 3 hours (adults) 15 mL/10 kg; PO q 2 to 3 hours (foals)	15 to 30 mL/45 kg; PO q 2 to 3 hours (cattle) 15 mL/10 kg; PO q 2 to 3 hours (calves)
Ketamine	1.5 to 2 mg/kg; IV Must be preceded with a sedative/hypnotic (see xylazine, diazepam, detomidine), or muscle relaxant (see guaifenesin) *Miniature pigs:* 5 to 20 mg/kg; IM (sedation) 20 to 30 mg/kg; IM (immobilization)	2 mg/kg; IV Must be preceded with a sedative/hypnotic (see xylazine, diazepam, detomidine), or muscle relaxant (see guaifenesin)

(continued)

Drug	Horses (and Miniature Pig Doses, Where Indicated)	Ruminants (Cattle, Sheep, and Goats)
Ketoconazole	1 to 2 mg/kg; IM; pre-medication with diazepam followed by 12 to 20 mg/kg; IM ketamine Topical shampoo for dermatophytosis	
Ketoprofen	2.2 mg/kg once daily; IV, IM for up to 5 days (musculoskeletal pain) 0.5 mg/kg; IV q 6 hours (endotoxemia)	3 mg/kg once daily; IV, IM for up to 3 days
Lactulose	150 to 200 mL qid; PO	
Lasalocid		250 mg/head per day; PO for cattle 200 to 299 kg, and 350 mg/head per day; PO for cattle > 300 kg (feed additive) 0.5 to 2 mg/kg; PO (30 g/ton of feed) (sheep)
Levamisole	8 mg/kg; PO (immuno-stimulant) *Miniature pigs:* 10 mg/kg; PO	3.3 to 8 mg/kg; SC (cattle) 8 mg/kg; SC (sheep and goats) 5.4 to 11 mg/kg; as drench or bolus 2.5 mL/50 kg; topically (pour-on) 100 g/100 kg feed (pellets)
Levothyroxine	35 to 100 mg/450 kg once daily; PO	
Lidocaine	2 to 50 mL local infiltration to effect (local anesthetic)	5 to 100 mL (cattle), 3 to 10 mL (sheep) local infil-

Drug	Horses (and Miniature Pig Doses, Where Indicated)	Ruminants (Cattle, Sheep, and Goats)
	0.5 mg/kg; as bolus IV q 5 minutes until 2 to 4 mg/kg total (antiarrhythmic) 1.3 mg/kg; slow IV bolus; then 0.05 mg/kg per minute; IV over 5 to 6 hours (ileus)	tration to effect (local anesthetic)
Lincomycin	May cause fatal colitis in horses. *Miniature pigs:* 11 mg/kg once daily; IM	May cause fatal colitis in ruminants
Luteinizing hormone (LH)	25 mg; IV, SC (mares)	25 mg; IV, SC (cows) 2.5 mg; IV, SC (ewes, does)
Magnesium hydroxide	200 to 250 mL (Milk of Magnesia) tid; PO (adults)	1 to 6 boluses; PO (1 bolus per 27 kg) 361 g (in 454 g powder) in 3.8 L water. Give 10 mL/kg orally by stomach tube. Gel: 108 g; PO per animal (mature cattle)
Magnesium sulfate	0.2 to 0.4 g/kg dissolved in 4 L warm water, once daily; PO	0.44 mg/kg of a 20% solution; IV, SC (grass tetany) 1 to 2 g/kg; PO (cathartic) 2.5 g/kg per day; PO (abomasal impaction)
Mannitol (20% w/v solution)	0.25 to 2 g/kg; slowly IV	1 to 3 g/kg; slowly IV
Marbofloxacin: See Fluoroquinolones	2 mg/kg once daily; PO	Fluoroquinolones are banned from extralabel use in food-producing *(continued)*

Drug	Horses (and Miniature Pig Doses, Where Indicated)	Ruminants (Cattle, Sheep, and Goats)
		animals in the United States
Meclofenamic acid	2.2 mg/kg per day; PO for 5 to 7 days	
Megestrol acetate	65 to 85 mg/kg once daily; PO	
Melengestrol acetate		0.25 to 0.5 mg/head per day in feed
Meperidine	0.2 to 0.4 mg/kg; IV 3 to 4 mg/kg; IM (pre-treat with xylazine or acepromazine) *Miniature pigs:* 2 to 10 mg/kg; IM q 4 hours	1 mg/kg; IV (cattle) Up to 2.5 mg/kg; IV (ewes)
Mepivicaine hydrochloride	Infiltration: 3 to 15 mL; nerve block 5 to 20 mL; epidural 10 to 15 mL; IA 25 to 40 mL topically for ventriculectomy	Infiltration: 3 to 5 mL; nerve block
Methionine	5 to 15 g/454 kg daily; in feed	
Methocarbamol	4.4 to 22 mg/kg; IV 22 to 55 mg/kg; IV (severe muscle spasms) 110 mg/kg; IV (convulsions)	110 mg/kg; IV (convulsions)
Methylcellulose flakes	0.25 to 0.5 kg/450 kg in 10 L water; PO 125 to 175 g daily; PO in feed	
Methylene blue	4.4 to 8.8 mg/kg; IV slow drip	4.4 to 8.8 mg/kg; IV slow drip
Methylprednisolone acetate	200 mg; IM 40 to 240 mg; IA	40 to 240 mg; IA
Methylprednisolone sodium succinate	0.5 mg/kg; IV or IM	

Drug	Horses (and Miniature Pig Doses, Where Indicated)	Ruminants (Cattle, Sheep, and Goats)
Methylsulfonomethane	10 g bid; PO for 4 days, then once daily	
Metoclopramide	0.1 to 0.25 mg/kg tid to qid; IM, SC, IV (slow)	1.1 to 0.25 mg/kg tid to qid; IM, SC, IV (slow) 0.3 mg/kg tid to qid; SC (sheep)
Metronidazole	10 to 25 mg/kg bid to qid; IV, PO	Banned from use in food animals
Miconazole	Apply cream to dermatophyte lesions once daily for 2 to 4 weeks.	
Midazolam	0.011 to 0.044 mg/kg; IV	
Mineral oil	2 to 4 L via nasogastric tube	1 to 4 L via nasogastric tube 500 mL via nasogastric tube (sheep and goats)
Monensin	Highly toxic to horses	11 to 33 g/ton feed (feed efficiency) 22 g/ton feed (coccidiosis) One controlled release capsule for cattle 200 to 350 kg One controlled release capsule to dairy cows 2 to 4 weeks prior to calving (Canada only) 20 g/ton feed (goats, coccidiosis) 0.75% in salt mixture (sheep, coccidiosis)
Morantel tartrate		10 mg/kg; PO in feed
Morphine	0.02 to 0.04 mg/kg; IV 0.2 to 0.4 mg/kg; IM	0.05 to 0.2 mg/kg; epidural (analgesia)

(continued)

Drug	Horses (and Miniature Pig Doses, Where Indicated)	Ruminants (Cattle, Sheep, and Goats)
	0.05 to 0.2 mg/kg; epidural (analgesia) *Miniature pigs* 0.2 mg/kg; IM q 4 hours (<20 mg total dose)	
Moxidectin	0.4 mg/kg; PO	1.2 mg/kg; SC (Canada) 0.5 mg/kg; topically (pour-on)
Naloxone	0.01 to 0.02 mg/kg; IV	
Natamycin (5% w/v suspension)	Apply topically to corneas every 2 to 4 hours	
Neomycin	7 to 12 mg/kg daily; PO for 3 to 5 days *Miniature pigs:* 7 to 12 mg/kg; PO	7 to 12 mg/kg daily; PO for 3 to 5 days (Canada) 4.5 mg/kg daily; PO for up to 14 days (United States)
Neostigmine	0.02 mg/kg; SC	0.02 mg/kg; SC
Niacin (nicotinic acid)		6 g/head bid; PO
Nitrofurazone: See Nitrofurans	2.5 to 4.5 mg/kg tid; PO (urinary tract infections) Intrauterine use (solution): 30 to 100 mL every day or every second day (metritis) Topical ointment, solution, and powder; apply to wounds once to several times per day for 5 to 7 days	Banned for use in food animals
Nizatidine	6.6 mg/kg tid; PO	
Norepinephrine bitartrate	0.01 mg/kg; IM	0.01 mg/kg; IM
Novobiocin		150 mg or 400 mg intramammary infusion per quarter (dry treatment)

Drug	Horses (and Miniature Pig Doses, Where Indicated)	Ruminants (Cattle, Sheep, and Goats)
Omeprazole	4 mg/kg daily; PO for 4 weeks to treat ulcers 2 mg/kg daily; PO to prevent recurrence	
Orbifloxacin (See Fluoroquinolones)	7.5 mg/kg once daily; PO	Fluoroquinolones are banned from extralabel use in food-producing animals in the United States
Oxfendazole	10 mg/kg; PO. May be repeated in 24 to 48 hours for early and late 4th stage larvae.	4.5 mg/kg; PO 5 mg/kg; PO (sheep, *Moniezia* spp.)
Oxibendazole	10 to 15 mg/kg; PO	
Oxymorphone hydrochloride	0.01 to 0.03 mg/kg; IM, IV	
Oxytetracycline	6.6 mg/kg bid; IV (short-acting formulations) 20 mg/kg every 48 hours; IM (long-acting formulations)	6 to 11 mg/kg once daily; IV, IM, SC 5 to 22 mg/kg once daily to bid; PO Long-acting products: 20 mg/kg every 48 hours; IM, SC (maximum dose at one site, 10 mL)
Oxytocin	Obstetrics: 50 to 100 U; IV, IM, SC Milk letdown: 10 to 20 U; IV, IM, SC Parturition Induction: 2.5 to 5 U/450 kg q 20 minutes; IV as a bolus **OR** 80 to 100 U; IV in 500 mL saline as a drip	Obstetrics: 50 to 100 U; IV, IM, SC (cattle); 30 to 50 U; IV, IM, SC (sheep) Milk letdown: 10 to 20 U; IV, IM, SC (cattle); 5 to 20 U; IV, IM, SC (sheep) Mastitis: 20 to 40 U; IV, IM, SC

(continued)

Drug	Horses (and Miniature Pig Doses, Where Indicated)	Ruminants (Cattle, Sheep, and Goats)
	Miniature pigs: 10 to 20 U; IM per animal	
Pancuronium	0.044 to 0.066 mg/kg; IV	
Paregoric	0.1 to 0.2 mg/kg tid to qid; PO (foals)	0.1 to 0.2 mg/kg tid to qid; PO (calves)
Paromomycin		50 mg/kg bid; PO (calves, cryptosporidiosis)
Penicillamine	3 to 4 mg/kg qid; PO for 10 days	12 to 25 mg/kg bid; PO
Penicillin G benzathine/ penicillin G procaine	2,000 IU/kg each of penicillin G benzathine and penicillin G procaine every 48 hours (United States) 6,000 IU/kg each of penicillin G benzathine and penicillin G procaine every 3 to 5 days; IM (Canada) *Miniature pigs:* 7,500 IU/kg each of penicillin G benzathine and penicillin G procaine	2,000 IU/kg each of penicillin G benzathine and penicillin G procaine every 48 hours; SC only (United States; cattle) 6,000 IU/kg each of penicillin G benzathine and penicillin G procaine (Canada; cattle) 7,500 IU/kg each of penicillin G benzathine and penicillin G procaine (Canada; sheep) Clinically effective doses of penicillin often exceed most label doses; consult a gFARAD center for appropriate withdrawal times
Penicillin G, potassium or sodium salt	10,000 to 50,000 IU/kg qid; IM, IV	10,000 to 50,000 IU/kg qid; IM, IV
Penicillin G procaine	21,000 to 50,000 IU/kg bid; IM *Miniature pigs:* 15,000 to 45,000 IU/kg daily for up to 5 days; IM	21,000 to 66,000 IU/kg daily for up to 5 days, IM

Drug	Horses (and Miniature Pig Doses, Where Indicated)	Ruminants (Cattle, Sheep, and Goats)
		Clinically effective doses of penicillin far exceed most label doses; consult a gFARAD center for appropriate withdrawal times
Penicillin V	110,000 mg/kg bid to qid; PO (foals)	
Pentobarbital	87 to 108 mg/kg; IV, IP or intracardiac (euthanasia)	87 to 108 mg/kg; IV, IP or intracardiac (euthanasia)
Pentoxifylline	4.4 mg/kg tid; PO (navicular disease) 7 to 8.5 mg/kg tid; PO (endotoxemia, laminitis)	
Pergolide	2 µg/kg daily; PO	
Phenobarbital	Loading dose: 12 mg/kg IV over 20 minutes, then 6.65 mg/kg bid; IV 11 to 25 mg/kg daily; PO Loading dose for foals: 20 mg/kg IV over 20 minutes, then 9 mg/kg tid; IV	
Phenoxybenzamine	0.7 to 1 mg/kg; IV in 500 mL saline twice at 12-hour intervals (acute laminitis, diarrhea) 0.7 mg/kg; PO q 6 hours (urinary incontinence)	
Phenylbutazone	4.4 mg/kg once daily; IV, PO Maintain on lowest possible dose and longest possible dosing interval	4.4 mg/kg every 48 to 72 hours; IV, PO

(continued)

Drug	Horses (and Miniature Pig Doses, Where Indicated)	Ruminants (Cattle, Sheep, and Goats)
	Miniature pigs: 4 to 8 mg/kg daily; PO	
Phenylephrine (10% solution)	Apply topically to corneas	
Phenytoin	5 to 10 mg/kg; IV (loading dose); 1 to 5 mg/kg q 4 hours; IM, IV, PO to maintain serum concentrations of 5 to 10 µg/mL (seizuring foals) 10 to 22 mg/kg bid; PO (digoxin-induced arrhythmias) 10 to 15 mg/kg per day; PO (Australian stringhalt) 6 to 8 mg/kg tid; PO (exertional rhabdomyolysis)	5 to 10 mg/kg; IV (loading dose); 1 to 5 mg/kg q 4 hours; IM, IV, PO to maintain serum concentrations of 5 to 10 µg/mL (seizures)
Pilocarpine	4% gel applied topically to corneas bid to tid	4% gel applied topically to corneas bid to tid
Piperazine	104 to 112 mg/kg; PO *Miniature pigs:* 200 mg/kg; PO	
Pirlimycin		Infuse into affected quarter; repeat in 24 hours
Poloxalene		110 mg/kg daily; PO 1 g/45 kg per day as a top dressing or in feed Double dose for severe bloat conditions
Polymixin B	1,000 to 6,000 U/kg bid diluted in 1 L of 0.9% w/v saline infused over 30 minutes (endotoxemia)	

Drug	Horses (and Miniature Pig Doses, Where Indicated)	Ruminants (Cattle, Sheep, and Goats)
Polysulfated glyco-saminoglycans	250 mg; IA once weekly for up to 5 weeks 500 mg every 4 days; IM for 7 treatments	250 mg; IA once weekly for up to 5 weeks 500 mg every 4 days; IM for 7 treatments
Ponazuril	5 mg/kg daily for 28 days; PO	
Potassium chloride	0.5 mEq/kg per hour; IV; not to exceed 2 mEq/kg per day (hypokalemia) 5 to 20 g; PO in divided doses (digitalis toxicity)	0.5 mEq/kg per hour; IV; not to exceed 2 mEq/kg per day (hypokalemia) 5 to 50 g; PO in divided doses
Pralidoxime (PAM)	10 to 40 mg/kg; slowly IV, may be repeated. Use in conjunction with atropine.	10 to 40 mg/kg; slowly IV, may be repeated. Use in conjunction with atropine.
Prednisolone	2.2 mg/kg daily to bid; PO	
Prednisolone acetate	1% ointment applied topically to corneas qid	1% ointment applied topically to corneas qid 100 to 200 mg; IM (ketosis)
Prednisolone sodium phosphate	5.5 to 11 mg/kg as initial dose, followed by maintenance doses at 1-, 3-, 6-, or 10-hour intervals as needed; IV	
Prednisolone sodium succinate	0.25 to 1 mg/kg bid; IV (slow) or IM (inflammation) 15 to 30 mg/kg; IV (slow), repeat in 4 to 6 hours (shock)	

(continued)

Drug	Horses (and Miniature Pig Doses, Where Indicated)	Ruminants (Cattle, Sheep, and Goats)
Pregnant mares' serum gonadotropin (PMSG)	1,000 U; SC, IM, IV	1,000 to 1,250 U; IM, IV, SC (cattle) 300 to 1,000 U; IM, IV, SC (sheep) 1,500 to 3,000 U; IM between day 8 and 13 of the cycle (superovulation in cattle) 500 to 1,000 U; IM (anestrus in cattle) 400 to 700 U; IM following vaginal progestagen sponge removal (estrus synchronization in sheep)
Procainamide	1 mg/kg per minute; IV infusion up to a total dose of 20 mg/kg (ventricular tachycardia) 25 to 35 mg/kg tid; PO	
Progesterone	50 to 100 mg/454 kg; IM 150 mg/450 kg once daily; IM (suppress estrus) 300 mg/450 kg once daily; IM (maintain pregnancy)	50 to 300 mg/450 kg; IM (cattle) 10 to 15 mg/animal daily; IM (sheep and goats) 0.125 mg/kg bid; SC in combination with estrogen (17β-estradiol) at 0.05 mg/kg bid; SC for 7 days (lactation induction in cattle)
Propantheline	30 to 45 mg/454 kg; IV (compounded from tablets; use with caution)	
Proparacaine (0.5% w/v solution)	Apply topically to corneas	Apply topically to corneas

Drug	Horses (and Miniature Pig Doses, Where Indicated)	Ruminants (Cattle, Sheep, and Goats)
Propionibacterium acnes	3.5 µg/kg; IV Repeat on days 4 and 7, then once weekly.	
Propofol	After premedication with xylazine (0.5 mg/kg; IV), give 2.4 mg/kg; IV for induction. Maintenance at 0.3 mg/kg per minute; IV	
Propranolol	0.05 to 0.16 mg/kg bid; IV (ventricular tachycardia) 0.38 to 0.78 mg/kg tid; PO	
Propylene glycol: See also cobalt-containing products		1 mg/kg; PO drench. As an aid in the prevention of acetonemia in dairy cattle. Feed at the rate of 0.11 to 0.22 kg per head per day beginning two weeks before freshening (ketosis prevention). Continue feeding for 6 weeks after freshening. Feed at the rate of 0.11 to 0.45 kg per head per day for 10 days (ketosis treatment).
Prostaglandin $F_{2\alpha}$	5 mg; SC *Miniature pigs:* 5 mg; IM (estrus synchronization); 10 to 25 mg; IM 2 to 6 days prior	25 mg; IM (cattle) 30 mg, combined with dexamethasone at 20 mg; IM if pregnancy is

(continued)

Drug	Horses (and Miniature Pig Doses, Where Indicated)	Ruminants (Cattle, Sheep, and Goats)
	to expected parturition (parturition induction)	beyond 150 days (abortifacient in cattle) 2 to 3 mg; IM (goats, pseudopregnancy) 8 to 10 mg; IM (sheep and goats)
Protamine sulfate (1% w/v solution)	Administer 1 mg by slow IV injection to antagonize each 100 U of heparin remaining in the patient; hence, the dose should be reduced as time between heparin administration and start of treatment increases (i.e., after 30 minutes give only 0.5 mg for q 100 U heparin) (heparin-induced hemorrhages).	100 mg/adult cow; IV (bracken fern toxicosis)
Psyllium mucilloid	0.5 kg in 6 to 8 L of water via nasogastric tube (add to water immediately prior to administration) 1 g/kg once daily to qid; PO	
Pyrantel pamoate	6.6 mg/kg; PO 13.2 mg/kg; PO (tapeworms) *Miniature pigs:* 6.6 mg/kg; PO	
Pyrantel tartrate	2.6 mg/kg daily; PO	25 mg/kg; PO (sheep, goats, llamas)
Pyrimethamine	1 mg/kg once daily; PO for a minimum of 3 months, in combination with a	

Drug	Horses (and Miniature Pig Doses, Where Indicated)	Ruminants (Cattle, Sheep, and Goats)
	sulfonamide (equine protozoal encephalomyelitis)	
Quinidine	1.1 to 2.2 mg/kg q 10 minutes; IV until conversion or desired effect [Gluconate]; total dose not to exceed 11 mg/kg 22 mg/kg q 2 hours; PO until conversion or desired effect [Sulfate]; do not exceed 132 mg/kg total dose	48 mg/kg; IV slowly over a 4-hour period [Sulfate]
Ranitidine	1.5 mg/kg bid to tid; IV 6.6 to 8 mg/kg tid; PO	45 mg/kg; PO (sheep)
Rifampin	5 to 10 mg/kg bid; PO	
Romifidine	0.04 to 0.1 mg/kg; IV	
Sevoflurane	Induction: 3% to 5% Maintenance: 1.5% to 2%	Induction: 3% to 6% Maintenance: 1.5% to 3%
Sodium bicarbonate	Emergency use: 2 to 5 mEq/kg; IV by rapid infusion of a 7.5% w/v solution; for less urgent metabolic acidosis: 2 to 5 mEq/kg of an isotonic (1.3% w/v solution) over 4 to 8 hours; IV 30 g bid; PO (acidosis in chronic renal failure)	Emergency use: 2 to 5 mEq/kg; IV by rapid infusion of a 7.5% w/v solution; for less urgent metabolic acidosis: 2 to 5 mEq/kg of an isotonic (1.3% w/v solution) over 4 to 8 hours; IV 30 g bid; PO (acidosis in chronic renal failure)
Sodium chloride	Isotonic (0.9% w/v): 40 mL/kg per day; IV (maintenance)	Isotonic (0.9% w/v): 40 mL/kg per day; IV (maintenance)

(continued)

Drug	Horses (and Miniature Pig Doses, Where Indicated)	Ruminants (Cattle, Sheep, and Goats)
	40 to 100 mL/kg per hour; IV (shock; if the higher dose is used, central venous pressure should be monitored) Hypertonic (7.5% w/v) saline: 4 to 5 mL/kg over 10 minutes; IV (hemorrhagic shock)	40 to 100 mL/kg per hour; IV (shock; if the higher dose is used, central venous pressure should be monitored) Hypertonic (7.5% w/v) saline: 4 to 5 mL/kg over 10 minutes; IV (hemorrhagic shock, abomasal disease) Feed to 4% w/w in ration (urolithiasis prevention)
Sodium cromoglycate	200 mg bid; via metered dose inhaler 80 mg daily; via jet nebulizer	
Sodium iodide	2 to 8 g; IV (20% w/v solution) as a mucolytic 20 to 40 mg/kg once daily; PO for several weeks	Not for use in lactating dairy cattle 80 mg/kg; IV (10% w/v solution for sheep, 20% w/v solution for cattle) at weekly intervals (*Actinobacillus*) 66 to 222 mg/kg; IV **OR** to 40 mL; IV (cattle), 5 to 20 mL; IV (sheep) as a mucolytic
Sodium sulfate		1 to 3 g/kg; PO (cathartic) 1 g/day for 4 weeks; PO (sheep, mobilize excessive hepatic copper)
Sodium thiosulfate; IV (25% w/v solution)	30 to 40 mg/kg; IV (cyanide toxicity)	660 mg/kg; IV

Drug	Horses (and Miniature Pig Doses, Where Indicated)	Ruminants (Cattle, Sheep, and Goats)

Spectinomycin	20 mg/kg tid; IM
	Miniature pigs:
	    10 mg/kg once daily
	    for 3 to 5 days; PO
		10 to 15 mg/kg daily
		    for 3 to 5 days;
		    SC in the neck

Stanozolol	0.55 mg/kg; IM once
	    weekly for up to
	    4 doses	

Sucralfate	2 to 4 g/450 kg bid-qid; PO	

Sulfachlorpyridazine		33 to 49.5 mg/kg bid
		    for 1 to 5 days;
		    IV, PO

Sulfadiazine-
    trimethoprim: See
    Sulfonamides;
    Potentiated
	15 mg/kg bid; IV
	30 mg/kg bid to tid; PO
	Miniature pigs: 25 to
	    50 mg/kg once
	    daily; PO	

Sulfadimethoxine	55 mg/kg; IV; then
	    27.5 mg/kg once
	    daily for up to
	    5 days; IV
		55 mg/kg; IV, PO;
		    then 27.5 mg/kg
		    once daily for up
		    to 5 days; IV, PO
		137.5 mg/kg every
		    4 days; PO
		    (sustained-release
		    boluses)

Sulfadoxine-
    trimethoprim: See
    Sulfonamides;
    Potentiated
		16 mg/kg daily; IV
		    (slow), IM

Sulfamethazine		247.5 mg/kg once; PO
		    then 123.75 mg/
		    kg daily for 3 days
		    (drinking water
		    solution)
		400 mg/kg once; PO
		    (sustained-release
		    bolus)

Terbutaline	0.02 to 0.06 mg/kg bid; IV	

(continued)

Drug	Horses (and Miniature Pig Doses, Where Indicated)	Ruminants (Cattle, Sheep, and Goats)
	1 : 1,000 to 1 : 100,000,000; intradermally (anhidrosis testing)	
Testosterone	6.6 to 11.1 mg/kg; IM once a week for 3 to 5 weeks	
Testosterone and estradiol		One implant (200 mg testosterone propionate, 20 mg estradiol benzoate) inserted under the skin of the ear in the center one third of the ear (cattle)
Tetanus antitoxin	Prevention: 1,500 U; IM, SC, IP can be repeated in 7 days Treatment: 30,000 to 100,000 U; IV, IM, SC (Note: label dose varies with product)	Prevention: 1,500 U; IM, SC Can be repeated in 7 days (cattle) 500 U; IM, SC (sheep, calves, and swine) 200 U; IM, SC (lambs) Treatment: 10,000 to 50,000 U; IM cattle) 3,000 to 15,000 U; IM (sheep and swine)
Tetracycline hydrochloride		11 mg/kg bid for up to 5 days; PO
Theophylline: See Aminophylline	5 to 15 mg/kg bid; PO	
Thiamine (Vitamin B$_1$)	0.5 to 5 mg/kg; IV, IM, PO	10 mg/kg diluted in 5% w/v dextrose; IV (slow) then 10 mg/kg bid for 2 to 3 days; IM (polioencephalomalacia)

Drug	Horses (and Miniature Pig Doses, Where Indicated)	Ruminants (Cattle, Sheep, and Goats)
		2 mg/kg qid; IM (concurrently with CaEDTA for lead poisoning)
Thiopental: See Thiobarbiturates	6 to 13 mg/kg (average 8.25 mg/kg); IV (with preanesthetic) 9 to 15.5 mg/kg (Pentothal) **OR** 4.4 to 10 mg/kg (Induthol); IV (without preanesthetic), up to 12.5 mg/kg for small ponies Maximum of 9 mg/kg; IV in horses > 545 kg 10 to 15 mg/kg; IV (maintenance) *Miniature pigs:* 10 mg/kg; IV (to effect)	8.2 to 10 mg/kg; IV (with premedication, bovine over 136 kg), not to exceed 22 mg/kg total dose 6.6 mg/kg; IV (unweaned calves) 10 to 14 mg/kg; IV (sheep) Induction: 3 to 5 mg/kg; IV (with preanesthetic) Maintenance: 15 to 22 mg/kg; IV over 4 to 5 minutes (calves) Maintenance: 20 to 22 mg/kg; IV over 4 to 5 minutes (goats)
Tilmicosin		10 mg/kg once; SC
Tobramycin	1 to 1.7 mg/kg tid; IV	
Tolazoline	4 mg/kg; IV (slow)	2 to 4 mg/kg; IV (slow)
Triamcinolone	0.02 to 0.1 mg/kg; IM, SC 6 to 18 mg; IA 0.02 to 0.1 mg/kg; IM 10 mg; subconjunctivally q 2 to 4 days	0.02 to 0.04 mg/kg; IM, SC 6 to 18 mg; IA
Trichloromethiazide/ dexamethasone	1.1 mL/100 kg bid; IM for the first day, then once daily for 2 additional days	1 to 2 boluses initially followed by ½ to 1 bolus a day to effect; PO (adult cattle)

(continued)

Drug	Horses (and Miniature Pig Doses, Where Indicated)	Ruminants (Cattle, Sheep, and Goats)
		20 mL; IM prior to, at the time of, or immediately following parturition (Canada only); follow up with bolus form in 12 to 36 hours
Trifluridine (1% w/v solution)	Apply q 2 to 3 hours to cornea	Apply q 2 to 3 hours to cornea
Triplennamine: See Antihistamines	0.4 to 1.1 mg/kg bid to tid; IM, IV	0.4 to 1.1 mg/kg; IM, IV
Tropicamide (0.5% to 1% w/v ophthalmic drops)	Apply once to cornea	Apply once to cornea
Tylosin	Do not administer to horses *Miniature pigs:* 5 to 8.8 mg/kg; IM	17.6 mg/kg once daily; IM 6.6 mg/kg once daily; IM (goats) 400 mg once daily; IM for 2 days (sheep, chlamydial abortion)
Vancomycin	20 to 40 mg/kg bid to qid; IV	
Vedoprofen	2 mg/kg; PO loading dose, followed by 1 mg/kg bid; PO	
Vitamin A	1,000 IU/kg in feed 2,000 IU/kg in feed (growth)	1,000 IU/kg feed 2 million IU per cow; IM (vitamin A deficiency) 2,200 IU/kg feed (growth in cattle) 400 IU/kg feed (growth in sheep) 3,200 to 3,800 IU/kg feed (lactating cattle) 750 IU/kg feed (pregnant sheep)

Drug	Horses (and Miniature Pig Doses, Where Indicated)	Ruminants (Cattle, Sheep, and Goats)
Vitamin D₃		10 million IU/adult cow; IM during the period from the 2nd to the 8th day preceding calving. When calving is delayed, a second dose can be given 8 days after the initial injection (prevention of parturient paresis in cows).
Vitamin E + selenium (E + Se)	1 mL E + Se (2.5 mg selenium) per 45 kg; by deep IM injection, may be repeated at 5- to 10-day intervals See individual products for further information.	See individual products for information.
Vitamin K₁	0.5 to 2.5 mg/kg; slowly IV, diluted in D₅W or 0.9% w/v saline (acute hypoprothrombinemia with severe hemorrhage) Not to exceed 10 mg/minute in mature animals or 5 mg/minute in newborn animals 0.5 to 2.5 mg/kg; SC, IM (nonacute hypoprothrombinemia) 0.5 to 1 mg/kg q 4 to 6 hours; SC (warfarin toxicosis) 1 to 2 mg/kg; SC divided at several sites (sweet clover poisoning)	0.5 to 2.5 mg/kg; slowly IV, diluted in D₅W or 0.9% w/v saline (acute hypoprothrombinemia with severe hemorrhage) Not to exceed 10 mg/minute in mature animals or 5 mg/minute in newborn animals 0.5 to 2.5 mg/kg; SC, IM (nonacute hypoprothrombinemia) 0.5 to 1 mg/kg q 4 to 6 hours; SC (warfarin toxicosis)

(continued)

Drug	Horses (and Miniature Pig Doses, Where Indicated)	Ruminants (Cattle, Sheep, and Goats)
		1 to 2 mg/kg; SC divided at several sites (sweet clover poisoning)
Xylazine	1.1 mg/kg; IV 2.2 mg/kg; IM 0.3 to 0.6 mg/kg; IV prior to sodium pentobarbital, sodium thiopental, nitrous oxide, ether, halothane, or glyceryl guaiacolate 0.33 mg/kg; IV followed by 0.033 to 0.066 mg/kg; IV butorphanol 1.1 mg/kg; IV followed by 1.76 to 2.2 mg/kg; IV ketamine 0.6 mg/kg; IV with 0.02 mg/kg acepromazine; IV 0.17 to 0.22 mg/kg diluted into 10 mL saline, epidurally *Miniature pigs:* 0.5 to 3 mg/kg; IM	0.05 to 0.33 mg/kg; IM 0.044 to 0.11 mg/kg; IV 0.01 to 0.22 mg/kg; IM (sheep and goats) Use extreme caution with xylazine administration to small ruminants
Yohimbine	0.12 mg/kg slowly IV (xylazine reversal) 0.15 mg/kg; IV q 3 hours (postoperative ileus) *Miniature pigs:* 0.12 mg/kg; IV (xylazine reversal)	0.12 mg/kg; slowly IV (xylazine reversal)
Zeranol		36 mg (all cattle), 72 mg (steers only) or 12 mg (feedlot lambs); SC in the ear

Handbook of Veterinary Drugs, Third Edition, edited by Dana Allen,
Lippincott Williams & Wilkins, Baltimore. © 2005

Section 5

Antimicrobial, Antiparasitic, and Anthelmintic Agents in Large Animals

TABLE 5-1 **Antimicrobial Agents in Large Animals Pending Microbial Culture**

Organism	Drugs of Choice	Alternative Drugs
Actinobacillus lignieresii	Sodium iodide and sulfas	Sodium iodide and oxytetracycline
Actinobacillus equuli, A. suis	Cephalosporins	Enrofloxacin Ampicillin/Sulbactam Trimethoprim/sulfa
Actinomyces	Penicillin G	Tetracyclines
Anaerobic organisms	Penicillins	Metronidazole (E) Ampicillin Cephalosporins Tilmicosin (R) Florfenicol (R) Oxytetracycline

(continued)

Organism	Drugs of Choice	Alternative Drugs
Archanobacterium pyogenes	Florfenicol	Penicillin G Tilmicosin
Bacillus anthracis	Penicillin G	Tetracyclines
Bacteroides spp.	Penicillin G	Metronidazole (E) Ampicillin Cephalosporins Tilmicosin (R) Florfenicol (R) Oxytetracycline
Bacteroides spp (penicillinase-producing)	Metronidazole	Chloramphenicol (E) Tilmicosin (R) Florfenicol (R)
Bordetella bronchiseptica	Ceftiofur	Gentamicin (E) Tetracyclines Trimethoprim/sulfa
Campylobacter (abortions)	Tetracyclines	
Chlamydia psittaci	Tetracyclines	Erythromycin
Clostridia spp.	Penicillin G	Metronidazole (E) Cephalosporins Oxytetracycline Tilmicosin (R) Florfenicol (R)
Coccidia	Sulfonamides	Amprolium Ionophores
Dermatophilus	Penicillin G	Cephalosporins Trimethoprim/sulfa
Enterobacter	Enrofloxacin	Gentamicin (E) Ceftiofur
Escherichia coli	Aminoglycosides (E)	Enrofloxacin Ceftiofur
Fusobacterium necrophorum	Penicillin G	Tetracyclines Ceftiofur Tilmicosin Florfenicol Tylosin
Haemophilus spp.	Ceftiofur	Danofloxacin ★ Enrofloxacin Florfenicol Oxytetracycline

Organism	Drugs of Choice	Alternative Drugs
		Spectinomycin Tilmicosin Trimethoprim/ sulfadoxine ♣
Klebsiella	Amikacin (E)	Ceftiofur Ampicillin/sulbactam Enrofloxacin Trimethoprim/ sulfadiazine (E)
Leptospira spp.	Tetracyclines	Dihydrostreptomycin ♣
Listeria monocyto- genes	Oxytetracycline	Penicillin G
Mannheimia (Pasteu- rella) haemolytica	Tilmicosin	Ceftiofur Danofloxacin ★ Enrofloxacin ★ Florfenicol Oxytetracycline Spectinomycin Trimethoprim/ sulfadoxine ♣
Mycoplasma spp.	Tiamulin (S) Tetracyclines	Tylosin Tilmicosin Enrofloxacin
Neorickettsia (Ehrlichia) risticii	Oxytetracycline	Erythromycin
Pasteurella spp. (in horses)	Ceftiofur	Ampicillin Ampicillin/sulbactam Enrofloxacin Gentamicin Erythromycin Oxytetracycline Trimethoprim/sulfa
Pasteurella multocida	Tilmicosin	Ceftiofur Danofloxacin ★ Enrofloxacin Florfenicol Oxytetracycline Spectinomycin Trimethoprim/ sulfadoxine ♣

(continued)

Organism	Drugs of Choice	Alternative Drugs
Proteus spp.	Ceftiofur	Amikacin (E) Enrofloxacin Gentamicin (E)
Pseudomonas spp.	Amikacin (E) Polymixin B (topical)	Enrofloxacin Gentamicin (E)
Rhodococcus equi	Azithromycin	Erythromycin/rifampin Enrofloxacin
Salmonella spp.	Enrofloxacin	Amikacin (E) Ampicillin Ceftiofur Gentamicin (E)
Sarcocystis neurona	Ponazuril	Pyrimethamine/ sulfadiazine
Staphylococcus aureus	Gentamicin (E) Tilmicosin (R)	Amikacin (E) Ampicillin/sulbactam Azithromycin (E) Ceftiofur Enrofloxacin Erythromycin
Streptococcus equi	Penicillin G	Ampicillin Ceftiofur Erythromycin Gentamicin Trimethoprim/sulfa
Streptococcus zooepi-demicus	Penicillin G	Ampicillin Ceftiofur Erythromycin Gentamicin

E, equine; R, ruminant; S, swine.

TABLE 5-2 **Anthelmintics and Parasiticides in Horses**[a]

Drug	Indications	Larvacidal
Febantel	Large and small strongyles *Parascaris* spp. *Oxyuris* spp.	+ for 4th stage *Oxyuris*
Fenbendazole	*Parascaris* spp. Large and small strongyles *Oxyuris* spp.	− at label dose, + at 10 mg/kg;PO for 5days, 50 mg/kg for 3 days
Ivermectin	*Parascaris* spp. Large and small strongyles *Onchocerca* *Habronema* *Draschia* (summer sores) Bots Lice	+ +
Moxidectin	*Parascaris* spp. Large and small strongyles *Onchocerca* *Habronema* *Draschia* (summer sores) Bots Lice	+ +
Oxibendazole	*Parascaris* spp. Large and small strongyles *Strongyloides* spp. *Oxyuris* spp.	
Piperazine	*Parascaris* spp. Large and small strongyles *Oxyuris* spp.	+
Ponazuril	*Sarcocystis neurona*	
Pyrantel	*Parascaris* spp. Large and small strongyles *Oxyuris* spp.	+ (when administered daily)

[a] Indications may include drugs not specifically approved for horses. Large strongyles include *Strongylus vulgaris*, *Strongylus edentatus*, and *Strongylus equinum*. Extra-label use may be based on anecdotal reports rather than on controlled clinical studies. The reader is directed to the section on drug descriptions.

TABLE 5-3   **Anthelmintics and Parasiticides in Ruminants**[a]

Drug	Indications	Larvacidal
Albendazole	*Fasciola* spp. (liver flukes) All gastrointestinal nematodes (except *Trichuris*) *Moniezia* (tapeworms) *Dictyocaulus* (lung worms)	+
Clorsulon	*Fasciola* spp. (liver flukes)	
Doramectin	All gastrointestinal nematodes (except *Nematodirus*) *Dictyocaulus* (lung worms) *Hypoderma* spp. Lice, mites, flies	+
Eprinomectin	All gastrointestinal nematodes Dictyocaulus (lung worms) *Hypoderma* spp. Lice, mites, flies	+
Fenbendazole	All gastrointestinal nematodes (except *Trichuris*) *Dictyocaulus* (lung worms) *Moniezia* (tapeworms)	±
Ivermectin	All gastrointestinal nematodes (except *Nematodirus*) *Dictyocaulus* (lung worms) *Hypoderma* spp. Lice, mites, flies, Oestrus ovis	+
Levamisole	All gastrointestinal nematodes (except *Trichuris*) *Dictyocaulus* (lung worms)	± variable
Morantel	All gastrointestinal nematodes (except *Trichuris*, *Bunostomum*)	
Moxidectin	All gastrointestinal nematodes (except *Trichuris*) *Dictyocaulus* (lung worms) *Hypoderma* spp. Lice, mites, flies	+

[a] Indications may include drugs not specifically approved for ruminants. Where ruminants are indicated, many products are not approved for sheep or goats. Extralabel use may be based on anecdotal reports rather than on controlled clinical studies. The reader is directed to the section on drug descriptions.

Handbook of Veterinary Drugs, Third Edition, edited by Dana Allen,
Lippincott Williams & Wilkins, Baltimore. © 2005

Section 6

Description of Drugs for Large Animals

ACEPROMAZINE

INDICATIONS: Acepromazine [formerly acetylpromazine] (AceProject ★, Acepro ✦ ★, Acevet ✦, Ace ✦, Atravet ✦, Atravet Soluble Granules ✦, Promace ★) is a phenothiazine tranquilizer approved for use in large animals to ease handling or trailering. When used as a preanesthetic, it markedly potentiates barbiturates. It also has antispasmodic effects through its partial blockade of α-adrenergic receptors and has been used in spasmodic colic. It is used to reduce muscle spasms in animals with tetanus and exertional rhabdomyolysis. Additionally, acepromazine is used to cause relaxation and protrusion of the penis for catheterization in the stallion or gelding. Acepromazine reduces the incidence of malignant hyperthermia in susceptible swine. Acepromazine is not approved for use in food animals in the United States, but it is approved in Canada.

ADVERSE AND COMMON SIDE EFFECTS: Tranquilization of dangerous animals may lead to a false sense of security; therefore, painful procedures should be avoided because acepromazine has no analgesic effect. Horses may react to sudden noises or movements despite appearing somnolent. The tranquilizing effect may last longer than the label indication of 8 hours. Even at high therapeutic doses, recumbency is unusual and the risk of the horse stepping or falling on attending personnel is minimal. An adequate blood volume and arterial blood pressure are necessary for the use of acepromazine because of its marked arterial hypotensive effects. The drug is extensively bound to plasma proteins (>99%); therefore, the dose should be reduced in hypoproteinemic animals. Acepromazine temporarily lowers the hematocrit of a horse by 25% and up to 50% in a dose-dependent manner via splenic sequestration. Penile protrusion occurs within 30 minutes following administration and can last for several hours; the extent and duration of penile protrusion are dose related. Priapism can occur in the horse, more commonly in stallions or recently castrated geldings. In cattle, acepromazine may induce only mild sedation or be ineffective in unmanageable or hyperexcited cattle. When used as a premedicant in cattle, regurgitation during induction may occur and recovery from general anesthesia may not be as smooth as when not administered. The central nervous system seizure threshold is decreased with phenothiazines, and acepromazine should not be used in susceptible animals such as foals with neonatal maladjustment or as a premedicant before myelography. Intracarotid injection may cause severe CNS excitement, seizures, and death.

DRUG INTERACTIONS: Toxicity of carbamates and organophosphates (e.g., physostigmine and trichlorfon) may be enhanced by the administration of phenothiazines; therefore, concurrent use is contraindicated. As phenothiazines are β-adrenergic receptor antagonists, concurrent administration of epinephrine may cause unopposed β-adrenergic effects. Benztropine mesylate (8 mg; IV for an adult horse) may reverse acepromazine-induced penile prolapse.

SUPPLIED AS VETERINARY PRODUCTS:
For injection containing 10 and 25 mg/mL
Tablets containing 10 and 25 mg
For oral use as soluble granules 1.25 mg/277 g

OTHER USES
Horses
STANDING CHEMICAL RESTRAINT
Acepromazine is often combined with sedatives and administered IV (0.02 mg/kg acepromazine plus 0.66 mg/kg xylazine) or opioids (acepromazine 0.04 mg/kg with 0.6 mg/kg meperidine IV or 0.02 mg/kg butorphanol; IV or 0.4 mg/kg pentazocine; IV).

ACUTE LAMINITIS
Acepromazine (0.044 mg/kg qid; IM) is also used for 4 to 5 days for α-adrenergic receptor blockade against presumed arterial hypertension during acute laminitis.

Ruminants
GENERAL ANESTHESIA
For procedures requiring short-acting general anesthesia, administer 0.05 to 0.1 mg/kg; IM or IV as a premedication, followed by ketamine at 2 to 5 mg/kg; IV.

ACETAZOLAMIDE

INDICATIONS: Acetazolamide (Acetazolam ✤, AK-Zol ★, Apo-Acetazolamide ✤, Dazamide ★, Diamox ✤ ★, Storzolamide ★) is a carbonic anhydrase inhibitor that increases the urinary excretion of bicarbonate and decreases extracellular potassium, reduces intraocular pressure, and reduces the rate of formation of cerebrospinal fluid, but transiently causes an increase in cerebrospinal fluid pressure. It is most commonly used to reduce intraocular pressure in glaucoma, a disease not common in large animals. Because it increases potassium excretion, acetazolamide is used to manage hyperkalemic periodic paralysis in horses.

ADVERSE AND COMMON SIDE EFFECTS: In humans, acetazolamide can cause somnolence, behavioral changes, and paresthesia. Hypersensitivity reactions are rare, manifesting as fever, skin rash, and bone marrow suppression. The drug depresses uptake of iodine by the thyroid gland. Teratogenic effects have been reported and the drug should not be used in pregnant animals.

DRUG INTERACTIONS: Because acetazolamide alkalinizes the urine, it may interfere with the renal elimination of other basic drugs (e.g., quinidine, procainamide, phenobarbital). Concurrent use with other diuretics may cause potassium depletion.

SUPPLIED AS HUMAN PRODUCTS:
Capsules (extended release) containing 500 mg
Tablets containing 125 mg and 250 mg

ACETIC ACID (5% w/v)

INDICATIONS: Acetic acid (vinegar) is used to treat nonprotein nitrogen-induced ammonia toxicosis in ruminants. The acetic acid administered lowers rumen pH, which favors the shift in uncharged ammonia to the charged ammonium ion, which reduces absorption of ammonia. Cold water is also administered to reduce the rumen temperature and hence the formation of ammonia. Acetic acid is also suggested for the prevention of enterolith formation in horses, by altering colonic pH.

ADVERSE AND COMMON SIDE EFFECTS: Acetic acid is irritating to mucous membranes and large quantities should be administered through a stomach tube.

DRUG INTERACTIONS: Unknown.

SUPPLIED AS:
Commercially available as a liquid

OTHER USES: Acetic acid is also used in solutions for udder washes and in proprietary preparations as a poultice.

ACETYLCYSTEINE

INDICATIONS: Acetylcysteine (Mucomyst ✤ ★, Mucosil ★, Parvolex ✤ ★) is available as a 10% or 20% w/v solution that can be nebulized to patients. Its mucolytic effect is due to the exposed sulfhydryl groups on the compound, which interact with disulfide bonds on mucoprotein. Acetylcysteine helps to break down respiratory mucus and enhance clearance. Acetylcysteine may also increase the levels of glutathione, which is a scavenger of oxygen-free radicals. Dilution to a less than 10% solution reduces the activity of acetylcysteine. Acetylcysteine is used to treat persistent meconium retention in foals, by breaking the disulfide bond of the mucoproteins in the meconium.

ADVERSE AND COMMON SIDE EFFECTS: Aerosolization of acetylcysteine can cause reflex bronchoconstriction due to irritant receptor stimulation, so its use should be preceded by bronchodilator therapy.

DRUG INTERACTIONS: Acetylcysteine inactivates ampicillin, amphotericin B, erythromycin lactobionate, and tetracycline antibiotics if used together as an aerosol.

SUPPLIED AS HUMAN PRODUCTS:
For oral inhalation or intratracheal instillation containing a 10% or 20% w/v sterile solution
Parvolex is also labeled for IV and oral use in humans.

OTHER USES
Horses
MECONIUM IMPACTION
As an enema for foals with meconium impaction, 120 to 240 mL of a 4% w/v solution is administered via a 30-gauge Foley catheter into the rectum and retained in place for 4 to 5 minutes. Repeat in 1 hour and with a slightly higher volume if necessary. The solution is made by mixing 8 g acetylcysteine powder and 20 g sodium bicarbonate (baking soda; to bring the pH to 7.6) in sufficient water to make 200 mL.

ALBENDAZOLE

INDICATIONS: Albendazole (Valbazen ✤ ★) is a broad-spectrum anthelmintic recommended for the treatment of internal parasites of cattle, including liver flukes (adult stage of *Fasciola hepatica, Fascioloides magna*), tapeworms (adult *Moniezia benedeni*), gastric worms (adult *Haemonchus placei, Trichostrongylus axei*, adult, 4th larval, and inhibited 4th larval stage of *Ostertagia ostertagi*), intestinal worms (adult stages of *Trichostrongylus colubriformis, Bunostomum phlebotomum, Nematodirus helvetianus,* and *Oesophagostomum radiatum*), and lungworms (adult and 4th larval stages of *Dictyocaulus viviparus*). Albendazole is also used in sheep and goats for most adult gastrointestinal nematodes and lungworms. Albendazole is the only broad-spectrum anthelmintic effective against adult liver flukes (*F. hepatica*) in sheep.

ADVERSE AND COMMON SIDE EFFECTS: The drug should not be used in female cattle in the first 45 days of pregnancy (21 days, Canada) or within 45 days (21 days, Canada) of removing bulls from the herd.

DRUG INTERACTIONS: None listed.

SUPPLIED AS VETERINARY PRODUCTS:
As a suspension containing 113.6 mg/mL
As a 30% w/w paste

OTHER USES
Sheep and Goats
MONIEZIA
3 to 8 mg/kg; PO
FLUKES
10 to 20 mg/kg; PO

ALBUTEROL

INDICATIONS: Albuterol (known as salbutamol in Canada and Europe) (Torpex ★, Proventil ★, Ventolin ✚ ★) is a short-acting β_2-receptor agonist delivered via metered dose inhaler in the treatment of acute bronchoconstriction. Stimulation of pulmonary β_2-adrenergic receptors increases activity of the enzyme adenylate cyclase, which increases cyclic adenosine monophosphate (AMP), and relaxes bronchial smooth muscle. Stimulation of β receptors decreases the release of inflammatory mediators from mast cells, but other inflammatory cells are not suppressed. The β_2-adrenergic receptor agonists also increase mucociliary clearance in the respiratory tract. Albuterol should always be used in conjunction with anti-inflammatory drugs in the treatment of inflammatory respiratory disease.

ADVERSE AND COMMON SIDE EFFECTS: With inhalation therapy, high drug concentrations are delivered directly to the lungs and systemic side effects are avoided or minimized. Chronic use of β_2-adrenergic receptor agonists may lead to down regulation of β_2-adrenergic receptors and decreased clinical efficacy. Despite being ideal for therapy of recurrent airway obstruction and inflammatory airway disease, the use of inhaled medications in performance horses is currently controversial and not permitted by most organizations. Albuterol can be detected by sport regulating authorities for a short period of time after administration by inhalation.

DRUG INTERACTIONS: The concurrent use of epinephrine and other sympathomimetic (adrenergic) agents and antihistamines may have additive effects and is not recommended. Monoamine inhibitors, possibly amitraz, may potentiate the action of the drug on the vascular system. Propranolol and other β-adrenergic receptor blocking agents may inhibit the effect of the drug. Theophylline or aminophylline may potentiate the bronchodilatory effects of albuterol.

SUPPLIED AS VETERINARY PRODUCT:
Aerosol drug delivery device (Torpex) delivering 120 µg/metered spray

HUMAN PRODUCTS
Inhalation aerosol delivering 90 µg (100 µg Canada) per metered spray (In the United States, metered dose inhalers [MDIs] are labeled according to the amount of drug delivered at the valve; while in Canada, they are labeled according to the amount of drug delivered to the mouthpiece of the actuator.)

ALTRENOGEST

INDICATIONS: Altrenogest (Regu-Mate ♣ ★) is a progestin used to suppress estrus in mares for a predictable occurrence of estrus following drug withdrawal. Suppression of estrus will encourage regular cycles following winter anestrus, facilitate scheduled breeding, and help manage mares exhibiting prolonged estrus. Ovulation will occur 5 to 7 days following the onset of estrus. Use of prostaglandin $F_2\alpha$ or a synthetic analog immediately following an 8- to 12-day course of altrenogest (label indication is 15 days) will induce estrus.

ADVERSE AND COMMON SIDE EFFECTS: Altrenogest is contraindicated in pregnant mares because higher doses have caused fetal abnormalities in laboratory animals. Pregnant women and women of childbearing age should use extreme caution when handling altrenogest as accidental dermal absorption could disrupt the menstrual cycle or prolong pregnancy.

DRUG INTERACTIONS: None listed.

SUPPLIED AS VETERINARY PRODUCT:
For oral administration, altrenogest solution containing 2.2 mg/mL and gel containing 2.15 mg/g syringe

AMIKACIN

INDICATIONS: Amikacin (Amiglyde-V ❀ ★, Amikacin sulfate ★, Amikin ❀ ★, Amifuse E ★, Amiject D ★, Amikacin C Injection ★, Am Tech AmiMax ★, Equi-Phar EquiGlide ★) was developed from kanamycin, and it has the broadest spectrum of activity among the aminoglycosides. It is effective against strains not susceptible to other aminoglycosides because it is more resistant to bacterial enzymatic inactivation and it is considered the least nephrotoxic. It is labeled for intrauterine treatment of genital tract infections such as endometritis, metritis, and pyometra in mares. Indications for parenteral use include bacteremia in neonatal foals and skin and soft tissue infections caused by *E. coli, Salmonella, Actinobacillus, Proteus, Pseudomonas,* or *Klebsiella* spp. Streptococci are often resistant, so a β-lactam antibiotic is usually administered concurrently. High-dose, once daily therapy is now recommended to maximize efficacy and minimize toxicity. Peak concentrations are targeted to achieve plasma concentrations that are 10 times the minimum inhibitory concentration (MIC) of the target pathogen. As the trough concentration is associated with nephrotoxicity, it is recommended that the amikacin concentration be less than 5 μg/mL before the next dose is administered.

ADVERSE AND COMMON SIDE EFFECTS: Amikacin should be used with caution in animals with compromised kidney function and is contraindicated in cases of severe renal impairment. High trough concentrations can cause renal tubular damage, which may be reversible once the drug is discontinued. Concurrent use with other nephrotoxic drugs should be avoided because of potential toxic additive effects. Ototoxicity can occur but is difficult to detect clinically. Neuromuscular blockade is a rare effect, related to blockade of acetylcholine at the nicotinic cholinergic receptor and is most often seen when anesthetic agents are administered concurrently with aminoglycosides. Affected patients should be treated promptly with parenteral calcium. Renal accumulation results in prolonged kidney residues; therefore, it should not be used in food animals. See also AMINOGLYCOSIDES.

DRUG INTERACTIONS: See AMINOGLYCOSIDES.

SUPPLIED AS VETERINARY PRODUCTS:
For injection containing 50 mg/mL
Solution for intrauterine infusion containing 250 mg/mL

SUPPLIED AS HUMAN PRODUCT:
For injection containing 50 and 250 mg/mL

AMINOGLYCOSIDES

INDICATIONS: The aminoglycoside antibiotics include streptomycin, neomycin, gentamicin, amikacin, tobramycin, and kanamycin. They are used for the treatment of gram-negative infections caused by staphylococci and enteric pathogens such as *E. coli*. They are often effective against enterococci, but therapy against streptococci is more effective when combined with a β-lactam antibiotic. Their action is bactericidal, and dose (concentration) dependent. The aminoglycosides are large polar antibiotics; therefore their distribution is limited to the extracellular fluid space. The volume of distribution is higher in neonates; therefore, they require higher doses than adults. Following parenteral administration, effective concentrations are obtained in synovial, perilymph, pleural, peritoneal, and pericardial fluid. Therapeutic concentrations are not achieved in bile, cerebrospinal fluid, respiratory secretions, prostatic and ocular fluids and aminoglycosides do not cross the placenta. The predominant site of drug accumulation is the renal cortex. High-dose, once-daily dosing of aminoglycosides has now become common in human and veterinary medicine; since it takes advantage of the concentration-dependent killing and long postantibiotic effect (PAE) of these drugs and avoids first exposure adaptive resistance and toxicity. Individuals can differ widely in the serum concentrations produced from the same aminoglycoside dosage regimen. When this relative unpredictability is combined with the often small difference between therapeutic and toxic serum concentrations, determining serum concentrations in a particular patient becomes very valuable. There is a tendency to underdose neonatal patients, especially those that are receiving aggressive fluid therapy. To maximize efficacy and minimize toxicity, therapeutic drug monitoring of gentamicin or amikacin is recommended.

ADVERSE AND COMMON SIDE EFFECTS: Nephrotoxicity, deafness, vestibular toxicity, respiratory paralysis, and cardiovascular depression have been reported with the use of these drugs. Endotoxemia predisposes to cardiovascular-induced depression. These drugs should be used with caution or avoided entirely in food-producing animals because they can persist for long periods of time as tissue residues. Neomycin is the most nephrotoxic aminoglycoside, followed in decreasing order of nephrotoxicity by gentamicin, tobramycin, kanamycin, amikacin, and streptomycin. The risk factors for aminoglycoside toxicity include: prolonged therapy (>7 to 10 days), acidosis and electrolyte disturbances (hypokalemia, hyponatremia), volume depletion (shock, endotoxemia), concurrent nephrotoxic drug therapy, preexisting renal disease, and elevated plasma trough concentrations. Calcium supplementation can reduce the risk of nephrotoxicity. The risk of nephrotoxicity can also be decreased by feeding the patient a high-protein/high-calcium diet such as alfalfa, as protein and calcium cations compete with aminoglycoside cations for binding to renal tubular epithelial cells. High dietary protein also increases glomerular filtration rate and renal blood flow, reducing aminoglycoside accumulation. The development of nephrotoxicity is detected by an increase in urine γ-glutamyltransferase (GGT) enzyme and an increase in the urine GGT:urine creatinine ratio. The UGGT:UCr may increase to 2 to 3 times baseline within 3 days of a nephrotoxic dose. If these tests are not available, the development of proteinuria is the next best indicator of nephrotoxicity and is easily determined in a practice setting. Elevations in serum urea nitrogen and creatinine confirm nephrotoxicity but are not seen for at least 7 days after significant renal damage has occurred.

DRUG INTERACTIONS: Aminoglycoside antibiotics can potentiate the action of neuromuscular blocking agents leading to respiratory depression, apnea, or muscle weakness, especially in animals with renal insufficiency. The neuromuscular blocking activity can be reversed with calcium. Furosemide may enhance the ototoxicity and nephrotoxicity of the aminoglycosides. IV calcium gluconate will reverse myocardial depression and restore blood pressure. Prolonged high oral doses of neomycin may cause diarrhea and malabsorption due to selective overgrowth of resistant indigenous intestinal flora. When administered concurrently with penicillin IV, precipitation will occur if the drugs are mixed.

SUPPLIED AS: See individual drug.

AMINOPHYLLINE

INDICATIONS: Aminophylline (theophylline ethylenediamine) (Aminophylline ♣ ★, Lufyllin ★, Dilor ★, Dyflex ★, Neothylline ★, Phyllocontin ♣ ★) is a theophylline salt that is 78% to 86% theophylline. It is more water soluble and produces less GI irritation than theophylline, so it is preferred for oral use in horses. Pharmacological effects of theophylline include increasing cyclic-AMP by inhibition of phosphodiesterase and antagonism of adenosine. Adenosine induces bronchoconstriction in asthmatic patients and antagonizes adenylate cyclase. Adenylate cyclase is responsible for the synthesis of cyclic-AMP, which is important for bronchial smooth muscle relaxation and inhibition of the release of inflammatory mediators from mast cells. Theophylline also inhibits prostaglandins, augments the release of catecholamines from storage granules, increases calcium availability to contractile proteins of the heart and diaphragm, and interferes with mobilization of calcium in smooth muscle cells. Theophylline (or aminophylline) is used in horses to treat recurrent airway obstruction by causing bronchial smooth muscle relaxation, decreasing the release of inflammatory mediators from mast cells, increasing diaphragmatic contraction, and increasing mucociliary transport. Theophylline (or aminophylline) can be used to accelerate recovery from benzodiazepine sedatives because it is an effective respiratory stimulant.

ADVERSE AND COMMON SIDE EFFECTS: Horses are sensitive to high concentrations of theophylline, especially following rapid IV administration. Cardiac arrhythmias, CNS excitement, tremors, convulsions, and gastrointestinal irritation may be seen.

DRUG INTERACTIONS: Hepatic metabolism of theophylline may be inhibited by erythromycin, cimetidine, propranolol, and fluoroquinolones, resulting in toxicity. Metabolism of theophylline may be induced by rifampin and phenobarbital, which may necessitate increasing the dose.

SUPPLIED AS HUMAN PRODUCTS:
For injection containing 25 and 50 mg/mL
Tablets containing 100, 200 mg

AMMONIUM CHLORIDE

INDICATIONS: Ammonium chloride (Uroeze ★) is used as a urinary acidifier in horses and ruminants for the prevention of urolithiasis caused by phosphate crystals. Urinary acidification can hasten excretion of strychnine in cases of strychnine toxicity. Ammonium chloride is reported to prevent parturient paresis, from dietary acidification causing increased intestinal calcium absorption and enhanced calcium resorption from bone. Ammonium chloride is also included in expectorant products, but its efficacy for this purpose is questionable.

ADVERSE AND COMMON SIDE EFFECTS: The ammonium ion is toxic at high concentrations. Metabolic acidosis can result from its administration. The drug is not to be used in animals with severe hepatic disease. High doses in sheep have been associated with increased coughing and associated rectal prolapse.

DRUG INTERACTIONS: Animals receiving large doses of salicylates (e.g., acetylsalicylic acid) may develop increased serum salicylate levels.

SUPPLIED AS VETERINARY PRODUCTS:
Small Animal Products

Tablets containing 200 mg in a protein base (Uroeze)
Powder containing 200 and 400 mg/0.65 g in a protein base (Uroeze)

OTHER USES
Cattle

PARTURIENT PARESIS
100 g/day; PO for 21 days prior to calving

AMOXICILLIN

INDICATIONS: Amoxicillin (Amoxi-Bol ★, Amoxi-Drop ★, Amoxi-Inject ★, Amoxi-Mast ★, Amoxi-Tabs ★, Amoxil ❦, Biomox ★, Robamox ★, Moxilean ❦) and ampicillin are aminopenicillins. The aminopenicillins are able to penetrate the outer layer of gram-negative bacteria better than penicillin G; therefore, they have activity against many of the gram-negative bacteria (*E. coli, Salmonella, Pasteurella* spp.) as well as gram-positive bacteria. However, resistance to the aminopenicillins is easily acquired by gram-negatives, so they are not usually effective against *Klebsiella, Proteus, Pseudomonas, and Staphylococcus aureus*. Most anaerobes are sensitive, except β-lactamase–producing strains of *Bacteroides*. Amoxicillin penetrates the gram-negative cell wall more easily than does ampicillin; therefore, it has greater activity against gram-negative bacteria. It is useful for treating soft tissue, respiratory, urinary tract, and intestinal infections caused by susceptible bacteria. It has been used successfully to treat experimental *Salmonella dublin* infections in 1-month-old calves. Amoxicillin is available in the United States for parenteral treatment of bovine pneumonia and foot rot, as an oral antibiotic for neonatal calf scours, and for intramammary treatment of mastitis in cattle. Because of low oral bioavailability, it cannot be administered orally to horses and postweaning ruminants.

ADVERSE AND COMMON SIDE EFFECTS: Abdominal discomfort and diarrhea can occur with oral medication in calves. Effectiveness of the intramuscular formulation may be limited by the relatively large injection volume and discomfort associated with administration. Penicillins are associated with autoimmune hemolytic anemia (Type II hypersensitivity), and anaphylaxis (Type I hypersensitivity). The immune-mediated anemia usually resolves with discontinuation of penicillin therapy. Anaphylaxis usually occurs after previous exposure to a penicillin and can be fatal. Intravenous epinephrine and oxygen administration and respiratory support are indicated.

DRUG INTERACTIONS: The β-lactam ring of the aminopenicillins is protected from bacterial enzyme degradation when they are combined with β-lactamase inhibitors such as clavulanic acid and sulbactam.

SUPPLIED AS VETERINARY PRODUCTS:
Oral suspension containing 50 mg/mL
Suspension for injection containing 250 mg/mL (25 g/vial)
Tablets containing 50, 100, 200, and 400 mg
Boluses containing 400 mg
Mastitis suspension containing 62.5 mg per disposable syringe

AMPHOTERICIN B

INDICATIONS: Amphotericin B (Fungizone ✤ ★) is an effective antifungal agent. Amphotericin B binds to sterols in the fungal cell membrane and alters the permeability of the membrane allowing intracellular potassium to "leak out." Because bacteria and rickettsia do not contain sterols, amphotericin B has no activity against them. However, mammalian cells do contain sterols (cholesterol, etc.), which accounts for the drug's toxicity. The drug has been used to treat the following infections: blastomycosis, histoplasmosis, cryptococcosis, coccidioidomycosis, *Sporothrix schenckii, Fusarium* species, and candidiasis. In horses, it has been used in the treatment of equine pythiosis caused by *Hyphomyces destruens* (aka. phycomycosis, swamp cancer, Florida horse leeches, Gulf Coast fungus).

ADVERSE AND COMMON SIDE EFFECTS: The most important side effect is renal dysfunction. Serum urea and creatinine levels and urinalysis should be monitored frequently throughout the treatment period. Administration of the drug is discontinued, at least temporarily, when the blood urea nitrogen (BUN) exceeds 30 to 40 mg/dL (10.7 to 14.3 mmol/L) or serum creatinine exceeds 3 mg/dL (265 μmol/L).

DRUG INTERACTIONS: The concurrent use of aminoglycosides, polymyxin B, cisplatin, methoxyflurane, or vancomycin may potentiate the nephrotoxicity of amphotericin B. When amphotericin B is combined with minocycline and flucytosine, serum concentrations of amphotericin B needed to inhibit growth of *Candida* or *Cryptococcus neoformans* are reduced. Rifampin enhances the effect of amphotericin B on *Aspergillus, Candida,* and *Histoplasma capsulatum.* Similarly, ketoconazole appears to potentiate the efficacy of amphotericin B against blastomycosis and histoplasmosis.

SUPPLIED AS HUMAN PRODUCT:
For injection containing 50 mg lyophilized amphotericin B per vial

AMPICILLIN

INDICATIONS: Ampicillin sodium (Ampicin ✤, Omnipen-N ★, Penbritin ✤, Polycillin-N ★, Totacillin-N ★), ampicillin trihydrate (Polyflex ✤ ★), ampicillin sulbactam (Synergistin ✤), and amoxicillin are aminopenicillins. The aminopenicillins are able to penetrate the outer layer of gram-negative bacteria better than penicillin G; therefore, they have activity against many of the gram-negative bacteria (*E. coli, Salmonella, Pasteurella* spp.) as well as gram-positive bacteria. However, resistance to the aminopenicillins is easily acquired by gram-negatives, so they are not usually effective against *Klebsiella, Proteus, Pseudomonas* and *Staphy-*

lococcus aureus. Most anaerobes are sensitive, except β-lactamase producing strains of *Bacteroides.* Ampicillin is useful for treating bacterial pneumonia, soft tissue and postsurgical infections, and mastitis caused by bacteria susceptible to ampicillin. The ampicillin trihydrate formulation is approved for treatment of pneumonia in cattle but may be ineffective at the label dose due to slow absorption and low peak concentrations. In Canada, ampicillin trihydrate is combined with sulbactam, the β-lactamase inhibitor. This extends the spectrum of ampicillin to include β-lactamase–producing *E. coli, Klebsiella, Proteus, Staphylococcus,* and most anaerobes, including *Bacteroides fragilis.* Sulbactam combines with the bacterial β-lactamase, an inactive enzyme complex is formed, and the coadministered ampicillin is then able to exert its effect.

ADVERSE AND COMMON SIDE EFFECTS: Penicillins are associated with autoimmune hemolytic anemia (Type II hypersensitivity) and anaphylaxis (Type I hypersensitivity). The immune-mediated anemia usually resolves with discontinuation of penicillin therapy. Anaphylaxis usually occurs after previous exposure to a penicillin and can be fatal. Intravenous epinephrine and oxygen administration and respiratory support are indicated.

DRUG INTERACTIONS: The β-lactam ring of the aminopenicillins is protected from bacterial enzyme degradation when they are combined with β-lactamase inhibitors such as clavulanic acid and sulbactam.

SUPPLIED AS VETERINARY PRODUCTS:
For injection in the trihydrate form in 10- and 25-g vials
For injection in the trihydrate-sulbactam form as 60 mg/mL sulbactam and 120 mg/mL ampicillin

SUPPLIED AS HUMAN PRODUCT:
For injection (sodium salt) in 125-, 250-, and 500-mg, and 1-, 2-, and 10-g vials

AMPROLIUM

INDICATIONS: Amprolium (Amprol ✤, Corid ★) is a coccidiostatic drug active against first-generation schizonts of developing coccidia. It is used in ruminants for prevention and treatment of coccidiosis caused by *Eimeria bovis* and *Eimeria zuernii.*

ADVERSE AND COMMON SIDE EFFECTS: Amprolium is a thiamine antagonist; therefore, high doses (321 to 880 mg/kg daily; PO) can cause polioencephalomalacia in ruminants.

DRUG INTERACTIONS: Amprolium is a thiamine analog; therefore, concurrent administration of thiamine or thiamine-containing products can antagonize the anticoccidial activity of amprolium.

SUPPLIED AS VETERINARY PRODUCTS:
Oral solution containing 96 mg/mL (9.6% w/v)
Soluble powder containing 20% w/w [Corid]
Feed mix containing 25% w/w [Amprol]
Feed additive crumbles containing 1.25% w/w [Corid]

ANTACIDS

INDICATIONS: Antacids containing aluminum and magnesium oxides and hydroxides, (Carmalax ★, Maalox ♣ ★, Magnalax ★, Milk of Magnesia ★, MVT Powder and MVT Boluses ★, Neighlox ♣, Oxamin Bolus ♣ and Oxamin Powder ♣, and Rumalax ★) are used to neutralize gastric acid. Combinations of the varying compounds are used to provide both a fast-acting and a persistent acid-neutralizing effect. Antacids are used to treat gastric ulcers in horses, abomasal ulcers in ruminants, and simple indigestion or grain overload in cattle. These products may also be ruminatoric.

ADVERSE AND COMMON SIDE EFFECTS: Excessive doses can cause metabolic alkalosis and electrolyte abnormalities such as hypermagnesemia. Aluminum-containing antacids can cause ileus, whereas magnesium-containing products may cause diarrhea.

DRUG INTERACTIONS: Antacids can chelate and decrease oral bioavailability of iron supplements, fluoroquinolones, and tetracyclines. Aluminum-containing antacid compounds decrease bioavailability of phenothiazines, digoxin, prednisone, prednisolone, ranitidine, and, possibly, cimetidine. Antacid-induced change in urine pH increases urinary excretion and decreases blood concentrations of salicylates.

SUPPLIED AS VETERINARY PRODUCT:
See individual products

ANTIHISTAMINES

INDICATIONS: Antihistamines (Antihist Solution ♣, Antihistamine Injection ♣ ★, Antihistamine Oral ♣, Antihistamine Powder ♣, Histavet-P ★, Pyrahist-10 ♣, Pyrilamine Maleate Injection ★, Re-Covr ★, Ved-Hist ★, Vetastim ♣) act as competitive antagonists for specific type-1 histamine receptors. Oral antihistamines are used for treatment of allergic and anaphylactic conditions in large animals. They are more effective when administered prior to mast cell degranulation. The powder form is labeled for oral use in horses for the relief of urticaria due to allergy and dyspnea due to recurrent airway obstruction, but it is poorly efficacious for the latter. Treatment of allergic reactions in large animals may be disappointing due to the influence of other mediators in addition to histamine. Injectable antihistamines (e.g., Re-Covr ★, Vetastim ♣) have also been advocated as adjunctive therapy along with IV calcium for milk fever in cattle.

ADVERSE AND COMMON SIDE EFFECTS: At low doses antihistamines can cause sedation. Higher doses and IV administration of antihistamines may cause extreme central nervous system (CNS) excitement, hyperpyrexia, and even death. Prolonged administration of oral antihistamines can cause constipation or diarrhea. Antihistamines should be used with caution in the pregnant animal because certain agents are teratogenic.

DRUG INTERACTIONS: Severe CNS depression can occur with concomitant use of barbiturates or chlorpromazine.

SUPPLIED AS VETERINARY PRODUCTS:
For injection containing 25 mg pyrilamine maleate and 10 mg ephedrine/mL
For injection containing 20 mg/mL pyrilamine maleate
For injection containing tripelennamine hydrochloride 20 mg/mL
Powder containing 50 mg pyrilamine maleate with 20 mg DL-ephedrine

OTHER USES: Antihistamines are also found in combination with antibiotics and glucocorticoid products (Azimycin ♣ ★, Dexamycin ♣).

ANTITUSSIVES

INDICATIONS: Antitussives should only be used in animals with a severe, nonproductive cough that deters eating or drinking or results in physical exhaustion, because the cough is a necessary defense mechanism for the respiratory tract. Proprietary products include Cough Aid ♣, Equintussi Cough Syrup ♣, Expectorant Compound II ★, Glytussin ★, and Heave Aid ♣. Most of the proprietary products act mainly as expectorants, some of the antihistamines being directly antitussive. Opioid analgesics (see BUTORPHANOL, MORPHINE, MEPERIDINE) also have potent antitussive properties.

ADVERSE AND COMMON SIDE EFFECTS: If productive coughing is suppressed, recovery from lower respiratory tract disease can be prevented or delayed.

DRUG INTERACTIONS: See individual products. Little information is available.

SUPPLIED AS VETERINARY PRODUCTS:

Syrup containing ammonium bicarbonate, ammonium chloride, chloroform, and menthol [Cough Aid, Equintussi Cough Syrup, Cough Aid]

Oral powder containing ammonium chloride, camphor, menthol, and ammonium bicarbonate [Heave Aid]

Oral powder containing ammonium chloride, guaifenesin, and potassium iodide [Expectorant Compound II, Glytussin]

APRAMYCIN

INDICATIONS: Apramycin (Apralan ✤, Apralan 75 ★) is an amino-cyclitol antibiotic used for the treatment of bacterial enteritis caused by *E. coli* in piglets. Oral absorption of apramycin decreases markedly with increasing age of the piglets. Single oral doses of 10, 30, and 100 mg/kg give peak blood levels 1 to 4 hours after administration, with detectable serum levels at 12 to 24 hours.

ADVERSE AND COMMON SIDE EFFECTS: None listed.

DRUG INTERACTIONS: None listed.

SUPPLIED AS VETERINARY PRODUCTS:

Soluble powder, 50-g activity container (containing 1.5 g/measure; Apralan)

Feed additive, 50 lb (containing 75 g/lb; Apralan 75)

ASPIRIN

INDICATIONS: Aspirin or acetylsalicylic acid (ASA Bolus ✤, Acetyl-salicylic Acid Tablets ✤, Asen 60 ✤, Aspirin 60 Grain ★, Aspirin 240 Grain Boluses ★, Aspirin Bolus ★, Aspirin Boluses ★, Aspirin Powder ★, Aspirin Tablets ★, Bexprin ✤, Centra ASA 60 ✤, Centra ASA 240 ✤, LA Aspirin Boluses ★) is a nonsteroidal anti-inflammatory drug (NSAID). NSAIDs block cyclooxygenase enzymes from forming thromboxane, prostacyclin, and the prostaglandins from arachidonic acid. This results in antipyretic action, mild analgesia, antiplatelet effects, and some anti-inflammatory effects. NSAIDs primarily are anti-inflammatory due to their inhibition of prostaglandin production. Therefore, NSAIDs do not resolve inflammation, but prevent its ongoing occurrence. Prostaglandin inhibition does not explain all of the anti-inflammatory activity of NSAIDs. NSAIDs are more lipophilic at a low pH, such is found in inflamed tissues. Some anti-inflammatory action appears to be related to their ability to insert into the lipid bilayer of cell and disrupt normal signals and protein–protein interactions in cell membranes. In the cell membrane of neutrophils, NSAIDs inhibit neutrophil aggregation, decrease enzyme release and superoxide generation, and inhibit lipoxygenase. NSAIDs act as analgesics by inhibiting cyclooxygenase and preventing the production of prostaglandins that sensitize the afferent nociceptors at peripheral sites of inflammation. However, there is increasing evidence that some NSAIDs have a central mechanism of action for analgesia and act synergistically with opioids. Platelet aggregation is classically inhibited by NSAIDs by preventing thromboxane production via the COX-1 pathway. Aspirin permanently modifies COX, so platelet function is only restored by the production of new platelets.

ASA is not used commonly in cattle because large doses must be administered frequently due to rapid excretion and dilution in the rumen. ASA is of low regulatory concern in food animals, but because of the epidemiological link between aspirin and Reye's syndrome in children, the gFARADs recommend minimum meat and milk withdrawal times of 24 hours. ASA is infrequently used in horses for antiplatelet activity or as an anti-inflammatory for recurrent uveitis. Nutritional supplements for older horses often contain yucca, which contains salicylates similar to ASA. Salicylates also occur in some grasses and hays and horse urine naturally contains large quantities of salicylates, therefore regulatory thresholds are quite high for salicylates and nutritional supplements are unlikely to cause positive drug tests.

ADVERSE AND COMMON SIDE EFFECTS: The most common adverse effect of ASA is gastric or intestinal irritation with varying degrees of gastrointestinal blood loss. ASA therapy should be discontinued one week prior to surgery. If used in pregnant animals, ASA may delay parturition. Acute aspirin overdose causes a severe metabolic acidosis. Administer sodium bicarbonate IV to treat acidosis and alkalinize urine to reduce reabsorption and administer a diuretic like mannitol to increase elimination.

DRUG INTERACTIONS: ASA competes for protein-binding sites with drugs such as penicillin, thiopental, and phenytoin. An ASA dose of 50 mg/kg increases serum digoxin levels up to 130% of normal. The early preload reducing effect of furosemide (independent of diuretic effect) is mediated by prostaglandins. A decrease in prostaglandin synthesis by NSAIDs may diminish the cardiovascular effects of furosemide.

SUPPLIED AS VETERINARY PRODUCTS:
As bolus containing 15.5 or 15.6 g/bolus (240 gr)
Tablets containing 3.9 g (60 gr)
Oral granules containing 14.5 g/20 g (Asen) or 5 g/15 g (Bexprin)

ATRACURIUM

INDICATIONS: Atracurium (Tracrium ✣ ★) is a neuromuscular blocking agent used as an adjuvant for surgical anesthesia. It is recommended for chemical restraint during mechanical ventilation in neonatal intensive care of foals, but it is very expensive.

ADVERSE AND COMMON SIDE EFFECTS: Atracurium should only be used in settings with facilities for assisted ventilation, and by highly trained personnel. Atracurium has no analgesic properties. If given rapidly, the drug can induce urticaria in humans by causing histamine release.

DRUG INTERACTIONS: Edrophonium or neostigmine can be used to reverse and decrease the duration of neuromuscular blockade. Inhalation anesthetics act synergistically with atracurium, allowing decreased doses. Concomitant use of aminoglycosides, tetracyclines, polymixins, and colistin will potentiate neuromuscular blockade by atracurium.

SUPPLIED AS HUMAN PRODUCT:
For injection containing 10 mg/mL

ATROPINE

INDICATIONS: Atropine (Atropine Sulfate Injectable ♣, Atropine Sulfate Injection ★, Atropine Sulfate ♣ ★, and others) is a belladonna alkaloid that is anticholinergic, antispasmodic, and mydriatic. Atropine inhibits structures innervated by the postganglionic parasympathetic nervous system. It decreases spasms of hyperperistalsis of diarrhea and inhibits salivary and respiratory secretions. The anticholinergic (parasympatholytic) drugs are effective bronchodilators by inhibiting vagally-mediated cholinergic smooth muscle tone in the respiratory tract. Cholinergic stimulation causes bronchoconstriction and asthmatic individuals appear to have excessive stimulation of cholinergic receptors. Atropine is used for acute bronchodilation in horses, where a low IV dose is more effective and less toxic than IV theophylline. A test dose of 5 to 7 mg may also be used to determine prognosis in horses with recurrent airway obstruction. Horses that fail to improve pulmonary function with a test dose of atropine are unlikely to be managed successfully. Atropine blocks vagal-induced bradycardia and bronchospasm induced by parasympathetic stimulation as found in organophosphate poisoning. It is used as a mydriatic in uveitis and corneal ulceration. Atropine is not used frequently as a preanesthetic in large animals because they only infrequently develop bradycardia and do not salivate excessively.

ADVERSE AND COMMON SIDE EFFECTS: Atropine has profound systemic pharmacological effects including ileus, xerostomia, urine retention, cycloplegia, tachycardia, and CNS excitement. Chronic administration may lead to serious bowel atony. Ocular administration in horses is associated with ileus and colic.

DRUG INTERACTIONS: None applicable in large animals.

SUPPLIED AS VETERINARY PRODUCT:
For injection containing 0.5, 0.54, and 15 mg/mL

AZAPERONE

INDICATIONS: Azaperone (Stresnil ♣ ★) is a potent sedative/tranquilizer for use in pigs. It has a rapid onset of action of approximately 5 to 10 minutes following IM injection, with a peak effect after 15 to 30 minutes and duration of action from 1 to 6 hours. During this time, the animal remains conscious but indifferent to the environment. Its main uses are to reduce aggression and fighting during weaning and mixing of pigs. Injections should be deep IM behind the neck, after which the animals should not be disturbed for 20 minutes.

ADVERSE AND COMMON SIDE EFFECTS: It is not to be used for castration because the period of hemorrhaging may be extended. The effects on breeding animals have not been determined. Do not inject the drug SC.

DRUG INTERACTIONS: None listed.

SUPPLIED AS VETERINARY PRODUCT:
For injection containing 40 mg/mL, in 50-mL vial

AZITHROMYCIN

INDICATIONS: Azithromycin (Zithromax ♣ ★) is an azalide antibiotic, similar to macrolide antibiotics such as erythromycin. Susceptible bacteria include staphylococci, streptococci, *Campylobacter jejuni, Clostridia, Rhodococcus equi, Mycoplasma* spp. and *Chlamydia* spp. Azithromycin is more active than the macrolides against gram-negative bacteria and anaerobes. Azithromycin is known for its high degree of lipid solubility. Peritoneal and synovial fluid concentrations of azithromycin parallel serum concentrations. Bronchoalveolar cell and pulmonary epithelial lining fluid concentrations are 15- to 170-fold and 1- to 16-fold higher than concurrent serum concentrations, respectively. Azithromycin is an attractive alternative to erythromycin for the treatment of *Rhodococcus equi* infections in foals due to its pharmacokinetic profile, which allows once a day or every other day dosing, and an apparent reduced incidence of adverse effects.

ADVERSE AND COMMON SIDE EFFECTS: No adverse reactions were detected during or after repeated intragastric administration of azithromycin in foals.

DRUG INTERACTIONS: None listed.

SUPPLIED AS HUMAN PRODUCTS:
For IV injection containing 100 mg/mL
Pediatric suspension containing 40 mg/mL
Tablets containing 250 mg and 600 mg

BACITRACIN ZINC, NEOMYCIN, POLYMIXIN B SULFATE

INDICATIONS: Bacitracin zinc, neomycin, and polymixin B (BNP Ointment ♣, Mycitracin ★, Neobacimyx ★, Trioptic-P ★, Triple Antibiotic Ointment ★, Vetropolycin ★) are antibiotic combinations for the broad-spectrum treatment of superficial bacterial infections of the conjunctiva and cornea. The combination product is also available with hydrocortisone (BNP-H Ointment ♣, Corticosporin ★, Neobacimyx-H ★, Trioptic-S ★, Vetropolycin-HC ♣). These drugs are not lipid soluble but penetrate the stroma when the corneal epithelium is disrupted. Neomycin is a typical bactericidal aminoglycoside with good activity against *Staphylococcus* spp. and gram-negative bacteria. *Pseudomonas* spp. are often resistant to neomycin, but polymixin B is rapidly bactericidal against gram-negative bacteria including *Pseudomonas* spp. Due to systemic toxicity, polymixin B is only used topically, so it is not typically included on susceptibility reports from microbiology services. Polymixin B also binds and inactivates endotoxin, reducing inflammation and tissue destruction. Like polymixin B, bacitracin is a topical product not routinely included on susceptibility reports. Bacitracin is active against gram-positive bacteria, with a mechanism of action similar to the β-lactam antibiotics. Penicillins and cephalosporins are not used as commercial ophthalmic formulations because of the risk of contact sensitization, so bacitracin is substituted as their antibacterial equivalent.

ADVERSE AND COMMON SIDE EFFECTS: Sensitivity to this combination is rare but may manifest as itching, burning, or inflammation at the site of medication.

DRUG INTERACTIONS: None listed.

SUPPLIED AS VETERINARY PRODUCTS:
Ointment; each contains 400 or 500 U bacitracin, 3.5 mg neomycin, and 5,000 U polymixin B sulfate or 10,000 U polymixin B sulfate [Trioptic-P]. Hydrocortisone is formulated with BNP products at 1% w/w.

SUPPLIED AS HUMAN PRODUCT:
Ocular solution

BAL (DIMERCAPROL)

INDICATIONS: BAL [British Anti-Lewisite] or dimercaprol (BAL: Dimercaprol in Oil ✿ ★) is a chelator used to treat toxicity due to arsenic or other heavy metals.

ADVERSE AND COMMON SIDE EFFECTS: Administration of dimercaprol causes a rise in systolic and diastolic arterial blood pressure accompanied by tachycardia. Conjunctivitis, blepharospasm, lacrimation, rhinorrhea, salivation, and abdominal pain have been noted in people receiving dimercaprol. Sterile abscesses at the site of injection occasionally occur. A transient reduction of polymorphonuclear leukocytes may occur after treatment. The drug is contraindicated in cases of hepatic insufficiency except when hepatopathy is the result of arsenic toxicity.

DRUG INTERACTIONS: Do not administer dimercaprol within 24 hours of iron or selenium compounds. Dimercaprol can form toxic complexes with iron and selenium.

SUPPLIED AS HUMAN PRODUCT:
For IM injection containing 100 mg/mL

BECLOMETHASONE

INDICATIONS: Beclomethasone (Beclovent ✿ ★) is a potent anti-inflammatory glucocorticoid available in a metered dose inhaler and administered to horses with a spacer device such as an AeroMask. Inhaled glucocorticoids are the most potent inhaled anti-inflammatory drugs currently available. Early intervention with inhaled glucocorticoids improves airway disease control and normalizes lung function and may prevent irreversible airway damage. The potential but small risk of adverse side effects is well balanced by their efficacy. Aerosol beclomethasone has been effective in treating horses for recurrent airway obstruction (aka heaves or chronic obstructive pulmonary disease). See GLUCOCORTICOID AGENTS.

ADVERSE AND COMMON SIDE EFFECTS: Oral candidiasis (thrush), dysphonia, and reflex cough and bronchospasm are the most common adverse effects in humans; all of these effects are reduced by the use of a spacer. At the currently recommended dose (500 µg q 12 hours), inhaled beclomethasone suppresses adrenocortical function in horses, but use is not associated with clinically apparent adverse effects.

DRUG INTERACTIONS: None listed.

SUPPLIED AS HUMAN PRODUCTS:
For aerosol administration containing 50 or 250 µg/accuation in a metered dose inhaler (Canada)
For aerosol administration containing 42 or 84 µg/accuation in a metered dose inhaler (United States)

BETAMETHASONE

INDICATIONS: Betamethasone (Betaject ✤, Betasone ✤ ★, Celestone Soluspan ✤ ★, Cel-U-Jec ★, Celestone Phosphate ★, Selectoject ★) is a potent glucocorticoid used for treating nonseptic inflammatory joint disease in horses and cattle. Its action is prolonged and injection can be repeated at 3-week intervals if clinical signs persist. It is combined with gentamicin and gentamicin and clotrimazole in a variety of topical products. See GLUCOCORTICOID AGENTS.

ADVERSE AND COMMON SIDE EFFECTS: Betamethasone is not to be used in animals with acute or chronic bacterial infections unless therapeutic doses of antibacterial agents are also used. Betamethasone should not be used in pregnant cattle. See GLUCOCORTICOID AGENTS for further information on adverse effects and drug interactions.

SUPPLIED AS VETERINARY PRODUCT:
For injection containing 5 mg/mL betamethasone diproprionate and 2 mg/mL betamethasone sodium phosphate [Betasone]

HUMAN PRODUCT
For injection containing 3 mg/mL betamethasone acetate with 3 mg/mL betamethasone sodium phosphate [Celestone, Betaject]

BETHANECHOL

INDICATIONS: Bethanechol (Duvoid ✤ ★, Bethanechol Chloride ✤ ★, Myotonachol ✤ ★, Urabeth ★, Urecholine ✤ ★) is a synthetic acetylcholine derivative used to stimulate gastrointestinal motility in postoperative gastrointestinal ileus and to stimulate urinary bladder contraction. Bethanechol has also been used to enhance gastric emptying and minimize gastroesophageal reflux for foals with gastric ulceration. It has also been advocated for stimulation of detrusor muscle activity to aid in bladder emptying in horses with urinary incontinence. Because the treatment produces varying results, clinicians should start with the lowest dose recommended.

ADVERSE AND COMMON SIDE EFFECTS: The drug should not be administered IM or IV because the incidence of serious toxic side effects, such as bronchoconstriction, colic, and hypotension, is greatly increased. Do not use in cases of obstruction of the urinary tract or intestinal tract.

DRUG INTERACTIONS: Do not administer bethanechol with other cholinergic or anticholinesterase agents (e.g., neostigmine) because of additive effects and toxicity. Administration with ganglionic blocking agents will produce a critical hypotension. Atropine, epinephrine, quinidine, and procainamide antagonize the effects of bethanechol.

SUPPLIED AS HUMAN PRODUCTS:
For injection containing 5 mg/mL
Tablets containing 10, 25, and 50 mg

BISMUTH SUBSALICYLATE

INDICATIONS: Bismuth subsalicylate (Pepto-Bismol ✤ ★, Bismo-Kote ★, Bismu-Kote ★, Bismusal Suspension ★, Corrective Suspension ★, Gastro-Cote ★) is a demulcent and gut protectant. Although other "mucosal protectants" have questionable efficacy, this product is considered by many gastroenterologists to be the symptomatic treatment of choice for acute diarrhea. Its efficacy has been proven in controlled clinical trials with humans with acute diarrhea (enterotoxigenic *E. coli* or "traveler's diarrhea"). Bismuth adsorbs bacterial enterotoxins, and the salicylate component is believed to have anti-inflammatory action. There are five sources of salicylate in this product accounting for approximately 9 mg of salicylate/mL. Two tablespoons (typical human dose) contains as much salicylate as one adult aspirin.

ADVERSE AND COMMON SIDE EFFECTS: Chronic use of bismuth salts can cause encephalopathy and osteodystrophy. Salicylate toxicity is possible if large amounts are administered. Administration causes the feces to turn black, making it difficult to assess gastrointestinal hemorrhage.

DRUG INTERACTIONS: Use may prevent the absorption of concurrently administered drugs.

SUPPLIED AS VETERINARY PRODUCT:
Oral liquid containing 17.5 mg/mL bismuth subsalicylate

SUPPLIED AS HUMAN PRODUCTS:
Liquid containing 17.47 mg/mL bismuth subsalicylate
Liquid containing 35 mg/mL bismuth subsalicylate

BOLDENONE UNDECYLENATE

INDICATIONS: Boldenone undecylenate (Equipoise ♣ ★) is a long-acting anabolic agent for horses used for treating debilitated animals and improving appetite, weight gain, and physical condition. Boldenone undecylenate is a steroid ester with marked anabolic properties and only small amounts of androgenic properties. The drug is not a substitute for a balanced diet. It is a controlled substance because of human abuse.

ADVERSE AND COMMON SIDE EFFECTS: Treatment may result in undesirable androgenic effects (masculinization, aggression, behavioral change), particularly in the case of overdose. Boldenone is not to be used in immature colts and fillies, stallions, pregnant mares, or brood mares in the breeding season.

DRUG INTERACTIONS: None listed.

SUPPLIED AS VETERINARY PRODUCT:
For injection containing 25 and 50 mg/mL

BOTULINUM ANTITOXIN

INDICATIONS: Botulinum antitoxin [polyvalent] is used for the early treatment of clinical cases of botulism in foals and horses. Once the toxin has entered the synaptic terminals and clinical signs are present, the antitoxin is ineffective; however, it will neutralize toxin not yet taken up at the nerve terminal. Botulinum antitoxin is extremely expensive, so vaccination with botulinum toxoid is recommended in endemic areas.

ADVERSE AND COMMON SIDE EFFECTS: None listed.

DRUG INTERACTIONS: None indicated.

SUPPLIED AS VETERINARY PRODUCT:
For injection containing antiserum 100 to 150 IU/mL
Sources: (a) New Bolton Center, Pennsylvania 1-610-444-5800 ext 2321; (b) Veterinary Dynamics, California 1-800-654-9743

BUPIVACAINE HYDROCHLORIDE

INDICATIONS: Bupivacaine hydrochloride (Marcaine ♣ ★, Sensorcaine ♣ ★) is a long-acting local anesthetic that is 2 to 4 times more potent than lidocaine and is used for local nerve blocks and epidural anesthesia. It has been used for prolonged regional analgesia in horses with diseases such as laminitis and experimentally in sheep for epidural anesthesia.

ADVERSE AND COMMON SIDE EFFECTS: As for most local anesthetics, the CNS may be stimulated, producing restlessness and tremor that may proceed to clonic convulsions. Certain local anesthetics may also cause sedation or behavioral changes. At high levels, which affect the CNS, the cardiovascular system is also affected by decreasing electrical excitability, conduction rate, and force of contraction of the myocardium. Hypersensitivity to local anesthetics can occur but is rare. The 0.75% w/v solution should not be used for obstetric anesthesia. Bupivacaine is more cardiotoxic than lidocaine and the toxicity seems to be aggravated by hypoxemia and acidemia. Hepatic disease may increase the potential for toxicity of local anesthetics.

DRUG INTERACTIONS: The addition of epinephrine to local anesthetics greatly prolongs and intensifies their action.

SUPPLIED AS HUMAN PRODUCT:
For injection containing 0.25%, 0.5%, and 0.75% w/v with or without epinephrine

BUTORPHANOL TARTRATE

INDICATIONS: Butorphanol tartrate (Torbugesic ❖ ★, Torbutrol ❖ ★) is a centrally-acting narcotic agonist–antagonist analgesic with potent antitussive properties. Butorphanol has a ceiling effect where doses above 0.11 mg/kg produce no increase in analgesia or side effects. Analgesia lasts approximately 4 hours. Butorphanol is synergistic when used in combination with sedatives (xylazine 0.6 mg/kg; IV with butorphanol 0.03 mg/kg; IV) for standing chemical restraint and colic pain in horses. It is used as an adjunct for sedation in cattle. Unlike classical narcotic agonists, butorphanol does not cause histamine release or significant ileus or constipation.

ADVERSE AND COMMON SIDE EFFECTS: Butorphanol should be used with caution with other sedative or analgesic agents because the effects are likely additive. There may be variable degrees of response to the same dose between individual animals and differing breeds of horses. Ataxia after administration is usually mild and temporary, lasting 3 to 10 minutes. Rapid IV injection of high doses (20 times recommended dose) can result in a short period of inability to stand, muscle fasciculations, or a brief convulsive seizure. Administration of 10 times the recommended dose may cause muscle fasciculations about the head and neck, ataxia, salivation, and nystagmus. Repeated administration at that dose may result in constipation. Butorphanol is a controlled substance and has human abuse potential.

DRUG INTERACTIONS: Butorphanol can be used as an antagonist to narcotic agonists, such as meperidine, morphine, and oxymorphone. As an antagonist, butorphanol is approximately equivalent to nalorphine and 30 times more potent than pentazocine. It is synergistic with α_2-adrenergic agonists (xylazine, detomidine) for colic pain. When used with other CNS depressants, such as the barbiturates and phenothiazine tranquilizers, additive respiratory depression may occur.

SUPPLIED AS VETERINARY PRODUCTS:
For injection containing 0.5 mg/mL and 10.0 mg/mL
Tablets containing 1, 5, and 10 mg

CALCIUM BOROGLUCONATE

INDICATIONS: Calcium borogluconate (Cal Aqua 25.75% ✹, Cal-Nate 23% Solution ✹, Cal-Nate 1069 ★, Cal-MPK 1234 ★, Cal-MP 1700 ★, Calciphos ★, Calcium 23% Solution ★, Calcium Gluconate ✹ ★, Calcium Borogluconate ✹, Calcium Borogluconate 23% ✹, Calcium Gluconate 23% ✹, Cal-Glu-Sol ✹, Cal Mag-K ✹, Cal Mag D Solution #2 ✹, Cal Mag Phos ✹, Mag Cal ✹, Cal Plus ✹, Calcium Magnesium Dextrose ✹, Maglucal Plus ✹, Cal-Dextro Solution No 2 ✹, Cal-Dextro ✹ ★, Norcalciphos ✹ ★, Calphos ★, Supercal ✹, and others) is used for the treatment of hypocalcemia in cattle, sheep, and horses. Products containing magnesium are also indicated for treatment of hypomagnesemic tetany (grass tetany) and transport tetany. Certain calcium products also contain phosphorus or potassium for treatment of related deficiencies or diseases complicated by hypokalemia. During IV administration, there is usually a positive inotropic effect. Intravenous atropine has been used to abolish cardiac arrhythmias associated with calcium administration.

ADVERSE AND COMMON SIDE EFFECTS: Administer IV slowly to prevent heart block. Administration should be stopped if arrhythmias or bradycardia occur. Animals with hypocalcemia and endotoxemia, such as cows with acute coliform mastitis, are especially prone to cardiac arrhythmias caused by IV calcium therapy.

DRUG INTERACTIONS: Magnesium antagonizes the cardioexcitatory effects of calcium. Calcium borogluconate is incompatible if mixed with cephalothin, prednisolone phosphate, tetracyclines, sodium bicarbonate, phenylbutazone, and sulfonamides.

SUPPLIED AS VETERINARY PRODUCTS:
For injection containing a 23% solution (w/v) of calcium borogluconate equivalent to 19.78 mg/mL calcium or 25.75% (w/v) equivalent to

21.42 mg/mL calcium; alone or combined with dextrose, magnesium, phosphorus, and/or potassium compounds (see individual products)

CALCIUM CHLORIDE

INDICATIONS: Calcium chloride ♣ ★ in solution is used as one form of calcium replacement therapy for IV treatment of hypocalcemic tetany in mares. The salt is usually given in a 10% w/v solution. A moderate fall in blood pressure due to peripheral vasodilation may occur with administration.

ADVERSE AND COMMON SIDE EFFECTS: Calcium chloride should not be injected into tissues. It is irritating to the gastrointestinal tract if given orally.

DRUG INTERACTIONS: Calcium chloride is incompatible if mixed before administration with cephalothin, chlorpheniramine, hydrocortisone, prednisolone phosphate, kanamycin sulfate, tetracyclines, or sodium bicarbonate.

SUPPLIED AS HUMAN PRODUCT:
For injection containing 100 mg/mL

CALCIUM DISODIUM EDETATE

INDICATIONS: Calcium disodium edetate ($CaNa_2EDTA$) is a chelating agent used to treat lead poisoning in horses and cattle. Commercial products are no longer available, but it may be formulated by compounding pharmacists. It removes free lead from bone and also from blood and soft tissues by forming lead chelate that is excreted by the kidneys. Treatment of lead poisoned cattle is questionable unless they can be tracked after remission of clinical symptoms in order to prevent lead from entering the human food chain. Due to prolonged depletion and variable pharmacokinetics, there are currently no guidelines to follow for assuring that such an animal will be safe for consumption when it reaches slaughter. It is difficult to determine when, or even if, treated animals should enter the food chain.

ADVERSE AND COMMON SIDE EFFECTS: Administer $CaNa_2$EDTA slowly to prevent tachycardia, dyspnea, and body tremors. Clinical symptoms may initially worsen with $CaNa_2EDTA$ due to transient increases in the concentration of lead in the blood following mobilization from the bone. Renal toxicity, intestinal irritation, and depletion of essential minerals are potential side effects of treatment. Adequate hydration should be ensured when using $CaNa_2EDTA$. Dilution in D_5W or 0.9% (w/v) saline will reduce the potential for thrombophlebitis.

DRUG INTERACTIONS: Avoid administering the drug simultaneously with barbiturates and sulfonamides.

SUPPLIED AS: Not commercially available. May be compounded by a pharmacy.

CARBACHOL

INDICATIONS: Carbachol (carbamylcholine chloride) (Carbachol ♣ ★) is an acetylcholine derivative that produces similar physiologic effects to acetylcholine but is more stable in the body. Carbachol is used to treat colic in horses caused by impactions, rumen atony and impaction in cattle, and to stimulate uterine contractions for obstetric procedures and treatment of retained placenta.

ADVERSE AND COMMON SIDE EFFECTS: Intravenous or IM injection may increase the risk of untoward effects. Carbachol may produce bronchoconstriction and hypotension. Profuse sweating may occur in the horse. It is contraindicated in old or cachectic animals and pregnant animals, in cases of mechanical obstruction of the intestinal tract, and in respiratory and cardiac disease. Carbachol is a very potent drug. Excessive peristaltic movements in animals with severe intestinal obstruction can cause rupture or intussusception. High doses in cattle (>4 mg/454 kg) may actually inhibit ruminoreticular activity.

DRUG INTERACTIONS: The prior administration of oils and saline cathartics is recommended if the drug is used for equine colic due to impaction or intestinal atony. Atropine can be used as an antidote.

SUPPLIED AS HUMAN PRODUCTS:
For injection containing 0.25 mg/mL
Ophthalmic drops containing 0.75%, 1.5%, 2.25%, or 3% w/v carbachol [Isopto Carbachol]
Ophthalmic injection for intraocular use only 0.01% w/v [Miostat]

OTHER USES
OPHTHALMIC
Carbachol is used for its brief miotic effects in cataract extractions and other anterior chamber procedures. It will also reduce intraocular pressure in animals that have become resistant to pilocarpine or physostigmine.

CARBARYL

INDICATIONS: Carbaryl (Dusting Powder ♣, Equi-Shield Fly Repellent Spray ★, Sevin ♣, and other combination products) is a moderate, reversible carbamate cholinesterase inhibitor. It is used to control external parasites of horses and cattle.

ADVERSE AND COMMON SIDE EFFECTS: Toxic effects are unlikely but may include bronchoconstriction, colic, salivation, and diarrhea. DO NOT apply before milking; only apply immediately after milking. Wash udder thoroughly before the next milking.

DRUG INTERACTIONS: Atropine can be used as an antidote.

SUPPLIED AS VETERINARY PRODUCT:
Powder or spray of varying concentrations (see individual products)

CEPHALOSPORINS

INDICATIONS: Cephalosporins (Cefa-Dri ♣ ★, Cefa-Lak ♣ ★, Cefa-Tabs ♣ ★, Cefa-Drops ♣ ★, Excenel ♣ ★, Excenel RTU ♣, Naxcel ★, and many human preparations) are antibiotics similar to penicillin in that their structure includes a β-lactam ring and they inhibit bacterial cell wall synthesis similar to the penicillins. Although widely used, cephalosporins tend to be expensive and should be reserved for diseases that require alternatives to penicillins. Cephalosporins are divided into first-, second-, and third-generation drugs. First-generation cephalosporins (cephalothin, cephapirin, cefazolin, cephalexin, cefadroxil) have good activity against gram-positive bacteria and modest activity against gram-negative bacteria. Second-generation cephalosporins (cefamandole, cefoxitin, cefaclor, cefuroxime axetil, cefonicid) have somewhat increased activity against gram-negative organisms, but less than third-generation cephalosporins (cefotaxime, moxalactam, ceftazidime, ceftizoxime, ceftriaxone, cefoperazone), which are more active against the Enterobacteriaceae, including β-lactamase–producing strains. However, third-generation cephalosporins are generally less active against gram-positive bacteria than first-generation agents. Various diseases have specific cephalosporins as drugs of choice, e.g., cephalothin for β-lactamase–producing staphylococcal infections, cefoxitin for treatment of aerobic and mixed aerobic-anaerobic infections such as lung abscesses, and cefotaxime for gram-negative meningitis. Absorption, body distribution, and half-lives vary greatly among the cephalosporins, but oral absorption is uniformly poor in horses and ruminants. Large animal veterinary products are used for treatment of mastitis (Cefa-Lak ♣ ★, Today ★), dry treatment of the mammary gland (Cefa-Dri ♣ ★, Tomorrow ★), and for bacterial pneumonia (Excenel ♣ ★, Excenel RTU ♣, Naxcel ★) in cattle. Ceftiofur is a new generation parenteral cephalosporin approved for use in cattle, swine, and horses. Ceftiofur is active against respiratory pathogens such as streptococci, *Pasteurella* spp. and *Haemophilus* spp., and most anaerobes, but has less activity against *Staphylococcus aureus* and Enterobacteriaceae. *Bacteroides* spp. and *Pseudomonas* spp. are resistant. It is approved in swine for respiratory disease and in cattle for respiratory disease and infectious pododermatitis. It is only approved in horses for treating respiratory tract infections caused by *Streptococcus zooepidemicus*. When administered, ceftiofur is rapidly metabolized to the active metabolite desfuroylceftiofur. Desfuroylceftiofur is less active than ceftiofur against *Staphylococcus aureus* and *Proteus* spp. Diagnostic laboratories use a ceftiofur disk for susceptibility testing because of the instability of desfuroylceftiofur, so susceptibility testing results for staphylococci and *Proteus* spp. may not be reliable for predicting the efficacy of ceftiofur therapy.

Cefazolin, cephalothin, and ceftiofur can be administered locally in the treatment of septic tendon sheaths or joints. Intravenous or intraosseous regional perfusion achieves extremely high local concentrations of antimicrobials and can be preformed standing in horses or in cattle restrained on a tilt table.

ADVERSE AND COMMON SIDE EFFECTS: In general, cephalosporins have a high therapeutic index. Ceftriaxone and cefepime cause gastrointestinal disturbances after administration to foals and horses. Ceftiofur is associated with injection site inflammation and diarrhea from altered gastrointestinal flora in horses. The currently available cephalosporins are considered to be potentially nephrotoxic via deposition of immune complexes in the glomerular basement membrane or from a direct toxic effect leading to acute tubular necrosis.

DRUG INTERACTIONS: In human medicine, it is recommended that cephalosporins not be used in conjunction with aminoglycosides; however, animal studies demonstrate a protective effect of the cephalosporins against nephrotoxicity. Like the penicillins, cephalosporins can be synergistic with aminoglycosides. Recent evidence shows in vitro antagonism between cephalosporins and chloramphenicol.

SUPPLIED AS VETERINARY PRODUCTS:
Intramammary products containing 300 mg cephapirin benzathine [Cefa-Dri ❦ ★, Tomorrow ★] or 200 mg cephapirin sodium [Cefa-Lak ❦ ★, Today ★]
For injection containing 50 mg/mL ceftiofur sodium [Naxcel ★, Excenel ❦] and 50 mg/mL ceftiofur hydrochloride [Excenel ★, Excenel RTU ❦]
Tablets (cefadroxil) containing 50, 100, 200, and 1,000 mg
Drops (cefadroxil) containing 50 mg/mL

CHARCOAL, ACTIVATED

INDICATIONS: Activated charcoal (Activated Charcoal Liquid ★, Actidote ★, Acta-Char ★, Acta-Char Liquid ★, Charcodote ❦ ★, Charcodote Aqueous ❦ ★, Charcodote TFS ❦ ★, Charcocaps ★, Liqui-Char ★, SuperChar ★, Toxiban ★) is an adsorbent for use in toxicities caused by ingested poisons, such as organophosphates. Activated charcoal may also adsorb free endotoxin in the lumen of the intestinal tract in animals with salmonellosis. Activated charcoal is neither metabolized nor absorbed by the intestine.

ADVERSE AND COMMON SIDE EFFECTS: None listed.

DRUG INTERACTIONS: None listed.

SUPPLIED AS VETERINARY PRODUCTS:
Granules containing 47.5 charcoal and 10.0 g kaolin per 100 g
Suspension containing 10.4% w/v charcoal and 6.25% w/v kaolin
Suspension containing 10.4% w/v charcoal and 6.25% w/v kaolin and 10% w/v sorbitol

SUPPLIED AS HUMAN PRODUCTS:
Suspension containing 50 g/250 mL, 30 g/240 mL, 30 g/120 mL, and others
Suspension (micronized) containing 200 mg/mL
Capsules containing 260 mg
Tablets containing 325 mg

CHLORAL HYDRATE

INDICATIONS: Chloral hydrate (Noctec ✤ ★, PMS Chloral Hydrate ✤) was one of the first central nervous system depressants to be used in veterinary surgery. Although still a valuable hypnotic for use in large animals, it is not a satisfactory anesthetic when used alone because it is a poor analgesic. Anesthetic doses severely depress the respiratory and vasomotor centers, approaching the LD_{50} for the drug. It is best used for its hypnotic effect in combination with local anesthetics, but the wide availability of potent tranquilizing agents has reduced its use in North America. There appears to be a latent period of action where further CNS depression occurs 10 to 15 minutes after injection of the drug.

ADVERSE AND COMMON SIDE EFFECTS: Perivascular injection can cause severe pain, tissue swelling, and destruction of the vein and sloughing of adjacent tissues. Chloral hydrate is irritating to the stomach, especially when empty.

DRUG INTERACTIONS: Chloral hydrate can be used in combination with magnesium sulfate and pentobarbital as a sedative or anesthetic agent for large animals.

SUPPLIED AS HUMAN PRODUCTS:
Capsules containing 500 mg
Syrup containing 250 mg or 500 mg/5 mL
Rectal suppositories containing 325, 500, or 650 mg

OTHER USES
Cattle

Chloral hydrate can also be used in cattle to depress nervous excitement that may accompany acetonemia. Given orally it increases the breakdown of starch in the rumen and influences rumen production of propionate; hence, it may also help correct the metabolic disturbance seen with clinical ketosis.

CHLORAMPHENICOL

INDICATIONS: Chloramphenicol (Amphicol Film Coated Tablets ★, Azramycine S125 ♣, Azramycine S250 ♣, Bemachol ★, Chlor 125 Palm ♣, Chlor Palm 250 ♣, Chlor Tablets ♣, Choralean Drops ♣, Chloramphenicol 1% ♣ ★, Chlorasone ★, Chlorbiotic ★, Chloricol ♣ ★, Karomycin Palmitate 125 ♣, Karomycin Palmitate 250 ♣, Medichol ★, Vedichol ★, Viceton ★, and others) is a bacteriostatic antibiotic that inhibits protein synthesis by binding to ribosomal subunits of susceptible bacteria, leading to the inhibition of peptidyl transferase and thereby preventing the transfer of amino acids to growing peptide chains and subsequent protein formation. It has a very wide spectrum of activity, with activity against streptococci, staphylococci, anaerobes, *Haemophilus, Salmonella, Pasteurella, Mycoplasma,* and *Brucella* spp. It is also active against *Rickettsia, Chlamydia,* and *Haemobartonella.* It is very lipid soluble and diffuses readily into most tissues. Highest concentrations are found in the liver and kidney. The lungs, heart, spleen, and skeletal muscle contain concentrations similar to that of blood. Chloramphenicol attains approximately 75% of blood levels in milk, pleural and ascitic fluid, and the placenta. It also diffuses readily into the cerebrospinal fluid, reaching 50% of serum levels within 3 to 4 hours of administration. Chloramphenicol palmitate is administered orally and the succinate form parenterally. Ophthalmic preparations are available for ocular bacterial infections. Chloramphenicol is used in horses with mixed bacterial infections, such as can occur in pleuritis and canker. It is banned for use in food animals in North America due to idiosyncratic human toxicity.

ADVERSE AND COMMON SIDE EFFECTS: Chloramphenicol is not to be administered to breeding animals, even though there were no reported associated problems during prior widespread use of the drug in food animals. Chloramphenicol is prohibited from use in food-producing animals because of rare, idiosyncratic (non–dose-dependent) human toxicity that results in fatal aplastic anemia and granulocytopenia. Toxic effects are related to the presence of the para-nitro group on the chloramphenicol molecule. This reaction does not occur with florfenicol, as it lacks the para-nitro group. Because it is a protein synthesis inhibitor, chronic use in animals may produce a dose-dependent bone marrow suppression, which is reversible upon discontinuing the drug. Chloramphenicol may suppress antibody production if given prior to an antigenic stimulus and may affect vaccination response.

DRUG INTERACTIONS: Chloramphenicol inhibits biotransformation of barbiturates, local anesthetics, phenytoin, phenylbutazone, xylazine, and dicumarol and may lower prothrombin levels. Chloramphenicol should not be administered in conjunction with or within 2 hours of pentobarbital anesthesia because it prolongs recovery time. Chloramphenicol should not be administered concurrently with penicillins, macrolides, aminoglycosides, or fluoroquinolones. Chloramphenicol may antagonize the activity of penicillins or aminoglycosides, and it acts on the same ribosomal site as the macrolides. Inhibition of protein synthesis by chloramphenicol interferes with the production of autolysins necessary for cell lysis after fluoroquinolones interfere with DNA supercoiling. Chloramphenicol may delay response to iron preparations.

SUPPLIED AS VETERINARY PRODUCTS:
Tablets containing 50, 100, 250, and 500 mg; 1 and 2.5 g
Capsules containing 100, 250, and 500 mg
Suspension containing 25, 50, 125, and 250 mg/mL
Ophthalmic preparations in solution containing 4 mg/mL
Ointment containing 10 mg/g

SUPPLIED AS HUMAN PRODUCTS:
Capsules containing 250 mg
Suspension containing 50 mg/mL (palmitate)
For injection containing 1 g (sodium succinate)

CHLORHEXIDINE

INDICATIONS: Chlorhexidine is a topical antiseptic used for surgical scrubs and for teat washing and dips in cattle (Bou-Matic Super Udder Wash ♣, Chlorasan ★, Della-Prep ♣, Dihexamin Udder Wash ♣, Hibitane Udder Wash ♣, Monarch Prep Udder Wash ♣, Nolvasan ★, Sani-Wash ♣, Virosan Solution ★, and many others). Used as a teat dip it controls and prevents the spread of mastitis-causing organisms. It is also included in ointment (Chlorasan Antiseptic Ointment ★, Hibitane Veterinary Ointment ♣) and in a powder for treatment of eye and wound infections (Eye and Wound Powder ♣). It is also used to disinfect inanimate objects in the veterinary clinic (ChlorHex Surgical Scrub ★, Hibitane Disinfectant ♣). Chlorhexidine is rapidly bactericidal to both gram-positive and most gram-negative bacilli. It is not virucidal. Chlorhexidine is effective in the presence of soaps, blood, and pus, although activity may be reduced. Chlorhexidine has a residual effect with up to 26% of the active ingredient remaining on the skin after 29 hours.

ADVERSE AND COMMON SIDE EFFECTS: Under ordinary use, chlorhexidine causes no adverse effects, but prolonged repetitive use may result in contact dermatitis and photosensitivity.

DRUG INTERACTIONS: Alcohols enhance the efficacy of chlorhexidine.

SUPPLIED AS VETERINARY AND HUMAN PRODUCTS:
See individual products

CHLORPROMAZINE

INDICATIONS: Chlorpromazine (Apo-Chlorpromazine ✤, Chlorprom ✤, Chlorpromanyl ✤, Largactil ✤ ★, Novo-Chlorpromazine ✤ ★, Ormazine ★, Thorazine ★) is a phenothiazine used for sedation and tranquilization in ruminants, but due to adverse CNS effects, it is contraindicated in horses. It is indicated for treatment of amphetamine toxicosis and has been considered by some as the neuroleptic drug of choice in cattle as a preanesthetic. Clinical effects are prominent for 4 to 5 hours but total effects may last 24 hours. Chlorpromazine is also indicated to treat clinical signs of tetanus in sheep and goats. Lack of a ready veterinary formulation and availability of other phenothiazines limits this drug's use in large animal practice.

ADVERSE AND COMMON SIDE EFFECTS: Tranquilization of dangerous animals with chlorpromazine may lead to a false sense of security. Painful procedures should be avoided because there is no analgesic effect. Horses may have episodes of violent excitement and incoordination following drug administration. An adequate blood volume and arterial blood pressure is necessary for the use of chlorpromazine because of its marked arterial hypotensive effects. Use in combination with epidural anesthesia is contraindicated because it potentiates arterial hypotension. Popular, albeit unethical, use in show cattle for tranquilization causes decreased adrenocorticotropic hormone (ACTH) and gonadotropin release and interferes with embryo transfer procedures for sometime after administration.

DRUG INTERACTIONS: Toxicity of carbamates and organophosphates may be enhanced by administration of phenothiazines. Concurrent use is contraindicated. Chlorpromazine potentiates the toxicity of the herbicide paraquat.

SUPPLIED AS HUMAN PRODUCTS:
Capsules containing 30, 75, and 150 mg
Tablets containing 10, 25, 50, 100, and 200 mg
Oral liquid containing 5 or 20 mg/mL
For injection containing 25 mg/mL
Suppositories containing 25 and 100 mg

CHORIONIC GONADOTROPIN

INDICATIONS: Chorionic gonadotropin [human chorionic gonadotropin, HCG] (A.P.L. ♣, Chorionad ♣, Chorionic Gonadotropin ★, Chorulon ♣ ★, Factrel ★) is a gonadal-stimulating hormone obtained from the urine of pregnant women. It is capable of supplementing or substituting for luteinizing hormone secreted by the anterior pituitary gland to promote follicle maturation and ovulation, and for the formation of the corpus luteum. In the male, chorionic gonadotropin stimulates the interstitial cells to produce testosterone. It is used for the treatment of cystic ovaries, nymphomania, impotence, and hypogenitalism due to pituitary hypofunction, and to hasten ovulation, particularly in the mare. Intravenous administration is satisfactory for a prompt effect, such as ovulation, but the IM route is more desirable when a prolonged effect such as Leydig cell stimulation is desired. For ovarian stimulation, other products (e.g., PMSG) are more effective.

ADVERSE AND COMMON SIDE EFFECTS: Chorionic gonadotropin is a foreign protein and can cause anaphylaxis when administered parenterally. Continued administration may result in antihormone antibody production, and the product may become ineffective in such animals.

DRUG INTERACTIONS: None listed.

SUPPLIED AS VETERINARY PRODUCT:
For injection containing 5,000 and 10,000 U

OTHER USES
Horses and Cattle
Cryptorchidism may respond to early injections of chorionic gonadotropin therapy, providing the inguinal canal is patent. Cryptorchid animals should not be used for breeding because cryptorchidism is a genetically influenced condition.

CIMETIDINE

INDICATIONS: Cimetidine (Apo-Cimetidine ♣, Novo-Cimetidine ♣, Nu-Cimet ♣, Peptol ♣, Tagamet ♣ ★) is an H_2-receptor antagonist that reduces gastric acid secretion in a dose-dependent competitive manner, by blocking histamine-induced gastric acid secretion. The H_2 blockers are highly selective in action and virtually without effect on H_1 receptors. The H_2 blockers also inhibit, at least partially, gastric secretion elicited by muscarinic agonists or gastrin. Cimetidine is used in horses to treat gastric ulcers. Cimetidine has been used experimentally in ruminants but only affected abomasal pH at extremely high oral doses.

ADVERSE AND COMMON SIDE EFFECTS: Adverse reactions are low in incidence and relatively minor and include skin rash, diarrhea, constipation, and loss of libido. Rapid IV injection may cause profound bradycardia. Cimetidine may increase serum creatinine through competition for sites of renal secretion.

DRUG INTERACTIONS: Cimetidine reduces metabolism of other drugs by inhibiting hepatic microsomal enzyme systems (warfarin, phenytoin, lidocaine, metronidazole, theophylline). Antacids should be given 1 hour before or after cimetidine to avoid interactions. Sucralfate may alter absorption of cimetidine.

SUPPLIED AS HUMAN PRODUCTS:
Tablets containing 200, 300, 400, 600, and 800 mg
Syrup containing 60 mg/mL
For injection containing 150 mg/mL

CIPROFLOXACIN OPHTHALMIC

INDICATIONS: Ciprofloxacin ophthalmic (Ciloxan ✤ ★) is a fluoro-quinolone antimicrobial solution. With its high lipid solubility, it is indicated in the treatment of infectious keratitis due to staphylococcal and gram-negative bacteria, including *Pseudomonas* spp. It has poor efficacy against streptococci, so culture is essential.

ADVERSE AND COMMON SIDE EFFECTS: White, crystalline precipitates may result from frequent administration. These precipitates are innocuous and do not affect therapeutic efficacy.

DRUG INTERACTIONS: None listed.

SUPPLIED AS HUMAN PRODUCT:
Ophthalmic solution containing 3.5 mg/mL

CISPLATIN

INDICATIONS: Cisplatin (Platinol ✤ ★) is an active cytotoxic drug with a narrow therapeutic range. Its usefulness as a systemic agent is limited by substantial neurotoxicity, nephrotoxicity, and toxicity to the gastrointestinal tract. It has been used intralesionally in horses with surface tumors, including equine sarcoids, squamous cell carcinomas, and squamous cell papillomas. A mean relapse-free interval of 21.6 months for sarcoids and 14 months for the carcinoma/papillomas has been reported. Treatment consists of a total of four sessions at 2-week intervals.

ADVERSE AND COMMON SIDE EFFECTS: Local toxicosis is reported to be minimal when used intralesionally in horses. In humans, even a single systemic dose can cause nephrotoxicity and ototoxicity. Nausea and vomiting are also common side effects.

DRUG INTERACTIONS: Cisplatin should not be used with other platinum-containing compounds.

SUPPLIED AS HUMAN PRODUCT:
For injection containing 0.5 and 1 mg/mL

CLENBUTEROL

INDICATIONS: Clenbuterol (Ventipulmin ✦ ★) is a sympatho-mimetic amine with a high degree of selectivity for β_2 sites in the body, with minimal binding propensity for β_1 (cardiac) receptors. Stimulation of β_2 sites causes relaxation of the smooth muscle of bronchi and the uterus. Clenbuterol is used for the treatment of bronchoconstriction in horses with recurrent airway obstruction (RAO) or inflammatory airway disease. Clenbuterol has a significant effect on increasing mucociliary transport in horses with RAO. Although recommended by some authors for facilitating obstetric manipulation in mares, strong abdominal contractions may negate any advantage gained through the effects of uterine relaxation. At therapeutic doses in horses, chronic clenbuterol administration is a repartitioning agent, increasing muscle mass while decreasing body fat. Human intoxication has occurred after ingestion of products from food animals treated with clenbuterol, so it is banned for use in any animal destined for human consumption. It may be detected in the retina of a treated animal for as long as 18 months after administration.

ADVERSE AND COMMON SIDE EFFECTS: Infrequently, transient sweating, muscle tremors, and tachycardia may occur. Clenbuterol should be discontinued in pregnant mares at the time of expected foaling because it can abolish uterine contractions.

DRUG INTERACTIONS: Clenbuterol antagonizes the effects of oxytocin and $PGF_{2\alpha}$. It is antagonized by β-blocking drugs.

SUPPLIED AS VETERINARY PRODUCTS:
Syrup containing 0.025 mg/mL
For injection containing 0.03 mg/mL (Canada only)

CLORSULON

INDICATIONS: Clorsulon (Curatrem ★) is a parasiticide used in cattle, sheep, and goats for the treatment and control of the liver fluke

Fasciola hepatica. The drug is effective against both immature and adult flukes and has a 10-fold margin of safety in ruminants.

ADVERSE AND COMMON SIDE EFFECTS: Because no milk withdrawal information is available, this product should not be used in dairy cattle of breeding age.

DRUG INTERACTIONS: None listed.

SUPPLIED AS VETERINARY PRODUCTS:
Oral liquid containing 85 mg/mL
10% injection in combination with 1% ivermectin [Ivomec Plus]

CLOXACILLIN

INDICATIONS: Cloxacillin (Dariclox ★, Dry-Clox ❦ ★, Orbenin Quick Release ❦, Orbenin-DC ★) is used for the treatment of mastitis in cattle caused by *Streptococcus agalactiae* and *Staphylococcus aureus* sensitive to penicillin, including penicillin-resistant strains. Cloxacillin is not destroyed by penicillinase produced by certain strains of *S. aureus*. Its antibacterial properties against nonpenicillinase-producing organisms are similar but less effective than penicillin G.

ADVERSE AND COMMON SIDE EFFECTS: As for other penicillins, allergic reactions can occur with cloxacillin. See PENICILLINS.

DRUG INTERACTIONS: See PENICILLINS.

SUPPLIED AS VETERINARY PRODUCTS:
Intramammary preparations containing 500 mg benzathine cloxacillin per 10-mL unit [Dry-Clox ❦ ★, Orbenin-DC ★]
    Intramammary preparations containing 200 mg cloxacillin sodium per 10-mL unit [Dariclox ★, Orbenin Quick Release ❦]

COBALT

INDICATIONS: Cobalt ❦ ★ is a component of vitamin B_{12}. Animals deficient in cobalt have reduced milk production, while severe deficiency causes emaciation, progressive inappetence, and anemia. Regions around the Great Lakes, as well as New England and Florida, are cobalt-deficient areas in North America. Australia, New Zealand, Great Britain, and portions of Africa are also cobalt-deficient areas. Cobalt sulfate or chloride is part of patent medicines in Canada (Ketamalt ❦, and others) used for the treatment and prevention of ketosis (acetonemia) in cows and sheep (pregnancy toxemia).

ADVERSE AND COMMON SIDE EFFECTS: Cobalt is relatively nontoxic.

DRUG INTERACTIONS: None listed.

SUPPLIED AS VETERINARY PRODUCTS:
Feed additive: in mineral or salt blocks, or as top dressing on pasture
Cobalt-containing acetonemia products (Canada only)

Liquid containing: cobalt chloride with choline chloride, ethylenediamine dihydroiodide, propylene glycol, and other compounds. See individual products.

COPPER INJECTABLE

INDICATIONS: Injectable copper (Caco Iron Copper ✽, Caco-Iron-Copper Solution ✽) is used as a hematinic for horses recovering from debilitating diseases, and for copper deficiency in large animals.

ADVERSE AND COMMON SIDE EFFECTS: Sheep are highly susceptible to copper toxicity. Administration of twice the recommended levels of soluble preparations can cause heavy mortalities in sheep and calves. Administration to cattle with liver disease or grazing plants containing toxic alkaloids that can induce liver damage, such as Tansy Ragwort, is contraindicated.

DRUG INTERACTIONS: None listed.

SUPPLIED AS VETERINARY PRODUCT:
For injection as copper gluconate (195 and 200 mg/mL) in combination with sodium cacodylate (6.4 and 6.5 mg/mL) and ferric chloride (1 and 1.13 mg/mL)

COPPER NAPHTHENATE

INDICATIONS: Copper naphthenate (Coppercure ✽, Copperox ✽, Coppersept ✽, Kopper Kare ✽, Kopertox ✽ ★) is a topical antifungal, antiseptic, and astringent, used for treating thrush, hoof punctures, cracked hooves, foot rot in cattle and sheep, and ringworm. It is also suggested for treating wounds after dehorning.

ADVERSE AND COMMON SIDE EFFECTS: Avoid direct contact with mucous membranes or the eyes. Do not apply to the teats of lactating animals.

DRUG INTERACTIONS: None listed.

SUPPLIED AS VETERINARY PRODUCT:
Solution containing copper naphthenate 37.5% w/v

COPPER SULFATE

INDICATIONS: Copper sulfate (Caustic Dressing Powder ★, Caustic Powder ★, Copper Sulfate-S ♣, Equi-Phar Caustic Powder ★, Proud-soff ★) is used as a caustic dressing for debridement and coagulation of wounds and in foot baths for the treatment of foot rot in cattle and sheep. Copper sulfate is also used in feeds or salt mixtures to prevent copper deficiency in cattle and sheep. Copper sulfate is included in topical preparations for treating ulcerative posthitis in sheep. Oral solutions of copper sulfate are reported to induce closure of the esophageal groove in ruminants.

ADVERSE AND COMMON SIDE EFFECTS: If the product is used in sheep as a foot bath, it may stain the wool. Sheep are highly susceptible to copper toxicity. Supplementation of copper in sheep diets should only be done where deficiency is known to exist.

DRUG INTERACTIONS: None listed.

SUPPLIED AS VETERINARY PRODUCTS:
Powder containing copper sulfate 50% w/w [Caustic Powder ★] or 51.5% w/w [Caustic Dressing Powder ★]
Powder containing 510 mg/g [Copper Sulfate-S ♣]
Granules containing copper sulfate 99% w/w
Chemical grade copper sulfate

CORTICOTROPIN

INDICATIONS: Corticotropin (A.C.T.H. 40 ♣, A.C.T.H. 40 I.U. ♣, H. P. Acthar Gel ★), also known as adrenocorticotropin, stimulates the adrenal cortex to secrete cortisol, corticosterone, aldosterone, and a number of weakly androgenic substances. ACTH is used in horses as a long-acting preparation for the treatment of musculoskeletal stiffness and arthritic conditions. ACTH is also used for bovine ketosis.

ADVERSE AND COMMON SIDE EFFECTS: Hypersensitivity may occur with repeated injections.

DRUG INTERACTIONS: Concurrent use of ketoconazole blunts the response of cortisol to the administration of ACTH.

SUPPLIED AS VETERINARY PRODUCT:
For injection containing 40 and 80 IU/mL in a repository preparation

SUPPLIED AS HUMAN PRODUCT:
For injection containing 80 IU/mL in a repository preparation

OTHER USES
Horses

The ACTH stimulation test is used in horses suspected of having functional pituitary adenoma and ACTH is given at 1 IU/kg ACTH gel; IM or, 100 IU of synthetic ACTH; IV.

COSYNTROPIN

INDICATIONS: Cosyntropin (Cortrosyn ♣ ★) is a synthetic subunit of corticotropin. It is preferable to ACTH for diagnosing primary adrenocortical insufficiency because it is less allergenic. It is not indicated in the treatment of glucocorticoid-responsive conditions. The maximal increase in plasma cortisol concentrations usually occurs one hour after injection. A normal response is a plasma cortisol concentration twice the baseline.

ADVERSE AND COMMON SIDE EFFECTS: Anaphylactic reactions may occur.

DRUG INTERACTIONS: None listed.

SUPPLIED AS HUMAN PRODUCT:
For injection containing 250 μg/vial

COUMAPHOS

INDICATIONS: Coumaphos (Co-Ral Dust Insecticide ★, Co-Ral 1% Dust ★, Co-Ral Equine and Livestock Insecticide Dust ★, KRS Spray ♣) is an organophosphate used mainly to treat external parasites of horses, swine, and cattle.

ADVERSE AND COMMON SIDE EFFECTS: Do not apply to sick, stressed, or convalescent animals. As for other organophosphates, atropine is used as the antidote for poisonings. For further information and drug interactions, see ORGANOPHOSPHATES in Description of Drugs for Small Animals. Treat lactating dairy cattle only after milking.

SUPPLIED AS VETERINARY PRODUCTS:
Topical powder containing 1% w/w and wettable powder containing 25% w/w coumaphos
Spray containing 3% w/v coumaphos

CROMOLYN SODIUM

INDICATIONS: Cromolyn sodium [sodium cromoglycate] (Novo-Cromolyn ♣, Intal Nebulizer Solution ♣ ★, Intal Spincaps ♣ ★, Intal

Inhaler ✤, Intal Syncroner ✤, Opticrom ✤ ★, PMS-Sodium Cromo-glycate ✤, Vistacrom ✤) is used for the treatment of horses with recurrent airway obstruction and inflammatory airway disease. Its exact mechanism of action is unknown, but it inhibits the release of histamine from pulmonary mast cells and other mediators (including leukotrienes) from the lung during allergic responses mediated by IgE. As such, it must be administered by inhalation and in advance of exposure to the allergen. Because cromolyn sodium has no inherent activity to relax bronchial smooth muscle, it has no place in the treatment of acute bronchospasm in horses.

ADVERSE AND COMMON SIDE EFFECTS: Rare but serious effects may include hypersensitivity to the drug, manifested by laryngeal edema, angioedema, urticaria, or anaphylaxis. When using a nebulizer to administer the drug, strict attention to cleanliness of the nebulizer is required to avoid bacterial contamination of the nebulized aerosol. This product should not be given by injection.

DRUG INTERACTIONS: None listed.

SUPPLIED AS HUMAN PRODUCTS:
Dry powder for inhalation containing 20 mg
Solution for nebulization containing 20 mg/mL
Pressurized metered-dose inhaler containing 1 mg/actuation (Canada), and 800 µg/actuation (United States)

CYPROHEPTADINE

INDICATIONS: Cyproheptadine (Periactin ✤ ★) is an antihistamine with anticholinergic and antiserotonergic action used in horses with photic headshaking. This headshaking behavior in horses exposed to bright sunlight is thought to be due to optic-infraorbital nerve summation and pain. Cyproheptadine appears to moderate infraorbital nerve sensation, but the mechanism of action is not known. Other antihistamines are not effective in eliminating headshaking behavior. Relief from the behavior is usually seen within 24 hours of beginning therapy.

ADVERSE AND COMMON SIDE EFFECTS: Mild side effects of depression, lethargy, and anorexia may be noted.

DRUG INTERACTIONS: None listed.

SUPPLIED AS HUMAN PRODUCT:
Tablets containing 4 mg

DANOFLOXACIN

INDICATIONS: Danofloxacin (A180 ★) is a fluoroquinolone antimicrobial for the treatment of bovine respiratory disease due to *Mannheimia haemolytica* and *Pasteurella multocida*. Because the fluoroquinolones are concentration-dependent killers with a long postantibiotic effect, the ideal dosage regimen is once-daily, high-dose therapy. Any extralabel use in food animals is strictly prohibited in the United States

ADVERSE AND COMMON SIDE EFFECTS: The danofloxacin formulation may cause transient local SC irritation. While fluoroquinolones are associated with arthropathies in a number of species, in clinical studies of up to 3X the label dose, danofloxacin did not cause cartilage damage in calves. The fluoroquinolones may cause adverse CNS effects in humans and animals due to a γ-aminobutyric acid (GABA) receptor antagonism. This has been associated with an increase in seizure incidence in humans and dogs.

DRUG INTERACTIONS: See FLUOROQUINOLONES.

SUPPLIED AS VETERINARY PRODUCT:
For injection containing 180 mg/mL

DANTROLENE

INDICATIONS: Dantrolene (Dantrium ♣ ★) is a skeletal muscle relaxant used in the prevention and treatment of malignant hyperthermia. Dantrolene has been advocated for use in preventing anesthetic-associated and exertional myopathy in horses but has not proven to be efficacious. Draft breeds may require lower than the recommended dose. Oral bioavailability is poor unless fasted.

ADVERSE AND COMMON SIDE EFFECTS: Sedation, nausea, vomiting, constipation, and, possibly, hypotension occur. Drug overdose may cause generalized muscle weakness. Hepatotoxicity has been documented in humans following long-term drug therapy.

DRUG INTERACTIONS: Concurrent use of CNS depressants may cause additive CNS depression. Concurrent use of β blockers in swine with malignant hyperthermia resulted in ventricular fibrillation and hyperkalemia.

SUPPLIED AS HUMAN PRODUCTS:
Capsules containing 25, 50, and 100 mg
For injection containing 20 mg/mL

DECOQUINATE

INDICATIONS: Decoquinate (Deccox Premix ♣, Deccox ★) is a feed additive coccidiostat for broiler chickens and ruminants. Decoquinate acts by preventing the sporozoite stage from developing once it has penetrated the host intestinal cell. It is to be fed for at least 28 days when coccidiosis is considered to be a hazard. Decoquinate is not effective for treating clinical coccidiosis.

ADVERSE AND COMMON SIDE EFFECTS: The drug should not be fed to ruminants producing milk for human consumption or hens laying eggs for human consumption.

DRUG INTERACTIONS: None listed.

SUPPLIED AS VETERINARY PRODUCTS:
Medicated premix containing 60 g/kg
Pellets containing 0.5% w/w in calf starter-grower
Medicated powder for whole milk containing 0.8% w/w decoquinate

DEMBREXINE

INDICATIONS: Dembrexine (Sputolysin Powder ♣) is a secretolytic with expectorant and secondary antitussive effects. It acts by altering the viscosity of respiratory mucus and improves the efficiency of respiratory tract clearance. Because of the effect on mucous production, there may be an initial increase in visible nasal discharge or cough before clinical improvement. It is reported to increase the concentrations of antibiotics in lung secretions. Dembrexine is used in horses with respiratory diseases such as chronic bronchitis or small airway disease in combination with other specific drugs for the underlying disease.

ADVERSE AND COMMON SIDE EFFECTS: No adverse effects have been reported. The effect on fertility in breeding stock has not been determined. This drug should not be used in horses intended for food.

DRUG INTERACTIONS: None listed.

SUPPLIED AS VETERINARY PRODUCT:
Powder containing 5 mg/g

DETOMIDINE

INDICATIONS: Detomidine (Dormosedan ♣ ★) is a synthetic α_2-adrenergic receptor agonist with potent sedative and analgesic properties. It is used in horses for chemical restraint of particularly fractious animals for procedures such as nasogastric intubation, bronchoscopy, and for pain relief for minor surgical procedures and colic. Detomidine produces profound lethargy, reduced sensitivity to environmental stimuli (sight, sound), and, after a short period of incoordination, a fixed, base-wide stance during the period of sedation. Its sedative and analgesic effects depend on the dose and route of administration and will last from 30 minutes to 2 hours. Sensitivity to touch is little affected and in some cases may be enhanced, in which case some horses that appear deeply sedated may respond excessively to sudden external stimuli.

ADVERSE AND COMMON SIDE EFFECTS: Bradycardia and partial atrioventricular block may occur. A diuretic effect may be observed within 45 to 60 minutes of treatment. The respiratory rate slows initially but returns to normal within 5 minutes. Piloerection, sweating, salivation, and partial, transient penile prolapse in males may be seen. This drug should not be used in horses with preexisting atrioventricular or sinoatrial block or in horses with severe cardiac insufficiency, cerebrovascular disease, respiratory disease, or chronic renal failure.

DRUG INTERACTIONS: Atropine (0.02 mg/kg; IV) will prevent the occurrence of the cardiac arrhythmias. Reversal of sedation can be accomplished with α_2-receptor blocking agents, such as yohimbine. Use the drug with caution if combining it with other sedatives. There are recent reports of the occurrence of fatal arrhythmias when detomidine has been administered to horses that were under treatment with trimethoprim/sulfa drugs. Because little is known of the predisposing conditions in these cases, an alternative sedative should be chosen if possible when trimethoprim/sulfas have been given to the horse.

SUPPLIED AS VETERINARY PRODUCT:
For injection containing 10 mg/mL

DEXAMETHASONE

INDICATIONS: Dexamethasone (Azium Solution ♣ ★, Azium Powder ♣ ★, Dexadreson ♣, Dexamethasone Injection ♣ ★, Dexamethasone Powder ♣, Dexamethasone 21 Phosphate Injection ♣, Dexamethasone Sodium Phosphate Injection ★, Dexaject ★, Dexamethasone 2 ♣, Dexamethasone 2 ★, Dexamethasone 5 ♣, Dexasone ★, Dexone ♣, Dextab ♣, Voren ★, and others) is a potent anti-inflammatory glucocorticoid, with 25 times the potency of cortisone and a long duration of action. All glucocorticoids have similar modes of action and effects, the difference being mainly in anti-inflammatory potency and duration of action. Glucocorticoids have numerous and widespread actions, influencing carbohydrate, lipid, and protein metabolism. The most important factor in their anti-inflammatory action is to inhibit the recruitment of neutrophils and monocyte-macrophages into affected tissues. Local heat, redness, and swelling is prevented or suppressed, but the underlying cause of disease remains. Anti-inflammatory effects of dexamethasone are beneficial in arthritis and inflammatory conditions in musculoskeletal injuries, and in immunologic diseases, such as purpura hemorrhagica, allergic rhinitis, and urticaria. Dexamethasone is also useful for the treatment of primary ketosis in cattle, the principal mechanism being mainly the reduction of milk production. Dexamethasone is advocated for treatment of shock, but the doses required for large animals are often impractical, and the beneficial effects have been seriously questioned in controlled clinical studies in human shock patients. Dexamethasone is used for treating cerebral edema, but its efficacy has been questioned. Ophthalmologic preparations are used to reduce uveal tract inflammation in diseases such as equine recurrent uveitis. Dexamethasone can induce premature parturition in cattle, sheep, and goats. It will also induce abortion in cattle when combined with prostaglandin $F_{2\alpha}$ in the last trimester of gestation.

ADVERSE AND COMMON SIDE EFFECTS: High, continued doses can cause adrenocortical suppression. Use of dexamethasone in horses under certain conditions has been associated with the occurrence of laminitis, possibly due to increased vascular reactivity to biogenic amines. Glucocorticoids should not be used in bacterial, viral, or parasitic infections unless concurrent anti-infective agents are used. Clinical signs may abate with their use, but with their sole use the underlying disease remains active. Topical use of glucocorticoids on the eye is contraindicated if corneal ulceration is present. If long-term therapy is undertaken, withdrawal should be gradual to avoid problems of iatrogenic hypoadrenocorticism. Glucocorticoids given to animals in the last trimester of pregnancy can induce premature parturition and predispose to retained placenta and metritis. Dexamethasone delays wound healing and reduces exuberant granulation tissue. Rapid IV administration may result in anaphylactic reactions. See also GLUCOCORTICOID AGENTS.

DRUG INTERACTIONS: See GLUCOCORTICOID AGENTS.

SUPPLIED AS VETERINARY PRODUCTS:
For injection containing 2, 4, and 5 mg/mL [sodium phosphate]
For injection containing 1 mg/mL [dexamethasone-21-isonicotinate]
Oral powder in packets containing 10 mg
Tablets containing 0.25 mg
In combination with other medications [Azimycin, Naquasone, Tresaderm]
See package label for specific details.

DEXTRAN

INDICATIONS: Dextran 70 (Macrodex ✤ ★) and Dextran 40 (Rheomacrodex ✤ ★) are polysaccharide solutions of high molecular weight that are used for plasma volume expansion and the treatment of hypovolemic shock (Dextran 70). Dextran 40, with its smaller molecular size, has a greater osmotic effect per gram. Dextran 70 has a particle size similar to that of albumin. A key role for its use in large animals is as a peritoneal lavage solution to prevent formation of adhesion in horses undergoing abdominal surgery. The proposed mechanism of this adhesion prevention is to increase surface separation of serosal surfaces.

ADVERSE AND COMMON SIDE EFFECTS: Administration should be avoided in horses with excessive contamination or leakage of bacteria during surgery because it increases the prevalence of peritonitis under these conditions. Thus, if the horse has evidence of moderate to severe serosal inflammation on the intestine, if any devitalized intestine appears present, or an enterotomy or anastomosis was performed, use of dextrans in the lavage fluid is contraindicated.

DRUG INTERACTIONS: None listed.

SUPPLIED AS HUMAN PRODUCTS:
Dextran 70

For injection containing 6 g dextran 70 and 900 mg sodium chloride per 100 mL [Macrodex-Saline]
For injection containing 6 g dextran 70 and 5 g dextrose per 100 mL [Macrodex-Dextrose]

Dextran 40

For injection containing 10 g dextran 40 and 900 mg saline per 100 mL [Rheomacrodex-Saline]
For injection containing 10 g dextran 40 and 5 g dextrose per 100 mL [Rheomacrodex-Dextrose]

DIAZEPAM

INDICATIONS: Diazepam (Valium ✤ ★, Valrelease ★) is a muscle relaxant, sedative, and anticonvulsive drug. Diazepam is used as a premedicant for general anesthesia to ensure smooth induction and recovery, particularly for foals and small ruminants, and for treating clinical tetanus. Diazepam is also indicated for behavior modification to treat novice stallions that appear anxious or fearful, or that pay more attention to the handler than the mare.

ADVERSE AND COMMON SIDE EFFECTS: Intravenous injection can be irritating. Teratogenic effects have been reported in humans.

DRUG INTERACTIONS: Metabolism may be decreased and excessive sedation may occur if diazepam is given with cimetidine, erythromycin, ketoconazole, or propranolol. Additive central nervous system effects may be anticipated if diazepam is given along with barbiturates, narcotics, or anesthetics. Antacids may slow the rate of oral drug absorption. The pharmacological effects of digoxin may be potentiated. Rifampin may induce hepatic microenzymal activity and decrease the efficacy of diazepam. An increase in the duration and intensity of respiratory depression may occur if diazepam is used with pancuronium or succinylcholine. Diazepam for injection should not be mixed with other drugs without consulting references. Diazepam must be stored in glass, as it will adsorb to plastics.

SUPPLIED AS HUMAN PRODUCTS:
Tablets containing 2, 5, and 10 mg
For injection containing 5 mg/mL

DICHLORVOS

INDICATIONS: Dichlorvos (Atgard Swine Dewormer ❦ ★, Disvap Spray and Fogging Solution ❦, Vapona Concentrate Insecticide ★) is a cholinesterase inhibitor used as an anthelmintic feed additive in swine against *Trichuris, Oesophagostomum,* and *Ascaris* spp. The pellets slowly release the drug, so it is absorbed over a 2- to 3-day period and toxicity reduced. Used as a fogging solution, it can be applied to premises or directly to dairy and beef cattle, and horses, to reduce the population of stable flies, horn flies, and house flies. Spray lightly on areas of the animal on which flies congregate.

ADVERSE AND COMMON SIDE EFFECTS: Toxicity can cause colic, excess salivation, diarrhea, bradycardia, and respiratory distress. Do not use in the milk room. The margin of safety is generally less than other broad-spectrum anthelmintics.

DRUG INTERACTIONS: Atropine is used as the antidote in poisonings. Praladoxime (2-PAM) will reactivate cholinesterase if given shortly after exposure.

SUPPLIED AS VETERINARY PRODUCTS:
Resin pellets containing 9.6% w/w in boxes of 836 g and pails of 4 kg
Powder in packets containing 78 g
Liquid concentrate containing 40.2% w/v for treatment of environment

DIETHYLCARBAMAZINE

INDICATIONS: Diethylcarbamazine (Decacide Tabs ♣, Diethylcarbamazine Citrate ★, Filaribits ★) is an antimicrofilarial compound that causes immobilization of the parasite and alters its surface membrane, rendering it more susceptible to destruction by host defenses. It is used in horses for the treatment of verminous myelitis and onchocerciasis.

ADVERSE AND COMMON SIDE EFFECTS: In humans, there may be mild, temporary malaise, weakness, and anorexia, or intense itching or skin rash in heavy *Onchocerca* infections. Similar effects may occur in horses.

DRUG INTERACTIONS: Pretreatment with glucocorticoids may be undertaken to minimize adverse reactions.

SUPPLIED AS VETERINARY PRODUCTS:
Small-Animal Products Only
Tablets containing 50, 60, 100, 180, 200, 300, and 400 mg

DIGOXIN

INDICATIONS: Digoxin (Lanoxin ★, Cardoxin ♣ ★) decreases sympathetic nerve activity and is a positive inotropic and negative chronotropic agent. Its chronotropic properties make it a popular choice in the management of supraventricular tachyarrhythmias, e.g., atrial flutter and fibrillation and sinus tachycardia associated with congestive heart failure. It is used in large animals in the treatment of congestive heart failure and for assisting the treatment of supraventricular tachycardia or arrhythmias, such as atrial fibrillation in horses, and for dilated cardiomyopathy in cattle. Digoxin is used before quinidine in the treatment of atrial fibrillation in horses and cattle with tachycardia (>60 and 100 beats/minute, respectively). Side effects of quinidine treatment may be decreased in animals pretreated with digoxin. Therapeutic drug monitoring can assist in initial therapy to optimize effect and to minimize toxicity. Peak concentrations should not exceed 2.5 ng/mL. Low oral bioavailability in cattle limits its use to IV treatment.

ADVERSE AND COMMON SIDE EFFECTS: Frequent electrocardiographic monitoring is indicated during digoxin administration. Signs of toxicity include depression, ataxia, and gastrointestinal upset, including diarrhea, weakness, and cardiac arrhythmias. Digoxin is contraindicated in ventricular arrhythmias and second- and third-degree heart block. Digoxin has no direct positive inotropic effect on the normal heart and may actually decrease cardiac output if administered to normal animals. Lidocaine and phenytoin are effective in managing digoxin-induced arrhythmias.

DRUG INTERACTIONS: Concurrent use with quinidine may increase plasma concentrations of digoxin, possibly by displacement of digoxin from binding sites in tissues. Phenylbutazone, phenobarbital, phenytoin, and rifampin may speed the metabolism of digoxin. Diuretics that deplete potassium (e.g., furosemide) potentiate digoxin toxicity.

SUPPLIED AS VETERINARY PRODUCT:
Elixir containing 0.05 and 0.15 mg/mL

HUMAN PRODUCTS
Capsules containing 0.05, 0.1, and 0.2 mg
Tablets containing 0.0625, 0.125, 0.25, and 0.5 mg
Elixir containing 0.05 mg/mL
For injection containing 0.05, 0.1, and 0.25 mg/mL

DIHYDROSTREPTOMYCIN

INDICATIONS: Dihydrostreptomycin (Ethamycin ✤) is an aminoglycoside antibiotic similar to streptomycin, which was produced initially for treatment of tuberculosis in humans. Resistance to this form of aminoglycoside has become widespread, but it remains useful for treating leptospirosis and actinomycosis. It is a suggested treatment for tuberculosis in the horse, although this disease is extremely rare in North America. The drug is also used in combination with long-acting tetracyclines for brucellosis in countries that have no eradication program. It is present in a number of combined products with other antibiotics, particularly penicillin G (Quartermaster ★, Special Formula 17900-Forte Suspension ✤).

ADVERSE AND COMMON SIDE EFFECTS: Overdose can cause renal tubular damage, which may be reversible once the drug is discontinued. Avoid use with other aminoglycosides because of potential additive toxic effects. The drug causes transient pain on injection. Ototoxicity can occur but is difficult to detect clinically. Dihydrostreptomycin has much higher ototoxic potential than streptomycin. Weakness from neuromuscular blockade can also occur. See also AMINOGLYCOSIDES.

DRUG INTERACTIONS: Concurrent use of furosemide can increase the ototoxic potential and predispose to renal tubular damage. See also AMINOGLYCOSIDES.

SUPPLIED AS VETERINARY PRODUCTS:
For injection containing 500 mg/mL
Mastitis tubes containing 100 mg combined with 100,000 U penicillin G procaine, 150 mg novobiocin, 50,000 U polymyxin B, 20 mg hydrocortisone, and 12.5 mg hydrocortisone sodium succinate (Canada)

Mastitis tubes containing 1 g combined with 1,000,000 U procaine penicillin G (United States)

DIMETHYL GLYCINE

INDICATIONS: Dimethyl glycine ♣ ★ is a nutritional supplement used in athletic horses in the hope that it delays fatigue or reduces lactate accumulation. Some studies suggest improvement in time trials for racing greyhounds over longer distances, but controlled crossover trials in exercising horses failed to identify beneficial effects on performance or in a number of related physiologic parameters. Unpublished reports also make claims that dimethyl glycine may reduce the incidence of recurrent exertional rhabdomyolysis.

ADVERSE AND COMMON SIDE EFFECTS: None listed.

DRUG INTERACTIONS: None listed.

SUPPLIED AS CHEMICAL PRODUCT:
As a powder containing free base dimethyl glycine

DIMETHYL SULFOXIDE

INDICATIONS: Dimethyl sulfoxide (Domoso Gel ♣ ★, Domoso Solution ♣ ★) is a potent organic solvent with a wide range of actions and proposed uses. It increases the penetration of low molecular weight compounds through intact skin. It has anti-inflammatory actions, analgesic properties, scavenges free radicals, interferes with neutrophil chemotaxis, and is a potent diuretic. It has been used topically to decrease inflammation in musculoskeletal injuries and for soft tissue inflammation such as may occur with thrombophlebitis. It has been proposed as a treatment for cerebral edema and acute central nervous system injury, such as spinal or head trauma, equine protozoal encephalomyelitis, West Nile Virus encephalitis or neonatal maladjustment syndrome of foals. However, the available literature concerning efficacy is conflicting. The IV route for therapy is common but is extralabel.

ADVERSE AND COMMON SIDE EFFECTS: The drug is not to be used in horses with ocular disease, liver or kidney problems, or animals with a history of allergy. Topical treatment may occasionally cause transient erythema and associated irritation of the area, possibly due to mast cell degranulation. Dryness of the skin and oyster-like breath odor have also been reported. Do not use more than 100 g or 100 mL daily or for longer than 30 days in the horse. It is not to be used in pregnant mares or mares intended for breeding. Subcutaneous injection results in a marked local necrotizing reaction. Intravenous injection of greater than 10% solutions can cause hemoglobinuria. Intravenous administration may also cause muscle fasciculations, sweating, intravascular hemolysis, and hemoglobinuria. Use caution when handling as it will penetrate rubber gloves and contact of dimethyl sulfoxide with human skin will result in malodorous breath and systemic side effects. It should be used in well ventilated areas as 70% of the product is excreted through the respiratory tract.

DRUG INTERACTIONS: Topical application may facilitate absorption of undesirable medications (such as mercury blisters) previously applied to the skin.

SUPPLIED AS VETERINARY PRODUCTS:
Topical gel preparation containing 90% w/w dimethyl sulfoxide
Solution containing 90% w/w medical grade dimethyl sulfoxide

DIOCTYL SODIUM SULFOSUCCINATE

INDICATIONS: Docusate sodium [dioctyl sodium sulfosuccinate, DSS, DOS] (Anti-Gaz Emulsion ❧, Anti-Bloat ❧, Bloat-Aid ❧, Bloat-Eze ❧, Bloat Treatment ★, Dioctynate ★, Disposable Enema Syringe ★, Docusate Solution ★, Docu-Soft Enema ★, Enema DSS ★, Enema SA ★, Tympanex Suspension ❧, Veterinary Surfactant ★) is a surface-acting anionic surfactant used as an aid in the treatment of frothy bloat in ruminants and for the treatment of large colon or gastric impactions in horses. At recommended dosages docusates have minimal laxative effects. The clinical usefulness is to hydrate intestinal contents by emulsifying feces, water, and fat in the intestinal lumen.

ADVERSE AND COMMON SIDE EFFECTS: Toxicity can occur at 3 to 5 times the recommended dose in horses; therefore, do not exceed a total dose of 200 mg/kg. Signs of toxicity include increased heart rate, respiratory rate, and intestinal sounds and severe watery diarrhea followed by dehydration, recumbency, and death.

DRUG INTERACTIONS: Docusates increase intestinal absorption of other drugs administered concurrently and may increase their toxicity.

SUPPLIED AS VETERINARY PRODUCTS:
Suspension containing 8 mg/mL or 50 mg/mL
Enema solution containing 5% w/v
Premeasured enema syringe containing 250 mg/12 mL

DIPHENHYDRAMINE

INDICATIONS: Diphenhydramine (Allerdryl ❧ ★, Benadryl ❧ ★, Hyrexin ★) is an antihistamine used to treat allergic reactions and anaphylactic reactions as an adjunct to epinephrine and supportive therapies. It is also used as an antidyskinetic in the case of extrapyramidal reaction in horses from metoclopramide and fluphenazine toxicity, where it provides central anticholinergic action and sedation.

ADVERSE AND COMMON SIDE EFFECTS: Adverse effects include CNS depression and anticholinergic effects (xerostomia, urine retention).

DRUG INTERACTIONS: In humans, antihistamines should be discontinued for 4 days before skin testing for allergies. Anxiolytic agents, sedatives, narcotics, and barbiturates may enhance CNS depression, and monoamine oxidase (MAO) inhibitors, possibly amitraz and selegiline, may prolong and intensify the anticholinergic (drying) effects of antihistamines. Concurrent use of chlorpheniramine with phenytoin may increase the pharmacological effects of phenytoin. In humans, normal doses of terfenadine when used in conjunction with ketoconazole or erythromycin, or in patients with severe liver disease, may cause severe and life-threatening cardiac arrhythmias. In addition, conditions that increase the risk of cardiac arrhythmias, e.g., electrolyte imbalance or the use of drugs that prolong the QT interval on an electrocardiogram, also may be associated with increased risk.

SUPPLIED AS HUMAN PRODUCTS:
Capsules containing 25 and 50 mg
Tablets containing 25 and 50 mg
Elixir and syrup containing 12.5 mg/mL
For injection containing 10 and 50 mg/mL
Solution and cream containing 1% and 2% w/v diphenhydramine

DIPYRONE

INDICATIONS: Dipyrone (Dipyrone 50% ♣) is an analgesic, antipyretic, anti-inflammatory, and antispasmodic used in large animals as a smooth muscle antispasmodic and analgesic, particularly in horses. It is indicated in conditions where pain is caused by hyperperistalsis, spasmodic colic, or esophageal contraction in choke. Its analgesic effect in cases of colic is poor. Due to extralabel use in food animals without data to support withdrawal times, dipyrone has been banned for sale in the United States.

ADVERSE AND COMMON SIDE EFFECTS: Overdosage can cause convulsions. Prolonged use can cause agranulocytosis and leukopenia. Subcutaneous or IM injections are highly irritating and associated with clostridial myositis in horses.

DRUG INTERACTIONS: Dipyrone is contraindicated for use in conjunction with phenylbutazone or barbiturates because of drug interactions involving the microsomal enzyme system. Dipyrone can interfere with or mask the presence of prohibited drugs in racehorses for up to 5 days. Concurrent use with chlorpromazine hydrochloride can result in clinically serious hypothermia.

SUPPLIED AS VETERINARY PRODUCT:
For injection containing 500 mg/mL

DOBUTAMINE

INDICATIONS: Dobutamine (Dobutrex ❦ ★, Dobutamine Hydrochloride Injection ❦ ★) is a positive cardiac inotrope similar in nature and action to dopamine used to improve peripheral perfusion. It has been advocated for neonatal foals suffering from asphyxia, for horses with circulatory shock caused by endotoxemia, and for severe hypotension that may occur in foals due to snake bite. It has no effect on the dopaminergic receptors of the renal vasculature.

ADVERSE AND COMMON SIDE EFFECTS: Before dobutamine is administered, hypovolemia must be corrected by appropriate fluid therapy. Tachycardia and arrhythmias may occur during infusion.

DRUG INTERACTIONS: Propranolol may negate the effects of dobutamine. Halothane may increase the likelihood of arrhythmias.

SUPPLIED AS HUMAN PRODUCT:
For injection containing 12.5 mg/mL

DOPAMINE

INDICATIONS: Dopamine (Intropin ❦ ★, Dopamine Hydrochloride and 5% Dextrose Injection ❦ ★) is the immediate metabolic precursor of norepinephrine and epinephrine. Its positive cardiac inotropic effects are used to improve peripheral perfusion. Its use has been advocated in neonatal foals suffering from asphyxia, horses with circulatory shock caused by endotoxemia, and for severe hypotension due to snake bite. It is also used in oliguric renal failure of foals as it can increase glomerular filtration rate via specific dopaminergic receptors in the kidney.

ADVERSE AND COMMON SIDE EFFECTS: Before dopamine is administered, the animal must have hypovolemia corrected by appropriate fluid therapy. Tachycardia and arrhythmias may occur during infusion. Extravasation of large amounts of dopamine during infusion can result in ischemic necrosis of the area.

DRUG INTERACTIONS: Phenytoin may decrease the effects of dopamine, leading to hypotension and bradycardia.

SUPPLIED AS HUMAN PRODUCTS:
For injection containing 40 mg/mL
For infusion containing 0.8, 1.6, or 3.2 mg/mL in 5% dextrose

DORAMECTIN

INDICATIONS: Doramectin (Dectomax Injectable Solution ♣ ★, Dectomax Pour-On ♣ ★) is an avermectin endectocide for cattle and swine (injectable formulation). It is used for the eradication of adult and most larval stages of most gastrointestinal roundworms and lungworms, and ectoparasites, such as lice, mites, and certain insect larva, including cattle grub (*Hypoderma bovis, Hypoderma lineatum*). Doramectin has no activity against tapeworms or flukes. The principle mechanism of action of the avermectins in parasitic nematodes is to increase membrane permeability to chloride ions. The parasiticidal action is likely to be mediated by interaction of avermectins with glutamate-gated chloride ion channels. These glutamate-gated chloride channels have not been reported in mammals.

ADVERSE AND COMMON SIDE EFFECTS: Doramectin has a wide margin of safety. Symptoms of overdose include ataxia, depression, salivation, mydriasis, and blindness. Treatment of overdose is symptomatic; neurologic signs usually resolve over several days. Do not administer CNS depressants such as diazepam or pentobarbital. Do not use in female dairy cattle over 20 months of age.

DRUG INTERACTIONS: None listed.

SUPPLIED AS VETERINARY PRODUCTS:
For injection containing 10 mg/mL
Pour-on containing 5 mg/mL (for use in cattle)

DOXAPRAM

INDICATIONS: Doxapram (Dopram-V Injectable ★) is a central respiratory stimulant used for hastening recovery from anesthesia, such as with pentobarbital and/or chloral hydrate, and for stimulating respiratory centers of neonatal animals following Cesarean section or dystocia. Onset of action is rapid and the dose should be adjusted according to clinical response. A patent airway should be ensured prior to drug administration. Doxapram can also be administered SC or sublingually in the neonate if the IV route is not available. Doxapram is indicated for treatment of poisonings in which there is depression of the respiratory center.

ADVERSE AND COMMON SIDE EFFECTS: Excessive doses can cause respiratory alkalosis. High doses can cause convulsions.

DRUG INTERACTIONS: Do not mix with alkaline solutions. Doxapram-stimulated respiration is severely depressed by morphine or meperidine.

SUPPLIED AS VETERINARY PRODUCT:
For injection containing 20 mg/mL

OTHER USES
Horses

Doxapram is also used as a respiratory stimulant to facilitate endoscopic examination of laryngeal motion in the horse.

ENILCONAZOLE

INDICATIONS: Enilconazole (Imaverol ♣, Clinafarm EC 13.8% ★) is a benzimidazole that inhibits fungal growth with potent antifungal action against dermatophytes. It is labeled in Canada as a topical wash for the treatment of dermatophytes. It has been used topically in horses to treat guttural pouch mycoses. In its diluted form it is nonirritating.

ADVERSE AND COMMON SIDE EFFECTS: The concentrated solution is irritating to the skin and eyes, but these are no longer problems if the solution is properly diluted.

DRUG INTERACTIONS: None listed.

SUPPLIED AS VETERINARY PRODUCTS:
Solution in concentrate at 100 mg/mL (Canada)
Chemical grade 13.8% w/w (United States)

ENROFLOXACIN

INDICATIONS: Enrofloxacin (Baytril 100 ♣ ★) is a synthetic fluoroquinolone. Enrofloxacin is effective in small animals against a broad range of microbes, including gram-positive and gram-negative bacteria, *Chlamydia*, *Rickettsia*, and *Mycoplasma* spp. It is approved for use for the treatment of bovine respiratory disease and is used extralabel in horses for the treatment of staphylococcal and gram-negative infections, including infections from *Salmonella* spp. and *Pseudomonas* spp. Enrofloxacin is not active against anaerobes and poorly effective against streptococci. Because the fluoroquinolones are concentration-dependent killers with a long postantibiotic effect, the ideal dosage regimen is once-daily, high-dose therapy. Any extralabel use in food animals is strictly prohibited in the United States. Enrofloxacin has a 50% oral bioavailability in horses, but must be given parenterally to ruminants. It is highly lipid soluble and achieves therapeutic concentrations in most tissues and abscesses.

ADVERSE AND COMMON SIDE EFFECTS: Enrofloxacin at clinical doses may cause arthropathies in neonatal foals, but this effect is not seen in adult horses, ruminants, or swine. Cartilage damage in foals is most severe with weight bearing and exercise; so if administered to foals because of life-threatening infections, they should be strictly stall rested. The enrofloxacin injectable solutions are irritating upon injection; therefore, the bovine formulation is labeled for SC administration and is given IV to horses. The small animal formulations may also be given IV to horses. The fluoroquinolones may cause adverse CNS effects in humans and animals due to a GABA receptor antagonism. This has been associated with an increase in seizure incidence in humans and dogs. Administration of enrofloxacin to humans results in hallucinations. Rapid IV administration of high doses of enrofloxacin to horses causes transient neurologic signs, including excitability and seizure-like activity.

DRUG INTERACTIONS: Oral absorption is hindered by antacid preparations as well as sucralfate. Nitrofurantoin, chloramphenicol, and rifampin are antagonistic to fluoroquinolone activity.

SUPPLIED AS VETERINARY PRODUCTS:
Tablets containing 22.7, 68, and 136 mg (United States) or 15, 50, and 150 mg (Canada)
For injection containing 22.7 mg/mL (United States), 50 mg/mL (Canada, small animal formulations), and 100 mg/mL (bovine formulation)

EPINEPHRINE

INDICATIONS: Epinephrine (Epichlor ♣, Epinject ★, Adrenalin ♣ ★) is the adrenergic receptor agonist drug of choice for cardiopulmonary resuscitation and anaphylaxis. Epinephrine stimulates both α- and β-adrenergic receptors, but its utility in CPR is primarily due to its α-adrenergic vasoconstrictor effects, rather than its effect on β_1 cardiac receptors. Epinephrine improves cerebral blood flow by dilating the cerebral microvasculature at the same time as supporting cerebral perfusion pressure by constricting the extracerebral portions of the carotid arteries. Peripheral vasoconstriction maintains arterial peripheral blood pressure. From β_1-receptor stimulation, epinephrine has a powerful inotropic effect and increases the vigor of ventricular fibrillation. Stimulation of β_2-adrenergic receptors increases activity of the enzyme adenylate cyclase, increasing cyclic AMP and relaxing bronchial smooth muscle. Epinephrine is also used as a local hemostatic for superficial mucosal bleeding and in combination with local anesthetics to localize their action and delay their absorption. Epinephrine is not absorbed to any extent by the oral route and has a very short half-life in the body. The 1:1000 strength is for SC or IM administration only. Further dilution to 1:10,000 is required for IV administration.

ADVERSE AND COMMON SIDE EFFECTS: Cardiac arrhythmias, including tachycardia and fatal ventricular fibrillation, can occur following inadvertent overdosage.

DRUG INTERACTIONS: Thyroid therapy, digitalis therapy, halogenated hydrocarbon anesthetics, and thiobarbiturates predispose to myocardial toxicity of catecholamines.

SUPPLIED AS VETERINARY PRODUCT:
For injection containing 1.0 mg/mL (1:1,000) epinephrine

SUPPLIED AS HUMAN PRODUCT:
For injection containing 0.1 mg/mL (1:10,000), 0.5 mg/mL (1:2000), and 1.0 mg/mL (1:1000)

ERGONOVINE

INDICATIONS: Ergonovine (Ergotrate ★, Ergonovine Maleate Solution ✤) is an ergot alkaloid with potent stimulatory activity on myometrial contraction in the periparturient animal. It is used mainly in the postpartum animal to enhance uterine contraction and involution, in prolapsed uterus after Cesarean section, and in cases of uterine hemorrhage. Following IM injection, clinical effects begin within 15 minutes and last 2 to 4 hours.

ADVERSE AND COMMON SIDE EFFECTS: Ergonovine should not be used prepartum because oxytocin is a superior myometrial stimulant for obstetrics. Prolonged or excessive use may cause dry gangrene, vascular damage, hypotension, and depression of the respiratory rate and volume.

DRUG INTERACTIONS: Ergonovine should not be mixed with any other medications.

SUPPLIED AS HUMAN PRODUCT:
For injection containing 0.2 mg/mL (United States) and 0.25 mg/mL (Canada)

ERYTHROMYCIN

INDICATIONS: Erythromycin (Alto-Erythromycin ✤, Apo-Erythro Base ✤, Erythro-36 ✤ ★, Erymycin-100 ★, Erythro-200 ✤ ★, Erythro-Dry ★, Erythro-Dry Cow ✤, Gallimycin-36 ✤ ★, Gallimycin ✤, Gallimycin-50 ✤, Gallimycin-200 ✤, Gallimycin-Dry Cow ★, Ilosone ✤ ★,

Ilotycin ✿ ★, Novo-Rythro Estolate ✿, and others) is a macrolide antibiotic with bacteriostatic activity primarily against gram-positive bacteria, bovine respiratory disease pathogens, and some strains of *Listeria*. Erythromycin diffuses well through most tissues and is useful for treating staphylococcal infections resistant to penicillin and for treating intracellular organisms, such as *Rhodococcus equi* in foals. Optimum antimicrobial activity of erythromycin is at an alkaline pH; therefore it has reduced activity in acidic environments (e.g., abscesses) but may be clinically effective because of high concentrations due to "iontrapping". Erythromycin also has nonantimicrobial effects on host cell metabolism, inflammatory mediators, and gastrointestinal motility. Erythromycin is also used in mastitis preparations for intramammary use. The estolate form of erythromycin is less susceptible to stomach acid than the base or stearate and is better absorbed through the gastrointestinal tract. In the horse, twice daily treatment with oral products provides sufficiently effective blood levels. The salt forms (phosphate and stearate) are better absorbed than the estolate form because of higher variability in gastric pH in horses than in humans. The routine use of the macrolides is limited because bacterial resistance develops quickly from repeated exposure.

ADVERSE AND COMMON SIDE EFFECTS: Macrolide antibiotics, including erythromycin and clarithromycin, are motilin receptor agonists. They also appear to stimulate motility via cholinergic and noncholinergic neuronal pathways. At microbially ineffective doses, they stimulate migrating motility complexes and antegrade peristalsis in the gastrointestinal tract. When used at antimicrobial doses in horses, erythromycin is associated with potentially fatal colitis from *Clostridia* spp.

Erythromycin is also associated with acute respiratory distress syndrome, hyperthermia, gastroenteritis, and hepatotoxicity in foals. The mechanism of hyperthermia in erythromycin-treated foals has not been elucidated, but likely results from derangement of the hypothalamic temperature "set-point." Extreme care should be taken when administering erythromycin to foals with respiratory disease during periods of hot weather. Foals should not be left outside on hot, sunny days while on erythromycin therapy.

Due to injection site irritation, IM administration of erythromycin is not recommended in horses and should only be done in the cervical muscles of cattle. The IM formulation can not be administered IV.

DRUG INTERACTIONS: Erythromycin inhibits the hepatic metabolism of a number of other drugs by interfering with cytochrome P450 enzymes, including theophylline, glucocorticoids, and digoxin. Theophylline toxicity readily occurs with concurrent administration of erythromycin. Kaolin impairs absorption of orally administered erythromycin. Erythromycin should not be used concurrently with chloramphenicol or lincomycin because of similar mechanisms of action.

At low doses, erythromycin may antagonize the antimicrobial action of the penicillins. Erythromycin lactobionate is incompatible if mixed with aminophylline, multiple vitamins, cephalothin, pentobarbital, sodium iodide, heparin, penicillin G, and tetracyclines.

SUPPLIED AS VETERINARY PRODUCTS:
For injection containing 100 and 200 mg/mL
Mastitis products containing 50 mg/mL
Tablets containing enteric-coated particles 33 and 500 mg
Feed additive containing 110 g/kg

SUPPLIED AS HUMAN PRODUCTS:
Tablets (enteric coated) containing 250, 333, and 500 mg (base)
Tablets containing 600 mg (ethylsuccinate salt)
Tablets (film coated stearate) containing 250, 333, and 500 mg
Oral suspension (estolate) containing 25 and 50 mg/mL
Oral suspension (ethylsuccinate) containing 20 mg/mL, 40 mg/mL, or 80 mg/mL
Oral suspension (stearate) containing 25 and 50 mg/mL (Canada)
For injection containing 500 and 1,000 mg (glucceptate salt)
For injection containing 500 and 1,000 mg (lactobionate)
Topical and ophthalmic preparations are also available

OTHER USES
Horses
PROKINETIC
A dose of 0.5 to 1.0 mg/kg IV tid of erythromycin lactobionate may increase gastrointestinal motility by mimicking the effects of the endogenous hormone motilin. Clinicians should be cautioned that even very low doses of oral erythromycin in adult horses are associated with fatal colitis.

ESTRADIOL

INDICATIONS: Estradiol (estradiol cypionate, ECP ♣ ★, Esnate ♣) is a synthetic estrogen that acts to stimulate and maintain normal physiologic processes of the female reproductive tract. Synthetic estrogens are more prolonged in action. Estrogen therapy in mares and cows may be used to treat uterine infections, atony, or poor uterine drainage, in combination with appropriate antimicrobial therapy. Estradiol cypionate has been used as an abortifacient for cows and mares in the first half of pregnancy, but prostaglandins are a more rational choice.

ADVERSE AND COMMON SIDE EFFECTS: Estradiol may cause prolonged estrus, precocious development, genital irritation, and reduction of milk yield. Large doses of estrogens can cause postparturient straining in cows with vaginal or uterine prolapse. Administration of estrogens to pregnant cows can induce abortion. Prolonged or excessive administration leads to ovarian suppression and hypoplasia, followed by ovarian cysts.

DRUG INTERACTIONS: None listed.

SUPPLIED AS VETERINARY PRODUCT:
For injection containing 1 (Canada) and 2 (United States) mg/mL

OTHER USES
Horses
URINARY INCONTINENCE
Estradiol is used for urinary incontinence of nonneurogenic origin in aged mares at 0.004 to 0.008 mg/kg IM every other day

Cattle
Estradiol is also used alone as an implant (Compudose ✤ ★), in the benzoate form in combination with testosterone (Synovex-H ✤ ★), trenbolone (Revalor-S ✤ ★, Synovex Plus ✤, Component TE-S ★), or progesterone (Component E-C ★, Component E-S ★, Synovex-C ✤ ★, Synovex-S ✤ ★), and in the valerate form with norgestomet (Syncro-Mate B ★) for growth promotion.

ETHYLENEDIAMINE DIHYDROIODIDE

INDICATIONS: Ethylenediamine dihydroiodide (EDDI-40 ✤, Edd-Iodine-42 ✤, Iodexine 42 ✤, Organic Iodide ★, Organic Iodide 20 ★, Organic Iodide 40 ★, Organic Iodine ★, Organic Iodine 20 ★, and others) is an oral iodine supplement used as an aid for treating iodine deficiencies, bovine foot rot, and infertility, and as an expectorant for respiratory disease.

ADVERSE AND COMMON SIDE EFFECTS: Signs of iodism, such as increased salivation, sneezing, eyelid swelling, and eye irritation, indicate the need for withdrawal of the supplement, after which clinical signs abate. Not to be fed to lactating dairy cattle.

DRUG INTERACTIONS: None listed.

SUPPLIED AS VETERINARY PRODUCT:
Powder to be mixed in feed or drinking water. See individual products for concentration and mixing instructions.

FAMOTIDINE

INDICATIONS: Famotidine (Apo-Famotidine ✤, Gen-Famotidine ✤, Novo-Famotidine ✤, Nu Famotidine ✤, Pepcid ✤ ★) is a histamine

(H_2)-receptor antagonist. Compared to cimetidine, famotidine is more potent, has a higher volume of distribution, oral absorption is not reduced by the presence of food, and it does not affect the hepatic metabolism of other drugs.

ADVERSE AND COMMON SIDE EFFECTS: In humans depression, anxiety, insomnia, conjunctival infection, nausea, vomiting, anorexia, dry mouth, diarrhea, arthralgia, bronchospasm, pruritus, fever, and thrombocytopenia have been reported. Famotidine is contraindicated in humans and animals with cardiovascular disease, as it is a negative inotrope.

DRUG INTERACTIONS: None listed.

SUPPLIED AS HUMAN PRODUCTS:
Tablets containing 10, 20, and 40 mg
For injection containing 10 mg/mL
Suspension containing 8 mg/mL

FENBENDAZOLE

INDICATIONS: Fenbendazole (MoorMan's MoorGuard Swine Dewormer ★, Panacur ♣ ★, Safe-Guard ♣ ★) is a broad-spectrum anthelmintic of the benzimidazole group used in horses for large strongyles, small strongyles, pinworms, and ascarids and for treating cattle parasitized by adult and 4th stage larvae of lungworm (*Dictyocaulus viviparus*), stomach worms (*Haemonchus contortus, Ostertagia ostertagi*), intestinal worms (*Cooperia* spp., *Trichostrongylus colubriformis, Nematodirus helvetianus, Bunostomum phlebotomum, Oesophagostomum radiatum, Moniezia benedeni*), arrested 4th stage larvae of *Ostertagia ostertagi*, and the adult stomach worm *Trichostrongylus axei*.

ADVERSE AND COMMON SIDE EFFECTS: Equine cyathastomes are frequently resistant to fenbendazole, limiting its usefulness in deworming programs. If administered at larvacidal doses, local or systemic hypersensitivity reactions may result from the release of dying parasite antigens.

DRUG INTERACTIONS: None listed.

SUPPLIED AS VETERINARY PRODUCTS:
Oral paste containing 100 mg/g
Granules containing 222 mg/g for use in horses
Suspension containing 100 mg/mL for use in horses and cattle

FENOTEROL

INDICATIONS: Fenoterol (Berotec ✿, Berotec Forte ✿) is a β_2-receptor agonist with bronchodilatory properties used for treatment of recurrent airway obstruction in horses. It is available in human metered-dose inhalers. When used in conjunction with specially equipped face masks (AeroMask), it has been shown to produce effective bronchodilation in horses.

ADVERSE AND COMMON SIDE EFFECTS: Adverse side effects can include tachycardia, nervousness, excitability, muscle tremor, or colic, but when used as an aerosol no such signs were observed.

DRUG INTERACTIONS: None listed.

SUPPLIED AS HUMAN PRODUCTS:
Metered-dose aerosol systems containing 100 or 200 µg per actuation
Inhalation solution containing 1.0 mg/mL

FENTHION

INDICATIONS: Fenthion (Lysoff ✿ ★, Spotton ✿ ★, Tiguvon ✿ ★) is a topical organophosphate antiparasiticide used to treat lice and grub infestations in cattle. Organophosphates act by inhibiting acetyl-cholinesterase, which interferes with neuromuscular transmission in the parasite. For grub control, fenthion should be applied soon after heel fly activity ceases. It is not for use in lactating dairy cattle or dry cows within 10 days of freshening. Do not use in calves under 3 months of age or in stressed or debilitated animals.

ADVERSE AND COMMON SIDE EFFECTS: Host-parasite reactions from dead parasites in the esophagus or spinal cord may cause bloat, hypersalivation, and posterior paralysis. These reactions are most common in the winter months when grubs are migrating through these tissues. Treatment of host-parasite reactions is symptomatic with anti-inflammatories. If necessary, relieve bloat by trocharization, as a stomach tube may traumatize swollen esophageal tissues. With overdose, cattle may exhibit tremors, lacrimation, miosis, hyperexcitability, hypersalivation, frequent urination and defecation, and muscular weakness or paralysis. Atropine and 2-PAM are the antidotes for organophosphate toxicity. Human exposure to this product should be avoided. If ingested, do not induce vomiting.

DRUG INTERACTIONS: Phenothiazines, dimethyl sulfoxide (DMSO), levamisole, pyrantel pamoate or tartrate, or other drugs with anti-cholinesterase activity should not be administered concurrently.

SUPPLIED AS VETERINARY PRODUCTS:
7.5% w/v fenthion pour-on solution
20% w/v fenthion topical solution
3% w/v fenthion pour-on solution

FLORFENICOL

INDICATIONS: Florfenicol (Nuflor ✽ ★) is a synthetic, broad-spectrum, long-acting antibiotic for use in bovine respiratory disease (shipping fever), infectious pododermatitis, and infectious keratoconjunctivitis. It has a very wide spectrum of activity, including streptococci, staphylococci, anaerobes, *Haemophilus, Pasteurella, Mycoplasma,* and *Brucella* spp. It is also active against *Rickettsia*, chlamydia, and *Hemobartonella*. The MIC values for Enterobacteriaceae are high and resistance to florfenicol readily develops.

ADVERSE AND COMMON SIDE EFFECTS: The idiosyncratic, dose-independent fatal aplastic anemia associated with chloramphenicol use does not occur with florfenicol, as it lacks the para-nitro group responsible for human toxicity in its structure. Both chloramphenicol and florfenicol are protein synthesis inhibitors, so a dose-dependent anemia may develop with chronic use. Use in horses by oral or parenteral routes is associated with alterations in fecal flora and diarrhea. Transient diarrhea or inappetence may be noted with its use in cattle. These signs should abate within a few days after the end of treatment. Because of the long-acting carriers in the cattle formulation, tissue irritation is seen with IM injection. Do not inject more than 10 mL at each site and administer only in the neck.

DRUG INTERACTIONS: Florfenicol should not be administered concurrently with penicillins, macrolides, aminoglycosides, or fluoroquinolones. It may antagonize the activity of penicillins or aminoglycosides, and it acts on the same ribosomal site as the macrolides.

SUPPLIED AS VETERINARY PRODUCT:
For injection containing 300 mg/mL in 100-, 250-, and 500-mL bottles

FLUMETHASONE

INDICATIONS: Flumethasone (Flucort Solution ✽ ★) is a long-acting glucocorticoid used in horses to treat musculoskeletal injuries and ketosis in cattle. Flumethasone is a modification of prednisolone and the most potent glucocorticoid formulation available. Flumethasone has 60 to 80 times the anti-inflammatory and gluconeogenic effects of prednisone, and 4 times that of dexamethasone. Anti-inflammatory effects of flumethasone are beneficial in arthritis and inflammatory conditions in musculoskeletal injuries and in immunologic diseases, such as purpura hemorrhagica, allergic rhinitis, and urticaria. Flumethasone is also useful in the treatment of primary ketosis in cattle. For more information see GLUCOCORTICOID AGENTS.

ADVERSE AND COMMON SIDE EFFECTS: High, continued doses of flumethasone can cause suppression of adrenocortical function. Glucocorticoids should not be used in bacterial, viral, or parasitic infections unless concurrent anti-infective agents are used. Clinical signs may abate with their use but the underlying disease remains active. Topical use of glucocorticoids on the eye is contraindicated if corneal ulceration is present. If long-term therapy is undertaken, withdrawal should be gradual to avoid problems of iatrogenic adrenal suppression. Glucocorticoids given to animals in the last trimester of pregnancy can induce premature parturition and predispose to retained placenta and metritis. Glucocorticoids may delay wound healing. See also GLUCOCORTICOID AGENTS.

DRUG INTERACTIONS: See GLUCOCORTICOID AGENTS.

SUPPLIED AS VETERINARY PRODUCT:
For injection containing 0.5 mg/mL

FLUNIXIN MEGLUMINE

INDICATIONS: Flunixin meglumine (Banamine ❀ ★, Cronyxin ❀, Equileve ★, Equi-Phar Equigesic ★, FluMeglumine ★, Suppressor ★) is an NSAID with analgesic and antipyretic properties similar to those of phenylbutazone. Flunixin meglumine has potent analgesic properties in the horse, especially in the management of colic pain. Flunixin is also advocated as a component of therapy for endotoxemia in horses and cattle and bovine respiratory disease. Flunixin meglumine has been found to reduce lung consolidation in experimentally induced viral pneumonia in calves. Parenteral flunixin is the NSAID of choice for managing inflammation in the equine eye, such as equine recurrent uveitis.

ADVERSE AND COMMON SIDE EFFECTS: Extremely high doses of flunixin may mask signs of surgical colic pain and interfere with treatment decisions. Flunixin has a good safety profile, but high doses or chronic dosing can cause anorexia, depression, renal damage, and gastrointestinal ulcers, especially in foals. Inadvertent intra-arterial injection may cause temporary ataxia, hysteria, hyperventilation, and muscle weakness. Intramuscular injections of flunixin are highly irritating to muscle and have been incriminated in cases of clostridial myositis in horses; therefore, IM use should be avoided when possible despite the label directions. If not treated promptly and aggressively, clostridial myositis causes severe tissue damage and may be rapidly fatal.

DRUG INTERACTIONS: Avoid concurrent use with other potentially nephrotoxic drugs.

SUPPLIED AS VETERINARY PRODUCTS:
Granules containing 25 mg/g
Paste containing 50 mg/g (United States)
For injection containing 50 mg/mL

OTHER USES
Horses
ENDOTOXEMIA
For prevention of fluid shifts and vascular damage during endotoxemia, a dose of 0.25 mg/kg qid; IV is suggested.

FLUOROQUINOLONES (SEE CIPROFLOXACIN, ENROFLOXACIN, AND DANOFLOXACIN)

INDICATIONS: Danofloxacin (A180 ★), enrofloxacin (Baytril ✿ ★), ciprofloxacin (Ciloxan ✿ ★), marbofloxacin (Zenequin ✿ ★), and orbifloxacin (Orbax ✿ ★) are fluoroquinolone antimicrobials used in large animals. These antimicrobials have activity against *Escherichia coli*, *Enterobacter*, *Klebsiella*, *Proteus*, *Pseudomonas*, some *Staphylococcus*, *Salmonella*, *Shigella*, *Vibrio*, *Yersinia*, and *Campylobacter* organisms. They have little activity against anaerobic cocci, *Bacteroides*, or clostridial organisms. Resistance does occur, especially with *Pseudomonas*, *Klebsiella*, *Acinetobacter*, and *Enterococcus* organisms. Streptococci (particularly enterococci) generally are resistant. This limits the use of fluoroquinolones in the treatment of equine respiratory infections, where streptococci often are present. Fluoroquinolones may be effective against atypical mycobacteria (*M. fortuitum* and *M. chelonei*), although higher dosages may be needed. The fluoroquinolones are effective in the treatment of respiratory tract infections, bronchopneumonia, enteric infections, bacterial infections of the reproductive tract, bacterial meningoencephalitis, osteomyelitis, skin, and soft tissue infections. Ciprofloxacin has more activity than other quinolones against *Pseudomonas* and *Acinetobacter*, but its oral absorption is very poor in horses and ruminants and the IV formulation is cost prohibitive. The human ophthalmic ciprofloxacin formulation is useful for staphylococcal and gram-negative corneal infections. Enrofloxacin and danofloxacin are approved for use in the treatment of bovine respiratory tract disease. Enrofloxacin, difloxacin, orbifloxacin, and marbofloxacin are used extralabel in horses for the treatment of staphylococcal and gram-negative infections, including infections from *Sal-*

monella spp. and *Pseudomonas* spp. Because the fluoroquinolones are concentration-dependent killers with a long postantibiotic effect, the ideal dosage regimen is once-daily, high-dose therapy. Any extralabel use in food animals is strictly prohibited in the United States.

ADVERSE AND COMMON SIDE EFFECTS: Fluoroquinolones at clinical doses may cause arthropathies in neonatal foals, but this effect is not seen in adult horses, ruminants, or swine. Cartilage damage in foals is most severe with weight bearing and exercise; so if administered to foals because of life-threatening infections, they should be strictly stall rested. The fluoroquinolones may cause adverse CNS effects in humans and animals due to a GABA receptor antagonism. This has been associated with an increase in seizure incidence in humans and dogs. Administration of enrofloxacin to humans results in hallucinations. Rapid IV administration of high doses of enrofloxacin to horses causes transient neurologic signs, including excitability and seizure-like activity.

DRUG INTERACTIONS: Oral absorption is hindered by antacid preparations as well as sucralfate. Nitrofurantoin, chloramphenicol, and rifampin are antagonistic to fluoroquinolone activity.

SUPPLIED AS VETERINARY PRODUCTS:
Tablets containing 22.7, 68, and 136 mg (United States) or 15, 50, and 150 mg (Canada) [Baytril]
For injection containing 22.7 mg/mL (United States), 50 mg/mL (Canada, small animal formulations) and 100 mg/mL (bovine formulation) [Baytril]
For injection containing 180 mg/mL [A180]
Tablets containing 5.7, 22.7, and 68 mg [Orbax]
Tablets containing 25, 50, 100, and 200 mg [Zenequin]

SUPPLIED AS HUMAN PRODUCT:
Ophthalmic solution containing 3.5 mg/mL [Ciloxan]

FLURBIPROFEN

INDICATIONS: Flurbiprofen sodium (Ocufen ✽ ★) is a propionic acid derivative similar to ibuprofen. These compounds are aspirin-like drugs that act to inhibit cyclooxygenase but are better tolerated by the patient than aspirin. Flurbiprofen is used as an ophthalmic medication to decrease ocular inflammation in the horse.

ADVERSE AND COMMON SIDE EFFECTS: Flurbiprofen may induce hypersensitivity and delay wound healing.

DRUG INTERACTIONS: Concurrent ophthalmic use of flurbiprofen with carbachol negates the desired actions of carbachol. Concurrent administration with some local anesthetics produces greater miotic inhibition.

SUPPLIED AS HUMAN PRODUCT:
Ophthalmic solution containing 0.03% w/v

FLUTICASONE

INDICATIONS: Fluticasone (Flovent ✤ ★) is a potent glucocorticoid administered by metered dose inhaler for chronic treatment of recurrent airway disease in horses. Glucocorticoids attenuate the inflammatory response, suppressing the generation of cytokines and recruitment of airway eosinophils and release of inflammatory mediators. Glucocorticoids reduce severity of symptoms, improve peak expiratory flow, diminish airway hyperresponsiveness, prevent exacerbations, and possibly prevent airway wall remodeling.

ADVERSE AND COMMON SIDE EFFECTS: The potential but small risk of adverse side effects from inhaled glucocorticoids is well balanced by their efficacy. Oral candidiasis (thrush), dysphonia and reflex cough, and bronchospasm are the most common adverse effects in humans; all of these effects are reduced by the use of a spacer. The risk of systemic side effects such as suppression of the hypothalamic-pituitary axis are less than with oral glucocorticoid therapy.

DRUG INTERACTIONS: None listed.

SUPPLIED AS HUMAN PRODUCT:
For aerosol administration containing 44, 110, and 220 µg (United States) or 25, 50, 125, and 250 µg (Canada) in a metered dose inhaler

FOLIC ACID

INDICATIONS: Folic acid (Apo-Folic ✤ ★, Folvite ✤ ★, Folic Acid Injection ★, Foldine ✤, Novo-Folacid ✤) is a member of the vitamin B complex group essential for the maintenance of normal erythropoiesis. Folic acid deficiency may occur due to blood loss, prolonged malabsorption, or sulfonamide administration. Therapy with folic acid may be indicated in cases where pyrimethamine is used on a long-term basis, such as in equine protozoal myeloencephalitis. Dietary deficiencies in large animals are rare but there is a suggestion that it may occur in horses fed rations lacking grass.

ADVERSE AND COMMON SIDE EFFECTS: The administration of oral folic acid to pregnant mares being treated for encephalomyelitis (EPM) may not protect the fetus from the effects of folate deficiency.

DRUG INTERACTIONS: Trimethoprim and pyremethamine act as folate antagonists and sulfonamides inhibit the absorption of folate. Chloramphenicol may antagonize the hematologic response anticipated with folic acid treatment.

SUPPLIED AS HUMAN PRODUCTS:
Tablets containing 0.1, 0.4, 0.8, 1 (United States), and 5 mg (Canada)
For injection containing 5 and 10 (United States) mg/mL

FOLLICLE-STIMULATING HORMONE

INDICATIONS: Follicle-stimulating hormone (Folltropin-V ✤, Lutropin-V ✤) is a purified pituitary extract with follicle-stimulating hormone (FSH) activity and luteinizing hormone (LH) activity. It is used primarily in sexually mature heifers and cows to induce superovulation. It is also used in mares, cows, sheep, and goats to assist ovulation.

ADVERSE AND COMMON SIDE EFFECTS: None listed.

DRUG INTERACTIONS: None listed.

SUPPLIED AS VETERINARY PRODUCT:
For injection containing 1, 5, 7.5, and 20 mg/mL

FUROSEMIDE

INDICATIONS: Furosemide (Disal ★, Equi-Phar Furosemide Injection ★, Furoject ★, Furotabs ★, Furosemide Injection 5% ★, Salix ✤ ★) is a potent loop diuretic that acts to prevent chloride reabsorption in the ascending loop of Henle. Furosemide is used for udder edema in cattle, edema of congestive heart failure, and edema of "stocking up" in horses. It is widely used in the race horse industry to prevent exercise-induced pulmonary hemorrhage, but its efficacy in prevention of such pulmonary hemorrhage and its potential for performance enhancement remain highly controversial. Furosemide is also indicated in oliguric renal failure because it is postulated to block the metabolic activity of tubular cells, thereby sparing the metabolic demands of the cells. Furosemide also enhances renal blood flow prior to its tubular effects.

ADVERSE AND COMMON SIDE EFFECTS: Metabolic alkalosis can occur from contraction of the extracellular fluid volume. Furosemide may cause electrolyte disturbances if used for more than 48 hours in cattle. Hypokalemia or hyponatremia may occur if used over prolonged periods. Furosemide may lower serum calcium.

DRUG INTERACTIONS: There is an increased risk of nephrotoxicity if furosemide is given concurrently with NSAIDs and/or aminoglycosides. Concurrent use with glucocorticoids increases the risk of hypokalemia. Hypokalemia increases the effects of digoxin and may result in digoxin toxicity despite "therapeutic" concentrations.

SUPPLIED AS VETERINARY PRODUCTS:
For injection containing 50 mg/mL
As a bolus containing 2 g
Tablets containing 12.5 and 50 mg

SUPPLIED AS HUMAN PRODUCTS:
Tablets containing 20, 40, and 80 mg
Oral solution containing 8 and 10 mg/mL
For injection containing 10 mg/mL

GENTAMICIN

INDICATIONS: Gentamicin (Garacin ★, Garasol Pig Pump ♣, GenGard ★, Gentaglyde Solution ★, Gentaject ★, GentaVed 100 ★, Gentamicin Sulfate Injection ★, Gentocin Ophthalmic ♣ ★, Gentocin Solution ♣ ★, Gentocin Spray ♣ ★, Tamycin ★) is a concentration-dependent aminoglycoside antibiotic effective against staphylococci and gram-negative bacteria such as *Escherichia coli* and *Pseudomonas*. It is used for soft tissue infections, bacterial keratitis, endometritis, metritis, and pyometra. It can be administered IV, IM, SC, IA, and by regional perfusion or incorporation into polymethylmethacrylate beads for the local treatment of osteomyelitis. It is also used in the treatment of bacteremia or septicemia in neonatal foals caused by *E. coli, Proteus, Pseudomonas,* or *Klebsiella*. It has no activity against anaerobes, and is ineffective in acidic, hyperosmolar environments, such as in abscesses. It is a large, polar compound so it remains largely confined to extracellular fluids, and does not reach therapeutic concentrations in milk, CSF, ocular tissues, and sex gland fluids. High-dose, once daily therapy is recommended to take advantage of concentration-dependent bacterial killing and a long postantibiotic effect and to avoid nephrotoxicity from accumulation in renal tubular epithelium. See also AMINOGLYCOSIDES.

ADVERSE AND COMMON SIDE EFFECTS: Gentamicin should be used with caution in animals with compromised kidney function. It is contraindicated in cases of severe renal impairment. Toxic levels can cause renal tubular damage, which may be reversible once the drug is discontinued. Avoid concurrent use with other aminoglycosides because of the potential additive toxic effects. Ototoxicity can occur but is difficult to detect clinically. Weakness from neuromuscular blockade can occur at high doses and is treated with calcium.

DRUG INTERACTIONS: Concurrent use of furosemide can increase the potential for toxicity. Dehydration can predispose to renal tubular damage. Gentamicin is not to be mixed with any other product.

SUPPLIED AS VETERINARY PRODUCTS:
For injection containing 5, 50, and 100 mg/mL
Oral solution containing 4.35 mg/mL
Intrauterine solution containing 10 mg/mL
Ophthalmic solution containing 3 mg/mL or spray containing 1 mg/mL
Soluble powder containing 5 g/75 g, 6 g/18 g, and 2 g/30 g

OTHER USES
Gentocin is also contained in combination with glucocorticoids for use in ophthalmic (Gentocin Durafilm ✿ ★) and topical (Gentocin Otic ✿ ★, Otomax Ointment ✿ ★, Topagen Spray ✿) preparations. Injectable products can be used subconjunctivally for the treatment of corneal ulcers when topical ointments or drops are not practical.

GLUCOCORTICOID AGENTS

INDICATIONS: Glucocorticoid agents are recommended for the treatment of allergic and immune-mediated diseases, cardiogenic and septic shock, and trauma and edema of the central nervous system and spinal cord. Beneficial effects include stabilization of lysosomal and capillary membranes, decrease in activation of the complement and clotting cascades, binding of endotoxin, positive inotropic effect, dilation of precapillary sphincters, prevention of gastrointestinal mucosal ischemia associated with shock, increase in glucogenesis, inhibition of the formation of vasoactive substances (kinins, prostaglandins), decrease in collagen and scar formation, and decrease in the accumulation of phagocytes at areas of inflammation. Analgesic activity is only related to prostaglandin inhibition. These agents do not possess direct analgesic activity.

The glucocorticoids are classified according to their duration of action. As biologic half-life increases, anti-inflammatory potency increases and mineralocorticoid potency decreases. Short-acting drugs (< 12 hours) include hydrocortisone and cortisone acetate. Intermediate-acting drugs (12 to 36 hours) include prednisone, prednisolone, methylprednisolone, and triamcinolone. The long-acting steroids (>48 hours) include paramethasone, flumethasone, betamethasone, and dexamethasone. Topical glucocorticoids are used for their local anti-inflammatory, antipruritic, and vasoconstrictive effects.

ADVERSE AND COMMON SIDE EFFECTS: Polyuria, polydipsia, polyphagia, panting, lethargy, weakness, and bilateral symmetrical alopecia are the most common clinical signs of glucocorticoid excess. Weight loss, anorexia, and diarrhea may also follow use of these drugs. Hemorrhagic gastroenteritis, pancreatitis, and hepatopathy have been reported with the use of glucocorticoids. Glucocorticoid drugs suppress inflammation, reduce fever, increase protein catabolism and their conversion to carbohydrates leading to a negative nitrogen balance, promote sodium retention and potassium diuresis, retard wound healing, lower resistance to infection, and cause a reduction in the number of circulating lymphocytes. Iatrogenic hyperadrenocorticism may follow prolonged use of parenteral as well as topical glucocorticoid agents. Glucocorticoids are contraindicated in animals with acute or chronic bacterial infections unless therapeutic doses of an effective bactericidal agent are used concurrently. Glucocorticoids may mask signs of infection such as elevation in body temperature. These drugs should be used with caution in animals with congestive heart failure, diabetes mellitus, and renal disease. Their use during the healing phase of bone fractures is not recommended. Glucocorticoids have been associated with increased incidence of cleft palate and other congenital malformations in offspring of treated dams. In addition, their use may be associated with the induction of the first stage of parturition when administered during the last trimester of pregnancy and may precipitate premature parturition followed by dystocia, fetal death, retained placenta, and metritis.

DRUG INTERACTIONS: Glucocorticoids may decrease the efficacy of bacteriostatic antibiotics by decreasing the inflammatory response and diminishing the phagocytic activity of leukocytes. Amphotericin B, furosemide, and the thiazide diuretics may potentiate hypokalemia. Hypokalemia may predispose to digitalis toxicity. Glucocorticoids may reduce serum salicylate levels. Phenytoin, phenobarbital, and rifampin may increase the metabolism of glucocorticoids, and insulin requirements of diabetic patients may increase. Hepatic metabolism of methylprednisolone may be inhibited by erythromycin. The concomitant use of glucocorticoids and cyclosporine may lead to increases in serum levels of both drugs. Live attenuated-virus vaccines should generally not be given to animals receiving glucocorticoid drugs. Concurrent use of NSAIDs may increase the potential for gastrointestinal ulceration. Estrogens may potentiate the effects of hydrocortisone and other glucocorticoids.

SUPPLIED AS: See specific product.

GLYCEROL

INDICATIONS: Glycerol [glycerin] (Glycerol ✿ ★) is an inert substance used to soothe and relieve inflammation primarily involving mucous membranes. In the horse, its anhydrous form has been advocated for oral use in the treatment of central nervous system trauma to manage cerebral edema. Glycerol is also nebulized into the respiratory tract to rehydrate and emulsify secretions. Glycerol [glycerin] is also used in many topical medications as a vehicle.

ADVERSE AND COMMON SIDE EFFECTS: At high concentrations glycerol will absorb water and is irritating and dehydrating to exposed tissue. If used as an aerosol, glycerol is irritating and can cause bronchoconstriction.

DRUG INTERACTIONS: None listed.

SUPPLIED AS CHEMICAL PRODUCT:
Anhydrous glycerin containing 99.95% w/v glycerol

GLYCOPYRROLATE

INDICATIONS: Glycopyrrolate (Glycopyrrolate Injection ★, Robinul ❀ ★, Robinul-V ❀ ★, Robinul Forte ❀ ★) is an anticholinergic drug similar in action to atropine. Relative to atropine, glycopyrrolate has more effective antisialogogue effects and is less likely to cause significant tachycardia while being more effective at blocking bradyarrhythmias. Glycopyrrolate is also more effective than atropine at blocking gastric acid secretion.

ADVERSE AND COMMON SIDE EFFECTS: Mydriasis and xerostomia may be noted with its use. Excretion of the drug may be prolonged in animals with impaired renal or gastrointestinal function. It should not be given to pregnant animals. Refer also to Adverse and Common Side Effects of ATROPINE, which would be expected to be similar.

DRUG INTERACTIONS: As for ATROPINE, which include enhancement of activity if used with antihistamines, procainamide, quinidine, meperidine, benzodiazepines, and phenothiazines. Adverse effects may be potentiated by primidone and long-term glucocorticoid use (via increasing intraocular pressure). Glycopyrrolate may enhance the actions of nitrofurantoin, thiazide diuretics, and sympathomimetic agents. The drug may antagonize the activity of metoclopramide.

SUPPLIED AS VETERINARY PRODUCT:
For injection containing 0.2 mg/mL (United States)

SUPPLIED AS HUMAN PRODUCTS:
Tablets containing 1 and 2 mg
For injection containing 0.2 mg/mL

GONADORELIN

INDICATIONS: Gonadorelin [GnRH] (Cystorelin ❀ ★, Factrel ❀ ★, Fertiline ❀, Fertagyl ❀) and its analog deslorelin (Ovuplant ❀ ★) are decapeptide hypothalamic-releasing factors responsible for stimulating the release of FSH and LH from the anterior pituitary gland. Gonadorelin is used to treat ovarian follicular cysts (cystic ovaries) in cattle with incomplete luteinization. Most cysts on the ovaries will clear within 3 days of injection. Deslorelin is used to induce ovulation in mares.

ADVERSE AND COMMON SIDE EFFECTS: None have been reported at 10 times the recommended dose.

DRUG INTERACTIONS: None reported.

SUPPLIED AS VETERINARY PRODUCTS:
For injection containing 50 and 100 µg/mL gonadorelin
Subcutaneous implant containing 2.1 mg deslorelin

OTHER USES
Horses and Cattle
Gonadorelin has also been used to induce ovulation at the time of breeding in both cattle and horses. It has also been advocated for treatment of stallions with lowered libido.

GRISEOFULVIN

INDICATIONS: Griseofulvin (Fulvicin U/F ✤ ★, Fulvicin U/F Powder ✤ ★) is an oral fungistatic antibiotic used in the treatment of infections by dermatophytic fungi of the skin, hair, and claws. Griseofulvin inhibits the growth of various species of *Microsporum, Epidermophyton,* and *Trichophyton* and is used primarily to treat ringworm in horses and calves. It is ineffective against other fungi, including *Candida.* Upon oral administration, griseofulvin is deposited in new epithelial cells that make up the skin, hair, and claws and prevents fungal infection of the newly formed tissues. The microsize formulation has a fine particle size with a greater surface area for absorption, resulting in higher blood levels in human studies.

ADVERSE AND COMMON SIDE EFFECTS: Griseofulvin may interfere with spermatogenesis. Although teratogenic effects have been seen in cats, griseofulvin has been fed to mares for alternating 30-day periods with no abnormal effects. The manufacturer, however, suggests it not be given to pregnant mares or breeding stock. Hepatotoxicity and photosensitization have also been reported but are rare.

DRUG INTERACTIONS: Phenobarbital decreases absorption of griseofulvin. Coumarin anticoagulant activity may be reduced by griseofulvin. Vaccination or viral infection induces interferon synthesis, which in turn inhibits hepatic enzyme systems and may prolong the elimination of griseofulvin.

SUPPLIED AS VETERINARY PRODUCTS:
Tablets (microsize) containing 250 and 500 mg (United States)
Powder containing 2.5 g/15-g packet

SUPPLIED AS HUMAN PRODUCTS:
Tablets (microsize or ultramicrosize) containing 125, 165, 250, 333, and 500 mg
Capsules containing 250 mg
Suspension containing 125 mg/5 mL

OTHER USES
Horses

Griseofulvin can also be used for the treatment of equine sporotrichosis.

GUAIFENESIN

INDICATIONS: Guaifenesin [formerly glyceryl guaiacolate] (Guaialaxin ★, Guaifenesin Injection ★, Guaifenesin ♣) is a centrally acting muscle relaxant with sedative and analgesic effects. It is used in large animals to treat convulsions, and for induction of general anesthesia, usually in combination with an ultrashort-acting barbiturate. The duration of action is brief, with a single muscle relaxant dose lasting 15 to 40 minutes. The primary disadvantage of guaifenesin is the large volume of parenteral solution required to produce sedation. Guaifenesin also has expectorant properties. It reduces the stickiness of mucus in chronic bronchitis and accelerates airway particle clearance.

ADVERSE AND COMMON SIDE EFFECTS: Inadvertent perivascular injection can result in tissue sloughing. If used at higher than recommended parenteral doses, guaifenesin can cause respiratory paralysis. Concentrations greater than 5% w/v can cause hemolysis. Females may have more rapid elimination of guaifenesin and require more frequent dosing to maintain effects.

DRUG INTERACTIONS: Concurrent use of physostigmine and other cholinesterase agents (e.g., neostigmine, pyridostigmine, and edrophonium) is contraindicated.

SUPPLIED AS VETERINARY PRODUCT:
For injection containing 50 g/1,000 mL (reconstitute 50 g with 954 mL sterile water) (United States)

SUPPLIED AS HUMAN PRODUCT:
Powder for reconstitution containing 2.27 kg (Canada)

OTHER USES
Horses and Cattle

Guaifenesin is also found in combination expectorant products (Quiex ♣) for use in large animals as an aid to liquefy respiratory secretions.

HALOTHANE

INDICATIONS: Halothane (Fluothane ✤ ★, Halothane USP ★) is an inhalant drug used for the induction of general anesthesia. It is a fast, potent anesthetic that allows for smooth induction without excitement and a quick, uneventful recovery.

ADVERSE AND COMMON SIDE EFFECTS: Dose-dependent hypotension has been documented with halothane use. Hepatic necrosis, although rare, may occur with the use of halothane, the incidence of which increases with each use of this agent. Should unexplained fever, jaundice, or other signs of liver dysfunction occur, its subsequent use in that animal is contraindicated. High doses of halothane may cause uterine atony and postpartum bleeding, and it is generally not recommended for obstetrical procedures unless uterine relaxation is required. Goats may be especially sensitive to halothane-induced liver disease, but this is poorly documented.

DRUG INTERACTIONS: Halothane is potentially arrhythmogenic, especially in the presence of epinephrine and the thiobarbiturates. Use with D-tubocurare can cause a reduction in blood pressure.

SUPPLIED AS HUMAN AND VETERINARY PRODUCTS:
Halothane is supplied in 250-mL bottles

HEPARIN

INDICATIONS: Heparin (Calcilean ✤, Calciparin ★, Heparin Sodium Injection ★, Hep-Lock ★, Hepalean-Lok ✤, Hepalean ✤, Heparin Leo ✤, Liquaemin Sodium ★) is a potent endogenous anticoagulant. It is used in horses at risk for thrombosis, such as in endotoxemia and animals at risk for developing disseminated intravascular coagulation (DIC). Heparin is also used empirically in acute laminitis because one proposed pathogenesis of the disease includes microthrombi formation in the vessels of the hoof. In the case of burn patients, heparin has been used to increase the effectiveness of repair mechanisms, to decrease thrombosis and the development of gangrene, and to protect against the development of DIC. In studies on an ischemic bowel model in horses, heparin has been shown to reduce abdominal adhesion formation. The mechanism is presumed to be interference with the formation of thrombin, thus preventing conversion of fibrinogen to fibrin.

ADVERSE AND COMMON SIDE EFFECTS: Bleeding and thrombocytopenia are the most common adverse effects of the drug, leading to prolonged activated partial thromboplastin time. Horses develop a temporary anemia, which is thought to occur from enhanced phagocytosis of red blood cells by the reticuloendothelial system. Protamine zinc may be used to reverse the adverse effects of bleeding. Intramuscular injection can result in hematoma formation and SC injection may result in edema at the injection site. Other side effects reported have included osteoporosis with long-term use, diminished renal function following long-term, high-dose therapy, rebound hyperlipidemia, hyperkalemia, alopecia, suppressed aldosterone synthesis, and priapism.

DRUG INTERACTIONS: Heparin may antagonize the action of glucocorticoids, insulin, and corticotropin and increase serum levels of diazepam. Antihistamines, IV nitroglycerin, digoxin, and tetracyclines may antagonize the effects of heparin. Heparin should be used with caution with other drugs that may adversely affect coagulation, such as aspirin, phenylbutazone, dextran, and warfarin.

SUPPLIED AS HUMAN PRODUCTS:
Sodium Salt

For injection containing 2, 10, 40, 50, 100, 1,000, 2,000, 2,500, 5,000, 7,500, 10,000, 20,000, 25,000, and 40,000 U/mL

Calcium Salt

For injection containing 25,000 U/mL

OTHER USES
Horses

ACUTE LAMINITIS
40 to 100 IU/kg; SC, IV

HYPERLIPEMIA
100 to 250 IU/kg; IV for use in ponies and horses with hyperlipemia to stimulate lipoprotein lipase. Lower doses of 40 IU/kg; IV have been beneficial and lessen the risk of inducing blood clotting problems.

ABDOMINAL ADHESION PREVENTION
40 IU/kg at surgery and 40 to 80 IU bid for 48 hours; IV for the first dose, then SC

HYALURONAN

INDICATIONS: Hyaluronan (HY-50 ✤ ★, Hy-50 Hylan ✤, Hyalovet 20 ✤ ★, Hyalovet Syringe Vials ★, Hylartil Vet ✤, Hyonate ✤, Hyvisc ★, Legend Injectable Solution ★) is a nonsulfated glycosaminoglycan (contains no sulfur molecules). It is produced by the membrane that lines the joint capsule and disperses into the joint fluid and taken up by the joint cartilage. Hyaluronan (HA) provides joint lubrication and protection of the joint cartilage from shear and compressive forces as the horse moves. It also reduces prostaglandin concentrations and scavenges free radicals in inflamed joints. Hyaluronan is primarily used in the treatment of degenerative joint disease of the carpal, fetlock, coffin, and hock joints of performance horses. Although cartilage damage is not always directly responsible for lameness, it is the limiting factor in rehabilitation of arthritic joints in the horse. It appears that HA concentration in joint fluid is reduced in degenerative joint disease. Injecting additional HA IV or directly into the joint appears to normalize the joint fluid and increase the production of HA by the joint membrane. The actual injected HA remains in the joint for only a few hours, but its effect on the joint appears to last days to months. It does not appear that HA has any direct effect on joint cartilage. Intra-articular HA can be used in combination with other intra-articular medications such as glucocorticoids. The combination therapy can result in a better and longer lasting improvement in lameness than either product alone.

ADVERSE AND COMMON SIDE EFFECTS: Transient heat or swelling may occur following intra-articular injection but should resolve spontaneously without treatment within 96 hours. This must be distinguished from iatrogenic septic arthritis, which can be a life-threatening complication of intra-articular injections.

DRUG INTERACTIONS: None listed.

SUPPLIED AS VETERINARY PRODUCT:
For injection containing 5, 10, and 17 mg/mL

HYDROCHLOROTHIAZIDE

INDICATIONS: Hydrochlorothiazide (Apo-Hydro ✤, Diaqua ★, Diuchlor H ✤, Esidrex ★, HydroDiuril ✤ ★, Hydrozide Injection ★, Mictrin ★, Neo-Codema ✤, Novo-Hydrazide ✤, Oretic ★, Urozide ✤) is a diuretic suggested for use as maintenance therapy for periodic paralysis in horses.

ADVERSE AND COMMON SIDE EFFECTS: Hypokalemia, hypochloremic alkalosis, dilutional hyponatremia, and loss of water-soluble vitamins may occur with chronic use. Other side effects may include diarrhea, polyuria, hyperglycemia, hyperlipidemia, hypotension, and hypersensitivity/dermatologic reactions.

DRUG INTERACTIONS: Concurrent use with glucocorticoids, corticotropin, or amphotericin B may predispose to hypokalemia. Thiazide hypokalemia, hypomagnesemia, or hypocalcemia predisposes to digitalis toxicity and hydrochlorothiazide may prolong the half-life of quinidine due to alkalinization of the urine. Sulfonamides may potentiate the action of hydrochlorothiazide. Diuretics may increase the risk of NSAID-induced renal failure secondary to decreased renal blood flow.

SUPPLIED AS VETERINARY PRODUCT:
For injection containing 25 mg/mL

SUPPLIED AS HUMAN PRODUCTS:
Tablets containing 25, 50, and 100 mg
Oral solution containing 10 mg/mL

HYDROCORTISONE SODIUM SUCCINATE

INDICATIONS: Hydrocortisone sodium succinate (Solu-Cortef ♣ ★, A-Hydrocort ♣ ★) is a glucocorticoid primarily used in cases of allergic reactions or shock or in animals suffering venomous snake bite. Use of this specific glucocorticoid drug for large animals is seldom essential and can be prohibitively expensive. For information concerning adverse and common side effects and drug interactions, see GLUCOCORTICOID AGENTS.

SUPPLIED AS HUMAN PRODUCT:
For injection containing 100, 250, 500, and 1,000 mg/vial

HYDROXYZINE

INDICATIONS: Hydroxyzine (Anxanil ★, Apo-Hydroxyzine ♣, Atarax ♣ ★, E-Vista ★, Hydroxacen ★, Hyzine-50 ★, Hy-Pan ★, Multipox ♣, Neucalm ★, Novo-Hydroxyzin ♣, Nu-Hydroxyzin ♣, PMS-Hydroxyzine ♣, Quiess ★, Vistaject-25 ★, Vistaril ★, Vistacon 50 ★, Vistaject-50 ★, Vistazine ★) is an anxiolytic, antihistaminic agent. The drug also has anticholinergic, antiemetic, and bronchodilator effects. It has been used in horses and ruminants for the treatment of urticaria.

ADVERSE AND COMMON SIDE EFFECTS: Transitory drowsiness is the most common side effect.

DRUG INTERACTIONS: Barbiturates and other sedatives may potentiate central nervous system depression. Hydroxyzine inhibits and reverses the vasopressor effect of epinephrine.

IMIPRAMINE

INDICATIONS: Imipramine (Apo-Imipramine ♣, Impril ♣, Norfranil ★, Novo-Pramine ♣, PMS-Imipramine ♣, Tipramine ★, Tofranil ♣ ★, Tofranil-PM ★) is a tricyclic antidepressant structurally related to phenothiazines that is used in horses for the treatment of narcolepsy. It has also been used to treat ejaculatory dysfunction in stallions.

ADVERSE AND COMMON SIDE EFFECTS: In humans, hypotension, tachycardia, arrhythmias, anxiety, ataxia, seizure, constipation, mydriasis, urinary retention, pruritus, anorexia, vomiting, diarrhea, icterus, and bone marrow suppression leading to granulocytopenia and thrombocytopenia have been documented. Experience with the drug in horses is minimal.

DRUG INTERACTIONS: Barbiturates potentiate adverse effects of imipramine but decrease serum levels of the drug. Cimetidine increases serum imipramine levels. Phenothiazines may enhance the drug's effects.

SUPPLIED AS HUMAN PRODUCTS:
Tablets containing 10, 25, 50, and 75 mg (hydrochloride and pamoate salts)
Capsules containing 75, 100, 125, and 150 mg
Injection containing 12.5 mg/mL

INSULIN

INDICATIONS: Insulin preparations ♣ ★ are used in the management of ketosis and hepatic lipidosis in cattle and hyperlipemia in horses and ponies. Insulin is also indicated for emergency treatment of hyperkalemia-associated electrocardiographic abnormalities that occur in foals with ruptured bladders and scouring calves. Most current large animal veterinary literature refers to use of protamine zinc insulin (PZI), a long-acting formulation that is only available in the United States as a pork/beef formulation (PZI VET ★). An ultralente type may also be used (Humulin U ♣ ★, Novolin ge Ultralente ♣).

ADVERSE AND COMMON SIDE EFFECTS: Overdose may cause hypoglycemia leading to disorientation, weakness, hunger, seizure, coma, and death. If overdose occurs, the animal should be fed sugar with water or food. If seizures occur, dextrose solutions should be given IV until seizure activity stops.

DRUG INTERACTIONS: Information regarding drug interactions with use of insulin in large animals is sparse. See INSULIN in Description of Drugs for Small Animals.

SUPPLIED AS VETERINARY PRODUCT:
For injection containing 40 U/mL of lente insulin (Caninsulin ♣)
For injection containing 40 U/mL of protamine zinc insulin (PZI VET ★)

SUPPLIED AS HUMAN PRODUCTS:
For injection containing 100 U/mL
Available in short-acting (regular), intermediate-acting, and long-acting formulations

Human semisynthetic and recombinant DNA formulations [Humulin or Novolin ge products]
Pork, beef and pork formulations [Iletin or Iletin II products]

IPRATROPIUM BROMIDE

INDICATIONS: Ipratropium bromide (Atrovent ♣ ★, Apo-Ipravent ♣, Kendral-Ipratropium ♣) is an anticholinergic agent that when administered by aerosol causes bronchodilation by blockade of M_3-muscarinic receptors on smooth muscle. The compound's quaternary structure discourages systemic absorption from the respiratory tract. Additionally, unlike other parasympatholytic agents, ipratropium bromide does not inhibit mucociliary clearance. It has been used for its bronchodilating effects in horses with recurrent airway obstruction (heaves or chronic obstructive pulmonary disease). Its onset of action is slower than β_2-adrenoceptor agonists, but the effects tend to be longer lasting at 4 to 6 hours.

ADVERSE AND COMMON SIDE EFFECTS: Ipratropium bromide should not be used for the treatment of acute bronchospasm because of its relatively slow onset of action. If ipratropium reaches the eye, there can be ocular complications of mydriasis, increased intraocular pressure, glaucoma, and eye pain.

DRUG INTERACTIONS: In humans, the bronchodilative effect is additive to theophylline and β-adrenoceptor agonists. Ipratropium should be used with caution in patients receiving other anticholinergic drugs because of possible additive effects.

SUPPLIED AS HUMAN PRODUCT:
Solution: each mL contains ipratropium 0.25% w/v in isotonic solution
Aerosol containing 20 µg/actuation

IRON DEXTRAN

INDICATIONS: Iron dextran (APA FER-100 ♣, Co-Op Injectable Iron ♣, Dexafer ♣, Injectable Iron ♣ ★, Iron Dextran Injectable ★, and others) is indicated for the treatment of iron deficiency anemia.

ADVERSE AND COMMON SIDE EFFECTS: Intramuscular injection can be irritating. Allergic reactions and anaphylaxis have occasionally been reported in people. High dosages may be embryotoxic and teratogenic.

DRUG INTERACTIONS: Clinical response may be delayed in patients concurrently receiving chloramphenicol, due to its dose-dependent bone marrow suppression.

SUPPLIED AS VETERINARY PRODUCT:
For injection containing 100 and 200 mg elemental iron/mL

ISOFLUPREDONE

INDICATIONS: Isoflupredone (Predef 2X Sterile Aqueous Suspension ♣ ★) is a potent glucocorticoid used for treatment of bovine ketosis and treatment of inflammatory conditions in horses and cattle. Isoflupredone has glycogen deposition activity and has 10 times more gluconeogenic activity than prednisone. Administration to ketotic cows causes blood glucose levels to return to normal levels, followed by a reduction in blood and urine ketones. Generally, there is a concomitant increase in appetite and rise in milk production to previous levels within 3 to 5 days following injection. Isoflupredone is also indicated for musculoskeletal injuries in cattle and horses and for treatment of allergic reactions.

ADVERSE AND COMMON SIDE EFFECTS: Isoflupredone should not be given for ketosis secondary to pneumonia, mastitis, or metritis unless accompanied by appropriate antimicrobial treatment. As for most glucocorticoids, suppression of signs of inflammation may mask signs of infection. Administration of multiple doses in cattle has been associated with a severe hypokalemia that may be fatal. Administration of glucocorticoids to horses has been associated with laminitis.

DRUG INTERACTIONS: See GLUCOCORTICOID AGENTS.

SUPPLIED AS VETERINARY PRODUCT:
For injection containing 2 mg/mL

ISOFLURANE

INDICATIONS: Isoflurane (Aerrane ♣, Forane ♣, IsoFlo ♣ ★, Isoflurane USP ★, Iso-Thesia ★) is an inhalant anesthetic agent. It is especially useful in horses because induction and recovery times are more rapid with isoflurane than with halothane. Cardiovascular status is better maintained with isoflurane, and isoflurane does not sensitize the heart to epinephrine-induced cardiac arrhythmias as does halothane.

ADVERSE AND COMMON SIDE EFFECTS: Dose-dependent cardiac and respiratory depression occurs. Hypotension, respiratory depression, arrhythmias, nausea, and postoperative ileus have been reported. Studies in ponies suggest that isoflurane may be more likely than halothane to produce anesthetic-associated myopathy even when arterial blood pressure is maintained above 60 mm Hg.

DRUG INTERACTIONS: Isoflurane potentiates the effects of muscle relaxants.

SUPPLIED AS HUMAN AND VETERINARY PRODUCT:
Supplied in 100-mL bottle

ISONIAZID

INDICATIONS: Isoniazid (Dom-Isoniazid ♣, Isotamine ♣, Isoniazid ♣ ★, Nydrazid ★, Laniazid ★, PMS-Isoniazid ♣) is used to treat actinomycosis of the mandible in cattle. It is inexpensive and readily consumed in small amounts of grain.

ADVERSE AND COMMON SIDE EFFECTS: Isoniazid appears nontoxic at the recommended dosage but may cause abortion and thus should not be used in pregnant cattle. In humans, isoniazid can cause severe liver damage. Peripheral neuritis is the most common side effect in humans.

DRUG INTERACTIONS: Isoniazid inhibits the breakdown of phenytoin if both drugs are administered concurrently. Aluminum hydroxide gel decreases gastrointestinal absorption of isoniazid and if used concurrently should be administered at least 1 hour after isoniazid.

SUPPLIED AS HUMAN PRODUCTS:
Tablets containing 50, 100, and 300 mg
Syrup containing 10 mg/mL
Injection containing 100 mg/mL

ISOPROTERENOL

INDICATIONS: Isoproterenol (Isuprel ♣ ★) is a β-adrenergic receptor agonist used for the short-term management of incomplete heart block, sinus bradycardia, and sick sinus syndrome, but is seldom used for these problems in large animals. It can be used as a bronchodilator in horses, but other more selective drugs are available.

ADVERSE AND COMMON SIDE EFFECTS: Nervous excitation, weakness, tachycardia, and ectopic beat formation are reported. The drug is considered more arrhythmogenic than dopamine or dobutamine, so it is rarely used in the treatment of heart failure or shock.

DRUG INTERACTIONS: Digitalis may have additive effects and lead to arrhythmias if used with isoproterenol. If used with theophylline or epinephrine, there is a possibility of increased cardiotoxic effects. Its effects are antagonized by propranolol.

SUPPLIED AS HUMAN PRODUCTS:
For injection containing 0.02 and 0.2 mg/mL
For inhalation delivering 125 (Canada) and 80, 120, or 131 μg/actuation (United States)

ISOXSUPRINE

INDICATIONS: Isoxsuprine (Vasodilan ★) is a β_2-adrenergic receptor agonist that relaxes myometrial and vascular smooth muscle. It is used orally in horses to treat navicular disease syndrome and acute laminitis, but pharmacokinetic/pharmacodynamic studies fail to demonstrate any vascular effects at the suggested dose.

ADVERSE AND COMMON SIDE EFFECTS: Side effects in humans include tachycardia, hypotension, abdominal distress, and severe rash.

DRUG INTERACTIONS: None listed.

SUPPLIED AS HUMAN PRODUCT:
Tablets containing 10 and 20 mg

ITRACONAZOLE

INDICATIONS: Itraconazole (Sporanox ♣ ★) is an imidazole derivative similar to ketoconazole used for treating superficial and systemic fungal infections. Imidazoles alter fungal membrane permeability by blocking synthesis of cellular sterols. Equine sporotrichosis and osteomyelitis associated with *Coccidioides immitis* have been successfully treated with this product. Additionally, mycotic nasal granulomas were eliminated in two horses with *Aspergillus* infections, but itraconazole was not successful in treating *Conidiobolus coronatus* rhinitis in another horse. Therapy is extremely expensive.

ADVERSE AND COMMON SIDE EFFECTS: Specific data are not available. In a recent report, three horses given 3 mg/kg bid; PO for 3 to 4.5 months showed no adverse side effects. See also KETOCONAZOLE.

DRUG INTERACTIONS: Itraconazole requires an acid environment for maximum absorption; therefore, do not administer concurrently with antacids, omeprazole, or H_2-receptor blockers (cimetidine, ranitidine, famotidine). Rifampin increases the hepatic metabolism of itraconazole.

SUPPLIED AS HUMAN PRODUCT:
Capsules containing 100 mg

IVERMECTIN

INDICATIONS: Ivermectin (AmTech Phoenectin ★, Bimectin ★, Double Impact ★, Equimectrin ★, Eqvalan ♣ ★, Ivercide ★, Ivomec ♣ ★, Privermectin ★, Produmec ★, and others) is a broad-spectrum endectocide. It is used in large animals for the eradication of adult and most larval stages of most gastrointestinal nematodes and lungworm of the *Dictyocaulus* spp. It is effective against ectoparasites such as lice, mites, and certain insect larva, including cattle grubs (*Hypoderma bovis, Hypoderma lineatum*), nasal bots (*Oestrus ovis*) of sheep, and nasal bots (*Gasterophilus intestinalis, Gasterophilus nasalis*) in horses. Ivermectin has no activity against flukes or tapeworms. In small ruminants ivermectin has close to 100% efficacy against gastrointestinal nematodes and certain lungworms and is effective for treatment of mange mites. It is not effective against *Muellerius capillaris, Trichuris* spp., or *Nematodirus* spp. Recent evidence suggests resistance to ivermectin is developing in some intestinal parasites affecting small ruminants. Ivermectin use in dairy cows at therapeutic doses may result in violative milk residues for prolonged time periods. Only the related compound, eprinomectin, is approved for use in lactating dairy cattle.

ADVERSE AND COMMON SIDE EFFECTS: Ivermectin has a wide margin of safety. Symptoms of overdose include ataxia, depression, salivation, mydriasis, and blindness. Treatment of overdose is symptomatic; neurologic signs usually resolve over several days. Do not administer CNS depressants such as diazepam or pentobarbital. Intramuscular injection in horses was associated with clostridial myositis at the site of injection, leading to withdrawal of the injectable product for horses. Horses occasionally develop transitory ventral edema due to death of microfilaria of *Onchocerca*. No treatment is usually required.

DRUG INTERACTIONS: None listed.

SUPPLIED AS VETERINARY PRODUCTS:
For injection containing 10 mg/mL (for use in cattle, swine, and sheep; NOT for injectable use in horses)
Premix for swine containing 6 mg/mL
Drench for sheep containing 0.8 mg/mL
Pour-on containing 5 mg/mL (for use in cattle)
Oral paste 1.87% w/w (for use in horses) containing 120 mg/6.42 g
Oral liquid for horses containing 10 mg/mL
Sustained-release bolus containing 1.72 g (★)

KAOLIN-PECTIN

INDICATIONS: Kaolin-pectin (Kaopectate Suspension ♣, Kaolin-Pectin ★, Kaolin Pectin Suspension ★, Kaolin-Pectin Plus ★, Kao-Pec ★, Kaopectolin ★, Kao-Pect + ★) is a gastrointestinal protectant used in the management of diarrhea. It coats the surface of the gut and exerts a mild demulcent and absorbent effect. It is ineffective in absorbing toxins produced by enteropathogenic bacteria. It appears to act by adding particulate matter to the feces, which serves to improve consistency until the disease spontaneously resolves. Kaolin is a potent coagulation activator and may be of some benefit in treating diarrhea associated with mucosal disruption and hemorrhage, such as coronavirus infection in calves.

ADVERSE AND COMMON SIDE EFFECTS: Kaolin-pectin may cause constipation, especially in poorly hydrated patients.

DRUG INTERACTIONS: None listed for large animals.

SUPPLIED AS VETERINARY PRODUCTS:
Oral suspensions containing 5.2 g kaolin and 260 mg pectin or 130 mg, or 90 g kaolin and 2 g pectin per fluid ounce (29.6 mL)
Oral suspension containing 197 mg kaolin and 4.33 mg pectin per mL

SUPPLIED AS HUMAN PRODUCT
Oral suspension containing kaolin 197 mg and pectin 4.33 mg/mL

KETAMINE

INDICATIONS: Ketamine (AmTech Ketamine Hydrochloride Injection ★, Ketaflo ★, Ketaject ★, Ketalean ♣, Ketaset ♣ ★, Keta-Sthetic ★, Keta-Thesia ★, Ketaved ★, Rogarsetic ♣, Vetaket ★, Vetalar ♣ ★) is a rapid-acting, nonbarbiturate general anesthetic. It is classified as a dissociative anesthetic and is accompanied by marked analgesia in most species. A major safety factor with ketamine is the lack of cardio-respiratory depression. Ketamine is used in combination with sedatives such as xylazine or detomidine for induction of general anesthesia. Ketamine combined with xylazine or detomidine is also an effective anesthetic for short procedures, such as surgical repair of minor wounds or castration of stallions. Muscle relaxation with ketamine alone is poor.

ADVERSE AND COMMON SIDE EFFECTS: Ketamine should not be used as the sole anesthetic agent in large animals. Intravenous injection is followed by extensor rigidity, a "dog-sitting" position, extreme muscle spasms and jerking purposeless movements, an excited facial expression, profuse sweating, and, occasionally, convulsions. If used alone, tremors and tonic spasticity will occur, and laryngeal reflexes remain active. Induction of general anesthesia should only be performed in combination with sedatives or tranquilizers and administered only after effects of the sedative or tranquilizer are clinically obvious (see ACEPROMAZINE, DETOMIDINE, DIAZEPAM, GUAIFENESIN, XYLAZINE). Because the eyes remain open and fixed, lubricant should be placed in the eyes during anesthesia. Eye position cannot be used as criteria for anesthetic depth. Sporadic reports of adverse reaction in horses have included turbulent recovery from anesthesia, or ineffective anesthesia, convulsions, and apparent hallucinations.

DRUG INTERACTIONS: Use of ketamine in humans taking thyroid replacement hormones has been associated with severe hypertension and tachycardia. Ketamine may also potentiate respiratory depression and/or paralysis following use of succinylcholine. Ketamine can be antagonized by administration of yohimbine or tolazoline.

SUPPLIED AS VETERINARY PRODUCT:
For injection containing 100 mg/mL

KETOCONAZOLE

INDICATIONS: Ketoconazole (Nizoral ♣ ★) is an imidazole derivative used for treating superficial and systemic fungal infections. Ketoconazole alters fungal membrane permeability by blocking synthesis of cellular sterols. Ketoconazole has been useful in treating histoplasmosis, coccidioidomycosis, and other systemic fungal infections in small animals, but the oral bioavailability in horses is too poor to be of clinical use. The shampoo formulation may be useful for treatment of dermatophytosis.

ADVERSE AND COMMON SIDE EFFECTS: Anorexia, photophobia, gingival bleeding, and paresthesia are untoward effects in people that should be monitored for in animals. Transient elevations in liver enzymes and jaundice have been reported. Gastrointestinal side effects may be prevented by administering the drug with food (which may also serve to increase its absorption) and by dividing the daily dose and administering the drug 2 to 4 times daily. Gynecomastia has also been associated with ketamine administration. The drug should not be given to pregnant animals because its use has been associated with stillbirths and mummified fetuses. In addition, decreased libido and impotence are reported in humans.

DRUG INTERACTIONS: Rifampin increases metabolic clearance of ketoconazole. Antacids, cimetidine, ranitidine, and sucralfate decrease the absorption of ketoconazole. It is recommended that these drugs be administered 2 hours after ketoconazole. Phenytoin may antagonize the actions of ketoconazole. Ketoconazole blunts the cortisol response to ACTH. Ketoconazole may increase the anticoagulant effects of warfarin. The duration of activity of methylprednisolone or prednisolone is prolonged with ketoconazole. Ketoconazole may decrease serum concentrations of theophylline in some patients.

SUPPLIED AS HUMAN PRODUCTS:
Tablets containing 200 mg
Suspension containing 20 mg/mL
Shampoo containing 2% w/v

KETOPROFEN

INDICATIONS: Ketoprofen (Anafen ✤, Ketofen ★) is an NSAID for the treatment of musculoskeletal inflammatory disorders in horses. It is approved in Canada for treatment of pain and inflammation associated with respiratory tract infections, mastitis, udder edema, downer cow syndrome, endotoxemia, simple gastrointestinal disorders, arthritis, and traumatic musculoskeletal injuries in cattle, including lactating dairy. It appears equally effective as flunixin meglumine in blocking endotoxin-stimulated cyclooxygenase-mediated inflammation. Onset of activity occurs within 2 hours of IV or IM administration, with peak response by 12 hours. Ketoprofen has a very short plasma elimination half-life, but due to high protein binding, it sequesters at sites of inflammation. The elimination half-life from inflamed tissues is approximately 24 hours.

ADVERSE AND COMMON SIDE EFFECTS: Adverse reactions as reported in horses include injection site swelling, collapse, fever, sweating, and neck swelling. Large overdoses (15- to 25-fold) can result in laminitis, inappetence, depression, icterus, recumbency, and abdominal swelling, but lesser overdoses (to 5-fold) appear well tolerated. Ketoprofen appears to cause fewer adverse gastrointestinal side effects than flunixin or phenylbutazone in horses. In cattle, it appears to cause less injection site irritation than other NSAIDs.

DRUG INTERACTIONS: Because ketoprofen is highly bound to plasma proteins, caution should be used when it is used concurrently with other highly protein bound drugs, such as warfarin, phenylbutazone, etc. Nonsteroidal anti-inflammatories in general may reduce the diuretic effects of furosemide. Use with caution with other drugs that may inhibit platelet aggregation or cause gastrointestinal ulceration.

SUPPLIED AS VETERINARY PRODUCT:
For injection containing 100 mg/mL, in 50-mL and 100-mL vials

OTHER USES
Horses
ENDOTOXEMIA

A dose of 0.5 mg/kg; IV every 6 hours appears to be as effective as low-dose flunixin meglumine for reduction of endotoxin-mediated circulatory problems.

LACTULOSE

INDICATIONS: Lactulose (Acilac ✚, Cephulac ✚ ★, Cholac ★, Chronulac ✚ ★, Comolose-R ✚, Constulose ★, Constilac ★, Duphalac ✚ ★, Enulose ★, Gen-Lac ✚, Lactulose PSE ★ Syrup, Lactulax ✚, Lactulose ✚, PMS-Lactulose ✚) is a synthetic nonabsorbable disaccharide used in the management of hepatic encephalopathy in horses. Enteric bacteria ferment lactulose to acidic by-products, decrease intraluminal pH, and favor the formation of ammonium ions, which are poorly absorbed. Lactulose also acts as a mild osmotic laxative, increases the rate of passage of ingesta, and leads to the reduction of bacterial production of ammonia. Lactulose is unlikely to be effective in the ruminant with hepatic encephalopathy because ruminal degradation of the drug can be expected.

ADVERSE AND COMMON SIDE EFFECTS: No adverse effects have been reported in horses. However, in humans, transient gastric distention, flatulence, and abdominal cramping may occur. Diarrhea may occur with excessive doses of lactulose.

DRUG INTERACTIONS: Antacids decrease the efficacy of the drug. Neomycin and other oral anti-infectives may inhibit lactulose activity by the reduction or removal of resident colonic bacteria. However, clinical evidence in humans suggests that combined therapy in hepatic encephalopathy may actually be synergistic.

SUPPLIED AS HUMAN PRODUCT:
Syrup containing 10 g/15 mL

LASALOCID

INDICATIONS: Lasalocid (Avatec ✚ ★, Bovatec ✚ ★) is an ionophore antibiotic used for enhancing feed efficiency in cattle and for the prevention of coccidiosis in cattle and sheep. It is not to be used in lactating dairy cattle.

ADVERSE AND COMMON SIDE EFFECTS: It may be fatal if ingested by horses or other equines. Lasalocid should not be fed to pigs or dogs. If fed undiluted to cattle, it could also be fatal. If fed at 5 times the recommended levels, transient diarrhea may occur. Lasalocid may cause rumenitis if given to newborn calves at a dose of 3 mg/kg; PO.

DRUG INTERACTIONS: None listed.

SUPPLIED AS VETERINARY PRODUCT:
Feed premix containing 150 g/kg
The premix is used in the formulation of medicated mineral blocks.

OTHER USES
Cattle
GRAIN BLOAT
1.32 mg/kg daily; PO for the prevention of grain bloat
INTERSTITIAL PNEUMONIA
200 mg/head per day; PO for the prevention of interstitial pneumonia associated with L-tryptophan/3-methyl indole

LEVAMISOLE

INDICATIONS: Levamisole (Levasole ★, Prohibit ★) is a broad-spectrum anthelmintic. It is not effective against *Muellerius capillaris.* Levamisole may help restore immune function, especially in old or debilitated animals, by increasing the number and function of T lymphocytes and macrophages. Levamisole has been shown to hasten recovery of calves with viral respiratory disease. It has also been reported to stimulate antibody production, increase macrophage phagocytosis, inhibit tumor growth, and stimulate suppressor cell activity, but the clinical applicability of such use in large animals remains poorly established. In cattle and sheep, the efficacy of levamisole is equal, regardless of whether the injectable, bolus, or pour-on formulation is used.

ADVERSE AND COMMON SIDE EFFECTS: Toxic doses produce signs suggestive of organophosphate toxicity, including diarrhea, anorexia, salivation, and muscular tremors. Mild toxicity may cause slight muzzle foam and licking of the lips in cattle. Death from toxicity in sheep and goats is the most commonly reported adverse drug reaction for these species. Such problems have occurred more commonly as a result of using the injectable form rather than oral dosing and use of products formulated for other species. Atropine is only partially effective as an antidote. If toxicity progresses to flaccid paralysis, respiratory assistance should be given until recovery has occurred. The pour-on formulation may cause occasional dermal irritation with scaling and fissures at the site of application. Other reports have included sudden death and injection site pain as adverse reactions to injections; pour-on reactions included frothing at the mouth, paddling, and death, as well as alopecia and exfoliation of the skin.

DRUG INTERACTIONS: Pyrantel, diethylcarbamazine, and organophosphate drugs may enhance the toxic effects of levamisole.

SUPPLIED AS VETERINARY PRODUCTS:
For injection containing 136.5 mg/mL
Soluble drench powder containing 11.7 g/packet

Soluble drench containing 13 g/packet
Soluble drench containing 52 g/packet
Soluble drench containing 544.5 g/packet
Soluble drench containing 93.6 g/100g
Oral tablets/boluses containing 184 mg and 2.19 g bolus
Wormer pellets containing 8 g/kg
Pour-on formulation containing 200 mg/mL
Medicated premix containing 500 g/kg

OTHER USES
Horses
RESPIRATORY DISEASE
Levamisole has been used empirically as an immunostimulant for horses with respiratory disease, based mainly on the drug's immuno-stimulant effects in laboratory animals.

LEVOTHYROXINE

INDICATIONS: Levothyroxine (AmTech Levothyroxine Sodium Tablets ★, Levo-Powder ★, Levoxine ★, Levotabs ★, NutriVed T-4 Chewables ★, Soloxine ❧ ★, Synthroid ❧ ★, Thyro-Tabs ★, Thyroxine-L ★, Thyrozine ★) is a synthetic form of T_4 used in the treatment of hypothyroid disease. Although hypothyroidism has been incriminated in a number of relatively common equine diseases, conclusive scientific data to substantiate its occurrence in horses are lacking.

ADVERSE AND COMMON SIDE EFFECTS: Thyroid replacement should be undertaken with caution in animals with hypoadreno-corticism, diabetes mellitus, or congestive heart failure. The increase in metabolism may place undue stress on the heart.

DRUG INTERACTIONS: With the use of thyroid medications, marked hypertension and tachycardia following induction with ketamine has been documented in people.

SUPPLIED AS VETERINARY PRODUCTS:
Tablets containing 0.1, 0.2, 0.3, 0.5, 0.6, and 0.8 mg
Tablets containing 0.4 and 0.7 mg (United States)
Powder (0.22%, United States) containing 1 g T_4 in 454 g powder, 2.3 g T_4 in 1050 g powder, 10 g T_4 in 4.53 kg powder

SUPPLIED AS HUMAN PRODUCTS:
Tablets containing 12.5, 25, 50, 75, 88, 100, 112, 125, 150, 175, 200, and 300 µg
Injection containing 200 or 500 µg/vial

LIDOCAINE

INDICATIONS: Lidocaine (Lidocaine Neat ✤, Lurocaine ✤, Anthracaine ★, Lidoject ★, Xylocaine ✤ ★) is one of the most commonly used local and topical anesthetics in large animals. It is also the drug of choice for the IV management of ventricular premature contractions or tachycardia. Because of a high first-pass effect it cannot be given orally. After IV administration, its onset of action is 2 minutes and its duration of action is 10 to 20 minutes.

ADVERSE AND COMMON SIDE EFFECTS: With drug overdose, drowsiness, tremors, nystagmus, seizure, hypotension, and increased atrioventricular conduction with atrial flutter and fibrillation have been reported. The neurologic signs can be controlled with diazepam. Hypokalemia reduces antiarrhythmic effects.

DRUG INTERACTIONS: Cimetidine, propranolol, and quinidine increase activity of lidocaine. Barbiturates decrease lidocaine action via enzyme induction. Phenytoin increases the cardiac depressant effect of lidocaine. High doses may prolong succinylcholine-induced apnea.

SUPPLIED AS VETERINARY PRODUCTS:
For injection containing 20 mg/mL
To prepare IV infusion using 2% veterinary solution, add 1 g (50 mL) of 2% solution to 1 L D_5W, thus providing 1 mg/mL (1,000 mg/mL). With a minidrop (60 drops/mL) IV set, each drop will contain approximately 17 µg.

OTHER USES
Horses

ILEUS

Horses with ileus can be administered an IV infusion of 1.3 mg/kg in a slow IV bolus, then 0.05 mg/kg per minute over a period of 5 to 6 hours. The mechanism of action may be the suppression of afferent neural pathways from the peritoneum, which induces analgesia. Lidocaine may also have some anti-inflammatory properties. It may also be directly stimulating to smooth muscle. Side effects at this dose are not common but may include trembling, muscle fasciculations, or ataxia, which are controlled by decreasing the infusion rate.

LINCOMYCIN

INDICATIONS: Lincomycin (Lincocin ✤ ★) is a lincosamide antibiotic with activity against gram-positive cocci, particularly *Streptococcus* spp. and *Staphylococcus* spp. It also is active against *Clostridium* *tetani* and *perfringens, Mycoplasma* spp., *Leptospira pomona,* and *Erysipelo-thrix insidiosa.* Lincomycin is effective against penicillinase-producing staphylococci. Significant concentrations of the drug are achieved in most tissues of the body other than CSF. The drug is excreted in the bile and urine. It is used in swine to treat infectious arthritis and mycoplasma pneumonia.

ADVERSE AND COMMON SIDE EFFECTS: Pain at the injection site is reported. Anal swelling, irritable behavior and skin reddening may also occur transiently in swine. Lincomycin may cause transient diarrhea in swine, while oral administration to ruminants and horses may cause severe gastrointestinal upset. Anorexia, decreased milk production, and ketosis have been reported in cattle given feed contaminated with 3 to 24 ppm of lincomycin.

DRUG INTERACTIONS: Kaolin, pectin, and bismuth subsalicylate decrease GI absorption. Chloramphenicol and erythromycin are mutually antagonistic with lincomycin. Lincomycin has intrinsic neuromuscular blocking properties and should be used with caution with other neuromuscular blocking agents.

SUPPLIED AS VETERINARY PRODUCTS:
Soluble powder for water medication in 40- or 80-g packets
Sterile solution containing 50 mg lincomycin and 100 mg spectinomycin for use in semen extenders
For injection containing 100 mg/mL (Canada) and 25 and 300 mg/mL (United States)

LUTEINIZING HORMONE

INDICATIONS: Luteinizing hormone (Lutrophin-V ♣) is an anterior pituitary extract that acts to stimulate follicular maturation and estrogen production in horses, cattle, sheep, and swine. Luteinizing hormone is used in cattle to correct ovarian cysts and in mares to treat ovulation failure.

ADVERSE AND COMMON SIDE EFFECTS: None listed.

DRUG INTERACTIONS: None listed.

SUPPLIED AS VETERINARY PRODUCT:
For injection containing 25 mg/5-mL vial

MAGNESIUM

INDICATIONS: Magnesium sulfate ♣ ★ (Epsom salts) is used in large animals mainly as an oral cathartic. There are many products that contain calcium, phosphorus, potassium, and dextrose in addition to magnesium, that are used to treat electrolyte deficiencies ("milk fever," "grass tetany") (Cal-Dextro ♣ ★, CMPK ♣ ★, Norcalciphos ♣ ★). Human IV formulations are available for IV use. Magnesium is used as adjunctive therapy of malignant hyperthermia in swine.

ADVERSE AND COMMON SIDE EFFECTS: Undiluted magnesium sulfate can cause osmotic damage to intestinal mucosal cells and may induce enteritis. Overdose of parenteral magnesium causes CNS depression, neuromuscular blockade, and cardiac arrest.

DRUG INTERACTIONS: Concurrent use of magnesium with anesthetics will increase CNS depression. Excessive neuromuscular blockade will result with concurrent use with nondepolarizing neuromuscular blocking agents.

SUPPLIED AS VETERINARY PRODUCTS:
Combination products containing varying amounts of calcium, potassium, magnesium, and phosphorus.

SUPPLIED AS CHEMICAL PRODUCT:
As salts containing 98% to 100% magnesium sulfate

SUPPLIED AS HUMAN PRODUCTS:
For injection containing 40, 80, 100, 125, 200, and 500 mg/mL
For injection containing 1% and 2% w/v magnesium in 5% dextrose

OTHER USES
EUTHANASIA
A concentrated magnesium sulfate solution can be administered IV as a euthanasia solution but only after the animal has been appropriately anesthetized.

MAGNESIUM HYDROXIDE

INDICATIONS: Magnesium hydroxide (Carmilax ★ Bolets, Carmilax Powder ★, InstaMag Bolus ★, Laxade Boluses ★, Laxade Powder ★, Magnalax Bolus ★, Magne-Lax ★, Milk of Magnesia ♣ ★, Polyox II Bolus ★, Polyox Powder ★, Rumalax ★, Rumalax Gel ★, and others) is an oral antacid and mild laxative. It is used in cattle to treat rumen acidosis and in horses for treatment of gastric ulceration.

ADVERSE AND COMMON SIDE EFFECTS AND DRUG INTERACTIONS: See ANTACIDS.

SUPPLIED AS VETERINARY PRODUCTS:
Oral boluses containing 6 and 17 g
Powder containing 361 g or 295 g per 454 g powder (United States)

Powder containing 106 g/340 g
Gel containing 216 g/454 g
Note: Three boluses contain the equivalent magnesium hydroxide to
946 mL of Milk of Magnesia.

SUPPLIED AS HUMAN PRODUCTS:
Oral suspension containing 77.5 mg/g
Tablets containing 300 and 600 mg

MANNITOL

INDICATIONS: Mannitol (Am-Vet Mannitol Injection ★, Manniject ★, Mannitol ♣ ★) is a potent osmotic diuretic. It is used for the prevention and treatment of oliguria and acute glaucoma and in the management of acute cerebral edema in diseases such as cranial trauma, polio-encephalomalacia, or equine neonatal maladjustment. The use of the drug in animals with intracranial injury is controversial. These patients may have a damaged blood–brain barrier, which would allow the drug to leak across into the damaged brain and cause the area to swell further. Mannitol has also been used to enhance the renal elimination of toxins such as aspirin, ethylene glycol, and some barbiturates.

ADVERSE AND COMMON SIDE EFFECTS: Volume overload and pulmonary edema may occur, especially in patients with compromised renal or cardiac disease. Hyponatremia and seizures have been reported with drug overdose. Mannitol is contraindicated in the case of cerebral hemorrhage.

DRUG INTERACTIONS: None established for large animals.

SUPPLIED AS VETERINARY PRODUCT:
For injection containing 180 mg/mL

SUPPLIED AS HUMAN PRODUCT (OSMITROL):
For injection containing 5%, 10%, 15%, 20%, and 25% w/v

OTHER USES
Horses and Ruminants
OLIGURIC RENAL FAILURE
0.25 to 1.0 g/kg as a 20% w/v solution; slowly IV

MECLOFENAMIC ACID

INDICATIONS: Meclofenamic acid (Arquel ♣ ★) is an NSAID used in the oral treatment of acute or chronic osteoarthritic disease in the horse. It has also been used experimentally to prevent respiratory distress in anaphylactic shock in conscious calves. Its onset of action is slow in horses, taking 36 to 96 hours to develop.

ADVERSE AND COMMON SIDE EFFECTS: Toxic signs in the horse (buccal erosions, anorexia, and gastrointestinal disturbances) can result from prolonged, high (12 to 16 mg/kg) daily doses. Higher than therapeutic doses can lower the packed cell volume. Horses with heavy bot infestation may develop mild colic and diarrhea following meclofenamic acid administration. The drug is contraindicated in animals with gastrointestinal, renal, or hepatic disorders.

DRUG INTERACTIONS: Meclofenamic acid binds to plasma proteins and may displace other drugs, such as warfarin, resulting in adverse reaction to the displaced drug.

SUPPLIED AS VETERINARY PRODUCTS:
Oral granules containing 500 mg in 10-g packet
Oral granules containing 50 mg/g in 100-g jar

MEGESTROL ACETATE

INDICATIONS: Megestrol acetate (Ovaban ♣ ★) is a progestational compound marketed for the postponement of estrus and the alleviation of false pregnancy in bitches. The drug is used in horses to treat behavioral problems such as aggression in stallions and nonpregnant mares.

ADVERSE AND COMMON SIDE EFFECTS: The drug should not be given to females with reproductive problems, during pregnancy, or to those with mammary tumors. Information on adverse effects in horses is scant, but in small animals, polyphagia, polydipsia, weight gain, and a change in behavior are common side effects.

DRUG INTERACTIONS: None established.

SUPPLIED AS VETERINARY PRODUCT: (small animal products only)
Tablets containing 5 and 20 mg

MELENGESTROL ACETATE

INDICATIONS: Melengestrol acetate (MGA ♣ ★) is a progestational compound used in feedlot heifers (>181 kg) to suppress estrus, enhance feed utilization, and to promote growth.

ADVERSE AND COMMON SIDE EFFECTS: Melengestrol should only be used in intact heifers as it is ineffective in steers or spayed heifers. The recommended withdrawal of the drug prior to shipping predisposes animals to heat at the time of loading for transport.

DRUG INTERACTIONS: Do not use the drug in feed containing pellet binding agents.

SUPPLIED AS VETERINARY PRODUCT:
Premix feed additive containing 200 or 500 mg/kg

MEPERIDINE

INDICATIONS: Meperidine/Pethidine (Demerol ♣ ★) is a short-acting narcotic sedative with pharmacological properties similar to morphine in that it binds to opiate receptors and raises the pain threshold. Unlike morphine, it is no more toxic to the newborn than adult animals. It is used to relieve pain associated with Cesarean section in the mare and for its analgesic and sedative properties during calving in cattle. It does not appreciably depress fetal respiration. It is a less potent analgesic than morphine. Meperidine can be used in place of morphine where an analgesic drug is required that does not also depress intestinal motility.

ADVERSE AND COMMON SIDE EFFECTS: The SC route of administration should be avoided because of local irritation and pain at the site of injection. It should be administered by slow IV injection, otherwise significant decreases in systemic blood pressure and bronchoconstriction can occur, possibly due to central vagal effects and histamine release.

DRUG INTERACTIONS: Naloxone antagonizes the respiratory depression and toxic effects of meperidine.

SUPPLIED AS HUMAN PRODUCTS:
Tablets containing 50 and 100 mg
Oral solution containing 10 mg/mL
For injection containing 10, 25, 50, 75, and 100 mg/mL

MEPIVACAINE HYDROCHLORIDE

INDICATIONS: Mepivacaine hydrochloride (Carbocaine-V 2% ♣ ★) is a rapid-acting local and topical anesthetic of similar potency to lidocaine, but with a more rapid onset and less toxicity. Its anesthetic effects last several hours and can be prolonged with the addition of epinephrine 1:100,000. It has been used in topical anesthesia of the laryngeal mucosa prior to ventriculectomy in horses.

ADVERSE AND COMMON SIDE EFFECTS: It should not be injected into infected tissues or regions that lack adequate blood circulation such as fibrosed areas. Epidural use should be avoided in hypovolemic animals.

DRUG INTERACTIONS: See LIDOCAINE.

SUPPLIED AS VETERINARY PRODUCT:
For injection containing 2% w/v

METHIONINE

INDICATIONS: Methionine (Ammonil ★, D-L-M Tablets ★, Equi-Phar DL-Methionine Powder ★, Methio-Tabs ★, Methigel ✤ ★, D-L-Methionine Powder ★, Methio-Form ✤ ★, Methio Tablets) is a urinary acidifying agent used in the treatment and prevention of struvite urolithiasis in small animals. In horses, it is used to promote keratinization and healing of hoof and sole defects, as in chronic laminitis.

ADVERSE AND COMMON SIDE EFFECTS: Methionine is contraindicated in patients with renal failure or pancreatic disease. It should only be used in the treatment of hepatic lipidosis caused by choline deficiency, as may occur with pancreatic exocrine insufficiency. It may, in fact, potentiate clinical signs of hepatic encephalopathy by leading to the increased production of mercaptan-like compounds.

DRUG INTERACTIONS: Methionine may increase the renal excretion of quinidine. The antibacterial efficacy of aminoglycosides and erythromycin may be decreased in the presence of acid urine produced by methionine.

SUPPLIED AS VETERINARY PRODUCTS:
Tablets containing 200 and 500 mg
Gel containing 80 mg/g
Powder as a feed additive containing 100% DL-methionine

METHOCARBAMOL

INDICATIONS: Methocarbamol (Carbacot ★, Robaxin-V ★, Skelex ★) is a centrally acting muscle relaxant used as adjunct therapy to rest and physical therapy in the treatment of musculoskeletal injury. It has also been used to reduce muscular spasm associated with tetanus and poisoning by strychnine.

ADVERSE AND COMMON SIDE EFFECTS: Excessive salivation, sedation, vomiting, muscular weakness, and ataxia have been reported in people. The CNS depressant effects will impair performance in horses. Extravascular injection may cause tissue necrosis. The injectable drug product contains polyethylene glycol 300, so it should not be given to animals with renal dysfunction. Methocarbamol should not be used in pregnant animals.

DRUG INTERACTIONS: Other CNS depressants may potentiate the CNS depressive effects of methocarbamol.

SUPPLIED AS VETERINARY PRODUCTS:
Tablets containing 500 mg (United States)
For injection containing 100 mg/mL (United States)

SUPPLIED AS HUMAN PRODUCTS:
Tablets containing 500 and 750 mg
For injection containing 100 mg/mL

METHYLCELLULOSE FLAKES

INDICATIONS: Methylcellulose flakes (Citrucel ❖ ★, Entrocel ❖, Methylcellulose Tablets ★) are hydrophilic, indigestible, nonabsorbable colloid derivatives of cellulose used to soften and bulk the stool and to formulate a lubricant for obstetrical use. They are also used for treatment of sand impaction in the horse, but psyllium mucilloid may be more effective.

ADVERSE AND COMMON SIDE EFFECTS: Fluid retention can occur with some forms of the flakes.

DRUG INTERACTIONS: None listed.

SUPPLIED AS: HUMAN PRODUCTS
Dry product containing 1 part methylcellulose flakes and 5 parts sugar
Tablets containing 500 mg
Liquid containing 18 mg/mL

METHYLENE BLUE

INDICATIONS: Methylene blue (Methylene Blue Injection ❖ ★, Methylene Blue Tablets ❖ ★, Urolene Blue ❖ ★) is used in the treatment of methemoglobinemia, from the ingestion of nitrate-accumulating plants in ruminants, and chlorate toxicosis in large animals. Although methemoglobinemia is a component of red maple leaf toxicity in horses, methylene blue is reported to be neither necessary nor beneficial for treatment of this specific toxicity. It is not approved for use in food animals and is suspected to be carcinogenic. Contact a gFARAD center prior to use for current withdrawal time information.

ADVERSE AND COMMON SIDE EFFECTS: The drug is contra-indicated in patients with renal insufficiency. Methylene blue may cause Heinz body hemolytic anemia and, possibly, acute renal failure. In people, additional side effects may include bladder irritation, nausea, vomiting, diarrhea, and abdominal pain. With large IV doses, fever, cardiovascular abnormalities, methemoglobinemia, and profuse sweating may also occur. Extravascular administration causes tissue necrosis.

DRUG INTERACTIONS: None reported.

SUPPLIED AS HUMAN PRODUCTS:
For injection containing 10 mg/mL
Tablets containing 65 mg
Methylene Blue, USP powder (from chemical supply companies)

METHYLPREDNISOLONE ACETATE OR SODIUM SUCCINATE

INDICATIONS: Methylprednisolone (A-Methpred ★, Depo-Medrol ❧ ★, Methysone 40 ❧, Solu-Medrol ❧ ★, Uni-Med ❧, Vetacortyl ❧) is a glucocorticoid used for its anti-inflammatory properties. It is available in a short-acting ester formulation and in a long-acting acetate formulation. Methylprednisolone sodium succinate is used for emergency management of shock and CNS trauma, but due to expense, its use is usually limited to neonatal large animals. Methylprednisolone acetate is most often used intra-articularly for nonseptic joint disease or IM for its anti-inflammatory properties.

ADVERSE AND COMMON SIDE EFFECTS: See GLUCOCORTI-COID AGENTS.

DRUG INTERACTIONS: See GLUCOCORTICOID AGENTS.

SUPPLIED AS VETERINARY PRODUCT:
For injection containing 20 and 40 mg/mL

SUPPLIED AS HUMAN PRODUCT:
For injection containing 20, 40, and 80 mg/mL

METHYLSULFONOMETHANE

INDICATIONS: Methylsulfonomethane ❧ ★ (MSM) is a nutriceutical derivative of dimethyl sulfoxide that has been claimed to promote healing and recovery from disease, athletic injuries, and stress. It is also used in horses to promote hoof keratinization in chronic laminitis.

ADVERSE AND COMMON SIDE EFFECTS: None listed.

DRUG INTERACTIONS: None listed.

SUPPLIED AS VETERINARY PRODUCT:
As feed additive powder 9.9 g/10 g

METOCLOPRAMIDE

INDICATIONS: Metoclopramide (Apo-Metoclop ♣, Maxeran ♣ ★, Maxolon ★, Metoclopramide Hydrochloride Intensol ★, Nu-Metoclopramide ♣, Octamide ★, Reglan ♣ ★) acts peripherally to enhance the action of acetylcholine at muscarinic synapses and in the central nervous system as a dopamine antagonist. It contributes to lower esophageal sphincter competence and promotes gastric emptying. It is useful in the management of gastric reflux and gastric motility disorders, as in sheep with abomasal emptying defect, and abomasal impaction in cattle. It is also used in horses to treat intestinal ileus. Rumen degradation, complexation, or binding reduces the amount of drug available that is administered orally by nearly 50%.

ADVERSE AND COMMON SIDE EFFECTS: Metoclopramide should not be used in patients with gastric outlet obstruction or those with a history of epilepsy. Intravenous administration in horses may result in violent CNS excitation, known as extrapyramidal effects. In case of such reactions, administer an anticholinergic antihistamine such as diphenhydramine at 2 mg/kg IV to restore the normal CNS balance of acetylcholine-dopamine. Oral administration in foals is associated with fewer side effects.

DRUG INTERACTIONS: Phenothiazine drugs potentiate CNS effects. Aspirin, diazepam, and tetracycline absorption may be accelerated in the presence of metoclopramide. Digoxin absorption may be decreased. Atropine will block the effects of the drug on gastrointestinal motility.

SUPPLIED AS HUMAN PRODUCTS:
Tablets containing 5 and 10 mg
Syrup containing 1 and 2 mg/mL
For injection containing 5 mg/mL

OTHER USES
Sheep
ABOMASAL EMPTYING DEFECT
0.3 mg/kg every 4 to 6 hours; SC

METRONIDAZOLE

INDICATIONS: Metronidazole (Apo-Metronidazole ♣, Flagyl ♣ ★, Metric 21 ★, Metro I.V. ★, Novo-Nidazol ♣, PMS-Metronidazole ♣, Protostat ★) is a synthetic antibacterial, antiprotozoal agent that has been used in the treatment of giardiasis, trichomoniasis, amoebiasis, balantidiasis, and trypanosomiasis. It is bactericidal to many anaerobic bacteria including *Bacteroides* spp., *Fusobacterium, Clostridium* spp., *Veillonella* spp., *Peptococcus* spp., and *Peptostreptococcus* spp., and has been used for treating anaerobic infections of the respiratory tract, as may occur in aspiration pneumonia and peritonitis. Metronidazole and other nitroimidazole compounds are banned for use in food animals due to carcinogenicity concerns.

ADVERSE AND COMMON SIDE EFFECTS: Limited information is available regarding adverse effects in large animals. Adverse CNS effects have been reported in small animals. It is potentially hepatotoxic and teratogenic.

DRUG INTERACTIONS: Blood levels may be decreased by concurrent use of phenobarbital or phenytoin, and blood levels may be increased by cimetidine use. The effects of oral anticoagulants are potentiated by metronidazole.

SUPPLIED AS HUMAN PRODUCTS:
Tablets containing 250 and 500 mg
Capsules containing 500 mg
For injection containing 500 mg/vial
For injection containing 5 mg/mL

MICONAZOLE

INDICATIONS: Miconazole (Conofite ♣, Micatin ♣ ★, Monistat ♣ ★) is an antifungal agent used for the treatment of dermatophytosis and fungal keratitis in large animals. It is no longer available in formulations suitable for systemic or ocular use.

ADVERSE AND COMMON SIDE EFFECTS: Reactions to topical application are rare but include mild pruritus and pain at the site of application.

DRUG INTERACTIONS: None listed.

SUPPLIED AS VETERINARY PRODUCTS:
Cream (2% w/w) for topical use

MIDAZOLAM

See MIDAZOLAM in Descriptions of Drugs for Small Animals.

MINERAL OIL

INDICATIONS: Mineral oil ♣ ★ (or liquid paraffin) is used for the relief of intestinal impaction, particularly in horses. It softens stools by coating the feces and preventing the colonic absorption of water. The agent works at the level of the colon and may take 6 to 12 hours to work effectively. It has also been used to hasten the transit of ingesta, as with grain overload in horses and ruminants, but other products (see MAGNESIUM SULFATE) are more appropriate.

ADVERSE AND COMMON SIDE EFFECTS: Mineral oil is contraindicated in patients with intestinal obstruction or dysphagia. Chronic administration may cause granulomatous reactions from mineral oil absorption and interference with absorption of fat soluble vitamins. Accidental aspiration causes severe lipid pneumonia.

DRUG INTERACTIONS: Increased absorption may occur if mineral oil is given concurrently with docusate sodium or docusate calcium. Mineral oil may interfere with the action of nonabsorbable sulfonamides.

SUPPLIED AS VETERINARY PRODUCT:
As a liquid for oral use

MONENSIN

INDICATIONS: Monensin (Coban ♣ ★, Rumensin ♣ ★, Rumensin CRC ♣) is an ionophore antibiotic used to enhance feed efficiency in cattle. It is also used in cattle and goats to prevent coccidiosis. Monensin is effective in reducing subclinical ketosis in dairy cattle, with additional benefits of increased milk production and increased protein content in the milk. The rumen bolus is approved for prevention of subclinical ketosis in Canada, with no milk withdrawal.

ADVERSE AND COMMON SIDE EFFECTS: Monensin can cause fatal cardiomyopathy if ingested by horses or other equines. Monensin also should not be fed to pigs or dogs. If fed undiluted to cattle, it could be fatal. If fed at 5 times the recommended levels to cattle, transient diarrhea may occur.

DRUG INTERACTIONS: None listed. Monensin can be mixed with melengestrol acetate (MGA ♣ ★) for heifer feeding programs.

SUPPLIED AS VETERINARY PRODUCTS:
Feed additive containing 132.2 or 176 g/kg
Block containing 880 mg/kg
Controlled-release bolus containing 32 g

OTHER USES
Cattle

BLOAT PREVENTION
1.32 mg/kg daily; PO

PNEUMONIA
200 mg/head per day; PO, for prevention of interstitial pneumonia associated with L-tryptophan/3-methyl indole

SUBCLINICAL KETOSIS PREVENTION
200 mg/head per day; PO to dairy cattle for prevention of subclinical ketosis coupled with an increase in milk production

MORANTEL TARTRATE

INDICATIONS: Morantel tartrate (Banminth ✤ ★, Rumatel ★) is a pyrimidine anthelmintic used for the removal and control of mature gastrointestinal nematode infections of dairy and beef cattle. Like pyrantel, morantel has nicotine-like properties and acts similarly to acetylcholine to cause a depolarizing neuromuscular blockade in susceptible nematodes.

ADVERSE AND COMMON SIDE EFFECTS: None listed.

DRUG INTERACTIONS: None listed. It may be administered concurrently with vaccines and other drugs without increased cholinesterase inhibition.

SUPPLIED AS VETERINARY PRODUCTS:
Pellets containing 10 g/kg
Premix containing 10 g/kg, 193.6 g/kg, or 200 mg/g
Bolus containing 2.5 g

OTHER USES
Sheep

OSTERTAGIA and *TRICHURIS* SPP.
10 mg/kg; PO. Morantel tartrate is 95% effective in removing gastrointestinal nematodes and 90% effective for *Ostertagia* and *Trichuris* spp.

MORPHINE

INDICATIONS: Morphine (Astramorph ★, Duramorph ★, Roxanol ★, M.S. Contin ✤ ★, M.O.S. ✤ ★, Morphitec ✤, Statex ✤) is a very effective analgesic narcotic agent. It is used for the management of acute pain and as a preanesthetic agent. In the horse, it has been used for treatment of pain associated with spasmodic colic or pleuritis, but many horses will show undesirable and dangerous CNS stimulation and excitement. Epidural administration of morphine alone or in combination with β_2-adrenergic receptor agonists, such as xylazine, provides long-lasting analgesia without CNS effects.

ADVERSE AND COMMON SIDE EFFECTS: In horses, systemic administration of morphine can cause excitement, restlessness, and loss of coordination. Pretreatment with acepromazine or xylazine may reduce behavioral changes. Overdose causes profound CNS and respiratory depression. Horses and ruminants may develop hyperthermia.

DRUG INTERACTIONS: Phenothiazines, antihistamines, fentanyl, and parenteral magnesium sulfate may potentiate the depressant effects of morphine.

SUPPLIED AS HUMAN PRODUCTS:
For injection containing 0.5, 1, 2, 3, 4, 5, 8, 10, 15, 25, and 50 mg/mL
Tablets containing 5, 10, 15, 20, 25, 30, 40, 50, 60, and 100 mg
Oral solution containing 1, 2, 4, 5, 10, 20, and 50 mg/mL
Capsules containing 10, 15, 20, 30, 50, 60, 100, and 200 mg
Suppositories containing 5, 10, 20, 30, 60, 100, and 200 mg

OTHER USES
EPIDURAL ANALGESIA
Morphine can be administered epidurally in small doses (0.05 to 0.2 mg/kg) to treat acute or chronic pain. Analgesia lasts from 6 to 24 hours. Adverse side effects are usually minimal but may include some CNS stimulation.

MOXIDECTIN

INDICATIONS: Moxidectin (Cyadectin Injectable ♣, Cydectin Pour-On ♣ ★, Quest ♣ ★) is a milbemycin endectocide synthesized from the bacterium *Streptomyces cyanogriseus* non *cyanogenus*. Compared to ivermectin, moxidectin is sequestered almost exclusively in fat, with an elimination half-life of 12 to 14 days following administration. It is used in large animals for the eradication of adult and most larval stages of most gastrointestinal nematodes and lungworm of the *Dictyocaulus* spp. It is effective against ectoparasites such as lice, mites, and certain insect larva, including cattle grubs (*Hypoderma bovis, Hypoderma lineatum*), nasal bots (*Oestrus ovis*) of sheep, and nasal bots (*Gasterophilus intestinalis, Gasterophilus nasalis*) in horses. Moxidectin has no activity against flukes or tapeworms. In horses, moxidectin has better activity than ivermectin against the encysted later third and fourth stage cyanthostome larvae, but is also ineffective against the hypobiotic third stages. Ivermectin has more activity against *Gasterophilus* (bots) than moxidectin, so the dose of moxidectin (0.4 mg/kg) is twice the dose of ivermectin (0.2 mg/kg) for this purpose. Moxidectin can be administered at the same dose as ivermectin for control of other parasites.

ADVERSE AND COMMON SIDE EFFECTS: When used according to label doses, adverse effects are minimal in cattle, but because of the increased dose and distribution to fat stores, moxidectin should not be given to young foals or severely debilitated animals with low fat stores. Dosing according to accurate body weight will greatly minimize the risk of toxicity. Moxidectin is not labeled for foals less than 4 months of age and neurotoxicity and deaths have been reported in young foals and miniature horses overdosed with moxidectin. Symptoms of overdose include ataxia, depression, salivation, mydriasis, and blindness. Treatment of overdose is symptomatic; neurologic signs usually resolve over several days. Do not administer CNS depressants such as diazepam or pentobarbital in case of moxidectin toxicity.

DRUG INTERACTIONS: None listed.

SUPPLIED AS VETERINARY PRODUCT:
For injection containing 10 mg/mL (Canada)
Pour-on containing 5 mg/mL (for use in cattle)
Oral gel containing 20 mg/mL (for horses)

NALOXONE

See NALOXONE, in Description of Drugs for Small Animals.

NATAMYCIN

INDICATIONS: Natamycin (Natacyn ★) is a broad-spectrum antifungal agent used in horses for treating ocular fungal infections. It is the only commercially available drug for the treatment of fungal keratitis. It is poorly lipid soluble and will not penetrate an intact cornea.

ADVERSE AND COMMON SIDE EFFECTS: Conjunctival chemosis and hyperemia have been reported in humans. The suspension is difficult to deliver through subpalpebral lavage systems.

DRUG INTERACTIONS: None listed.

SUPPLIED AS HUMAN PRODUCT:
Ophthalmic 5% w/v suspension

NEOMYCIN

INDICATIONS: Neomycin (Biosol ♣ ★, Neomed 325 ♣, Neomix ♣ ★, Neo-Ved 200 ★, Neovet ★, Neomycin ♣ ★) is an aminoglycoside antibiotic. It is generally less effective than amikacin or gentamicin against many bacteria. It is commonly used as a topical antibiotic and in over the counter oral antidiarrheal preparations for ruminants and swine. There is widespread *E. coli* resistance to neomycin, so its efficacy for scours is questionable. Neomycin can be used orally in horses with hepatic encephalopathy to reduce nitrogen breakdown by bacterial flora of the gut. Parenteral use of the drug is toxigenic and has been implicated as a major cause of renal failure in cattle. Oral bioavailability is poor in normal animals, but with enteritis, significant amounts may be absorbed and accumulate in renal tissues. Neomycin is a very common cause of violative tissue residues in veal calves in the United States and Canada.

ADVERSE AND COMMON SIDE EFFECTS: Neomycin is the most nephrotoxic aminoglycoside. The drug is also potentially toxic to the vestibular and auditory nerves. Prolonged oral administration of neomycin to horses can induce diarrhea. See AMINOGLYCOSIDES.

DRUG INTERACTIONS: Orally administered neomycin may decrease the absorption of digitalis, penicillin V and K, and vitamin K.

SUPPLIED AS VETERINARY PRODUCTS:
Oral liquid containing 50 and 140 mg/mL
Soluble powder containing 500, 715, and 812 mg/g

OTHER USES
Horses
HEPATIC ENCEPHALOPATHY
50 to 100 mg/kg qid; PO

NEOSTIGMINE

INDICATIONS: Neostigmine methylsulfate (PMS-Neostigmine Methylsulfate ✤, Prostigmin ✤ ★, Stimuline ✤) is an anticholinesterase used for the treatment of atony of the rumen, uterine inertia, paralyzed bowel, paralyzed urinary bladder, posterior paralysis, posttraumatic paralysis, curare overdose, larkspur poisoning, and muscle rigidity or spasticity. There is marked clinical variability in response to dose.

ADVERSE AND COMMON SIDE EFFECTS: Overdose may cause a cholinergic crisis characterized by salivation, urination, diarrhea, bradycardia or tachycardia, miosis, lacrimation, bronchospasm, and hypotension. A cholinergic crisis should be treated with atropine (0.4 mg/kg; IM, IV). Neostigmine may precipitate atrial fibrillation in cattle.

DRUG INTERACTIONS: Glucocorticoids may decrease the anticholinesterase activity of neostigmine. Neostigmine antagonizes the action of pancuronium and tubocurarine. Atropine antagonizes the muscarinic effects of neostigmine and is often used to treat adverse effects of the drug. Neostigmine may effectively reverse neuromuscular blockade caused by aminoglycosides. Dexpanthenol may have additive effects if given with neostigmine.

SUPPLIED AS VETERINARY PRODUCT:
For injection containing 2 mg/mL

SUPPLIED AS HUMAN PRODUCTS:
Tablets containing 15 mg neostigmine bromide
For injection containing 0.5, 1, and 2.5 mg/mL neostigmine methylsulfate

NIACIN

INDICATIONS: Niacin (nicotinic acid) and nicotinamide are included in the dry cow ration of dairy cows and early lactating cows to help prevent hepatic lipidosis and ketosis. Niacin (Nu-Keto ★) alone, or in commercially available compounds (Bovi Plus ♣, Lipotinic Boluses ★, Ketopro Oral Gel ★) is used as a nutritional supplement for animals off feed. Niacin decreases blood ketones and free fatty acids and increases blood glucose. Niacin is proposed to decrease ketosis and increase milk production, but supporting evidence is not strong.

ADVERSE AND COMMON SIDE EFFECTS: None listed.

DRUG INTERACTIONS: Niacin has been used in conjunction with monensin for prevention of ketosis, the latter being recently licensed in Canada for use in lactating dairy cows.

SUPPLIED AS VETERINARY PRODUCTS:
As a feed additive 100% w/w
Boluses containing 6 g niacin/15 g

SUPPLIED AS HUMAN PRODUCTS:
Tablets containing 25, 50, 100, 250, 500, 750, and 1,000 mg
Capsules containing 125, 250, 300, 400, and 500 mg
Elixir containing 10 mg/mL

NITROFURANS

INDICATIONS: Nitrofurans are synthetic compounds with antibacterial properties against gram-positive and gram-negative bacteria, although they are used primarily for their gram-negative activity. Nitrofurans have also been used as antifungal and antiprotozoal drugs. Although their exact antibacterial mechanism is not known they may inhibit an enzymatic oxidative process. A number of nitrofurans are available for clinical use, including furazolidone (Furall ★, Furazolidone Aerosol Powder ★, Topazone ♣), nitrofurantoin (Equifur ♣), nitrofurazone (Fura-Dressing ♣, Fura Ointment ♣ ★, Fura-Sweat ♣, Furacin Soluble Dressing ♣, Furacin Solution ♣, Fura Septin Soluble Dressing ★, Fura-Zone Ointment ★, Intrafur Solution ♣, Niderm Ointment ♣, Nitro Ointment ♣ NFZ ★, Nitro-Fur Solution ♣, Nitrozone Ointment ★, Nitrofurazone Ointment ♣ ★, Nitrofurazone Soluble Dressing ★, Pinkaway Powder ♣), and nitrofuraldezone. The antibacterial activities of nitrofurans are reduced in the presence of blood, pus, and milk. The toxic and chemical properties of nitrofurans have limited their widespread use as systemic anti-infective drugs. Nitrofurazone is used locally but is of little value systemically. Nitrofurantoin is rapidly and completely absorbed from the intestinal tract, and it is used as a urinary antiseptic.

Because of the carcinogenic activity of nitrofurazone in rats and mice, nitrofuran drugs, including nitrofurantoin, furaltadone, furazolidone, nitrofuraldezone, and nitrofurazone, are banned for use in food animals. The gravity of this restriction for use in food animals is similar to that of chloramphenicol.

ADVERSE AND COMMON SIDE EFFECTS: None seen with topical use.

DRUG INTERACTIONS: Concurrent use of nitrofurantoin with probenecid may raise plasma levels of nitrofurantoin to undesirable levels and impair its action as a urinary antiseptic.

SUPPLIED AS VETERINARY PRODUCTS:
Nitrofurans are available as oral and parenteral medications and in wound dressing medications. See individual product for detailed information.

NIZATIDINE

INDICATIONS: Nizatidine (Axid ♣ ★) is an H_2-receptor antagonist and acetylcholinesterase inhibitor that has been used in the horse to treat gastric ulcers. In small animals, it is used for its prokinetic effects. Effective doses for use in horses are yet to be established.

ADVERSE AND COMMON SIDE EFFECTS: Side effects are few in humans but may include somnolence and elevated liver enzymes.

DRUG INTERACTIONS: None listed.

SUPPLIED AS HUMAN PRODUCT:
Capsules containing 150 and 300 mg

NOREPINEPHRINE BITARTRATE

INDICATIONS: Norepinephrine (Levophed ♣ ★) is a potent β$_1$- and α-adrenergic receptor agonist. Its practical use in large animals is limited mainly for the treatment of hypotension due to shock.

ADVERSE AND COMMON SIDE EFFECTS AND DRUG INTERACTIONS: SEE EPINEPHRINE.

SUPPLIED AS HUMAN PRODUCT:
For injection containing 1 mg/mL

NOVOBIOCIN

INDICATIONS: Novobiocin is an antibiotic active against gram-positive cocci including staphylococci and some streptococci. Variable effectiveness has been found against *Proteus, Pseudomonas,* and *Pasteurella multocida*. It is marketed in large animals as mastitis preparations as the sole agent (Albadry ♣, Biodry ★) or in combination with penicillin G (Albacillin Suspension ★, Albadry Plus ★, Novodry Plus Suspension ♣) and with penicillin G, polymixin B, dihydrostreptomycin and hydrocortisone (Special Formula 17900-Forte ♣).

ADVERSE AND COMMON SIDE EFFECTS: There are no adverse effects listed for mastitis preparations.

DRUG INTERACTIONS: None listed.

SUPPLIED AS VETERINARY PRODUCTS:
Mastitis tubes containing 150 mg
Dry treatment tubes containing 400 mg

OMEPRAZOLE

INDICATIONS: Omeprazole (GastroGuard ★) is a proton pump-inhibitor used for the treatment of esophagitis, erosive gastritis, and gastric ulcers in horses. The drug is 5 to 10 times more potent than cimetidine in inhibiting gastric acid secretion and has a long duration of action (24 hours or more). It has cytoprotective (by enhancing mucosal cell prostaglandin production) and acid-reducing properties and decreases gastric hyperacidity. While ulcers will heal while horses are on omeprazole therapy, they tend to recur once therapy is discontinued.

ADVERSE AND COMMON SIDE EFFECTS: In humans, nausea, flatulence, vomiting, and diarrhea are reported. Headaches and dizziness have also been reported. Suppression of gastric acid secretion by omeprazole in humans leads to hypergastrinemia, which causes mucosal cell hyperplasia, rugal hypertrophy, and eventually development of carcinoids. Omeprazole is also a microsomal enzyme inhibitor (to a similar extent as cimetidine). Omeprazole is specifically formulated for horses in the GastroGuard product. Compounded products from human formulations are clinically ineffective.

DRUG INTERACTIONS: The elimination times of diazepam, phenytoin, and warfarin are increased with chronic administration of omeprazole.

SUPPLIED AS VETERINARY PRODUCTS:
Adjustable dose syringe that contains 2.28 g of omeprazole paste

OXFENDAZOLE

INDICATIONS: Oxfendazole (Benzelmin ✤ ★, Synanthic ✤ ★) is a broad-spectrum anthelmintic effective for the removal of ascarids (*Parascaris equorum),* mature and immature pinworms (*Oxyuris equi*), large strongyles including the 4th stage larvae of *Strongylus vulgaris,* and small strongyles of horses. It is effective in cattle for removal and control of lungworms, roundworms (including inhibited forms of *Ostertagia ostertagi*), and adult tapeworms.

ADVERSE AND COMMON SIDE EFFECTS: None listed.

DRUG INTERACTIONS: None listed.

SUPPLIED AS VETERINARY PRODUCTS:
Oral paste containing 4.5 g/dose syringe
Suspension containing 90.6 or 225 mg/mL

OTHER USES
Sheep
MONIEZIA
5 mg/kg; PO

OXIBENDAZOLE

INDICATIONS: Oxibendazole (Anthelcide ✤, Anthelcide EQ ★) is an equine anthelmintic effective for the removal and control of threadworms (*Strongyloides westeri),* large roundworms (*Parascaris equorum*), mature and L_4 larval stages of pinworms (*Oxyuris equi*), and large and small strongyles. Of the benzimidazole anthelmintics, oxibendazole has the most efficacy against small strongyles.

ADVERSE AND COMMON SIDE EFFECTS: The drug should not be used in debilitated horses or horses suffering from infectious disease, toxemia, or colic. Repeated dosing is not recommended in breeding stallions or pregnant mares.

DRUG INTERACTIONS: None listed.

SUPPLIED AS VETERINARY PRODUCTS:
Oral paste containing 22.7% w/w
Suspension containing 100 mg/mL

OXYMORPHONE

See OXYMORPHONE, in Description of Drugs for Small Animals.

OXYTETRACYCLINE

See TETRACYCLINES.

OXYTOCIN

INDICATIONS: Oxytocin ✤ ★ is a synthetic pituitary hormone used to stimulate uterine muscle contraction and milk letdown. Because of its action on the uterus, oxytocin is used to speed the normal process of parturition. It is also used to promote postoperative uterine contraction following Cesarean section and to control uterine hemorrhage, to aid in the replacement of the prolapsed uterus, and/or evacuation of uterine debris such as retained placenta or pyometra. Oxytocin is also used to treat associated agalactia with acute udder edema in the cow. It is also indicated for evacuation of residual milk and inflammatory secretions in mastitis but is of questionable efficacy. Oxytocin will not stimulate milk formation by the mammary glands. Oxytocin is 10 to 40 times more effective when administered IV as compared to other routes of administration.

ADVERSE AND COMMON SIDE EFFECTS: For prepartum use, the cervix should be fully relaxed. Pretreatment with estrogen before oxytocin may facilitate cervical relaxation. Large doses can produce a marked fall in arterial blood pressure, uterine spasm, and abdominal discomfort.

DRUG INTERACTIONS: Concurrent use of sympathomimetics may result in postpartum hypertension.

SUPPLIED AS VETERINARY PRODUCT:
For injection containing 20 IU/mL

PANCURONIUM

INDICATIONS: Pancuronium (Gen-Pancuronium ❦, Pancuronium Bromide Injection ★, Pavulon ❦ ★) is a synthetic nondepolarizing neuromuscular blocking agent. It can be used to facilitate mechanical ventilation during the intensive care of large-animal neonates.

ADVERSE AND COMMON SIDE EFFECTS: The drug should be used with caution in patients with compromised renal function and in those in whom tachycardia may be hazardous. Drug toxicity may be treated with mechanical support of ventilation and the use of atropine followed by neostigmine.

DRUG INTERACTIONS: Neuromuscular blockade may be potentiated by aminoglycoside antibiotics (amikacin, gentamicin, kanamycin, neomycin, streptomycin), bacitracin, halothane, isoflurane, lincomycin, magnesium sulfate, polymyxin B, and quinidine. Succinylcholine may hasten the onset of action of pancuronium and potentiate neuromuscular blockade. The action of pancuronium is antagonized by acetylcholine, anticholinesterases, and potassium ion. Theophylline may inhibit or reverse the neuromuscular blocking effect of pancuronium and precipitate arrhythmias.

SUPPLIED AS HUMAN PRODUCT:
For injection containing 1 and 2 mg/mL

PAREGORIC

INDICATIONS: Paregoric (opium tincture ★) is a camphorated tincture of opium, used to treat diarrhea in foals and calves. It also has analgesic and sedative properties. It inhibits gastrointestinal motility and intestinal secretion and may enhance intestinal absorption.

ADVERSE AND COMMON SIDE EFFECTS: Opiates should be used with caution in animals with renal insufficiency, adrenocortical insufficiency, hypothyroid disease, and in severely debilitated or geriatric patients. These drugs are contraindicated in cases of diarrhea likely caused by toxins. Cautious use of these drugs is also recommended in cases with trauma to the head or with suspected increased cerebrospinal fluid pressure and in those with significant respiratory disease or hepatic disease. Sedation, constipation, and bloat may occur from paregoric use. Ileus, pancreatitis, and CNS effects are also reported. Naloxone may be used to reverse adverse effects.

DRUG INTERACTIONS: Antihistamines, phenothiazines, barbiturates, and anesthetic agents may exacerbate CNS or respiratory depression.

SUPPLIED AS HUMAN PRODUCT:
Paregoric (opium tincture; camphorated) containing 2 mg morphine
equivalent per 5 mL

PAROMOMYCIN

INDICATIONS: Paromomycin (Humatin ♣ ★) is used for the treatment of *Giardia* and *intestinal amoeba*. Recent research has shown it
to be highly effective and nontoxic when treating calves for cryptosporidiosis. It reduces the duration and severity of diarrhea and eliminates oocyst shedding in experimentally infected neonatal calves.

ADVERSE AND COMMON SIDE EFFECTS: None listed for large
animals.

DRUG INTERACTIONS: None known for large animals.

SUPPLIED AS HUMAN PRODUCT:
Capsules containing 250 mg

PENICILLAMINE

INDICATIONS: Penicillamine (Cuprimine ♣ ★, Depen ♣ ★) is a
thiol compound that chelates cystine, lead, iron, mercury, and copper
and promotes their excretion in the urine. It is principally used in
large animals for the management of lead or mercury poisoning and
for hepatitis in ruminants associated with progressive copper accumulation. In the case of copper-associated hepatic disease, clinical
improvement may take months to years. High cost restricts its use in
large animals.

ADVERSE AND COMMON SIDE EFFECTS: Lethargy, oral lesions,
anorexia, proteinuria, and thrombocytopenia have been reported. The
drug decreases the strength of skin wound closure by its effect on collagen and should only be used after wound healing is complete.

DRUG INTERACTIONS: Phenylbutazone may potentiate hematologic
and renal toxicity of the drug. Oral iron or zinc may inhibit absorption
of the drug.

SUPPLIED AS HUMAN PRODUCTS:
Tablets containing 250 mg penicillamine
Capsules containing 125 and 250 mg penicillamine

PENICILLIN

INDICATIONS: Penicillin is a widely used antibiotic in large animal
practice. It is available as the potassium and sodium salts for IV use, the

procaine salt for IM or SC administration (Agri-Cillin ★, Depocillin ♣, Derapen SQ/LA ♣, Hi-Pencin 300 ♣, Microcillin ★, Pen G Injection ♣, Pen-Aqueous ♣ ★, Pen-G ★, Pen-G Procaine ★, Penicillin G Procaine ♣ ★, Penmed ♣, Penpro ♣, Procaine Penicillin G ♣, Propen LA ♣, Ultrapen LA ♣), the benzathine salt for long-acting use [combined with procaine penicillin] (Ambi-Pen ★, Benzapro ♣, Combicillin ★, Duplocillin LA ♣, Duo Pen ★, Dura-Pen ★, Durapen ★, Longisil ♣, PenMed ♣, Sterile Penicillin G Benzathine-Penicillin G ★, Twin-Pen ★), or for oral administration as the phenoxymethyl derivative of penicillin, penicillin V (Beepen-VK ★, Betapen-VK ★, Ledercillin VK ★, Pen-Vee K ★, V-Cillin K ★, Veetids ★). Aerobic bacteria susceptible to penicillin G include most β-hemolytic streptococci, β-lactamase–negative staphylococci, *Actinomyces species*, some *Bacillus anthracis*, *Corynebacterium* spp., and *Erysipelothrix rhusiopathiae*. Most species of anaerobes are susceptible, excluding β-lactamase–producing *Bacteroides* spp. *Penicillin G is* easily inactivated by β-lactamases and has little efficacy against organisms that can produce these enzymes.

The rate of absorption from intramuscular injections of procaine penicillin G varies depending on the injection site, with injections into the neck muscle producing more rapid absorption and higher plasma concentrations than with injections into the hindquarters. Subcutaneous injection of benzathine and/or procaine penicillin G may cause irritation and necessitate prolonged withdrawal periods in food animals. Long-acting products typically contain a 50:50 mixture of benzathine penicillin G and procaine penicillin G. Benzathine penicillin does not produce therapeutic blood concentrations and leaves detectable residues at the injection site even after the label withdrawal time. Procaine penicillin G formulations alone provide effective therapy with less risk of violative drug residues than benzathine/procaine combinations.

ADVERSE AND COMMON SIDE EFFECTS: Hypersensitivity reactions to penicillins are the most common untoward reaction and can occur with any penicillin group. Penicillin is associated with autoimmune hemolytic anemia (Type II hypersensitivity), and anaphylaxis (Type I hypersensitivity) in horses. The immune-mediated anemia usually resolves with discontinuation of penicillin therapy. Anaphylaxis usually occurs after previous exposure to penicillin and can be fatal. Intravenous epinephrine and oxygen administration and respiratory support are indicated. Although widely assumed that penicillin and cephalosporins are cross reactive in sensitive individuals, the actual incidence in humans is low. Only the potassium or sodium salt formulations should be administered IV. Veterinary formulations contain higher concentrations of procaine than human formulations and high temperatures increase the solubility of procaine. Therefore, penicillin procaine G should be kept refrigerated and administered by careful IM injection. Violent CNS reactions may occur if procaine-containing formulations are inadvertently administered IV. There is no treatment for such procaine reactions, but most animals will recover quickly unless they injure themselves. Procaine is slowly eliminated and commonly causes violative residues in racehorses and performance horses given procaine penicillin G.

DRUG INTERACTIONS: Various penicillins can inactivate aminoglycosides in vitro. Probenecid markedly decreases the tubular secretion of the penicillins.

SUPPLIED AS VETERINARY PRODUCTS:
For injection as the procaine salt containing 300,000 IU/mL
For injection as a long-acting procaine suspension containing 300 mg/mL (Canada)
For injection as the benzathine salt containing 100,000 to 150,000 IU/mL combined with the procaine salt containing 100,000 to 150,000 IU/mL (Note: For European formulations, 1,000 IU is equivalent to 1 mg penicillin.)

SUPPLIED AS HUMAN PRODUCTS:
For injection, potassium or sodium penicillin containing 1, 5, and 10 million units
Tablets of penicillin V containing 125, 250, and 500 mg
Suspension containing 125, 250, and 300 mg/5 mL

OTHER USES
Penicillin is found in numerous combination products with other antibiotics (see DIHYDROSTREPTOMYCIN/STREPTOMYCIN) in mastitis preparations and in combination with glucocorticoids or antihistamines for systemic or intramammary use.

PENTOBARBITAL

INDICATIONS: Pentobarbital (Beuthanasia-D ★, Euthansol ❧, Euthanyl ❧, Euthanyl Forte ❧, Fatal Plus ★, Nembutal Sodium ❧ ★, Pentobarbital Sodium Injection ★, Sleepaway ★, Socumb ★, Sodium Pentobarbital Injection ★, Somnotol ❧) is classified as a short-acting barbiturate that acts to depress the central nervous system. Pentobarbital is used in large animals for the treatment of convulsions, for sedation in most large animals at low doses, and as a humane method of euthanasia. Pentobarbital suppresses sensitivity of the motor endplate of skeletal muscle to acetylcholine, but does not fully relax the abdominal muscles. Ruminants, particularly sheep and goats, metabolize pentobarbital from the plasma at a high rate, which may explain the need for supplemental increments of pentobarbital in anesthesia every 15 to 30 minutes. Barbiturates are potent depressants of cerebral oxygen consumption and depress respiratory centers, particularly when given by IV injection. Most barbiturates can cross the placenta and result in depression of fetal respiration. Caesarean section performed solely with pentobarbital anesthesia results in 100% fetal mortality. Doses of barbiturates 4 times that producing respiratory arrest may be administered before cardiac arrest occurs. Pentobarbital is not suitable for use alone as a general anesthetic in large animals. Pentobarbital can be used at a low dose for standing sedation in cattle.

ADVERSE AND COMMON SIDE EFFECTS: If used alone for IV anesthesia in the horse or cow, pentobarbital may cause initial excitement. Some horses may rear and fall backward, injuring the poll. Additionally, the animal may injure itself during the prolonged period of recovery while attempting to stand. Barbiturate anesthesia in the horse should not be prolonged for longer than 1 hour, and no more than 5 g of any barbiturate should be given, even to draft breeds. Because the liver metabolizes pentobarbital, it should not be administered to animals with hepatic disease.

DRUG INTERACTIONS: Pentobarbital may induce a severe cardiodepressant effect if used with streptomycin. Use of chloramphenicol within 25 days of pentobarbital can decrease the rate of pentobarbital metabolism and predispose to overdose of the barbiturate. Duration of sleeping time with pentobarbital is prolonged with concurrent use of sulfonamides, acetylsalicylic acid, or doxycycline.

SUPPLIED AS VETERINARY PRODUCTS:
For injection containing 65 mg/mL for general anesthesia
For injection containing 200, 240, 340, 390, and 540 mg/mL for euthanasia

OTHER USES
Cattle
STANDING SEDATION
2 mg/kg IV will give moderate sedation of up to 30 minutes and mild sedation to 60 minutes after administration.

PENTOXIFYLLINE

INDICATIONS: Pentoxifylline (Trental ♣ ★, Navicon ♣) is a xanthine derivative that improves peripheral blood flow and tissue oxygenation. It also decreases blood viscosity and improves red blood cell flexibility by inhibiting phosphodiesterase. Oral bioavailability in horses is highly variable, but it is approved for use in Canada for treatment of navicular disease.

ADVERSE AND COMMON SIDE EFFECTS: Information in humans indicates that pentoxifylline should not be used in patients with marked liver or kidney impairment. It is also contraindicated in humans with peptic ulcers or intolerance to other xanthines, such as theophylline. Arrhythmias, edema, hypertension, hypotension, and abdominal discomfort are reported in humans. Additionally, occasional and transient sweating, behavioral change, conjunctival congestion, edema, pruritus, and epiphora are also reported.

DRUG INTERACTIONS: Erythromycin, cimetidine, and fluoroquinolones may decrease hepatic metabolism of pentoxifylline.

SUPPLIED AS VETERINARY PRODUCT:
Oral powder containing 2 g/28.4-g pouch

SUPPLIED AS HUMAN PRODUCT:
Tablets containing 400 mg

PERGOLIDE

INDICATIONS: Pergolide (Permax ✤ ★) is an ergot alkaloid derivative that acts as a potent dopamine receptor agonist. In the horse, adenomata of the pars intermedia of the pituitary gland causes excessive secretion of adrenocorticotropin (ACTH) or other proopiomelanocortin (POMC) peptides and causes equine Cushing's disease. Pars intermedia peptide secretion is under dopaminergic control and dopamine agonists such as pergolide palliate the clinical signs. In horses, pergolide is superior to cyproheptadine (a serotonin antagonist) in lowering plasma ACTH concentrations and controlling clinical signs.

ADVERSE AND COMMON SIDE EFFECTS: None reported in horses.

DRUG INTERACTIONS: Drugs known to affect protein binding should be used with caution due to pergolide's high binding to plasma proteins. In humans, interaction may occur with metoclopramide, phenothiazines, reserpine, and other hypotension-producing medications.

SUPPLIED AS HUMAN PRODUCT:
Tablets containing 0.05, 0.25, and 1 mg

PHENOBARBITAL

INDICATIONS: Phenobarbital (Luminal ★, Solfoton ★) is used in large animals to treat convulsions of cerebrocortical diseases, such as head trauma, neonatal maladjustment of foals, idiopathic Arabian epilepsy, lead poisoning, nervous coccidiosis, polioencephalomalacia, and others.

ADVERSE AND COMMON SIDE EFFECTS: Phenobarbital can cause liver damage, either due to drug allergy or toxic metabolism. See BARBITURATES and PHENOBARBITAL, in Descriptions of Drugs for Small Animals.

DRUG INTERACTIONS: See BARBITURATES and PHENOBARBITAL, in Descriptions of Drugs for Small Animals.

SUPPLIED AS HUMAN PRODUCTS:
For injection containing 30, 60, 65, 120, and 130 mg/mL
Tablets containing 15, 16, 30, 32, 60, 65, and 100 mg
Elixir containing 3 and 4 mg/mL

PHENOXYBENZAMINE

INDICATIONS: Phenoxybenzamine is a long-acting α-adrenergic receptor blocking agent. The drug may be of use in reducing α-adrenergic–induced arterial spasm in acute laminitis. Its α-adrenergic receptor blocking effects have also been used for treating presumed intestinal hypermotility in horses with diarrhea. However, this can also result in severe hypotension in a volume-depleted animal.

ADVERSE AND COMMON SIDE EFFECTS: In humans, hypotension, reflex tachycardia, weakness, miosis, increased intraocular pressure, nausea, and vomiting are reported. In horses, mild sedation has been reported.

DRUG INTERACTIONS: Phenoxybenzamine antagonizes the effects of α-adrenergic receptor agonists such as phenylephrine.

SUPPLIED AS HUMAN PRODUCT:
Commercial formulations are no longer available but compounded products are available from pharmacies.

OTHER USES
Horses
URINARY INCONTINENCE
0.7 mg/kg qid; PO to decrease urethral tone and aid in bladder emptying. Phenoxybenzamine should be given along with bethanechol at 0.04 to 0.08 mg/kg tid; SC.

PHENYLBUTAZONE

INDICATIONS: Phenylbutazone (Bizolin 200 ★, Butaject ★, Butasone 400 ✿, Butasone Conc ✿, Butequin ✿, Butezole ✿, Buzone Concentrate ✿, Buzone Injectable ✿, Buzone Powder ✿, Equipalazone ✿, Equi-Phar ★, Equiphen Paste ★, Phenybutazone ✿, Phenybutazone

Tablets ❧ ★, Phenylbutazone Injectable ❧, Phenylbutazone Injection ❧ ★, Phenylbutazone Powder ❧, Phenylzone Paste ★, Pro-Bute Injection ★, Pro-Bute Tablets ★, and others) is a synthetic, NSAID. NSAIDs block cyclooxygenase (COX), which blocks formation of thromboxane, prostacyclin, and the prostaglandins from arachidonic acid. This results in antipyretic action, mild analgesia, antiplatelet effects, and some anti-inflammatory effects. NSAIDs primarily are anti-inflammatory due to inhibition of prostaglandin production. Therefore, NSAIDs do not resolve inflammation, but prevent its ongoing occurrence. So while prostaglandin production will rapidly diminish, any previously present prostaglandin must be removed before inflammation will subside. NSAIDs act as analgesics by inhibiting COX and preventing the production of prostaglandins that sensitize the afferent nociceptors at peripheral sites of inflammation. However, there is increasing evidence that some NSAIDs have a central mechanism of action for analgesia and act synergistically with opioids. Phenylbutazone is particularly useful for alleviating musculoskeletal lameness in horses. The drug is also used to reduce fever from viral infection. Following oral administration, it is well absorbed, but time to peak concentration may be delayed by feeding. The drug is distributed throughout the body, with highest concentrations in the liver, heart, kidney, lungs, and plasma. Plasma protein binding in horses is greater than 99%. Phenylbutazone and its metabolite cross the placenta and are excreted in milk. Phenylbutazone is metabolized in the liver to oxyphenbutazone, an active metabolite that is eliminated slower from the body than phenylbutazone. The capacity of the liver to metabolize phenylbutazone becomes overwhelmed at relatively low drug doses. Therefore, increasing doses of phenylbutazone result in disproportionately increasing plasma concentrations, which can easily result in toxicity. These pharmacokinetics also lead to prolonged residues in tissues of food animals; so if used, consult a gFARAD center for appropriate withdrawal times for meat and milk.

ADVERSE AND COMMON SIDE EFFECTS: The adverse effects of the NSAIDs are related to cyclooxygenase inhibition in tissues where prostaglandins are beneficial and protective. Because of its prolonged elimination half-life, phenylbutazone is more toxic in horses and ruminants than the other commonly used NSAIDs such as flunixin meglumine and ketoprofen. Reduction in protective prostaglandins results in blood vessel constriction and tissue necrosis in the kidney and reduction in blood flow and protective mucous production in the gastrointestinal tract resulting in ulcers. Phenylbutazone has a higher incidence of toxicity in neonates because kidney function is not fully developed. When indicated in neonates, it should be administered at the lowest possible dose. Phenylbutazone should be administered very cautiously to dehydrated animals. Since it predominately distributes in extracellular water, plasma concentrations will be greater than normal in the dehydrated animal and more likely to cause toxicity. Signs of toxicity include anorexia, depression, oral and gastrointestinal ulcers (including the cecum and colon), protein-losing enteropathy, and death from shock. Neutropenia and severe depletion of bone marrow neutrophils also occur. Ponies may be more susceptible to phenylbutazone toxicity than horses. Renal papillary necrosis is also a consequence of toxicity, being more likely to occur in states of reduced renal blood flow such as dehydration. Although phenylbutazone therapy causes a high incidence of agranulocytosis in humans, this does not appear to be a problem in the horse. Treatment of NSAID gastrointestinal toxicity is intensive and mainly symptomatic. The hypoproteinemia that results from loss of plasma proteins into the ulcerated gastrointestinal tract can be corrected with intravenous infusions of plasma. The fluid and electrolyte losses that accompany the diarrhea are managed with commercially available intravenous fluids. Broadspectrum antibiotics are indicated when there is evidence of bacterial septicemia. Pain must be managed with opioid analgesics. Antiulcer medications may be beneficial and speed recovery. Surgical removal of damaged sections of stomach or intestine may be necessary in some cases. Recovery is usually slow and in severe cases the prognosis is always guarded. Extravascular administration of the injectable formulation results in severe tissue necrosis.

DRUG INTERACTIONS: Phenylbutazone is highly bound to plasma proteins and can displace other drugs that bind to plasma proteins, such as other anti-inflammatory drugs, sulfonamides, or anticoagulants such as warfarin, leading to increased pharmacological effect or toxicity of the displaced drug. Concurrent administration of penicillin G with phenylbutazone in horses increases plasma concentrations of penicillin G, but lowers tissue concentrations. Displacement of plasma protein-bound thyroid hormone complicates interpretation of thyroid function tests. NSAIDs reduce the prostaglandin-mediated action of furosemide and ACE-inhibitors.

SUPPLIED AS VETERINARY PRODUCTS:
For injection containing 200 mg/mL
Powder containing 1, 1.5, and 4 g phenylbutazone per 15 g powder
Tablets containing 100 and 200 mg and 1 g
Paste form (apple flavor) containing 1 g/3 mL paste, 6 g/30 g
Granules containing 1 g/pouch
Gel containing 4 g/30 g

OTHER USES
Cattle
MUSCULOSKELETAL PAIN
4.4 to 10 mg/kg; IV, PO for alleviating chronic musculoskeletal pain such as in laminitis, arthritis, or spondylitis. The long elimination half-

life of 36 to 65 hours in cattle necessitates dosing at approximately 2-day intervals. Consult a gFARAD center for withdrawal times.

PHENYLEPHRINE

INDICATIONS: Phenylephrine (AK-Dilate ♣ ★, AK-Nefrin ★, Dionephrine ♣, IsoptoFrin ★, Minums Phenylephrine ♣, Mydfrin ♣ ★, Neo-Synephrine ♣ ★, Ocu-Nephrin ★, Ocu-Phrin ★, Phenylephrine ♣ ★, Prefrin ♣ ★, Relief ★) is an α-adrenergic receptor agonist used in ophthalmic preparations to enhance pupillary dilation poorly responsive to parasympatholytic drugs. Phenylephrine has been used as a mydriatic in equine recurrent uveitis.

ADVERSE AND COMMON SIDE EFFECTS: Prolonged topical use of phenylephrine has been associated with the development of corneal ulcers.

DRUG INTERACTIONS: Phenylephrine may be ineffective if combined with a parasympatholytic agent.

SUPPLIED AS HUMAN PRODUCT:
Ophthalmic solution containing 0.12%, 2.5%, and 10% w/v

PHENYTOIN

INDICATIONS: Phenytoin or diphenylhydantoin (Dilantin ♣ ★, Diphenylan Sodium ★, Novo-Phenytoin ♣, Phenytoin Sodium Injection ♣ ★, Phenytoin Oral Suspension ★) is an anticonvulsant. Phenytoin stops the propagation and spread of neural excitation. The drug is used for management of digitalis-induced tachyarrhythmias. Phenytoin prevents the myotonia that occurs with hyperkalemic periodic paralysis of horses and is suggested for treatment of Australian Stringhalt. Absorption, distribution, and elimination of oral phenytoin in horses are highly variable, making it difficult to determine an appropriate dosage regimen.

ADVERSE AND COMMON SIDE EFFECTS: Vomiting, ataxia, tremors, depression, hypotension, and atrioventricular block are reported in the dog. Only mild tranquilization has been reported in horses.

DRUG INTERACTIONS: Antacids (aluminum, calcium, and magnesium compounds), antihistamines, cisplatin, vinblastine, bleomycin, barbiturates, calcium gluconate, carbamazepine, folic acid, oxacillin, and rifampin decrease serum levels of phenytoin. Serum levels are increased (and the potential for toxicity and loss of seizure control) by chloramphenicol, cimetidine, allopurinol, theophylline, anticoagulants, benzodiazepines, dexamethasone, estrogens, methylphenidate, nitrofurantoin, pyridoxine, phenothiazines, sulfonamides, salicylates, and phenylbutazone. Phenytoin may decrease the activity of glucocorticoids, disopyramide, doxycycline, estrogens, quinidine, dopamine, and furosemide. The analgesic properties of meperidine may be decreased and its toxicity enhanced by phenytoin. Additive hepatotoxicity may occur if phenytoin is used in conjunction with primidone or phenobarbital. Pyridoxine (vitamin B_6) may decrease serum phenytoin levels. Lidocaine and propranolol may have additive cardiac depressant effects. Valproic acid may increase or decrease serum concentrations.

SUPPLIED AS HUMAN PRODUCTS:
Capsules (extended release) containing 30 and 100 mg
Oral suspension containing 6 and 25 mg/mL
Tablets containing 50 mg
For injection containing 50 mg/mL

OTHER USES
Horses
EXERTIONAL RHABDOMYOLYSIS
Begin with 6 to 8 mg/kg; PO for 3 to 5 days and increase by 1 mg/kg increments until rhabdomyolysis is prevented. Doses should be adjusted to achieve serum levels of 5 to 10 µg/mL. Reduce the dose if the horse appears drowsy.

PILOCARPINE

INDICATIONS: Pilocarpine (Adsorbocarpine ★, Akarpine ✽ ★, Diocarpine ✽, Isopto Carpine ★, Miocarpine ✽, Ocu-Carpine ★, Pilopine HS ✽ ★, Pilocar ★, Piloptic ★, Pilostat ★) is a cholinergic agent used to treat open-angle glaucoma in humans. Although primary glaucoma in large animals is rare, secondary or acquired glaucoma may occur following periodic ophthalmia of horses or as a sequela to melanoma or squamous cell carcinoma of the eye.

ADVERSE AND COMMON SIDE EFFECTS: Frequent intraconjunctival instillation of pilocarpine can result in sufficient absorption to produce systemic effects. Tolerance may develop with prolonged use. Poisoning from pilocarpine is characterized by exaggeration of parasympathetic effects. See ORGANOPHOSPHATES in Description of Drugs for Small Animals.

DRUG INTERACTIONS: None listed.

SUPPLIED AS HUMAN PRODUCTS:
Ophthalmic solution containing 0.25%, 0.5%, 1%, 2%, 3%, 4%, 5%, and 6% w/v

Inserts releasing 20 and 40 µg/hour
Ophthalmic gel containing 4% w/w

PIPERAZINE

INDICATIONS: Piperazine (Alfalfa Pellet Horse Wormer ★, Co-op Wormer 52% ♣, Piperazine ♣ ★, Worazine 53% ♣, Wonder Wormer for Horses ★) is an old, safe dewormer for horses and swine that acts by anticholinergic action at the myoneural junction in nematodes, leading to flaccid paralysis. Worms then lose motility and ability to maintain their position in the GI tract and are swept along by intestinal peristalsis and passed alive in the feces. Mature worms are more susceptible to the action of piperazine than are lumen-dwelling larvae and immature adults. Migrating larval stages are unaffected by piperazine; therefore, treatments are repeated in 2 to 4 weeks. Piperazine's greatest activity is against ascarids in most veterinary species. In horses, it has some activity against cyanthostomes (including benzimidazole-resistant cyanthostomes) and pinworms. Piperazine is used in swine because of excellent efficacy against ascarids and nodular worms.

ADVERSE AND COMMON SIDE EFFECTS: The most common clinical signs of toxicity in decreasing order of frequency are tremors, ataxia, seizures, and weakness. For recent ingestion, activated charcoal and a saline or osmotic cathartic are recommended. The drug should not be given to animals with chronic liver or renal disease. Rapid kill of ascarids in highly parasitized foals may result in small intestinal blockage and rupture.

DRUG INTERACTIONS: Piperazine and chlorpromazine may precipitate seizure activity if used at the same time. Piperazine may exaggerate the extrapyramidal effects of phenothiazines. Pyrantel/morantel antagonize the efficacy of piperazine. The concurrent use of laxatives is not recommended because these agents may cause elimination of the drug before it has had an opportunity to work effectively.

SUPPLIED AS VETERINARY PRODUCTS:
Alfalfa pellets containing 50% w/w piperazine
Water additive dewormer containing 17 g/100 mL
Feed additive of 106 g/package
Feed or water additive containing 50% and 52.5% w/w piperazine as soluble powder

PIRLIMYCIN

INDICATIONS: Pirlimycin (Pirsue ♣ ★) is a lincosamide antibiotic approved for the treatment of gram-positive mastitis in dairy cows. Pirlimycin functions by binding to the 50s ribosomal subunit of bacterial ribonucleic acid (RNA), which interferes with protein synthesis within the bacteria. Pirlimycin has activity against staphylococcal organisms such as *Staphylococcus aureus* and *streptococcal organisms* such as *Streptococcus agalactiae, Streptococcus dysgalactiae,* and *Streptococcus uberis.*

ADVERSE AND COMMON SIDE EFFECTS: The use of any mastitis therapy with limited or strain dependent activity against the common gram-negative environmental bacteria (*E. coli, Klebsiella* spp.) may be associated with infections caused by these organisms if proper infusion techniques are not followed. Thus, proper aseptic teat preparation prior to use of an intramammary infusion product and proper aseptic infusion techniques are highly recommended to reduce the risk of postinfusion infection with environmental bacteria because of teat end contamination.

DRUG INTERACTIONS: None listed.

SUPPLIED AS VETERINARY PRODUCT:
Disposable 10 mL intramammary syringes containing 5 mg/mL of pirlimycin

POLOXALENE

INDICATIONS: Poloxalene (Bloat Guard ★, Sweet Lix Bloat Guard Block medicated ★, Therabloat Drench Concentrate ★) is used in the prevention of bloat in ruminants due to legume feeding. It can be top dressed for feed or mixed in the feed. Under severe bloat-producing conditions, the dose can be doubled.

ADVERSE AND COMMON SIDE EFFECTS: The expiration date should be strictly observed. If poloxalene is subjected to high environmental temperatures (>37°C, or 98.6°F) for longer than 6 months, spontaneous combustion can occur.

DRUG INTERACTIONS: None listed.

SUPPLIED AS VETERINARY PRODUCTS:
Block containing 6.6% w/w poloxalene
Multiwall bags containing 530 g poloxalene/kg
Oral concentrate containing 25 g/fluid ounce (833 mg/mL)
Liquid containing 99.5% w/w poloxalene

POLYMYXIN B

INDICATIONS: Polymyxin B (Aerosporin ❀ ★) is used in the treatment of gram-negative infections, especially those caused by *Pseudo-*

monas, Pasteurella, Klebsiella, Salmonella, Bordetella, and *Shigella* organisms. *Proteus* and *Brucella* organisms are frequently resistant. Due to systemic toxicity, polymyxin B is only used topically, so it is not typically included on susceptibility reports from microbiology services; however, in a recent study, 100% of *Pseudomonas aeruginosa* veterinary isolates were susceptible to polymyxin B. Polymyxin B also binds and inactivates endotoxin, reducing inflammation and tissue destruction. The drug is frequently used as a topical preparation in combination with other antimicrobials for treating localized infections of the ears or eyes (BNP ♣, Mycitracin ★, Neobacimyx ★, TriOptic-P ★, Vetropolycin ♣ ★) or for instillation in mastitis (Special Formula 17900 ♣). It is being investigated as a lipid-encapsulated formulation for treatment of endotoxemia in horses. There is a human bladder irrigation solution available that also contains neomycin (Neosporin Irrigating Solution ♣ ★) that is used to prevent gram-negative infections from indwelling urinary catheters.

ADVERSE AND COMMON SIDE EFFECTS: Pain at the site of injection, nephrotoxicity, central nervous system signs, and neuromuscular blockade have been reported with systemic use. Contact hypersensitivity and urticaria can occur at the site of contact with neomycin and polymyxin B.

DRUG INTERACTIONS: Aminoglycoside antibiotics, bacitracin, and quinidine intensify the nephrotoxic and neurotoxic potential of polymyxin B. Succinylcholine and anesthetics may prolong the neuromuscular blockade and precipitate respiratory paralysis associated with the use of polymyxin B.

SUPPLIED AS HUMAN PRODUCT:
For injection containing 500,000 U/20 mL vial, equivalent to 50 mg polymyxin
Irrigating solution containing 40 mg of neomycin and 200,000 U/mL of polymyxin

SUPPLIED AS VETERINARY PRODUCTS:
Combined in various ophthalmic and otic preparations

POLYSULFATED GLYCOSAMINOGLYCAN (PSGAG)

INDICATIONS: Polysulfated glycosaminoglycan (Adequan I.A. ♣ ★, Adequan I.M. ♣ ★) is a potent proteolytic enzyme inhibitor that diminishes or reverses the processes that result in the loss of cartilaginous mucopolysaccharides. It is recommended for the treatment of noninfectious degenerative and/or traumatic joint dysfunction and associated lameness in the horse. PSGAG improves joint function by stimulating synovial membrane activity, reducing synovial protein levels, and increasing synovial fluid viscosity. Parenteral administration (IM) has been effective for reducing joint inflammation attributable to degenerative joint disease and has the added advantage of minimizing the risk of joint sepsis or postinjection inflammation associated with intra-articular administration.

ADVERSE AND COMMON SIDE EFFECTS: Postinjection joint inflammation may result from hypersensitivity to PSGAG, traumatic injection technique, increased dose or frequency of administration, or combination with other drugs. Joint sepsis is a rare complication of intra-articular injection, but is difficult to distinguish from the nonseptic inflammatory reaction.

DRUG INTERACTIONS: PSGAG should not be mixed with other drugs. Concomitant use with steroids or NSAIDs may mask signs of joint sepsis.

SUPPLIED AS VETERINARY PRODUCT:
For injection containing 100 and 250 mg/mL

PONAZURIL

INDICATIONS: Ponazuril (Marquis ★) is a triazine antiprotozoal used for the treatment of equine protozoal encephalomyelitis (EPM) caused by *Sarcocystis neurona* in horses. Prior to treatment, EPM should be distinguished from other diseases that may cause ataxia in horses. Clearance of the parasite by ponazuril may not completely resolve the clinical signs attributed to the natural progression of EPM. The prognosis for animals treated for EPM depends upon the severity of disease and the duration of the infection prior to treatment.

ADVERSE AND COMMON SIDE EFFECTS: The safe use of ponazuril in horses used for breeding purposes, during pregnancy, or in lactating mares has not been evaluated. In field trials, some horses developed oral blisters and skin reactions. Loose feces were seen in horses given higher than label doses.

DRUG INTERACTIONS: The safety of ponazuril with concomitant therapies in horses has not been evaluated.

SUPPLIED AS VETERINARY PRODUCT:
Oral paste syringes containing 150 mg of ponazuril

POTASSIUM CHLORIDE

INDICATIONS: Potassium chloride ♣ ★ (Potassiject ★) is used for the treatment of digitalis toxicity and for the treatment of hypokalemia commonly associated with diarrhea, electrolyte depletion with exhausted horse syndrome, or metabolic alkalosis as may occur with abomasal disease in cattle. It is also available in mixed electrolyte solutions with dextrose for the treatment of milk fever, grass tetany, and secondary ketosis in cattle.

ADVERSE AND COMMON SIDE EFFECTS: If administered IV, potassium chloride should not exceed 0.5 mEq/kg per hour or 2 mEq/kg per day. Oral administration is the preferred route of supplementation. Potassium chloride has an unpleasant taste; therefore, gastric intubation for administration may be indicated. Excessively rapid administration can result in fatal cardiac arrhythmias. Electrocardiographic monitoring is advised if IV administration at rates above the guidelines indicated are deemed necessary. Signs of cardiotoxicity include prolongation of the QRS and PR intervals, loss of P waves, peaked T waves, and bradycardia.

DRUG INTERACTIONS: The concurrent use of penicillin G potassium with potassium chloride may cause severe hyperkalemia.

SUPPLIED AS VETERINARY PRODUCT:
For injection containing 2 mEq/mL

SUPPLIED AS HUMAN PRODUCTS:
For injection containing 2 mEq/mL in 10-mL (20 mEq) and 20-mL (40 mEq) vials
For injection containing 10, 20, 30, 40, 60, and 90 mEq

PRALIDOXIME

INDICATIONS: Pralidoxime [pyridine-2-aldoxime-methiodide] (Protopam Chloride ♣ ★), or PAM, is part of a group of compounds known as oximes. It is a reactivator of cholinesterase and is used as an antidote for organophosphate poisoning. PAM significantly reverses the combination of organophosphate with cholinesterase. Delay of treatment may be less effective as the phosphorylated enzyme complex of organophosphate to cholinesterase becomes resistant to reactivation by oximes. Atropine should be administered first to block muscarinic receptor sites.

ADVERSE AND COMMON SIDE EFFECTS: High doses of pralidoxime can cause neuromuscular blockade and inhibition of acetylcholinesterase. Rapid IV injection may cause tachycardia and weakness.

DRUG INTERACTIONS: Oximes should not be used in carbamate toxicity because they are ineffective in antagonizing carbamate cholinesterase inhibitors, and because they have weak anticholinesterase properties, may act synergistically with carbamates.

SUPPLIED AS HUMAN PRODUCT:
Cake to be diluted for injection containing 1 g

PREDNISONE, PREDNISOLONE

INDICATIONS: Prednisone (Predsone-5 ✿) and Prednisolone (Prednisolone Sodium Succinate ✿ ★, Solu-Delta-Cortef ✿ ★, Uni-Pred 50 ✿) are intermediate-acting glucocorticoid agents. Prednisone is readily metabolized by the liver to prednisolone in most species, but not the horse. After oral administration of prednisone to horses, only negligible amounts of prednisone can be detected in plasma and prednisolone is undetectable. In contrast, oral prednisolone has a high oral bioavailability in horses and should be used preferentially for treatment. Prednisolone is indicated for the treatment of inflammatory conditions of the skin and joints and for supportive care during periods of stress. Prednisolone sodium succinate is also beneficial for the treatment of acute hypersensitivity reactions, atopic and contact dermatitis, summer eczema, and conjunctivitis. This drug is also used in animals with severe overwhelming infections (in combination with appropriate antibiotic therapy) and for the prevention and treatment of adrenal insufficiency and shock (in conjunction with fluid support).

ADVERSE AND COMMON SIDE EFFECTS AND DRUG INTERACTIONS: See GLUCOCORTICOID AGENTS.

SUPPLIED AS VETERINARY PRODUCTS:
Prednisolone
For injection containing 20 mg/mL prednisolone sodium phosphate
For injection containing 10 and 50 mg/mL prednisolone acetate
Tablets containing 5 mg prednisolone
For injection containing 10 and 50 mg/mL prednisolone sodium succinate

Prednisone
Tablets containing 5 mg prednisone

SUPPLIED AS HUMAN PRODUCTS:
Oral solution containing 5 and 15 mg/5 mL prednisolone
Oral solution containing 1 and 5 mg/mL prednisone
Tablets containing 1, 2.5, 5, 10, 20, 25, and 50 mg prednisone
For injection containing 25 and 50 mg/mL prednisolone acetate, 20 mg/mL prednisolone phosphate

PREGNANT MARE'S SERUM GONADOTROPIN (PMSG)

INDICATIONS: Pregnant mare's serum gonadotropin [PMSG] (Folligon ✿) is a complex glycoprotein produced by the endometrial cups of the pregnant mare's uterus. PMSG has high follicle-stimulating hormone (FSH) properties and luteinizing hormone (LH) actions. Due to its FSH activity, it stimulates growth of the interstitial cells of the ovaries as well as growth and maturation of the follicles; hence it is used to induce superovulation for embryo transfer in cows. In the mare, PMSG administration may produce out-of-season estrus (fall and late winter) followed by ovulation if a follicle is palpable on the ovary at the time of injection.

ADVERSE AND COMMON SIDE EFFECTS: Anaphylaxis can occur after administration of PMSG. Repeated administration may decrease efficacy due to the production of antihormone antibodies.

DRUG INTERACTIONS: None listed.

SUPPLIED AS VETERINARY PRODUCT:
For injection containing 5,000 U/25 mL

OTHER USES
Sheep and Goats
OVULATION INDUCTION
The LH activity of PMSG (400 to 700 IU; IM) will induce ovulation and thus is used along with intravaginal progestagens for out-of-season breeding or estrus synchronization in sheep and goats.

PROGESTERONE

INDICATIONS: Progesterone ✤ ★ is a gonadal hormone from the corpus luteum that favors the maintenance of pregnancy. Other actions include induction of mammary tissue growth and secretory changes to the endometrium, which only occur after suitable priming of the target tissue by estrogen. Progesterone inhibits the action of follicle-stimulating hormone (FSH), preventing the development of follicles and blocking ovulation. A number of commercially available drugs have progesterone activity (Centra Progestin ✤, Progesterone ✤, CIDR ✤) or similar-acting progestagens [altrenogest] (Regu-Mate ✤ ★), [medroxyprogesterone acetate] (Veramix Sponges ✤), [melengestrol acetate] (MGA Premix ✤ ★), [megestrol acetate] (Ovaban Tablets ✤ ★, Ovarid Tablets ✤). Progesterone is used to treat habitual or threatened abortion and has been used empirically to prevent embryonic death in horses and cattle. Other suggested uses are nymphomania and mammary underdevelopment. As nymphomania is likely due to the presence of cystic ovaries, progesterone is not indicated in such cases. Possibly the most widespread and effective use of progesterone or similar acting compounds has been to control estrus cycles. Progesterone will suppress estrus in large animals and subsequent withdrawal yields a predictable occurrence of estrus. Specific progestagen products, such as intravaginal sponges for sheep (Veramix Sponges ♣), intravaginal devices for cattle (CIDR ♣), implants for cattle (Synchro-Mate ★), and oral solution for horses (ReguMate ♣ ★), assist in timed induction of estrus. Suppression of estrus will also facilitate regular cycles following winter anestrus in mares and facilitate scheduled breeding and help manage mares exhibiting prolonged estrus. Ovulation will occur 5 to 7 days after the onset of estrus. The progestin melengestrol acetate (MGA Premix ♣ ★) has been used as a feed additive to suppress heat in feedlot heifers and for stimulation of growth and improved feed utilization.

ADVERSE AND COMMON SIDE EFFECTS: Progesterones favor closure of the cervix, preventing infections of the uterus draining. Overdosage of progesterone can cause cystic ovaries in cattle. The drug should not be used in lactating dairy cattle.

DRUG INTERACTIONS: None listed.

SUPPLIED AS VETERINARY PRODUCTS:
Medroxyprogesterone-impregnated   intravaginal   polyurethane sponges containing 60 mg/sponge
Intravaginal device containing 1.9 g progesterone (Canada)
Feed additive containing 17.6, 220, 440, and 1,100 mg/kg melengestrol acetate
Tablets containing 5 and 20 mg megestrol acetate
Injection containing 50 mg/mL
Solution containing 2.2 mg/mL altrenogest
Gel containing 2.15 mg/g altrenogest

OTHER USES
Cattle
GROWTH PROMOTION
Progesterone is a component of growth implants combined with estradiol benzoate (Steer-Oid ♣ ★, Synovex-C ♣ ★, Synovex-S ♣ ★).

INDUCE LACTATION
Progesterone can be administered to open heifers or cows to induce lactation at 0.125 mg/kg bid; SC, in combination with estrogen (17β-estradiol) at 0.05 mg/kg bid; SC, for 7 days.

PROCAINAMIDE

See PROCAINAMIDE, in Description of Drugs for Small Animals.

PROPANTHELINE

INDICATIONS: Propantheline bromide (Pro-Banthine ♣ ★) is an anticholinergic agent. It is used in horses to decrease intestinal spasm to facilitate rectal examination. At this time no commercial product is available for parenteral use, but it may be compounded by a pharmacist.

ADVERSE AND COMMON SIDE EFFECTS: Tachycardia, weakness, nausea, constipation, pupillary dilation, and dryness of the mucous membranes may occur. Signs of drug overdose include urinary retention, excitement, hypotension, respiratory failure, paralysis, and coma.

DRUG INTERACTIONS: Antihistamines, procainamide, quinidine, meperidine, benzodiazepines, and the phenothiazines may enhance the activity of propantheline and primidone, and long-term glucocorticoid use may potentiate the adverse effects of the drug. Propantheline may enhance the activity of nitrofurantoin, thiazide diuretics, and sympathomimetic drugs. Propantheline delays the gastrointestinal absorption of, but increases serum levels of, ranitidine and it may decrease the gastrointestinal absorption of cimetidine.

SUPPLIED AS HUMAN PRODUCT:
Tablets containing 7.5 and 15 mg

PROPARACAINE

INDICATIONS: Proparacaine (AK-Taine ★, Alcaine ❧ ★, Diocaine ❧, Kainair ★, Ocu-Caine ★, Ophthetic ❧ ★, Ophthaine ★, Spectro-Caine ★) is a local anesthetic used for desensitization of the cornea and conjunctiva. Unlike some topical anesthetics, proparacaine produces little or no initial irritation.

ADVERSE AND COMMON SIDE EFFECTS: Proparacaine is generally safe for patients with hypersensitivities to other local anesthetics. However, in humans there are rare occurrences of immediate hyperallergic corneal reactions with development of diffuse epithelial keratitis.

DRUG INTERACTIONS: None listed.

SUPPLIED AS HUMAN PRODUCT:
Ophthalmic solution containing 0.5% w/v

PROPIONIBACTERIUM ACNES

INDICATIONS: *Propionibacterium acnes* (EqStim ❧ ★) is a nonspecific immunostimulant used as adjuvant therapy for respiratory disease in horses. It activates macrophages, induces lymphokine production, increases natural killer cell activity, and enhances cell-mediated immunity.

ADVERSE AND COMMON SIDE EFFECTS: Fever, tremors, anorexia, and lethargy may occur a few hours after injection. Anaphylactic reactions may occur after administration.

DRUG INTERACTIONS: Do not use in conjunction with glucocorticoids or other immune suppressors. Steroid therapy should be withdrawn at least 7 days before initiating this therapy.

PROPOFOL

INDICATIONS: Propofol (Diprivan ♣ ★, Propoflo ★, Rapinovet ♣ ★) is a hypnotic agent given IV to induce and maintain anesthesia. The drug is rapidly metabolized by the liver, which results in rapid recovery from anesthesia. It has been used satisfactorily in foals premedicated with xylazine to induce anesthesia for restraint during magnetic resonance imaging. Some respiratory depression does occur during the anesthesia.

ADVERSE AND COMMON SIDE EFFECTS: See PROPOFOL in Description of Drugs for Small Animals.

DRUG INTERACTIONS: See PROPOFOL in description of Drugs for Small Animals.

SUPPLIED AS VETERINARY PRODUCT:
For injection containing 10 mg/mL

SUPPLIED AS HUMAN PRODUCT:
For injection containing 10 mg/mL

PROPRANOLOL

INDICATIONS: Propranolol (Inderal ♣ ★ and generics) is a nonselective β_1- and β_2-adrenergic receptor blocking agent. Its use in large animals is restricted to the management of tachycardia in the horse.

ADVERSE AND COMMON SIDE EFFECTS: Propranolol is contraindicated in patients with congestive heart failure unless it is secondary to a tachyarrhythmia responsive to β-blockade. The drug is also contraindicated in those patients with second- or third-degree heart block and sinus bradycardia and with bronchoconstrictive lung disease, for example, horses with recurrent airway obstruction. Adverse effects including bradycardia, central nervous system effects, gastrointestinal effects, and dermatologic and hematologic effects are common in humans.

DRUG INTERACTIONS: Antacids delay GI absorption of propranolol. Antiarrhythmic effects of quinidine, procainamide, and lidocaine are enhanced by propranolol, but toxic effects may be additive. Serum levels of propranolol are increased by cimetidine. The hypotensive effects of propranolol are enhanced by chlorpromazine, cimetidine, furosemide, phenothiazines, and hydralazine. Propranolol increases the serum levels of lidocaine. It also increases the effects of tubocurarine and succinylcholine. The action of terbutaline, epinephrine, and phenylpropanolamine may be antagonized by propranolol. Concurrent use of digitalis may potentiate bradycardia. Concurrent use of salicylates may inhibit the antihypertensive effects of propranolol. The effect of propranolol may be decreased by the concurrent use of thyroid hormone supplementation, and the dose of propranolol may need to be decreased in animals receiving methimazole. The bronchodilatory effects of theophylline may be antagonized by propranolol.

SUPPLIED AS HUMAN PRODUCTS:
Tablets containing 10, 20, 40, 60, 80, 90, and 120 mg
Tablets (extended release) containing 60, 80, 120, and 160 mg
For injection containing 1 mg/mL
Solution containing 4, 8, and 80 mg/mL

PROPYLENE GLYCOL

INDICATIONS: Propylene glycol is used alone (Propylene Glycol ✽ ★) or combined with other medications (Domcol Solution ✽, Ketoban Oral Solution and Gel ★, Keto Plus Gel ★, PCE Glycol ✽, Co-op Ketox ✽, Co-op Ketox Liquid Plus ✽, Glycol-P ✽, Ketopar ✽ Ketoroid ✽) for the treatment and prevention of ketosis (acetonemia) in cows and sheep (pregnancy toxemia). Given orally, propylene glycol is a glucose precursor in ruminants. The drug is also administered to ruminants in combination with other medications (Bloat-Pac7 ★, Veterinary Surfactant ★) for the management of pasture bloat.

ADVERSE AND COMMON SIDE EFFECTS: Overuse may have a deleterious effect on rumen flora, decrease rumen motility, and cause diarrhea.

DRUG INTERACTIONS: None listed.

SUPPLIED AS VETERINARY PRODUCTS:
Liquid as propylene glycol 100%
Propylene glycol in combination with other products such as cobalt, choline chloride ethylenediamine dihydroiodide, and potassium iodide for ketosis therapy (Canada), or with dioctyl sodium succinate for treatment of bloat (United States).

OTHER USES

Horses

MUCOLYTIC

Propylene glycol can be used in horses as a mucolytic for disrupting respiratory mucus. This requires use of a nebulizer and can cause airway irritation and bronchoconstriction. Propylene glycol is also used as a base for many products. See DIOCTYL SODIUM SULFOSUCCINATE.

PROSTAGLANDIN F$_{2\alpha}$

INDICATIONS: Prostaglandin F$_{2\alpha}$ (PGF$_{2\alpha}$) is available as a number of natural (dinoprost tromethamine; Lutalyse ✤ ★) or synthetic compounds such as cloprostenol (Estrumate ✤ ★, Planate ✤), fluprostenol (Equimate ★), and fenprostalene (Synchrocept B ✤, Bovilene ★). Prostaglandin F$_{2\alpha}$ administration causes functional and morphologic regression of the corpus luteum if it is at least 4 or 5 days old. Estrus usually follows 2 to 5 days after treatment, followed by ovulation and normal fertility. PGF$_{2\alpha}$ is used to manipulate the estrus cycle for planned breeding, to aid in evacuation of pyometra, and in cattle to induce abortion. It is also used in goats to treat hydrometra (pseudopregnancy). Due to the seasonal polyestrous nature of the mare, the efficacy of PGF$_{2\alpha}$ in the mare may vary with the time of year it is administered.

ADVERSE AND COMMON SIDE EFFECTS: Specific products are available for horses and for cattle. PGF$_{2\alpha}$ should not be given to cows that may be pregnant unless to induce abortion. Data show that 95% of cows up to 4½ months into pregnancy will abort, as will some cattle in later gestation when treated with PGF$_{2\alpha}$. Because PGF$_{2\alpha}$ can be absorbed through the skin, care should be taken in handling the product, particularly for women of childbearing age and asthmatics. Some products used in mares may cause sweating, increased heart rate, and abdominal discomfort. These signs abate within 30 minutes to 1 hour. A low incidence of clostridial infection at the site of injection has been reported following prostaglandin administration. Only cattle with functional corpus luteum can be expected to respond to cloprostenol.

DRUG INTERACTIONS: None listed.

SUPPLIED AS VETERINARY PRODUCTS:

For injection containing 5 mg/mL prostaglandin F$_{2\alpha}$ (dinoprost tromethamine) [Lutalyse ✤ ★]

For injection containing 88 mg cloprostenol/mL [Planate ✤, for swine] and 250 mg/mL cloprostenol [Estrumate ✤ ★]

For injection containing 50 mg/mL fluprostenol [Equimate ★]

For injection containing 0.5 mg/mL fenprostalene [Synchrocept B ✹, Bovilene ★]

PROTAMINE SULFATE

INDICATIONS: Protamine sulfate ✹ ★ is a low-molecular-weight protein that antagonizes the anticoagulant effects of heparin. It is used to reverse severe bleeding associated with excessive anticoagulation caused by heparin. It may also be used to treat braken fern toxicity in cattle.

ADVERSE AND COMMON SIDE EFFECTS: It must be given only by the IV route and administered slowly. Rapid administration may cause dyspnea, bradycardia, and hypotension, possibly from the release of endogenous histamine. Hypersensitivity reactions may also occur after administration of protamine sulfate. These effects are minimized if the drug is injected slowly over a 3- to 10-minute period. A rebound effect leading to prolonged bleeding may occur several hours after heparin has apparently been neutralized. The cause may be due to release of heparin from the heparin–protamine complex or release of additional heparin from extravascular spaces. Protamine sulfate given in the absence of heparin has its own anticoagulant activity.

DRUG INTERACTIONS: None reported.

SUPPLIED AS HUMAN PRODUCT:
For injection containing 10 mg/mL

OTHER USES
Cattle

BRACKEN FERN TOXICITY
For bracken fern (*Pteridium* sp.) poisoning, administer protamine (100 mg) IV in combination with whole blood (2.25 to 4.5 L).

PSYLLIUM MUCILLOID

INDICATIONS: Psyllium mucilloid (Equine Psyllium ★, Equi-Phar Sweet Psyllium ★, Sandex Crumbles ★, Vetasyl ✹ ★, Metamucil ✹ ★, Novo-Mucilax ✹, and others) is a hydrophilic substance that forms a gelatinous mass when mixed with water. It is used for the treatment of sand impaction colic in horses. The gel lubricates and binds the sand, moving it distally, clearing the impaction. After initial doses are mixed with water, the mucilloid can be mixed with sweet feed.

ADVERSE AND COMMON SIDE EFFECTS: Once in contact with water, the mucilloid quickly forms a gel and becomes difficult to pump through a nasogastric tube. Side effects are minimal. Temporary cramping, flatulence, and bloating may occur. It should, however, not be used in patients with abdominal pain, vomiting, nausea, or fecal impaction.

DRUG INTERACTIONS: None established.

SUPPLIED AS VETERINARY PRODUCTS:
Capsules containing 250, 400, and 495 mg
Powder containing 2 or 3.75 oz/scoop (100%)

SUPPLIED AS HUMAN PRODUCT:
Powder containing 3, 3.4, or 6 g/rounded teaspoonful

PYRANTEL

INDICATIONS: Pyrantel [pyrantel pamoate] (AmTech Anthelban V ★, Equi-Phar ProTal ★, Nemex Tabs ★, Nemex-2 ★, Pyran ✤, Pyr-A-Pam ✤, Rotectin 2 ★, Strongid-P Paste ✤ ★, Strongid-T ✤ ★, Sure Shot Liquid Wormer ★), [pyrantel tartrate] (Banminth Premix ✤, Banminth For Horses & Colts ★, Continuex ★, P Equi-Phar Colt and Horse Wormer ★, Strongid-C ✤ ★) is an anthelmintic effective against the adult forms of the large and small strongyles and ascarids of horses. It is also an effective broad-spectrum anthelmintic for swine and ruminants, including the adult forms of *Haemonchus contortus* in sheep and goats. Pyrantel is a cholinesterase inhibitor and has a wide margin of safety. The tartrate salt is generally administered dry in the feed rather than in solution to minimize absorption of this highly soluble form.

ADVERSE AND COMMON SIDE EFFECTS: Cautious use of the drug is advised in patients with liver dysfunction, malnutrition, dehydration, or anemia.

DRUG INTERACTIONS: Because of its cholinergic properties, it has been suggested that pyrantel should not be used concurrently with levamisole, organophosphates, or diethylcarbamazine. However, there appears to be no clinical evidence to substantiate this and labeling for pyrantel products indicates safety for simultaneous use with insecticides, tranquilizers, muscle relaxants, and central nervous system depressants. Piperazine and pyrantel have antagonistic actions and should not be used together.

SUPPLIED AS VETERINARY PRODUCTS:
Paste containing 3.58 g/premeasured syringe
Liquid containing 2.27, 4.54, and 50 mg/mL
Tablets containing 22.7, 35, 113.5, and 125 mg
Granules containing 10.6 g/kg
Premix containing 10.8% w/w (swine) and 1.25% w/w (equine)

OTHER USES
Horses

TAPEWORMS
13.2 mg/kg; PO

PYRIMETHAMINE

INDICATIONS: Pyrimethamine (Daraprim ♣ ★, Quinnoxine-S ♣) is used in combination with the sulfonamides, such as sulfadiazine, in the treatment of equine protozoal encephalomyelitis (EPM). Pyrimethamine inhibits folic acid metabolism in the parasite and appears to increase the activity of the sulfonamide against the sporozoan parasite.

ADVERSE AND COMMON SIDE EFFECTS: Problems are rare at the recommended dose, but depression, anorexia, vomiting, and reversible bone marrow suppression (anemia, leukopenia, and thrombocytopenia) may occur within 4 to 6 days of initiation of therapy with the pyrimethamine–sulfonamide combination. The nonregenerative anemias seen in response to long-term administration of potentiated sulfonamides are believed to be related to folate reduction. Supplementation with oral folic acid is often recommended for horses on long-term potentiated sulfonamide therapy. The administration of oral folic acid to pregnant mares being treated for EPM may not protect the fetus from the effects of folate deficiency. Mares have delivered foals with congenital defects after oral administration of potentiated sulfonamides while supplemented with oral folic acid and vitamin E. The risk of congenital defects should be considered when treating pregnant mares with pyrimethamine and sulfonamides.

DRUG INTERACTIONS: Pyrimethamine is synergistic in antimicrobial activity with sulfonamides. Concurrent therapy with trimethoprim and pyrimethamine does not increase the efficacy against protozoa, and is suspected to increase the incidence of side effects due to folate reduction. Pyrimethamine is highly bound to plasma protein and may displace other drugs, such as phenylbutazone or warfarin, thereby increasing their free blood concentrations.

SUPPLIED AS VETERINARY PRODUCT:
Water additive for poultry containing 9.8 g/L, combined with sulfaquinoxaline 32.5 g/L [Quinnoxine-S ♣]

SUPPLIED AS HUMAN PRODUCT:
Tablets containing 25 mg

QUINIDINE

INDICATIONS: Quinidine bisulfate (Biquin ♣ ★), quinidine gluconate (Quinaglute ★, Quinate ♣), quinidine polygalacturonate (Cardioquin ✤ ★) and quinidine sulfate (Apo-Quinidine ✤, Quinidex ✤ ★, Quinora ★) is used in the management of atrial fibrillation in horses and cattle. The IV route has recently been advocated as a more rapid mode of treatment in horses, using the gluconate form, but is considerably more expensive and less likely to be effective in long-standing atrial fibrillation. Although quinidine is also useful in treating atrial fibrillation in cattle, they will usually convert to normal sinus rhythm without treatment once the initiating disease (e.g., gastrointestinal problems) is resolved.

ADVERSE AND COMMON SIDE EFFECTS: The drug is contraindicated in patients with myasthenia gravis, digitalis intoxication, heart block, and escape beats. Anorexia, nasal edema, diarrhea, vagolytic response, urine retention, weakness, hypotension, laminitis, and decreased cardiac contractility are reported. Sinus node suppression, ventricular tachycardia, atrioventricular block, and prolongation of the PR, QRS, and QT intervals are also reported. A paradoxical acceleration in ventricular rate may occur, especially when the drug is used to treat patients with atrial flutter or fibrillation. In these cases it is often used after patients have first been given a digitalis glycoside. Quinidine intoxication can be antagonized by rapid alkalinization of the blood with sodium bicarbonate. Drug dose should be decreased in cases with liver disease, congestive heart failure, hyperkalemia, or hypoalbuminemia.

DRUG INTERACTIONS: Quinidine increases serum digoxin levels. Cimetidine increases serum quinidine levels. Phenothiazines potentiate the cardiac depressive effects of quinidine. Quinidine potentiates the neuromuscular blocking effects of curariform and depolarizing blocking agents as well as those induced by neomycin and kanamycin. Anticholinergic drugs have additive vagolytic effects. Phenobarbital and phenytoin decrease the half-life of quinidine, necessitating readjustment of drug dose. Sodium bicarbonate, antacids, and thiazide diuretics prolong the half-life of quinidine, predisposing to toxicity. Quinidine may enhance the hypotensive effects of β-adrenergic receptor blocking agents and vasodilators.

SUPPLIED AS HUMAN PRODUCTS:
Tablets containing 200 and 300 mg quinidine sulfate
Tablets containing 275 mg quinidine polygalacturonate (200 mg quinidine sulfate)
Tablets (sustained release) containing 300 mg quinidine sulfate
Tablets containing 250 mg quinidine bisulfate (200 mg quinidine sulfate)
For injection containing 190 mg/mL quinidine sulfate
Tablets containing 325 mg quinidine gluconate
Tablets (sustained release) containing 324 mg quinidine gluconate
For injection containing 80 mg/mL quinidine gluconate

Guidelines for Conversion of Atrial Fibrillation (AF) in Horses:

For horses with recent onset (<7 days) of AF or if AF develops during anesthesia:

1.1 to 2.2 mg/kg IV every 10 minutes to a total dose of 8.8 to 11 mg/kg or conversion occurs

For horses with chronic AF:

22 mg/kg administered via NG tube every 2 hours to a total dose of 88 to 132 mg/kg or conversion occurs. If neither conversion nor toxicity occurs, continue this dose every 6 hours for up to 4 days.

Discontinue therapy if QRS duration exceeds 125% of pretreatment values, rapid supraventricular tachycardias (>100 beats/minute) or ventricular arrhythmias develop.

RANITIDINE

INDICATIONS: Ranitidine (Alti-Ranitidine HCl ✹, Apo-Ranitidine ✹, Novo-Ranitidine ✹, Nu-Ranit ✹, Zantac-C ✹, Zantac ✹ ★) is an H_2-receptor antagonist that reduces gastric acid secretion in a dose-dependent competitive manner by blocking histamine-induced gastric acid secretion. The H_2 blockers (see also CIMETIDINE) are highly selective in action and virtually without effect on H_1 receptors. Although the H_2 receptors are widely distributed throughout the body, the extragastric receptors appear to be of only minor physiologic importance. The H_2 blockers also inhibit, at least partially, gastric secretion elicited by muscarinic agonists and gastrin. Ranitidine is used in horses to treat gastric ulcers and as a preventive measure for animals considered at risk for the development of gastric ulcers, such as sick neonatal foals. Unlike cimetidine, ranitidine increases the passage of ingesta through the gut by stimulating gastric, small intestinal and colonic motility, and it may stimulate pancreatic exocrine secretion. It is more potent than cimeditine and only minimally (10%) inhibits hepatic metabolism of some drugs. Ranitidine lacks the antiandrogenic activity that may occur with cimetidine and can be usually substituted for cimetidine.

Ranitidine has been shown experimentally to increase abomasal pH in sheep. The IV route caused a greater increase and for a longer period of time than oral dosing. Peak increase in abomasal pH with IV dosing occurred at 4 to 6 hours, with pH remaining above baseline for 24 to 36 hours. From this information it may be possible to use this drug in the treatment of abomasal ulceration in ruminants on a once-daily dosage regimen.

ADVERSE AND COMMON SIDE EFFECTS: Adverse reactions are low in incidence and relatively minor, and include skin rash, diarrhea, constipation, and loss of libido. Rapid IV injection may cause profound bradycardia. Lower than recommended doses will alleviate clinical signs of gastric ulceration, but significant ulceration may continue unabated.

DRUG INTERACTIONS: Ranitidine has fewer effects on hepatic drug metabolism through the cytochrome P-450 system than does cimetidine. Propantheline delays ranitidine absorption and increases peak concentration, thus increasing its bioavailability. Theophylline absorption from controlled-release formulations is decreased by ranitidine-induced achlorhydria. Antacids decrease gastrointestinal absorption of ranitidine, and concurrent use should be spaced by at least 2 hours. Ranitidine may delay the renal clearance of procainamide, the clinical significance of which remains unclear.

SUPPLIED AS HUMAN PRODUCTS:
Tablets containing 150 and 300 mg
Capsules containing 150 and 300 mg
Oral syrup containing 15 mg/mL
For injection containing 25 mg/mL

RIFAMPIN

INDICATIONS: Rifampin (Rifadin ✤ ★, Rofact ✤, Rimactane ✤ ★) is an antimicrobial effective against a variety of mycobacterium species and *Staphylococcus aureus, Haemophilus,* and *Rhodococcus equi.* Rifampin is considered especially active in the treatment of staphylococcal and rhodococcal infections and is used in the eradication of pathogens located in difficult to reach target areas, such as inside phagocytic cells. It is active at an acid pH, making it a rational choice for the treatment of septic foci and granulomatous infections. It can be used alone for treatment of bacterial endocarditis or osteomyelitis in large animals or in combination with other agents such as erythromycin to reduce the frequency of acquired resistance. Rifampin is very lipophilic and penetrates most tissues including milk, bone, abscesses, and the CNS.

ADVERSE AND COMMON SIDE EFFECTS: If given IV to horses, even slowly over 10 minutes, adverse reactions such as weakness, slight to profuse sweating, defecation, and apprehension may occur. Adverse reactions have not been reported with oral use. Feces, saliva, sweat, tears, and urine may be discolored red-orange by rifampin and its metabolites. In humans and dogs, hepatopathy are reported. Although rare, anorexia, vomiting, diarrhea, thrombocytopenia, hemolytic anemia, interstitial nephritis, and bloody/cloudy urine, as well as death have also been reported.

DRUG INTERACTIONS: Combination with halothane or isoniazid may cause hepatotoxicity. Microsomal enzyme induction from rifampin may shorten the elimination half-life and decrease plasma drug concentrations of chloramphenicol, corticosteroids, theophylline, itraconazole, ketoconazole, warfarin, and barbiturates.

SUPPLIED AS HUMAN PRODUCTS:
Capsules containing 150 and 300 mg
Injection containing 600 mg

ROMIFIDINE

INDICATIONS: Romifidine (Sedivet ♣) is a potent, semisynthetic α_2-adrenergic receptor agonist with sedative effects like xylazine and detomidine, but is longer lasting and produces less ataxia. Its use in horses is indicated to facilitate handling, examination, and minor treatments. It provides dose-dependent sedation and tolerance to pain. Lowering of the head is the first sign of sedation, followed by lethargy, reduced sensitivity to environmental stimuli, and immobility. The onset of sedation occurs within 1 to 2 minutes and lasts 40 to 80 minutes. When used as a premedicant agent, it is given 8 to 10 minutes prior to general anesthesia. Clinically useful sedation of 60 minutes duration occurs with the concurrent administration of butorphanol.

ADVERSE AND COMMON SIDE EFFECTS: A prolonged reduction in blood pressure and heart rate with partial atrioventricular (AV) block occur following administration. This can be prevented by the IV administration of atropine at 0.01 mg/kg 3 to 5 minutes before romifidine administration. Following administration, occasional sweating and diuresis may occur. As with the other α_2-sympathomimetics, sedated horses may show increased skin sensitivity to the hind legs. Its use is contraindicated in horses with preexisting AV block, respiratory disease, advanced liver or kidney disease, or endotoxic or traumatic shock. Its safety has not been established for use in breeding horses.

DRUG INTERACTIONS: None listed.

SUPPLIED AS VETERINARY PRODUCT:
For injection containing 10 mg/mL in 20-mL multidose vials.

SEVOFLURANE

See SEVOFLURANE, under Description of Drugs for Small Animals.

SODIUM BICARBONATE

INDICATIONS: Sodium bicarbonate ♣ ★ (Bicarboject ★, Neutralyzer ★) is indicated for the treatment of metabolic acidosis as occurs commonly in neonatal diarrhea of large animals. It is also indicated for the management of hyperkalemia and hypercalcemia.

ADVERSE AND COMMON SIDE EFFECTS: The agent is contraindicated in cases with alkalosis, significant chloride loss associated with gastric or abomasal reflux, or with hypocalcemia where infusion of this agent will predispose to hypocalcemic tetany. Sodium bicarbonate should be used with caution in those patients with potential volume overload, for example, congestive heart failure and renal disease. Hypercapnia predisposing to ventricular fibrillation may occur in patients during cardiopulmonary resuscitation if adequate ventilatory support is not given. The use of this drug may cause metabolic alkalosis, hypokalemia, hypocalcemia, hypernatremia, volume overload, and paradoxical cerebrospinal fluid (CSF) acidosis leading to respiratory arrest. Myocardial depression and peripheral vasodilation leading to hypotension, hyperosmolality, CSF acidosis, increased intracranial pressure, and intracranial hemorrhage have been reported.

DRUG INTERACTIONS: If sodium bicarbonate is mixed with calcium-containing fluids, insoluble complexes may form. The action of epinephrine is impaired if it is mixed with sodium bicarbonate. Oral sodium bicarbonate may reduce the absorption of anticholinergic agents, cimetidine, ranitidine, iron products, ketoconazole, and tetracycline antibiotics and reduce the efficacy of sucralfate. Orally administered drugs are best given 2 hours before or after sodium bicarbonate.

SUPPLIED AS VETERINARY PRODUCTS:
For injection containing 8.4% w/v (1 mEq/mL)
For injection containing 7.5% w/v (0.89 mEq/mL)
Paste containing 2.27 g/454-g tube
A 1.3% w/v (13 g/L) solution of sodium bicarbonate is approximately isotonic. One gram of sodium bicarbonate contains 12 mEq of sodium and 12 mEq of bicarbonate.

SUPPLIED AS HUMAN PRODUCTS:
Tablets containing 325 mg (5 grain) and 650 mg (10 grain)
Tablets containing 500 mg
For injection containing 4% (0.48 mEq/mL), 4.2% (0.5 mEq/mL), 5% (0.595 mEq/mL), 7.5% (0.9 mEq/mL), and 8.4% (1 mEq/mL)

SODIUM CHLORIDE

INDICATIONS: Sodium chloride (Hypersaline E ★, Hyper Saline Solution 8X ★, Hypertonic Saline ★, Physiologic Saline ❀, Physiological Saline Solution ❀, Physiologic Saline Solution ★, Saline 0.9% ★, Saline Solution ★, Sterile Saline Solution ★) is recommended for the treatment of hyponatremia, hypochloremic metabolic alkalosis, and the restoration of normovolemia and the promotion of urinary calcium excretion. Isotonic sodium chloride (0.9% w/v) remains in the extracellular space (two-thirds in the interstitial space, one-third in the intravascular space) after IV injection. Half-strength saline (0.45% w/v) is directed into the intracellular space (one-third) and extracellular space (two-thirds) after IV administration and is a suggested treatment for animals with hypernatremia. Hypertonic saline (7.5% w/v) has been successfully used to reverse the pathologic effects of hemorrhagic/hypovolemic shock in ruminants and the horse. It is a suggested treatment for abomasal metabolic alkalosis associated with abomasal problems in ruminants. It has also been advocated as adjunctive treatment for corneal ulceration in horses.

ADVERSE AND COMMON SIDE EFFECTS: Excessive volumes of 0.9% saline may cause hyperchloremic metabolic acidosis and hypokalemia, especially in patients with diarrhea in which sodium loss is greater than chloride and in those patients in whom the kidney can not excrete the excess chloride load. Volume overload and pulmonary edema is a potential concern in animals with cardiac or renal insufficiency. Hypernatremia may also occur and lead to irritability, lethargy, weakness, ataxia, stupor, coma, and seizure.

DRUG INTERACTIONS: Glucocorticoids and corticotropin may predispose to sodium retention and volume overload especially in patients with congestive heart failure.

SUPPLIED AS HUMAN AND VETERINARY PRODUCTS:
For injection containing 0.45% (77 mEq/L) sodium and chloride
For injection containing 0.9% (154 mEq/L) sodium and chloride
For injection containing 5% and 7.2% sodium chloride (Hypertonic Saline ✤ ★)

OTHER USES
Horses and Ruminants
HYPOVOLEMIC SHOCK
7.2% saline: 4 to 5 mL/kg slowly over 8 to 10 minutes or longer; IV

SODIUM CROMOGLYCATE

INDICATIONS: Sodium cromoglycate (Intal ✤ ★) is reported to inhibit degranulation of mast cells and release of proinflammatory mediators. It is used as an aerosol to inhibit both the immediate and nonimmediate bronchoconstriction reactions to inhaled allergens. It has no intrinsic bronchodilator or anti-inflammatory activity. Inhalation of sodium cromoglycate 20 to 30 minutes before antigen inhalation challenge prevents the induction of airway obstruction in horses with recurrent airway obstruction (heaves, chronic obstructive pulmonary disease). Four consecutive daily treatments ameliorated clinical signs of heaves in horses for over 3 weeks. Thus, it is advocated for prevention of occurrence of clinical signs of airway obstruction in horses, by administration in advance of a predictable antigen exposure. However, clinical experience suggests that only selected horses will respond to the treatment, possibly because of variations in type and stage of immune hyperreactivity between horses.

ADVERSE AND COMMON SIDE EFFECTS: The most frequently reported adverse effects in humans were irritation to the throat, coughing, wheezing, and nausea. Bronchospasm, nasal congestion, and laryngeal and pharyngeal irritation have been reported. Other adverse reactions that occur infrequently include anaphylaxis, angioedema, dizziness, dysuria, joint swelling, lacrimation, urticaria, and myopathy. Adverse effects in horses have not been described.

DRUG INTERACTIONS: None reported.

SUPPLIED AS HUMAN PRODUCTS:
As aerosol in spincaps, containing 20 mg/dose
As solution for nebulization containing 10 mg/mL

SODIUM IODIDE

INDICATIONS: Sodium iodide (AmTech Sodium Iodide 20% Injection ★, Iodoject ★, Sodide ❧, Sodium Iodide 20% Injection ❧ ★, Sodium Iodide Solution 20% ❧ ★, Sodium Iodine 20% ❧) has antimicrobial activity and is used in the treatment of actinomycosis or actinobacillosis in cattle, and sporotrichosis in horses.

ADVERSE AND COMMON SIDE EFFECTS: Adverse effects include anorexia, lacrimation, depression, cardiomegaly, and cutaneous reactions that are generally reversible when the drug dose is decreased. The drug is contraindicated in hyperthyroidism, advanced pregnancy, and acute metal poisoning. Administer sodium iodide by slow IV injection; avoid SC or IM injection. Sodium iodide should not be used in lactating dairy cattle.

DRUG INTERACTIONS: None reported.

SUPPLIED AS VETERINARY PRODUCT:
For injection containing 200 mg/mL [20%]

SODIUM SULFATE

INDICATIONS: Sodium sulfate ❧ ★ [Glauber's salt] is used in ruminants as a preventive for urolithiasis. It is also administered as a cathartic for large animals. When administered it should be mixed as a 6% w/v solution and given by stomach tube. Sodium sulfate is also indicated to help mobilize excessive hepatic copper in sheep.

ADVERSE AND COMMON SIDE EFFECTS: Excessive doses can result in profuse diarrhea and abdominal discomfort.

DRUG INTERACTIONS: None listed.

SUPPLIED AS: Commercially available as Glauber's salt.

SODIUM THIOSULFATE

INDICATIONS: Sodium thiosulfate (Rexolate ★) is used as an antidote for cyanide poisoning, heavy metal poisoning, and has been used to treat cattle in field outbreaks of copper poisoning in combination with sodium molybdate.

ADVERSE AND COMMON SIDE EFFECTS: None listed.

DRUG INTERACTIONS: None listed.

SUPPLIED AS HUMAN PRODUCT:
For injection containing 25% w/v sodium thiosulfate

SPECTINOMYCIN

INDICATIONS: Spectinomycin (Adspec ♣ ★, Spectam ♣, Spectam Injectable ♣, Spectam Oral Solution ♣, Spectam Scour-Halt ♣ ★, Spectam Soluble Powder ♣, Spectam Water Soluble ★, Spectinomycin Oral ♣ ★, Trobicin ♣ ★) is an aminocyclitol antibiotic similar in action to aminoglycosides and is used in swine to treat diarrhea due to *Escherichia coli* and in cattle to treat bovine respiratory disease complex. It has broad spectrum activity against gram-positive and gram-negative bacteria including *E. coli*, *Klebsiella*, *Proteus*, *Enterobacter*, *Salmonella*, *Streptococcus*, *Staphylococcus*, and *Mycoplasma*.

ADVERSE AND COMMON SIDE EFFECTS: Neuromuscular blockade is a rare side effect that can be reversed by parenteral calcium administration. Spectinomycin is less nephrotoxic and ototoxic than other aminocyclitol antibiotics. In cattle, mild swelling may occur at the injection site. Discoloration at the injection site may persist beyond 11 days after injection. This may necessitate trimming of the injection site and surrounding tissues at slaughter. Anaphylactic reactions may occur in animals previously sensitized to aminocyclitols.

DRUG INTERACTIONS: Antagonism may occur if the drug is used concurrently with chloramphenicol or tetracycline. Spectinomycin combined with lincomycin acts synergistically against mycoplasma organisms.

SUPPLIED AS VETERINARY PRODUCTS:
For injection containing 100 mg/mL
Oral solution containing 50 mg/mL
Soluble powder containing 500 mg/g

SUPPLIED AS HUMAN PRODUCT:
For injection containing 2 g

OTHER USES: Spectinomycin can also be found in combination with lincomycin (Linco-Spectin, L-S20, L-S100 ✤), but lincomycin has been associated with lethal complications in horses and sheep, and thus this formulation should be strictly avoided in these species.

STANOZOLOL

INDICATIONS: Stanozolol (Winstrol-V ✤ ★) is an anabolic steroid with strong anabolic and weak androgenic activity. It is potentially useful as an adjunct to the management of catabolic disease states. The drug has been recommended to stimulate erythropoiesis, arouse appetite, promote weight gain, and increase strength and vitality. The efficacy of promoting these positive changes is questionable and prolonged treatment (3 to 6 months) may be required before a response in the erythron is seen. The drug is most commonly used in horses to enhance athletic performance. Also see ANABOLIC STEROIDS, under Description of Drugs for Small Animals.

ADVERSE AND COMMON SIDE EFFECTS: The drug should be used with caution in animals with cardiac or renal insufficiency and those with hypercalcemia. It may promote sodium and water retention and exacerbate azotemia; it may also promote hypercalcemia, hyperphosphatemia, and hyperkalemia. The drug is potentially hepatotoxic. Stanozolol should not be used in animals intended for breeding or in pregnant animals because of possible masculinization of fetuses.

DRUG INTERACTIONS: Anabolic agents may potentiate the effect of anticoagulants.

SUPPLIED AS VETERINARY PRODUCTS:
Tablets containing 2 mg
For injection containing 50 mg/mL

SUCRALFATE

INDICATIONS: Sucralfate (Apo-Sucralfate ✤, Carafate ★, Novo-Sucralfate ✤, Nu-Sucralfate ✤, Sulcrate ✤, Sucrate Suspension Plus ✤) accelerates the healing of oral, esophageal, gastric, and duodenal ulcers. Sucralfate disassociates in the acid environment of the stomach to sucrose octasulfate and aluminium hydroxide. Sucrose octasulfate polymerizes to a viscous, sticky substance that creates a protective effect by binding to ulcerated mucosa. This prevents back diffusion of hydrogen ions, inactivates pepsin, and adsorbs bile acid. In addition, sucralfate increases the mucosal synthesis of prostaglandins, which have a cytoprotective role in the gastric mucosa. Sucralfate may be useful for the prevention of nonsteroidal anti-inflammatory-induced ulceration.

ADVERSE AND COMMON SIDE EFFECTS: Side effects are rare. Constipation is the only significant problem reported in small animals.

DRUG INTERACTIONS: Antacids and H_2-receptor blocking agents decrease gastric pH and reduce the efficacy of sucralfate; therefore, they should be given at least one-half hour after giving sucralfate. Sucralfate decreases the bioavailability of digoxin, cimetidine, ranitidine, ketoconazole, phenytoin, theophylline, and tetracycline antibiotics. Concurrent oral drug administration should be separated by 2 hours. Sucralfate also decreases gastrointestinal absorption of ciprofloxacin and norfloxacin.

SUPPLIED AS HUMAN PRODUCTS:
Tablets containing 1 g sucralfate
Suspension containing 1 g/5 mL

SULFACHLORPYRIDAZINE

INDICATIONS: Sulfachlorpyridazine (Vetasulid ★) is a sulfonamide antimicrobial used to treat colibacillosis in swine and calves. It is also used parenterally as a general purpose sulfonamide in cattle.

ADVERSE AND COMMON SIDE EFFECTS: See SULFONAMIDES.

DRUG INTERACTIONS: Intramuscular injection is associated with pain and poor blood concentrations and is not recommended. See SULFONAMIDES.

SUPPLIED AS VETERINARY PRODUCTS:
Oral boluses containing 2 g (for calves)
Oral powder containing 54 g/bottle
Oral suspension containing 50 mg/mL (for swine)

SULFADIMETHOXINE

INDICATIONS: Sulfadimethoxine (Albon ★, Albon SR ★, Bactrovet ★, Di-Methox ★, S-125 Tablets ♣, S-250 Tablets ♣, Sulfadimethoxine

Injection-40% ★) is a sulfonamide antimicrobial used for the treatment of respiratory, genitourinary, enteric, and soft tissue infections caused by susceptible organisms including *Streptococcus, Staphylococcus, Escherichia, Salmonella, Klebsiella, Proteus,* and *Shigella*. It is the only sulfonamide approved for use in lactating dairy cattle in the United States.

ADVERSE AND COMMON SIDE EFFECTS: See SULFONAMIDES.

DRUG INTERACTIONS: Intramuscular injection is associated with pain and poor blood drug levels and is not recommended. See SULFONAMIDES.

SUPPLIED AS VETERINARY PRODUCTS:
Tablets containing 125, 250, and 500 mg
Oral suspension containing 50 and 125 mg/mL
Injection containing 400 mg/mL (United States)
Boluses containing 5 and 15 g
Slow-release boluses containing 12.5 g
Premix containing 6.6% w/w

SULFAMETHAZINE

INDICATIONS: Sulfamethazine (CalfSpan ♣, Sodium Sulfamethazine 25% ♣, Sodium Sulfamethazine Solution 12.5% and 25% ♣, Sulfa-Max III Cattle Bolus ★, Sulfa-Max III Calf Bolus ★, SulfaSure SR ★, SulfaSure SR Calf Bolus ★, Sulfamethazine Bolus ♣, Sulfa 25 ♣, Sulmet ★, SustainIII ♣ ★, SustainIII Cattle Bolus ★, SustainIII Calf Bolus ★, and others) is a sulfonamide antimicrobial used for the treatment of a wide variety of bacterial infections in large animals. Various formulations can be used for addition to water for mass medication (e.g., Sodium Sulfamethazine 25% ♣, Sulmet ★) and others for individual treatment with sustained-release products (e.g., Sustain III ♣ ★).

ADVERSE AND COMMON SIDE EFFECTS: See SULFONAMIDES.

DRUG INTERACTIONS: See SULFONAMIDES.

SUPPLIED AS VETERINARY PRODUCTS:
Water additive containing 12.5 and 25 g/100 mL
Bolus containing 2.5, 5, 15, and 15.6 g
Sustained-release bolus form containing 8, 8.25, 22.5, 27, 30, and 32.1 g
Powder in 1-lb (454-g) packets

OTHER USES: Sulfamethazine is also found in combination with a number of medications, either with other sulfa drugs (Sulfalean ♣,

Triple Sulfa ✤), or other antibacterials (AureoS-700 ✤ ★), or vitamins and minerals (Super Chlor 250 ✤).

SULFONAMIDES

INDICATIONS: The sulfonamides are bacteriostatic drugs that are effective against streptococci, *Bacillus, Corynebacterium, Nocardia, Brucella, Campylobacter, Pasteurella,* and *Chlamydia. Pseudomonas, Serratia,* and *Klebsiella* are generally resistant. The sulfonamides readily enter the CSF and are effective in treating meningeal infections. Sulfonamides substitute for *p*-aminobenzoic acid (PABA), preventing its conversion to dihydrofolic acid. Alone, this action is considered bacteriostatic. Since the antimicrobial mechanism of action is by competitive substitution, the sulfonamide tissue concentration must be kept high enough to prevent bacterial access to PABA. Therefore, the sulfonamides are ineffective in pus and necrotic tissue, which provide additional sources of PABA to the bacteria. The sulfonamides are nontoxic to mammalian cells because they utilize dietary folate for synthesis of dihydrofolic acid and do not require PABA. Sulfonamides are classified according to their duration of effect. Short-acting sulfonamides require dosing at 8-hour intervals and include sulfadiazine, sulfamerazine, sulfamethazine, and sulfamethoxazole. These short-acting sulfas are generally indicated in the treatment of systemic and urinary tract infections. Intermediate-acting sulfonamides require dosing every 12 to 24 hours and include sulfisoxazole and sulfadimethoxine, which are primarily indicated in the treatment of urinary tract infections. The long-acting sulfonamides, such as sulfasoxine, require dosing every few days; they have been primarily used in people for the treatment of chronic bronchitis and urinary tract infections.

ADVERSE AND COMMON SIDE EFFECTS: Precipitation in urine and crystalluria are not generally a problem in veterinary patients, but sulfonamides should be used with caution in patients with preexisting renal disease, especially if complicated by dehydration or metabolic acidosis. Pruritus and photosensitization have been reported and alopecia may occur with long-term use. Other reported conditions associated with the use of these drugs include polyarthritis, urticaria, facial swelling, fever, hemolytic anemia, polydipsia, polyuria, hepatitis, diarrhea, anorexia, and seizure activity. Hypersensitivity, including anaphylaxis, although rare, has also been documented.

DRUG INTERACTIONS: Antacids decrease the absorption of sulfonamides. Methenamine and other acidifying agents increase the risk of sulfonamide crystallization in the urine. *p*-Aminobenzoic acid and local anesthetics may antagonize sulfonamide action. Phenothiazines may increase the toxic effects of sulfonamide.

SUPPLIED AS VETERINARY PRODUCT:
See individual product.

SULFONAMIDES, POTENTIATED

INDICATIONS: The combinations of a sulfonamide with trimethoprim or pyrimethamine are referred to as "potentiated sulfonamides," such as trimethoprim-sulfadiazine (Di-Trim ★, Tribrissen ♣ ★, Uniprim ♣ ★) or trimethoprim-sulfadoxine (Trivetrin ♣, Borgal ♣, Biotrim ♣, Trimadox ♣). Pyrimethamine-sulfonamides are compounded by pharmacists. Potentiated sulfonamides are bactericidal antibacterial combinations recommended for the treatment of alimentary tract, respiratory, and urinary tract infections and skin and soft tissue infections caused by susceptible organisms including *E. coli, Enterobacter, Klebsiella, Streptococcus, Staphylococcus, Pasteurella, Proteus, Clostridia, Salmonella, Shigella, Brucella, Actinomyces, Corynebacterium, Bordetella, Neisseria,* and *Vibrio* organisms. Other significant organisms that are susceptible to potentiated sulfonamides include protozoa (*Toxoplasma gondii, Sarcocystis neurona*) and coccidia. Parenteral trimethoprim-sulfadoxine formulations are available for treating food animals in Canada but not in the United States. Potentiated sulfonamides are readily absorbed from the gastrointestinal tract of horses, but absorption may be affected by feeding. Trimethoprim is degraded in the rumen, so oral potentiated sulfonamides are not used in ruminants.

ADVERSE AND COMMON SIDE EFFECTS: The drug should not be used in animals with marked liver disease or blood dyscrasias or in those with sulfonamide sensitivity. Anemia, leukopenia, thrombocytopenia, anorexia, and ataxia have been noted at higher doses. Trimethoprim may cause increases in serum creatinine via competition for sites of renal excretion. The nonregenerative anemias seen in response to long-term administration of potentiated sulfonamides are believed to be related to folate reduction. Supplementation with oral folic acid is often recommended for horses on long-term potentiated sulfonamide therapy. The administration of oral folic acid to pregnant mares being treated for EPM may not protect the fetus from the effects of folate deficiency. Mares have delivered foals with congenital defects after oral administration of potentiated sulfonamides while supplemented with oral folic acid and vitamin E. The risk of congenital defects should be considered when treating pregnant mares with potentiated sulfonamides. Local infusion of potentiated sulfonamides into the uterus of mares causes irritation of the endometrium and a decreased pregnancy rate. Avoid intramuscular administration because of tissue irritation from the organic solvents, high concentration and high pH of the formulations. Intravenous administration must be done by slow and careful injection. Rapid administration is associated with thrombophlebitis and anaphylaxis.

DRUG INTERACTIONS: Antacids may decrease the bioavailability of trimethoprim-sulfonamides if administered concurrently. Trimethoprim-sulfadiazine may prolong clotting times in patients receiving warfarin. Sulfonamides may increase the effects of phenylbutazone, phenytoin, salicylates, thiazide diuretics, and probenicid. The concurrent use of potentiated sulfonamides with detomidine is contraindicated, as it appears that the potentiated sulfonamide sensitizes the myocardium and results in cardiac dysrhythmias and hypotension that may be fatal. The procaine in procaine penicillin G is a PABA analog and may reduce efficacy if used concurrently with potentiated sulfonamides.

SUPPLIED AS VETERINARY PRODUCTS:
For injection containing 40 mg/mL trimethoprim and 200 mg/mL sulfadiazine or sulfadoxine
For injection containing 80 mg/mL trimethoprim and 400 mg/mL sulfadiazine
Bolus containing 200 mg trimethoprim and 1 g sulfadiazine
Oral paste containing 67 mg/g trimethoprim and 333 mg/g sulfadiazine
Oral suspension containing 9.1 mg trimethoprim and 45.5 mg sulfadiazine
Oral powder containing 67 mg/g trimethoprim and 333 mg/g sulfadiazine

SYNERGISTIN

INDICATIONS: Synergistin ♣ is a combination of ampicillin trihydrate and sulbactam benzathine, a β-lactamase enzyme inhibitor. Sulbactam has poor intrinsic antimicrobial activity, but binds to β-lactamase enzymes, preventing the destruction of ampicillin. It is approved for use in cattle for the treatment of bacterial pneumonia and pneumonic pasteurellosis and is indicated in the treatment of bacterial infections resistant to ampicillin alone because of production of β-lactamase by pathogenic bacteria.

ADVERSE AND COMMON SIDE EFFECTS: See Ampicillin.

DRUG INTERACTIONS: None listed.

SUPPLIED AS VETERINARY PRODUCT:
For injection containing 120 mg ampicillin trihydrate with 60 mg sulbactam benzathine/mL

OTHER USES
Horses

Synergistin is also used in horses for the treatment of bacterial infections such as pneumonia, although it is not approved for use in this species. The drug combination has been effective in treating experimentally induced gram-negative pneumonia in foals at 6.6 mg/kg ampicillin and 3.3 mg/kg sulbactam IM q 24 hours.

TERBUTALINE

INDICATIONS: Terbutaline (Bricanyl ❧ ★, Brethane ★, Brethine ★) is a synthetic adrenergic stimulant with selective β_2- and negligible β_1-adrenergic receptor agonist activity. It is useful as a bronchodilator and has been used for testing for anhidrosis in horses by assessing sweat response to intradermal injections of gradually reducing concentrations.

ADVERSE AND COMMON SIDE EFFECTS: The drug should not be given to patients with tachycardia associated with digitalis intoxication. The drug should be used with caution in patients with hypertension, cardiac arrhythmias, or renal or hepatic dysfunction. Side effects may include tachycardia, hypotension or hypertension, tremor, fatigue, or seizure activity.

DRUG INTERACTIONS: Propranolol antagonizes the bronchodilating effect of terbutaline. Use with other sympathetic agents may potentiate the risk of arrhythmias.

SUPPLIED AS HUMAN PRODUCTS:
Tablets containing 2.5 and 5 mg
For injection containing 1 mg/mL
Aerosol containing 0.20 mg/actuation
Turbuhaler containing 0.5 mg/inhalation

TESTOSTERONE AND ESTRADIOL

INDICATIONS: Testosterone and estradiol (Component E-H ★, Synovex-H ❧ ★, Uni-Bol ❧) are used in large animals to improve weight gain and muscle mass. Equine products (Uni-Bol ❧) are used as anabolic agents where the potential adverse masculinizing effects of testosterone alone are undesirable. Implant pellets are used in heifers to stimulate weight gain and feed efficiency. Use is recommended for heifers weighing 185 to 365 kg. Maximal growth will be attained with good quality stock free of parasitism and disease.

ADVERSE AND COMMON SIDE EFFECTS: Testosterone is not recommended for use in stallions. Treatment in mares should not occur within 6 months prior to the breeding season. Implants are not intended for use in dairy heifers or breeding animals. The drug is not recommended for use in ovariectomized heifers. Bulling, vaginal and rectal prolapse, udder development, ventral edema, and elevated tail heads are occasional reported side effects. Implants should only be placed in the ear. Implantation at other sites may result in condemnation of the carcass.

DRUG INTERACTIONS: None listed.

SUPPLIED AS VETERINARY PRODUCTS:
For injection containing 100 mg/mL testosterone, 7.5 mg/mL estradiol enanthate, and 1 mg/mL estradiol benzoate
Implant pellets containing 200 mg testosterone propionate and 20 mg estradiol benzoate

TESTOSTERONE

INDICATIONS: Testosterone (Anatest ✤, Uni-Test ✤, Uni-Test Suspension ✤) is a potent anabolic hormone used in horses to improve weight gain, strength, and performance. It is used in other animals to treat impotence and cryptorchidism and to suppress lactation.

ADVERSE AND COMMON SIDE EFFECTS: Testosterone is not recommended for use in stallions. Stop treatment in mares at least 6 months prior to the breeding season.

DRUG INTERACTIONS: None listed.

SUPPLIED AS VETERINARY PRODUCT:
For injection containing 100 mg/mL in propionate or aqueous suspension.

OTHER USES
Sheep
ULCERATIVE POSTHITIS
Testosterone propionate is useful for reducing the incidence and severity of ulcerative posthitis in sheep at an implant dose of 100 mg every 3 months.

Cattle

To create estrus-detector animals (cull cows, heifers, steers): give 200 mg testosterone propionate q 24 hours for 9 days, and then give a 1 gram booster every 10 to 14 days.

TETANUS ANTITOXIN

INDICATIONS: Tetanus antitoxin ❖ ★ is prepared from the blood of horses hyperimmunized with the toxin of *Clostridium tetani*. It is used for the prevention of tetanus in animals that have suffered a penetrating wound and are of unknown immune status. Preventive doses confer immediate passive immunity that lasts 7 to 14 days. The antitoxin will not affect toxin already bound in the nervous system but may bind to circulating toxin. Concurrent treatment of the site of infection is necessary. Animals that survive tetanus remain susceptible to the disease, as the dose of toxin required for clinical disease is less than that necessary to prime the immune system.

ADVERSE AND COMMON SIDE EFFECTS: Biologics of equine origin have been associated with the development of hepatitis (Theiler's disease) in horses.

DRUG INTERACTIONS: None listed.

SUPPLIED AS VETERINARY PRODUCT:
For injection containing 1,500 U

TETRACYCLINE

INDICATIONS: Tetracyclines and its derivatives that are used in large animals include oxytetracycline, chlortetracycline, and doxycycline (Action 200 ★, Agrimycin ★, Alamycin LA ❖, Aureomycin ❖ ★, Biocyl ★, Bio-Mycin ❖ ★, Chlorosol-50 ❖, Chlora-cycline ★, CLTC 100 MR ★, CTC ★, Duramycin ★, Fermycin Soluble ★, Intracin ❖, Kelamycin Intrauterine Suspension ❖, Liquamycin LA-200 ❖ ★, Liquamycin/LP ❖, Maxim-200 ★, Medamycin ★, Onycin ❖, Oxy 1000 ❖, Oxysol ❖, Oxy LA ❖, Oxy LP ❖, Oxy-Mycin ★, OT200 ★, Oxytet ❖ ★, Oxy-Tet ★, Oxytetracycline ❖ ★, Oxymycine LP ❖, Oxymycine LA ❖, Oxytetracycline ❖ ★, Oxyvet ❖, Oxyject 100 ★, Oxy Tetra Forte ❖, Oxyshot LA ★, Panamycin 500 Bolus ★, Promycin ❖, Procure 200 ★, Solu-Tet ★, Terramycin ❖ ★, Terra-Vet ★, Tetracycline Hydrochloride ❖ ★, Tetra ❖, Tetrabol ❖, Tetrachel 250 ❖, Tetradure ❖, Tetralean ❖, Tetramed ❖, Tetraject ❖, Vibramycin ❖ ★, and many others) are broad-spectrum antibiotics that inhibit most gram-positive bacteria, some gram-negative bacteria, *Chlamydia, Mycoplasma, Rickettsia,* and some protozoa (*Haemobartonella, Anaplasma*). Tetracyclines are used for the treatment of a number of bacterial infections in large animals, including pneumonia, metritis, mastitis, tetanus, and foot rot, as well as systemic diseases such as anaplasmosis, leptospirosis, and brucellosis. Long-acting products have been effective in treating infectious pododermatitis and infectious bovine keratoconjunctivitis caused by *Moraxella bovis* and for prophylaxis in the reduction of incidence and severity of pneumonic pasteurellosis (shipping fever) in feedlot cattle. Tetracyclines are found in highest concentration in the kidney, liver, spleen, and lung and are deposited at sites of ossification. Tetracyclines are most effective against rapidly growing organisms. Bacterial resistance to tetracyclines develops rapidly. Tetracycline is the generic name for these compounds and also the name of the specific semisynthetic compound. Tetracycline and oxytetracycline are available as oral and parenteral products. Chlortetracycline is available as an oral product. Doxycycline is used orally in horses. High doses of oxytetracycline have been used with some success to treat flexural limb deformities in foals and calves. Objective evaluation of this treatment has recently shown its value in obtaining short-term moderate decrease in metacarpophalangeal joint angle in newborns within 36 hours of birth. The possible mechanism of action is unknown; however, chelation of calcium, or alternatively, a neuromuscular blocking effect has been suggested.

ADVERSE AND COMMON SIDE EFFECTS: Tetracycline is irritating if administered IM. Chlortetracycline causes severe tissue irritation if injected IM. Oral administration of tetracyclines to cattle may cause bloat or digestive upset. The clinical use of oxytetracycline in horses is controversial because of reports of adverse gastrointestinal effects. However, adverse effects were also associated with excessive dosage, concomitant use of other antimicrobials, and stressors such as surgery and transport. Anecdotally, oxytetracycline therapy has been used successfully in equine practice, and the recognition of the equine ehrlichial diseases has increased oxytetracycline use in horses. In a chronic dosing study using a long-acting formulation of oxytetracycline, no deleterious effects on fecal flora were detected and treated horses remained clinically normal. Doxycycline is less likely to cause adverse gastrointestinal effects as it is bound in an inactive form in the intestines. High doses of tetracyclines have been incriminated in causing renal failure in feedlot cattle. Infusion of chlortetracycline into the udder of cows during the dry period may cause udder damage. Occasional hypersensitivity reactions may occur after administration of tetracyclines. Renal tubular necrosis from oxytetracycline is associated with high doses, outdated parenteral products, endotoxemia, dehydration and hypovolemia, and concurrent pigment nephropathy. Rapid IV administration of oxytetracycline results in hypotension and collapse. This is attributed to intravascular chelation of calcium and/or decreased blood pressure from the drug vehicle (propylene glycol). Pretreatment with calcium borogluconate IV prevents collapse. Rapid intravenous administration of doxycycline to horses causes tachycardia, systemic arterial hypertension, collapse, and death. This reaction is likely due to chelation of intracellular calcium, resulting in neuromuscular blockade of the myocardium.

DRUG INTERACTIONS: Absorption of oral tetracycline products is impaired by milk products, aluminum hydroxide gels, sodium bicarbonate, calcium and magnesium salts, and iron preparations.

SUPPLIED AS VETERINARY PRODUCTS:
Chlortetracycline
Powders for administering in feed or water containing 25, 50, and 100 g/lb; 55, 110, and 220 g/kg
Boluses containing 500 mg
Tablets containing 25 mg

Oxytetracycline
For injection containing 50 mg/mL, 100 mg/mL
For injection in long-acting formulation containing 200 mg/mL
Premix containing 110, 220, 250, and 440 g/kg
Powder for water additive containing 10, 22, 25, 25.6, 88, 100, 102.4, 204.8, and 500 g/packet
Tablets containing 250 mg

Tetracycline
Water additive containing 25, 102.4, and 324 g/lb; 55, 62.5, 250, and 1,000 mg/g
Liquid containing 100 mg/mL
Bolus containing 500 mg

SUPPLIED AS HUMAN PRODUCT:
Doxycycline
Tablets and capsules containing 20, 50, and 100 mg
Powder for oral suspension containing 5 mg/mL

OTHER USES
Horses
FLEXURAL LIMB DEFORMITIES
3 g (44 mg/kg) oxytetracycline to foals younger than 1 week; IV once, or repeated in 24 hours

Sheep
LEPTOSPIROSIS
200 to 400 mg/head per day chlortetracycline in the feed for 2 to 3 weeks for leptospirosis outbreaks

THIAMINE

INDICATIONS: Thiamine or vitamin B_1 (B-1 ★, T-Dex ♣, Thiamine Hydrochloride Injection ♣ ★, Thiamine HCl Injection ♣ ★, T Sol ♣, Ultra-B_1 ♣) is used for the treatment of vitamin B_1 deficiencies in animals. In ruminants the most common manifestation of vitamin B_1 deficiency is polioencephalomalacia. Response to treatment of polio-encephalomalacia in ruminants is rapid. There is usually insufficient thiamine in multiple vitamin injectables for treatment of polioencepha-lomalacia.

ADVERSE AND COMMON SIDE EFFECTS: Rapid IV administra-tion can result in anaphylaxis. Dilution of commercial products in D_5W OR 0.9% saline is advised.

DRUG INTERACTIONS: None listed.

SUPPLIED AS VETERINARY PRODUCTS:
For injection containing 100, 200, and 500 mg/mL
Powder containing 16,677 mg/kg, 17,600 mg/kg, or 1,000 mg/30 g
Liquid containing 1 g/30 mL

OTHER USES
Ruminants

LEAD TOXICITY
20 mg/kg daily; SC for 15 days

THIOBARBITURATES

INDICATIONS: Thiobarbiturates [thiopental] (Induthol ♣, Pentothal ♣ ★, Pentothal Sodium ♣) are ultrashort-acting barbiturate anesthet-ics used for induction of anesthesia in large animals and for short sur-gical procedures, such as castration. Duration of anesthesia is 10 to 25 minutes with recovery in 30 to 90 minutes. During the period of induction, a brief period of excitement may occur. The brief period of anesthetic action is due to rapid distribution of the drug from the plasma into various tissues. Large or repeated doses will prolong anes-thesia as plasma levels remain near that of fat and tissues. Metabolism of thiobarbiturates is slow and repeated doses will prolong the time to recovery. Barbiturate anesthesia in the horse should not be prolonged for longer than 1 hour and no more than 5 g of any barbiturate should be given, even to draft breeds. Thiobarbiturates are reconstituted with water to form a solution for IV use. Once reconstituted, the solution quality deteriorates within 1 week or less, depending on a number of storage factors. Ponies may require higher doses than horses. In goats, thiobarbiturates are useful for short procedures, such as castration or tattooing.

ADVERSE AND COMMON SIDE EFFECTS: Respiratory centers are depressed after thiobarbiturate administration, but approximately 16 times as much drug is required to stop the myocardium as to paralyze respiration. Subcutaneous or perivascular injection with thiobarbiturates, particularly at a 5% or 10% w/v concentration, is irritating and may result in severe tissue reactions, including abscess formation and tissue slough. Areas of perivascular injection should be treated with saline for dilution and hyaluronidase to promote dispersion. Thiobarbiturates can trigger cardiac arrhythmias such as ventricular fibrillation. Pretreatment with acepromazine or chlorpromazine will considerably lessen this risk. Intracarotid injection can result in cerebrovascular endothelial injury and subsequent brain necrosis. Recovery from anesthesia in horses is often accompanied by violent excitement, which can be prevented with premedication with a phenothiazine tranquilizer.

DRUG INTERACTIONS: Reinduction of thiobarbiturate anesthesia can occur with administration of high doses of phenylbutazone or aspirin through displacement of thiobarbiturates from plasma proteins. These products are physically unstable with acids, acidic salts, and oxidizing agents.

SUPPLIED AS VETERINARY PRODUCT:
For injection containing 5 g thiopental

SUPPLIED AS HUMAN PRODUCTS:
For injection containing 1, 2.5, and 5 g
Vials for injection containing 0.5 and 1 g

TIAMULIN

INDICATIONS: Tiamulin (Denagard ✦ ★) is an antibiotic used in swine for the treatment of pneumonia caused by *Haemophilus pleuropneumonia*, for control of porcine proliferative enteropathies (ileitis) associated with *Lawsonia intracellularis*, and for swine dysentery caused by *Brachyspira hyodysenteriae*. It is well absorbed orally and high levels are achieved in lung tissue.

ADVERSE AND COMMON SIDE EFFECTS: Erythema has been observed that resolves with discontinuation of the drug. Overdose can cause transient salivation, vomiting, and CNS depression.

DRUG INTERACTIONS: Do not administer concurrently with ionophores (monensin, lasalocid, narasin, or salinomycin) as adverse reactions will occur.

SUPPLIED AS VETERINARY PRODUCTS:
Medicated premix with 10 g/lb
Concentrate solution containing 12.3% w/v tiamulin

TILMICOSIN

INDICATIONS: Tilmicosin (Micotil ❤ ★, Pulmotil ❤ ★) is a long-acting macrolide antibiotic used for the treatment of and mortality reduction in bovine respiratory disease caused by *Pasteurella haemolytica* and *Pasteurella multocida*. It is also approved for treatment of pneumonic pasteurellosis in lambs associated with *P. haemolytica*. Tilmicosin is indicated for the control of swine respiratory disease associated with *Actinobacillus pleuropneumoniae* and *P. multocida*. Its spectrum of activity is predominantly gram-positive organisms, with some gram-negative organisms and several mycoplasmas.

ADVERSE AND COMMON SIDE EFFECTS: Avoid contact with eyes. Intravenous injection in cattle and parenteral administration to swine has been fatal from cardiovascular toxicity. Treatment of lactating dairy cattle results in prolonged milk residues. Do not use in lambs less than 15 kg. Do not inject more than 25 mL per site. Swelling at the site of injection may occur under normal conditions but is mild and transient. Reports of sudden death, injection site swelling, collapse, anaphylaxis, and lameness have been associated with reactions to parenteral injections in cattle. Human injection may result in severe adverse reactions, particularly if doses are large. Do not use in automatically powered syringes. Exercise extreme caution to avoid accidental self-injection. In case of human injection, consult a physician immediately. Emergency medical telephone numbers are 1-800-722-0987 or 1-317-276-2000. The cardiovascular system appears to be the target of toxicity. This antibiotic persists in tissues for several days. The cardiovascular system should be monitored closely and supportive treatment provided. Dobutamine partially offsets the negative inotropic effects of tilmicosin. β-Adrenergic receptor antagonists, such as propranolol, exacerbate the negative inotropy of tilmicosin-induced tachycardia in dogs. Epinephrine potentiates lethality of tilmicosin in pigs.

DRUG INTERACTIONS: None listed.

SUPPLIED AS VETERINARY PRODUCT:
For injection containing 300 mg/mL (for cattle)
Premix containing 200 g/kg (for swine)

TOBRAMYCIN

INDICATIONS: Tobramycin (Nebcin ❤ ★) is an aminoglycoside antibiotic. It is closely related to gentamicin in spectrum, activity, and pharmacological properties, but it is more active against some strains of *Pseudomonas* that are resistant to gentamicin. Tobramycin is less nephrotoxic than gentamicin. Also see AMINOGLYCOSIDES.

ADVERSE AND COMMON SIDE EFFECTS: See AMINOGLYCO-SIDES.

DRUG INTERACTIONS: Tobramycin should not be mixed with other drugs. Also see AMINOGLYCOSIDES.

SUPPLIED AS HUMAN PRODUCTS:
For injection containing 10 and 40 mg/mL
For injection in premeasured syringes containing 60 and 80 mg
Bulk vials containing 1.2 g

TOLAZOLINE

INDICATIONS: Tolazoline (Priscoline ★, Tolazine ✚ ★) is an α_2-adrenergic receptor antagonist that has been used to reverse xylazine-induced (via caudal epidural administration) rumen hypomotility, and partially antagonize xylazine-induced cardiopulmonary depression without affecting sedation or local (S3 to coccyx) analgesic effects. It has also been used in horses (7.5 mg/kg; IV) to antagonize ventricular bradycardia and atrioventricular conduction disturbances and central nervous system depression associated with xylazine administration. Tolazoline in this instance may cause a persistent, mild systemic hypertension.

ADVERSE AND COMMON SIDE EFFECTS: Tachycardia, peripheral vasodilation, and hyperalgesia of the lips may occur. Piloerection may be noted on the rump and neck. Clear lacrimal and nasal discharges may be noted, as well as signs of apprehension. Overdose causes gastrointestinal hypermotility and colic symptoms. Intraventricular conduction is slowed and ventricular arrhythmias and death may occur with excessive doses.

DRUG INTERACTIONS: Hypotension may occur followed by an exaggerated rebound hypertension if tolazoline is administered concurrently with epinephrine or norepinephrine.

SUPPLIED AS VETERINARY PRODUCT:
For injection containing 100 mg/mL

SUPPLIED AS HUMAN PRODUCT:
For injection containing 25 mg/mL

TRIAMCINOLONE

INDICATIONS: Triamcinolone (Aristocort ✚ ★, Aristospan ★, Amcort ★, Articulose ★, Centracort ★, Cortalone ★, Kenaject ★,

Kenalog ❧ ★, Scheinpharm Triamcine-A ❧, Tac-3 ★, Tac-40 ★, Triam-A ★, Triamonide 40 ★, Tri-Kort ★, Trilog ★, Triam-Forte ★, Triamolone ★, Trilone ★, Tristoject ★, Vetalog ★) is a potent long-acting glucocorticoid. The drug is indicated for the treatment of arthritic and related disorders and for the treatment of allergic and dermatologic conditions responsive to glucocorticoids. It is used predominantly for horses with noninfectious soft tissue injuries and arthritis and for allergic respiratory disease. Also see GLUCOCORTICOID AGENTS.

ADVERSE AND COMMON SIDE EFFECTS: Subconjunctival injection may be associated with granuloma formation requiring surgical excision. High doses have been associated with laminitis in horses when concentrated human formulations have been substituted for veterinary formulations. Also see GLUCOCORTICOID AGENTS.

DRUG INTERACTIONS: See GLUCOCORTICOID AGENTS.

SUPPLIED AS VETERINARY PRODUCTS:
Tablets containing 0.5 and 1.5 mg
Suspension for injection containing 2 and 6 mg/mL

SUPPLIED AS HUMAN PRODUCTS:
Tablets containing 1, 2, 4, and 8 mg
Syrup containing 2 mg/5 mL and 4 mg/mL
For injection containing 3, 10, and 40 mg/mL
For intralesional injection containing 25 mg/mL

OTHER USES
Horses

RECURRENT AIRWAY OBSTRUCTION
Triamcinolone is used by some clinicians for reducing the clinical signs of small airway disease. However, as with other glucocorticoids, iatrogenic induction of laminitis can occur.

TRICHLORMETHIAZIDE/DEXAMETHASONE

INDICATIONS: Naquasone ❧ ★ is a combination of the benzothiadiazide diuretic trichlormethiazide and dexamethasone. This combination of drugs is complementary in the reduction of prepartum and postpartum udder edema in cattle. The diuretic action of trichlormethiazide is to inhibit reabsorption of sodium and chloride in the renal tubules, thereby enhancing excretion of sodium, chloride, and water. Effects on potassium and bicarbonate exchange in the tubules are much less and temporary. In contrast to other benzothiadiazide diuretics, potassium supplementation is not usually necessary. Dexamethasone may enhance the reduction of udder edema through its anti-inflammatory properties. The injectable form has been used for treatment of inflammatory conditions such as musculoskeletal injuries in the horse.

ADVERSE AND COMMON SIDE EFFECTS: Electrolyte depletion may occur with prolonged or overzealous therapy. Because of trichlormethiazide, Naquasone is contraindicated in severe renal impairment. Naquasone should not be given to animals with bacterial infections unless they are being treated with appropriate antibiotics. The dexamethasone portion of Naquasone may mask signs of infection such as elevation in body temperature. Administration of the injectable product to prepartum cows may cause premature parturition and retained placenta. Do not administer Naquasone to pregnant mares.

DRUG INTERACTIONS: None listed.

SUPPLIED AS VETERINARY PRODUCTS:
For injection containing 10 mg/mL trichlormethiazide and 0.5 mg/mL dexamethasone acetate
Boluses containing 200 mg trichlormethiazide and 5 mg dexamethasone

TRIFLURIDINE

INDICATION: Trifluridine (Viroptic Ophthalmic Solution ♣ ★) is a halogenated pyrimidine used in humans for the treatment of ocular herpes viral infections. Although this may have theoretical use for treatment of bovine herpes virus-I or equine herpes virus ocular manifestations, resolution of both conditions generally occurs without drug treatment.

ADVERSE AND COMMON SIDE EFFECTS: Burning or stinging on instillation or palpebral edema are reported. Rarely, superficial punctate keratopathy, epithelial keratopathy, stromal edema, keratitis sicca, hyperemia, or increased intraocular pressure has been reported in humans.

DRUG INTERACTIONS: None listed.

SUPPLIED AS HUMAN PRODUCT:
Ophthalmic solution containing 1% w/v

TROPICAMIDE

INDICATIONS: Tropicamide (Diotrope ♣, L-Picamide ★, Mydriacyl ♣ ★, Ocu-TropiC ★, PMS-Tropicamide ♣, Tropicacyl ♣ ★) is a synthetic tertiary amine antimuscarinic compound with properties similar to atropine. Tropicamide is a short-acting ophthalmic preparation used to dilate the pupil for short-acting relief of pain of ciliary spasm associated with uveitis and for funduscopic examination.

ADVERSE AND COMMON SIDE EFFECTS AND DRUG INTER-ACTIONS: See ATROPINE.

SUPPLIED AS HUMAN PRODUCT:
Ophthalmic solution containing 0.5% and 1.0% w/v

TYLOSIN

INDICATIONS: Tylosin (Tylan ✤ ★, Tylocine ✤, Tylosin ✤ ★) is a macrolide antibiotic with activity against gram-negative and gram-positive bacteria, spirochetes, chlamydiae, and mycoplasma organisms. This drug is frequently used in large animals for the treatment of swine dysentery. However, tylosin is also effective in the treatment of bovine respiratory disease complex, foot rot, diphtheria and metritis in cattle, pneumonia, arthritis, chlamydial abortion in sheep, and other infectious problems caused by tylosin-susceptible organisms.

ADVERSE AND COMMON SIDE EFFECTS: Anorexia, diarrhea, and local pain with IM injection are reported. Do not inject more than 10 mL per site. Injection of tylosin in horses has been fatal.

DRUG INTERACTIONS: Tylosin may increase serum digitalis levels.

SUPPLIED AS VETERINARY PRODUCTS:
For injection containing 50 and 200 mg/mL
Soluble powder water additive containing 100 g/jar as tylosin tartrate
Soluble powder for feed additive containing 22, 88, and 220 g/kg as tylosin phosphate

VANCOMYCIN

INDICATIONS: Vancomycin (Lyphocin ★, Vancocin ✤ ★, Vancoled ★) is an antibiotic primarily effective against gram-positive organisms, including methicillin-resistant strains. It acts at the bacterial cell wall and is unrelated chemically to any other available antibiotics. Oral absorption is poor. Although a dosage has been published for use in horses, little information is available on its efficacy or safety. Because of its valuable role in the treatment of resistant infections in humans, its use in veterinary medicine should be limited.

ADVERSE AND COMMON SIDE EFFECTS: Hypersensitivity, flushing, neutropenia, and thrombocytopenia have been reported, as have phlebitis and pain at the site of injection. Vancomycin is ototoxic and nephrotoxic.

DRUG INTERACTIONS: Avoid concurrent administration of other nephrotoxic drugs.

SUPPLIED AS HUMAN PRODUCTS:
For injection containing 500 mg and 1, 5, and 10 g
Capsules containing 125 and 250 mg

VEDOPROFEN

INDICATIONS: Vedoprofen (Quadrisol 100 ♣) is an NSAID for horses with anti-inflammatory, analgesic, and antipyretic action. It is structurally related to ketoprofen and carprofen. It is well absorbed orally and accumulates in inflammatory exudates for a prolonged duration of action. It is for the control of inflammation and relief of pain associated with musculoskeletal disorders and soft tissue lesions. It can be given prophylactically to horses prior to surgery.

ADVERSE AND COMMON SIDE EFFECTS: At high doses or prolonged administration, side effects are typical of other NSAIDs. See PHENYLBUTAZONE.

DRUG INTERACTIONS: Vedoprofen is highly bound to plasma proteins and may displace other drugs that bind to plasma proteins, such as other anti-inflammatory drugs, sulfonamides, or anticoagulants such as warfarin, leading to increased pharmacological effect or toxicity of the displaced drug. NSAIDs reduce the prostaglandin-mediated action of furosemide and ACE-inhibitors.

SUPPLIED AS VETERINARY PRODUCT:
Dose syringe with gel containing 100 mg/mL

VITAMIN A

INDICATIONS: Vitamin A (A-500 ♣) is a generic term for compounds possessing the biologic activity of retinol. It is present in considerable amounts in green forage plants. Vitamin A functions to maintain normal structure and function of epithelial cells and ocular structures such as the retina and cornea that are important for normal vision. Deficiency in large animals on forage diets is uncommon, but signs may manifest as increased keratinization of epithelial surfaces and keratinization of mucous-secreting surfaces such as the respiratory or gastrointestinal tract. Night blindness, excessive lacrimation, and corneal keratinization may also occur with Vitamin A deficiency. A single injection may last several months and the liver can store approximately a 3- to 6-month supply of vitamin A. For parenteral use the drug is combined with vitamin D (Co-op A-D Injectable ♣, Poten A.D. ♣, Vitamin A-D-500 ★, Vita-Ject A-D 500 ★, Vitamin A-D ♣, Vitamin A-D

Injectable ❀ ★, Vitamin AD Injection ★, Vitamin AD-500 ❀, Vitamin AD Injectable ❀).

ADVERSE AND COMMON SIDE EFFECTS: Toxicity can occur with excess dietary or parenteral supplementation, with clinical signs resembling deficiency states. Administration of combination products of vitamin A and D has been associated with cardiovascular collapse and abortion in cattle.

DRUG INTERACTIONS: None listed.

SUPPLIED AS VETERINARY PRODUCT:
For injection containing 500,000 IU/mL combined with 75,000 IU/mL vitamin D_3

VITAMIN D₃

INDICATIONS: Vitamin D_3 (High-D Dispersible ★, Hydro-Vit D_3 ❀, Soln-Vit D_3 ❀, Vita-D ❀, Poten-D ❀, Downer-D ❀) increases intestinal and renal calcium absorption and mobilizes calcium from the bone. It is used in pregnant cows to prevent milk fever. Knowledge of the exact date of expected calving is essential because vitamin D must be administered between 2 and 8 days prepartum for optimal effect. Maximal effect occurs between 48 to 96 hours and wanes during the following 96 hours. The drug is also contained in combination with vitamin A (Vitamin A-D-500 ★, Vitamin AD 500 ❀, Vitamin A-D Injectable ★, Vitamin AD Injection ★, and others), but the concentration of vitamin D is insufficient for use as a preventive for parturient paresis. Vitamin D is also available in combination with calcium chloride (Cal Oral Plus ★) for oral calcium supplementation.

ADVERSE AND COMMON SIDE EFFECTS: Administration to cows not in the immediate prepartum state and at high dosages can result in vascular calcification and/or renal calcium deposition.

DRUG INTERACTIONS: None listed.

SUPPLIED AS VETERINARY PRODUCTS:
Water additive containing 66,667, 80,000, or 160,000 IU/kg
For injection containing 500,000 and 1,000,000 IU/mL
For injection containing 75,000 IU/mL combined with 500,000 IU/mL vitamin A
Oral suspension containing 2,400 IU combined with 400 mg/mL calcium chloride

VITAMIN E + SELENIUM

INDICATIONS: Vitamin E + selenium (Alphasel Powder ❀, Bo Se Injectable ★, Dystosel ❀, Dystosel DS ❀, Equ-SeE ★, E-Se Injectable

♣ ★, E-Sel ♣, Mu-Se Injectable ♣ ★, Selenium-E ♣, Selepherol ♣, Selon-E ♣, Super SeE ★, Ultra-Sel ♣, Vetre-Sel-E ♣) is a combination product used in the treatment and prevention of white muscle disease (nutritional myopathy) in calves and sheep and for myositis due to selenium and tocopherol deficiency in horses.

ADVERSE AND COMMON SIDE EFFECTS: Selenium is toxic if given in excess. Vitamin E has low toxicity. Administer only to animals known to be ingesting subnormal levels of selenium. Anaphylactic reactions have occurred occasionally, particularly if the drug is given by IV injection in horses. Treat the animal immediately with epinephrine if anaphylaxis occurs. Some products will cause transitory local muscle soreness. Injection site abscess and clostridial myositis have also been reported in cattle and horses. Additionally, abortion, diarrhea, and bloat have been noted in cattle, while dyspnea, abdominal pain, polypnea, head shaking or swelling, and tachycardia have been described in horses.

DRUG INTERACTIONS: None indicated.

SUPPLIED AS VETERINARY PRODUCTS:
For injection containing 2.5 mg selenium and 68 IU vitamin E/mL
For injection containing 3 mg selenium and 136 IU vitamin E/mL
For injection containing 5 mg selenium and 68 IU vitamin E/mL
For injection containing 6 mg selenium and 136 IU vitamin E/mL
Feed additive containing 90.7 mg selenium and 20,000 IU vitamin E/lb
Feed additive containing 40 mg selenium and 35,000 IU vitamin E/kg
Powder containing 85 µg sodium selenite and 35 IU vitamin E/g

OTHER USES
Horses

Vitamin E is also advocated for treatment and prevention of equine degenerative myelopathy. The optimal success of this treatment has been through recognition and treatment at early stages of the disease, especially in horses less than 12 months of age.
Treatment: 6,000 IU/250 to 500 kg; PO daily
Prophylaxis: 1,500 to 2,000 IU; PO daily per foal

For the equine athlete, vitamin E has been advocated in feed supplementation at 80 to 100 IU/kg dry matter feed.

Cattle

Vitamin E-selenium given 1 month prior to calving (2.5 to 3.75 mg selenium content of the combination; SC or IM) has reduced the incidence of retained placentas in selenium-deficient herds.

VITAMIN K$_1$

INDICATIONS: Vitamin K$_1$ [phytonadione] (Veta-K1 ♣, Vita-Ject Vitamin K$_1$ Injectable ★, Vitamin K$_1$ ★) is a naturally occurring vitamin K compound used for the treatment of prolonged bleeding due to vitamin K deficiency states, as occur in cattle fed moldy sweet clover containing anti–vitamin K compounds such as bishydroxycoumarin, or from toxicity from ingested rodenticides containing dicoumarol. The drug is also indicated in horses receiving excess warfarin and in animals with hepatocellular disease. The primary function of vitamin K is to promote hepatic biosynthesis of prothrombin (factor II), as well as factors VII, IX, and X. Vitamin K_1 is more effective than menadione (vitamin K_3) in countering bleeding problems associated with vitamin K deficiency. The prothrombin time should be shortened within 1 to 2 hours of administration and can be monitored for response to therapy. Bleeding should be controlled in 3 to 6 hours and the prothrombin time may be normal in 12 to 24 hours. The smallest effective dose should be used to minimize the risk of allergic reaction. In severe bleeding, whole blood transfusion or plasma transfusion may also be warranted.

ADVERSE AND COMMON SIDE EFFECTS: Severe, sometimes fatal, reactions can occur if given IV, even if precautions such as dilution of vitamin K and slow infusions have been observed. Hypersensitivity can also occur from other ingredients of this product. Pain or swelling at the site of injection may occur. Keep the drug out of sunlight at all times.

DRUG INTERACTIONS: Vitamin K_1 will not counteract the anticoagulant effects of heparin.

SUPPLIED AS VETERINARY PRODUCTS:
For injection containing 10 mg/mL phytonadione
Oral capsule containing 25 mg

XYLAZINE

INDICATIONS: Xylazine (AmTech Xylazine HCl ★, Anased ❤ ★, Cervizine ★, Rompun ❤ ★, Sedazine Injection ★, Tranquived ★, Xyla-Ject ★, Xylamax ❤, Xylazine Injection ★, Xylazine HCL ★) is a tranquilizing agent characterized in the horse by a rapid onset, good to excellent sedation, excellent analgesia of 15 to 30 minutes duration, and a smooth recovery. Xylazine is particularly potent as a short-acting analgesic in horses with colic. Ruminants are particularly sensitive to the sedative effects of xylazine, so they are dosed using small animal formulations. The duration of sedation in ruminants is longer than in horses.

ADVERSE AND COMMON SIDE EFFECTS: Temporary salivation, diuresis, ruminal stasis, and diarrhea have been observed in cattle. Use of the drug is contraindicated in animals receiving epinephrine or those with ventricular arrhythmias. It should be used with caution in animals with heart disease, hypotension, shock, respiratory dysfunction, severe hepatic or renal disease, a history of seizure activity, or those severely debilitated. Bradycardia may be prevented by the administration of atropine or glycopyrrolate. Xylazine induces a modest catecholamine release and may result in patchy sweating and elevated blood glucose in the horse. The drug may precipitate early parturition and retained placenta if used in the last trimester of pregnancy. Repeated doses of xylazine in tympanic colic should be avoided because it can have detrimental effects by decreasing intestinal motility. Draft breeds of horses may be more sensitive to the effects of xylazine. Movement in response to sharp auditory stimuli may be observed. Occasionally, parenteral administration to equines may not induce effective sedation.

DRUG INTERACTIONS: Xylazine sensitizes the heart to epinephrine-induced arrhythmias, especially in the face of halothane anesthesia. Other CNS depressants, including barbiturates, narcotics, and phenothiazines may potentiate CNS and respiratory depression. Yohimbine (0.12 mg/kg; slowly IV) or tolazoline (4 mg/kg; slowly IV) can be used in horses to antagonize the effects of xylazine, shorten recovery times, and reduce anesthetic-related complications. Avoid perivascular or intracarotid injection.

SUPPLIED AS VETERINARY PRODUCT:
For injection containing 20 and 100 mg/mL

OTHER USES
Horses
EPIDURAL ANALGESIA
0.17 to 0.22 mg/kg diluted to a 10-mL volume using 0.9% saline, given epidurally into the first or second coccygeal space. Analgesia duration is approximately 3.5 hours and at the lower dose hind end ataxia is not reported to occur.

YOHIMBINE

INDICATIONS: Yohimbine (Antagonil ♣ ★, Yobine ♣ ★) is a competitive α_2-adrenergic receptor blocking agent used for reversal of the effects of xylazine and detomidine. It is also used empirically in horses in combination with parasympathomimetics such as bethanechol to treat ileus caused by adrenergic stimulation.

ADVERSE AND COMMON SIDE EFFECTS: Signs of sympathomimetic stimulation, including sweating, increased heart rate and blood pressure, muscle tremors, and irritability, have been noted in humans and laboratory animals. Adverse effects are yet to be described in large animals.

DRUG INTERACTIONS: None listed.

SUPPLIED AS VETERINARY PRODUCT:
For injection containing 2 (approved in dogs) and 5 mg/mL (approved in deer)

OTHER USES
Horses
GASTROINTESTINAL ILEUS
Slow IV administration (0.075 mg/kg) of yohimbine has been used to counteract negative propulsive effects of endotoxin on the gastro-intestinal tract, presumed mediated through α_2-adrenoreceptors. This regimen has restored intestinal electromechanical activity after induced ileus in Shetland ponies.

ZERANOL

INDICATIONS: Zeranol (Ralgro ♣ ★) is a hormone implant used in cattle for growth promotion and improving feed efficiency. Zeranol acts by stimulating increased secretion of endogenous somatotropin.

ADVERSE AND COMMON SIDE EFFECTS: None listed. Zeranol may not be as effective if used in animals with poor husbandry or parasite control.

DRUG INTERACTIONS: None listed.

SUPPLIED AS VETERINARY PRODUCT:
Implants containing 36 mg zeranol

SUPPLIED AS HUMAN PRODUCTS:
Tablets and capsules containing 10, 25, 50, and 100 mg (hydrochlo-ride and pamoate salts)
Syrup containing 10 mg/5 mL
For injection containing 25 and 50 mg/mL

OTHER USES
Sheep
Zeranol can be used in rams to reduce the incidence of ulcerative posthitis, but it is not as effective as testosterone.

Part III

Exotics

Handbook of Veterinary Drugs, Third Edition, edited by Dana Allen,
Lippincott Williams & Wilkins, Baltimore. © 2005

Section 7

Introduction: Chemotherapeutics in Avian and Exotic Pet Practice

Provision of optimum medical care to avian and the less traditional, or exotic, pet species requires both the art and the science of veterinary medicine. Very few drugs are licensed or specifically formulated for use in birds, small mammals, or reptiles. Despite increasing research on the pharmacokinetics and efficacy of medications in these species, the majority of dosage regimes are still empirical and derived, sometimes very roughly, from other species. It is essential that the veterinarian be knowledgeable about the mode of action and reported side effects of a given drug to assess its appropriateness for a novel patient or treatment situation. Owners must be aware that the majority of medications are off-label and that a guarantee of either safety or efficacy is impossible in all situations. Veterinarians must remain abreast of the current literature pertaining to the treatment of exotic pets and adjust or discard recommendations that are shown to be inappropriate. Contributions to the literature by practitioners, particularly on observed efficacy, adverse effects, or applications of new drugs to exotic animal practice, assist in promoting rational, effective, and safe treatment regimens. The dosages in this book are derived from information in the published literature, including texts, refereed journal articles, and less formal communications such as letters to the editor or "In My Experience" style comments. Nonrefereed material often provides the first information on the application of new drugs and on adverse or unexpected side effects.

The Drug Description section provides information on the use of a particular drug in a given group of animals. Summarized pharmacokinetic details are provided to help the reader judge the applicability of research results to a particular clinical situation. Drug dosages derived from pharmacokinetic work or efficacy trials in exotic species are marked with an asterisk in the dosage tables. Because of the format of this book, specific references are not included, but are available from the author on request. Readers are referred to the Small Animal or Large Animal sections for general information on the characteristics and use of particular drugs in the more common domestic species and for the commercial availability of drugs used in standard veterinary practice.

ALLOMETRIC SCALING

Allometric scaling is a mathematical technique used to adapt drug dosage and frequency of administration from one species of animal to another. Metabolic rates and many other physiologic processes that affect pharmacokinetic parameters are exponentially rather than linearly associated with body weight or mass. Hence, the direct application of a mg/kg dose from a small animal, or species with a high metabolic rate, to a large animal, or species with a slower metabolic rate, may result in a considerable overdosage. Underdosage could occur if the calculation is reversed, that is, from a large to a small species of animal. Allometric scaling formulas multiply an exponential function of lean body weight by a constant (K). Vertebrates are placed in five very broad K groups, the value of K reflecting mean core body temperature and basal energy requirements, as follows:

Reptiles (at 37°C): 10

Marsupials: 49

Placental mammals: 70

Nonpasserine birds: 78

Passerine birds: 129

Although metabolic scaling has been used to determine treatment protocols, it is important to recognize the underlying assumptions. It is assumed that all animals absorb, distribute, and metabolize a given drug in the same manner. This is untrue in many instances, for example, the absorption of an orally administered compound is likely to be very different among a herbivorous reptile, a carnivorous mammal, and a granivorous bird. Quantitative differences in excretory pathways make allometric scaling of aminoglycoside and penicillin doses from mammals to birds inappropriate. Physiologic mechanisms vary even within a vertebrate class, for example, between aquatic and terrestrial reptiles, or temperate and highly xerophilic birds. The half-life of gentamicin correlates with body size for some, but not all, avian species. It is well recognized that pharmacokinetic parameters in reptiles are significantly affected by changes in ambient, and hence body, temperature. The K value used to scale allometric doses for reptiles was determined for an ambient temperature of 37°C and may be inappropriate for other environmental situations. It is, therefore, likely that the most valid allometric extrapolations will be between species with similar basic physiologic mechanisms and for drugs metabolized and excreted by processes that are closely related to basal metabolic rate. Allometric scaling is no replacement for pharmacokinetic studies in the species of concern and, for reptile patients, held at the appropriate ambient temperature.

The following calculations incorporate the K value of 70 (appropriate for placental mammals) and illustrate how to use allometric scaling to extrapolate drug dosage rate and frequency of administration from a control species in which this information is known, to one in which it is not.

1. The specific minimum energy cost (SMEC) is calculated for both the animal in which drug dosage is known (control) and the patient to be treated.

$$\text{SMEC} = 70 \, (W_{kg}^{-0.25})$$

2. The SMEC dose rate (dose per metabolic energy unit) for the control animal is calculated by dividing the drug's dose rate (mg/kg) for that species by its SMEC ($\text{SMEC}_{control}$).

$$\text{SMEC} = \text{dose rate (mg/kg)} = \text{Dose}_{control}(\text{mg/kg})/\text{SMEC}_{control}$$

3. The dose rate for the patient is calculated by multiplying the $\text{SMEC}_{patient}$ by the SMEC dose rate.

$$\text{Dose}_{patient}(\text{mg/kg}) = \text{SMEC}_{patient} \times \text{SMEC dose rate (mg/kg)}$$

4. Treatment frequency is allometrically scaled in a similar fashion to determine the frequency of administration within a 24-hour period, or the number of times the dose should be administered.

$$\text{SMEC frequency} = \text{treatment frequency}_{control}/\text{SMEC}_{control}$$

5. The frequency of administration for a 24-hour period for the patient is calculated by multiplying the SMEC frequency by the $\text{SMEC}_{patient}$.

$$\text{Frequency}_{patient} = \text{SMEC frequency} \times \text{SMEC}_{patient}$$

Handbook of Veterinary Drugs, Third Edition, edited by Dana Allen,
Lippincott Williams & Wilkins, Baltimore. © 2005

Section 8

The Use of Chemotherapeutic Agents in Rodents and Rabbits

The table in Section 9 lists drugs and doses recommended for use in rodents and rabbits in clinical practice. This information is derived from the published literature pertaining to pet and laboratory animals. Almost all doses are empirical, as only a few efficacy and pharmacokinetic trials have been carried out with the intention of providing clinically oriented recommendations, and these are primarily in rabbits. This is despite the extensive use of these species in research and in pharmaceutical toxicity testing. Less information is available for the treatment of chinchillas, which have not been used in research as frequently as rabbits and smaller rodents. Drug administration in species included in this section is virtually always extralabel, and therefore, the veterinarian must select medications with caution. When treating rabbits intended for human consumption, drug residue issues must also be considered.

Small rodent species other than those specifically listed are also seen in veterinary practice. The veterinarian should attempt to match these animals with a species listed in this table in order to most safely extrapolate drug dosage regimens. Matching should be particularly based on similar gastrointestinal form and function in order to minimize the possibility of antimicrobial toxicity.

The small body size of many of the species discussed in this chapter limits the routes of medication available, and makes careful calculations of doses and dilutions essential.

Direct oral dosing by syringe into the diastema of the mouth is a commonly utilized technique. Some animals may lick medication directly from the syringe if it is sufficiently palatable, otherwise careful restraint and slow infusion are required. Small volumes of palatable products can also be placed in or on favorite foodstuffs. Oral preparations registered for use in children may be useful, although further dilution is often necessary. Rabbits and rodents are difficult to medicate with intact tablets or capsules.

For commercial groups of animals, medication of food or water may be appropriate. Food and water consumption are affected by a variety of factors, including species, state of health, and environmental conditions. Since maintenance of therapeutic drug levels is dependent on reliable and consistent ingestion of the treated food or water, it is difficult to ensure that each individual animal receives a correct dose, particularly in groups. Some medications for oral consumption can be made into flavored gelatin blocks using products such as Jell-O. The formulation should be made up with half the amount of water suggested and the drug added once the mixture has cooled but before it sets. This type of formulation is particularly useful to administer analgesics to animals in laboratory situations. For many medications placed in drinking water, it is necessary to add sugar or another sweetener to mask any unpleasant taste.

Intramuscular injections are best given in the muscles of the hind limb, taking care to avoid the sciatic nerve, and in the lumbar area. As most species have little muscle mass, only small volumes of drug can be administered in this fashion. The subcutaneous route of administration is often the preferred route as increased volumes can be administered to a greater variety of sites. Injection of irritating substances in either location may lead to sloughing or self-mutilation. Use of appropriately sized needles and syringes is necessary in tiny patients. The intraperitoneal route of drug administration is frequently used in laboratory settings for anesthetic administration. Larger drug volumes can be administered in this way; however, the risk of visceral injury and peritonitis does exist.

The intravenous route of drug administration is rarely used in clinical practice in species other than rabbits owing to the difficulty in venous access. Intraosseous administration of fluids and medications has also been described. Caution should be taken when applying topical products, as toxicity can result from self-grooming and product ingestions or from overdosage relating to the greater surface to body mass ratio of smaller creatures.

WARNING: The susceptibility of rabbits and certain rodents, especially chinchillas, guinea pigs, and hamsters, to antibiotic-induced enterotoxemia is well recognized. Rats and mice are less susceptible to this disruption of the normal intestinal flora, or dysbiosis. Overgrowth of gram-negative and anaerobic gram-positive bacteria results in enteritis, toxin production and enterotoxemia, diarrhea, and death. *Clostridium difficile* and *Clostridium spiroforme,* which produces an iota toxin, are particularly implicated in this phenomenon. Narrow spectrum penicillins (e.g., ampicillin, amoxicillin), β-lactams, and macrolide antibiotics (e.g., clindamycin, lincomycin, and erythromycin) are most frequently implicated in causing dysbiosis and mortality. Other drugs of particular concern include: cephalosporins in hamsters and guinea pigs (toxic); oral tetracyclines in guinea pigs (diarrhea and dysbiosis); procaine especially in gerbils and possibly mice; streptomycin and dihydrostreptomycin in rats, mice, hamsters, and guinea pigs (flaccid paralysis); and griseofulvin in guinea pigs (*Penicillium* derived). Use of the offending antibiotic should be stopped immediately if diarrhea develops, and the use of broad-spectrum antibiotics, metronidazole, and cholestyramine considered along with supportive care and possibly refaunation. Trimethoprim-sulfonamide combinations, enrofloxacin, chloramphenicol, and aminoglycosides are unlikely to cause gastrointestinal dysbiosis.

Handbook of Veterinary Drugs, Third Edition, edited by Dana Allen,
Lippincott Williams & Wilkins, Baltimore. © 2005

Section 9

Common Dosages for Rodents and Rabbits

Drug	Rabbits	Guinea Pigs	Chinchillas	Hamsters	Gerbils	Rats	Mice
Acepromazine	0.5 to 2 mg/kg; SC, IM	0.5 to 5 mg/kg; SC, IM	0.5 to 1 mg/kg; SC, IM	0.5 to 5 mg/kg; SC, IM	DO NOT USE	0.5 to 2.5 mg/kg; SC, IM, IP	0.5 to 5 mg/kg; SC, IM
Acetaminophen	200 to 500 mg/kg; PO 1 to 2 mg/mL of drinking water					100 to 300 mg/kg q 4 hours; PO 1 to 2 mg/mL of drinking water	200 to 300 mg/kg q 4 hours; PO 1 to 2 mg/mL of drinking water
Acetaminophen + codeine						1 to 2 mg acetaminophen + 0.1 to 0.2 mg codeine/mL of drinking water	1 to 2 mg acetaminophen + 0.1 to 0.2 mg codeine/mL of drinking water
Acetylsalicylic acid	100 mg/kg q 4 to 6 hours; PO	80 to 90 mg/kg q 4 hours; PO 20 mg/kg; SC		240 mg/kg q 4 hours; PO	240 mg/kg q 4 hours; PO	100 to 120 mg/kg q 4 hours; PO 20 mg/kg; SC	120 to 300 mg/kg q 4 hours; PO 20 mg/kg; SC

Drug							
Albendazole	7.5 to 20 mg/kg once daily; PO to treat *Encephalitozoon cuniculi*	50 to 100 mg/kg or 25 mg/kg once daily for 3 days to treat *Giardia*; PO					
Aluminum hydroxide/magnesium hydroxide/simethicone antacids (Diovol Plus)	1 to 2 mL as needed; PO	0.5 to 1 mL as needed; PO	1 mL as needed; PO	0.1 to 0.3 mL as needed; PO	0.1 to 0.3 mL as needed; PO	0.1 to 0.3 mL as needed; PO	0.1 to 0.3 mL as needed; PO
Amikacin	8 to 16 mg/kg total daily dose, once daily to divided tid; SC, IM, IV	10 to 15 mg/kg total daily dose, once daily to divided tid; SC, IM, IV	10 to 15 mg/kg total daily dose, once daily to divided tid; SC, IM, IV; 2 to 5 mg/kg bid to tid; SC, IM	10 to 20 mg/kg total daily dose, once daily to divided tid; IM, SC	10 to 20 mg/kg total daily dose, once daily to divided tid; IM, SC	10 to 20 mg/kg total daily dose, once daily to divided tid; IM, SC	10 to 20 mg/kg total daily dose, once daily to divided tid; IM, SC

(continued)

Drug	Rabbits	Guinea Pigs	Chinchillas	Hamsters	Gerbils	Rats	Mice
Aminophylline	4 mg/kg bid; IM, PO						
Amitraz (Mitaban) make up as per package directions		Make up as per package directions Apply topically 3 to 6 treatments 14 days apart		Make up as per package directions Apply topically 3 to 6 treatments 14 days apart			
Amoxicillin	DO NOT USE	6 mg/kg tid for 5 days; SC (do not increase dose)	DO NOT USE	DO NOT USE		150 mg/kg bid; IM	100 mg/kg bid; SC
Ampicillin	DO NOT USE (see drug description of topical use)	6 mg/kg tid for 5 days; SC (do not increase dose)	DO NOT USE	DO NOT USE	10 to 33 mg/kg tid; PO, SC	10 to 33 mg/kg tid; PO, SC	10 to 33 mg/kg tid; PO, SC

Drug					
Amprolium 9.6% solution	1 mL/7 kg once daily for 5 days; PO 0.5 mL/500 mL of drinking water for 10 days				
Ascorbic acid (see vitamin C)					
Aspirin (see acetylsalicylic acid)					
Atipamezole	1 mg/kg; IM, IP, SC, IV			1 mg/kg; IM, IP, SC, IV	1 mg/kg; IM, IP, SC, IV
	0.05 to 2 mg/kg; IM, SC (see drug description of atropinase, glycopyrrolate is preferred) 0.05 to 0.2 mg/kg; SC	0.04 to 0.05 mg/kg; SC, IM	0.04 to 0.05 mg/kg; SC, IM	0.04 to 0.05 mg/kg; SC, IM (see also glycopyrrolate)	0.02 to 0.05 mg/kg; SC, IM

(continued)

Drug	Rabbits	Guinea Pigs	Chinchillas	Hamsters	Gerbils	Rats	Mice
Atipamezole (cont.)	2 to 10 mg/kg q 20 minutes as necessary for organo-phos-phate toxicity; IM, SC						
	1% atropine oph-thalmic drops to dilate eyes in albino animals (see drug descrip-tion of atropinest-erase)	1% atropine oph-thalmic drops to dilate eyes in albino animals	1% atropine oph-thalmic drops to dilate eyes in albino animals	1% atropine oph-thalmic drops to dilate eyes in albino animals	1% atropine oph-thalmic drops to dilate eyes in albino animals	1% atropine ophthalmic drops to dilate eyes in albino animals	1% atropine ophthalmic drops to dilate eyes in albino animals

Drug						
Atropine Atropine + phenylephrine	1 drop of 1% atropine plus 1 drop of 10% phenylephrine ophthalmic drops 3 to 4 times over 15 minutes to dilate eyes in animals with ocular pigmentation (see drug description of atropinesterase)	1 drop of 1% atropine plus 1 drop of 10% phenylephrine ophthalmic drops 3 to 4 times over 15 minutes to dilate eyes in animals with ocular pigmentation	1 drop of 1% atropine plus 1 drop of 10% phenylephrine ophthalmic drops 3 to 4 times over 15 minutes to dilate eyes in animals with ocular pigmentation	1 drop of 1% atropine plus 1 drop of 10% phenylephrine ophthalmic drops 3 to 4 times over 15 minutes to dilate eyes in animals with ocular pigmentation	1 drop of 1% atropine plus 1 drop of 10% phenylephrine ophthalmic drops 3 to 4 times over 15 minutes to dilate eyes in animals with ocular pigmentation	1 drop of 1% atropine plus 1 drop of 10% phenylephrine ophthalmic drops 3 to 4 times over 15 minutes to dilate eyes in animals with ocular pigmentation
Barium sulfate	10 to 15 mL/kg; PO	3 to 10 mL/kg; PO	3 to 10 mL/kg; PO	3 to 10 mL/kg; PO	3 to 10 mL/kg; PO	3 to 10 mL/kg; PO

(continued)

Drug	Rabbits	Guinea Pigs	Chinchillas	Hamsters	Gerbils	Rats	Mice
Buprenorphine	0.01 to 0.05 mg/kg bid to qid; SC, IM, IV	0.05 to 0.1 mg/kg bid to tid; SC, IM	0.05 to 0.1 mg/kg bid to tid; SC, IM	0.05 to 0.1 mg/kg bid to tid; SC, IM	0.05 to 0.1 mg/kg bid to tid; SC, IM	0.01 to 0.1 mg/kg bid to tid; SC, IM	0.05 to 0.1 mg/kg bid to tid; SC, IM
Butorphanol	0.1 to 0.5 mg/kg q 2 to 4 hours; SC, IM, IV	2 mg/kg q 2 to 4 hours; SC, IM	0.2 mg/kg; SC, IM	2 mg/kg q 2 to 4 hours; SC, IM	2 mg/kg q 2 to 4 hours; SC, IM	0.5 to 5 mg/kg q 4 to 6 hours; SC, IM	1 to 5 mg/kg q 4 to 6 hours; SC, IM
Calcium EDTA	27.5 mg/kg bid to qid for 5 days; SC; dilute to 10 mg/mL with saline. Repeat if necessary.		25 to 30 mg/kg bid to qid for 5 days; SC			2.1 mg/kg; PO	5 to 10 mg/kg; PO

Drug					
Captan			1 teaspoon per 2 cups of dust bath		
Carbaryl 5% powder	Dust lightly once weekly	Dust lightly once weekly	Dust lightly once weekly	Dust lightly once weekly	Dust lightly once weekly
Carprofen	1 to 1.5 mg/kg bid; PO 1 to 5 mg/kg once daily; PO, SC			5 mg/kg once daily; PO, SC	5 mg/kg once daily; PO, SC
Cefazolin	20 to 30 mg/kg once daily; IM				
Ceftiofur	2 g lyophilized drug/20 g PMMA (local treatment in abscess cavities)				

(continued)

Drug	Rabbits	Guinea Pigs	Chinchillas	Hamsters	Gerbils	Rats	Mice
Cephalexin						60 mg/kg bid; PO 15 mg/kg bid; SC	60 mg/kg bid; PO 30 mg/kg bid; SC
Cephalothin	15 to 30 mg/kg once daily; SC, IM						
Chloramphenicol palmitate	50 mg/kg bid; PO	30 to 50 mg/kg bid to tid; PO	50 mg/kg bid; PO	50 to 200 mg/kg tid; PO	50 to 200 mg/kg tid; PO	50 to 200 mg/kg tid; PO	50 to 200 mg/kg tid; PO
Chloramphenicol succinate	30 to 50 mg/kg bid to tid; IM, SC	30 to 50 mg/kg bid; IM, SC	30 to 50 mg/kg bid; IM, SC	30 to 50 mg/kg bid to tid; IM, SC	30 to 50 mg/kg bid to tid; IM, SC	30 to 50 mg/kg bid to tid; IM, SC	30 to 50 mg/kg bid to tid; IM, SC
Chlorpromazine		25 mg/kg; SC				20 to 30 mg/kg; SC	
Chlortetracycline	50 mg/kg bid; PO	May cause dysbiosis	50 mg/kg bid; PO	20 mg/kg bid; IM, SC		6 to 10 mg/kg bid; SC, IM	25 mg/kg bid; SC, IM

Drug						
Cholestyramine	2 g in 20 mL water once daily by gavage (2.5 to 3.8 kg animal)					
Chorionic gonado-tropin	100 IU once, repeat in 10 to 14 days; IM					
Cimetidine	5 to 10 mg/kg bid to tid; PO, SC, IM, IV	5 to 10 mg/kg bid to tid; PO, SC, IM, IV	5 to 10 mg/kg bid to qid; PO, SC, IM	5 to 10 mg/kg bid to qid; PO, SC, IM	5 to 10 mg/kg bid to qid; PO, SC, IM	5 to 10 mg/kg bid to qid; PO, SC, IM
Ciprofloxacin	5 to 15 mg/kg bid; PO	5 to 15 mg/kg bid; PO	10 mg/kg bid; PO	10 mg/kg bid; PO	10 mg/kg bid; PO	10 mg/kg bid; PO
	15 to 20 mg/kg once daily to tid; PO	15 to 20 mg/kg once daily; PO	15 to 20 mg/kg once daily; PO	15 to 20 mg/kg once daily; PO	15 to 20 mg/kg once daily; PO	15 to 20 mg/kg once daily; PO
Cisapride	0.5 mg/kg once daily to tid; PO, SC			0.5 mg/kg tid; PO		

(continued)

Drug	Rabbits	Guinea Pigs	Chinchillas	Hamsters	Gerbils	Rats	Mice
Clotrimazole	Topical application to clipped skin as needed						
Codeine						60 mg/kg q 4 to 6 hours; SC	10 to 20 mg/kg q 4 to 6 hours; SC; 60 to 90 mg/kg q 4 hours; PO
Copper sulfate	1% topically applied as a dip						
Cyproheptadine	1 mg/rabbit once daily to bid; PO						
Dexamethasone	0.5 to 2 mg/kg bid; PO, SC, IM. Wean off dosage at end of treatment.	0.1 to 0.6 mg/kg; IM		0.1 to 0.6 mg/kg; IM	0.1 to 0.6 mg/kg; IM	0.1 to 0.6 mg/kg; IM	0.1 to 0.6 mg/kg; IM

Drug							
Diazepam	1 to 5 mg/kg; IM, IV	1 to 5 mg/kg; IM	1 to 5 mg/kg; IM 5 mg/kg; IP	3 to 5 mg/kg; IM 5 mg/kg; IP	3 to 5 mg/kg; IM 5 mg/kg; IP	2.5 to 5 mg/kg; IM 2.5 mg/kg; IP	3 to 5 mg/kg; IM 5 mg/kg; IP
Dichlorvos impregnated resin strip	Follow package directions for room size, hang in room for 24 hours once weekly for 6 weeks			1-inch square laid on cage for 24 hours once weekly for 6 weeks	1-inch square laid on cage for 24 hours once weekly for 6 weeks	1-inch square laid on cage for 24 hours once weekly for 6 weeks	1-inch square laid on cage for 24 hours once weekly for 6 weeks
Diethylstilbestrol	0.5 mg/kg PO once to twice per week as needed						
Dimetridazole	0.2 mg/mL of drinking water		0.8 mg/mL of drinking water	0.5 mg/mL of drinking water	0.5 mg/mL of drinking water	1 mg/mL of drinking water	1 mg/mL of drinking water
Dipyrone	6 to 12 mg/kg bid to tid; PO, SC, IM						

(continued)

Drug	Rabbits	Guinea Pigs	Chinchillas	Hamsters	Gerbils	Rats	Mice
Doxapram	2 to 5 mg/kg as needed; SC, IV		5 to 10 mg/kg; SC, IV	5 to 10 mg/kg; SC, IV	5 to 10 mg/kg; SC, IV	5 to 10 mg/kg; SC, IV	5 to 10 mg/kg; SC, IV
Doxycycline	2.5 to 5 mg/kg bid; PO 4 mg/kg once daily, PO 100 to 200 mg/L of drinking water for 14 days	2.5 to 5 mg/kg bid; PO	2.5 to 5 mg/kg bid; PO	2.5 to 5 mg/kg bid; PO	2.5 to 5 mg/kg bid; PO	2.5 to 5 mg/kg bid for 7 to 21 days; PO	2.5 to 5 mg/kg bid; PO
Enilconazole	Apply topically as required 2 mg/mL solution, rinse twice weekly for 3 weeks	Apply topically as required 2 mg/mL solution, rinse twice weekly for 3 weeks					

Enrofloxacin (see text re SC use)	*5 mg/kg bid; PO, SC	2.5 to 10 mg/kg bid; PO, SC, IM	2.5 to 10 mg/kg bid; PO, SC, IM	10 mg/kg bid for 5 to 7 days; PO, IM		2.5 to 10 mg/kg bid; PO, SC, IM	2.5 to 10 mg/kg bid; PO, SC, IM
	5 to 15 mg/kg bid; PO, SC, IM (general range)	5 to 10 mg/kg once daily; PO, IM	5 to 10 mg/kg once daily; PO, IM	5 to 10 mg/kg once daily; PO, IM	5 to 10 mg/kg once daily; PO, IM	5 to 10 mg/kg once daily; PO, IM	5 to 10 mg/kg once daily; PO, IM
	50 to 200 mg/L of drinking water for 14 days	50 to 200 mg/L of drinking water for 14 days	50 to 200 mg/L of drinking water for 14 days	50 to 200 mg/L of drinking water for 14 days	50 to 200 mg/L of drinking water for 14 days	50 to 200 mg/L of drinking water for 14 days	50 to 200 mg/L of drinking water for 14 days
Enrofloxacin (Baytril Otic)	Apply topically as directed, adjust dose to body size of patient						

(continued)

Drug	Rabbits	Guinea Pigs	Chinchillas	Hamsters	Gerbils	Rats	Mice
Erythromycin	DO NOT USE	DO NOT USE	DO NOT USE	500 mg/gal (United States) [132 mg/L] of drinking water continuously 20 mg/kg bid; PO			
Fenbendazole	20 mg/kg once daily for 5 days; PO; also used once daily or divided bid long term for Rx of Encephalitozoon cuniculi	20 mg/kg once daily for 5 days; PO	20 mg/kg once daily for 5 days; PO	20 mg/kg once daily for 5 days; PO	20 mg/kg once daily for 5 days; PO	20 mg/kg once daily for 5 days; PO	20 mg/kg once daily for 5 days; PO

	10 to 20 mg/kg; PO once, repeat in 10 to 14 days	50 to 100 mg/kg once; PO	50 mg/kg once daily for 3 days, repeat in 2 and 4 weeks; PO	50 mg/kg once daily for 3 days, repeat in 2 and 4 weeks; PO	50 mg/kg once daily for 3 days, repeat in 2 and 4 weeks; PO	50 mg/kg once daily for 3 days, repeat in 2 and 4 weeks; PO	50 mg/kg once daily for 3 days, repeat in 2 and 4 weeks; PO
Fentanyl + droperidol (see Innovar-Vet)							
Fentanyl + fluanisone (see Hypnorm)							
Fipronil	DO NOT USE						
Flumazenil	0.1 mg/kg; IV						
Flunixin	0.3 to 2 mg/kg once daily to bid for no more than 3 days; PO, deep IM	2.5 mg/kg once daily to bid; IM	2.5 mg/kg once daily to bid; IM	2.5 mg/kg once daily to bid; IM	2.5 mg/kg once daily to bid; IM	2.5 mg/kg once daily to bid; IM	2.5 mg/kg once daily to bid; IM
Furosemide	2 to 5 mg/kg bid; PO, SC, IM, IV	2 to 5 mg/kg bid; PO, SC	2 to 5 mg/kg bid; PO, SC	2 to 5 mg/kg bid; PO, SC	2 to 5 mg/kg bid; PO, SC	2 to 5 mg/kg bid; PO, SC	2 to 5 mg/kg bid; PO, SC (continued)

Drug	Rabbits	Guinea Pigs	Chinchillas	Hamsters	Gerbils	Rats	Mice
Gentamicin	5 to 8 mg/kg total dose; once daily or divided bid for 28 to 40 days; SC, IM	5 to 8 mg/kg total dose; once daily to divided tid; SC, IM, IV	5 to 8 mg/kg total dose; once daily to divided tid; SC, IM, IV	5 to 8 mg/kg total dose; once daily to divided tid; SC, IM, IV	5 to 8 mg/kg total dose; once daily to divided tid; SC, IM, IV	5 to 8 mg/kg total dose; once daily to divided tid; SC, IM, IV	5 to 8 mg/kg total dose; once daily to divided tid; SC, IM, IV
		5 mg/kg once daily; SC, IM	5 mg/kg once daily; SC, IM	5 mg/kg once daily; SC, IM	5 mg/kg once daily; SC, IM	5 mg/kg once daily; SC, IM	5 mg/kg once daily; SC, IM
Glycopyrrolate	0.01 to 0.1 mg/kg; SC, IM	0.01 to 0.1 mg/kg; SC, IM		0.01 to 0.1 mg/kg; SC, IM	0.01 to 0.1 mg/kg; SC, IM	0.01 to 0.1 mg/kg; SC, IM	0.01 to 0.1 mg/kg; SC, IM
Griseofulvin	25 mg/kg once daily or divided bid for 28 to 40 days; PO	25 mg/kg once daily for 3 to 5 weeks; PO	25 mg/kg once daily for 3 to 5 weeks; PO	25 mg/kg once daily for 2 to 4 weeks; PO	25 mg/kg once daily for 2 to 4 weeks; PO	25 mg/kg once daily for 2 to 4 weeks; PO	25 mg/kg once daily for 2 to 4 weeks; PO
		300 g/ton guinea pig pellets					

Halothane	Inhalant anesthetic	Inhalant anesthetic	Inhalant anesthetic	Inhalant anesthetic	Inhalant anesthetic	Inhalant anesthetic	Inhalant anesthetic	Inhalant anesthetic
Hypnorm	0.2 to 0.5 mL/kg; IM	0.5 to 2 mL/kg; SC, IM, IP	0.5 to 1 mL/kg; IM	0.5 to 1 mL/kg once; IP, SC	0.5 to 1 mL/kg; IM	0.3 to 0.6 mL/kg once; SC, IP	0.3 to 0.6 mL/kg once; SC, IP	0.2 to 0.5 mL/kg once; IM
Hypnorm + diazepam	0.3 mL/kg; IM + 2 mg/kg; IV	0.3 mL/kg; IM + 2 mg/mL; IP 1 mL/kg + 2.5 mg/kg; IP	1 mL/kg + 2.5 mg/kg; IP			0.3 to 0.4 mL/kg + 2.5 mg/kg; IM, IP	0.3 to 0.4 mL/kg + 2.5 mg/kg; IM, IP	0.4 mL/kg + 5 mg/kg; IP
Hypnorm + midazolam (Versed)	0.3 mL/kg; IM + 0.5 to 2 mg/kg; IV	8 mL/kg; IP (1 part Hypnorm + 1 part Versed + 2 parts sterile water)	4 mL/kg; IP (1 part Hypnorm + 1 part Versed + 2 parts sterile water)	8 mL/kg; IP (1 part Hypnorm + 1 part Versed + 2 parts sterile water)		8 mL/kg; IP (1 part Hypnorm + 1 part Versed + 2 parts sterile water)	2.7 mL/kg; IP (1 part Hypnorm + 1 part Versed + 2 parts sterile water)	10 mL/kg; IP (1 part Hypnorm + 1 part Versed + 2 parts sterile water)
Ibuprofen	10 to 20 mg/kg q 4 hours; IV	10 mg/kg q 4 hours; IM					10 to 30 mg/kg q 4 hours; PO	7 to 15 mg/kg q 4 hours; PO

(continued)

Drug	Rabbits	Guinea Pigs	Chinchillas	Hamsters	Gerbils	Rats	Mice
Ibuprofen (cont.)	7.5 to 20 mg/kg q 4 hours; PO					15 mg/kg once daily; PO	30 mg/kg once daily; PO
Imidacloprid	Treat as per cats						
Innovar-Vet 10% solution	0.1 to 0.3 mL/kg; SC, IM	0.44 to 0.8 mL/kg; SC, IM		DO NOT USE	DO NOT USE	0.1 to 0.5 mL/kg; SC, IM	0.1 to 0.5 mL/kg; SC, IM
Innovar-Vet 10% solution + xylazine		0.2 to 0.4 mL/kg + 20 mg/kg IM				0.1 to 0.15 mL/kg + 20 mg/kg; IM	
Isoflurane	Anesthetic of choice	Anesthetic of choice	Anesthetic of choice	Anesthetic of choice	Anesthetic of choice	Anesthetic of choice	Anesthetic of choice
Itraconazole	5 to 10 mg/kg daily for 3 to 4 weeks; PO						
Ivermectin	200 to 400 µg/kg once, repeat in	300 to 500 µg/kg once, repeat in	200 to 400 µg/kg once, repeat in	200 to 400 µg/kg once, repeat in	200 to 400 µg/kg once, repeat in	200 to 400 µg/kg once, repeat in 7 to 10 days; PO, SC	200 to 400 µg/kg once, repeat in 7 to 10 days; PO, SC

10 to 14 days for a total of 2 to 3 treatments as needed; PO, SC. For ear mites dose can be divided in two and applied topically into each ear. Use at least two doses, up to 18 days apart.	7 to 10 days; PO, SC	7 to 10 days; PO, SC	7 to 10 days; PO, SC		200 µg/kg once daily for 5 days (for pinworms)	2 mg/kg once, repeat in 10 days **OR** 1 mg/kg once daily for 2 days; PO, SC (for pinworms)
Ketamine 20 to 50 mg/kg; IM	20 to 60 mg/kg; IM, IP	20 to 60 mg/kg; IM, IP	40 to 80 mg/kg; IP	40 to 100 mg/kg; IP	40 to 80 mg/kg; IP	40 to 80 mg/kg; IP
Ketamine + acepromazine 25 to 50 mg/kg + 0.25 to 1 mg/kg; IM	20 to 50 mg/kg + 0.5 to 1 mg/kg; IM	20 to 40 mg/kg + 0.5 mg/kg; IM (surgical anesthesia)	50 to 150 mg/kg + 2.5 to 5 mg/kg; IM	DO NOT USE	50 to 75 mg/kg + 2.5 to 5 mg/kg; IM, IP	50 to 100 mg/kg + 2.5 to 5 mg/kg; IM

(continued)

Drug	Rabbits	Guinea Pigs	Chinchillas	Hamsters	Gerbils	Rats	Mice
Ketamine + diazepam	20 to 40 mg/kg + 5 to 10 mg/kg; IM	20 to 50 mg/kg + 3 to 5 mg/kg; IM	20 to 40 mg/kg + 1 to 5 mg/kg; IM (light anesthesia)	40 to 70 mg/kg + 2 to 5 mg/kg; IM	40 to 50 mg/kg + 3 to 5 mg/kg; IM, IP	40 to 75 mg/kg + 3 to 5 mg/kg; IM	40 to 100 mg/kg + 3 to 5 mg/kg; IM
Ketamine + medetomidine	25 to 35 mg/kg + 0.5 mg/kg; IM	40 mg/kg + 0.5 mg/kg; IM, IP	40 mg/kg + 0.5 mg/kg; IM, IP	100 mg/kg + 0.25 mg/kg; IP	40 mg/kg + 1 to 2 mg/kg; IM	75 mg/kg + 0.5 mg/kg; IP	65 to 75 mg/kg + 1 mg/kg; IP
Ketamine + xylazine	20 to 40 mg/kg + 3 to 5 mg/kg; IM	20 to 50 mg/kg + 2 to 5 mg/kg; IM	35 to 40 mg/kg + 1 to 8 mg/kg; IM	50 to 150 mg/kg + 1 to 10 mg/kg; IM	50 to 70 mg/kg + 1 to 2 mg/kg; IM, IP	75 to 100 mg/kg + 1 to 5 mg/kg; IM, IP	50 to 100 mg/kg + 1 to 10 mg/kg; IM
	10 mg/kg + 3 mg/kg; IV						
Ketoconazole	10 to 15 mg/kg once daily for 3 to 4 weeks						

Ketoprofen	1 mg/kg bid to tid; IM 3 to 5 mg/kg once daily; SC		5 mg/kg once daily; SC, PO
Leuprolide acetate	100 to 200 µg/guinea pig; IM		
Lime sulfur 2.5% solution	Apply once weekly for 4 to 6 weeks	Apply once weekly for 4 to 6 weeks	
Lindane (0.03% solution)	Dip once weekly for 3 weeks	Dip once weekly for 3 weeks	Dip once per week for 3 weeks
Loperamide (Immodium)	0.1 mg/kg tid for 3 days, then once daily for 2 days; PO (coliform diarrhea) 0.1 to 0.2 mg/kg q 4 hours for 2 to 3 doses; PO (gastric stasis)		Dip once per week for 3 weeks

(continued)

Drug	Rabbits	Guinea Pigs	Chinchillas	Hamsters	Gerbils	Rats	Mice
Lufenuron	Treat as per cat						
Malathion (2% solution)	Dip once q 10 days for 3 weeks	Dip once q 10 days for 3 weeks				Dip once q 10 days for 3 weeks	Dip once q 10 days for 3 weeks
MECA	1 part MECA: 1 part activator: 10 parts water; applied topically as a dip or spray						
Meclizine	12.5 to 25 mg/kg bid to tid; PO						
Medetomidine (see also Ketamine + medetomidine)	0.5 mg/kg; SC			0.1 mg/kg; SC		0.03 to 0.1 mg/kg; SC	0.03 to 0.1 mg/kg; SC

Meloxicam	0.1 to 0.3 mg/kg once daily, taper to lowest dose possible after 2 to 3 days; PO, SC					1 mg/kg once daily, taper to lowest dose possible after 2 to 3 days; PO, SC 0.2 mg/kg; SC
Meperidine	5 to 20 mg/kg q 2 to 6 hours as needed; SC, IM 0.2 mg/mL of drinking water	10 to 20 mg/kg q 2 to 6 hours as needed; SC, IM 0.2 mg/mL of drinking water	10 to 20 mg/kg q 2 to 6 hours as needed; SC, IM 0.2 mg/mL of drinking water	10 to 20 mg/kg q 2 to 6 hours as needed; SC, IM 0.2 mg/mL of drinking water	10 to 50 mg/kg q 2 to 3 hours as needed; SC, IM 0.2 mg/mL of drinking water	10 to 20 mg/kg q 2 to 3 hours as needed; SC, IM 0.2 mg/mL of drinking water
Metoclopramide	0.5 mg/kg tid to qid; PO, SC					

(continued)

Drug	Rabbits	Guinea Pigs	Chinchillas	Hamsters	Gerbils	Rats	Mice
Metronidazole	20 to 60 mg/kg bid for 3 to 5 days or as needed; PO	20 to 60 mg/kg bid to tid; PO	20 to 60 mg/kg bid to tid; PO	20 to 60 mg/kg bid to tid; PO	20 to 60 mg/kg bid to tid; PO	10 to 60 mg/kg bid to tid; PO	10 to 60 mg/kg bid to tid; PO
	25 mg/kg bid for up to 21 days; PO for anaerobic dental infections		10 to 40 mg/kg once daily to bid; PO	7.5 mg/70 to 90 g hamster tid; PO; 210 mg/kg per day; PO (protection against C. difficile enterocolitis)		10 to 40 mg/rat once daily; PO	2.5 mg/mL of drinking water for 5 days
Miconazole (cream or 2% shampoo)	Apply topically as required	Apply topically as required	Apply topically as required				

Drug							
Midazolam	0.5 to 2 mg/kg; IM	1 to 5 mg/kg; SC, IM		1 to 2 mg/kg; SC, IM 5 mg/kg; IP	1 to 2 mg/kg; SC, IM 5 mg/kg; IP	1 to 2 mg/kg; SC, IM 2.5 mg/kg; IP	1 to 2 mg/kg; SC, IM 5 mg/kg; IP
Moxidectin	0.2 mg/kg every 10 days for 2 treatments						
Nalbuphine	1 to 2 mg/kg q 4 hours as required; SC, IM, IV	1 to 4 mg/kg q 3 hours as required; SC, IM		4 to 8 mg/kg q 3 hours as required; SC, IM	4 to 8 mg/kg q 3 hours as required; SC, IM	1 to 4 mg/kg q 3 hours as required; SC, IM	2 to 8 mg/kg q 3 hours as required; SC, IM
Naloxone (titrate to effect)	0.2 mg/kg; IM, IV	0.01 to 0.2 mg/kg; IM, IV		0.01 to 0.2 mg/kg; IM, IP, IV	0.01 to 0.2 mg/kg; IM, IP, IV	0.01 to 0.2 mg/kg; IM, IP, IV	0.01 to 0.2 mg/kg; IM, IP, IV
Neomycin	30 mg/kg once daily to bid; PO 0.2 to 0.8 mg/mL of drinking water	30 to 50 mg/kg once daily; PO	15 mg/kg bid; PO	100 mg/kg once daily; PO 0.44 mg/mL of drinking water	100 mg/kg once daily; PO 2.6 mg/mL of drinking water	50 mg/kg once daily; PO ~2.6 mg/mL of drinking water	50 mg/kg once daily; PO ~2.6 mg/mL of drinking water

(continued)

Drug	Rabbits	Guinea Pigs	Chinchillas	Hamsters	Gerbils	Rats	Mice
Oxymorphone	0.05 to 0.2 mg/kg bid to tid; SC, IM	0.2 to 0.5 mg/kg bid to qid; SC, IM		0.2 to 0.5 mg/kg bid to qid; SC, IM	0.2 to 0.5 mg/kg bid to qid; SC, IM	0.2 to 0.5 mg/kg bid to qid; SC, IM	0.2 to 0.5 mg/kg bid to qid; SC, IM
Oxytetracycline	15 mg/kg tid; SC, IM	Caution: may result in dysbiosis	10 mg/kg bid; IM	16 mg/kg once daily; SC	20 mg/kg once daily; SC	6 to 10 mg/kg bid; IM	
	50 mg/kg bid; PO		50 mg/kg bid; PO		10 mg/kg tid; PO	10 to 20 mg/kg tid; PO	10 to 20 mg/kg tid; PO
	1 mg/mL of drinking water	1 mg/mL of drinking water	1 mg/mL of drinking water	0.25 to 1 mg/mL of drinking water	0.8 mg/mL of drinking water	0.4 mg/mL of drinking water	0.4 mg/mL of drinking water
Oxytocin	1 to 2 U/rabbit; SC, IM	0.2 to 3 U/kg; IM 1 U/guinea pig; SC, IM	0.2 to 3 U/kg; SC, IM, IV 1 U/chinchilla; SC, IM	0.2 to 3 U/kg; IM, SC	0.2 to 3 U/kg; IM, SC	1 U/kg; SC, IM	5 to 10 mg/kg q

Pancreatic enzyme replacement	1 teaspoon + 3 tablespoons yogurt; let stand 15 minutes, then give 2 to 3 mL bid
Penicillin G, procaine	20,000 to 60,000 U/kg once daily for 5 to 7 days; SC, IM
Penicillin G, benzathine + procaine	47,000 to 84,000 U/kg once per week for 3 treatments; SC, IM (*Treponema cuniculi*)

(continued)

Drug	Rabbits	Guinea Pigs	Chinchillas	Hamsters	Gerbils	Rats	Mice
Penicillin G, benzathine + procaine (cont.)	75,000 U/rabbit < 2.5 kg; 150,000 U/rabbit > 2.5 kg; q 48 hours for 8 weeks; then q 72 hours for 4 weeks; SC (for treatment of abscesses)						
Pentazocine	5 to 10 mg/kg q 4 hours; SC, IM, IV	5 to 10 mg/kg q 2 to 4 hours; SC, IM		5 to 10 mg/kg q 2 to 4 hours; SC, IM	5 to 10 mg/kg q 2 to 4 hours; SC, IM	5 to 10 mg/kg q 2 to 4 hours; SC, IM	2 to 4 hours; SC, IM
Piperazine adipate	500 mg/kg once daily for 2 days; PO	4 to 7 mg/mL of drinking water for 3 to 10 days	500 mg/kg once daily for 2 days; PO	3 to 5 mg/mL of drinking water for 7 days, off 7 days, on 7 days	3 to 5 mg/mL of drinking water 7 days, off 7 days, on 7 days	4 to 7 mg/mL of drinking water for 3 to 10 days	4 to 7 mg/mL of drinking water for 3 to 10 days

| Piperazine citrate | 1 mg/mL of drinking water for 1 day, repeat in 10 to 14 days 3 mg/mL of drinking water for 14 days on, 14 days off, repeat 100 to 200 mg/kg once daily for 2 days, or once and repeat in 10 to 14 days; PO | 10 mg/mL of drinking water for 7 days, off 7 days, on 7 days | 100 mg/kg once daily for 7 days; PO | 10 mg/mL of drinking water for 7 days, off 7 days, on 7 days | 4 to 5 mg/mL of drinking water for 7 days, off 7 days, on 7 days | 4 to 5 mg/mL of drinking water for 7 days, off 7 days, on 7 days | 4 to 5 mg/mL of drinking water for 7 days, off 7 days, on 7 days |

(continued)

Drug	Rabbits	Guinea Pigs	Chinchillas	Hamsters	Gerbils	Rats	Mice
Polysulfated glycosamino-glycans	2.2 mg/kg q 3 days for 21 to 28 days, then q 14 days; SC, IM						
Praziquantel	5 to 10 mg/kg once, repeat in 10 days; PO, SC, IM	5 to 10 mg/kg once, repeat in 10 days; PO, SC, IM	5 to 10 mg/kg once, repeat in 10 days; PO, SC, IM	5 to 11 mg/kg once, repeat in 10 days; PO, SC, IM	5 to 11 mg/kg once, repeat in 10 days; PO, SC, IM	5 to 11 mg/kg once, repeat in 10 days; PO, SC, IM	25 mg/kg once, repeat in 10 days; PO, SC, IM
						30 mg/kg, 3 doses @ 2-week intervals; PO	30 mg/kg, 3 doses @ 2-week intervals; PO
Prednisone	0.5 to 2 mg/kg; PO	0.5 to 2 mg/kg; PO, SC	.0.5 to 2 mg/kg; PO, SC	0.5 to 2 mg/kg; PO	0.5 to 2 mg/kg; PO	0.5 to 2 mg/kg; PO	0.5 to 2 mg/kg; PO
Propofol	10 mg/cg; IV slowly					10 mg/kg induction, 0.6 mg/kg per minute constant infusion; IV	26 mg/kg induction, 2.2 mg/kg per minute constant infusion; IV

Pyrethrin products (0.05% shampoo) or use as directed for cats	Once weekly for 4 weeks	Once weekly for 4 weeks	Once weekly for 4 weeks	Once weekly for 4 weeks	Once weekly for 4 weeks	Once weekly for 4 weeks	Once weekly for 4 weeks	Once weekly for 4 weeks
Selamectin	Treat as per cat							
Sevoflurane	Inhalant anesthetic used to effect	Inhalant anesthetic used to effect	Inhalant anesthetic used to effect	Inhalant anesthetic used to effect	Inhalant anesthetic used to effect	Inhalant anesthetic used to effect	Inhalant anesthetic used to effect	
Simethicone	1 to 2 mL (20 mg/0.3 mL product) as needed; PO							
Stanozolol	1 to 2 mg/rabbit; PO, once							

(continued)

Drug	Rabbits	Guinea Pigs	Chinchillas	Hamsters	Gerbils	Rats	Mice
Sulfadimethoxine	25 to 50 mg/kg once daily, or 50 mg/kg loading dose followed by 25 mg/kg for 5 days; PO 12.5 to 15 mg/kg bid for 10 to 14 days; PO	25 to 50 mg/kg once daily for 10 to 14 days; PO	25 to 50 mg/kg once daily for 10 to 14 days; PO	25 to 50 mg/kg once daily for 10 to 14 days; PO			
Sulfamerazine	0.2 to 1 mg/mL of drinking water	1 mg/mL of drinking water	1 mg/mL of drinking water	1 mg/mL of drinking water	1 mg/mL of drinking water	1 mg/mL of drinking water or 0.25 mg/g of diet	1 mg/mL of drinking water or 0.25 mg/g of diet
Sulfamethazine	1 to 5 mg/mL of drinking water 5 to 10 mg/g of diet	1 to 5 mg/mL of drinking water	1 to 5 mg/mL of drinking water	1 to 5 mg/mL of drinking water	1 to 5 mg/mL of drinking water	1 to 5 mg/mL of drinking water	1 to 5 mg/mL of drinking water

Drug							
Sulfaquinoxaline	0.25 to 1 mg/mL of drinking water 0.6 mg/g of diet	1 mg/mL of drinking water	1 mg/mL of drinking water	1 mg/mL of drinking water	1 mg/mL of drinking water	1 mg/mL of drinking water	1 mg/mL of drinking water
T-61	0.3 mL/kg; IV	0.3 mL/kg; IV	0.3 mL/kg; IV	0.3 mL/kg; IV	0.3 mL/kg; IV	0.3 mL/kg; IV	0.3 mL/kg; IV
Terbinafine	8 to 20 mg/kg once daily for 3 to 4 weeks; PO	*4 to 12.5 mg/kg once daily; PO					
Tetracycline	50 mg/kg bid to tid; PO	10 to 20 mg/kg bid to tid; PO	50 mg/kg bid to tid; PO	10 to 20 mg/kg tid; PO	10 to 20 mg/kg tid; PO	10 to 20 mg/kg tid; PO	10 to 20 mg/kg tid; PO
	1 mg/mL of drinking water	0.7 mg/mL of drinking water (may cause dysbiosis)	0.3 to 2 mg/mL of drinking water	0.4 mg/mL of drinking water	2 to 5 mg/mL of drinking water	2 to 5 mg/mL of drinking water OR 1 to 5 mg/g of diet	2 to 5 mg/mL of drinking water

(continued)

Drug	Rabbits	Guinea Pigs	Chinchillas	Hamsters	Gerbils	Rats	Mice
Thiabendazole	50 to 100 mg/kg once daily for 5 days; PO *110 mg/kg once, then 70 mg/kg q 4 hours for 8 doses; PO (versus *Obeliscoides cuniculi*)	100 mg/kg once daily for 5 days; PO	50 to 100 mg/kg once daily for 5 days, PO	100 mg/kg once daily for 5 days; PO	100 mg/kg once daily for 5 days; PO	100 mg/kg once daily for 5 days; PO	100 mg/kg once daily for 5 days; PO
Thiopental	15 to 20 mg/kg; IV	20 to 55 mg/kg; IP	40 mg/kg; IP	40 mg/kg; IP		30 to 40 mg/kg; IV, IP	25 to 50 mg/kg; IP
Tiletamine-zolazepam	DO NOT USE	20 to 60 mg/kg; IM (anesthesia) [see	20 to 44 mg/kg; IM (light anesthesia)	50 to 80 mg/kg; IM (anesthesia)	50 to 80 mg/kg; IM (anesthesia)	10 to 40 mg/kg; IM (anesthesia)	50 to 80 mg/kg; IM, IP (anesthesia)

	description of drug before use in guinea pigs]				
	3 mg/kg; IM (sedation)	3 mg/kg; IM (sedation)	3 mg/kg; IM (sedation)	3 mg/kg; IM (sedation)	3 mg/kg; IM (sedation)
Tilmicosin	15 to 25 mg/kg; SC (may be toxic—see drug description)				
Tresaderm (dexamethasone, neomycin, thiabendazole)	Install 3 drops in ear bid for 7 days, stop for 7 days, then repeat (for ear				

(continued)

Drug	Rabbits	Guinea Pigs	Chinchillas	Hamsters	Gerbils	Rats	Mice
Tresaderm (cont.)	mites; may be used alone or in combination with ivermectin)						
Trimethoprim sulfadiazine	30 mg/kg once daily to bid; SC	30 mg/kg once daily to bid; SC, IM	30 mg/kg once daily to bid; SC, IM	30 mg/kg once daily; SC	30 mg/kg once daily; SC	30 mg/kg once daily; SC	30 mg/kg once daily; SC
Trimethoprim-sulfamethoxazole	15 to 30 mg/kg bid; PO	15 to 50 mg/kg bid; PO	15 to 30 mg/kg bid; PO	15 to 30 mg/kg bid; PO	15 to 30 mg/kg bid; PO	15 to 30 mg/kg bid; PO	15 to 30 mg/kg bid; PO
Tropicamide 1% eye drops	Topically to dilate eyes in albino animals (see drug description of atropinesterase)	Topically to dilate eyes in albino animals	Topically to dilate eyes in albino animals	Topically to dilate eyes in albino animals	Topically to dilate eyes in albino animals	Topically to dilate eyes in albino animals	Topically to dilate eyes in albino animals

Tylosin	10 mg/kg once daily to bid; SC, IM, PO	10 mg/kg once daily, SC, IM, PO	10 mg/kg once daily, SC, IM, PO	2 to 8 mg/kg bid; SC, IM, PO	10 mg/kg once daily to bid; SC, IM, PO	10 mg/kg once daily to bid; SC, IM, PO
				10 mg/kg once daily; SC, IM, PO		
	0.5 mg/mL of drinking water (toxicity reported)			0.5 mg/mL of drinking water (toxicity reported)	0.5 mg/mL of drinking water	~0.5 mg/mL of drinking water
Verapamil	200 µg/kg at surgery and tid for 9 doses total; IV, IP					

(continued)

Drug	Rabbits	Guinea Pigs	Chinchillas	Hamsters	Gerbils	Rats	Mice
Vitamin B complex	Dose to thiamine content at 1 to 2 mg/kg as needed; IM	Dose to thiamine content at 1 to 2 mg/kg as needed; IM	Dose to thiamine content at 1 to 2 mg/kg as needed; IM	Dose to thiamine content at 1 to 2 mg/kg as needed; IM	Dose to thiamine content at 1 to 2 mg/kg as needed; IM	Dose to thiamine content at 1 to 2 mg/kg as needed; IM	Dose to thiamine content at 1 to 2 mg/kg as needed; IM
Vitamin C		10 to 30 mg/kg once daily for maintenance; up to 50 mg/kg for treatment of deficiency; SC, IM, PO 200 to 1,000 mg/mL of drinking water					

Drug							
Vitamin K₁	1 to 10 mg/kg as needed; IM	1 to 10 mg/kg as needed; IM	1 to 10 mg/kg as needed; IM	1 to 10 mg/kg as needed; IM	1 to 10 mg/kg as needed; IM	1 to 10 mg/kg as needed; IM	1 to 10 mg/kg as needed; IM
Xylazine (see Ketamine + xylazine)							
Yohimbine	0.2 mg/kg; IV 0.5 mg/kg; IM		0.2 mg/kg; IV 0.5 mg/kg; IM	0.2 mg/kg; IV 0.5 mg/kg; IM	0.2 mg/kg; IV 0.5 mg/kg; IM	0.2 mg/kg; IV 0.5 mg/kg; IM	0.2 mg/kg; IV 0.5 mg/kg; IM

*, drug dosages derived from pharmacokinetic work or efficacy trials in exotic species; PMMA, polymethylmethacrylate.

Handbook of Veterinary Drugs, Third Edition, edited by Dana Allen,
Lippincott Williams & Wilkins, Baltimore. © 2005

Section 10

Description of Drugs for Rodents and Rabbits

ACEPROMAZINE

INDICATIONS: Acepromazine (formerly Acetylpromazine) (Atravet
✤ ★, PromAce ★) is a phenothiazine drug used as a sedative and pre-
anesthetic agent. For more information, see ACEPROMAZINE in the
Small Animal section.

ADVERSE AND COMMON SIDE EFFECTS: The use of acepromazine may precipitate seizures in gerbils. Hypotension may occur
at the higher dosages.

ACETAMINOPHEN

INDICATIONS: Acetaminophen (Atasol ✤, Tempra ✤ ★, Tylenol ✤ ★)
is an antipyretic, analgesic agent with weak anti-inflammatory properties. See ACETAMINOPHEN in the Small Animal section.

ADVERSE AND COMMON SIDE EFFECTS: Acetaminophen has not
been used extensively in rabbits and rodents; therefore, little information is available regarding toxicity. Published dosages are very high as
compared to those for the dog and the cat. See ACETAMINOPHEN in
the Small Animal section for details on toxicity in these species.

DRUG INTERACTIONS: Human acetaminophen plus codeine elixirs
can be used in drinking water for enhanced analgesia in rodents. Dex-

trose or other sweeteners should be added to the water to increase palatability.

ACETYLSALICYLIC ACID

INDICATIONS: Acetylsalicylic acid (ASA) or aspirin (ArthriCare ★, Entrophen ✚, and many others) is an effective analgesic, antipyretic, and nonsteroidal anti-inflammatory agent. Aspirin should not be used for deep visceral or acute, intense pain. In rabbits, aspirin has a wide volume of tissue distribution and a half-life of 9.7 hours when administered orally. Oral doses can be dissolved in drinking water. For more information, see ASPIRIN in the Small Animal section.

ADVERSE AND COMMON SIDE EFFECTS: Gastric upset may occur after several treatments.

ALBENDAZOLE

INDICATIONS: Albendazole (Valbazen ✚ ★) is an anthelmintic marketed for use in cattle and sheep against all stages of liver flukes, tapeworms, gastric and intestinal nematodes, and lungworms. The drug has been used in small animals for the treatment of filaroidiasis, capillariasis, giardiasis, and paragonimiasis. Albendazole is safer and more effective than metronidazole or quinacrine for the treatment of giardiasis. For more information, see ALBENDAZOLE in the Small Animal section.

Albendazole has been used to treat giardiasis in chinchillas, and may be useful for the treatment of *Encephalitozoon cuniculi* infection in rabbits.

SUPPLIED AS VETERINARY PRODUCTS:
Suspension containing 113.6 mg/mL
Oral paste containing 30% albendazole

ALUMINUM HYDROXIDE

INDICATIONS: Aluminum hydroxide (Amphojel ✚ ★, Dialume ★) is an antacid, antiflatulent medication useful in the treatment of gastric ulcers and hyperphosphatemia associated with renal failure. Aluminum hydroxide may be combined with magnesium hydroxide and with simethicone (Diovol Plus ✚). The addition of magnesium hydroxide (Amphojel 500 ★, Maalox ✚ ★) optimizes the extent and rate of acid neutralization.

These products have been used to reduce excess gas production in gastrointestinal disturbances in rabbits and rodents. For more information, see ANTACIDS and ALUMINUM HYDROXIDE in the Small Animal section.

ADVERSE AND COMMON SIDE EFFECTS: These compounds are contraindicated in animals with alkalosis. The aluminum component may predispose to constipation. Aluminum-containing antacids may delay gastric emptying and should be used with caution in patients with gastric outlet obstruction. This would be particularly relevant to rabbits with poor gastric motility.

DRUG INTERACTIONS: Antacid products may interfere with or promote the absorption of a variety of other medications, including tetracycline antibiotics. For more information, see ANTACIDS and ALUMINUM HYDROXIDE in the Small Animal section.

AMIKACIN

INDICATIONS: Amikacin (Amiglyde-V ✿ ★, Amikin ✿ ★, Amiject D ★) is an aminoglycoside antibiotic indicated for the treatment of infections caused by many gram-negative bacteria including susceptible strains of *Escherichia coli*, *Klebsiella* spp., *Proteus* spp., and *Pseudomonas* spp. For more information, see AMIKACIN and AMINOGLYCOSIDE ANTIBIOTICS in the Small Animal section.

ADVERSE AND COMMON SIDE EFFECTS: Nephrotoxicity may occur, especially in animals that are dehydrated, have electrolyte imbalances, or have preexisting renal disease. Concurrent administration of fluids is recommended, especially in gerbils.

AMINOPHYLLINE

INDICATIONS: Aminophylline (Phyllocontin ✿ ★ and generics) is a bronchodilator principally used for the management of cough caused by bronchospasm. It has mild inotropic properties and mild, transient diuretic activity. The drug has been used via nebulization as well as the standard routes of administration.

Aminophylline has been recommended for the treatment of respiratory disease using protocols similar to those in dogs and cats.

ADVERSE AND COMMON SIDE EFFECTS: See AMINOPHYLLINE and THEOPHYLLINE in the Small Animal section for information on effects and usage in dogs and cats. The drug should be used with caution in patients with gastrointestinal tract ulcers or impaired renal or hepatic function.

DRUG INTERACTIONS: See AMINOPHYLLINE and THEOPHYLLINE in the Small Animal section. Aminophylline should not be mixed in a syringe with other drugs.

AMITRAZ

INDICATIONS: Amitraz (Mitaban ✤ ★) is indicated for the eradication of demodicosis in hamsters and sarcoptic mange in guinea pigs. Amitraz has also been used in rabbits for tick removal and to treat *Demodex cuniculi,* a rarely diagnosed clinical problem. The drug is used topically. For more information, see AMITRAZ in the Small Animal section.

ADVERSE AND COMMON SIDE EFFECTS: Use amitraz with caution because application has resulted in death, which was most likely due to overdosage.

AMPICILLIN, AMOXICILLIN

INDICATIONS: Ampicillin (Omnipen ★, Polyflex ✤ ★) and amoxicillin (Amoxi-Tabs ★, Amoxi-Drop ★, Amoxi-Inject ★, Amoxil ✤ ★, Moxilean ✤, Robamox-V ★) are indicated in the treatment of bacterial diseases, including some *Pasteurella* infections. Ampicillin is used topically (e.g., impregnated into gauze strips) to treat dental abscesses in rabbits (see caution below). For more information, see AMPICILLIN, AMOXICILLIN, and PENICILLIN ANTIBIOTICS in the Small Animal section.

ADVERSE AND COMMON SIDE EFFECTS: These drugs are used occasionally in mice and rats, but are contraindicated in most other species of rodents and in rabbits because their administration can cause a reduction of intestinal flora (anaerobes, lactobacilli, and streptococci) followed by clostridial and coliform overgrowth and fatal enterotoxemia. This condition is seen most commonly in hamsters, guinea pigs, and rabbits. Mice, rats, and gerbils may also be affected. Oral therapy with one of these penicillins is more likely to cause this toxic syndrome than parenteral administration.

AMPROLIUM

INDICATIONS: Amprolium (Amprol ✤, Corid ★) is an antiprotozoal agent placed in the drinking water as a coccidiostat and for the treatment of hepatic and intestinal coccidiosis in rabbits. For more information, see AMPROLIUM in the Small or Large Animal sections.

ADVERSE AND COMMON SIDE EFFECTS: Amprolium is a thiamine inhibitor and may rarely cause thiamine deficiency.

ASCORBIC ACID

See VITAMIN C

ASPIRIN

See ACETYLSALICYLIC ACID

ATIPAMEZOLE

INDICATIONS: Atipamezole (Antisedan ✤ ★) is a synthetic α-adrenergic receptor antagonist marketed for the reversal of the sedative and analgesic effects of medetomidine hydrochloride. Atipamezole is generally given on a volume per volume (v/v) basis (milliliter for milliliter) of medetomidine administered, which is equivalent to a dosage of 5 times the medetomidine given on a milligram to milligram basis. In dogs, calculated dosages of atipamezole are based on body surface rather than body weight. The recommended route of administration is intramuscularly; however, the drug has been administered IM, IP, SC, and IV. For more information, see ATIPAMEZOLE in the Small Animal section.

ATROPINE

INDICATIONS: Atropine ✤ ★ is an anticholinergic, antispasmodic, and mydriatic drug used as a preanesthetic to reduce salivation and reduce bronchial secretions, and to treat organophosphate toxicity. For more information, see ATROPINE in the Small Animal section.

In small rodents, an anticholinergic drug such as atropine is generally used as a preanesthetic to reduce salivation. Rats and guinea pigs are particularly prone to excessive salivation following the administration of sialogogic drugs; e.g., ketamine, or inhalation of pungent or irritating gases. Anticholinergic drugs also stabilize the heart rate when α_2-receptor agonist drugs are used.

Atropine ophthalmic drops are used to induce mydriasis, but are more effective in albino animals as compared to animals with pigmented eyes. For the latter, a combination of atropine plus phenylephrine is more effective. In rabbits, atropinesterase may reduce the mydriatic effect of atropine.

ADVERSE AND COMMON SIDE EFFECTS: Because many rabbits and rats possess serum atropinesterase, atropine may be ineffective or effective only at very high doses in these species. Glycopyrrolate is, therefore, a more effective choice. In guinea pigs, atropine may cause hypertension, thereby increasing the tendency for hemorrhage during surgery.

OTHER USES: Atropine is used to treat organophosphate toxicity at doses up to 10 mg/kg every 20 minutes. One fourth of the dose is given IV, if possible, and the remainder IM or SC.

BARIUM SULFATE

INDICATIONS: Barium sulfate ♣ ★ is an inert radiopaque material, which provides positive contrast during x-ray or fluoroscopic examination. Barium sulfate is not absorbed or metabolized and is eliminated intact from the body through the feces as a function of gastrointestinal transit time. Caution should be taken not to overfill the stomachs of rodents or rabbits as these animals cannot vomit. The barium should be slowly administered orally through the diastema of the mouth as passing a stomach tube is extremely difficult in these species. The rate of gastrointestinal emptying varies with species as well as the presence of anesthetic or sedative agents.

ADVERSE AND COMMON SIDE EFFECTS: The most common side effects reported in humans are constipation or diarrhea and cramping. The use of barium sulfate is contraindicated when the possibility of gastric or intestinal perforation exists. Aspiration of barium sulfate can lead to significant pneumonia and possibly death.

SUPPLIED AS HUMAN PRODUCTS:
Numerous barium sulfate suspensions from 1.2 to 98 % w/w and 4.9 to 220 % w/v (♣ ★)

BUPRENORPHINE HYDROCHLORIDE

INDICATIONS: Buprenorphine hydrochloride (Buprenex ★) is a partial opiate agonist used for its analgesic properties. Buprenorphine can also be used to reverse the effects of μ opioids such as fentanyl, yet still provide postprocedural analgesia. For further information, see BUPRENORPHINE in the Small Animal section.
   Buprenorphine's 6 to 12 hour duration of effect makes this drug particularly useful in small rodents. The drug can be given preoperatively or postoperatively for analgesia.

ADVERSE AND COMMON SIDE EFFECTS: Gastric distention associated with pica has been noted in rats given larger doses (0.5 mg/kg; SC) of buprenorphine. Respiratory depression may occur after administration. Opiates should be used with caution in animals with severe renal insufficiency, head trauma, central nervous system (CNS) dysfunction, and in debilitated or geriatric patients. Buprenorphine is resistant to antagonism by naloxone. For further information, see BUPRENORPHINE in the Small Animal section.

BUTORPHANOL

INDICATIONS: Butorphanol (Torbugesic ♣ ★, Torbutrol ♣ ★) is a narcotic agonist/antagonist analgesic with potent antitussive activity in some species. In rabbits, the elimination half-life is 3.16 hours after SC administration and 1.64 hours after IV administration of a 0.5 mg/kg dose. Butorphanol can also be used to reverse the effects of μ opioids such as fentanyl, yet still provide postprocedural analgesia. For more information, see BUTORPHANOL in the Small Animal section.

ADVERSE AND COMMON SIDE EFFECTS: Butorphanol is contraindicated in pregnant and lactating rats because it increases nervousness and decreases newborn caretaking behavior. Butorphanol may result in respiratory depression, and therefore, it is often given upon recovery of anesthetized animals, which have not been intubated.

CALCIUM EDTA

INDICATIONS: Calcium disodium EDTA (Calcium Disodium Versenate ✤ ★) is a chelating agent used for the treatment of lead toxicity in rabbits and chinchillas. Prior to administration, calcium EDTA is diluted to a 1% v/v solution using 5% dextrose in water or saline. Two 5-day courses of treatment 1 week apart may be necessary.

ADVERSE AND COMMON SIDE EFFECTS AND DRUG INTERACTIONS: See CALCIUM EDTA in the Small Animal section.

CAPTAN

INDICATIONS: Captan (Orthocide ✤ ★, Captan 10 ✤) is an agricultural fungicide used on a variety of commercial and garden plants. Captan powder, mixed in the sand or dust used by chinchillas for dustbathing, has been used to control dermatophyte infections.

ADVERSE AND COMMON SIDE EFFECTS: Captan is considered to have low toxicity, with very high doses required to produce adverse effects. The LD50 in mice is 7,000 mg/kg PO. Guinea pigs are moderately sensitive to skin sensitization caused by captan. Studies in several animal species have shown that captan is rapidly absorbed from the GI tract and rapidly metabolized; with residues excreted primarily in the urine. Captan should not be used in pregnant animals and some studies have shown embryo toxicity at very high doses.

SUPPLIED AS COMMERCIAL GARDEN PRODUCT:
Powder containing 50% captan

CARBARYL

INDICATIONS: Carbaryl (Dusting Powder ✤, Equi-Shield Fly Repellent Spray ★, Happy Jack Flea and Tick Powder II ★, Mycodex Pet Shampoo with carbaryl ★, Prozap Garden & Poultry Dust ★, Sevin ✤, Zodiac Flea and Tick Power ✤), a carbamate insecticide and cholinesterase inhibitor, is used in the eradication of arthropod ectoparasites including *Cheyletiella, Chirodiscoides, Myobia, Myocoptes, Radfordia, Psorergates,* and *Liponyssus* spp. For more information, see CARBAMATE INSECTICIDES in the Small Animal section or CARBARYL in the Large Animal section.

ADVERSE AND COMMON SIDE EFFECTS: Carbaryl is the least toxic of the carbamate insecticides; however, caution against overdosage should be taken, especially in young rodents. Even low doses of this drug may inhibit breeding. Atropine will counter toxic effects produced by carbaryl. Diazepam may also help reduce the severity of clinical signs related to toxicity.

SUPPLIED AS VETERINARY PRODUCTS:
Numerous dusting powders containing 5% w/w carbaryl ✚ ★
Shampoo containing 0.5% w/v carbaryl (Mycodex Pet Shampoo ★)

CARPROFEN

INDICATIONS: Carprofen (Rimadyl ✚ ★) is a carboxylic acid non-steroidal anti-inflammatory agent with analgesic, anti-inflammatory and antipyretic properties. Carprofen has been used for the treatment of both acute postoperative pain and chronic arthritic or painful conditions. Carprofen has been described for use in rabbits, rats and mice, and is likely effective in other small rodents. For more information, see CARPROFEN in the Small Animal section.

CEFAZOLIN

INDICATIONS: Cefazolin (Ancef ✚ ★, Kefzol ✚ ★) is a rapidly acting, first-generation cephalosporin. Of the cephalosporins, it achieves the greatest serum concentrations at equal doses on a mg/kg basis, has the longest elimination half-life, and is the most active against *Escherichia coli, Klebsiella,* and *Enterobacter.* For additional information, see CEFAZOLIN and CEPHALOSPORIN ANTIBIOTICS in the Small Animal section.

Cefazolin has been used in rabbits for the treatment of infections by susceptible organisms.

ADVERSE AND COMMON SIDE EFFECTS: Cephalosporin antibiotics are intermediate in their ability to cause dysbiosis, and should be used with caution in rabbits and rodents. Thrombocytopenia is a recognized adverse effect of cefazolin in humans.

CEFTIOFUR

INDICATIONS: Ceftiofur (Excenel ✚, Naxcel ★, Excenel RTU ✚, Excenel ★) is a third-generation, broad spectrum cephalosporin active against gram-positive and gram-negative bacteria, including β-lacta-mase–producing strains. The drug is marketed for use in a variety of domestic animal species. For more information, see CEFTIOFUR in the Large Animal section and CEPHALOSPORIN ANTIBIOTICS in the Small Animal section.

In rabbits, ceftiofur has been used parenterally and impregnated into polymethylmethacrylate beads for the treatment of localized infections such as dental abscesses.

ADVERSE AND COMMON EFFECTS: Cephalosporin antibiotics are intermediate in their ability to cause dysbiosis, and should be used with caution in rabbits and rodents. Thrombocytopenia and anemia, which may be reversible, can occur in mammals given 3 to 5 times the recommended dose of ceftiofur.

SUPPLIED AS:
For injection containing 50 mg/mL ceftiofur sodium (Excenel ♣, Naxcel ★)
For injection containing 50 mg/mL ceftiofur hydrochloride (Excenel RTU ♣, Excenel ★)

CEPHALEXIN

INDICATIONS: Cephalexin (Keflex ♣ ★, Keftab ★, Novo-Lexin ♣, Nu-Cephalex ♣) is a broad-spectrum, first-generation cephalosporin antibiotic available for oral use. For more information, see CEPH-ALEXIN and CEPHALOSPORIN ANTIBIOTICS in the Small Animal section.

Cephalexin has been used for dermatitis in rats and mice. Ceph-alosporin antibiotics are intermediate in their ability to cause dysbio-sis, and should be used with caution in rabbits and in small rodent species other than mice and rats. Parenteral cephalothin and ceftiofur have been used successfully in rabbits by some practitioners.

CEPHALOTHIN

INDICATIONS: Cephalothin (Keflin ♣, Ceporacin ♣) is a broad-spec-trum first-generation cephalosporin antibiotic for parenteral use. First-generation drugs are active against gram-positive bacteria, including penicillin-resistant staphylococci, and against some gram-negative bac-teria, including *E. coli, Proteus,* and *Klebsiella* spp. For more information, see CEPHALOSPORIN ANTIBIOTICS in the Small Animal section.

Cephalothin has been used in rabbits for the treatment of suscep-tible infections.

ADVERSE AND COMMON SIDE EFFECTS: Cephalosporin anti-biotics are intermediate in their ability to cause dysbiosis, and should be used with caution in rabbits and rodents. Cephalothin is irritating; large or repeated IM injection may cause pain and result in local inflammatory reactions or sterile abscesses. Thrombophlebitis has been associated with IV use in humans. In humans, cephalothin is potentially nephrotoxic and should not be used in conjunction with an aminoglycoside. This parenteral product is not acid stable and should not be given orally.

CHLORAMPHENICOL

INDICATIONS: Chloramphenicol (Azramycine ♣, Chlor Palm ♣, Chlor Tablets ♣, Chloromycetin ♣ ★, Karomycin Palmitate ♣, and many others) is a bacteriostatic antibiotic with activity against a number of pathogens. It has been one of the most common first-line drugs for the treatment of bacterial infections in rabbits and rodents until recently because its availability has been reduced, based on concerns over human safety. Chloramphenicol has also been used in rabbits for the treatment of *Treponema* sp. infections. Disruption of intestinal microflora has not been associated with the use of this drug in rabbits or small rodents. For more information, see CHLORAMPHENICOL in the Small Animal section.

ADVERSE AND COMMON SIDE EFFECTS: Administration of the drug through drinking water has been recommended for colony situations, but this may cause reduced water intake, especially in chinchillas, rabbits, and guinea pigs, due to the bitter taste. Chloramphenicol in drinking water at 500 mg/L resulted in 25% to 50% reduction in water intake in rabbits in one study. Owners should be warned to take precautions to avoid contact with the drug.

CHLORPROMAZINE

INDICATIONS: Chlorpromazine (Largactil ♣, Thorazine ★) is a phenothiazine derivative used as a preanesthetic, sedative, and antiemetic agent. For more information, see CHLORPROMAZINE in the Small Animal section.

ADVERSE AND COMMON SIDE EFFECTS: Chlorpromazine may precipitate seizures in gerbils. It is hypotensive and may cause hypothermia and hyperglycemia.

DRUG INTERACTIONS: A number of drug interactions exist. See CHLORPROMAZINE in the Small Animal section for further details.

CHLORTETRACYCLINE

INDICATIONS: Chlortetracycline (Aureomycin ♣ ★, Fermycin Soluble ★, Aureomix ★, and many others) is a broad-spectrum bacteriostatic antibiotic with activity against gram-positive and gram-negative organisms, chlamydiae, rickettsiae, mycoplasmas, and many anaerobes. For more information, see TETRACYCLINE ANTIBIOTICS in the Small Animal section.

ADVERSE AND COMMON SIDE EFFECTS: Chlortetracycline may induce dysbiosis, particularly in guinea pigs.

DRUG INTERACTIONS: Oral absorption is inhibited by calcium-, magnesium-, and iron-containing substances.

SUPPLIED AS VETERINARY PRODUCTS:
Water-soluble powders and agricultural feed additives containing various concentrations of chlortetracycline (Aureomycin ❀ ★, Fermycin Soluble ★, Aureomix ★, and many others)
Tablets containing 25 mg (Aureomycin Tablets ★)

CHOLESTYRAMINE

INDICATIONS: Cholestyramine (Novo-Cholamine ❀, PMS-Cholestyramine ❀, Questran ❀ ★, Prevalite Powder ★) is a quaternary amine ion resin capable of binding bacterial toxins, including those produced by *Clostridium difficile* and *spiroforme*. In human medicine, this resin has shown only modest activity and is not recommended for use in patients with severe cases of *C. difficile* colitis. Cholestyramine has been used experimentally in rabbits and hamsters to prevent mortality after administration of clindamycin, an antibiotic known to result in disturbance of the normal enteric bacterial flora and fatal enterotoxemia. Rabbits treated with cholestyramine for 21 days after a dose of clindamycin did not show any evidence of gastrointestinal disease, in contrast with control animals. With a similar experimental protocol, hamsters remained healthy while receiving cholestyramine, but died after discontinuation of cholestyramine treatment. This suggests that their enteric flora had not regained a normal balance, as compared to that of treated rabbits. In a separate, but similar experiment, treatment of hamsters with 1,000 mg of cholestyramine per kg per day protected only 10% of the animals through day 7. The use of cholestyramine in clinical practice has not been well documented.

SUPPLIED AS HUMAN PRODUCT:
Powder for oral suspension containing 4 g/packet (Novo-Cholamine ❀, PMS-Cholestyramine ❀, Questran ❀, Prevalite ★)

CHORIONIC GONADOTROPIN

INDICATIONS: Chorionic gonadotropin (Human), or HCG (Veterinary Products: A.P.L. ❀, Chorionad ❀, Chorionic Gonadotropin ★, Chorulon ❀ ★; Human Products: Follutein ★, Progon 10,000 ❀) is produced in the human placenta. The commercial product is obtained from the urine of pregnant women. The action of HCG is virtually identical to that of pituitary luteinizing hormone (LH), although HCG appears to have a small degree of follicle-stimulating hormone (FSH) activity as well. HCG has been used to stimulate ovulation in rabbits and to reduce the size of ovarian cysts in guinea pigs prior to surgical removal. For more information, see CHORIONIC GONADOTROPIN in the Large Animal section.

ADVERSE AND COMMON SIDE EFFECTS: Chorionic gonadotropin is a foreign protein and can cause anaphylaxis when administered parenterally. Continued administration may result in antihormone antibody production and loss of effectiveness. Side effects described for humans include fluid retention, headache, irritability, restlessness, fatigue, edema, and pain at the site of injection.

CIMETIDINE

INDICATIONS: Cimetidine (Novo-Cimetine ✹, Tagamet ✹ ★), a histamine (H_2)-receptor blocking agent, reduces gastric acid secretion and is used in the treatment of gastric ulceration. For more information, see CIMETIDINE in the Small Animal section.

CIPROFLOXACIN

INDICATIONS: Ciprofloxacin (Cipro ✹ ★) is a fluoroquinolone antibiotic with activity against a range of gram-negative and gram-positive bacteria (e.g., *E. coli, Klebsiella, Proteus, Pseudomonas, Staphylococcus, Salmonella, Shigella, Yersinia, Campylobacter,* and *Vibrio* spp.) and some spirochetes. The drug is available for oral, IV, and ophthalmic use and is produced *in vivo* as a metabolite after the administration of enrofloxacin. It has little activity against anaerobic cocci or *Clostridia* or *Bacteroides* organisms. Ciprofloxacin has not been associated with disruption of the normal enteric flora. Ciprofloxacin ophthalmic drops can be used in rabbits in combination with systemic antibiotic therapy for the treatment of ocular and upper respiratory infections by *Pasteurella multocida.* See also CIPROFLOXACIN and FLUOROQUINOLONE ANTIBIOTICS in the Small Animal section.

ADVERSE AND COMMON SIDE EFFECTS: See FLUOROQUINOLONE ANTIBIOTICS in the Small Animal section. Ciprofloxacin tablets are commonly used as the basis of an oral suspension; however, the stability of the resulting product has not been thoroughly investigated.

DRUG INTERACTIONS: Absorption is hindered by antacid preparations. See CIPROFLOXACIN and FLUOROQUINOLONE ANTIBIOTICS in the Small Animal section.

CISAPRIDE

INDICATIONS: Cisapride (Propulsid ★, Prepulsid ✤) was marketed in North America for the treatment of heartburn in humans, but has been removed from general access due to its association with cardiac arrhythmias. The drug was used in small animal practice to stimulate GI motility in cases of primary motility disorders and in cases of gastro-esophageal reflux. Cisapride acts by increasing acetylcholine release, which stimulates GI motility. The drug generally is given 15 to 30 minutes before a meal. For more information, see CISAPRIDE in the Small Animal section.

Cisapride has been used to stimulate gastrointestinal motility in anorexic and sick rabbits, particularly in animals with gastric impaction, gastric stasis, or gastric trichobezoars. Cisapride has also been used for the treatment of constipation in chinchillas. Metoclopramide would be an alternate choice of medication.

ADVERSE AND COMMON SIDE EFFECTS: Use of the drug is contraindicated in animals with gastrointestinal hemorrhage, complete gastric or intestinal obstruction, or perforation.

DRUG INTERACTIONS: Because cisapride increases gastric emptying, absorption of drugs from the stomach may be decreased, whereas absorption from the small bowel may be increased.

CLOTRIMAZOLE

INDICATIONS: Clotrimazole (Canesten ✤, Lotrimin ★, Mycelex ★) is a topical imidazole useful in the treatment of localized dermatophytosis, particularly in rabbits. For more information, see CLOTRIMAZOLE in the Small Animal section.

CODEINE

INDICATIONS: Codeine (Codeine Phosphate ✤, Paveral ✤ ★, Tylenol No. 1 ✤) is an analgesic with antitussive and antidiarrheal properties. For more information, see CODEINE in the Small Animal section.

ADVERSE AND COMMON SIDE EFFECTS: Codeine depresses the respiratory drive, increases airway resistance, and dries respiratory secretions. Treatment with this drug may precipitate respiratory insufficiency.

SUPPLIED AS HUMAN PRODUCTS:
For injection containing 30 and 60 mg codeine phosphate (generic ✤ ★)
Caplets containing 8 mg (#1), 15 mg (#2), 30 mg (#3), and 60 mg (#4) codeine with 300 mg acetaminophen and caffeine (Tylenol with codeine ✤ ★)

Elixir containing 8 mg/5 mL codeine with 160 mg/5 mL acetaminophen (Tylenol with Codeine Elixir ♣) and containing 12 mg/5 mL codeine with 120 mg/5 mL acetaminophen (Tylenol with Codeine Elixir ★)

COPPER SULFATE

INDICATIONS: Copper sulfate (chemical grade ♣ ★, Copper Sulfate-S ♣) has been used topically to control dermatophytosis caused by *Trichophyton mentagrophytes* in a commercial rabbitry where treatment of individual animals with griseofulvin was not feasible. Animals were dipped in a 1% w/v solution 6 times over a 26-day period. The number of carriers and extent of clinical signs were greatly reduced, but the infection was not completely eliminated. Also see COPPER SULFATE in the Large Animal section.

ADVERSE AND COMMON SIDE EFFECTS: The animal's eyes should be protected by a compound such as petroleum jelly during the dipping procedure.

CYPROHEPTADINE

INDICATIONS: Cyproheptadine (Periactin ★, generics ♣ ★) is an antihistamine–antiserotonin, and acetylcholine antagonist. The drug has been used in rabbits to stimulate appetite. For further information, see CYPROHEPTADINE in the Small Animal section.

ADVERSE AND COMMON SIDE EFFECTS: Excitability and aggressive behavior have been documented in some cats. Other adverse effects sometimes noted in people include nausea, vomiting, jaundice, and drowsiness. The drug is contraindicated in patients with glaucoma, pyloric or duodenal obstruction, urinary retention, and acute asthma.

DRUG INTERACTIONS: Monoamine oxidase inhibitors, possibly amitraz and selegiline, prolong and intensify the anticholinergic effects of the drug. Central nervous system depressant drugs may have an additive effect if used concurrently with cyproheptadine.

SUPPLIED AS HUMAN PRODUCTS:
Tablets containing 4 mg ♣ ★
Syrup containing 2 mg/5 mL (Periactin ★, generics ♣ ★)

DEXAMETHASONE

INDICATIONS: Dexamethasone (Azium ♣ ★, Azium SP ♣ ★, Dex-5 ♣) is a glucocorticoid anti-inflammatory agent. For more information, see DEXAMETHASONE in the Small Animal section. Rabbits and rodents are felt to be more susceptible to the immunosuppressive effects of glucocorticoids than some other mammals. Nonsteroidal anti-inflammatory drugs (NSAIDs) may be more appropriate choices in many instances, particularly for long-term therapy.

ADVERSE AND COMMON SIDE EFFECTS: Dexamethasone may cause gastrointestinal irritation and ulceration. The drug must be used with extreme caution in small rodents to avoid overdosage. It is best to begin treatment with a low dose and increase over time if necessary.

DIAZEPAM

INDICATIONS: Diazepam (Valium ♣ ★, Valrelease ★) is a benzodiazepine tranquilizer used as a preanesthetic and anticonvulsant. For more information, see DIAZEPAM in the Small Animal section. Diazepam has been suggested as a premedication before surgery for urolithiasis in rabbits to relax urethral muscle tone. Diazepam is formulated for oral and intravenous use, although it has been used intramuscularly. Midazolam is a similar drug intended for intramuscular use.

DRUG INTERACTIONS: Diazepam is commonly used in combination with ketamine for sedation and anesthesia.

DICHLORVOS IMPREGNATED RESIN STRIPS

INDICATIONS: Dichlorvos (Vapona No Pest Strip and others ♣ ★) is a cholinesterase inhibitor anthelmintic and insecticide. It is used as an impregnated resin strip that is hung in the animal's environment to eliminate arthropod ectoparasites including *Myobia, Myocoptes, Radfordia, Liponyssus, Cheyletiella,* and *Chirodiscoides* spp. Sections of strip should be placed inside the cage within a ventilated container, such as a perforated plastic vial, to prevent direct contact or ingestion. The dose or length of strip used is empirical. For more information, see DICHLORVOS and CHLORINATED HYDROCARBONS in the Small Animal section.

ADVERSE AND COMMON SIDE EFFECTS: This product may be hazardous for humans as headache and nausea have been reported after breathing Vapona-laden air. Persons handling the strips should wear gloves. In addition, the strips should be allowed to breathe outside for several hours before use. It is essential to follow manufacturer's instructions in order to prevent excessive air concentrations and overdosage.

SUPPLIED AS COMMERCIAL PRODUCTS:
Impregnated resin strips containing 20% w/w dichlorvos (Vapona No Pest Strip ♣ ★, Black Flag Insect Strip, and many others)

DIETHYLSTILBESTROL

INDICATIONS: Diethylstilbestrol (Stilboestrol ✤, Stilbestrol ✤, Stilphostrol ★, Honvol ✤) is used in the management of estrogen-responsive reproductive problems. The drug has been used to treat urinary incontinence in spayed rabbits. See DIETHYLSTILBESTROL in the Small Animal section.

SUPPLIED AS VETERINARY PRODUCT:
Tablets containing 1 mg DES (Stilboestrol ✤)

SUPPLIED AS HUMAN PRODUCTS:
Tablets containing 0.1, 0.5, and 1 mg DES (Stilbestrol ✤); 5 mg (diethylstilbestrol ★), 50 mg (Stilphostrol ★), and 100 mg (Honvol ✤) For injection containing 250 mg/5 mL (Honvol ✤) and 50 mg/mL (Stilphostrol ★)

DIMETRIDAZOLE

INDICATIONS: Dimetridazole (Dimetridazole ✤, Emtryl ✤) is an antimicrobial agent effective against anaerobic bacteria and protozoa. The drug has been used for the prevention of clostridial enterotoxemia in rabbits, and for the treatment of enteric protozoal infections including giardiasis.

SUPPLIED AS VETERINARY PRODUCT:
Water-soluble powder with 40% w/w (Dimetridazole 40% ✤, Emtryl Soluble ✤)

   Feed additives (Dimetridazole 30% w/w Premix ✤, Emtryl Premix ✤)

DIPYRONE

INDICATIONS: Dipyrone (Dipyrone 50% ✤) is an anti-inflammatory, antipyretic drug and an antispasmodic and analgesic agent. It is prescribed for the relief of pain, reducing fever, and relaxing smooth muscle. For more information, see DIPYRONE in the Small Animal section.

SUPPLIED AS VETERINARY PRODUCT:
For injection containing 500 mg/mL (Dipyrone 50% ✤)

DOXAPRAM

INDICATIONS: Doxapram (Dopram-V ✤ ★) is used to stimulate respiration during anesthesia, to reduce anesthetic recovery time in patients with postanesthetic respiratory depression, and to stimulate respiration in neonates. Doxapram is intended for intravenous use, but will have an effect when given by other parenteral routes if venous access cannot be obtained. For more information, see DOXAPRAM in the Small Animal section.

DOXYCYCLINE

INDICATIONS: Doxycycline (Vibramycin ❦ ★, Vibra-Tabs ❦ ★, and others) is a long-acting, lipid-soluble tetracycline antibiotic used in the treatment of bacterial, rickettsial, chlamydial, and mycoplasmal infections. Doxycycline has greater activity against anaerobes and facultative intracellular bacteria than other tetracyclines. It is useful in patients with renal failure because it is excreted by the intestine. For more information, see TETRACYCLINE ANTIBIOTICS in the Small Animal section. Doxycycline is particularly useful for the treatment of mycoplasmal infections in mice and rats.

DRUG INTERACTIONS: Combined oral therapy with doxycycline (5 mg/kg) and enrofloxacin (10 mg/kg) has been recommended for the treatment of *Mycoplasma pulmonis* pneumonia in mice and rats.

ADVERSE AND COMMON SIDE EFFECTS: Doxycycline may induce enterotoxemia, particularly in guinea pigs.

SUPPLIED AS VETERINARY PRODUCTS:
Water-soluble powder containing 50 mg/g (Vibravet 5% ❦)
Oral suspension containing 5 mg/mL after reconstitution (Vibravet ❦)

SUPPLIED AS HUMAN PRODUCTS:
Tablets and capsules containing 50 mg (Monodox ★) and 100 mg (Monodox ★, Alti-Doxycycline ❦, Apo-Doxy ❦, Doxycin ❦, Doxytec (lactose) ❦, Novo-Doxylin ❦, Nu-Doxycycline ❦, Vibramycin ❦, Vibra-Tabs ❦ ★)
Oral suspension containing 5 mg/mL after reconstitution (Vibramycin ★)
Oral suspension containing 50 mg/5 mL (Vibramycin calcium syrup ★)
For injection in 100 mg and 200 mg vials (Vibramycin ★)
For IV injection in vials of 100 and 200 mg (Doxy 100 ★, Doxy 200 ★, Vibramycin hyclate ★, doxycycline hyclate ★, Vibramycin-IV ❦)

ENILCONAZOLE

INDICATIONS: Enilconazole (Imaverol ❦) is a topical imidazole antifungal agent that is marketed as a topical preparation for the treatment of dermatophytosis. See ENILCONAZOLE in the Small Animal section.
    Enilconazole has been recommended for the treatment of dermatophytes in rabbits and guinea pigs, either topically applied to lesions or as a rinse or dip (100 mg/mL solution diluted 1:50 = 0.2% = 2 mg/mL).

ADVERSE AND COMMON SIDE EFFECTS: See ENILCONAZOLE in the Small Animal section.

ENROFLOXACIN

INDICATIONS: Enrofloxacin (Baytril ✤ ★) is a fluoroquinolone antibiotic with activity against a variety of gram-positive and gram-negative bacteria and mycoplasmas. Relevant susceptible bacteria affecting rabbits and rodents include *Escherichia coli, Klebsiella pneumoniae, Staphylococcus aureus* and *epidermidis, Pasteurella multocida,* and *Proteus mirabilis* as well as *Mycoplasma* spp. in mice and rats. For more information, see ENROFLOXACIN in the Small Animal section.

Pharmacokinetic studies have been carried out in rabbits. In a single dose study using 5 mg/kg administered IM and IV, enrofloxacin was rapidly absorbed from the IM injection site reaching maximum plasma levels of 3.04 µg/mL at 10 minutes after drug administration with a bioavailability of 92% versus IV administration. The elimination half-life for both routes of administration was 131.5 minutes. There was a high volume of distribution suggesting good tissue penetration. A second study used the same 5 mg/kg dose administered orally, SC, and IV. Subcutaneous absorption was rapid with a peak concentration of 2.07 µg/mL 20 minutes after drug administration. The elimination half-life after SC administration was 1.71 hours, and the bioavailability 77% versus IV administration. Oral absorption was slower and less efficient than SC administration, with an average maximum serum concentration of 0.45 µg/mL reached at 2.3 hours and a bioavailability of 61% versus IV drug administration. Enrofloxacin was detectable in serum for 10 hours after IV, 6 hours after SC, and 24 hours after PO administration. The authors recommended dosages of 5 mg/kg orally or SC each 12 hours for 14 days to provide enrofloxacin tissue concentrations effective against *P. multocida.*

In a clinical trial involving rabbits naturally infected with *P. multocida,* animals were given 5 mg/kg SC twice daily or 200 mg/L of drinking water, changed daily, ad lib for 14 days. Animals were observed for 3 weeks after therapy was completed and then were euthanized for necropsy. The SC treatment regimen resulted in resolution of clinical signs and elimination of *Pasteurella* organisms from the respiratory tract. *P. multocida* was still isolated from the tympanic bulla of one animal suggesting a higher dose may be necessary for the treatment of infections at this site. Oral treatment also resolved clinical signs of respiratory infection, but organisms could still be cultured from the respiratory tract at necropsy. Enrofloxacin at the above dosages did not eliminate *Bordetella bronchiseptica* from the nasal passages. In another study, enrofloxacin in the water at 100 mg/L significantly reduced mortality resulting from inoculation with a septicemic form of *P. multocida* without adversely affecting water consumption. Long-term treatment (i.e., months) may be necessary to treat chronic severe pasteurellosis. Enrofloxacin has not been associated with disruption of enteric microflora in rabbits.

Enrofloxacin has also been recommended for the treatment of hamsters with proliferative enteritis caused by *Lawsonia intracellularis.* The injectable product can be compounded into an oral formulation using a palatable liquid syrup base.

Baytril Otic is a canine antimicrobial and antifungal product, which has been used to good effect to treat bacterial otitis in rabbits. The product contains enrofloxacin (5 mg/mL) and silver sulfadiazine (10 mg/mL) in an aqueous alcohol base. Baytril Otic has not been evaluated for use in dogs with perforated tympanic membranes; if hearing or vestibular dysfunction occur during treatment, it is recommended that therapy be discontinued.

ADVERSE AND COMMON SIDE EFFECTS: Parenteral enrofloxacin injection may result in tissue necrosis and sloughing. The manufacturers suggest switching to oral administration after no more than three IM injections. Although some references provide doses for SC administration, the canine product is licensed only for IM use. Enrofloxacin has been reported to cause cartilage damage and arthropathy in young guinea pigs and rabbits. Enrofloxacin should be used with caution in rabbits with CNS disorders as the drug has, rarely, been associated with CNS stimulation and convulsive seizures in some species.

DRUG INTERACTIONS: Combined oral therapy with doxycycline (5 mg/kg) and enrofloxacin (10 mg/kg) has been recommended for the treatment of *Mycoplasma pulmonis* pneumonia in mice and rats.

ERYTHROMYCIN

INDICATIONS: Erythromycin (Erythro-100 ★, Gallimycin ✤ ★) is a bacteriostatic macrolide antibiotic with a predominantly gram-positive spectrum of activity. It has been placed in drinking water or administered orally in hamster colonies for the prevention and treatment, respectively, of enteritis, which is presumed to be caused by *Campylobacter jejuni.* For further information on the injectable use of erythromycin, see ERYTHROMYCIN in the Small Animal section.

ADVERSE AND COMMON SIDE EFFECTS: Dosages greater than 500 mg/gallon can cause dysbiosis and enteropathy. Erythromycin is not safe for administration to rabbits, guinea pigs, and chinchillas since disruption of enteric microflora may result.

FENBENDAZOLE

INDICATIONS: Fenbendazole (Panacur ❀ ★) is an anthelmintic recommended for the elimination of nematodes and some tapeworms. It is also effective against *Giardia* and some trematodes and microfilaria. For more information, see FENBENDAZOLE in the Small Animal section.

Fenbendazole has been used to treat giardiasis in chinchillas and pinworms in a variety of small rodents. The drug appears to have some promise for the treatment of *Encephalitozoon cuniculi* infections in rabbits. Fenbendazole appears to be well tolerated in rabbits and rodents.

ADVERSE AND COMMON SIDE EFFECTS: Veterinarians should be aware that fenbendazole toxicity, manifested as leukopenia resulting from bone marrow necrosis, has been reported in a variety of species. Routine monitoring of complete blood cell counts (CBCs) is recommended for rabbits on long-term therapy for encephalitozoonosis.

FENTANYL-DROPERIDOL

See INNOVAR-VET

FENTANYL-FLUANISONE

See HYPNORM

FIPRONIL

INDICATIONS: Fipronil (Frontline ★, Top Spot ★) is a phenyl pyrazole pesticide, which acts as an insecticide by disruption of the insect's central nervous system (CNS) via the γ-aminobutyric acid (GABA)-regulated chloride channel. Fipronil has been marketed to control fleas, ticks, and mites on domestic animals and as a pour-on or dip for cattle to control ticks.

ADVERSE AND COMMON SIDE EFFECTS: Fipronil should NOT be used in rabbits as there are several anecdotal reports of deaths following administration to this species. The safety in small rodent species is not known.

SUPPLIED AS VETERINARY PRODUCT:
Spray containing 0.29% w/v (Frontline Spray Treatment ★)
Solution containing 9.7% w/v (Frontline Top Spot for Cats and Kittens ★, Frontline Top Spot for Dogs and Puppies ★)

FLUMAZENIL

INDICATIONS: Flumazenil (Romazicon ★, Anexate ♣) is a benzo-diazepine receptor antagonist that can be used to reverse the sedative effects of diazepam or midazolam.

ADVERSE AND COMMON SIDE EFFECTS: Flumazenil has a wide margin of safety and few adverse effects. In dogs with CNS disease, it is recommended that the drug should be used with caution as seizures may occur.

DRUG INTERACTIONS: None of significance.

SUPPLIED AS HUMAN PRODUCT:
For injection containing 0.1 mg/mL (Romazicon ★, Anexate ♣)

FLUNIXIN MEGLUMINE

INDICATIONS: Flunixin meglumine (Banamine ♣ ★) is a potent anti-prostaglandin with anti-inflammatory and antipyretic properties that make it useful in the treatment of inflammation and pain associated with musculoskeletal disease. Its analgesic properties are considered superior to those of aspirin, meperidine, pentazocine, codeine phosphate, and phenylbutazone. The injectable product has been compounded with flavored syrups to make an oral suspension. The stability of this oral suspension has not been formally assessed. See FLUNIXIN MEGLUMINE in the Small Animal section.

ADVERSE AND COMMON SIDE EFFECTS: Parenteral injection can be irritating; therefore, injections should be made deep into the largest muscle mass available. This can be a significant problem in small rodents with minimal muscle mass. The efficacy of flunixin in rabbits and rodents has been questioned by clinicians; the use of newer NSAIDs such as meloxicam and carprofen is preferred.

FUROSEMIDE

INDICATIONS: Furosemide (Lasix ♣ ★) is a potent loop diuretic that is effective in reducing pulmonary edema of cardiac origin and promoting diuresis. For more information, see FUROSEMIDE in the Small Animal section.

GENTAMICIN

INDICATIONS: Gentamicin (Gentocin ♣ ★, Gentasul ♣, Garagen ★) is an aminoglycoside antibiotic used in the treatment of bacterial infections, especially infections with gram-negative organisms. For more information, see GENTAMICIN in the Small Animal section.

The elimination half-life of gentamicin administered to rabbits was found to be approximately 1 hour in several studies, suggesting that therapeutic blood levels are not maintained with commonly recommended dosage schedules. However, suppression of bacterial growth appears to continue after blood levels drop below the minimum inhibitory concentration, thus extending the effect of the drug.

ADVERSE AND COMMON SIDE EFFECTS: Concurrent administration of fluids is recommended to prevent renal toxicity, especially in gerbils. A dose of 40 mg/kg of gentamicin, administered IM once daily to rabbits for 5 days, resulted in mild to moderate acute renal tubular necrosis. This damage was prevented by concurrent dosage with 10 or 100 mg of vitamin B_6 (pyridoxine HCl), which also reduced gentamicin serum levels although not below therapeutic levels. Gentamicin is also ototoxic, especially in albino guinea pigs. For more information concerning adverse effects and DRUG INTERACTIONS, see AMINO-GLYCOSIDE ANTIBIOTICS in the Small Animal section.

OTHER USES: Gentamicin has been used to prevent or treat enterotoxemia caused by the administration of inappropriate antibiotics. Since the drug is not absorbed through intact intestinal mucosa, oral administration will result in intraluminal activity.

GLYCOPYRROLATE

INDICATIONS: Glycopyrrolate (Robinul-V ★, Robinul ♣ ★) is an anticholinergic agent used in preanesthetic regimens to reduce salivary, tracheobronchial, and pharyngeal secretions during anesthetic induction and intubation. The drug is also used to reduce the volume and acidity of gastric secretion and to inhibit vagal influences on cardiac function, particularly when α_2-receptor agonist drugs are co-administered. Guinea pigs and rats are particularly prone to excessive salivation. Experimental work using a relatively high dose (0.1 mg/kg; IM) has shown glycopyrrolate to be an effective anticholinergic agent in rabbits by preventing bradycardia associated with xylazine administration. In rats, 0.5 mg/kg glycopyrrolate was also shown to be a more potent vagolytic agent and to have a more prolonged effect than atropine. For more information, see GLYCOPYRROLATE and ATROPINE in the Small Animal section.

GRISEOFULVIN

INDICATIONS: Griseofulvin (Fulvicin U/F ♣ ★) is used for the treatment of dermatophyte infections, including *Trichophyton* and *Microsporum* spp. Absorption of griseofulvin in enhanced by dietary fat and is affected by the particle size of the product. Griseofulvin is fungistatic. Treatment is usually continued for at least 2 to 4 weeks. For more information, see GRISEOFULVIN in the Small Animal section.

ADVERSE AND COMMON SIDE EFFECTS: Griseofulvin is teratogenic and should not be used in pregnant animals. Diarrhea, leukopenia, and anorexia have been reported in guinea pigs on long-term therapy. Topical enilconazole has been suggested as an alternative to griseofulvin therapy.

HALOTHANE

INDICATIONS: Halothane (Fluothane ✤ ★, Halothane ✤ ★) is an inhalant drug used for the induction of general anesthesia. Concentrations in common use are of 3% to 4 % for induction and 1 to 2 % for maintenance. For more information, see HALOTHANE in the Small Animal section. Isoflurane is preferred in the small species described in this section due to its more rapid induction and recovery periods, and reduced cardiac effects.

ADVERSE AND COMMON SIDE EFFECTS: Halothane sensitizes the myocardium to the effects of catecholamines. This effect is of particular concern when anesthetizing nervous rabbits.

HYPNORM

INDICATIONS: Hypnorm (fentanyl + fluanisone) is a neuroleptic analgesic combination used in rabbits and a variety of rodent species in laboratory situations. The drug combination produces good analgesia but poor muscle relaxation, and will cause significant respiratory depression. For more information, see FENTANYL in the Small Animal section.

ADVERSE AND COMMON SIDE EFFECTS: See FENTANYL in the Small Animal section.

DRUG INTERACTIONS: The addition of diazepam or midazolam produces surgical anesthesia with improved muscle relaxation and only mild to moderate respiratory depression. The fentanyl portion of the combination can be reversed with an opioid antagonist. The use of a mixed agonist/antagonist, such as butorphanol, buprenorphine, or nalbuphine, will reduce the degree of respiratory depression and of sedation while still providing analgesia. The use of a μ agonist such as naloxone also removes all analgesic effect.

SUPPLIED AS: Fentanyl 0.2 mg/mL + fluanisone 10 mg/mL (Hypnorm, Janssen Pharmaceuticals, not currently registered in North America)

IBUPROFEN

INDICATIONS: Ibuprofen (Advil ♣ ★, Motrin ♣ ★) is a nonsteroidal anti-inflammatory agent with antipyretic and analgesic properties. Its use has been described in rabbits and, to a limited extent, in small rodents. Use of the drug may prevent adhesion formation after abdominal surgery. See IBUPROFEN in the Small Animal section.

ADVERSE AND COMMON SIDE EFFECTS: The drug can cause gastric irritation and ulceration, the severity of which varies among species. See IBUPROFEN in the Small Animal section.

SUPPLIED AS HUMAN PRODUCT:
Oral suspension containing 20 mg/mL (Children's Motrin Suspension ♣, Children's Advil ★, Motrin ★, Ibuprofen ★) or 40 mg/mL (Advil Pediatric Drops ♣, Infant's Motrin Suspension Drops ♣)

IMIDACLOPRID

INDICATIONS: Imidacloprid (Advantage ♣ ★) is a systemic, chloronicotinyl insecticide, which has been used in agriculture for the control of sucking insects such as fleas, aphids, whiteflies, termites, turf insects, soil insects, and some beetles. Imidacloprid is now available as a topical product for flea control in dogs and cats, and has been recommended as a replacement for carbaryl and pyrethrin for the control of fleas and lice in rabbits.

ADVERSE AND COMMON SIDE EFFECTS: The oral LD50 dose of technical grade imidacloprid is 450 mg/kg body weight in rats and 131 mg/kg in mice. The 24-hour dermal LD50 in rats is >5,000 mg/kg. Imidacloprid is considered nonirritating to eyes and skin (tested in rabbits) and nonsensitizing to skin (tested in guinea pigs).

SUPPLIED AS VETERINARY PRODUCT:
Individual one dose tubes for topical use containing 0.4 mL of 9.1% w/w (Advantage Orange/9 For Cats and Kittens 8 Weeks and Older and 9 lbs and Under ♣ ★)

INNOVAR-VET

INDICATIONS: Innovar-Vet ♣ ★ is a combination of fentanyl citrate (0.628 mg/mL) and droperidol (20 mg/mL). The drug has tranquilizing and analgesic properties and is used as a preanesthetic sedative or as an anesthetic induction agent for rabbits and rodents. This combination provides good analgesia but very poor muscle relaxation and is thus best used for providing restraint for minor surgical procedures. For more information, see INNOVAR-VET in the Small Animal section.

ADVERSE AND COMMON SIDE EFFECTS: This drug combination can cause marked respiratory depression, especially at high doses. The drug is very irritating to tissues and may induce self-mutilation when given IM, particularly in guinea pigs and rats. Innovar-Vet is not recommended for use in hamsters or gerbils. Deaths, lameness, and self-mutilation have been reported in guinea pigs at doses of 0.88 mL/kg. Naloxone (0.2 mg/kg) and nalorphine (2 mg/kg) can be used to reverse the effects of fentanyl.

DRUG INTERACTIONS: Innovar-Vet is commonly used in combination with xylazine.

ISOFLURANE

INDICATIONS: Isoflurane (Aerrane ♣ ★, Forane ♣ ★, IsoFlo ♣ ★, Iso-Thesia ★) is the inhalant anesthetic agent of choice for rabbits and rodents because of its rapid induction and recovery times and cardiovascular stability. Concentrations in common use are of 3% to 5% for induction and 1.5% to 3% for maintenance. For more information, see ISOFLURANE in the Small Animal section.

ITRACONAZOLE

INDICATIONS: Itraconazole (Sporanox ♣ ★) is a triazole antifungal agent active against histoplasmosis, blastomycosis, aspergillosis, cryptococcosis, dermatophytosis, and candidiasis. The drug is used orally and is best absorbed with a fatty meal. For more information, see ITRACONAZOLE in the Small Animal section.

Itraconazole has been suggested for the treatment of dermatophytosis in rabbits. The drug is incorporated into keratinocyte basal membranes with continuous release to skin for 3 to 4 weeks after treatment. A topical product would also be necessary to remove spores from the hair shafts. Use of topical enilconazole may be safer and more effective.

ADVERSE AND COMMON SIDE EFFECTS: None described in rabbits at this time. Monitoring of hepatic function would be appropriate.

IVERMECTIN

INDICATIONS: Ivermectin (Heartgard ♣ ★, Ivomec ♣ ★, Eqvalan ♣ ★, and others) is used for the eradication of a variety of endo- and ectoparasites including *Myobia musculi, Myocoptes musculinus, Radfordia* spp., lice and mites in guinea pigs (*Trixacarus caviae* and *Chirodiscoides caviae,* respectively), and *Psoroptes cuniculi* in rabbits. Routes of administration include orally, parenterally, and topically.

Several research reports have detailed the effectiveness of ivermectin against ear mites (*Psoroptes cuniculi*) in rabbits and *Myocoptes musculinus* and *Myobia musculi* in mice. Ivermectin also has been used successfully in rabbits to treat *Cheyletiella parasitovorax* and *Obeliscoides cuniculi*, but was found to be relatively ineffective against pinworms (*Passalurus ambiguus*). A very high dose, 2.0 mg/kg (2,000 μg/kg) orally twice at a 10-day interval, was necessary to eliminate pinworms in mice. A single dose of ivermectin can also be used to kill maggots developing in contaminated wounds. Injectable ivermectin formulations can be diluted in propylene glycol for more accurate dosing in small species. For more information, see IVERMECTIN in the Small Animal section.

ADVERSE AND COMMON SIDE EFFECTS: Toxicity has not been seen after oral administration of the recommended dose. Parenteral administration may result in discomfort at the site of injection.

KETAMINE

INDICATIONS: Ketamine (Ketalean ♣, Ketaject ★, Ketaved ★, Rogarsetic ♣, Vetaket ★, Vetamine ★, Vetame ★, Ketaset ♣ ★, Vetalar ♣ ★) is a nonbarbiturate dissociative anesthetic best used in combination with other agents. Ketamine is not used alone in small rodents as extremely high doses are required for immobility and adequate analgesia is not attained. Sedation and loss of righting reflex may be obtained in rabbits with ketamine alone, but analgesia is again insufficient for even minor surgical procedures. For more information, see KETAMINE in the Small Animal section.

ADVERSE AND COMMON SIDE EFFECTS: Ketamine is a tissue irritant when given IM. Its use has been associated with nerve damage and self-mutilation in guinea pigs. In rabbits, ketamine should be diluted and injected with caution to avoid the sciatic nerve. In small rodents, the drug is best diluted and administered intraperitoneally into the left lower abdominal quadrant. The animal's forequarters should be tilted down during injection to move the abdominal organs forward and avoid injection into a loop of bowel.

DRUG INTERACTIONS: Ketamine can be used at a reduced dose in combination with xylazine, diazepam, medetomidine, and acepromazine. The use of xylazine and medetomidine provides the greater analgesia required for surgical anesthesia. Bedding animals on aromatic softwood shavings may induce hepatic microsomal enzymes that can alter metabolism of the drug and reduce the duration of anesthesia.

KETOCONAZOLE

INDICATIONS: Ketoconazole (Nizoral ✝ ★) is an antifungal agent used for the treatment of deep fungal and yeast infections. Ketoconazole is fungistatic at low concentrations, and fungicidal at higher levels. Absorption of ketoconazole is enhanced in an acid environment and with a high-fat meal. High levels of dietary carbohydrate reduce absorption in humans. For more information, see KETOCONAZOLE in the Small Animal section.

Ketoconazole has been suggested as a treatment for dermatophytosis in rabbits that are intolerant to griseofulvin. The drug is incorporated into skin and hair follicles after systemic use. Concurrent treatment with a topical product would be necessary to remove spores from the hair shafts.

ADVERSE AND COMMON SIDE EFFECTS: Do not use in breeding animals as ketoconazole may disrupt normal steroidogenesis.

KETOPROFEN

INDICATIONS: Ketoprofen (Anafen ✝, Ketofen ★) is an NSAID with potent analgesic and antipyretic properties. The drug inhibits the cyclooxygenase and lipoxygenase inflammatory pathways. Ketoprofen is used in the management of fever and acute, subacute, and chronic pain associated with musculoskeletal disease. In small animals, onset of activity of the drug occurs within 30 minutes of parenteral administration and 1 hour after oral administration. Ketoprofen has been described for use in rabbits and rats and is likely effective in other small rodents. For more information, see KETOPROFEN in the Small Animal section.

LEUPROLIDE ACETATE

INDICATIONS: Leuprolide acetate (Lupron ✝ ★) is a synthetic gonadotropin-releasing hormone (GnRH) analog. The drug binds to GnRH receptors in the anterior pituitary with high specificity, affinity, and activity. It initially induces hormonal upregulation, but receptors are downregulated after prolonged exposure to continued rapid pulses of GnRH levels. There is an initial stimulation of FSH and LH production and release, which may induce ovulation. Shortly after, there is a decrease in LH and, in some species, FSH. In humans, leuprolide acetate is used to treat prostate cancer, endometriosis, and central precocious puberty. For more information, see LEUPROLIDE ACETATE in the Ferret section.

Leuprolide acetate has been used in the treatment of cystic ovaries in guinea pigs.

LIME SULFUR

INDICATIONS: Lime sulfur, or calcium polysulfide, is an agricultural chemical with insecticidal and fungicidal properties that has been used topically in the treatment of ectoparasites including *Trixacarus caviae* in guinea pigs and *Cheyletiella* sp., *Sarcoptes* sp., and *Notoedres* sp. mites in rabbits. For use in cats, a combination of 1 part 23% lime sulfur (liquid), 5 parts shampoo, and 2 parts water has been suggested for dermatophyte infection.

ADVERSE AND COMMON SIDE EFFECTS: Although lime sulfur is generally described as a very safe preparation, the MSDS sheets for calcium polysulfide (chemical name) provide cautions against ingestion, inhalation, and contact with skin and eyes. Lime sulfur is yellow and has a strong odor. Transient pruritus may result from a hypersensitivity reaction to the dead mites and their antigens after treatment. Short-acting corticosteroids may help relieve this pruritus. Oral toxic doses of the active sulfur for rats and rabbits are as follows: rats—oral LD50 > 8437 mg/kg; rabbits—oral lowest lethal dose = 175 mg/kg.

DRUG INTERACTIONS: None reported.

SUPPLIED AS AGRICULTURAL CHEMICAL:
Lime sulfur (calcium polysulfide) liquid or powder

LINDANE

INDICATIONS: Lindane (Kwellada ♣, Lindane ♣, Hexit ♣, Happy Jack Kennel Dip ★, generics) is a chlorinated hydrocarbon insecticide used topically for the treatment of ectoparasites including *Trixacarus caviae* in guinea pigs and *Notoedres* and *Sarcoptes* spp. in rabbits. For more information, see CHLORINATED HYDROCARBONS in the Small Animal section.

SUPPLIED AS VETERINARY PRODUCTS:
Topical insecticidal compounds containing 12.89% w/v lindane (Happy Jack Kennel Dip ★)

SUPPLIED AS HUMAN PRODUCTS:
Topical lotions and shampoos containing 1% w/v lindane (Hexit ♣, Kildane ★, Kwell ★, Kwildane ★, Kwellada ♣, PMS Lindane ♣, Scabene ★, Thionex ★, GBH ♣, and others)

LOPERAMIDE

INDICATIONS: Loperamide (Imodium ♣ ★) is a human antidiarrheal agent with high affinity for both peripheral and central opioid receptors. It also has been used in the treatment of acute colitis and malabsorption/maldigestion.

The use of loperamide has been described, in conjunction with oral rehydration therapy, for the treatment of *E. coli* diarrhea in a colony of rabbits. The drug has also been suggested for more general use in rabbits with gastrointestinal disease and motility disturbances. Repeated dosage over a short period of time (i.e., 2 to 3 doses over 12 to 24 hours) appears to promote gastric motility in rabbits with gastric stasis.

ADVERSE AND COMMON SIDE EFFECTS: The drug is relatively safe in humans and dogs. Sedation, constipation, and ileus are described. For more information, see LOPERAMIDE in the Small Animal section.

LUFENURON

INDICATIONS: Lufenuron (Program ♣ ★) is a chitin synthesis inhibitor and insect growth regulator, which inhibits insect development within the insect egg, preventing maturation to an adult insect. Lufenuron is marketed for flea control in dogs and cats.

This product has been reported to be safe for flea control in rabbits at standard doses. Based on evidence from dogs and cats, lufenuron may also have activity against dermatophytes by inhibiting chitin synthesis in fungal cell walls.

ADVERSE AND COMMON SIDE EFFECTS: Side effects reported with the use of the injectable product in cats include injection site reactions, gastrointestinal reactions, inactivity, and loss of appetite. In dogs, vomiting, depression/lethargy, pruritus, urticaria, diarrhea, anorexia, and skin congestion have been described in animals treated with Program.

DRUG INTERACTIONS: None described.

SUPPLIED AS VETERINARY PRODUCTS:
For injection containing 100 mg/mL (Program ♣ ★)
Oral suspension containing 133 mg and 266 mg/dose (Program ♣)
and 90 and 204.9 mg/syringe (Program ★)
Tablets containing 45, 90, 204.9, and 409.8 mg (Program ♣ ★)

MALATHION

INDICATIONS: Malathion (Ovide ★, Co-op Backrubber Concentrate ♣, IPCO Malathion EC ♣, Malathion 50 ♣, Prozap malathion 57 EC ★) is an organophosphate insecticide used for the treatment of ectoparasites including *Cheyletiella, Chirodiscoides, Myobia, Myocoptes, Radfordia, Psorergates,* and *Liponyssus* spp. For more information, see ORGANOPHOSPHATE INSECTICIDES in the Small Animal section.

ADVERSE AND COMMON SIDE EFFECTS: Malathion is rapidly absorbed, biotransformed, and excreted in the urine and, to a lesser extent, the feces. Caution must be taken against overdose, particularly when diluting highly concentrated large animal products and in young rodents. Toxicity has been anecdotally reported in rabbits after treatment with a 2% w/v dip, although the published threshold for acute toxicity after dermal exposure is extremely high in this species. Breeding may be inhibited after treatment with this chemical. In rabbits, malathion is described as a mild ocular irritant. The threshold for dermal irritation is lethal concentration (LC$_{50}$) > 5.2 mg/L. In guinea pigs, malathion is described as a mild ocular and dermal irritant but is not sensitizing.

SUPPLIED AS HUMAN PRODUCT:
Lotion containing 0.5% w/v (Ovide ★)

SUPPLIED AS VETERINARY PRODUCTS:
Topical insecticidal compounds containing 50 % w/v malathion (Co-op Backrubber Concentrate ♣, IPCO Malathion EC ♣), 53.4% w/v malathion (Malathion 50 ♣) and 57% w/v (Prozap malathion 57 EC ★)

MECA (METASTABILIZED CHLOROUS ACID/CHLORIDE DIOXIDE)

INDICATIONS: MECA is a commercial disinfectant that has been used topically to control dermatophytosis caused by *Trichophyton mentagrophytes* in a commercial rabbitry where treatment of individual animals with griseofulvin was not feasible. Animals were dipped in or sprayed with a solution of 1 part base compound, 1 part activator, and 10 parts water 6 times over a 26-day period. The number of carriers and extent of clinical signs were greatly reduced, but the infection was not completely eliminated. Spraying was more effective than dipping, perhaps because the compound was massaged into the fur after the spray was applied.

ADVERSE AND COMMON SIDE EFFECTS: The animal's eyes should be protected by a compound such as petroleum jelly during the dipping procedure.

SUPPLIED AS COMMERCIAL PRODUCT:
Chemical product, LD disinfectant (Alcide Corp. ★)

MECLIZINE

INDICATIONS: Meclizine (Bonamine ♣, Antivert ★, Meclizine HCl ★) is a human drug used for the prevention and treatment of nausea, vomiting, and dizziness associated with motion sickness and for the symptomatic treatment of vertigo associated with diseases affecting the vestibular system.

Meclizine has been used in rabbits to reduce torticollis and rolling associated with otitis and with infection by *Encephalitozoon cuniculi.*

ADVERSE AND COMMON SIDE EFFECTS: The most common side effects in humans are drowsiness, blurred vision, and anticholinergic effects including dryness of the mouth, nose, and throat, constipation, and dysuria. Meclizine should be used with caution in patients with asthma, glaucoma, urinary tract blockage, enlargement of the prostate gland, and heart failure. High plasma levels of meclizine, such as can occur with hepatic impairment, can result in the development of extrapyramidal neurologic signs.

DRUG INTERACTIONS: Additive CNS depression can occur with the use of medications such as antihistamines, sedatives, tranquilizers, analgesics, and anesthetics. Concurrent use of tricyclic antidepressants may increase the adverse effects of either medication.

SUPPLIED AS HUMAN PRODUCTS:
Chewable tablet containing 25 mg (Bonamine ♣, Antivert ★, Meclizine HCl ★)
Tablets containing 12.5, 25, and 50 mg (Meclizine HCl ★, Antivert ★)

MEDETOMIDINE

INDICATIONS: Medetomidine (Domitor ♣ ★) is an α_2-receptor agonist agent with sedative and analgesic properties. Medetomidine has been reported in combination with ketamine for sedation and anesthesia in guinea pigs, rats, and mice. Atipamezole is used to reverse the effects of medetomidine. For more information, see MEDETOMIDINE and ATIPAMEZOLE in the Small Animal section.

DRUG INTERACTIONS: In mammals, atropine or glycopyrrolate given at the same time as or after medetomidine may induce bradycardia, heart block, premature ventricular contraction, and sinus tachycardia.

MELOXICAM

INDICATIONS: Meloxicam (Metacam ♣, Mobic ★, Mobicox ♣) is a nonsteroidal anti-inflammatory agent with analgesic and antipyretic properties. The drug inhibits prostaglandin synthesis and is primarily, but not specifically, a COX-2 inhibitor. Meloxicam is indicated for the relief of inflammation and pain in acute and chronic musculoskeletal disease, including postoperative pain. Meloxicam has been described for use in rats and rabbits, and is likely effective in other small rodents. For more information, see MELOXICAM in the Small Animal section.

SUPPLIED AS VETERINARY PRODUCTS:
For injection containing 5 mg/mL (Metacam ✤)
Oral suspension containing 1.5 mg/mL (Metacam ✤)

SUPPLIED AS HUMAN PRODUCT:
Tablets containing 7.5 mg and 15 mg (Mobic ★, Mobicox ✤)

MEPERIDINE

INDICATIONS: Meperidine (Demerol ✤ ★) is a short-acting narcotic analgesic used for the relief of moderate to severe pain and as a pre-anesthetic. Meperidine oral syrup can be used to medicate drinking water for ongoing analgesia of moderate pain. For more information, see MEPERIDINE in the Small Animal section.

METHOXYFLURANE

INDICATIONS: Methoxyflurane (Metofane ✤ ★) is used for induction and maintenance of general anesthesia. Concentrations in common use are of 3% to 3.5% for induction and 0.4% to 1% for maintenance. For more information, see METHOXYFLURANE in the Small Animal section.

Isoflurane is now considered the anesthetic of choice for rabbits and small rodents due to its rapid induction and recovery periods and cardiovascular and respiratory stability.

ADVERSE AND COMMON SIDE EFFECTS: "Squirming" is seen in guinea pigs in stage 3, or deep anesthesia, giving a false impression of insufficient anesthetic depth. Other clinical indicators of anesthetic level, such as jaw tone and toe pinch reflex, should also be monitored in this species.

METOCLOPRAMIDE

INDICATIONS: Metoclopramide (Reglan ★, generics ✤ ★) is an anti-emetic agent that contributes to lower esophageal sphincter competence and promotes gastric emptying. It is useful in the management of gastric impaction, gastric stasis, and gastric trichobezoars in rabbits and is likely useful in the management of similar conditions in rodents. For more information, see METOCLOPRAMIDE in the Small Animal section.

ADVERSE AND COMMON SIDE EFFECTS: Metoclopramide should not be used in animals with gastrointestinal hemorrhage, obstruction, or perforation, particularly as rabbits and rodents do not vomit.

DRUG INTERACTIONS: Metoclopramide may decrease gastric and increase small intestinal absorption of drugs.

METRONIDAZOLE

INDICATIONS: Metronidazole (Flagyl ❦ ★) is a synthetic antibacterial, antiprotozoal agent with activity against anaerobic bacteria. It has been used to treat giardiasis and enteric infections, including enteric clostridial disease and dysbiosis, in rabbits and rodents and to treat dental abscesses in rabbits, which often involve anaerobic organisms. For more information, see METRONIDAZOLE in the Small Animal section.

In experimentally induced *Clostridium difficile* colitis, hamsters treated with metronidazole at 210 mg/kg per day for 5 days were completely protected from mortality and disease symptoms during active treatment with clindamycin. However, within 72 hours of cessation of metronidazole therapy, the hamsters began to develop disease and die, with only 20% survival by day 14.

ADVERSE AND COMMON SIDE EFFECTS: An anecdotal report links the use of metronidazole in chinchillas to subsequent liver failure.

MICONAZOLE

INDICATIONS: Miconazole (Conofite ❦ ★, Micazole ★, Micatin ❦, Monistat ❦, and numerous others) is a topical synthetic imidazole-derived antifungal agent useful in the treatment of localized dermatophytosis and active against most pathogenic fungi, gram-positive bacteria, and some *Acanthamoeba* spp. In human medicine, miconazole products are used topically for fungal infections of skin and mucous membranes (e.g., candidiasis).

The use of miconazole in rabbits and guinea pigs has been described in the literature; however, there is no reason it should not be equally effective in other species. Miconazole shampoo may be a better formulation than creams, lotions, or ointments, which do not penetrate infected hair shafts or follicles.

ADVERSE AND COMMON SIDE EFFECTS AND DRUG INTERACTIONS: None reported in rabbits.

SUPPLIED AS VETERINARY PRODUCTS:
Cream: 2% w/w (Conofite ❦ ★)
Lotion: 1% (Conofite ★, Miconosol ★)

Shampoo: 2% w/w (Dermazole ❦)
Spray: 1% (Miconazole Nitrate Spray ★, Miconosol ★)

SUPPLIED AS HUMAN PRODUCTS:
Cream, powder, and aerosol formulations for topical use (Micatin ❦, Monistat ❦, numerous others ★)

MIDAZOLAM

INDICATIONS: Midazolam (Versed ❦ ★) is a short-acting parenteral benzodiazepine, central nervous system depressant with sedative-hypnotic, amnestic, anxiolytic, muscle-relaxing, and anticonvulsant properties. It is used as a preanesthetic, in combination with ketamine for anesthesia, and alone as an anticonvulsant agent. The drug is 2 to 3 times more potent than diazepam and has a shorter elimination half-life. For more information, see MIDAZOLAM in the Small Animal section. Midazolam is administered intramuscularly, in contrast to diazepam, and is preferred in rodents and rabbits for this reason.

ADVERSE AND COMMON SIDE EFFECTS: No significant cardiovascular effects are noted. Respiratory depression and dose-dependent sedation occur.

MOXIDECTIN

INDICATIONS: Moxidectin (ProHeart 6 ❦ ★, Guardian ❦, Cydectin ❦, Quest ❦ ★) is a new second-generation macrocyclic lactone parasiticide in the milbemycin family. Moxidectin is administered orally or by injection to dogs and topically in cattle and deer against a variety of nematodes, biting and sucking lice, mange mites, and ticks. Moxidectin also appears to have macrofilaricidal activity, killing adult filarial worms in clinical trials. For more information, see MOXIDEC-TIN in the Small Animal section.

Moxidectin has been used in rabbits for the treatment of mites, including *Psoroptes cuniculi* and *Notoedres cati var cuniculi.*

NALBUPHINE

INDICATIONS: Nalbuphine (Nubain ❦ ★, Nalbuphine HCl ★) is a mixed opioid agonist/antagonist used as an analgesic agent. Nalbuphine can also be used to reverse the effects of μ opioids such as fentanyl, yet still provide postprocedural analgesia.

SUPPLIED AS HUMAN PRODUCTS:
For injection containing 10 and 20 mg/mL (Nubain ❦ ★, Nalbuphine HCl ★)

NALOXONE

INDICATIONS: Naloxone (Naloxone ♣ ★, Narcan ♣ ★) is an opioid antagonist with sympathomimetic actions used to reverse narcotic-induced depression, including respiratory depression induced by morphine, oxymorphone, meperidine, or fentanyl plus droperidol (Innovar-Vet). Naloxone should be titrated to effect in order to maintain the analgesic properties of the initially administered opioid. For more information, see NALOXONE in the Small Animal section.

ADVERSE AND COMMON SIDE EFFECTS: Use of a fixed dose of naloxone may result in a relative "over-dosage" causing loss of analgesia and, potentially, sympathomimetic effects including increased peripheral vascular resistance and pulmonary edema.

NEOMYCIN

INDICATIONS: Neomycin (Biosol ♣, Mycifradin ♣ ★) is an amino-glycoside antibiotic used topically and orally for its local antibiotic effects in the gut. Neomycin can be used to treat enteritis including that caused by inappropriate antibiotic use and dysbiosis. For more information, see NEOMYCIN in the Small Animal section.

ADVERSE AND COMMON SIDE EFFECTS: Neomycin is highly toxic when absorbed systemically. Neomycin is the most nephrotoxic aminoglycoside. The drug is also potentially toxic to the vestibular and auditory nerves, especially if the drug is instilled into external ear canals with ruptured tympanic membranes. It may also cause a contact hypersensitivity and otitis externa. Neomycin may decrease cardiac output and produce hypotension. Increased absorption of orally administered neomycin occurs in the presence of inflammatory or ulcerative disease of the gastrointestinal tract (GIT).

DRUG INTERACTIONS: Neomycin has a neuromuscular blocking action that enhances the activity of skeletal muscle relaxants and general anesthetics.

SUPPLIED AS VETERINARY PRODUCT:
Oral liquid containing 140 mg/mL (Biosol ♣)

SUPPLIED AS HUMAN PRODUCTS:
Tablets containing 500 mg (Mycifradin ♣, Generic ★)
Oral suspension containing 125 mg per 5 mL (Mycifradin ♣ ★)

OXYMORPHONE

INDICATIONS: Oxymorphone (Numorphan ♣ ★, P/M Oxymorphone ★) is a narcotic agent used for sedation, preanesthesia, and the management of pain. Pain relief lasts 2 to 4 hours following IM or IV injection. Oxymorphone is about 10 times more potent an analgesic than morphine, causes less sedation, and does not suppress the cough reflex. For more information, see OXYMORPHONE in the Small Animal section.

ADVERSE AND COMMON SIDE EFFECTS: Respiratory depression and bradycardia have been reported after oxymorphone administration. Overdosage and adverse effects of the drug can be reversed with naloxone.

OXYTETRACYCLINE

INDICATIONS: Oxytetracycline (Liquamycin ♣ ★, Terramycin ♣ ★) is a short-acting, water-soluble tetracycline with activity against a broad range of gram-positive and gram-negative organisms as well as chlamydiae, rickettsiae, and mycoplasmas. For more information, see OXYTETRACYCLINE and TETRACYCLINE ANTIBIOTICS in the Small Animal section.

Oxytetracycline has been used IM in chinchilla colonies to reduce the impact of listeriosis. In a pharmacokinetic study in "mixed breed" rabbits, a dose of 15 mg IM q 8 hours was recommended to maintain a minimum plasma concentration of slightly >3 μg/mL and did not cause toxicosis.

ADVERSE AND COMMON SIDE EFFECTS: Oxytetracycline may induce dysbiosis, particularly in guinea pigs. In a pharmacokinetic study of oxytetracycline in healthy rabbits, depression, diarrhea, and anorexia resulted within 1 day of the administration of 30 mg/kg, IM, given every 8 hours. No toxic effects were seen in animals given 15 mg/kg in the same manner. This suggests a very narrow safety margin in this species.

OXYTOCIN

INDICATIONS: Oxytocin (Pitocin ★, Syntocinon ♣ ★) has been used for the induction of parturition and to stimulate milk letdown, particularly in rabbits and the larger rodents. Pretreatment of the patient with calcium gluconate (5 to 10 mL of 10% w/v) 30 minutes before oxytocin administration may increase effectiveness in uterine inertia. In guinea pigs, one must ensure that dystocia due to a fused pelvis is not present. If this is the case, Caesarian section would be warranted. For more information, see OXYTOCIN in the Small Animal section.

DRUG INTERACTIONS: The activity of oxytocin on the uterus is strongly influenced by circulating levels of estrogen and progesterone. The response of the uterus to oxytocin is greatest when estrogen levels are high. Epinephrine reduces the effect of oxytocin. If uterine inertia is suspected, the animal should be pretreated with calcium gluconate 30 minutes before administration of oxytocin.

PANCREATIC ENZYME REPLACEMENT

INDICATIONS: These products (Pancrease-V ♣, Pancrezyme ★, Creon ♣ ★, Ultrase ♣ ★, Viokase ♣ ★) are mixtures containing standardized activities of the pancreatic enzymes lipase, amylase, and protease used for the management of pancreatic exocrine insufficiency. For further information, see PANCREATIC ENZYME REPLACEMENT in the Small Animal section.

These products have been used in rabbits to help dissolve gastric trichobezoars and in the treatment of nonspecific gastric slowing. Although their effectiveness is controversial, they would be expected to be most effective early in the clinical course of the disease.

ADVERSE AND COMMON SIDE EFFECTS: These products may cause mucosal irritation or dermatitis if allowed to remain on the skin around the mouth after oral administration.

PENICILLIN G
PENICILLIN, BENZATHINE
PENICILLIN, PROCAINE

INDICATIONS: Procaine penicillin G and the combination of benzathine and procaine penicillin G are the repository forms of penicillin G. For more information, see PENICILLIN ANTIBIOTICS in the Small Animal section.

Injectable penicillin is the most common treatment for facial and genital lesions in rabbits caused by *Treponema paraluis-cuniculi*. The drug has also been used for the treatment of bacterial infections including pasteurellosis, necrobacillosis, and dental and other abscesses in rabbits. Treatment of abscesses requires long-term therapy, often in conjunction with surgical debridement. One regimen involves 12 weeks of SC injections initially every second day and then every third day. Despite this, penicillin has the potential to cause dysbiosis and enterocolitis in rabbits. Penicillin should not be used in rodents due to concerns over dysbiosis and procaine toxicity.

ADVERSE AND COMMON SIDE EFFECTS: The use of penicillin antibiotics can result in a reduction in intestinal anaerobes, lactobacilli, and streptococci allowing overgrowth of clostridial or coliform agents and the development of enteritis and enterotoxemia. Hamsters and guinea pigs are the most susceptible to this condition while mice, rats, gerbils, and rabbits are somewhat more resistant. The threshold for procaine toxicity is particularly low in gerbils.

PENTAZOCINE

INDICATIONS: Pentazocine (Talwin-V ★, Talwin ♣ ★) is an opioid agonist-antagonist used in the management of moderate to severe pain. Pentazocine can also be used to reverse the effects of μ opioids such as fentanyl, yet still provide postprocedural analgesia. For more information, see PENTAZOCINE in the Small Animal section. Use of pentazocine has been reported in rabbits and a variety of small rodents.

PHENYLEPHRINE

INDICATIONS: Phenylephrine (Ak-Dilate ♣ ★, Minims Phenylephrine ♣, Dilatair ★, and many others) is a sympathomimetic agent with effects mainly on adrenergic receptors that is used ophthalmically as a mydriatic agent. The drug also has a local vasoconstrictor effect.

ADVERSE AND COMMON SIDE EFFECTS: Side effects associated with systemic absorption of the drug in humans include bradycardia, cardiac irregularities, hypertension, and irregular respiration.

DRUG INTERACTIONS: Phenylephrine is used in combination with atropine for mydriasis in rabbits and rodents with pigmented eyes.

SUPPLIED AS HUMAN DRUG:
Ophthalmic drops containing 10% phenylephrine (Ak-Dilate ♣ ★, Minims Phenylephrine ♣, Dilatair ★, and many others)

PIPERAZINE

INDICATIONS: Piperazine (Hartz Once a Month ★, Once a Month Roundworm Treatment ♣, Pipa-Tabs ★, Purina Liquid Dog Wormer ★) is an anthelmintic used for the eradication of ascarids and some nodular worms. It is moderately effective against pinworms, and is used most often in rabbits for this purpose. Piperazine can be used in the drinking water to treat large groups of animals. For more information, see PIPERAZINE in the Small Animal section.

POLYSULFATED GLYCOSAMINOGLYCANS

INDICATIONS: Polysulfated glycosaminoglycans (Adequan IM ♣ ★, Cosequin ★) may be beneficial in the treatment of osteoarthritis through a variety of mechanisms. To maximize therapeutic benefit, treatment should begin soon after the inciting traumatic event. For more information, see POLYSULFATED GLYCOSAMINOGLYCANS in the Small Animal section.

Polysulfated glycosaminoglycans have been used to treat osteoarthritis in rabbits.

PRAZIQUANTEL

INDICATIONS: Praziquantel (Droncit ♣ ★, Prazarid ♣) is an anthelmintic used for the elimination of cestodes and trematodes, including liver flukes, in rabbits and small rodents. For more information, see PRAZIQUANTEL in the Small Animal section.

PREDNISONE

INDICATIONS: Prednisone (Deltasone ♣, Meticorten ★) is an intermediate-acting glucocorticoid used as an anti-inflammatory agent. For more information, see PREDNISONE and GLUCOCORTICOID AGENTS in the Small Animal section. Rabbits and rodents are felt to be more susceptible to the immunosuppressive effects of glucocorticoids than some other mammals. Nonsteroidal anti-inflammatory drugs may be more appropriate choices in many instances.

ADVERSE AND COMMON SIDE EFFECTS: Prednisone must be used with extreme caution in small rodents to prevent overdosage. Overdosage may result in gastrointestinal irritation and ulceration, depression of the immune system, polyuria, polydipsia, polyphagia, and hepatic lipidosis.

PROPOFOL

INDICATIONS: Propofol (Diprivan ♣ ★, PropoFlow ★, Rapinovet ♣ ★) is a sedative/hypnotic IV anesthetic agent used for the induction and maintenance of general anesthesia. It is indicated to provide general anesthesia for procedures lasting less than 5 minutes and for induction and maintenance of general anesthesia using incremental doses or continued rate infusion to effect. It is particularly useful for cases in which a short recovery is desired. For more information, see PROPOFOL in the Small Animal section.

Propofol must be administered intravenously, hence its use has been described most frequently in rabbits or under laboratory conditions. Hypoventilation and apnea may occur after propofol administration, particularly upon initial induction and with rapid IV injection. In rabbits, high dose rates are required to produce surgical anesthesia, thus increasing the likelihood of apnea.

PYRETHRIN-CONTAINING PRODUCTS

INDICATIONS: Pyrethrin-containing products (Happy Jack ★, Mycodex ★, Ovitrol ♣, Zodiac ♣, and others) are naturally occurring insecticides derived from the plant *Chrysanthemum cinerariae-folium*, and are commonly used for control of ectoparasites including fleas and, in rabbits, *Cheyletiella parasitovorax*. These drugs are GABA agonists that stimulate the insect's central nervous system causing muscular excitation, convulsions, and paralysis. Insect mortality is enhanced when pyrethrin is combined with piperonyl butoxide (e.g., Sectrol and Ovitrol). Piperonyl butoxide inhibits pyrethrin metabolism.

Flea powders and shampoos containing 0.05% to 0.15% pyrethrin are the products most frequently used to treat rabbits and rodents. Insecticidal shampoos are effective against various ectoparasites in rabbits and rodents, including fur mites and lice. For more information, see PYRETHRIN-CONTAINING PRODUCTS in the Small Animal section.

ADVERSE AND COMMON SIDE EFFECTS: These products are relatively nontoxic to mammals. Some products may be irritating to the patient's eyes; therefore, instillation of eye ointment is recommended before bathing.

SUPPLIED AS VETERINARY PRODUCTS:
Powder, spray, and shampoo formulations containing varying percentages of pyrethrin and piperonyl butoxide are available on the marketplace. Some products also contain carbaryl and other insecticidal compounds.

SELAMECTIN

INDICATIONS: Selamectin (Revolution ♣ ★) is a macrocytic lactone long-acting antiparasitic agent used topically to control a variety of ectoparasites and endoparasites in dogs and cats. For more information, see SELAMECTIN in the Small Animal section.

Selamectin has been suggested for the control of fleas in rabbits as a replacement for carbaryl and pyrethrins. There is no published information on its effectiveness against other parasites in this species.

SEVOFLURANE

INDICATIONS: Sevoflurane (Sevoflurane ♣, Ultane ★) is a nonflammable, halogenated inhalation anesthetic agent for induction and maintenance of general anesthesia. Recovery time is faster than that for halothane and isoflurane and time for anesthetic induction is quicker. The higher maximum allowable concentration (MAC) value means that sevoflurane is less potent than isoflurane and will require a higher inspired concentration to maintain anesthesia. One of the major benefits of this agent is that the depth of anesthesia can be changed rapidly enabling more precise control.

Sevoflurane is being used with increasing frequency in veterinary practice for the anesthesia of small exotic pet species, including rabbits and rodents.

ADVERSE AND COMMON SIDE EFFECTS AND DRUG INTERACTIONS: For more information, see SEVOFLURANE in the Small Animal section.

SIMETHICONE

INDICATIONS: Simethicone (Mylicon ★, Phazyme ♣ ★, Ovol ♣, and others) is an over-the-counter human antiflatulent product. The drug reduces the surface tension of gas bubbles in the stomach or lower bowel making them more likely to be belched or passed rectally. Simethicone does not prevent the formation of gas by intestinal bacteria.

Simethicone has been used in rabbits with gastrointestinal motility abnormalities including bloat and ileus. Simethicone is also available in combination with antacid products. See ALUMINUM HYDROXIDE in this section for more information.

ADVERSE AND COMMON SIDE EFFECTS: Simethicone is not absorbed from the intestine and is not contraindicated in the presence of any particular disease condition. Minor side effects in humans include bloating, constipation, diarrhea, gas, and heartburn.

DRUG INTERACTIONS: None

SUPPLIED AS HUMAN PRODUCTS:
Oral liquid containing 20 mg/0.3 mL (Mylicon ★)
Chewable tablets containing 60, 95, and 125 mg (Phazyme ♣ ★), and 80 mg (Mylicon ★)

STANOZOLOL

INDICATIONS: Stanozolol (Winstrol-V ♣ ★) is an anabolic steroid with strong anabolic and weak androgenic activity. It is potentially useful as an adjunct to the management of catabolic disease states. See STANOZOLOL and ANABOLIC STEROIDS in the Small Animal section. Stanazolol has been recommended for use in rabbits and in rats with chronic renal disease.

SULFADIMETHOXINE
SULFAMERAZINE
SULFAMETHAZINE
SULFAQUINOXALINE

INDICATIONS: The sulfonamides are orally administered bacteriostatic antibiotics and coccidiostats. They are used for the prevention and treatment of intestinal coccidiosis and, in rabbits, hepatic coccidiosis due to *Eimeria stiedae*. Sulfadimethoxine may be active against renal coccidia in guinea pigs, however, this condition is generally not treated. For more information, see SULFADIMETHOXINE and SULFONAMIDE ANTIBIOTICS in the Small Animal section.

ADVERSE AND COMMON SIDE EFFECTS: Sulfamerazine depresses thyroid activity in rats. Crystalluria may occur in acidic urine. Chronic treatment with sulfamerazine may result in alterations in intestinal flora leading to malnutrition and vitamin deficiency, especially vitamin K.

SUPPLIED AS VETERINARY PRODUCTS:
Sulfamethazine:
Various formulations for oral use in drinking water (Sulmet ★, Purina Sulfa ★, Sulfamethazine ★, Sulfamethazine 25 ❦, Sulfa-25 ❦, and others)
Sulfaquinoxaline products:
Liquid concentrate for use in drinking water at 19% (Sulfaquinoxaline 19.2% Liquid Concentrate ❦), 20% (20% Sulfaquinoxaline Sodium Solution ★, Sulfa Q 20% Concentration ★), and 31.92% (31.92% Sul-Q-Nox ★)

T-61

INDICATIONS: T-61 Euthanasia Solution ❦ is a nonnarcotic euthanasia agent that has a narcotic-like action while causing paralysis of the respiratory center and striated skeletal and respiratory muscles. To ease euthanasia, most rabbits and rodents are anesthetized with an inhalant anesthetic and then T-61 is administered IV or via intracardiac injection.

ADVERSE AND COMMON SIDE EFFECTS: Vocalization and muscular activity are seen in some species.

SUPPLIED AS COMMERCIAL PRODUCT:
Solution for IV and intrapulmonary injection containing 255 mg combined drugs per mL (T-61 Euthanasia Solution ❦)

TERBINAFINE

INDICATIONS: Terbinafine hydrochloride (Lamisil ✤ ★ and generics) is a new, synthetic allylamine-available antifungal agent used in human medicine primarily for the treatment of dermatophyte infections, particularly when there is chronic nail involvement. Topical cream and tablet formulations are available. Terbinafine is highly lipophilic in nature and tends to accumulate in skin, nails, and fatty tissues. Terbinafine is considered more effective, as well as being significantly less toxic than griseofulvin, while requiring a shorter duration of therapy. Terbinafine has *in vitro* activity against a wide variety of dermatophytes, molds, and dimorphic fungi, including most *Candida* spp. and *Aspergillus* spp.

Terbinafine has been suggested as a better drug than ketoconazole or griseofulvin for treating *Trichophyton mentagrophytes* ringworm in guinea pigs. The drug has been used successfully in guinea pigs experimentally infected with *Tinea pedis,* a human pathogen.

ADVERSE AND COMMON SIDE EFFECTS: The most commonly reported adverse effects in humans are skin rash, headache, and GI upset.

SUPPLIED AS HUMAN PRODUCT:
Tablets containing 125 mg (Novo-Terbinafine ✤) and 250 mg (Apo-Terbinafine ✤, Gen-Terbinafine ✤, Lamisil ✤, Novo-Terbinafine ✤, PMS-Terbinafine ✤, Lamisil Tablets ★)
Topical spray containing 10 mg terbinafine per g (Lamisil Spray ✤)

TETRACYCLINE

INDICATIONS: Tetracycline (Panmycin Aquadrops Liquid ★, Tetrachel-Vet Syrup ★, Novo-tetra suspension ✤) is a bacteriostatic antibiotic effective against many aerobic and anaerobic gram-positive and gram-negative bacteria, spirochetes, mycoplasmas, and rickettsial organisms. For more information, see TETRACYCLINE ANTIBIOTICS in the Small Animal section.

Tetracycline has been recommended for the treatment of treponemiasis and listeriosis in rabbits, and for the treatment of diarrhea caused by *Lawsonia intracellularis* in hamsters (see caution below). Although tetracycline has also been suggested for the treatment of mycoplasmal pneumonia in mice and rats, doxycycline may be a better treatment choice.

In rabbits, a single oral dose of 150 mg/kg resulted in peak blood concentrations of 1.54 µg/mL and 2.71 µg/mL in fed and fasted rabbits, respectively, within 30 to 50 minutes after drug administration. Bioavailability was only about 10% of that achieved by intravenous injection, and was reduced by the presence of food in the stomach.

Since the calculated volume of distribution was large and high tissue levels have been seen in liver, lung, and kidney, serum levels might not truly reflect the therapeutic effectiveness of the drug at the disease biophase.

ADVERSE AND COMMON SIDE EFFECTS: Involution of lymphoid tissue and impairment of the immune response are concerns in rabbits receiving oral tetracycline long term. Tetracycline may cause dysbiosis in guinea pigs and chinchillas. Tetracycline should also be used with caution in hamsters, although it has been recommended for the treatment of young hamsters with proliferative ileitis caused by *Lawsonia intracellularis.* Tetracycline is added to the drinking water for many purposes; however, antibiotic blood levels are often below minimum inhibitory concentration levels for relevant bacteria. Even a dose of 1,600 mg/L did not result in significant blood levels in rabbits. Daily water consumption may decrease due to the taste of the medication.

SUPPLIED AS VETERINARY PRODUCTS:
For oral administration containing 25 mg/mL (Tetrachel-Vet Drops ★) and 100 mg/mL (Panmycin Aquadrops Liquid ♣ ★, Tetrachel-Vet Syrup ★)

SUPPLIED AS HUMAN PRODUCT:
Oral suspension containing 125 mg/5 mL (Novo-tetra suspension ♣)

THIABENDAZOLE

INDICATIONS: Thiabendazole (Equizole ★, Mintezol ★, Thibenzole ★) is a broad-spectrum anthelmintic drug with antipyretic and anti-inflammatory effects and fungicidal activity. It is well tolerated by rabbits and rodents and has been highly effective for the treatment of *Obeliscoides cuniculi* in rabbits. A dose of 110 mg/kg once, followed by 70 mg/kg q 4 hours for 8 doses showed 99% efficacy in the treatment of this parasite with no adverse effects. For more information, see THIABENDAZOLE in the Small Animal section and TRESADERM in this section.

THIOPENTAL SODIUM

INDICATIONS: Thiopental sodium (Veterinary Pentothal kit ★, Pentothal ♣ ★) is an ultrashort-acting thiobarbiturate used for procedures requiring general anesthesia of short duration. Thiopental has been used intravenously in rabbits and intraperitoneally in rodents, primarily under laboratory conditions. The drug should be diluted to a concentration of 1.25% or less to allow accurate dosage. The use of an inhalant anesthetic such as isoflurane has a greater margin of safety in general practice. For more information, see THIOPENTAL SODIUM and BARBITURATES in the Small Animal section.

TILETAMINE + ZOLAZEPAM

INDICATIONS: Tiletamine zolazepam (Telazol ★) is an injectable combination useful for sedation and restraint, and anesthetic induction or anesthesia of short duration (30 minutes) requiring mild to moderate analgesia. Tiletamine is a dissociative anesthetic similar to ketamine with the benzodiazepine tranquilizer zolazepam reducing muscle rigidity and seizure-like activity. The tiletamine fraction has a shorter duration than zolazepam and; therefore, recoveries may be quite delayed because of continued tranquilization. Telazol has been used primarily in rats and mice, although CNS excitation may occur.

ADVERSE AND COMMON SIDE EFFECTS: This combination is contraindicated in rabbits because the tiletamine fraction is nephrotoxic, particularly at high doses. CNS depression and poor anesthesia occur in guinea pigs.

TILMICOSIN

INDICATIONS: Tilmicosin (Micotil ❋ ★) is a macrolide antibiotic used to treat cattle and sheep for respiratory disease. The drug has good effectiveness against *Pasteurella multocida*. For more information, see TILMICOSIN in the Large Animal section.

Tilmicosin has been used for the treatment of pasteurellosis in rabbits, and several experimental studies have been carried out evaluating its use. A single injection of 25 mg/kg tilmicosin SC resulted in peak serum levels of 1.91 µg/mL at 2 hours and the drug had an elimination half-life of 6 hours. Overall, serum levels were below the MIC for *P. multocida* by 24 hours. Concentrations in lung and uterus were higher than those in serum at a number of time points within the 72 hours of evaluation. A separate study looked at the hematologic effects of a SC single dose of 25 mg/kg over a 4-day period. A temporary decrease in red and white blood cell counts was noted but this was not considered significant. Multidose pharmacokinetic work providing scientific information on the frequency of administration is not available.

ADVERSE AND COMMON SIDE EFFECTS: There are a number of anecdotal reports of sudden death associated with the use of tilmicosin in rabbits. A number of veterinarians will not use this drug in rabbits. The cardiovascular system appears to be the target of toxicity in laboratory animals and domestic livestock. Some tissue swelling and necrosis can occur at the site of SC injection. It is essential to calculate drug dosage carefully, as the therapeutic index may be low.

SUPPLIED AS VETERINARY PRODUCT:
For injection containing 300 mg/mL (Micotil ♣ ★)

TRESADERM

INDICATIONS: Tresaderm ♣ ★ is a dermatologic solution containing thiabendazole, dexamethasone, and neomycin sulfate that is indicated for the treatment of chronic dermatoses and otitis externa of bacterial, mycotic, and parasitic origin. In rabbits, the drug is used to treat otitis externa caused by *Psoroptes cuniculi* infestation, often in combination with topical or systemic ivermectin.

ADVERSE AND COMMON SIDE EFFECTS: In dogs, transient discomfort has been reported when the drug is applied to denuded areas. Hypersensitivity to neomycin has also been described. Tresaderm should be used with caution in small rodents to avoid overdosage with dexamethasone.

SUPPLIED AS VETERINARY PRODUCT:
Topical otic solution (Tresaderm ♣ ★)

TRIMETHOPRIM-SULFADIAZINE
TRIMETHOPRIM-SULFADOXINE
TRIMETHOPRIM-SULFAMETHOXAZOLE

INDICATIONS: Trimethoprim plus sulfadiazine (or sulphadiazine), sulfadoxine, and sulfamethoxazole (Tribrissen ♣ ★, Trivetrin ♣, Borgal ♣, Septra ♣ ★, Bactrim ♣ ★, and many others) are bactericidal antibiotic combinations used commonly as first-line drugs for the treatment of rabbits and small rodents. They have been recommended for the treatment of *Lawsonia intracellularis* induced enteritis in hamsters, and *Streptococcus zooepidemicus* abscesses in guinea pigs. They are also effective in the treatment of hepatic coccidiosis in rabbits. For more information, see TRIMETHOPRIM-SULFADIAZINE in the Small Animal section or SULFONAMIDES, POTENTIATED in the Large Animal section.

ADVERSE AND COMMON SIDE EFFECTS: The use of trimethoprim-sulfonamide combinations may depress thyroid activity in rats.

SUPPLIED AS VETERINARY PRODUCTS:
For injection containing 40 mg/mL trimethoprim and 200 mg/mL sulfadiazine (Tribrissen 24% ♣)
For injection containing 40 mg/mL trimethoprim and 200 mg/mL sulfadoxine (Bimotrin ♣, Borgal ♣, Trimidox ♣, Trivetrin ♣)

For injection containing 80 mg/mL trimethoprim and 400 mg/mL sulfadiazine (Tribrissen 48% ♣)
Tablets containing trimethoprim plus sulfadiazine in the following combinations: 5 + 25, 20 + 100, 80 + 400 (DiTrim ★, Tribrissen ♣ ★)
Oral suspension containing approximately 10 mg trimethoprim and 50 mg sulfadiazine/mL (Tribrissen ★, Tribrissen Piglet Suspension ♣)
Oral paste containing 67 mg/g trimethoprim and 333.3 mg/g sulfadiazine (Tribrissen 400 Oral Paste ★)

SUPPLIED AS HUMAN PRODUCTS:
Oral suspensions containing 8 mg trimethoprim and 40 mg sulfamethoxazole per mL (Bactrim ♣ ★, Coptin ♣, Septra ♣ ★, and others)

TROPICAMIDE

INDICATIONS: Tropicamide (Diotrope ♣, L-Picamide ★, Mydriacyl ♣ ★, Ocu-Tropic ★, PMS-Tropicamide ♣, Tropicacyl ♣ ★) is a short-acting synthetic tertiary amine antimuscarinic compound similar to atropine used to induce mydriasis in animals that lack ocular pigmentation. Animals with pigmented eyes may require administration of a combination of atropine and phenylephrine. In rabbits, atropinesterase may reduce the mydriatic effect of tropicamide.

SUPPLIED AS HUMAN PRODUCTS:
For topical ophthalmic use containing 0.5% w/v (Mydriacyl ★, Ocu-Tropic ★, and others) and 1.0% w/v (Mydriacyl ♣ ★, I-Picamide ★, Minims Tropicamide ♣, Mydriafair ★, Ocu-Tropic ★, Opticyl ★, Spectro-Cyl ★, Tropicacyl ♣ ★)

TYLOSIN

INDICATIONS: Tylosin (Tylan ♣ ★, Tylocine ♣, Tylosin ♣ ★) is a bacteriostatic macrolide antibiotic with activity against some gram-negative and gram-positive bacteria, spirochetes, chlamydiae, and mycoplasmal organisms. The drug has been used in drinking water to treat *Mycoplasma pulmonis* pneumonia in rats. For more information, see TYLOSIN in the Small Animal section.

ADVERSE AND COMMON SIDE EFFECTS: The use of tylosin may result in colonic overgrowth of nonsusceptible bacteria and diarrhea.

VERAPAMIL

INDICATIONS: Verapamil (Isoptin ♣ ★) is a calcium channel-blocking agent used in the management of atrial flutter, atrial fibrillation, and atrial tachycardia. The drug has been used experimentally and, to a limited extent, clinically to decrease adhesion formation after abdominal surgery in rabbits. No adverse effects on cardiopulmonary function or wound healing were noted.

SUPPLIED AS HUMAN PRODUCT:
For injection containing 2.5 mg/mL (Isoptin ✤ ★)
Various tablet and capsule formations ✤ ★

VITAMIN B COMPLEX

INDICATIONS: Vitamin B complex ✤ ★ is used as a component of supportive therapy, particularly in animals with digestive disturbances. Published doses are quite variable, and are often quoted in mL without accompanying details on the formulation or concentration of the product(s) used.

ADVERSE AND COMMON SIDE EFFECTS AND DRUG INTER-ACTIONS: See THIAMINE in the Small Animal section.

SUPPLIED AS VETERINARY PRODUCTS:
Numerous products for injection and use in drinking water containing various vitamin level combinations ✤ ★
Oral syrup (V.A.L. Syrup ★)

VITAMIN C

INDICATIONS: Vitamin C, or ascorbic acid, is a water-soluble vitamin necessary for a variety of metabolic processes, which must be provided in adequate amounts on a daily basis to guinea pigs to prevent the development of clinical scurvy. Vitamin C supplementation is used prophylactically and for the treatment of vitamin C deficiency in these animals, and as a supportive measure in anorectic or ill guinea pigs. For more information, see ASCORBIC ACID in the Small Animal section.

ADVERSE AND COMMON SIDE EFFECTS: Overdosage with vitamin C may cause diarrhea. Precipitation of urate, oxalate, or cysteine crystals in urine has been reported.

DRUG INTERACTIONS: The urinary acidification that results from vitamin C administration may decrease the excretion of other drugs, such as sulfonamides. The potency of vitamin C in both feed and water declines over time. Medicated drinking water should be made fresh daily. Contact with metal watering systems accelerates deterioration; therefore, glass or plastic containers are suggested.

SUPPLIED AS HUMAN PRODUCTS:
For injection containing 222 mg/mL (Generic ★), 250 mg/mL (Generic ★), and 500 mg/mL (Generic ★, Cecore 500 ★, Cee-500 ★, Mega-C/A Plus ★)
Tablets containing 100, 250, 500, or 1,000 mg ✤ ★

SUPPLIED AS VETERINARY PRODUCTS:
For injection containing 250 mg/mL (Ascorbic Acid Injection ✤, Ascorbic Acid Inj. USP ✤, Centravite-C ✤, Sodium Ascorbate ✤)

OTHER USES: Vitamin C has also been used at a dose of 30 mg/kg per day to induce urinary acidification in the treatment of struvite urolithiasis. It is not indicated for the treatment of other forms of urolithiasis.

VITAMIN K

INDICATIONS: Vitamin K_1 or phytonadione (Aqua-Mephyton ★, Mephyton ★, Veta-K1 ✤ ★) is used to treat coagulopathies due to fat-soluble vitamin malabsorption such as occurs with long-term use of antibacterial agents. It is also used to treat vitamin K antagonism caused by salicylates, coumarins, and indanediones, including warfarin and brodifacoum poisoning. Treatment is recommended for 4 to 6 days or as needed for warfarin poisoning, and for 3 to 4 weeks or as needed, for brodifacoum toxicity. For more information, see VITAMIN K in the Small Animal section.

XYLAZINE

INDICATIONS: Xylazine (Anased ✤ ★, Rompun ✤ ★, and others) is an injectable α_2-receptor agonist sedative used in conjunction with ketamine for anesthesia of rodents and rabbits. For more information, see XYLAZINE in the Small Animal section. The use of an inhalant anesthetic such as isoflurane has a greater margin of safety in general practice than the use of xylazine.

ADVERSE AND COMMON SIDE EFFECTS: The negative cardio-vascular effects of xylazine can be particularly significant in small patients. A pharmacological study in rats showed that low-dose intravenous boluses of xylazine (0.1 to 5 mg/kg) resulted in significant and prolonged dose-dependent increases in urine flow rate and sodium excretion, as well as short-lasting effects on blood pressure, heart rate, and glomerular filtration rate. Provision of concurrent fluid replacement therapy was suggested. In two animals, yohimbine administered at 1 mg/kg IV blocked the side effects described.

YOHIMBINE

INDICATIONS: Yohimbine (Yobine ✤ ★, Antagonil ✤ ★) can be used to antagonize the effects of xylazine to shorten anesthetic recovery times and reduce anesthetic-related complications. For more information, see XYLAZINE in the Small Animal section or YOHIMBINE in the Large Animal section.

SUPPLIED AS VETERINARY PRODUCTS:
For injection containing 2 mg/mL (Yobine ✤ ★) and 5 mg/mL (Antagonil ✤ ★)

Handbook of Veterinary Drugs, Third Edition, edited by Dana Allen,
Lippincott Williams & Wilkins, Baltimore. © 2005

Section 11

The Use of Chemotherapeutic Agents in Ferrets

Medical therapy for ferrets has generally been derived from recommendations for domestic cats. Similarities in body size and gastrointestinal form and function make feline dosages reasonable starting points for extrapolation. Administration of oral liquids is generally simpler than pilling. The ferret should be firmly scruffed to ensure that the owner is not bitten and that the full dose of medication is administered. Small volumes of liquid preparations and some ground tablets or capsule contents can be mixed with food; however, palatability and taste preferences vary significantly among products and individuals, respectively. Strong-tasting malt products, such as feline nutritional supplement pastes and fatty acid/oil supplements (e.g., Ferretone and Furotone), can be good vehicles for disguising the taste of medications.

Parenteral injections are given via the subcutaneous and intramuscular routes. As ferrets have relatively little muscle mass for their size, subcutaneous injection may be preferred when large volume injections or repeated injections are required. The muscles of the hind legs or lumbar area can be used as sites for intramuscular injection; however, special attention must be paid to the position of the sciatic nerve. Intravenous injections can be made into the cephalic, lateral saphenous, and sometimes jugular veins; but excellent restraint or even general anesthesia will be required.

The information in this chapter has been limited to that pertaining to the indications and use of medications specifically in ferrets. To avoid duplication of material among chapters, and as most information describing general indications, drug interactions, and adverse and common side effects is based on what is known in dogs and cats, the reader is referred to the Small Animal section for more detailed descriptions. In North America, there are no medications (excluding vaccines) specifically licensed for use in ferrets.

Handbook of Veterinary Drugs, Third Edition, edited by Dana Allen,
Lippincott Williams & Wilkins, Baltimore. © 2005

Section 12

Common Dosages for Ferrets

Drug	Dosage	Indication
Acepromazine	0.01 to 0.3 mg/kg; SC, IM, IV	Sedation
Acepromazine + butorphanol + glycopyrrolate	0.1 mg/kg + 0.2 mg/kg (butorphanol) + 0.01 mg/kg (glyco-pyrrolate); IM	Moderate to deep sedation
Acetylsalicylic acid	10 to 20 mg/kg bid to q 48 hours; PO	Analgesia, anti-inflammatory, anticoagulant
Aluminum hydroxide	30 to 90 mg/kg once daily to tid; PO	Treatment of hyperphos-phatemia due to chronic renal failure
Amikacin	8 to 16 mg/kg total per day, once daily or divided bid to tid; SC, IM, IV 10 to 15 mg/kg bid; SC, IM	General antibiotic ther-apy. See precautions for aminoglycosides.
Aminophylline	4 to 6.5 mg/kg bid; PO, IM	Bronchodilation

(continued)

Drug	Dosage	Indication
Amitraz	Apply to affected skin 3 to 6 times, at 14-day intervals	Ectoparasite control, especially mites
Amoxicillin	10 to 20 mg/kg once daily to tid; PO, SC	General antibiotic therapy
	30 mg/kg bid + metronidazole (20 mg/kg bid) + bismuth sub-salicylate (17.5 mg/kg bid, Pepto-Bismol original formula); PO	Treatment of *Helico-bacter pylori* gastri-tis, can be combined with H_2-receptor blockers
Amoxicillin + clavulanic acid	10 to 20 mg/kg bid to tid; PO	General antibiotic therapy (dose of combined drugs)
	13 to 25 mg/kg bid; PO, SC, IM	Dose is for amoxicillin portion
	0.5 mL/ferret bid; PO (Clavamox = 50 mg amoxicillin + 12.5 mg clavu-lanic acid/mL)	General antibiotic therapy
Amphotericin B	0.4 to 0.8 mg/kg once weekly to a total cumulative dose of 7 to 25 mg; IV	Systemic antifungal therapy
	0.25 to 1 mg/kg daily or on alternate days until total cumulative dose of 7 to 25 mg given; IV	
	0.15 mg/kg 3 times weekly for 2 to 4 mos; IV	Cryptococcosis
	OR Follow published canine protocols	
Ampicillin	5 to 20 mg/kg bid; PO, SC, IM, IV	General antibiotic therapy
Apomorphine	5 mg/kg single dose; SC	To stimulate emesis

Drug	Dosage	Indication
Ascorbic acid	See vitamin C	
Asparaginase	400 IU; IP	Chemotherapy for lymphoma; see text for entire dosing protocol
Aspirin	See acetylsalicylic acid	β-Adrenergic receptor blocker used in treatment of cardiomyopathy
Atenolol	6.25 mg/kg once daily; PO	
Atipamezole	0.4 to 1 mg/kg; IM	Reversal agent for medetomidine
	5 times dose of medetomidine on a milligram to milligram basis	
	2 to 10 mg/kg as needed; SC, IM	Treatment for organophosphate toxicity
Atropine	0.02 to 0.05 mg/kg; SC, IM, IV	Preanesthetic and parasympatholytic
Azathioprine	0.9 mg/kg q 24, 48, or 72 hours (for severe, moderate, or mild gastro-enteritis, respectively); PO	For the treatment of inflammatory bowel disease
Barium sulfate	10 to 15 mL/kg; PO	GI contrast radiography (dilute as per product directions for varying opacity)
Bismuth subsalicylate	0.25 to 1 mL/kg tid to qid; PO	Gastric protectant
	17.5 mg/kg bid (Pepto-Bismol original formula) + amoxicillin (30 mg/kg bid) + metronidazole (20 mg/kg bid); PO	Treatment of *Helicobacter pylori* gastritis, can be combined with H_2-receptor blockers
	24 mg/kg ranitidine bismuth citrate + 12.5 mg/kg clarithromycin tid, for 14 days; PO	Treatment of *Helicobacter pylori* gastritis

(continued)

Drug	Dosage	Indication
Buprenorphine	0.01 to 0.05 mg/kg bid to qid as needed; SC, IM, IV	Analgesic
Butorphanol	0.05 to 0.5 mg/kg q 2 to 12 hours as needed; SC, IM, IV	Analgesic
Carbaryl (0.5 % w/v shampoo, 5.0 % w/w powder)	Treat once weekly for 3 to 6 weeks	Ectoparasite control
Captopril	⅛ of a 12.5-mg tablet q 48 hours to start; PO	Vasodilator as part of therapy for congestive heart failure
Cefadroxil	10 to 20 mg/kg bid; PO	General antibiotic therapy
Cephalexin	15 to 30 mg/kg bid to tid; PO	General antibiotic therapy
Chloramphenicol	50 mg/kg bid; PO (palmitate), SC, IM (succinate)	General antibiotic therapy; treatment of choice for proliferative bowel disease with minimum treatment period of 14 days
	10 to 40 mg/kg tid for 2 weeks; PO (palmitate)	Proliferative bowel disease
Chlorpheniramine	1 to 2 mg/kg bid to tid; PO	Antihistamine
Chorionic gonadotropin	100 IU once after 2nd week of estrus, repeat in 2 weeks if needed; IM	To terminate estrus
Cimetidine	10 mg/kg tid; PO, SC, IM, slow IV	Histamine (H_2)-receptor blocking agent for gastric ulcer therapy
Ciprofloxacin	5 to 15 mg/kg bid; PO	General antibiotic therapy
Cisapride	0.5 mg/kg tid; PO	Gastrointestinal motility stimulant

Drug	Dosage	Indication
Clarithromycin	12.5 mg/kg tid + 24 mg/kg ranitidine bismuth, for 14 days; PO	Treatment of *Helicobacter pylori* gastric infection
Clavulanic acid and amoxicillin	See Amoxicillin + clavulanic acid	
Clindamycin	5.5 to 10 mg/kg bid; PO	General antibiotic therapy
Cloxacillin	10 mg/kg qid; PO, IM, IV	General antibiotic therapy
Cyclophosphamide		Chemotherapy for lymphomas; see text for entire dosing protocol
Dexamethasone	0.2 to 1 mg/kg once daily; IM, IV	Therapy for shock, anti-inflammatory, after bilateral adrenalectomy
Dexamethasone sodium phosphate	0.2 to 1 mg/kg once daily; IM, IV	As above, also prior to blood transfusion
Dextrose	0.5 to 2 mL of 50% in slow IV bolus to effect Continuous IV infusion of 5% dextrose in crystalloid fluids	Hypoglycemia caused by insulinoma
Diazepam	0.2 to 1 mg/kg as needed; IV	For sedation or seizure control
Diazoxide	5 mg/kg daily dose initially, divided bid to tid as necessary, increasing up to 60 mg/kg daily total dose; PO	For treatment of insulinoma, in combination with prednisone
Diethylcarbamazine	5 to 11 mg/kg once daily; PO	Daily heartworm preventive

(continued)

Drug	Dosage	Indication
Digoxin elixir	0.005 to 0.01 mg/kg once daily to bid; PO. Adjust dose as necessary	Management of congestive heart failure and cardiomyopathy
Diltiazem	1.5 to 7.5 mg/kg once daily to qid; PO. Adjust dose as necessary	Management of congestive heart failure and cardiomyopathy
Diphenhydramine	0.5 to 2 mg/kg bid to tid; PO; or bid; IM	Antihistamine
Doxapram	5 to 11 mg/kg; IV	Respiratory stimulant
Doxorubicin	1 mg/kg q 21 days; IV	Chemotherapy for lymphoma; see text for entire dosing protocol
Doxycycline	2.5 to 5 mg/kg bid; PO	General antibiotic therapy
Enalapril	0.5 mg/kg q 48 hours initially, increase dose as clinically appropriate; PO	Management of congestive heart failure and cardiomyopathy
Enilconazole	Apply topically as required	
Enrofloxacin	5 to 15 mg/kg bid; PO, SC, IM	General antibiotic therapy
Erythromycin	10 mg/kg qid; PO	General antibiotic therapy
Famotidine	0.25 to 0.5 mg/kg once daily; PO, IV	Histamine (H_2)-receptor blocking agent for gastric ulcer therapy
Fenbendazole	20 mg/kg once daily for 5 days; PO	Endoparasites
Fludrocortisone	0.025 mg once daily; PO. Adjust according to patient's response	Adrenal steroid support after bilateral adrenalectomy
Flunixin meglumine	0.3 to 2 mg/kg once daily to bid; PO, SC, deep IM, IV; maximum of 3 days treatment	Nonsteroidal anti-inflammatory

Drug	Dosage	Indication
	0.3 to 1 mg/kg every 2 to 4 days long term; PO	Nonsteroidal anti-inflammatory
Furosemide	1 to 4 mg/kg bid to tid; PO, SC, IM, IV	Diuretic, initial management of congestive heart failure
	1 to 2 mg/kg bid; PO	Long-term maintenance therapy of congestive heart failure
Gentamicin	4 to 8 mg/kg total per day, once daily or divided bid to tid; SC, IM, IV	General antibiotic therapy; see precautions for aminoglycosides
	2 mg/kg bid for 10 to 14 days; PO	Treatment of proliferative colitis (*Lawsonia intracellularis*)
Glycopyrrolate	0.01 to 0.02 mg/kg; SC, IM, IV	Anticholinergic preanesthetic
GnRH	20 µg once after 2nd week of estrus, repeat in 2 weeks if needed; SC, IM	To terminate estrus
Griseofulvin	25 mg/kg once daily for 3 to 6 weeks; PO	Systemic antifungal therapy
Halothane	3% to 5% induction, 0.5% to 2.5% maintenance	Inhalant anesthetic
HCG	100 IU once; IM	To induce ovulation and terminate estrus
Hydrocortisone	25 to 40 mg/kg single dose; IV	Treatment of shock, adrenal insufficiency
Hydroxyzine hydrochloride	2 mg/kg tid; PO	Antihistamine
Imidacloprid	Treat as for small cat (see Small Animal section)	Flea control
Insulin, NPH	0.5 to 5 U/kg bid; SC, IM; start with low dose and increase according to patient's response	For treatment of diabetes mellitus; monitor blood/urine glucose

(continued)

Drug	Dosage	Indication
Iron dextran	10 mg/kg once weekly as needed; IM	For iron deficiency anemia
Isoflurane	3% to 5% for induction, 0.5% to 2.5% or as required for maintenance	Inhalant anesthetic of choice
Itraconazole	5 to 10 mg/kg daily for 3 to 4 weeks; PO	Dermatophytosis
	25 to 33 mg once daily with food; PO	Case report of cryptococcal rhinitis
Ivermectin	200 to 400 µg/kg twice at 14-day intervals; PO, SC	General parasite control
	500 to 1,000 µg/kg; half of dose to be placed in each ear; massage in well	Control of ear mites
	*6 µg/kg once monthly; PO	Heartworm prevention
	20 to 22 µg/kg once monthly; PO	Heartworm prevention
	¼ of a 68-µg canine Heartgard tablet	Heartworm prevention
Kaolin-pectin products	1 to 2 mL/kg q 2 to 6 hours as needed; PO	Gastrointestinal protectant
Ketamine + acepromazine	10 to 40 mg/kg + 0.05 to 0.5 mg/kg; IM, IV	Anesthesia
Ketamine + acepromazine + butorphanol	10 to 15 mg/kg + 0.05 to 0.1 mg/kg + 0.1 to 0.2 mg/kg; IM	Moderate to deep sedation, anesthesia
Ketamine + butorphanol	15 mg/kg + 0.2 mg/kg; IM	Anesthesia
Ketamine + diazepam	10 to 35 mg/kg + 1 to 3 mg/kg; IM	Anesthesia
	5 to 10 mg/kg + 0.5 to 1 mg/kg; IV	Anesthesia
	10 to 35 mg/kg + 0.1 to 0.5 mg/kg; IV	Anesthesia

Drug	Dosage	Indication
Ketamine + diazepam + butorphanol	15 mg/kg + 3 mg/kg + 0.2 mg/kg; IM	Anesthesia
Ketamine + medetomidine	5 to 8 mg/kg + 60 to 80 µg/kg; IM	Anesthesia
Ketamine + medetomidine + butorphanol	5 mg/kg + 80 µg/kg + 0.1 mg/kg; IM	Anesthesia (use separate syringe for butorphanol)
Ketamine + midazolam	10 to 35 mg/kg + 0.1 to 0.5 mg/kg; IM	Anesthesia
Ketamine + xylazine	10 to 30 mg/kg + 1 to 2 mg/kg; IM	Anesthesia (see caution under description for xylazine)
Ketoconazole	10 to 30 mg/kg once daily to bid; PO	Systemic antifungal therapy
Lactulose (syrup— 15 mg/10 mL)	0.1 to 0.75 mL/kg bid; PO	In hepatic disease to decrease blood ammonia levels; laxative
Leuprolide acetate (Lupron)	100 to 500 µg/ferret once monthly; IM	Hyperadrenocorticism (1-month depot formulation)
	2 g/ferret each 4 months; IM	Hyperadrenocorticism (4-month depot formulation)
Lime sulfur	Dilute 1:40 in water, wash once weekly for 6 weeks	Ectoparasite control (especially mites)
Lincomycin	10 to 15 mg/kg tid; PO	General antibiotic therapy
	10 mg/kg bid; IM	General antibiotic therapy
Megestrol acetate	DO NOT USE	
Meloxicam	0.2 mg/kg initial dose, then 0.1 mg/kg once daily for 2 to 3 days. Reduce to 0.025 mg/kg q 24 to 48 hours for long-term use; PO, SC, IM, IV	Analgesic and anti-inflammatory

(continued)

Drug	Dosage	Indication
Meperidine	3 to 10 mg/kg as needed q 2 to 4 hours; SC, IM, IV	Analgesic
Methotrexate		Chemotherapy for lymphoma; see text for entire dosing protocol
Metoclopramide	0.2 to 1 mg/kg bid to qid; PO, SC	Gastric motility disorders, vomiting and nausea associated with gastritis
Metronidazole	10 to 20 mg/kg bid; PO	Antibacterial agent with good anaerobic spectrum
	20 mg/kg bid; PO for 10 days	Giardiasis
	20 mg/kg bid + amoxicillin (30 mg/kg bid) + bismuth subsalicylate (17.5 mg/kg bid, Pepto-Bismol original formula); PO	Treatment of *Helicobacter pylori* gastritis, can be combined with H_2-receptor blockers
Medetomidine	See Ketamine + medetomidine	
	0.08 to 0.2 mg/kg; SC, IM	Dose dependent sedation and immobilization
Melarsomine	Follow canine protocol (Small Animal section)	Treatment of heartworm disease
Midazolam	0.2 to 0.5 mg/kg; IM	Sedation
Midazolam + oxymorphone ι glycopyrrolate	0.5 mg/kg + 0.1 mg/kg (oxymorphone) + 0.01 mg/kg (glycopyrrolate); IM	Moderate to deep sedation
Milbemycin oxime	1.15 to 2.33 mg/kg once monthly; PO	Heartworm prevention
Mitotane	50 mg once daily; PO, for 7 days, then q 72 hours as needed	Management of adrenal neoplasia when other medical therapy unsuccessful and surgical removal not possible

Drug	Dosage	Indication
Morphine	0.1 to 2 mg/kg q 4 to 6 hours as needed; SC, IM	Analgesia
Nalbuphine	0.03 to 1.5 mg/kg q 2 to 4 hours; IM, IV	Analgesia
Naloxone	0.01 to 0.1 mg/kg or to effect; SC, IM, IV	Opioid reversal by titration
Neomycin	10 to 20 mg/kg bid to qid; PO	Local antibiotic therapy in the gastrointestinal tract
Nitroglycerin	⅛-in. length of 2% ointment applied topically; once daily to bid	Management of congestive heart failure
Oxymorphone	0.05 to 0.2 mg/kg q 2 to 6 hours as needed; SC, IM, IV	Analgesia
Oxytetracycline	20 mg/kg tid; PO	General antibiotic therapy
	10 mg/kg bid; IM	General antibiotic therapy
Oxytocin	0.2 to 3 U/kg once; SC, IM	Stimulate uterine motility or milk letdown
Penicillin G, Procaine	40,000 U/kg once daily or divided bid; IM	General antibiotic therapy
Penicillin G, Na or K	20,000 U/kg q 4 hours; SC, IM, IV	General antibiotic therapy
	40,000 U/kg qid; PO	General antibiotic therapy
Pentazocine	1 to 3 mg/kg q 2 to 4 hours; SC, IM, IV	Analgesia
	5 to 10 mg/kg q 4 hours; IM	Analgesia
Phenobarbital elixir	1 to 2 mg/kg bid to tid for seizure control, titrate dose for maintenance; PO	Control and prevention of seizures

(continued)

Drug	Dosage	Indication
Piperazine	50 to 100 mg/kg once, repeat in 2 weeks; PO	Gastrointestinal parasitism (especially nematodes)
Praziquantel	12.5 mg (½ of 23-mg tablet) once, repeat in 2 weeks; PO	Gastrointestinal cestodes
	5 to 10 mg/kg once, repeat in 2 weeks; SC	Gastrointestinal cestodes
Prednisone, prednisolone	0.5 to 2.0 mg/kg once daily to bid, reduce dose and frequency for long-term therapy; PO, IM	Anti-inflammatory
	0.5 to 2.5 mg/kg bid; PO, IM; start at low dose, increase as necessary	Treatment of hypoglycemia due to insulinoma; reduce dosage if combined with diazoxide therapy
	1 mg per ferret once daily for 3 mos; PO; taper dose to wean animal at completion of therapy	In conjunction with adulticide treatment for heartworm disease
	1 to 2 mg/kg once daily; PO	Chemotherapy for lymphoma; see text for entire dosing protocol
Propofol	2 to 10 mg/kg; IV	Anesthetic induction, titrate additional doses to effect
Propranolol	0.5 to 2 mg/kg bid to tid; PO, SC	Medical management of cardiomyopathy
Prostaglandin $F_{2\alpha}$	0.5 mg as needed; IM	Treatment of metritis
Pyrantel pamoate	4.4 mg/kg once, repeat in 2 weeks; PO	Treatment of gastrointestinal nematodes
Pyrethrin products	Use topically as directed; treat once weekly as needed	Treatment of ectoparasites, especially fleas

Drug	Dosage	Indication
Ranitidine	3.5 mg/kg bid; PO	Nonspecific gastric ulceration and gastritis
	See drug description	Histamine (H_2)-receptor blocking agent for gastric ulcer therapy
Selamectin	Treat topically with 15 mg (1×2.5 mL tube of puppy/kitten Revolution) as directed	Treatment of ectoparasites and endoparasites, heartworm prevention
	6 to 18 mg/kg topically as directed, once monthly	
Stanozolol	10 mg/kg once weekly as required; IM	Anabolic steroid
	0.5 mg/kg bid; PO, SC, IM	Anabolic steroid (see note in text re frequency of dosage)
Sucralfate	25 mg/kg to 125 mg/ferret bid to qid; PO	Treatment of gastric ulceration and gastritis
	⅛ of 1-g tablet/ferret qid; PO	Treatment of gastric ulceration and gastritis
Sulfadimethoxine	25 mg/kg once daily; PO, SC, IM	General antibiotic therapy
	50 mg/kg once, then 25 mg/kg daily for 9 days; PO	Treatment of gastrointestinal coccidiosis
Sulfasalazine	10 to 20 mg/kg bid; PO	Inflammatory bowel disease
Tetracycline	25 mg/kg bid to tid; PO	General antibiotic therapy
Theophylline (elixir)	4.25 mg/kg bid to tid; PO	Bronchodilation
Thiacetarsamide	2.2 mg/kg bid for 2 days; IV	Adulticide for heartworm treatment (see precautions)
Tiletamine + zolazepam	5 to 22 mg/kg; IM	Sedation to anesthesia *(continued)*

Drug	Dosage	Indication
Trimethoprim-sulfonamide combinations	15 to 30 mg/kg bid; PO, SC	General antibiotic therapy
	30 mg/kg once daily for 2 weeks; PO	Treatment of gastro-intestinal coccidiosis
Tylosin	10 mg/kg once daily to bid; PO	General antibiotic therapy
Ursodiol	15 to 20 mg/kg once daily to bid; PO	Treatment of cholangio-lar and gallbladder disorders
Vincristine		Chemotherapy for lym-phoma; see text for entire dosing protocol
Vitamin B complex	Dose to thiamine content at 1 to 2 mg/kg as needed; IM	Vitamin B supple-mentation
Vitamin C	50 to 100 mg/kg bid; PO	Supportive therapy, as an antioxidant
Xylazine	See Ketamine + xylazine	
Yohimbine	0.5 mg/kg; IM	Reversal agent for xylazine
	0.2 mg/kg; IV	Reversal agent for xylazine

*, drug dosages derived from pharmacokinetic work or efficacy trials in exotic species.

Handbook of Veterinary Drugs, Third Edition, edited by Dana Allen,
Lippincott Williams & Wilkins, Baltimore. © 2005

Section 13

Description of Drugs for Ferrets

ACEPROMAZINE

INDICATIONS: Acepromazine (formerly acetylpromazine) (Atravet
✚ ★, PromAce ★) is a phenothiazine drug used as a sedative and preanesthetic agent, or combined with ketamine for anesthesia. Many of
the doses published for acepromazine are considerably higher than
more recent recommendations for the drug's use in dogs and cats. As
there is no specific reversal agent for acepromazine, the dose must be
matched to the condition of the patient. For more information, see
ACEPROMAZINE in the Small Animal section.

ADVERSE AND COMMON SIDE EFFECTS: Profound sedation and
hypotension may occur at higher dosages. In ferrets, excitation was
reported to last for 4 hours after a dose of 5 mg/kg SC.

ACETYLSALICYLIC ACID

INDICATIONS: Aspirin (ASA) or acetylsalicylic acid (ArthriCare ★,
Entrophen ✚, and many others) is an effective analgesic for the management of mild to moderate nonvisceral pain, and an antipyretic and
anti-inflammatory agent. It has been used in conjunction with thiacetarsamide in the treatment of heartworm disease because of its antiplatelet activity. For more information, see ASPIRIN in the Small
Animal section.

ADVERSE AND COMMON SIDE EFFECTS: Specific toxic effects have not been described in the ferret. See ASPIRIN in the Small Animal section for general information.

DRUG INTERACTIONS: See ASPIRIN in the Small Animal section for general information, with particular reference to treatment of cardiac disease and interactions with insulin preparations. Nonsteroidal anti-inflammatory drugs (NSAIDs) and glucocorticoid agents should not be used concurrently.

ALUMINUM HYDROXIDE

INDICATIONS: Aluminum hydroxide (Amphojel ♣ ★, Dialume ★, Mylanta ★) is an antacid, antiflatulent medication useful for its cytoprotective effect on gastrointestinal tract (GIT) mucosa and buffering capacity, as well as in reducing hyperphosphatemia associated with renal failure. In ferrets, aluminum hydroxide has been used primarily in the treatment of chronic renal failure. For further information, see ALUMINUM HYDROXIDE and ANTACIDS in the Small Animal section.

ADVERSE AND COMMON SIDE EFFECTS: See ALUMINUM HYDROXIDE in the Small Animal section.

DRUG INTERACTIONS: Antacid products may increase or decrease the absorption of a variety of other medications taken orally. See ALUMINUM HYDROXIDE in the Small Animal section.

AMIKACIN

INDICATIONS: Amikacin (Amiglyde-V ♣ ★, Amikin ♣ ★, Amiject D ★) is an aminoglycoside antibiotic indicated for the treatment of various soft tissue infections. Measurement of serum amikacin levels is helpful in dogs and cats to ensure appropriate dosage rate and interval. The recommended peak and trough levels for amikacin in dogs and cats are likely adequate approximations of those for ferrets. See also AMIKACIN and AMINOGLYCOSIDE ANTIBIOTICS in the Small Animal section.

ADVERSE AND COMMON SIDE EFFECTS: Like other aminoglycosides, amikacin has nephrotoxic, neurotoxic, and ototoxic potential. An increase in the efficacy and a decrease in toxicity may occur when the total dose is given once daily. Neuromuscular blockade and acute renal failure can occur after IV injection. Aminoglycosides administered IV should be diluted with saline or sterile water and administered over 20 minutes.

AMINOPHYLLINE

INDICATIONS: Aminophylline (Phylloconton ✷ ★ and generics) is a bronchodilator principally used for the management of cough caused by bronchospasm. It has mild inotropic properties and mild, transient diuretic activity.

In ferrets, aminophylline has been used to treat dyspnea associated with cardiac disease. The drug has been used via nebulization as well as the standard routes of administration.

ADVERSE AND COMMON SIDE EFFECTS: See AMINOPHYL-LINE and THEOPHYLLINE in the Small Animal section for information on effects and usage in dogs and cats. The drug should be used with caution in ferrets with cardiac disease, as well as in patients with systemic hypertension, cardiac arrhythmias, gastrointestinal tract ulcers, impaired renal or hepatic function, diabetes mellitus, hyperthyroid disease, and glaucoma.

DRUG INTERACTIONS: See AMINOPHYLLINE and THEOPHYL-LINE in the Small Animal section. Aminophylline should not be mixed in a syringe with other drugs.

AMITRAZ

INDICATIONS: Amitraz (Mitaban ✷ ★) is indicated for the eradication of demodicosis and sarcoptic mange. The drug is classified as a monoamine oxidase (MAO) enzyme inhibitor (causes a buildup of biological amines in the central nervous system) although the exact mechanism of its action as a pesticide is unknown. It also inhibits prostaglandin synthesis and is an α-adrenergic receptor agonist.

ADVERSE AND COMMON SIDE EFFECTS: The most common toxic side effects are ataxia and depression. Other side effects may include transient sedation, mydriasis, hypersalivation, transient pruritus (due to the effect of dead mites), hypothermia or hyperthermia, vomiting, diarrhea, and occasionally bradycardia. Clinical signs of severe toxicosis may include hypotension, hyperglycemia, mydriasis, and hypothermia. See AMITRAZ in the Small Animal section.

DRUG INTERACTIONS: In small animals, atropine potentiates the pressor effects of amitraz and may cause hypertension and cardiac arrhythmias, and potentiate ileus and gastric distention. Yohimbine (0.1 mg/kg; IV) is a safe and effective antidote in cases of amitraz toxicosis. See AMITRAZ in the Small Animal section.

AMOXICILLIN

INDICATIONS: Amoxicillin (Amoxi-Tabs ★, Amoxi-Drop ★, Amoxi-Inject ★, Amoxil ♣ ★, Moxilean ♣, Robamox-V ★) is a penicillin antibiotic indicated for the treatment of genitourinary, gastrointestinal, respiratory, and skin/soft tissue infections. In ferrets, amoxicillin is specifically indicated for the treatment of gastritis and gastric ulcers caused by *Helicobacter mustelae* in combination with metronidazole, gastric protectants (e.g., bismuth subsalicylate), and H$_2$-receptor blockers (e.g., cimetidine). This combination was effective in eradicating *H. mustelae* from 71% of ferrets in one study. No abnormalities were found in kits born to jills that were medicated while pregnant.

Amoxicillin has the same antibacterial spectrum as ampicillin but is better absorbed from the gastrointestinal tract and has a more rapid bactericidal activity and a longer duration of action. For more information, see PENICILLIN ANTIBIOTICS in the Small Animal section.

ADVERSE AND COMMON SIDE EFFECTS: None specifically described in the ferret; see PENICILLIN ANTIBIOTICS in the Small Animal section for general information.

DRUG INTERACTIONS: See PENICILLIN ANTIBIOTICS in the Small Animal section for general information.

AMOXICILLIN + CLAVULANIC ACID

INDICATIONS: Clavamox (Clavamox Drops ♣ ★, Clavamox Tablets ♣ ★) is an amoxicillin and clavulanic acid combination. See CLAVAMOX and see PENICILLIN ANTIBIOTICS in the Small Animal section for information on antibacterial spectrum and tissue distribution.

ADVERSE AND COMMON SIDE EFFECTS: The drug combination is contraindicated in animals with sensitivity to the penicillins or the cephalosporin antibiotics. See also PENICILLIN ANTIBIOTICS in the Small Animal section.

DRUG INTERACTIONS: See PENICILLIN ANTIBIOTICS in the Small Animal section.

SUPPLIED AS VETERINARY PRODUCTS:
Tablets containing 50, 100, 200, and 300 mg amoxicillin and 12.5, 25, 50, and 75 mg clavulanic acid, respectively, for a total of 62.5, 125, 250, and 375 mg (Clavamox ♣ ★)

Oral suspension containing amoxicillin 50 mg/mL and clavulanic acid 12.5 mg/mL (Clavamox ♣ ★)

SUPPLIED AS HUMAN PRODUCTS:
Chewable tablets containing 125, 200, 150, and 400 mg amoxicillin and 31.25, 28.5, 62.5, and 57 mg clavulanic acid, respectively for a total of 156.25, 228.5, 312.5, and 457 mg of combined drug (Augmentin ★)

AMPHOTERICIN B

INDICATIONS: Amphotericin B (Fungizone ♣ ★) is an effective systemically administered antifungal agent whose use has been described for the treatment of blastomycosis and cryptococcosis in ferrets.

ADVERSE AND COMMON SIDE EFFECTS: The most important adverse effect is renal dysfunction. Serum urea and creatinine levels and urinalyses should be monitored frequently throughout the treatment period. See AMPHOTERICIN B in the Small Animal section for details on dosing regimens designed to reduce nephrotoxicity. In the ferret, it may be difficult to obtain IV access over a prolonged treatment period.

DRUG INTERACTIONS: A number of significant drug interactions exist; see AMPHOTERICIN B in the Small Animal section. Ketoconazole appears to potentiate the efficacy of amphotericin B against blastomycosis and histoplasmosis. Combined therapy has been recommended for the treatment of blastomycosis in ferrets.

SUPPLIED AS HUMAN PRODUCT:
For IV injection containing 50 mg/vial (Amphocin ★, Fungizone ♣ ★)
For IV injection (liposome formulation) containing 50 mg/vial (AmBisome ★)
For IV injection containing 2.5 mg/mL (Fungizone ♣) and 5 mg/mL (Albelcet ♣ ★)

AMPICILLIN

INDICATIONS: Ampicillin (Omnipen ★, Polyflex ♣ ★, Principen ♣) is a penicillin antibiotic indicated in the treatment of urinary tract, gastrointestinal tract, and respiratory tract infections. Ampicillin has increased antibacterial activity against many gram-negative bacteria not susceptible to the natural penicillins or penicillinase-resistant penicillins, including some strains of *Escherichia coli* and *Klebsiella*. Ampicillin also has activity against anaerobic bacteria, including clostridial organisms. Ampicillin is susceptible to β-lactamase–producing bacteria (e.g., *Staphylococcus aureus*).

ADVERSE AND COMMON SIDE EFFECTS:
See PENICILLIN ANTIBIOTICS in the Small Animal section.

DRUG INTERACTIONS: Do not administer ampicillin with bacterio-static drugs (e.g., chloramphenicol, erythromycin, or tetracyclines) because the combination may reduce the bactericidal activity of the ampicillin.

APOMORPHINE HYDROCHLORIDE

INDICATIONS: Apomorphine ★ (Britaject ♣) is a useful and effective centrally acting emetic agent for dogs. Use of the drug in cats is controversial. Xylazine or syrup of ipecac is safer and more effective in this species. Apomorphine produces vomiting by directly stimulating the chemoreceptor trigger zone and possibly by excitation of the vestibular apparatus. For more information, see APOMORPHINE HYDROCHLORIDE in the Small Animal section. In ferrets, excitation is reported to last for 4 hours after a dose of 5 mg/kg SC.

ADVERSE AND COMMON SIDE EFFECTS: Respiratory depression, sedation, bradycardia, hypotension, salivation, and protracted vomiting have been reported in small animals. See APOMORPHINE HYDROCHLORIDE in the Small Animal section for further details.

SUPPLIED AS HUMAN PRODUCTS:
Note: Apomorphine is difficult to obtain. In Canada, it only can be obtained on an emergency drug-release basis.
Tablets containing 6 mg ★
Ampules containing 10 mg/mL (Britaject ♣)

ASCORBIC ACID

See VITAMIN C.

ASPARAGINASE

INDICATIONS: Asparaginase (Elspar ★, Kidrolase ♣) is a chemotherapeutic agent used in the treatment of a variety of neoplastic conditions in small animals, including lymphoma, and idiopathic thrombocytopenia. For more information, see ASPARAGINASE in the Small Animal section.

In ferrets, asparaginase has been used for the treatment of lymphoma in combination with other chemotherapeutic drugs. The following protocol has been published:

Week 1: vincristine (0.07 mg/kg; IV) + asparaginase (400 IU/kg; IP) + prednisone (1 mg/kg; PO; q 24 hours; continued throughout therapy). Week 2: cyclophosphamide (10 mg/kg; SC). Week 3: doxorubicin (1 mg/kg; IV). Weeks 4 to 6: repeat weeks 1 to 3 without asparaginase. Week 8: vincristine (0.07 mg/kg; IV). Week 10: cyclophosphamide (10 mg/kg; SC). Week 12: vincristine

(0.07 mg/kg; IV). Week 14: methotrexate (0.5 mg/kg; IV). Continue protocol at biweekly intervals after week 14.

ADVERSE AND COMMON SIDE EFFECTS: Because this drug is a foreign protein, repeated use can lead to immediate hypersensitivity and urticaria, vomiting, diarrhea, dyspnea, hypotension, pruritus, and collapse. The drug should be used with caution in patients with liver disease, diabetes mellitus, infection, or a history of urate calculi. For more information, see ASPARAGINASE in the Small Animal section.

DRUG INTERACTIONS: Several drug interactions exist, including those with other chemotherapeutic agents. For more information, see ASPARAGINASE in the Small Animal section.

ASPIRIN

See ACETYLSALICYLIC ACID.

ATENOLOL

INDICATIONS: Atenolol (Novo-Atenol ✚, Tenormin ✚ ★) is a selective β_1-receptor blocking agent equal in potency to propranolol. It is the preferred drug in patients with pulmonary disease, e.g., asthma. Atenolol may be useful in the treatment of hypertrophic cardiomyopathy in ferrets.

ADVERSE AND COMMON SIDE EFFECTS: The drug is excreted through the kidneys and should be used with caution in animals with compromised renal function. For additional details, see ATENOLOL in the Small Animal section.

DRUG INTERACTIONS: A number of significant drug interactions exist.

ATIPAMEZOLE

INDICATIONS: Atipamezole (Antisedan ✚ ★) is a synthetic β-adrenergic receptor antagonist marketed for the reversal of the sedative and analgesic effects of medetomidine hydrochloride. Atipamezole is generally given on a volume per volume (v/v) basis (milliliter for milliliter) of medetomidine administered, which is equivalent to a dosage of 5 times the medetomidine given on a milligram to milligram basis. In dogs, calculated dosages of atipamezole are based on body surface area rather than body weight. The recommended route of administration is intramuscularly. For more information, see ATIPAMEZOLE in the Small Animal section.

ATROPINE

INDICATIONS: Atropine ♣ ★ is an anticholinergic, antispasmodic, and mydriatic drug. It is indicated in the treatment of sinus brady-cardia, sinus block or arrest, and incomplete atrioventricular block. It is a parasympatholytic agent that causes relaxation of the gastro-intestinal, biliary, and genitourinary tracts and suppresses salivary, gastric, and respiratory tract secretions when given preoperatively. Atropine is a mydriatic and cycloplegic agent, making it useful in the management of ocular inflammation. It is also used in the treatment of organophosphate and carbamate poisoning.

ADVERSE AND COMMON SIDE EFFECTS, DRUG INTER-ACTIONS: See ATROPINE in the Small Animal section.

AZATHIOPRINE

INDICATIONS: Azathioprine (Imuran ♣ ★) is a thiopurine anti-metabolite immunosuppressive agent used primarily in the treatment of autoimmune disease. It suppresses primary and secondary antibody responses and has significant anti-inflammatory activity. In ferrets, azathioprine is used alone or in conjunction with glucocorticoid agents for the treatment of inflammatory bowel disease. Response to therapy is gradual, with improvement possibly taking several months. A fla-vored oral suspension can be compounded for use in ferrets. For more information, see AZATHIOPRINE in the Small Animal section.

ADVERSE AND COMMON SIDE EFFECTS: A range of adverse effects has been described in dogs and cats, the latter being particu-larly sensitive to bone marrow toxicity. For more information, see AZATHIOPRINE in the Small Animal section.

DRUG INTERACTIONS: See AZATHIOPRINE in the Small Animal section.

BARIUM SULFATE

INDICATIONS: Barium sulfate ♣ ★ is an inert radiopaque material that provides positive contrast during x-ray or fluoroscopic examina-tion. Barium sulfate is not absorbed or metabolized and is eliminated intact from the body through the feces as a function of gastrointestinal transit time. The rate of gastrointestinal emptying will vary with the presence of anesthetic or sedative agents.

ADVERSE AND COMMON SIDE EFFECTS: The most common side effects reported in humans are constipation or diarrhea and cramp-ing. The use of barium sulfate is contraindicated when the possibility of gastric or intestinal perforation exists. Aspiration of barium sulfate can lead to significant pneumonia and possibly death.

SUPPLIED AS HUMAN PRODUCTS:
Numerous barium sulfate suspensions from 1.2% to 98 % w/w and 4.9% to 220 % w/v (✤ ★)

BISMUTH SUBSALICYLATE

INDICATIONS: Bismuth subsalicylate (Pepto-Bismol ✤ ★) is used in the treatment of diarrhea and, in combination with amoxicillin and metronidazole, for the treatment of gastritis and gastric ulcers associated with infection by *Helicobacter mustelae*. It inhibits the synthesis of prostaglandins responsible for gastrointestinal tract hypermotility and inflammation. The drug may also have antibacterial and antisecretory properties. Bismuth subsalicylate relieves indigestion by forming insoluble complexes with offending noxious agents and by forming a protective coating.

Experimentally, a combination of enrofloxacin (8.5 mg/kg per day divided twice daily; PO) + colloidal bismuth subcitrate (12 mg/kg per day divided twice daily; PO) cleared 100% of ferrets of infection by *H. mustelae*. Other researchers investigated the effectiveness of a salt formed from the H_2-receptor antagonist ranitidine and bismuth citrate (ranitidine bismuth citrate). Doses of 12 mg/kg PO or 24 mg/kg PO q 12 hours for 28 days eradicated infection in 50% and 69% of ferrets, respectively. All animals at the lower dose were positive for *Helicobacter* by 3 weeks after administration ended, while 10% of high-dose ferrets remained clear of infection. In another study, clarithromycin (12.5 mg/kg q 8 hours for 14 days; PO) + ranitidine bismuth citrate (24 mg/kg q 8 hours for 14 days; PO) was completely effective in eradicating *H. mustelae* from 6/6 infected ferrets. The organism could not be isolated from treated ferrets for up to 43 weeks after the termination of treatment. Treatment with ranitidine bismuth citrate alone was not effective. The combined treatment with these two drugs was recommended as a slightly simpler alternative to the amoxicillin + metronidazole + bismuth subsalicylate regimen.

ADVERSE AND COMMON SIDE EFFECTS: See BISMUTH SUBSALICYLATE and ASPIRIN in the Small Animal section.

DRUG INTERACTIONS: The antimicrobial action of tetracyclines may be reduced if bismuth subsalicylate is used concurrently. It is advised that tetracycline be given at least 2 hours before or after bismuth administration.

BUPRENORPHINE HYDROCHLORIDE

INDICATIONS: Buprenorphine hydrochloride (Buprenex ★) is a partial opiate agonist with analgesic properties. Analgesia lasts 4 to 8 hours in dogs and cats.

ADVERSE AND COMMON SIDE EFFECTS: Respiratory depression may occur after administration. Opiates should be used with caution in animals with severe renal insufficiency, head trauma, central nervous system (CNS) dysfunction, and in debilitated or geriatric patients. The drug is resistant to antagonism by naloxone.

DRUG INTERACTIONS: The concurrent use of other CNS depressants (anesthetics, antihistamines, tranquilizers) may potentiate CNS and respiratory depression. This drug may inhibit the analgesic effects of opiate agonists (e.g., morphine).

BUTORPHANOL

INDICATIONS: Butorphanol (Torbugesic ♣ ★, Torbutrol ♣ ★) is a narcotic agonist/antagonist analgesic that is also used as a preanesthetic. Butorphanol has potent antitussive activity in dogs. See BUTORPHANOL in the Small Animal section for further information.

ADVERSE AND COMMON SIDE EFFECTS: Butorphanol has minimal cardiovascular effects and causes only slight respiratory depression. When used as a single agent it generally causes little sedation; however, some ferrets appear to be affected to a greater degree. All opiates should be used with caution in debilitated animals and those with head trauma, increased cerebrospinal fluid pressure, hypothyroidism, severe renal disease, or adrenocortical insufficiency.

DRUG INTERACTIONS: See BUTORPHANOL in the Small Animal section. Butorphanol should not be added to the same syringe as sedative or anesthetic agents with which it is being used in combination.

CARBARYL

INDICATIONS: Carbaryl (Dusting Powder ♣, Equi-Shield Fly Repellent Spray ★, Happy Jack Flea and Tick Powder II ★, Mycodex Pet Shampoo with carbaryl ★, Prozap Garden & Poultry Dust ★, Sevin ♣, Zodiac Flea and Tick Power ♣) is a carbamate insecticide and cholinesterase inhibitor used topically in ferrets for the eradication of arthropod ectoparasites, including mites, lice, fleas, and ticks.

ADVERSE AND COMMON SIDE EFFECTS: Toxicity results from cholinesterase inhibition and is treated by administration of atropine. Clinical signs include miosis, salivation, frequent urination and defecation, vomiting, bronchoconstriction, ataxia, incoordination, muscle tremors, convulsions, respiratory depression, paralysis, and possibly death. Carbamate products should not be used on immature ferrets or in pregnant or nursing animals. See CARBAMATE INSECTICIDES in the Small Animal or CARBARYL in the Large Animal section.

DRUG INTERACTIONS: See CARBAMATE INSECTICIDES in the Small Animal section.

SUPPLIED AS VETERINARY PRODUCTS:
Numerous dusting powders containing 5% w/w carbaryl ✤ ★
Shampoo containing 0.5% w/v carbaryl (Mycodex Pet Shampoo ★)

CAPTOPRIL

INDICATIONS: Captopril (Capoten ✤ ★) is an angiotensin-converting enzyme (ACE) inhibitor. It significantly increases cardiac output while reducing systemic vascular resistance, pulmonary capillary wedge pressure, and right atrial pressure. Heart rate usually is unaffected in patients receiving captopril. Captopril is useful in conditions of congestive heart failure and in the management of systemic hypertension. The drug has been used in the treatment of cardiac disease in ferrets. For more information see CAPTOPRIL in the Small Animal section.

ADVERSE AND COMMON SIDE EFFECTS: Ferrets are very susceptible to the hypotensive effects of captopril and most treated animals become lethargic. Animals may not tolerate administration more frequently than every other day, and, therefore, treatment should be started with this schedule.

CEFADROXIL

INDICATIONS: Cefadroxil (Cefa-Tabs ✤ ★, Cefa-Drops ✤ ★) is a broad-spectrum, first-generation cephalosporin antibiotic. For more information see CEFADROXIL and CEPHALOSPORIN ANTIBIOTICS in the Small Animal section.

CEPHALEXIN

INDICATIONS: Cephalexin (Keflex ✤ ★, Keftab ★, Novo-Lexin ✤, Nu-Cephalex ✤) is a broad-spectrum, first-generation cephalosporin antibiotic. For more information, see CEPHALOSPORIN ANTIBIOTICS in the Small Animal section. In ferrets, cephalexin has been particularly recommended for the treatment of respiratory and urinary tract infections and pyoderma.

ADVERSE AND COMMON SIDE EFFECTS: In addition to the side effects noted for the CEPHALOSPORIN ANTIBIOTICS, cephalexin has been reported to cause salivation, tachypnea, and excitability in dogs and vomiting and fever in cats. See CEPHALOSPORIN ANTIBIOTICS in the Small Animal section.

DRUG INTERACTIONS: See CEPHALOSPORIN ANTIBIOTICS in the Small Animal section.

CHLORAMPHENICOL

INDICATIONS: Chloramphenicol (Azramycine ♣, Chlor Palm ♣, Chlor Tablets ♣, Chloromycetin ♣ ★, Karomycin Palmitate ♣, and many others) is a bacteriostatic antibiotic with activity against a wide range of pathogens. It is well absorbed following oral administration and widely distributed throughout the body. See CHLORAMPHENI-COL in the Small Animal section for further details.

Chloramphenicol is the treatment of choice for proliferative bowel disease in ferrets, which is currently believed to be caused by *Lawsonia intracellularis,* a *Campylobacter*-like organism. Treatment may be curative, but some animals remain carriers and may relapse.

ADVERSE AND COMMON SIDE EFFECTS: The most common side effect in dogs and cats following oral administration is gastrointestinal upset manifested by transient depression, anorexia, nausea, vomiting, or diarrhea. Adverse reactions may also include a reversible bone marrow suppression and nonregenerative anemia, thrombocytopenia, and leukopenia; however, these adverse effects have not been specifically described in the ferret.

DRUG INTERACTIONS: A number of significant drug interactions exist. See CHLORAMPHENICOL in the Small Animal section.

CHLORPHENIRAMINE MALEATE

INDICATIONS: Chlorpheniramine (Chlor-Trimeton ★, Chlor-Tripolon ♣) is an antihistamine used in the ferret to control sneezing and coughing resulting from influenza-virus infection. For additional information see CHLORPHENIRAMINE MALEATE and ANTIHISTAMINES in the Small Animal section.

ADVERSE AND COMMON SIDE EFFECTS: The most common adverse effects in dogs and cats are lethargy and somnolence. Anorexia, vomiting, and diarrhea may also occur. For additional information see CHLORPHENIRAMINE MALEATE and ANTIHISTAMINES in the Small Animal section.

DRUG INTERACTIONS: See CHLORPHENIRAMINE MALEATE and ANTIHISTAMINES in the Small Animal section.

CHORIONIC GONADOTROPIN

INDICATIONS: Chorionic gonadotropin (Human), or HCG (Veterinary Products: A.P.L. ♣, Chorionad ♣, Chorionic Gonadotropin ★, Chorulon ♣ ★; Human Products: Follutein ★, Progon 10,000 ♣) is a gonadal-stimulating hormone obtained from the urine of pregnant women. The action of HCG is virtually identical to that of pituitary LH, although HCG appears to have a small degree of FSH activity as well. For more information, see CHORIONIC GONADOTROPIN in the Large Animal section.

HCG is used in ferrets to terminate estrus. A single dose of 100 IU IM most closely simulated copulation-induced ovulation in experimental trials. Treatment is most effective if administered after the second week of estrus. Ovulation should occur within 35 hours after treatment, and signs of estrus such as vulvar swelling should disappear within 21 to 30 days. Restoration of bone marrow activity after persistent estrus may require several weeks. The drug may not terminate estrus in ferrets that have been in heat for a prolonged period (i.e., a month or more).

ADVERSE AND COMMON SIDE EFFECTS: Chorionic gonadotropin is a foreign protein and can cause anaphylaxis when administered parenterally. Continued administration may result in antihormone antibody production and loss of effectiveness. As androgens may cause fluid retention, HCG should be used with caution in patients with cardiac or renal disease. Other side effects described for humans include headache, irritability, restlessness, fatigue, edema, and pain at the site of injection.

CIMETIDINE

INDICATIONS: Cimetidine (Novo-Cimetine ✤, Tagamet ✤ ★) is a histamine (H_2)-receptor blocking agent that reduces gastric acid secretion and is useful in the management of gastric and duodenal ulceration. In ferrets, cimetidine is most often used in combination with antibiotics (i.e., amoxicillin and metronidazole) and gastric protectants in the treatment of gastritis and gastric ulceration associated with infection by *Helicobacter mustelae*. See CIMETIDINE in the Small Animal section for further details on indications.

ADVERSE AND COMMON SIDE EFFECTS: Adverse effects in small animals appear rare. Ferrets dislike the taste of the oral elixir. See CIMETIDINE in the Small Animal section.

DRUG INTERACTIONS: When using combined therapy in ferrets, it is important to note that antacids may reduce gastrointestinal absorption of cimetidine and if used should be given no less than 1 hour before or after cimetidine. Because sucralfate can interfere with gastrointestinal absorption of drugs, it is recommended that cimetidine be given parenterally or that dosage times be staggered by about 2 hours. Cimetidine also decreases the metabolism and/or absorption of many drugs by interfering with hepatic microenzyme systems and altering gastric pH. See CIMETIDINE in the Small Animal section.

CIPROFLOXACIN

INDICATIONS: Ciprofloxacin (Cipro ❀ ★) is a fluoroquinolone antibiotic with activity against a range of gram-negative and gram-positive bacteria (e.g., *Escherichia coli, Klebsiella, Proteus, Pseudomonas, Staphylococcus, Salmonella, Shigella, Yersinia, Campylobacter,* and *Vibrio* spp.) and some spirochetes. The drug is available for oral, IV, and ophthalmic use and is produced *in vivo* as a metabolite after the administration of enrofloxacin. For more information, see CIPROFLOXACIN and FLUOROQUINOLONE ANTIBIOTICS in the Small Animal section.

ADVERSE AND COMMON SIDE EFFECTS: See FLUOROQUINOLONE ANTIBIOTICS in the Small Animal section. Some reports describe the use of ciprofloxacin tablets to formulate an oral suspension; however, the stability and potency of this suspension over time have not been described.

DRUG INTERACTIONS: Absorption of ciprofloxacin is hindered by antacid preparations. See FLUOROQUINOLONE ANTIBIOTICS in the Small Animal section.

CISAPRIDE

INDICATIONS: Cisapride (Prepulsid ❀, Propulsid ★) was marketed in North America for the treatment of heartburn in humans but has been removed from general access due to its association with cardiac arrhythmias. The drug was used in Small Animal practice to stimulate GI motility in cases of primary motility disorders and in cases of gastroesophageal reflux. The drug generally is given 15 minutes before a meal. For more information, see CISAPRIDE in the Small Animal section. Cisapride is chemically related to metoclopramide, which would be an alternative drug for similar conditions.

ADVERSE AND COMMON SIDE EFFECTS: See CISAPRIDE in the Small Animal section.

DRUG INTERACTIONS: Because cisapride increases gastric emptying, absorption of drugs from the stomach may be decreased, whereas absorption from the small bowel may be increased. See CISAPRIDE in the Small Animal section.

CLARITHROMYCIN

INDICATIONS: Clarithromycin (Biaxin ❀ ★) is a semi-synthetic macrolide antibiotic used to treat a variety of bacterial infections in people. It is specifically marketed for respiratory infections in adults and children, *Helicobacter pylori* gastritis, and prevention and therapy of *Mycobacterium avium* complex disease in HIV patients in combination with ethambutol plus ciprofloxacin or rifabutin. It may also be useful alone or in combination with azithromycin for the prevention and treatment of toxoplasmosis.

In ferrets, clarithromycin has been evaluated for the treatment of *Helicobacter mustelae* infections. In one study, clarithromycin alone (12.5 mg/kg q 8 hours for 14 days; PO) was effective in clearing infection in 4/6 ferrets. Combining treatment with ranitidine bismuth citrate (24 mg/kg q 8 hours for 14 days; PO) resulted in the eradication of infection in all six ferrets evaluated; the organism could not be isolated from treated ferrets for up to 43 weeks after the termination of treatment. This combination treatment was recommended as a slightly simpler alternative to the amoxicillin + metronidazole + bismuth subsalicylate regimen. See also BISMUTH SUBSALICYLATE in this section.

ADVERSE AND COMMON SIDE EFFECTS: In humans, infrequent side effects include diarrhea, nausea, and abnormal taste.

DRUG INTERACTIONS: A number of drug interactions exist as clarithromycin inhibits cytochrome P-450 enzymes. Concurrent treatment with cisapride is contraindicated.

SUPPLIED AS HUMAN PRODUCTS:
Pediatric granules for suspension at 125 mg/5 mL and 250 mg/5 mL (Biaxin ♣)
Tablets containing 125 mg and 500 mg (Biaxin ♣, Biaxin BID ♣ ★, Biaxin XL Filmtab Tablets ★)
Oral suspension containing 125 mg/5 mL, 187.5 mg/5 mL, 250 mg/ 5 mL after reconstitution (Biaxin ★)

CLAVULANIC ACID + AMOXICILLIN

See AMOXICILLIN + CLAVULANIC ACID.

CLINDAMYCIN

INDICATIONS: Clindamycin (Antirobe ♣ ★, Cleocin ★) is a lincosamide antibiotic with activity against a wide variety of pathogenic bacteria including many anaerobes and some sporozoan organisms. See CLINDAMYCIN in the Small Animal section for information on antibacterial spectrum and tissue distribution. Clindamycin has been recommended for the treatment of bone and dental disease in ferrets.

ADVERSE AND COMMON SIDE EFFECTS: Adverse effects may include vomiting and diarrhea (sometimes hemorrhagic) following oral use of the drug and local pain after IM injection. See CLINDAMYCIN in the Small Animal section for further details.

DRUG INTERACTIONS: See CLINDAMYCIN in the Small Animal section.

CLOXACILLIN

INDICATIONS: Cloxacillin (Cloxapen ★, Orbenin ♣) is a penicillin antibiotic used primarily against gram-positive, β-lactamase–producing bacteria, especially *Staphylococcus* spp. For further information, see PENICILLIN ANTIBIOTICS in the Small Animal section.

ADVERSE AND COMMON SIDE EFFECTS: See PENICILLIN ANTIBIOTICS in the Small Animal section.

DRUG INTERACTIONS: See PENICILLIN ANTIBIOTICS in the Small Animal section.

CYCLOPHOSPHAMIDE

INDICATIONS: Cyclophosphamide (Cytoxan ♣ ★, Procytox ♣) is an alkylating agent with potent immunosuppressive properties that has been used in small animals in the treatment of autoimmune disorders and neoplasia, including lymphosarcoma. For more information, see CYCLOPHOSPHAMIDE in the Small Animal section.

In ferrets, cyclophosphamide has been used for the treatment of lymphoma, in combination with other chemotherapeutic drugs. Several protocols have been published, with varying success.

Week 1: vincristine (0.07 mg/kg; IV) + asparaginase (400 IU/kg; IP) + prednisone (1 mg/kg; PO, q 24 hours; continued throughout therapy). Week 2: cyclophosphamide (10 mg/kg; SC). Week 3: doxorubicin (1 mg/kg; IV). Weeks 4 to 6: repeat weeks 1 to 3 without asparaginase. Week 8: vincristine (0.07 mg/kg; IV). Week 10: cyclophosphamide (10 mg/kg; SC). Week 12: vincristine (0.07 mg/kg; IV). Week 14: methotrexate (0.5 mg/kg; IV). Continue protocol at biweekly intervals after week 14.

OR

Cyclophosphamide (1/4 of a 25 mg tablet once every 3 weeks for 3 doses; PO) + vincristine (0.05 mg for ferrets up to 1 kg; 0.1 mg for ferrets 1 kg and over; once weekly for 4 weeks; IV) + prednisone (2 mg/kg q 24 hours; PO). Continue daily treatment with prednisone for 4 to 5 weeks, then discontinue gradually with a tapering dose.

ADVERSE AND COMMON SIDE EFFECTS: Bone marrow depression, hemorrhagic cystitis, and an association with the induction of transitional cell carcinoma of the bladder have been documented in other species. For more information, see CYCLOPHOSPHAMIDE in the Small Animal section.

DRUG INTERACTIONS: A number of significant interactions exist, see CYCLOPHOSPHAMIDE in the Small Animal section.

DEXAMETHASONE

INDICATIONS: Dexamethasone (Azium ❤ ★, Azium SP ❤ ★, Dex-5 ❤) is a glucocorticoid used in small animal medicine for its anti-inflammatory effects and in the treatment of a variety of disease conditions. Dexamethasone sodium phosphate does not require hepatic biotransformation and is active immediately upon injection. The most frequently published indications for its use in ferrets include: 1) to treat shock (although newer treatment protocols for shock do not include dexamethasone), 2) to prevent allergic reaction(s) prior to blood transfusion, and 3) immediately after unilateral or bilateral adrenalectomy to supplement glucocorticoid levels. However, as hyperplastic or neoplastic adrenal glands in ferrets appear to produce increased amounts of steroid hormones rather than glucocorticoids, there is likely little indication for the use of dexamethasone after removal of a single adrenal gland. Fludrocortisone is a more appropriate drug for the long-term medical management of ferrets that have undergone bilateral adrenalectomy.

Published doses of dexamethasone for ferrets (e.g., up to 8 mg/kg; IM or IV) are often much higher than those currently recommended for use in dogs and cats (i.e., 0.125 to 1 mg/kg). For further information, see DEXAMETHASONE and GLUCOCORTICOID AGENTS in the Small Animal section.

ADVERSE AND COMMON SIDE EFFECTS AND DRUG INTERACTIONS: See DEXAMETHASONE and GLUCOCORTICOID AGENTS in the Small Animal section. NSAIDs and glucocorticoid agents should not be used concurrently.

DEXTROSE

INDICATIONS: Dextrose ❤ ★ is used to treat hypoglycemia in ferrets with insulinomas. Dextrose is administered IV during hypoglycemic episodes that are not responsive to oral therapy, and during and for several days after surgical removal of an insulinoma. Blood glucose levels should be monitored postoperatively to determine when therapy should be discontinued.

ADVERSE AND COMMON SIDE EFFECTS: When 50% dextrose is used as an IV bolus, it is important to cease administration once clinical signs resolve because rapid elevations in blood glucose can result in rebound hyperinsulinemia.

DRUG INTERACTIONS: None described.

SUPPLIED AS VETERINARY PRODUCT:
For IV or intraperitoneal injection containing 50% dextrose

DIAZEPAM

INDICATIONS: Diazepam (Valium ✚ ★, Valrelease ★) is an effective anticonvulsant for the control of seizure in status epilepticus. The drug is also used as a preanesthetic and may stimulate appetite in ferrets at low doses. Published dosage ranges vary by approximately 10x; therefore, practitioners must ensure they match the dose to the clinical stability of the patient. See DIAZEPAM in the Small Animal section for further information.

ADVERSE AND COMMON SIDE EFFECTS: Diazepam is registered for IV use and causes pain when administered IM. Midazolam is a similar benzodiazepine drug that is formulated for IM administration. The benzodiazepines are generally safe drugs. They have minimal cardiopulmonary effects and are short-acting agents. Dose-related sedation, ataxia, excitement, and sometimes paradoxical aggression may occur. In some ferrets administered 35 mg ketamine + 3 mg/kg diazepam, paddling motions of the limbs occurred within the first 5 minutes of injection or for a 25-minute period starting approximated 25 minutes after injection. Cutaneous analgesia with this combination was less than that obtained with ketamine + xylazine. The benzodiazepines should not be used for more than 2 days to stimulate appetite. See DIAZEPAM in the Small Animal section for further information.

DRUG INTERACTIONS: See DIAZEPAM in the Small Animal section.

DIAZOXIDE

INDICATIONS: Diazoxide (Proglycem ✚ ★) is an antihypertensive agent used in ferrets in conjunction with prednisone for the management of hypoglycemia resulting from islet cell tumors (insulinomas). It inhibits pancreatic insulin secretion, enhances epinephrine-induced glycogenolysis, and inhibits peripheral glucose utilization. In ferrets, medical therapy for insulinoma-induced hypoglycemia is used when the tumor(s) cannot be removed surgically. Prednisone is used initially to prevent hypoglycemic episodes. Diazoxide is added to the regimen when prednisone is no longer efficacious.

ADVERSE AND COMMON SIDE EFFECTS: The most common side effects in ferrets are anorexia, vomiting, and diarrhea. Other possible side effects include diabetes mellitus, anemia, agranulocytosis, thrombocytopenia, sodium and fluid retention, and cardiac arrhythmias.

DRUG INTERACTIONS: The dose of prednisone can be decreased when diazoxide is used in combination. Medical treatment should be used in conjunction with dietary manipulation (i.e., frequent high-protein/low-carbohydrate meals). For more information, see DIAZOXIDE in the Small Animal section.

DIETHYLCARBAMAZINE

INDICATIONS: Diethylcarbamazine (DEC) (Carbam ★, Decacide Tabs ❖ ★, Diethylcarbamazine Citrate ★, Filaribits ❖ ★, Nemacide ★) is an antiparasitic agent that has been recommended for the prevention of heartworm disease in ferrets.

ADVERSE AND COMMON SIDE EFFECTS: Vomiting and diarrhea are occasionally noted in dogs. Administration with food reduces this problem. Do not use in microfilaremic animals because hypersensitivity or anaphylaxis and death may occur.

DRUG INTERACTIONS: Levamisole and pyrantel may enhance the toxic effects of DEC and vice versa.

DIGOXIN

INDICATIONS: Digoxin (Lanoxin ★, Cardoxin ❖ ★) decreases sympathetic nerve activity and is a positive inotropic and negative chronotropic agent. Digoxin is used in ferrets to improve cardiac output in conditions of congestive heart failure and cardiomyopathy. For dilative cardiomyopathy, digoxin can be combined with furosemide and enalapril, as for cats. Therapeutic blood digoxin levels for ferrets have not been specifically defined; however, those for dogs and cats provide approximate guidelines. See DIGOXIN in the Small Animal section for further information.

ADVERSE AND COMMON SIDE EFFECTS: A variety of toxic effects have been described in dogs and cats. Serum levels should be monitored to evaluate dose and dosing frequency. See DIGOXIN in the Small Animal section for further information.

DRUG INTERACTIONS: Interactions exist with a number of drugs, which, for example, affect potassium levels and hepatic and gastric function. See DIGOXIN in the Small Animal section for further information.

DILTIAZEM

INDICATIONS: Diltiazem (Cardizem ✤ ★) is a calcium channel-blocking agent whose use has been described in ferrets for the treatment of hypertrophic cardiomyopathy. Published dosages vary in amount and frequency and should be adjusted to the response of the individual patient. See DILTIAZEM in the Small Animal section for further information.

ADVERSE AND COMMON SIDE EFFECTS: See DILTIAZEM in the Small Animal section.

DRUG INTERACTIONS: Diltiazem is reported to increase serum digoxin levels in humans. See DILTIAZEM in the Small Animal section for further information.

DIPHENHYDRAMINE

INDICATIONS: Diphenhydramine (Benadryl ✤ ★) is an antihistamine that has been used in ferrets to reduce coughing and sneezing associated with influenza-viral infection, to guard against the effects of histamine release from mast cell tumors at surgery, and before or after vaccination or administration of chemotherapeutic agents to prevent or treat urticaria and other allergic reactions. Diphenhydramine topical cream may reduce local reaction associated with mast cell tumors. For further information, refer to DIPHENHYDRAMINE and ANTIHISTAMINES in the Small Animal section.

DOXAPRAM

INDICATIONS: Doxapram (Dopram-V ✤ ★) is used to stimulate respiration in patients with postanesthetic respiratory depression or apnea and to encourage the return of laryngopharyngeal reflexes in patients with mild to moderate respiratory and central nervous system depression due to anesthetic overdose. In the neonate, doxapram may be used to stimulate respiration following dystocia or Cesarean section. Doxapram is intended for intravenous use, but will have an effect when given by other parenteral routes if venous access cannot be obtained.

ADVERSE AND COMMON SIDE EFFECTS: See DOXAPRAM in the Small Animal section.

DRUG INTERACTIONS: Halothane and enflurane may precipitate arrhythmias when used with doxapram. It is recommended that doxapram use be delayed about 10 minutes after discontinuation of these anesthetic agents. See DOXAPRAM in the Small Animal section.

DOXORUBICIN

INDICATIONS: Doxorubicin (Adriamycin ✿ ★, Rubex ★) is a chemo-therapeutic agent used in the treatment of a variety of neoplasms in small animal practice. In ferrets, doxorubicin has been used for the treatment of lymphoma, in combination with other chemotherapeutic drugs.

One published protocol includes:

Week 1: vincristine (0.07 mg/kg; IV) + asparaginase (400 IU/kg; IP) + prednisone (1 mg/kg; PO; q 24 hours; continued throughout therapy). Week 2: cyclophosphamide (10 mg/kg; SC). Week 3: doxorubicin (1 mg/kg; IV). Weeks 4 to 6: repeat weeks 1 to 3 without asparaginase. Week 8: vincristine (0.07 mg/kg; IV). Week 10: cyclophosphamide (10 mg/kg; SC). Week 12: vincristine (0.07 mg/kg; IV). Week 14: methotrexate (0.5 mg/kg; IV). Continue protocol at biweekly intervals after week 14.

ADVERSE AND COMMON SIDE EFFECTS: In dogs, it has been suggested that dose based on body weight, as opposed to body surface area, results in more uniform therapeutic effect and predictable toxic responses. Acute, short-term, and chronic toxic effects are described in the dog and cat. Diphenhydramine (Benadryl) given at a dose of 2.2 mg/kg intramuscularly 20 minutes before doxorubicin use has been recommended to prevent acute toxicity including head-shaking, pruritus, erythema, and occasionally acute collapse. For more information, see DOXORUBICIN in the Small Animal section.

DOXYCYCLINE

INDICATIONS: Doxycycline (Vibramycin ✿ ★) is a second-generation, long-acting, lipid-soluble tetracycline antibiotic used in the treatment of bacterial, rickettsial, chlamydial, and mycoplasmal infections. As compared to other tetracyclines, doxycycline and minocycline are rapidly and almost completely absorbed by the gastrointestinal system and have greater activity against anaerobes and facultative intracellular bacteria. For more information, see DOXYCYCLINE and TETRACYCLINE ANTIBIOTICS in the Small Animal section.

DRUG INTERACTIONS: A number of oral preparations interfere with the absorption of tetracyclines. See DOXYCYCLINE and TETRACYCLINE ANTIBIOTICS in the Small Animal section for further details.

ENALAPRIL

INDICATIONS: Enalapril (Enacard ✿ ★, Vasotec ✿ ★) is an angiotensin-converting enzyme (ACE) inhibitor used for its vasodilatory properties in the treatment of congestive heart failure. For more information, see ENALAPRIL in the Small Animal section.

In ferrets, treatment should be initiated with a low dose every 48 hours. Frequency and dose can be increased according to the patient's response providing no adverse effects are noted. Treatment protocols should be similar to those used in cats (e.g., furosemide + enalapril + digoxin for dilative cardiomyopathy, and furosemide + enalapril + nitroglycerin [as necessary] for hypertrophic cardiomyopathy). Enalapril tablets can be compounded into a suspension to facilitate administration. One method described for doing this involves dissolving the tablet in distilled water plus a methylcellulose suspending agent and cherry syrup.

ADVERSE AND COMMON SIDE EFFECTS: Lethargy, anorexia, and weakness resulting from hypotension have been reported in the ferret, which seems sensitive to the side effects of this product. A range of other effects has been described in small animals. For more information, see ENALAPRIL in the Small Animal section.

DRUG INTERACTIONS: See ENALAPRIL in the Small Animal section for further information, especially with respect to concurrent use of diuretic agents.

ENILCONAZOLE

INDICATIONS: Enilconazole (Imaverol ✤) is a topical imidazole antifungal agent that is marketed as a topical preparation for the treatment of dermatophytosis. See ENILCONAZOLE in the Small Animal section.

Enilconazole has been recommended for the treatment of dermatophytes in ferrets, either topically on lesions or as a rinse or dip.

ADVERSE AND COMMON SIDE EFFECTS: Unpredictable toxicity has been reported in the cat. See ENILCONAZOLE in the Small Animal section.

ENROFLOXACIN

INDICATIONS: Enrofloxacin (Baytril ✤ ★) is a fluoroquinolone antibiotic with activity against a wide range of pathogenic agents. The injectable product can be compounded into an oral formulation using a palatable liquid syrup base. See ENROFLOXACIN in the Small Animal section for further details on antibacterial spectrum.

Enrofloxacin has been recommended for the treatment of a variety of bacterial infections in ferrets, including hepatitis (in conjunction with metronidazole) and *Helicobacter mustelae* gastritis. Enrofloxacin (4.25 mg/kg q 12 hours; PO) + colloidal bismuth subcitrate (6 mg/kg q 12 hours; PO) was successful in eradicating *H. mustelae* from 100% of treated ferrets.

ADVERSE AND COMMON SIDE EFFECTS: Induction of cartilage damage in growing ferrets has not been specifically described; however, caution should be applied when prescribing this drug for young growing kits or pregnant females. Enrofloxacin administered by injection can cause marked myonecrosis; therefore, oral treatment is preferred whenever possible. For more information on adverse effects in dogs and cats, see ENROFLOXACIN and FLUOROQUINOLONE ANTIBIOTICS in the Small Animal section.

DRUG INTERACTIONS: Absorption is hindered by antacid preparations as well as sucralfate. See ENROFLOXACIN and FLUORO-QUINOLONE ANTIBIOTICS in the Small Animal section for details on other interactions.

ERYTHROMYCIN

INDICATIONS: Erythromycin (Erythro-100 ★, Gallimycin ❈ ★) is a macrolide antibiotic with primary activity against gram-positive bacteria. It is effective against streptococci, staphylococci, *Erysipelothrix, Clostridium, Bacteroides, Borrelia,* and *Fusobacterium,* as well as *Pasteurella* and *Bordetella* organisms. The drug also has activity against *Campylobacter fetus,* mycoplasmas, chlamydiae, rickettsiae, spirochetes, some atypical mycobacteria, *Leptospira,* and amoebae. For more information, see ERYTHROMYCIN in the Small Animal section.

In ferrets, erythromycin has been suggested for the treatment of proliferative colitis caused by *Lawsonia intracellularis,* a *Campylobacter*-like organism.

ADVERSE AND COMMON SIDE EFFECTS: Adverse effects are rare but have been reported in small animals. See ERYTHROMYCIN in the Small Animal section for more details. All parenteral preparations are irritating at the site of injection.

DRUG INTERACTIONS: Kaolin, pectin, and bismuth decrease gastrointestinal tract absorption of the drug. A number of significant drug interactions exist. See ERYTHROMYCIN in the Small Animal section for details on other drug interactions.

FAMOTIDINE

INDICATIONS: Famotidine (Pepcid ❈ ★) is a histamine (H$_2$)-receptor antagonist used in human medicine. Although it is more potent than cimetidine, studies have not indicated that it actually is more efficacious than cimetidine or ranitidine in the management of gastric hyperacidity and gastrointestinal ulcers. For more information, see FAMO-TIDINE in the Small Animal section.

Famotidine has been suggested as an alternative to cimetidine for the treatment of gastritis and gastric ulceration in ferrets.

FENBENDAZOLE

INDICATIONS: Fenbendazole (Panacur ♣ ★) is an anthelmintic recommended for the elimination of nematodes and some tapeworms. It is also effective against *Giardia* and some trematodes and microfilaria. For more information, see FENBENDAZOLE in the Small Animal section.

ADVERSE AND COMMON SIDE EFFECTS: See FENBENDAZOLE in the Small Animal section.

FLUDROCORTISONE

INDICATIONS: Fludrocortisone (Florinef ♣ ★) is a long-acting steroid with potent mineralocorticoid and moderate glucocorticoid activity. It is indicated in the treatment of hypoadrenocorticism, where it promotes sodium retention and urinary potassium excretion. In ferrets, fludrocortisone is used to support animals that have undergone bilateral adrenalectomy.

ADVERSE AND COMMON SIDE EFFECTS: In dogs and cats adverse effects are rare. See FLUDROCORTISONE in the Small Animal section for further details.

DRUG INTERACTIONS: Several drug interactions exist that may be relevant in the treatment of ferrets. See FLUDROCORTISONE in the Small Animal section for further details.

FLUNIXIN MEGLUMINE

INDICATIONS: Flunixin meglumine (Banamine ♣ ★) is a potent antiprostaglandin with anti-inflammatory and antipyretic properties that make it useful in the treatment of inflammation and pain associated with musculoskeletal disease. More recent NSAIDs, such as meloxicam, have fewer potential adverse effects. For further information, see FLUNIXIN MEGLUMINE in the Small Animal section.

In ferrets, frequency of recommended dosing varies from several times daily for short-term therapy to once each 2 to 4 days for long-term use. Doses described are similar for the two protocols. The injectable product can be formulated into an oral preparation using a palatable syrup.

ADVERSE AND COMMON SIDE EFFECTS: Flunixin should be administered for no more than 3 consecutive days. Gastric ulceration may be exacerbated by the concurrent use of prednisone. As injection of flunixin meglumide is irritating, it is recommended that injection be made deep into large muscle bundles. For further information, see FLUNIXIN MEGLUMINE in the Small Animal section.

DRUG INTERACTIONS: Concurrent use of methoxyflurane may predispose to acute renal tubular necrosis. NSAIDs and glucocorticoid agents should not be used concurrently.

FUROSEMIDE

INDICATIONS: Furosemide (Lasix ✤ ★) is a potent loop diuretic used in ferrets to reduce preload and pulmonary edema in patients with congestive heart failure and cardiomyopathy. For further information, see FUROSEMIDE in the Small Animal section.

ADVERSE AND COMMON SIDE EFFECTS: A number of adverse effects have been described in dogs and cats. See FUROSEMIDE in the Small Animal section for further information.

DRUG INTERACTIONS: A number of drug interactions exist. See FUROSEMIDE in the Small Animal section for further information.

GENTAMICIN

INDICATIONS: Gentamicin (Gentocin ✤ ★, Gentasul ✤, Garagen ★) is an aminoglycoside antibiotic. See GENTAMICIN in the Small Animal section for details on drug pharmacokinetics in the dog and cat.
  Oral treatment with gentamicin has been suggested as a treatment for cases of proliferative colitis caused by *Lawsonia intracellularis* that do not respond to treatment with chloramphenicol. The parenteral product can be diluted with an aqueous solution and administered orally.

ADVERSE AND COMMON SIDE EFFECTS AND DRUG INTERACTIONS: Gentamicin can be nephrotoxic and ototoxic. See GENTAMICIN and AMINOGLYCOSIDE ANTIBIOTICS in the Small Animal section.

GLYCOPYRROLATE

INDICATIONS: Glycopyrrolate (Robinul-V ★, Robinul ✤ ★) is an anticholinergic agent used in preanesthetic regimens to reduce salivary, tracheobronchial, and pharyngeal secretions during anesthetic induction and intubation. The drug is also used to reduce the volume and acidity of gastric secretion and to inhibit vagal influences on cardiac function, particularly when α_2-receptor agonist drugs are used. For more information, see GLYCOPYRROLATE and ATROPINE in the Small Animal section.

GONADORELIN (GnRH)

INDICATIONS: Gonadorelin (Cystorelin ♣ ★, Factrel ♣ ★, Fertagyl ♣ ★, Fertiline ♣) is used in ferrets to terminate persistent estrus. It is most effective if administered after the second week of estrus. Vulvar swelling should regress in 2 to 3 weeks, while restoration of bone marrow activity after persistent estrus may require several weeks. See GONADORELIN in the Small Animal section for information on use in dogs and cats, as well as GONADORELIN in the Large Animal section.

ADVERSE AND COMMON SIDE EFFECTS: None have been reported in the ferret.

GRISEOFULVIN

INDICATIONS: Griseofulvin (Fulvicin U/F ♣ ★) is used for the treatment of dermatophyte infections. The drug is fungistatic, binding to keratin and disrupting fungal growth by inhibiting mitosis. Griseofulvin is detectable in the skin within 4 to 8 hours of oral administration. Absorption of griseofulvin in enhanced by dietary fat and is affected by the particle size of the product. Treatment of dermatophytosis usually lasts for at least 2 to 4 weeks. Topical enilconazole has been suggested as an alternative to griseofulvin therapy.

ADVERSE AND COMMON SIDE EFFECTS: Nausea, vomiting, and diarrhea are the most common side effects of griseofulvin therapy. Hepatotoxicity and photosensitization also have been reported but are rare. Griseofulvin may inhibit spermatogenesis and is teratogenic and mutagenic in a number of species; therefore, the drug should not be used in pregnant animals.

HALOTHANE

INDICATIONS: Halothane (Fluothane ♣ ★, Halothane ♣ ★) is an inhalant drug used for the induction of general anesthesia. For more information, see HALOTHANE in the Small Animal section. Isoflurane is generally the preferred gaseous anesthetic in small species due to its more rapid induction and recovery periods, and reduced cardiotoxic effects.

ADVERSE AND COMMON SIDE EFFECTS: Halothane sensitizes the myocardium to the effects of catecholamines.

HYDROCORTISONE

INDICATIONS: Hydrocortisone (Uni-Cort ❧, Cortef Tablets ❧, Hydrocortone Tablets ★) is a short-acting glucocorticoid agent with indications in human medicine including the treatment of adrenal insufficiency, congenital adrenal hyperplasia, allergic reaction, and septic shock. In ferrets, the drug has been used for the same purposes, although newer treatment protocols for shock do not include the use of corticosteroids. Some products are composed of purified extracts of the adrenal glands of domestic animals, rather than synthetic chemicals. For more information, see GLUCOCORTICOID AGENTS in the Small Animal section. NSAIDs and glucocorticoid agents should not be used concurrently.

SUPPLIED AS VETERINARY PRODUCT:
For injection 200 μg/mL (Uni-Cort ❧)

SUPPLIED AS HUMAN PRODUCTS:
Tablets containing 5 mg (Cortef ★), 10 mg (Cortef ❧ ★, Hydrocortone ★), 20 mg (Cortef ❧ ★)
Oral suspension containing 10 mg/5 mL (Cortef ★)
For injection containing 25 mg/mL and 50 mg/mL (Generic ★)

HYDROXYZINE

INDICATIONS: Hydroxyzine (Atarax ❧ ★) is an anxiolytic, antihistaminic agent. The drug also has anticholinergic, antiemetic, and bronchodilatory effects. It has been used in small animals primarily for its antihistaminic properties. For more information, see HYDROXYZINE and ANTIHISTAMINES in the Small Animal section.

ADVERSE AND COMMON SIDE EFFECTS: Transitory drowsiness is the most common side effect with the use of hydroxyzine. Other adverse effects may include fine rapid tremors, seizures, xerostomia, hypotension, diarrhea, and decreased appetite.

DRUG INTERACTIONS: Barbiturates and other sedatives may potentiate central nervous system depression.

IMIDACLOPRID

INDICATIONS: Imidacloprid (Advantage ❧ ★) is a systemic, chloronicotinyl insecticide that has been used in agriculture for the control of sucking insects such as fleas, aphids, whiteflies, termites, turf insects, soil insects, and some beetles. Imidacloprid is now available as a topical product for flea control in dogs and cats, and has been recommended for the control of fleas in ferrets.

SUPPLIED AS VETERINARY PRODUCT:
Individual one-dose tubes for topical use containing 0.4 mL of 9.1% w/w (Advantage Orange/9 For Cats and Kittens 8 Weeks and Older and 9 lbs. and Under ♣ ★)

INSULIN

INDICATIONS: Insulin preparations ♣ ★ are used in the management of diabetes mellitus. The various types of beef-pork insulin and their properties are described under INSULIN in the Small Animal section. NPH insulin, now discontinued, was the form most commonly prescribed for use in ferrets. Starting dosages ranged from 0.25 to 0.5 units/kg, with up to 5 to 6 units/kg needed daily in some cases.

ADVERSE AND COMMON SIDE EFFECTS AND DRUG INTERACTIONS: See INSULIN in the Small Animal section.

IRON DEXTRAN

INDICATIONS: Iron dextran (Ferrodex ★, Ironol-100 ♣, and others) is indicated for the treatment of iron deficiency anemia.

ADVERSE AND COMMON SIDE EFFECTS: Intramuscular injections can be irritating. Allergic reactions and anaphylaxis have occasionally been reported in humans.

DRUG INTERACTIONS: Clinical response may be delayed in patients concurrently receiving chloramphenicol.

SUPPLIED AS VETERINARY PRODUCTS:
For injection containing 100 and 200 mg elemental iron/mL (Ferrodex ★, Ironol-100 ♣, and generic products)

ISOFLURANE

INDICATIONS: Isoflurane (Aerrane ♣ ★, Forane ♣ ★, IsoFlo ♣ ★, Iso-Thesia ★) is a halogenated inhalant anesthetic agent with a low blood:gas partition coefficient that results in rapid induction and recovery periods. Cardiovascular status is better maintained with isoflurane than with halothane, and isoflurane does not sensitize the heart to epinephrine-induced cardiac arrhythmias as does halothane. For more information, see ISOFLURANE in the Small Animal section.
    Isoflurane is currently the inhalant anesthetic of choice for ferrets.

ADVERSE AND COMMON SIDE EFFECTS: Isoflurane is a cardiac and respiratory depressant. Dose dependent hypotension has been described in the ferret. Because splenic sequestration of red blood cells occurs under isoflurane anesthesia in ferrets, caution should be taken when anesthetizing severely anemic animals.

ITRACONAZOLE

INDICATIONS: Itraconazole (Sporanox ♣ ★) is a triazole antifungal agent active against histoplasmosis, blastomycosis, aspergillosis, cryptococcosis, dermatophytosis, and candidiasis. The drug is used orally and is best absorbed with a fatty meal. For more information, see ITRACONAZOLE in the Small Animal section.

Itraconazole has been suggested for the treatment of dermatophytosis in ferrets. The drug is incorporated into keratinocyte basal membranes with continuous release to skin for 3 to 4 weeks after treatment. A topical product should also be used concurrently to remove spores from the hair shafts.

Itraconazole has been used to successfully treat a ferret with rhinitis caused by *Cryptococcus neoformans* var. *gattii*. The animal was initially given 33 mg orally once daily for 171 days, and then the dose was reduced to 25 mg daily. At the time the article was written a total of 10 months of treatment had been completed. Treatment was to continue until the animal's LCAT titer was 0.

SUPPLIED AS HUMAN PRODUCT:
Capsules containing 100 mg (Sporanox ♣ ★)
Oral solution containing 10 mg/mL (Sporanox ♣ ★)
For IV injection containing 10 mg/mL (Sporanox ★)

IVERMECTIN

INDICATIONS: Ivermectin (Heartgard ♣ ★, Ivomec ♣ ★, Eqvalan ♣ ★, and others) is used for the eradication of parasites including enteric nematodes and ectoparasites, especially sarcoptic mange. The injectable product has also been applied topically to the inner ear to treat ear mites.

Ivermectin is also used for the prevention of infection by *Dirofilaria immitis* and as a microfilaricide. Experimental work has suggested that doses of 3 and 6 µg/kg are capable of preventing maturation of *D. immitis* larvae, whereas, in another study the minimum effective dose was between 12.5 and 50 µg/kg. The American Heartworm Association recommends a monthly oral dose of 6 µg/kg beginning 1 month before the onset of the transmission season and continuing throughout the period of exposure. Higher doses are generally used in practice. Ivermectin liquid can be diluted in propylene glycol to make an oral solution of convenient volume. One commonly cited recipe is as follows: 0.3 mL of 1% bovine ivermectin mixed in 30 mL of propylene glycol resulting in a 0.1 mg/mL solution. The diluted suspension must also be protected from light. Ferrets have commonly been treated for heartworm prophylaxis with ¼ tablet of the smallest canine Heartgard product (68 µg/tablet) or with the feline Heartgard Fx (165 µg/tablet).

One report in the literature describes the successful treatment of eosinophilic gastroenteritis with two doses of ivermectin (400 µg/kg) administered SC at a 2-week interval.

ADVERSE AND COMMON SIDE EFFECTS: Ivermectin has a wide margin of safety.

KAOLIN-PECTIN

INDICATIONS: Kaolin-pectin (Kaopectate ♣ ★ and others) is a gastro-intestinal protectant used in the management of diarrhea. It coats the surface of the gut and exerts a mild demulcent and absorbent effect. It is actually relatively ineffective in absorbing toxins produced by enteropathogenic bacteria. It appears to act by adding particulate matter to the feces, which improves consistency until the disease spontaneously resolves. Kaolin is a potent coagulation activator and may be of some benefit in treating diarrhea associated with mucosal disruption and hemorrhage. Some antidiarrheal products registered for use in humans, including Kaopectate Oral Suspension, contain attapulgite (magnesium aluminum silicate) rather than kaolin (aluminum silicate).

ADVERSE AND COMMON SIDE EFFECTS: Kaolin-pectin may cause constipation, especially in poorly hydrated patients.

DRUG INTERACTIONS: The absorption of lincomycin is decreased if given concurrently with kaolin-pectin. Administer kaolin-pectin 2 hours before or 3 to 4 hours after lincomycin. Absorption of digoxin may also be hindered by kaolin-pectin.

SUPPLIED AS VETERINARY PRODUCT:
Oral suspension containing kaolin 197 mg and pectin 4.33 mg per mL (large animal preparation) (Kaopectate ♣), 5.85 g kaolin and 130 mg pectin/30 mL (Kaopectolin ★, Kaolin Pectin ★, Kaolin-Pectin Plus ★, Kao-Pec ★, Kao-Pect ★), and kaolin 5.8 g and pectin 268 mg/30 mL (Kaolin-Pectin Suspension ★)

SUPPLIED AS HUMAN PRODUCTS:
Oral suspension containing kaolin 5.2 g and 260 mg pectin/30 mL (Kao-Spen ★), 5.85 g kaolin and 130 mg pectin/30 mL (Kaopectolin ★), 7 g kaolin and 143 mg pectin/30 mL (Donnagel-MB ♣)
Oral suspension containing attapulgite (Kaopectate Oral Suspension ♣ ★) in 600 mg/15 mL (Children's, Regular) and 750 mg/15 mL (Extra-strength)

KETAMINE

INDICATIONS: Ketamine (Ketaset ♣ ★, Vetalar ♣ ★) is a nonbarbiturate dissociative anesthetic best used in combination with other agents. For more information, see KETAMINE in the Small Animal section.

In ferrets, ketamine has been used to induce deep sedation and anesthesia in combination with sedatives, opioids, and tranquilizers including xylazine, medetomidine, diazepam, midazolam, butorphanol, and acepromazine to improve muscle relaxation and/or increase analgesia. In small animal practice, mask induction (with or without prior sedation) and maintenance on isoflurane is a much more common anesthetic protocol.

ADVERSE AND COMMON SIDE EFFECTS: Ketamine is a tissue irritant when given IM. Muscle relaxation is poor when ketamine is administered by itself.

KETOCONAZOLE

INDICATIONS: Ketoconazole (Nizoral ♣ ★) is used in the treatment of a variety of topical and systemic mycotic infections, sometimes in combination with amphotericin B. For a time the drug was recommended for the treatment of hyperadrenocorticism when surgical removal of the affected adrenal gland was not possible; however, clinical cases have responded poorly. Ketoconazole effectively blocks cortisol synthesis in dogs with pituitary-dependent hyperadrenocorticism as well as those with adrenocortical tumors; hence, it has been used for this purpose. As adrenal disease in ferrets is not associated with increased cortisol production, the rationale for treatment may not be appropriate, although the drug does also affect production of other steroid hormones. The GnRH analog, leuprolide acetate, is now used for the medical treatment of adrenal disease in ferrets.

ADVERSE AND COMMON SIDE EFFECTS: Gastrointestinal side effects in dogs may be prevented by administering the drug with food (which may also serve to increase its absorption) and by dividing the daily dose and administering the drug 2 to 4 times daily. Ketoconazole should not be used in breeding animals.

DRUG INTERACTIONS: See KETOCONAZOLE in the Small Animal section.

LACTULOSE

INDICATIONS: Lactulose (Cephulac ♣ ★, Chronulac ♣ ★) is a synthetic nonabsorbable disaccharide. It acts as a mild osmotic laxative, increases the rate of passage of ingesta, and reduces bacterial production of ammonia, making it useful in the management of hepatic encephalopathy. Enteric bacteria ferment lactulose to acidic by-products, which decrease intraluminal pH, and favor the formation of ammonium ions, which are poorly absorbed.

ADVERSE AND COMMON SIDE EFFECTS AND DRUG INTERACTIONS: See LACTULOSE in the Small Animal section.

LEUPROLIDE ACETATE

INDICATIONS: Leuprolide acetate (Lupron ✿ ★) is a synthetic GnRH analog. The drug binds to GnRh receptors in the anterior pituitary with high specificity, affinity, and activity. It initially induces hormonal upregulation, but receptors are downregulated after prolonged exposure to continued rapid pulses of GnRH levels. There is an initial stimulation of FSH and LH production and release, which may induce ovulation. Shortly after, there is a decrease in LH and, in some species, FSH. In humans, leuprolide acetate is used to treat prostate cancer, endometriosis, and central precocious puberty.

In ferrets, leuprolide acetate is used for the treatment of clinical syndromes resulting from excess steroid production by the adrenal cortex in adrenal hyperplasia and neoplasia. In most ferrets, clinical signs including hair loss, vulvar swelling, and prostatic hyperplasia respond well to treatment. Improvement should be noted within several weeks, while full regrowth of the hair coat may take several months. If the adrenal glands are functioning independently of GnRH stimulation, e.g., adrenal carcinoma, this drug is not expected to be effective. As this treatment suppresses adrenal steroid output without directly affecting the adrenal gland, it must be continued for the life of the ferret.

Leuprolide acetate is available in several injectable depot formulations with different durations of action and is intended for human use. The drug can be reconstituted according to manufacturer's directions and then further diluted in sterile water for injection, often to a concentration of 0.5 to 1 mg/mL. Under sterile conditions, the final solution is divided into aliquots of appropriate dose (generally 0.1 mg), and kept frozen (freezing at –70°C is preferred; however, anecdotally –20°C appears adequate for periods of up to one year). When handled correctly, the product should remain effective until the manufacturer's expiry date. The choice of product and total dose are based on the number of days for which the clinical effect is intended. Treatment is initiated and most commonly maintained with the one month depot formulation; however, some practitioners may switch to a longer acting product. Some ferrets appear to respond better to the one month depot formulation than to the other formulations.

ADVERSE AND COMMON SIDE EFFECTS: Few side effects have been described in ferrets, especially if the drug is administered as directed via deep intramuscular injection. Nodular lesions and erythema at the site of injection have been rarely reported. A large number and wide range of effects have been reported in people, to the extent that a "National Lupron Victims Network" has been established.

SUPPLIED AS HUMAN PRODUCTS:
Lupron Depot for injection:
For monthly use containing 3.75 mg ♣ ★ and 7.5 mg ♣ ★ per vial
For use every 3 months containing 11.25 mg ♣ ★ and 22.5 mg ♣ per vial
For use every 4 months containing 30 mg ♣ ★ per vial

LIME SULFUR

INDICATIONS: Lime sulfur, or calcium polysulfide, is an agricultural chemical with insecticidal and fungicidal properties that has been used topically in the treatment of sarcoptic mange and dermatomycosis. Lime sulfur may be safer than ivermectin for the treatment of young kits. For use in cats, a combination of 1 part 23% lime sulfur (liquid), 5 parts shampoo, and 2 parts water has been suggested for dermatophyte infection.

ADVERSE AND COMMON SIDE EFFECTS: Although lime sulfur is generally described as a very safe preparation, the material safety data sheets (MSDSs) for calcium polysulfide (chemical name) provide cautions against ingestion, inhalation, and contact with skin and eyes. Lime sulfur is yellow and has a strong odor.

SUPPLIED AS AGRICULTURAL CHEMICAL:
Lime sulfur (calcium polysulfide) liquid or powder

LINCOMYCIN

INDICATIONS: Lincomycin (Lincocin ♣ ★) is a lincosamide antibiotic. For information on antibacterial spectrum and indications for use in dogs, see LINCOMYCIN in the Small Animal section.

ADVERSE AND COMMON SIDE EFFECTS: Vomiting and loose stools may occur after administration. Hemorrhagic diarrhea has been reported in dogs, as well as pain upon injection.

DRUG INTERACTIONS: Kaolin, pectin, and bismuth subsalicylate decrease gastrointestinal absorption. For further information, see LINCOMYCIN in the Small Animal section.

MEGESTROL ACETATE

INDICATIONS: Megestrol acetate or MGA (Ovaban ♣ ★, Ovarid ♣) is a progestational compound used in some species to prevent or postpone estrus. Use of the drug is contraindicated in ferrets because it predisposes to pyometra. See also MEGESTROL ACETATE in the Small Animal section.

MELARSOMINE

INDICATIONS: Melarsomine (Immiticide ★) is indicated in the treatment of heartworm disease caused by immature (4-month-old, stage L₅) to mature adult infections of *Dirofilaria immitis* in dogs. The drug causes greater worm mortality than thiacetarsamide and is associated with fewer complications.

Malarsomine has been used successfully to treat heartworm disease in ferrets according to canine protocols. Oral prednisolone (1 mg/kg q 24 hours) should be administered concurrently and for 4 months or until the ferret is negative on an occult heartworm test.

ADVERSE AND COMMON SIDE EFFECTS: Melarsomine has a low margin of safety. For more information, see MELARSOMINE in the Small Animal section. In ferrets, deaths attributed to worm embolism have occurred within 12 hours of treatment with melarsomine.

MELOXICAM

INDICATIONS: Meloxicam (Metacam ♣, Mobic ★, Mobicox ♣) is a nonsteroidal anti-inflammatory agent with analgesic and antipyretic properties. The drug inhibits prostaglandin synthesis and is primarily, but not exclusively, a COX-2 inhibitor. Meloxicam is indicated for the relief of inflammation and pain in acute and chronic musculoskeletal disease, including postoperative pain. Meloxicam is used in ferrets for the above mentioned purposes. For more information, see MELOXICAM in the Small Animal section.

DRUG INTERACTIONS: NSAIDs and glucocorticoid agents should not be used concurrently.

SUPPLIED AS VETERINARY PRODUCTS:
For injection containing 5 mg/mL (Metacam ♣)
Oral suspension containing 1.5 mg/mL (Metacam ♣)

SUPPLIED AS HUMAN PRODUCTS:
Tablets containing 7.5 mg (Mobic ★, Mobicox ♣) and 15 mg (Mobicox ♣)

MEPERIDINE

INDICATIONS: Meperidine (Demerol ♣ ★) is a short-acting narcotic analgesic used for the relief of moderate to severe pain or as a preanesthetic. Meperidine has only minimal sedative effects. For more information, see MEPERIDINE in the Small Animal section.

ADVERSE AND COMMON SIDE EFFECTS: Meperidine is the only narcotic with depressant effects on the heart, and it also may cause histamine release. A number of adverse effects have been described. Do not administer meperidine IV. See MEPERIDINE in the Small Animal section for further details. The drug is quite irritating when given by SC administration.

DRUG INTERACTIONS: Central nervous system depression or stimulation induced by meperidine may be potentiated by amphetamines, barbiturates, or cimetidine. See MEPERIDINE in the Small Animal section for further details.

METHOTREXATE

INDICATIONS: Methotrexate ♣ ★ is an antimetabolite chemotherapeutic agent that has been recommended for the treatment of a variety of neoplastic conditions in dogs, including lymphoreticular neoplasms. For more information, see METHOTREXATE in the Small Animal section.

In ferrets, methotrexate has been used for the treatment of lymphoma, in combination with other chemotherapeutic drugs. The following protocol has been published.

Week 1: vincristine (0.07 mg/kg; IV) + asparaginase (400 IU/kg; IP) + prednisone (1 mg/kg; PO; q 24 hours; continued throughout therapy). Week 2: cyclophosphamide (10 mg/kg; SC). Week 3: doxorubicin (1 mg/kg; IV). Weeks 4 to 6: repeat weeks 1 to 3 without asparaginase. Week 8: vincristine (0.07 mg/kg; IV). Week 10: cyclophosphamide (10 mg/kg; SC). Week 12: vincristine (0.07 mg/kg; IV). Week 14: methotrexate (0.5 mg/kg; IV). Continue protocol at biweekly intervals after week 14.

ADVERSE AND COMMON SIDE EFFECTS: A number of acute and delayed toxic effects have been reported in other species. For more information, see METHOTREXATE in the Small Animal section.

DRUG INTERACTIONS: A variety of drug interactions exist. For more information, see METHOTREXATE in the Small Animal section.

METOCLOPRAMIDE

INDICATIONS: Metoclopramide (Reglan ★, generics ♣ ★) is an antiemetic agent with central (chemoreceptor trigger zone) and peripheral activity. It contributes to lower esophageal sphincter competence and promotes gastric emptying. It is useful in the management of vomiting, gastroesophageal reflux, and gastric motility disorders. For more information, see METOCLOPRAMIDE in the Small Animal section.

Metoclopramide has been recommended for use in ferrets to treat vomiting and nausea associated with gastric ulceration and gastritis.

ADVERSE AND COMMON SIDE EFFECTS: Metoclopramide should not be used in patients with gastric outlet obstruction or those with a history of epilepsy. Renal disease may increase blood levels of the drug. Central nervous system (CNS) reactions include increased frequency of seizure activity, vertigo, hyperactivity, depression, and disorientation.

DRUG INTERACTIONS: Phenothiazine drugs may potentiate CNS effects. Digoxin, cimetidine, tetracycline, narcotic agents, and sedatives enhance CNS effects. Digoxin absorption may also be decreased, whereas acetaminophen, aspirin, diazepam, and tetracycline absorption may be accelerated. Atropine will block the effects of the drug on gastrointestinal tract motility.

METRONIDAZOLE

INDICATIONS: Metronidazole (Flagyl ✽ ★) is a synthetic antibacterial agent particularly useful for its bactericidal effects on many anaerobic bacteria. Metronidazole also has antiprotozoal activity and is used to treat giardiosis in ferrets.

Metronidazole is specifically indicated, in combination with amoxicillin, gastric protectants (e.g., bismuth subsalicylate), and H_2-receptor blockers (e.g., cimetidine), for the treatment of gastritis and gastric ulcers caused by *Helicobacter mustelae.* This combination was effective in eradicating *H. mustelae* from 71% of ferrets in one study. No abnormalities were found in kits born to jills that were medicated while pregnant. Metronidazole has also been recommended for the treatment of hepatitis, in combination with a broad-spectrum antibiotic, and as an adjunct to chloramphenicol therapy for proliferative bowel disease. It has been suggested that the addition of sucrose to oral preparations reduces the aftertaste. Tablets can also be crushed and mixed in a highly palatable substance such as a cat hairball laxative. For further information, see METRONIDAZOLE in the Small Animal section.

ADVERSE AND COMMON SIDE EFFECTS: See METRONIDAZOLE in the Small Animal section for details on adverse effects reported in dogs. The tablets have a bitter taste and should not be crushed before use. The drug may also be mutagenic and should not be given to pregnant animals.

DRUG INTERACTIONS: See METRONIDAZOLE in the Small Animal section.

MICONAZOLE

INDICATIONS: Miconazole (Conofite 🍁 ★, Micazole ★, Micatin 🍁, Monistat 🍁, numerous others) is a topical synthetic imidazole-derived antifungal agent useful in the treatment of localized dermatophytosis and active against most pathogenic fungi, gram-positive bacteria, and some *Acanthamoeba* spp. In human medicine, miconazole products are used topically for fungal infections of skin and mucous membranes (e.g., candidiasis).

Miconazole has been suggested for the treatment of dermatophytosis in ferrets. Miconazole shampoo may be a better formulation than creams, lotions, or ointments, which do not penetrate infected hair shafts or follicles.

ADVERSE AND COMMON SIDE EFFECTS AND DRUG INTERACTIONS: None reported in ferrets.

SUPPLIED AS VETERINARY PRODUCTS:
Cream: 2% w/w (Conofite 🍁 ★)
Lotion: 1% (Conofite ★, Miconosol ★)
Shampoo: 2% w/w (Dermazole 🍁)
Spray: 1% (Miconazole Nitrate Spray ★, Miconosol ★)

SUPPLIED AS HUMAN PRODUCTS:
Cream, powder, and aerosol formulations for topical use (Micatin 🍁, Monistat 🍁, numerous others ★)

MIDAZOLAM

INDICATIONS: Midazolam (Versed 🍁 ★) is a short-acting parenteral benzodiazepine, central nervous system depressant with sedative-hypnotic, anxiolytic, muscle-relaxing, and anticonvulsant properties. It is used as a preanesthetic, in combination with ketamine for anesthesia, and alone as an anticonvulsant agent. The drug is 2 to 3 times more potent than diazepam and has a shorter elimination half-life. Midazolam is formulated for intramuscular use, in contrast to diazepam. Midazolam can be reversed with flumazenil. For more information, see MIDAZOLAM in the Small Animal section.

ADVERSE AND COMMON SIDE EFFECTS: No significant cardiovascular effects have been noted in ferrets. Respiratory depression and dose-dependent sedation occur.

MILBEMYCIN

INDICATIONS: Milbemycin oxime (Interceptor ✤ ★) is an anthelmintic, insecticidal, and acaricidal compound. Milbemycin has been used in the prevention of heartworm disease caused by *Dirofilaria immitis*, as a microfilaricide, and for the control of gastrointestinal parasites. For more information, see MILBEMYCIN in the Small Animal section.

ADVERSE AND COMMON SIDE EFFECTS: None described in ferrets. See MILBEMYCIN in the Small Animal section.

MITOTANE

INDICATIONS: Mitotane or o,p'-DDD (Lysodren ✤ ★) is indicated in the treatment of pituitary-dependent hyperadrenocorticism in dogs. It causes selective necrosis of the zona fasciculata and reticularis in the adrenal gland. Damage to the zona glomerulosa is minimal. For further information, see MITOTANE in the Small Animal section.

Mitotane has been used with variable success to treat ferrets with hyperadrenocorticism when surgical removal is not possible. Leuprolide acetate is now the preferred therapeutic agent.

ADVERSE AND COMMON SIDE EFFECTS: The most significant side effect described in ferrets is the development of severe hypoglycemia, presumably due to a reduction in negative feedback from an undetected insulinoma. The possible emergence of this problem should be addressed when mitotane is dispensed. See also MITOTANE in the Small Animal section.

DRUG INTERACTIONS: See MITOTANE in the Small Animal section.

SUPPLIED AS HUMAN PRODUCT:
Tablets containing 500 mg (a pharmacist can reformulate into capsules to produce the required dosage) (Lysodren ✤ ★)

MORPHINE

INDICATIONS: Morphine (Astramorph ★, Duramorph ★, Roxanol ★, M.S. Contin ✤ ★, M.O.S. ✤ ★, Morphitec ✤, Statex ✤) is a very effective analgesic narcotic agent. It is increasingly used for the management of acute pain and as a preanesthetic agent in small animal practice. In dogs and cats analgesia lasts 4 to 6 hours after IM injection. Morphine also increases cardiac output and decreases pulmonary edema associated with congestive heart failure and cardiomyopathy. For more information, see MORPHINE in the Small Animal section.

ADVERSE AND COMMON SIDE EFFECTS: In addition to analgesia, morphine produces CNS depression with sedation or sleep. A number of adverse effects have been described in dogs and cats; see MORPHINE in the Small Animal section for further details. The depressive effects of the drug are antagonized by naloxone (0.1 mg/kg; IV). Morphine should not be used in animals with renal failure, a history of seizures, or in hypovolemic shock. Administration of morphine by the IV route may result in adverse effects related to histamine release.

DRUG INTERACTIONS: Phenothiazines, amitriptyline, antihistamines, fentanyl, and parenteral magnesium sulfate may potentiate the depressant effects of morphine.

NALBUPHINE

INDICATIONS: Nalbuphine (Nubain ✤ ★, Nalbuphine HCl ★) is a mixed opioid agonist/antagonist used as an analgesic agent. Nalbuphine can also be used to reverse the effects of μ opioids such as fentanyl, yet still provide postprocedural analgesia.

SUPPLIED AS HUMAN PRODUCTS:
For injection containing 10 and 20 mg/mL (Nubain ✤ ★, Nalbuphine HCl ★)

NALOXONE

INDICATIONS: Naloxone ✤ ★ is a narcotic antagonist. It is the preferred agent for reversal of narcotic-induced depression, including respiratory depression induced by morphine, oxymorphone, meperidine, or fentanyl. For more information, see NALOXONE in the Small Animal section.

ADVERSE AND COMMON SIDE EFFECTS: At recommended doses, the drug is relatively free of adverse effects. At high doses, seizure activity has been reported. The duration of its action may be less than that of the opioid it is antagonizing; consequently, animals should be monitored for signs of returning narcosis. The safety of the drug in pregnant animals has not been established, although reproductive studies in rats did not reveal any adverse effects.

DRUG INTERACTIONS: Naloxone also reverses the effects of butorphanol and pentazocine. One milliliter (0.4 mg) of P/M Naloxone counteracts the following narcotic dosages: 1.5 mg oxymorphone, 15 mg morphine sulfate, 100 mg meperidine, and 0.4 mg fentanyl.

SUPPLIED AS HUMAN PRODUCT:
For injection containing 0.2, 0.4, and 1 mg/mL (Canada, United States)

NEOMYCIN

INDICATIONS: Neomycin (Biosol ✤, Mycifradin ✤ ★), an aminogly-coside antibiotic, is used topically and orally for its local antibiotic effects in the gastrointestinal tract. It is generally less effective against many bacteria than either amikacin or gentamicin. The drug is very toxic when used systemically.

ADVERSE AND COMMON SIDE EFFECTS: Neomycin is the most nephrotoxic aminoglycoside. The drug is also potentially toxic to the vestibular and auditory nerves. Ototoxicity is especially a concern if the drug is instilled into external ear canals with ruptured tympanic membranes. It may also cause a contact hypersensitivity and otitis externa. Neomycin may decrease cardiac output and produce hypotension. Increased absorption of orally administered neomycin occurs in the presence of inflammatory or ulcerative disease of the GIT.

DRUG INTERACTIONS: Orally administered neomycin may decrease the absorption of digitalis, methotrexate, penicillin V and K, and vitamin K.

SUPPLIED AS VETERINARY PRODUCT:
Oral liquid containing 140 mg/mL (Biosol ✤)

SUPPLIED AS HUMAN PRODUCTS:
Tablets containing 500 mg (Mycifradin ✤, Generic ★)
Oral suspension containing 125 mg/5 mL (Mycifradin ✤ ★)

NITROGLYCERIN

INDICATIONS: Nitroglycerin (Nitro-Bid ✤ ★, Nitrol ✤ ★) is a venous vasodilator used in the medical management of congestive heart failure and cardiomyopathy in ferrets, especially when pulmonary edema is present. Nitroglycerin, furosemide, and enalapril are used together to treat hypertrophic cardiomyopathy. Apply the ointment to a relatively hairless or shaved area of skin. For more information, see NITROGLYCERIN in the Small Animal section.

ADVERSE AND COMMON SIDE EFFECTS: Rash and hypotension are reported.

DRUG INTERACTIONS: Use of calcium channel-blocking agents (e.g., verapamil and diltiazem), β-blocking agents (e.g., propranolol, atenolol, or metoprolol), and phenothiazine drugs may potentiate hypotension.

OXYMORPHONE

INDICATIONS: Oxymorphone (Numorphan ❦ ★, P/M Oxymorphone ★) is a narcotic agent used for sedation, preanesthesia, and the management of pain. See OXYMORPHONE in the Small Animal section for further details.

ADVERSE AND COMMON SIDE EFFECTS AND DRUG INTERACTIONS: See OXYMORPHONE in the Small Animal section for further details. Adverse effects of the drug can be reversed with naloxone.

OXYTETRACYCLINE

INDICATIONS: Oxytetracycline (Liquamycin ❦ ★, Terramycin ❦ ★) is a short-acting, water-soluble tetracycline. For more information, see OXYTETRACYCLINE and TETRACYCLINE ANTIBIOTICS in the Small Animal section.

ADVERSE AND COMMON SIDE EFFECTS: Oxytetracycline may cause discoloration of the teeth in young animals. High doses or prolonged use may cause delayed bone growth and healing. Tetracyclines cause nausea, anorexia, vomiting, and diarrhea in small animals. Irritation and necrosis can occur at sites of parenteral injections.

DRUG INTERACTIONS: A number of oral preparations interfere with the absorption of tetracyclines. See OXYTETRACYCLINE and TETRACYCLINE ANTIBIOTICS in the Small Animal section for further details.

OXYTOCIN

INDICATIONS: Oxytocin (Pitocin ★, Syntocinon ❦ ★) is a hormone of the posterior pituitary gland used in ferrets to stimulate milk letdown and help expel retained fetuses.

ADVERSE AND COMMON SIDE EFFECTS: The drug is contraindicated in animals with dystocia due to abnormal presentation of the fetus or in those with a closed cervix. See OXYTOCIN in the Small Animal section.

DRUG INTERACTIONS: See OXYTOCIN in the Small Animal section.

PENICILLIN G AND V

INDICATIONS: Penicillin antibiotics, including penicillin G and V, are effective bactericidal antibiotics used for the treatment of gram-positive and gram-negative infections. Penicillin drugs are widely distributed throughout the body to most body fluids and bone with the exception of the brain and cerebrospinal fluid (unless inflamed). Penicillin G is effective against most gram-positive organisms. Penicillin V has the same spectrum but is more reliably absorbed from the gastrointestinal tract into the systemic circulation.

ADVERSE AND COMMON SIDE EFFECTS: Toxicity is rare in dogs and cats. See PENICILLIN ANTIBIOTICS in the Small Animal section. Sensitivity to one penicillin implies sensitivity to all penicillins.

DRUG INTERACTIONS: See PENICILLIN ANTIBIOTICS in the Small Animal section. Food and antacids decrease the absorption of orally administered penicillins. The drug should be given 1 hour before or 2 hours after feeding.

PENTAZOCINE

INDICATIONS: Pentazocine (Talwin-V ★, Talwin ✿ ★) is a narcotic agonist/antagonist with κ_1 receptor activity used in the management of moderate to severe pain. The drug does not depress respiration and produces little or no sedation at therapeutic doses. See PENTAZOCINE in the Small Animal section for further details.

ADVERSE AND COMMON SIDE EFFECTS: See PENTAZOCINE in the Small Animal section for further details. Overdosage and side effects of the drug can be reversed with naloxone.

DRUG INTERACTIONS: Do not mix pentazocine with soluble barbiturates because precipitation will occur.

PHENOBARBITAL

INDICATIONS: Phenobarbital ✿ ★ is the drug of choice for the control of seizure activity in small animals. Therapeutic blood phenobarbital levels for ferrets have not been specifically defined; however, those for dogs and cats provide approximate guidelines. See PHENOBARBITAL and BARBITURATES in the Small Animal section for further indications and information on pharmacokinetics.

ADVERSE AND COMMON SIDE EFFECTS: Initially, sedation and ataxia may be noted, especially at higher doses. These effects tend to resolve with continued treatment. For further information on treatment of drug overdose, see PHENOBARBITAL in the Small Animal section.

DRUG INTERACTIONS: Interactions exist with a number of compounds. See PHENOBARBITAL in the Small Animal section.

PIPERAZINE

INDICATIONS: Piperazine (Hartz Once a Month ★, Once a Month Roundworm Treatment ✤, Pipa-Tabs ★, Purina Liquid Dog Wormer ★) is an anthelmintic used for the eradication of roundworms.

ADVERSE AND COMMON SIDE EFFECTS: See PIPERAZINE in the Small Animal section.

DRUG INTERACTIONS: See PIPERAZINE in the Small Animal section. The concurrent use of laxatives is not recommended because these agents may cause elimination of the drug before it has had an opportunity to work effectively.

PRAZIQUANTEL

INDICATIONS: Praziquantel (Droncit ✤ ★) is an anthelmintic used to eliminate tapeworms. After drug administration, the parasite loses its ability to resist digestion by the host and because of this, it is common to see only disintegrated and partially digested pieces of tapeworm in the stool. For more information, see PRAZIQUANTEL in the Small Animal section.

ADVERSE AND COMMON SIDE EFFECTS: The drug is very safe but is not recommended for use in puppies or kittens younger than 4 weeks of age. Drug overdose may be associated with anorexia, vomiting, salivation, diarrhea, and depression.

DRUG INTERACTIONS: None reported.

PREDNISOLONE
PREDNISOLONE SODIUM SUCCINATE
PREDNISONE

INDICATIONS: Prednisolone (Delta-Cortef ★, Solu-Delta-Cortef ✤) and prednisone (Deltasone ✤ ★, Meticorten ★, and others) are intermediate-acting glucocorticoid agents. Prednisone is converted by the liver to prednisolone. Except for cases of liver failure, the drugs can essentially be used interchangeably. These drugs are indicated for the treatment of a number of medical problems including inflammatory and allergic conditions, acute hypersensitivity reactions, severe overwhelming infections with toxicity (in combination with appropriate antibiotic therapy), for supportive care during periods of stress, and for the prevention and treatment of adrenal insufficiency and shock (in conjunction with fluid support). Fludrocortisone is a more appropriate drug for the long-term medical management of ferrets that have undergone bilateral adrenalectomy. For further information, see PREDNISOLONE/PREDNISOLONE SODIUM SUCCINATE/PREDNISONE in the Small Animal section.

OTHER USES

POSTADRENALECTOMY

Glucocorticoid administration has been described during and immediately after adrenalectomy in the ferret; however, it has also been stated that routine treatment is likely unnecessary. Published dosing regimens include a dose of 0.25 to 0.5 mg/kg bid orally for 5 to 10 days, after which the dose is gradually tapered over a period of several weeks to several months. Steroid administration should be based on evidence of clinical need. As adrenal neoplasms do not generally produce excess glucocorticoids, it is unlikely that insufficiency will occur after removal of a single affected gland.

INSULINOMA

In ferrets, prednisone is used for the initial management of hypoglycemia associated with islet cell neoplasia (insulinoma). Diazoxide is added to the drug regimen when prednisone alone is no longer efficacious. Medical treatment should be in conjunction with dietary manipulation—frequent high-protein/low-carbohydrate meals.

DIROFILARIA IMMITIS

It is recommended that oral prednisolone (1 mg/kg q 24 hours) be administered concurrently with thiacetarsamide or melarsomine in order to reduce complications and death associated with embolism of dead worms. Treatment should continue for 3 to 4 months or until the ferret is negative on an occult heartworm test. This runs contrary to the statement that glucocorticoids may have a protective effect on adult heartworms, decreasing the efficacy of the parasiticides.

EOSINOPHILIC GASTROENTERITIS

Prednisone is one of the recommended treatments for eosinophilic gastroenteritis in ferrets. Treatment is initiated with doses ranging from 1.5 to 2.5 mg/kg orally once daily until clinical signs abate (usually in approximately 7 days), and then the ferret is gradually weaned off therapy. Some animals may require long-term or even permanent therapy.

LYMPHOSARCOMA

Prednisone can be used palliatively in ferrets with lymphoma to reduce the size of tumor masses and reduce clinical signs such as diarrhea. An oral dose of 2 mg/kg once daily is most commonly recommended. Several combination chemotherapeutic protocols have been published with varying success. Two of them are as follows:

1. Week 1: vincristine (0.07 mg/kg; IV) + asparaginase (400 IU/kg; IP) + prednisone (1 mg/kg; PO; q 24 hours; continued throughout therapy). Week 2: cyclophosphamide (10 mg/kg; SC). Week 3: doxorubicin (1 mg/kg; IV). Weeks 4 to 6: repeat weeks 1 to 3 without asparaginase. Week 8: vincristine (0.07 mg/kg; IV). Week 10: cyclophosphamide (10 mg/kg; SC). Week 12: vincristine (0.07 mg/kg; IV). Week 14: methotrexate (0.5 mg/kg; IV). Continue protocol at biweekly intervals after week 14.

2. Cyclophosphamide (1/4 of a 25 mg tablet once every 3 weeks for 3 doses; PO) + vincristine (0.05 mg for ferrets up to 1 kg; 0.1 mg for ferrets 1 kg and over; once weekly for 4 weeks; IV) + prednisone (2 mg/kg q 24 hours; PO). Continue daily treatment with prednisone for 4 to 5 weeks, then discontinue gradually with a tapering dose.

ADVERSE AND COMMON SIDE EFFECTS: Long-term therapy with prednisone at immunosuppressive doses (e.g., 1 mg/kg or higher; q 24 hours) can result in muscle wasting, a potbellied appearance, and elevations in hepatic enzymes.

DRUG INTERACTIONS: NSAIDs and glucocorticoid agents should not be used concurrently.

PROPOFOL

INDICATIONS: Propofol (Diprivan ✤ ★, PropoFlow ★, Rapinovet ✤ ★) is a sedative/hypnotic IV anesthetic agent used for the induction and maintenance of general anesthesia. It is indicated to provide general anesthesia for procedures lasting less than 5 minutes and for induction and maintenance of general anesthesia using incremental doses to effect. It is particularly useful for cases in which a short recovery period is desired. For more information, see PROPOFOL in the Small Animal section.

ADVERSE AND COMMON SIDE EFFECTS: As in other species, rapid administration of propofol may result in apnea.

PROPRANOLOL

INDICATIONS: Propranolol (Inderal ✤ ★) is a nonselective β_1- and β_2-receptor blocking agent. It has been used in ferrets primarily for the medical management of hypertrophic cardiomyopathy. Diltiazem may be a more effective choice. For more information, see PROPRANOLOL in the Small Animal section.

ADVERSE AND COMMON SIDE EFFECTS: Propranolol may cause lethargy and lack of appetite in ferrets.

DRUG INTERACTIONS: See PROPRANOLOL in the Small Animal section.

PROSTAGLANDIN F$_{2\alpha}$

INDICATIONS: Prostaglandin F$_{2\alpha}$ (Lutalyse ❦ ★) has been used in the treatment of metritis in the ferret. The drug causes contraction of the myometrium and relaxation of the cervix. Reduction in uterine size and improvement in clinical signs are not evident for at least 48 hours after the start of therapy. It also has been used as an abortifacient in small animals.

ADVERSE AND COMMON SIDE EFFECTS: See PROSTAGLANDIN F$_{2\alpha}$ in the Small Animal section.

DRUG INTERACTIONS: The concurrent use of estrogens is not recommended because estrogens enhance the effects of the drug on the uterus.

PYRANTEL PAMOATE

INDICATIONS: Pyrantel pamoate (Pyr-A-Pam ❦, Pyran ❦, Nemex ★) is an anthelmintic used to eradicate enteric nematodes. Pyrantel is a cholinesterase inhibitor.

ADVERSE AND COMMON SIDE EFFECTS: Cautious use of the drug is advised in patients with liver dysfunction, malnutrition, dehydration, and anemia. Although the drug is considered safe, vomiting may occur.

DRUG INTERACTIONS: The drug should not be used concurrently with levamisole because of similar mechanisms of action and potential toxicity. Adverse effects may be potentiated by the concurrent use of organophosphates or diethylcarbamazine. Piperazine and pyrantel have antagonistic actions and should not be used together.

PYRETHRIN-CONTAINING PRODUCTS

INDICATIONS: Pyrethrin-containing products (Happy Jack ★, Mycodex ★, Ovitrol ❦, Zodiac ❦, and others) are naturally occurring insecticides derived from the plant *Chrysanthemum cinerariae-folium,* and are commonly used for flea control. These drugs are γ-aminobutyric acid (GABA) agonists that stimulate the insect's central nervous system, causing muscular excitation, convulsions, and paralysis. Insect mortality is enhanced when these products are combined with piperonyl butoxide (e.g., Sectrol and Ovitrol). Piperonyl butoxide inhibits pyrethrin metabolism.

ADVERSE AND COMMON SIDE EFFECTS: These products are relatively nontoxic to mammals. See PYRETHRIN-CONTAINING PRODUCTS in the Small Animal section.

DRUG INTERACTIONS: See PYRETHRIN-CONTAINING PRODUCTS in the Small Animal section.

SUPPLIED AS VETERINARY PRODUCTS:
Powder, spray, and shampoo formulations containing varying percentages of pyrethrin and piperonyl butoxide are available on the marketplace. Some products also contain carbaryl and other insecticidal compounds.

RANITIDINE

INDICATIONS: Ranitidine (Zantac ✿ ★) is a histamine (H_2)-receptor antagonist that is used for the treatment of GI ulceration. It is more potent (5 to 12 times) in inhibiting gastric acid secretion than cimetidine, but it clinically is no more effective. For more information, see RANITIDINE in the Small Animal section.

In ferrets, ranitidine is used in the treatment of gastritis and gastric ulceration. The drug can be compounded as a flavored suspension. Researchers have investigated the effectiveness of a salt formed from ranitidine and bismuth citrate (ranitidine bismuth citrate) against gastric *Helicobacter mustelae*. Doses of 12 mg/kg PO or 24 mg/kg PO every 12 hours for 28 days eradicated infection in 50% and 69% of ferrets, respectively. All animals treated with the lower dose had recrudescence of infection by 3 weeks after administration ended, while 10% of the high-dose group remained clear of infection. Clarithromycin (12.5 mg/kg q 12 hours for 14 days; PO) + ranitidine bismuth citrate (24 mg/kg q 12 hours for 14 days; PO) was completely effective in eradicating *H. mustelae* from infected ferrets.

SELAMECTIN

INDICATIONS: Selamectin (Revolution ✿ ★) is a macrocytic lactone long-acting antiparasitic agent used topically to control a variety of ectoparasites and endoparasites in dogs and cats. For more information, see SELAMECTIN in the Small Animal section.

In ferrets, selamectin has been suggested for the control of fleas and ear mites and the prevention of heartworm disease.

STANOZOLOL

INDICATIONS: Stanozolol (Winstrol-V ✿ ★) is an anabolic steroid with strong anabolic and weak androgenic activity. It is potentially useful as an adjunct to the management of catabolic disease states. The drug has been recommended to stimulate erythropoiesis, arouse appetite, promote weight gain, and increase strength and vitality. The efficacy of promoting these positive changes is variable and prolonged treatment (3 to 6 months) may be required before a response in the erythron is seen. Dosage regimens in the literature range from twice daily, by oral or parenteral routes, to once weekly IM. In human medicine, stanazolol is administered once daily PO or once each 2 weeks by IM injection. See also STANOZOLOL and ANABOLIC STEROIDS in the Small Animal section.

ADVERSE AND COMMON SIDE EFFECTS AND DRUG INTER-ACTIONS: See STANOZOLOL in the Small Animal section.

SUCRALFATE

INDICATIONS: Sucralfate (Carafate ★, Sulcrate ✤) is a magnesium-containing complex that accelerates the healing of oral, esophageal, gastric, and duodenal ulcers and has been used in ferrets for the treatment of gastritis and gastric ulcers. Sucralfate may be useful for the prevention of NSAID-induced ulceration. See SUCRALFATE in the Small Animal section.

ADVERSE AND COMMON SIDE EFFECTS: Constipation is the only significant problem reported in small animals.

DRUG INTERACTIONS: Antacids and H_2-receptor blocking agents decrease gastric pH and reduce the efficacy of sucralfate and; therefore, drug delivery should be spaced apart by at least 30 minutes. See SUCRALFATE in the Small Animal section.

SULFADIMETHOXINE

INDICATIONS: Sulfadimethoxine (Albon ★, SULFA 125 and 250 ✤) is a sulfonamide antibiotic used most commonly in ferrets for the eradication of coccidiosis. See SULFADIMETHOXINE in the Small Animal section for further information.

ADVERSE AND COMMON SIDE EFFECTS: See SULFONAMIDE ANTIBIOTICS in the Small Animal section.

DRUG INTERACTIONS: Although injectable formulations are available, IM injection is associated with pain and poor blood drug levels and; therefore, is not recommended. See SULFONAMIDE ANTIBIOTICS in the Small Animal section.

SULFASALAZINE

INDICATIONS: Sulfasalazine (Azulfidine ★, Salazopyrin ✤) has been used in the treatment of inflammatory bowel disease in the ferret. In the colon, bacteria degrade the drug to release aminosalicylic acid, which has an anti-inflammatory effect, and sulfapyridine. See SULFASALAZINE in the Small Animal section for further details on mode of action.

ADVERSE AND COMMON SIDE EFFECTS: A number of adverse effects have been described in small animals. See SULFASALAZINE in the Small Animal section for details.

DRUG INTERACTIONS: Antibiotics may alter metabolism of sulfasalazine by altering intestinal flora. See SULFASALAZINE in the Small Animal section for specific drug interactions.

TETRACYCLINE

INDICATIONS: The tetracycline antibiotics exert a bacteriostatic effect against many aerobic and anaerobic gram-positive and gram-negative bacteria, spirochetes, mycoplasmas, and rickettsial organisms. They are also used in the treatment of protozoan infections. Tetracycline (Panmycin Aqua-drops Liquid ✤ ★, Tetrachel-Vet ★) itself is short-acting and water soluble.

Tetracycline has been suggested for the treatment of proliferative bowel disease in ferrets; however, chloramphenicol is thought to be more effective.

ADVERSE AND COMMON SIDE EFFECTS AND DRUG INTER-ACTIONS: See TETRACYCLINE ANTIBIOTICS in the Small Animal section.

SUPPLIED AS VETERINARY PRODUCTS:
For oral administration containing 25 mg/mL (Tetrachel-Vet Drops ★) and 100 mg/mL (Panmycin Aqua-drops liquid ✤ ★, Tetrachel-Vet Syrup ★)

SUPPLIED AS HUMAN PRODUCT:
Oral suspension containing 125 mg/5 mL (Novo-tetra suspension ✤)

THEOPHYLLINE

INDICATIONS: Theophylline (Theo-Dur ✤ ★, Theolair ★, Quibron-T/SR ✤ ★, Slo-Bid ✤ ★) is a bronchodilator indicated for the management of cough due to bronchospasm. See THEOPHYLLINE in the Small Animal section.

ADVERSE AND COMMON SIDE EFFECTS: A number of contra-indications to treatment and side effects have been noted in small animals. See THEOPHYLLINE in the Small Animal section.

DRUG INTERACTIONS: A number of interactions exist. See THEO-PHYLLINE in the Small Animal section.

THIACETARSAMIDE

INDICATIONS: Thiacetarsamide (Caparsolate ✦ ★) was taken off the North American market in 2000, but was previously used to a limited extent and with variable effect in ferrets for the eradication of adult heartworms (*Dirofilaria immitis*). An alternative drug is melarsomine.

ADVERSE AND COMMON SIDE EFFECTS: A number of adverse effects have been described in dogs and cats, and risks associated with treatment are also fairly high in ferrets. Concurrent treatment with prednisolone (see below under DRUG INTERACTIONS) or heparin has been recommended to reduce the occurrence of death due to thromboembolism, a significant posttreatment complication in ferrets. Heparin should be subcutaneously administered as follows: 100 U per ferret once daily for up to 5 days before and for 14 to 21 days after administration of thiacetarsamide. After 3 weeks of heparin therapy, aspirin (22 mg/kg once daily; PO) can be administered for an additional 3 months.

DRUG INTERACTIONS: Glucocorticoids may have a protective effect on adult heartworms, thus decreasing the efficacy of thiacetarsamide. In addition, glucocorticoids may cause increased pulmonary vascular intimal proliferation, predisposing the pulmonary vessels to obstruction. Despite this, prednisone or prednisolone (1 mg/kg once daily; PO for 7 to 14 days or until the ferret is negative on a heartworm test) has been suggested as alternatives to posttreatment heparin therapy.

TILETAMINE + ZOLAZEPAM

INDICATIONS: Tiletamine + zolazepam (Telazol ★) is an injectable combination useful for sedation and restraint. It is also used as an anesthetic for procedures of short duration (30 minutes) requiring mild to moderate analgesia. Tiletamine is a dissociative anesthetic similar to ketamine while the benzodiazepine tranquilizer, zolazepam, reduces muscle rigidity and seizure-like activity. The tiletamine fraction has a shorter duration than zolazepam; therefore, recoveries may be quite delayed because of continuing tranquilization. Ketamine should be used to extend anesthesia rather than the tiletamine + zolazepam combination. Telazol has been used in combination with butophanol to improve analgesia, and at a lower dose with xylazine to deepen the plane of anesthesia.

ADVERSE AND COMMON SIDE EFFECTS: The use of Telazol in ferrets was evaluated experimentally utilizing single doses of 12 mg/kg and 22 mg/kg IM. While the combination resulted in excellent immobilization and generally smooth induction and recovery, muscle relaxation and analgesia were dose dependent and adequate for only minor procedures at the lower dose. Administration of the higher dose did not result in achievement of a plane of deep surgical anesthesia. At both doses, a moderate increase in nasal secretions and salivation resulted in increased sneezing. This could be ameliorated by concurrent use of atropine. Ferrets administered 12 mg/kg had shallow rapid respiration, sometimes >60 breaths/minute, while at the higher dose there was inspiratory breath holding and a much lower respiratory rate (i.e., 12 to 18/minute). Paddling or swimming movements were common during induction and recovery, which could be quite prolonged. At a dose of 12 mg/kg the mean recovery time (the time at which the righting reflex returned) was 1 hour 57 minutes, with a range from 35 minutes to 3 hours 17 minutes. Ten of 12 ferrets administered the higher dose required more than 4 hours to recover.

TRIMETHOPRIM-SULFONAMIDE COMBINATIONS

INDICATIONS: Trimethoprim-sulfonamide combinations, i.e., sulfadiazine and sulfamethoxazole (Tribrissen ❤ ★, Trivetrin ❤, Borgal ❤, Septra ❤ ★, Bactrim ❤ ★, and others) are bactericidal antibiotics recommended for the treatment of infections caused by susceptible organisms in a variety of soft tissues, especially the respiratory and urinary tracts, and for the treatment of intestinal coccidiosis.

ADVERSE AND COMMON SIDE EFFECTS: None are specifically described in the ferret. Excessive salivation may occur in animals given uncoated tablets.

DRUG INTERACTIONS: Antacids may decrease the bioavailability of oral trimethoprim-sulfa if administered concurrently.

SUPPLIED AS VETERINARY PRODUCTS:
For injection containing 40 mg/mL trimethoprim and 200 mg/mL sulfadiazine (Tribrissen 24% ❤)
For injection containing 40 mg/mL trimethoprim and 200 mg/mL sulfadoxine (Bimotrin ❤, Borgal ❤, Trimidox ❤, Trivetrin ❤)
For injection containing 80 mg/mL trimethoprim and 400 mg/mL sulfadiazine (Di-Biotic 48% Injection ★, Tribrissen 48% ❤)
Suspension containing 10 mg/mL trimethoprim and 50 mg/mL sulfadiazine (Tribrissen Piglet Suspension ❤)
Oral paste containing 67 mg/g trimethoprim and 333.3 mg/g sulfadiazine) (Tribrissen 400 Oral Paste ★)
Tablets containing trimethoprim and sulfadiazine in the following mg combinations: 5 + 25, 20 + 100, 80 + 400, 160 + 800 (Tribrissen ★)

SUPPLIED AS HUMAN PRODUCTS:
For injection containing 16 mg trimethoprim and 80 mg sulfamethoxazole per mL (Sulfamethoxazole & Trimethoprim Concentrate for Injection ★, Septra Injection ♣)
Tablets containing 80 mg trimethoprim and 400 mg sulfamethoxazole (Apo-Sulfatrim ♣, Novo-Trimel ♣, Septra ♣, Bactrim ★, Cotrim ★, Sulfatrim ★), 160 mg trimethoprim and 800 mg sulfamethoxazole (Apo-Sulfatrim DS ♣, Novo-Trimel DS ♣, Septra DS ♣, Bactrim DS ★, Cofatrim Forte★, Cotrim DS ★, Septra DS ★, Sulfatrim DS ★), and 90 mg trimethoprim and 410 mg sulfadiazine (Coptin ♣)
Oral suspensions containing 40 mg trimethoprim and 200 mg sulfamethoxazole per 5 mL (Apo-Sulfatrim ♣, Novo-Trimel Oral Suspension ♣, Septra Pediatric Suspension ♣, Bactrim Pediatric ★, Septra Grape Suspension ★, Cotrim Pediatric ★, Sulfatrim Pediatric ★, Sulfatrim Suspension ★) and 45 mg trimethoprim and 205 mg sulfadiazine per 5 mL (Coptin ♣)

TYLOSIN

INDICATIONS: Tylosin (Tylan ♣ ★, Tylocine ♣, Tylosin ♣ ★) is a bacteriostatic macrolide antibiotic with activity against gram-negative and gram-positive bacteria, spirochetes, chlamydiae, and mycoplasmal organisms. The drug has been used to manage canine and feline colitis and has been recommended for the treatment of proliferative bowel disease in the ferret. For more information, see TYLOSIN in the Small Animal section.

ADVERSE AND COMMON SIDE EFFECTS: Anorexia, diarrhea, and local pain with IM injection are reported in dogs and cats.

DRUG INTERACTIONS: Tylosin may increase serum digitalis levels.

URSODIOL

INDICATIONS: Ursodiol, or ursodeoxycholic acid (UDCA) (Urso ♣, Actigall ★), is a chloretic agent used to treat chronic inflammatory cholestatic liver disease, bile sludging, dissolution of radiolucent noncalcified gallstones smaller than 20 mm in diameter, primary biliary cirrhosis, chronic persistent hepatitis, cirrhosis, and biliary atresia. The drug promotes biliary flow and has anti-inflammatory properties. Total endogenous bile acids are reduced. It will not dissolve calcified or bile pigment gallstones.
  In ferrets, ursodiol has been used in the treatment of cholangiohepatitis and cholestasis, and disorders of the gallbladder.

ADVERSE AND COMMON SIDE EFFECTS: None have been reported in dogs or cats. For information on adverse effects in humans, see URSODIOL in the Small Animal section.

DRUG INTERACTIONS: Aluminum-based antacids absorb bile acids and interfere with ursodiol by decreasing its absorption. For more information, see URSODIOL in the Small Animal section.

VINCRISTINE

INDICATIONS: Vincristine (Oncovin ★, generics ♣) is a chemotherapeutic agent used in the management of a variety of neoplasms in dogs and cats, including lymphoproliferative disease. The drug often is used in conjunction with other chemotherapeutic agents. For more information, see VINCRISTINE in the Small Animal section.

In ferrets, asparaginase has been used in combination therapy for the treatment of lymphoma. Several protocols have been published, with varying success. Two are as follows:

1) Week 1: vincristine (0.07 mg/kg; IV) + asparaginase (400 IU/kg; IP) + prednisone (1 mg/kg; PO, q 24 hours, continued throughout therapy). Week 2: cyclophosphamide (10 mg/kg; SC). Week 3: doxorubicin (1 mg/kg; IV). Weeks 4 to 6: repeat weeks 1 to 3 without asparaginase. Week 8: vincristine (0.07 mg/kg; IV). Week 10: cyclophosphamide (10 mg/kg; SC). Week 12: vincristine (0.07 mg/kg; IV). Week 14: methotrexate (0.5 mg/kg; IV). Continue protocol at biweekly intervals after week 14.

2) Cyclophosphamide (1/4 of a 25 mg tablet once every 3 weeks for 3 doses; PO) + vincristine (0.05 mg for ferrets up to 1 kg; 0.1 mg for ferrets 1 kg and over; once weekly for 4 weeks; IV) + prednisone (2 mg/kg q 24 hours; PO). Continue daily treatment with prednisone for 4 to 5 weeks, then discontinue gradually with a tapering dose.

ADVERSE AND COMMON SIDE EFFECTS: Vincristine should be used with caution in animals with liver disease, leukopenia, bacterial infection, or preexisting neuromuscular disease. The WBC count should be monitored during treatment.

DRUG INTERACTIONS: See VINCRISTINE in the Small Animal section.

VITAMIN B COMPLEX

INDICATIONS: Vitamin B complex ♣ ★ is used as a component of supportive therapy.

ADVERSE AND COMMON SIDE EFFECTS AND DRUG INTER-ACTIONS: See THIAMINE in the Small Animal section.

SUPPLIED AS VETERINARY PRODUCTS:
Numerous products for injection and use in drinking water containing various vitamin level combinations ❧ ★
Oral syrup (V.A.L. Syrup ★)

VITAMIN C

INDICATIONS: Ascorbic acid or vitamin C (Apo-C ❧, Redoxon ❧) is essential for the synthesis and maintenance of collagen and intercellular ground substance of body tissue cells, blood vessels, bone, cartilage, tendons, and teeth. It is also important in wound healing and resistance to infection. It may influence the immune response. For more information, see ASCORBIC ACID in the Small Animal section.

In ferrets, administration of ascorbic acid has been recommended for general support in immunosuppressive diseases and during chemotherapy for lymphoma.

ADVERSE AND COMMON SIDE EFFECTS: See ASCORBIC ACID in the Small Animal section. Chelated, buffered, or ester forms of ascorbic acid may cause less gastrointestinal irritation. Ascorbic acid is bitter and must be mixed with strongly flavored food treats to disguise the taste.

DRUG INTERACTIONS: See ASCORBIC ACID in the Small Animal section.

XYLAZINE

INDICATIONS: Xylazine (Anased ❧ ★, Rompun ❧ ★, and others) is an injectable α_2-receptor agonist sedative used in conjunction with ketamine to improve muscle relaxation and provide anesthesia. For more information, see XYLAZINE in the Small Animal section.

ADVERSE AND COMMON SIDE EFFECTS: Hypoxemia, bradycardia, and EKG abnormalities can occur in ferrets administered ketamine + xylazine combinations. The use of an inhalant anesthetic such as isoflurane is likely safer when dealing with clinical patients whose health status may not be totally understood.

DRUG INTERACTIONS: Yohimbine can be used to antagonize the effects of xylazine.

YOHIMBINE

INDICATIONS: Yohimbine (Yobine ✤ ★, Antagonil ✤ ★) can be used to antagonize the effects of xylazine to shorten anesthetic recovery times and reduce bradycardia and other anesthetic-related complications. For more information, see XYLAZINE in the Small Animal section or YOHIMBINE in the Large Animal section.

SUPPLIED AS VETERINARY PRODUCT:
For injection containing 2 mg/mL (Yobine ✤ ★) and 5 mg/mL (Antagonil ✤ ★)

Handbook of Veterinary Drugs, Third Edition, edited by Dana Allen,
Lippincott Williams & Wilkins, Baltimore. © 2005

Section 14

The Use of Chemotherapeutic Agents in Reptilian Medicine

CHOICE OF MEDICATION

With the exception of a small number of antibiotics, recommendations for the use of chemotherapeutic agents in reptiles are primarily based on clinical experience rather than on controlled or pharmacokinetic studies. Many are derived from mammalian and avian doses and have not been specifically adapted for the variations in body size and generally slower metabolic rate that occur in reptiles. Information on safety and efficacy is likewise derived. For a given drug, suggested dosage and frequency and routes of administration often vary widely from one report to another. Generalizations are often made across the classes of reptiles; however, wide variations in anatomy, physiology, and behavioral ecology make these likely to be inappropriate. Because reptiles are ectothermic, ambient or body temperature has a significant effect on absorption, distribution, excretion, and toxicity of administered medications. Only a few of the existing pharmacokinetic studies evaluate the effects of varying ambient temperature. No medications are specifically designed or registered for use in reptiles; therefore, all treatments are "extralabel" and require the discretion and experience of the veterinarian. Despite these problems, chemotherapeutic agents are widely and effectively used for the treatment of disease in reptiles.

The compounds listed in this text are those recommended in the literature and currently available in Canada or the United States. Unfortunately, for most species/drug combinations, there is no single "right" dose. Where a particular drug has been recommended for use in a particular species, or for a particular medical condition, this has been noted. Dosages based on pharmacokinetic or controlled efficacy trials are noted with an asterisk in the table. General information and drug availability are provided in the Small or Large Animal sections, as noted, or in the reptile section itself.

ROUTES OF ADMINISTRATION

Medications are administered to reptiles primarily via the oral, subcutaneous, and intramuscular routes. Intravenous and, because venous access in many species or specimens is difficult or impossible to obtain, the intraosseous and intracoelomic routes are also utilized. Oral medications can be administered in the food (e.g., by injection into a prey species), by mixing with a prepared diet, directly into the oral cavity (especially in some lizards), or by direct gastric or esophageal intubation. Ill animals may not eat or drink sufficiently to obtain reliable amounts of medications delivered in food or water. Opening the mouth to pass a stomach tube may not be possible in some turtles or tortoises. As there is little known about the rate or efficiency of uptake of most orally administered medications, parenteral administration is preferable when rapid or high concentrations of drug are required.

It is generally advised that parenteral injections be administered to the anterior half of the body in order to prevent nephrotoxicity or accelerated renal excretion of the therapeutic agent. Reptiles have a renal portal system: blood from the posterior portions of the body passes through renal peritubular venous plexi before entering the general circulation. It has traditionally been thought that this circulatory pattern could result in the immediate excretion of a drug filtered or secreted through the kidney or, because of high local drug concentrations, in increased nephrotoxicity. These concerns have not been substantiated by the very few studies that have touched on renal physiology in relation to drug therapy; however, most reptile clinicians will continue the practice of using the anterior half of the body in preference when feasible. Additional work in a greater range of species is still necessary to fully understand the effects of renal portal blood flow on therapeutic blood concentrations.

In snakes, intramuscular injections are made into the epaxial muscles on either side of the dorsal spinous processes. In lizards and chelonians, the muscles of the forelegs are generally used. Small specimens may not have adequate muscle mass for repeated or large volume injections and other routes must be considered. Subcutaneous administration is a common alternative. Injection of irritant substances may result in local sloughing of skin or subcutaneous tissue. Some injectable compounds (e.g., calcium) can be diluted in saline or other isotonic fluids and administered intracoelomically. Caution must be taken to avoid injuring the coelomic viscera with the needle or catheter.

ENVIRONMENTAL TEMPERATURE

Provision of appropriate environmental conditions is an essential part of any therapeutic plan. As ectotherms, reptiles rely on external means to maintain body temperature. It has been shown that metabolism, the immune system, healing, and resistance to infection are all highly influenced by temperature. It is, therefore, essential that animals are held at appropriate ambient temperatures during treatment. The upper end of the preferred optimum temperature zone (POTZ) is generally recommended; the specific temperature zone will vary considerably among species. Between 25°C and 30°C is commonly selected for many temperate and tropical reptiles. Ambient temperature also affects drug pharmacokinetics and the blood concentration of the antibiotic necessary for successful bacterial elimination. The *in vitro* minimum inhibitory concentration values for some reptile pathogens have been shown to decrease with increasing environmental temperature. Unfortunately, there has been insufficient research to allow these factors to be adjusted on a routine clinical basis.

Handbook of Veterinary Drugs, Third Edition, edited by Dana Allen,
Lippincott Williams & Wilkins, Baltimore. © 2005

Section 15

Common Dosages for Reptiles

Drug	Dosage	Indication/Species
Acyclovir	5% topical cream for several weeks 80 mg/kg q 24 hours until symptoms are gone; PO	Herpes virus infections of tortoises Herpes virus infections of tortoises
Albendazole	50 to 75 mg/kg once; PO	Nematodiasis and possibly other parasites including trematodes and *Giardia*
Allopurinol	10 to 20 mg/kg q 24 hours; PO	To reduce uric acid production in cases of gout
Aluminum hydroxide	1 mL/kg q 24 hours; PO	To reduce blood phosphorus levels in green iguanas with renal disease
Amikacin	*5 mg/kg loading dose, then 2.5 mg/kg q 72 hours; IM	Gopher snakes kept at 25°C and 37°C

(continued)

Drug	Dosage	Indication/Species
Amikacin (cont.)	*3.5 mg/kg once; IM	Ball pythons kept at 25°C and 37°C
	*5 mg/kg q 48 hours; IM	Gopher tortoises kept at 30°C
	*2.25 mg/kg q 72 to 96 hours; IM	Juvenile American alligators kept at 22°C
	2.5 or 5 mg/kg initial dose, then 2.5 mg/kg q 72 hours; IM	Common recommendation for snakes and lizards
	2 mg/10 mL saline	For nebulization
Aminophylline	2 to 4 mg/kg; IM	To induce bronchodilation in treatment of respiratory disease
Amitraz	2 mL/L water as pour on	Ticks on mountain tortoises (see details under drug description)
Amoxicillin	22 mg/kg q 12 to 24 hours; PO 10 to 20 mg/kg q 24 h; IM	General antibacterial use
Amphotericin B	5 mg nebulized in 150 mL in sterile water q 12 hours for 1 hour for 7 days	For mycotic pneumonia
	1 mg/kg diluted with sterile water q 24 hours for 14 to 28 days; intratracheally	For mycotic pneumonia
	0.1 mg/kg of a 5 mg/mL solution in sterile water q 24 hours for 34 days; intrapulmonary	Greek tortoise with pulmonary candidiasis
	0.5 to 1 mg/kg; IC, IV q 1 to 3 days for 14 to 28 days; routes at end	For the treatment of aspergillosis combined with fluid therapy
Ampicillin	*50 mg/kg q 12 hours; IM	Spur-tailed tortoises kept at 27°C

Drug	Dosage	Indication/Species
	10 to 20 mg/kg q 12 to 24 hours; PO, SC, IM	Reported range of dosages for multiple indications
Ascorbic acid	10 to 25 mg/kg; PO, SC, IM 100 to 250 mg/kg; PO, IM	
Atipamezole	*5 times the dose of medetomidine administered (milligram to milligram basis); IM, IV	Reversal of medetomi- dine induced sedation
Atropine sulfate	0.01 to 0.04 mg/kg; SC, IM	Preanesthetic
	0.02 to 0.04 mg/kg q 12 hours for at least 10 days; SC	Excess oral/respiratory mucus in boid snakes
	0.04 to 0.1 mg/kg as needed	Organophosphate toxicity
Azithromycin	*10 mg/kg q 3 days (skin), 5 days (res- piratory tract), or 7 days (liver, kidney); PO	Ball pythons held at 30°C
Barium sulfate	*25 mL/kg 25% w/v suspension	GI contrast radiography in green iguanas
	10 to 15 mL/kg; PO	General recommendation
Buprenorphine	0.01 to 0.1 mg/kg as needed; IM	Analgesia or premedica- tion, reported range of dosage
Butorphanol	0.04 to 2 mg/kg as needed; IM	Analgesia or premedica- tion, reported range of dosage
Calcitonin	50 U/kg once, repeat in 1 to 2 weeks; IM	Metabolic bone disease
Calcium products— oral	23 mg/kg q 12 hours; PO as long as con- dition persists	Calcium deficiency and metabolic bone disease

(continued)

Drug	Dosage	Indication/Species
Calcium products—parenteral	10 to 150 mg/kg (diluted to from 1% to 10%) q 12 to 24 hours or as needed; SC, IM, IV	Calcium deficiency, metabolic bone disease, before oxytocin or vasotocin to treat hypocalcemic egg binding
	100 mg/kg q 6 to 12 hours: IM, SC	Green iguanas
	400 to 500 mg/kg (diluted to 10%) once or at 12- to 48-hour intervals as necessary; intracoelomic, IV or intraosseously by slow infusion over 24 hours	
Calcium EDTA	2 mg/kg; IM	Lead poisoning in a snapping turtle
Carbaryl	2.5% w/v solution in alcohol; apply topically	Ectoparasites
	5% w/w dusting powder; rinse after 30 minutes	Ectoparasites
Carbenicillin	*400 mg/kg q 24 hours; IM	Snakes kept at 30°C
	*400 mg/kg q 48 hours; IM	Tortoises kept at 30°C
	*115 or 120 mg/kg (forelimb versus hindlimb) q 24 hours; IM	Red-eared slider turtles kept at 28°C
	100 to 400 mg/kg q 24 hours; IM	Commonly reported range of dosage for multiple indications
Carprofen	2 to 4 mg/kg once, then 1 to 2 mg/kg q 24 to 72 hours; PO, IV, SC	Analgesia
Cefoperazone	125 mg/kg q 24 hours	Tegu lizard
	100 mg/kg q 96 hours	False water cobra

Drug	Dosage	Indication/Species
Cefotaxime	20 to 40 mg/kg q 24 to 72 hours; IM	Commonly reported range of dosage for multiple indications
Ceftazidime	*20 mg/kg q 72 hours; IM	Snakes kept at 30°C
	*20 to 22 mg/kg q 72 hours; IM	*Pseudomonas* infections in juvenile logger-head sea turtles at 24°C
	20 mg/kg q 72 hours; IM	Commonly reported dosage
Ceftiofur	20 mg/kg q 24 hours; IM	Tortoises
	4 mg/kg q 24 hours; IM	Tortoises, upper respiratory infection
	2.2 mg/kg q 24 hours; IM	Turtles
	2.2 mg/kg q 48 hours; IM	Snakes
	4 mg/kg q 24 h; IM	Osteomyelitis (treat for 2 to 6 months)
Cefuroxime	50 mg/kg q 48 hours; IM	Snakes kept at 30°C
	100 mg/kg q 24 hours; IM	
Cephalexin	20 mg/kg q 24 hours for 7 days; IM	Green iguanas
Cephalothin	20 to 40 mg/kg q 12 hours; IM	
Chloramphenicol palmitate	100 mg/kg q 24 hours; PO	
Chloramphenicol succinate	*40 mg/kg q 24 hours; SC	Gopher snakes kept at 24°C
	*50 mg/kg; SC	Snakes kept at 26°C; dosing frequency from 14 to 99 hours, depending on species of snake; see description of drug for details

(*continued*)

Drug	Dosage	Indication/Species
Chloramphenicol succinate (cont.)	20 to 50 mg/kg q 24 hours or 7 to 20 mg/kg q 12 hours; SC, IM	Commonly reported range of dosage for multiple indications
Chlorhexidine (2% solution)	1:20 or 1:30 dilution in water, swab on affected area q 12 hours for at least 10 to 14 days	Mouth rot in snakes
	20 mL/U.S. gallon water (5.3 mL/L)	Topically for bacterial shell disease in chelonians or mycotic dermatitis in iguanas
Chlortetracycline	200 mg/kg q 24 hours; PO	
Cimetidine	4 mg/kg q 6 to 12 hours; PO	For gastric irritation and ulceration
Ciprofloxacin	5 mg/kg q 24 hours; PO	Common kingsnakes
	2.5 mg/kg q 48 to 72 hours; PO 10 mg/kg q 48 hours; PO	Reticulated pythons, snakes
Cisapride	0.5 to 2 mg/kg q 24 hours; PO	To stimulate gastro-intestinal motility
	4 mg/kg q 12 hours; IM	To reduce hyperphosphatemia in green iguanas with renal failure
Clarithromycin	*15 mg/kg q 2 to 3 days; PO	Desert tortoises at 30°C to 33.3°C, potential for treatment of mycoplasmal infection
Clindamycin	5 mg/kg q 24 hours; PO	Common kingsnakes
Clotrimazole	Topically as needed	Localized fungal infections
Cyfluthrin	*Apply topically, effective up to dilutions of 1:10,000	To kill *Amblyomma marmoreum* ticks from leopard tortoises

Drug	Dosage	Indication/Species
Dexamethasone	62.5 to 250 μg/kg; IM, IV	Septic shock, trauma
	30 to 150 μg/kg; IM, IV, intraosseously	Shock, inflammation
Diazepam	0.2 to 0.6 mg/kg; IM	Alligators
	*0.37 mg/kg; IM	Tranquilization in American alligators
	0.3 to 2 mg/kg; IM	General range of reported dosage for sedation
Dichlorvos impregnated resin strip	0.5 to 6.0 mm/10 ft³ of cage space; treat for 2 to 5 days and repeat in 14 days if required	Ectoparasites, keep out of direct contact with animals
	6 mm/10 ft³ of cage space for 3 hours, 3 × per week for 2 weeks	Ectoparasites, keep out of direct contact with animals
	2.5 cm² of strip/25 cm³ cage space for 2 to 3 days each week	Ectoparasites
	1 cm² of strip/30 cm³ cage space for 28 days	Ectoparasites, decontamination of empty cages
Diethylcarbamazine	50 mg/kg once, repeat at 2- to 3-week intervals; PO	Ascarids
	3 mg/kg q 24 hours for 1 to 2 mo; PO	Microfilaria
Dihydrostreptomycin	5 to 10 mg/kg q 12 hours; IM, topically	Cutaneous wounds and infections
Diloxanide	0.5 g/kg single dose; PO	Amebiasis
Dimetridazole	100 mg/kg single dose, repeat in 2 weeks; PO	Amebae and flagellates
	60 to 100 mg/kg q 24 hours for 5 days, repeat in 2 weeks; PO	

(continued)

Drug	Dosage	Indication/Species
Dimetrizadole (cont.)	40 mg/kg single dose, repeat in 2 weeks; PO	Sensitive snake species (e.g., tricolor king, indigo, milk, Uracoan rattler)
	20 to 40 mg/kg q 24 hours for 5 days; repeat in 2 weeks; PO	
	20 mg/kg q 24 hours for 10 days; PO	
Doxapram	0.25 mL/kg; IV (Dopram-V, 20 mg/mL)	To stimulate respiration during anesthesia and anesthetic recovery
	5 to 10 mg/kg; IV, intraosseously	
Doxycycline	*50 mg/kg once, then 25 mg/kg in 78 hours if necessary; IM (note: original paper also describes time interval as "8 days")	Spur-tailed tortoises kept at 27°C
	50 mg/kg q 72 hours; IM	Spur-tailed tortoises
	5 to 10 mg/kg q 24 hours for 10 to 45 days; PO	Respiratory syndrome of desert tortoises
Emetine HCl	0.5 mg/kg q 24 hours for 10 days; SC, IM	Tissue amebiasis
	2.5 or 5.5 mg/kg q 24 hours for 5 to 7 days; SC, IM	
Enrofloxacin	*10 mg/kg loading dose, then 5 mg/kg q 48 hours; IM	For sensitive gram-negative bacteria, juvenile Burmese pythons kept at 26°C
	*10 mg/kg q 48 hours; IM	For *Pseudomonas* spp., juvenile Burmese pythons kept at 26°C

Drug	Dosage	Indication/Species
	*5 mg/kg q 24 to 48 hours	For respiratory pasteurellosis and other infections in gopher tortoises kept at 30°C
	*5 mg/kg q 24 hours; IM	For susceptible gram-negative organisms, Indian star tortoises kept at 26°C to 30°C
	*5 mg/kg q 12 hours; IM	For *Pseudomonas* and *Citrobacter* spp., Indian star tortoises kept at 26°C to 30°C
	*10 mg/kg q 24 hours for 14 days; PO	Reducing salmonella prevalence in green iguanas
	*5 mg/kg q 36 hours; IM	For mycoplasmal infection in American alligators kept at 27°C
	10 mg/kg q 24 hours; IM	Hermann's tortoises
	2.5 to 5 mg/kg q 96 to 120 hours; IM	Box turtles
	15 mg/kg q 3 days; IM	Upper respiratory tract disease in tortoises
	5 mg/kg q 48 hours; IM + 50 mg enrofloxacin/ 250 mL sterile water or saline, flush each nostril with 1 to 3 mL q 24 to 48 hours until no nasal discharge is visible	Upper respiratory disease in desert tortoises (combined parenteral and topical administration)
	5 or 10 mg/kg q 24 or 48 hours; PO, SC, IM	Commonly reported range of dosage for multiple indications
Febantel + praziquantel (Vercom)	0.5 to 1 mL/kg once, repeat in 14 days; PO	Nematodes in prehensile-tailed skinks

(*continued*)

Drug	Dosage	Indication/Species
Fenbendazole	*10 to 100 mg/kg q 14 days for a maximum of 4 treatments; PO	Nematodiasis in ball pythons
	50 to 100 mg/kg once, repeat in 2 weeks; PO	Commonly reported range of dosage for nematodiasis in snakes, lizards, and chelonians
	50 to 100 mg/kg q 24 hours for 3 days, repeat the 3 treatments in 3 weeks; PO	Ascarids in box turtles
	100 mg/kg once; infused into the cloaca	Oxyurid infestations in tortoises
Fipronil	Topically by spray or wipe, q 7 to 10 days; rinse well after approx. 5 minutes of application	Mites and ticks (see drug description re toxicity)
Fluconazole	*Loading dose of 21 mg/kg, then 10 mg/kg q 5 days; SC	Loggerhead sea turtles at 23°C to 26.5°C
Flunixin meglumine	0.1 to 0.5 mg/kg q 12 to 24 hours for 1 to 3 days; SC, IM, IV	Analgesia, anti-inflammatory
	2 mg/kg q 24 hours; IM, SC	
Furosemide	2 to 5 mg/kg q 12 to 24 hours; IM, IV	Diuresis
Gentamicin sulfate	*2.5 mg/kg at a minimum of 72-hour intervals; SC	Gopher snakes kept at 24°C
	*2.5 to 3 mg/kg loading dose, then 1.5 mg/kg q 96 hours; IM	Blood pythons at 28°C to 30°C

Drug	Dosage	Indication/Species
	*10 mg/kg q 48 to 72 hours for no more than 2 weeks; IM	Red-eared slider and western painted turtles kept at 26°C
	*6 mg/kg q 3 to 5 days; IM	Red-eared slider turtles kept at 24°C
	*3 mg/kg q > 96 hours; IM	Eastern box turtles kept at 29°C
	*2.3 or 2.5 mg/kg (forelimb versus hindlimb) q 72 hours; IM	Red-eared slider turtles kept at 28°C
	*3 mg/kg q 72 hours	Box turtles kept at 21°C to 29°C
	*5 mg/kg q 48 hours; IM	Gopher tortoises
	*1.75 mg/kg q 96 hours; IM	Juvenile American alligators kept at 22°C
	2.5 to 4 mg/kg q 72 to 96 hours; IM	Commonly reported range of dosage for multiple indications
	10 to 20 mg/15 mL saline; nebulize for 30 min q 12 hours	Respiratory disease in tortoises
	2 mg/10 mL saline for nebulization	Respiratory disease
Gentian violet	Topical treatment as needed	Mycotic shell infections in chelonians
Glucose	3 g/kg; PO	Hypoglycemia in crocodilians
Glycopyrrolate	0.01 mg/kg once; SC	Preanesthetic
	0.01 mg/kg q 24 hours; SC	To reduce oral and respiratory mucus in boid snakes
Griseofulvin	20 to 40 mg/kg q 3 days; PO	Fungal dermatitis
Iodine	2 to 4 mg/kg q 7 days; PO	Prophylaxis for goitrogenic diet in chelonians
	0.005% solution povidone iodine topically as needed	Fungal dermatitis

(continued)

Drug	Dosage	Indication/Species
Isoflurane	3% to 5% induction, 1% to 3% maintenance	Inhalant anesthetic of choice
Itraconazole	*23.5 mg/kg; PO with food	Spiny lizards (see drug description for dosing interval)
	*5 mg/kg q 24 hours; PO	Kemp's Ridley sea turtles at 25°C to 28°C
	*15 mg/kg q 72 hours; PO	Kemp's Ridley sea turtles at 25°C to 28°C
Ivermectin	*200 µg/kg, repeat in 2 weeks, maximum of 4 treatments; PO	Ball pythons for GI nematodes
	200 to 400 µg/kg, repeat in 2 weeks; SC, PO, IM	Commonly reported range of dosage for endo- and ectoparasites
	200 µg/kg weekly for 3 weeks; SC	Skin mites in snakes
	5 to 20 mg/L water sprayed on the skin once or q 7 to 10 days as needed	Skin mites in snakes and lizards
	1,000 µg/kg once, or repeat in 14 to 16 days; PO	To eliminate shedding of pentastome eggs in Tokay and Standings day geckos
	Ivermectin can be toxic to chelonians even at low dosage; use with extreme care and with knowledge of species sensitivity; toxicity is reported in non-chelonian species as well	
Kanamycin sulfate	10 to 15 mg/kg q 24 hours; IM, IV, wound flush	

Drug	Dosage	Indication/Species
Ketamine	10 to 100 mg/kg; IM	General range of dosage; results in sedation or immobilization at lower doses (e.g., <50 mg/kg) and anesthesia at higher doses
	2 to 10 mg/kg; IV	Tortoises, iguanas
	*30 mg/kg; IM	Surgical anesthesia in agamid lizards at 30°C
	*15 to 20 mg/kg; IM	Venom collection in colubrid snakes > 500 g
	*60 mg/kg; IM	Venom collection in colubrid snakes < 500 g
	91 to 131 mg/kg; IM	Venom collection in rattlesnakes
Ketamine + medetomidine	*10 mg/kg + 160 µg/kg; IM	Anesthesia in American alligators
	*5 mg/kg + 50 µg/kg; IV	Anesthetic induction in loggerhead sea turtles
	*5 mg/kg + 100 µg/kg; IM	Sedation and anesthesia for minor procedures in red-eared slider turtles
	*10 mg/kg + 200 µg/kg; IM	Sedation and anesthesia in red-eared slider turtles
	5 mg/kg + 100 µg/kg; IV	Sedation and anesthesia for minor procedures in leopard and yellow-footed tortoises, held at 29.5°C
	3 to 8 mg/kg + 25 to 80 µg/kg; IV	Sedation and anesthesia for minor procedures in Aldabra tortoises, held between 24°C and 29.5°C
	5 to 15 mg/kg + 50 to 150 µg/kg; IM	Sedation and anesthesia, general range of dosage

(*continued*)

Drug	Dosage	Indication/Species
Ketamine + medetomidine + butorphanol	5 to 20 mg/kg + 100 to 300 μg/kg + 0.4 mg/kg in same syringe; IV	Short-term anesthesia in aquatic chelonians
Ketamine + midazolam	*20 to 40 mg/kg + 2 mg/kg; IM	Sedation and anesthesia in snapping turtles kept at 21°C
Ketoconazole	*15 mg/kg q 24 hours; PO	Gopher tortoises kept at 27°C
	15 to 50 mg/kg q 24 hours for 14 to 28 days; PO	Commonly reported range of dosage
	25 mg/kg q 24 hours for 2 weeks; PO	Mycotic dermatitis and pneumonia in chelonians
	50 mg/kg q 24 hours for 2 weeks; PO	Mycotic dermatitis in crocodilians
	50 mg/kg + 50 mg/kg thiabendazole q 24 hours for 2 weeks; PO	Mycotic pneumonia in juvenile green sea turtles
Ketoprofen	0.5 to 2 mg/kg q 24 to 48 hours; SC, IM	Analgesia
Levamisole	5 to 20 mg/kg once, repeat in 2 to 3 weeks; SC, IM, intracoelomically	Ascarids, acanthocephalans, pentastomes, rhabdias
	400 mg/kg single dose; PO	Roundworms in snakes and lizards
Levothyroxine	20 μg/kg on alternate days; PO	Hypothyroidism in tortoises
Lincomycin	5 to 10 mg/kg q 12 to 24 hours; IM	Commonly reported range of dosage for multiple indications
Mebendazole	20 to 25 mg/kg once, repeat in 2 weeks; PO	Nematodes; commonly reported range of dosage
	50 to 100 mg/kg once, repeat in 2 weeks; PO	Nematodes; skinks, snakes, and other species
Medetomidine	*150 μg/kg; IM	Sedation in desert tortoises at 24°C

Drug	Dosage	Indication/Species
Meloxicam	0.1 to 0.2 mg/kg q 24 hours; PO; reduce to a minimum effective dose after 2 to 3 days	Analgesia and anti-inflammatory
Meperidine	*2 to 4 mg/kg; intracoelomically	Pain reduction in Nile crocodiles
Metoclopramide	60 µg/kg q 24 hours for 7 days; PO	Stimulation of gastric emptying in tortoises
Metronidazole	*20 mg/kg q 48 hours; PO	Anaerobic bacterial infections in yellow rat snakes
	*20 mg/kg q 24 to 48 hours; PO	Anaerobic bacterial infections in green iguanas
	40 to 100 mg/kg once, repeat in 2 weeks; PO	Amebiasis, trichomoniasis, and other flagellates; commonly reported range of dosage
	40 mg/kg once, repeat in 2 weeks; PO	Sensitive snake species (e.g., tricolor king, indigo, milk, whip-snakes, racers, Uracoan rattlers)
	25 to 40 mg/kg once, repeat in 3 to 4 days; PO	Protozoal infections
	250 mg/kg, single dose; PO	Protozoal infections, maximum dose per animal of 400 mg
	75 to 275 mg/kg q 24 hours for 3 days, or weekly; PO	Reported range of dosage for protozoal infections
	150 mg/kg q 7 days; PO	Antibacterial therapy, maximum dose per animal of 400 mg
	20 mg/kg q 24 to 48 hours; PO	Antibacterial therapy including long-term treatment for osteomyelitis

(continued)

Drug	Dosage	Indication/Species
Metronidazole (cont.)	50 to 100 mg/kg once; PO	To stimulate appetite in snakes
	60 to 80 mg/kg q 24 hours for 3 treatments; SC	Chelonians less than 1 kg
Miconazole	Topically as needed	Localized fungal infections
Midazolam	*1.5 to 2.5 mg/kg; IM	Sedation in red-eared slider turtles kept at 24°C to 27°C
	1 to 2 mg/kg; IM	Commonly reported range of dosage
Milbemycin	0.25 to 0.5 mg/kg once, repeat in 8 days if necessary; PO, SC	Nematodiasis in red-eared slider, Gulf coast box, and ornate box turtles
Neomycin	2.5 mg/kg q 12 to 24 hours; PO	With methscopalamine (Biosol-M)
	10 mg/kg q 24 hours; PO	Enteric infections
Nystatin	100,000 U/kg q 24 hours (or more frequently) for 10 days; PO	Oral candidiasis and gastrointestinal yeast infections
Oil, olive, or vegetable spray	Topically by wipe or spray	For treatment of skin mites
Oxfendazole	66 mg/kg once; PO	Roundworms
Oxytetracycline HCl	6 to 12 mg/kg q 24 hours; PO, IM	General recommendation
	10 mg/kg IV; q 4 days	American alligators
Oxytocin	1 to 10 IU/kg; IM; repeat in 2 to 4 hours as necessary	Commonly reported range of dosage to stimulate oviposition; chelonians
	10 to 30 IU/kg; IM; repeat in 2 to 4 hours as necessary	Commonly reported range of dosage to stimulate oviposition; lizards and snakes
	10 IU/kg q 6 hours, 1 hour after calcium gluconate	Egg retention in green iguanas

Drug	Dosage	Indication/Species
	5 to 10 IU/kg; slow IV or IO drip	Egg retention in green iguanas
Paromomycin	25 to 110 mg/kg q 24 hours for up to 4 weeks; PO	Amebiasis in snakes
	25 or 55 mg/kg once, repeat in 7 or 14 days, respectively; PO	
	100 mg/kg q 24 hours for 7 days and then twice a week for 3 months; PO	To reduce shedding and severity of cryptosporidiosis in snakes
Penicillin G	10,000 to 20,000 U/kg q 6 to 8 hours; SC, IM	
	20,000 to 80,000 U/kg, IM, as a wound flush	
Penicillin, benzathine	10,000 U/kg q 48 to 96 hours; IM	
Penicillin, benzathine/ procaine	10,000 U/kg q 24 to 72 hours; IM	
Permethrin	*Apply topically, effective up to dilutions of 1:10,000	To kill *Amblyomma marmoreum* ticks from leopard tortoises
	*Use as directed (Provent-A-Mite spray)	For ticks and mites on snakes
	Up to 0.1 mg active ingredient/kg, topically	Ticks and mites on snakes and lizards
Piperacillin	*100 mg/kg q 48 hours; IM	Blood pythons kept at 28°C to 30°C
	100 to 200 mg/kg q 24 to 48 hours; IM	Commonly reported range of dosage for multiple indications
	100 mg/kg q 24 hours; IM	Osteomyelitis (treat for 2 to 6 months)

(continued)

Drug	Dosage	Indication/Species
Piperazine	40 to 60 mg/kg q 24 hours, repeat in 10 to 14 days; PO	Nematodes
Polymyxin B	1 to 2 mg/kg q 24 hours; IM	
Praziquantel	3.5 to 8 mg/kg, repeat in 14 and, if needed, 28 days; PO, SC, IM	Cestodes, trematodes
	30 mg/kg single dose; PO	
	*150 mg/kg (50 mg/kg at times 0, 7, and 9 hours); PO once	Cardiovascular spirorchid flukes in green sea turtles
	*75 mg/kg (25 mg/kg at times 0, 3, and 6 hours); PO once	Loggerhead sea turtles
Praziquantel plus febantel (Vercom)	0.5 to 1 mL/kg, repeat in 2 weeks; PO	Nematodes in prehensile tailed skinks
Prednisolone	1 to 2 mg/kg; PO	Anti-inflammatory
Prednisolone sodium succinate	5 to 10 mg/kg as required; IM, IV	Septic shock (with appropriate antibiotic therapy)
Propofol	*5 mg/kg; IV or intraosseously	Anesthetic induction in green iguanas
	*5 mg/kg, IV or intracardiac	Anesthesia of short duration in brown tree snakes
	5 to 15 mg/kg; IV	Commonly reported range of dosage
Propranolol	1 mg/kg; intracoelomically	To stimulate egg laying, in conjunction with vasotocin and prostaglandin, in plateau lizards
Prostaglandin E_2	0.09 mg/kg intracloacally, applied near the uterovaginal opening	To stimulate oviposition in a spotted python, in conjunction with prostaglandin $F_{2\alpha}$

Drug	Dosage	Indication/Species
Prostaglandin $F_{2\alpha}$	25 µg/kg; intra-coelomically	To stimulate nesting behavior and egg laying, in conjunction with vasotocin and propranolol, in plateau lizards
	500 µg/kg once; IM	Egg retention in snakes
Pyrethrin	0.03 to 0.09% spray; saturate animal for 5 min, then soak in water for 30 min or otherwise rinse well	Treatment of ectoparasites, especially mites on snakes and lizards
	1% permethrin; spray lightly then blot off excess; wash animals and repeat in 10 days if required	Mites on snakes
Selenium	25 to 500 µg/kg; IM	Deficiency in lizards
Silver sulfadiazine	Topically as needed (oral and cutaneous)	Mouth rot in snakes, burns, and bacterial infections
Spiramycin	160 mg/kg q 24 hours for 10 days; PO	To reduce shedding and severity of cryptosporidiosis in snakes
Streptomycin sulfate (see Dihydrostreptomycin)		
Sucralfate	0.5 to 1 g/kg q 6 to 8 hours; PO	Gastric protectant for gastritis and gastric ulceration
Sulfadiazine	75 mg/kg once on day 1, then 45 mg/kg on days 2 to 6; PO	Intestinal and biliary coccidia
	25 mg/kg q 24 hours for 7 to 21 days; PO	
Sulfadimethoxine	90 mg/kg once on day 1, then 45 mg/kg q 24 hours for an additional 4 to 6 days; PO, IM	Intestinal and biliary coccidia

(continued)

Drug	Dosage	Indication/Species
Sulfadimethoxine (cont.)	90 mg/kg q 48 hours for 3 treatments; PO 30 mg/kg once on day 1, then 15 mg/kg q 24 hours for an additional 3 days; IM 75 mg/kg once on day 1, then 40 mg/kg q 24 hours for an additional 5 days; PO, IM	
Sulfadimidine (33% w/v)	0.3 to 0.6 mL/kg once on day 1, then the same or one-half the dose q 24 hours for an additional 9 days; PO	Intestinal and biliary coccidia
Sulfamerazine	25 mg/kg q 24 hours for 21 days; PO	Intestinal and biliary coccidia
Sulfamethazine	75 or 90 mg/kg once on day 1, then 40 or 45 mg/kg q 24 hours for an additional 4 to 5 treatments; PO 25 mg/kg q 24 hours for 7 to 21 days; PO	Intestinal and biliary coccidia
Sulfamethoxydiazine	80 mg/kg once, then 40 mg/kg q 24 hours for an additional 4 treatments; SC, IM	Intestinal and biliary coccidia
Sulfamethoxypyridazine	80 mg/kg once, then 40 mg/kg q 24 hours for 4 days; SC	Coccidial infections
	50 mg/kg q 24 hours for 3 days, repeat after an interval of 3 days; PO	Coccidial infections

Drug	Dosage	Indication/Species
Sulfaquinoxyline	75 mg/kg once on day 1, then 40 mg/kg q 24 hours for an additional 6 treatments; PO, IM	Intestinal and biliary coccidia
Tetracycline	10 mg/kg q 24 hours; PO	Snakes and crocodilians
	25 to 50 mg/kg q 12 to 24 hours; PO, SC, IM	
Thiabendazole	50 to 100 mg/kg once, repeat in 2 weeks; PO	Nematodiasis (also antifungal)
Tiletamine-zolazepam (Telazol)	*15 mg/kg; IM	For minor chemical restraint in American alligators
	2 to 8 mg/kg; IM	Sedation, chemical restraint for minor procedures
	10 to 30 mg/kg; IM	Chemical restraint, anesthesia
Tobramycin	2 mg/kg q 24 hours; IM	Chelonia, snakes, and lizards
	2.5 mg/kg q 12 hours; IM	Chameleons
	2.5 mg/kg q 72 hours; IM	General dose
	10 mg/kg q 24 hours; IM	Turtles
	10 mg/kg q 24 to 48 hours; IM	Tortoises and terrapins
Tolnaftate	1% w/v cream q 12 hours; topically	Mycotic dermatitis
Trimethoprim-sulfadiazine, sulfadoxine, sulfamethoxazole	15 to 30 mg/kg q 12, 24, or 48 hours; PO, SC, IM	Antibacterial therapy
	15 to 30 mg/kg q 24 hours for 2 days, then q 48 hours; PO, SC, IM	Antibacterial therapy

(continued)

Drug	Dosage	Indication/Species
Trimethoprim-sulfadiazine, sulfadoxine, sulfamethoxazole (cont.)	30 mg/kg q 24 hours for 7 days; PO, SC, IM	Enteric coccidia
	30 mg/kg; PO or IM once on day 1, then 15 mg/kg; IM or 30 mg/kg; PO q 48 hours for up to 14 additional treatments	Enteric coccidia
	30 to 60 mg/kg q 24 hours for 2 mo; PO	To reduce shedding and severity of cryptosporidiosis in snakes
	30 mg/kg q 24 hours for 14 days, then 1 to 3 × per week for several months; PO	To reduce shedding and severity of cryptosporidiosis in snakes
Tylosin	5 mg/kg q 24 hours for up to 60 days; IM	General range of dosage for multiple indications
	25 mg/kg q 24 hours; PO, IM	General range of dosage for multiple indications
Vasotocin	0.01 to 1 µg/kg; intra-coelomically	To stimulate egg laying
Vitamin A	1,000 to 2,000 IU/kg	Vitamin A deficiency in chelonians
	2,000 IU/kg once weekly for 4 to 6 weeks; SC	Box turtles
	2,000 IU/kg each third day for 2 weeks, then once weekly for 2 treatments; SC, IM	
	Up to 10,000 IU/kg once; PO	Vitamin A deficiency
	10,000 IU/300 g loading dose, then 2,000 IU/300 g every 7 days for 2 to 3 treatments; PO	Box turtles

Drug	Dosage	Indication/Species
	2,000 IU/30 g every 7 days for 2 treatments; PO	Chameleons
Vitamin B complex (various products, components often unspecified in literature)	0.25 to 0.5 mL/kg; PO, SC, IM	Nutritional supplement and appetite stimulant
	OR dose by thiamine content (see below)	
Vitamin B$_1$ (Thiamine)	1.5 to 2 mg/kg q 24 hours for 2 weeks; IM	Thiamine supplementation
	50 to 100 mg/kg; IM	Thiamine deficiency
Vitamin B$_{12}$ (Cyanocobalamin)	50 µg/kg; SC, IM	Supplementation and general nutritional support
Vitamin C (see Ascorbic Acid)		
Vitamin D$_3$	100 to 200 IU/kg once or weekly; IM	Metabolic bone disease in iguanas
	1,000 to 1,650 IU/kg single dose; IM	Hypovitaminosis D
	7,500 IU q 2 weeks as needed; IM	Tortoises
Vitamin E	50 to 100 mg/kg as needed; IM	Nutritional muscular dystrophy
	50 to 800 IU/kg 1 to 3 times/week	Steatitis in aquatic chelonians and crocodilians
Vitamin K	0.25 to 0.5 mg/kg; IM	Vitamin K deficiency in crocodilians and to aid in coagulation factor production
Xylazine	1 to 2 mg/kg; IM	In conjunction with ketamine for anesthesia

*indicates dosages based on pharmacokinetic or controlled efficacy trials.

Handbook of Veterinary Drugs, Third Edition, edited by Dana Allen,
Lippincott Williams & Wilkins, Baltimore. © 2005

Section 16

Description of Drugs for Reptiles

ACYCLOVIR

INDICATIONS: Acyclovir (Avirax ✤, Zovirax ✤ ★) is an antiviral drug with activity against various herpes viruses and cytomegalovirus. Acyclovir has been used orally and topically in tortoises to treat herpes virus infections. It is also available as an intravenous formulation.

ADVERSE AND COMMON SIDE EFFECTS: IM injection of the sodium salt can result in hemorrhage and muscle necrosis. Phlebitis commonly follows IV administration. In humans, headaches, vomiting, and diarrhea are the most common adverse reactions reported. Nephrotoxicity and, rarely, neurologic signs can occur with parenteral administration. Because acyclovir is incompletely absorbed from the gastrointestinal system, oral overdosage and toxicity is unlikely.

DRUG INTERACTIONS: Amphotericin B and ketoconazole increase the effectiveness of acyclovir against some viral diseases in humans.

SUPPLIED AS HUMAN PRODUCTS:
Capsules containing 200 mg (Acyclovir ★, Zovirax ★)
Tablets containing 200 mg (Avirax ✤, Gen-Acyclovir ✤, Nu-Acyclovir ✤, Zovirax ★, Zovirax Oral ✤), 400 mg (Acyclovir ★, Apo-Acyclovir ✤, Avirax ✤, Gen-Acyclovir ✤, Nu-Acyclovir ✤, Zovirax ★, Zovirax Oral ✤), and 800 mg (Acyclovir ★, Apo-Acyclovir ✤, Avirax ✤, Gen-Acyclovir ✤, Nu-Acyclovir ✤, Zovirax Oral ✤)

Suspension containing 200 mg/5 mL (Zovirax ✦ ★)
For injection containing 500 mg or 1 g of acyclovir sodium (Zovirax
✦ ★)
Cream containing 50 mg/g (Zovirax ✦)
Ointment containing 50 mg/g (Zovirax ✦ ★)
Suspension containing 200 mg/5 mL (Zovirax ✦ ★)
For injection containing 500 mg or 1 g of acyclovir sodium (Zovirax
✦ ★)

ALBENDAZOLE

INDICATIONS: Albendazole (Valbazen ✦ ★) is an anthelmintic marketed for use in cattle, which has activity against all stages of liver flukes, tapeworms, gastric and intestinal nematodes, and lungworms. The drug has been used in small animals for the treatment of filaroidiasis, capillariasis, giardiasis, and paragonimiasis. Albendazole is safer and more effective than metronidazole or quinacrine for the treatment of giardiasis. For more information, see ALBENDAZOLE in the Small Animal section. In reptiles, albendazole is used for the treatment of enteric nematodiasis.

SUPPLIED AS VETERINARY PRODUCTS:
Suspension containing 113.6 mg/mL
Oral paste containing 30% albendazole

ALLOPURINOL

INDICATIONS: Allopurinol (Aloprim ★, Purinol ✦, Zyloprim ✦ ★) inhibits the enzyme xanthine oxidase and blocks the formation and urinary excretion of uric acid. Its use has been suggested to reduce uric acid production and prevent or treat cases of gout (uric acid accumulation). For more information, see ALLOPURINOL in the Small Animal section.

ADVERSE AND COMMON SIDE EFFECTS: In birds, there appears to be considerable variability in efficacy and toxicity among species and individuals.

DRUG INTERACTIONS: A number of significant drug interactions exist. See ALLOPURINOL in the Small Animal section.

ALUMINUM HYDROXIDE

INDICATIONS: Aluminum hydroxide (Amphojel ✦ ★, Dialume ★) is an antacid, antiflatulent medication used in mammals for the treatment of gastric ulcers and of hyperphosphatemia associated with renal failure. Aluminum hydroxide is often combined with magnesium hydroxide and with simethicone (Diovol Plus ✦).

In reptiles, aluminum hydroxide has been used in the treatment of hyperphosphatemia associated with renal failure. For more information, see ANTACIDS and ALUMINUM HYDROXIDE in the Small Animal section.

ADVERSE AND COMMON SIDE EFFECTS: These compounds are contraindicated in animals with alkalosis. The aluminum component may predispose to constipation. Aluminum-containing antacids may delay gastric emptying and should be used with caution in patients with gastric outlet obstruction.

DRUG INTERACTIONS: Antacid products may interfere with or promote the absorption of a variety of other medications, including tetracycline antibiotics. For more information, see ANTACIDS and ALUMINUM HYDROXIDE in the Small Animal section.

AMIKACIN

INDICATIONS: Amikacin (Amiglyde-V ♣ ★, Amikin ♣ ★, Amiject D ★) is an aminoglycoside antibiotic indicated in the treatment of superficial and systemic bacterial infections, especially those caused by gram-negative organisms such as *Pseudomonas* and *Aeromonas* spp. Amikacin is a drug of choice for initial antimicrobial therapy while awaiting bacterial culture results. The drug can also be nebulized in saline for treatment of pneumonia. For more information, see AMIKACIN in the Small Animal section.

Experimental pharmacokinetic studies have been carried out in several species of reptiles. In gopher snakes kept at environmental temperatures of 25°C and 37°C, the rate of absorption and the elimination half-life (71.9 and 75.4 hours, respectively) of amikacin were similar after administration of 5 mg/kg of body weight IM. At the higher temperature, greater volume of distribution and renal clearance resulted in lower serum concentrations of the drug.

In studies of ball pythons held at 25°C or 37°C there was no effect of environmental temperature on amikacin clearance. The median elimination half-life was 4.5 days. A dose of 3.5 mg/kg IM was recommended to achieve serum minimal inhibitory concentration values effective against most gram-negative bacteria, but it was felt that a much higher dosage, i.e., 12 mg/kg, would be required for *Pseudomonas aeruginosa*. Amikacin serum concentrations remained above recommended therapeutic trough concentrations of 2 μg/mL for more than 6 days, resulting in the authors' suggestion that treatment consist of a single dose to avoid amikacin accumulation.

In gopher tortoises held at 30°C, a pharmacokinetic study suggested a dose of 5 mg/kg IM every 48 hours. Tortoises acclimated to 20°C had a similar volume of distribution for amikacin; however, slower elimination of the drug resulted in amikacin accumulation.

The pharmacokinetics of amikacin were also studied in juvenile American alligators held at a water temperature of 22°C. The elimination half-life of amikacin administered at 1.75 and 2.25 mg/kg IM was shorter than that reported in gopher snakes, suggesting that more frequent dosing is necessary in alligators. The higher dose (2.25 mg/kg) was recommended to achieve serum levels effective against *Pseudomonas* spp.

ADVERSE AND COMMON SIDE EFFECTS: Nephrotoxicity is reputed to be of concern; however, its occurrence has not been reported. Snakes necropsied 6 days after being administered a single dose of 5 mg/kg did not show histologic evidence of renal disease. During amikacin treatment, it is essential to maintain hydration by ensuring the availability of fresh water or through the administration of oral, intracoelomic, or SC isotonic fluids. If prolonged therapy is expected, monitoring of plasma or serum uric acid levels may be appropriate. The monitoring of blood amikacin levels would be helpful to protect against toxicity and ensure therapeutic blood levels. Neurotoxicity has been reported. It has been suggested that a single high dose may give therapeutic levels for several weeks and be less toxic than multiple small doses. Most recent pharmacokinetic studies suggest that the majority of currently published dosage regimens may result in the accumulation of amikacin over time.

DRUG INTERACTIONS: Amikacin is often used in combination with penicillins and cephalosporins such as ampicillin, amoxicillin, carbenicillin, piperacillin, ceftazidime, and cefotaxime. *In vitro* studies have shown that carbenicillin causes less inactivation of amikacin than it does gentamicin; therefore, amikacin may be a better choice for combination therapy.

AMINOPHYLLINE

INDICATIONS: Aminophylline (Phylloconton ✤ ★ and generics) is a bronchodilator principally used for the management of cough caused by bronchospasm. It has mild inotropic properties and mild, transient diuretic activity. Aminophylline has been suggested as an adjunct therapy in the treatment of respiratory disease in reptiles when bronchodilation is required. For more information, see AMINOPHYLLINE in the Small Animal section.

AMITRAZ

INDICATIONS: Amitraz (Mitaban ✤ ★) is a monoamine oxidase (MAO) inhibitor (causes a buildup of norepinephrine in the central nervous system [CNS]) and is used for the treatment of ectoparasites. It also inhibits prostaglandin synthesis and is an α-adrenergic receptor agonist. For more information, see AMITRAZ in the Small Animal section.

Amitraz has been described for the removal of *Amblyomma* ticks from leopard tortoises (*Geochelone pardalis*). The emulsion was poured over the tortoises' front and rear carapace openings while they were on their backs, left for a few minutes, then allowed to drain. The ticks detached and died over 3 to 4 days, and then the residual amitraz was washed off the tortoises. In a more recent study evaluating the effectiveness of acaricides *in vitro*, amitraz was found to be completely ineffective in killing *Amblyomma marmoreum* ticks.

ADVERSE AND COMMON SIDE EFFECTS: The most common side effects of amitraz toxicity in dogs are ataxia and depression. The safety of amitraz was evaluated in leopard tortoises. Twice the recommended mammalian dosage was applied to all accessible skin surfaces, then experimental animals were observed for side effects for 72 hours. This treatment was carried out 3 times at weekly intervals. Several minor side effects lasting for under 1 hour were observed and included: decreased food consumption, reduced defecation, diarrhea, and eye irritation.

DRUG INTERACTIONS: Atropine potentiates the pressor effects of amitraz and may cause hypertension and cardiac arrhythmias.

AMOXICILLIN

INDICATIONS: Amoxicillin (Amoxi-Tabs ★, Amoxi-Drop ★, Amoxi-Inject ★, Amoxil ♣ ★, Moxilean ♣, Robamox-V ★) is indicated for the treatment of superficial and systemic bacterial infections. Amoxicillin has the same antibacterial spectrum as ampicillin but is better absorbed from the gastrointestinal tract (GIT) and has a more rapid bactericidal activity and a longer duration of action. For more information, see AMOXICILLIN in the Small Animal section.

Amoxicillin has been suggested for long-term treatment (i.e., 2 to 6 months) in cases of osteomyelitis. There are no pharmacokinetic data available describing a rational dosing strategy for reptiles.

AMPHOTERICIN B

INDICATIONS: Amphotericin B (Amphocin ★, Fungizone ♣ ★) is an effective fungicidal agent active against a variety of systemic mycotic infections. The drug has been used in reptiles for the treatment of mycotic pneumonia via nebulization or intratracheal infusion. Direct intrapulmonary injection of the drug via a transcarapacial catheter was used successfully to treat a Greek tortoise with a pulmonary infection by *Candida albicans*.

Crystalline amphotericin B is insoluble in water. The drug is combined with sodium desoxycholate to form a mixture that provides a colloidal dispersion for intravenous infusion following reconstitution. The drug is reconstituted using sterile water into a 3% suspension with a pH of 6 to 8. The resulting suspension is sensitive to light and is inactivated at low pH. Once reconstituted, amphotericin B has a shelf life of only a few hours at room temperature and approximately 1 week if refrigerated. The drug can be frozen in aliquots, then diluted in 5% dextrose or water as necessary for IV use or nebulization, respectively. More stable water-based suspensions have been compounded using products such as cellulose gum. Amphotericin B should not be combined with saline or other electrolyte solutions to prevent precipitation and crystal formation. Intratracheal and intranasal administration of improperly prepared products has been associated with severe tissue reactions in birds. Liposomal formulations are also available.

ADVERSE AND COMMON SIDE EFFECTS: When used parenterally, amphotericin B is highly nephrotoxic in most species. For more information, see AMPHOTERICIN B in the Small Animal section.

SUPPLIED AS HUMAN PRODUCTS:
For IV injection containing 50 mg/vial (Amphocin ★, Fungizone ❀ ★)
For IV injection (liposome formulation) containing 50 mg/vial (AmBisome ★)
For IV injection containing 2.5 mg/mL (Fungizone ❀) and 5 mg/mL (Albelcet ❀ ★)

AMPICILLIN

INDICATIONS: Ampicillin (Omnipen ★, Polyflex ❀ ★, Principen ★) has been recommended for the treatment of bacterial infections including *Pasteurella testudinis* pneumonia in tortoises and ulcerative shell disease in chelonians. For more information, see AMPICILLIN in the Small Animal section.

One experimental study looked at the pharmacokinetics of 50 and 100 mg/kg of ampicillin administered IM into the gluteal muscles of spur-tailed tortoises held at 27°C, and compared blood levels with minimal inhibitory concentrations for a range of bacteria isolated from reptiles. Although the maximum plasma level was much greater with the dose of 100 mg/kg (421.8 versus 159.1 µg/mL), by 6.5 to 7 hours after injection plasma levels had dropped below the "therapeutic limit" of 3 µg/mL. A dose of 50 mg/kg q 12 hours was considered the regimen of choice for the treatment of infections by *Staphylococcus* spp. In two animals, secondary peaks of blood antibiotic levels were noted; these were attributed to reabsorption of water and ampicillin from the bladder. A range of doses for ampicillin in reptiles has been published in formularies and case reports, and most are substantially lower than

50 mg/kg. There are no pharmacokinetic data on oral absorption of the drug in reptiles.

DRUG INTERACTIONS: Ampicillin is frequently used in combination with aminoglycosides to increase antibacterial spectrum and effectiveness. In addition, lizards and tortoises have been reported to be cleared of enteric *Salmonella* spp. after oral treatment with 250 mg chloramphenicol combined with 75 mg ampicillin daily for 10 days.

ASCORBIC ACID

INDICATIONS: Vitamin C (Apo-C ♣, Redoxon ♣, generics, and many others) is used as a general supplement for sick reptiles. Vitamin C is sometimes recommended in addition to antibiotic therapy for the treatment of mouth rot in snakes; however, the efficacy is unknown. Vitamin C has also been used in the treatment of splitting skin syndrome in some large constrictors. Because snakes can manufacture vitamin C in their kidneys and intestines, a true deficiency may not occur and treatment is somewhat controversial. Published dosages vary by a 10-fold range; however, the drug is generally very safe.

SUPPLIED AS VETERINARY PRODUCTS:
For injection containing 250 mg/mL (Ascorbic Acid Injection ♣, Ascorbic Acid Inj. U.S.P. ♣ Centravite-C ♣, Sodium Ascorbate ♣)

SUPPLIED AS HUMAN PRODUCTS:
Tablets containing 100, 250, 500, or 1,000 mg
For injection containing 222 mg/mL (Generic ★), 250 mg/mL (Generic ★), and 500 mg/mL (Generic ★, Cecore 500 ★, Cee-500 ★, Mega-C/A Plus ★)

ATIPAMEZOLE

INDICATIONS: Atipamezole (Antisedan ♣ ★) is a synthetic α-adrenergic antagonist marketed for the reversal of the sedative and analgesic effects of medetomidine hydrochloride. It has been used to reverse the sedative effects of medetomidine in a variety of reptilian species, but may not completely reverse medetomidine's cardiopulmonary depressive effects. For more information on the use of atipamezole in reptiles, see MEDETOMIDINE in this section. For general information, see ATIPAMEZOLE in the Small Animal section. Atipamezole is generally given on a volume-per-volume basis (milliliter for milliliter) of medetomidine (Domitor) administered, which is equivalent to a dosage of 5 times the medetomidine given on a milligram to milligram (mg:mg) basis. In dogs, calculated dosages of atipamezole are based on body surface rather than body weight.

ADVERSE AND COMMON SIDE EFFECTS: Immediate and severe hypotension with no identifiable cardiac or arterial flow detectable for 30 to 90 seconds was described in 4 of 6 gopher tortoises given atipamezole IV at a dose of 500 µg/kg. The authors recommended that atipamezole not be administered IV in turtles and tortoises. Atipamezole was used IV to reverse medetomidine + ketamine anesthesia in leopard, yellow-footed, and Aldabra tortoises without clinical evidence of diminished cardiac function. Doses used ranged from 100 to 400 µg/kg. Two of the leopard tortoises did, however, vomit after the atipamezole was administered.

ATROPINE

INDICATIONS: Atropine ♣ ★ is an anticholinergic and antispasmodic agent used as a preanesthetic and in the treatment of vagally induced bradycardia and organophosphate toxicity. Its use has also been recommended, in combination with antibiotic therapy, to reduce oral and respiratory mucus in boid snakes with infectious stomatitis or respiratory disease. For more information, see ATROPINE in the Small Animal section.

AZITHROMYCIN

INDICATIONS: Azithromycin (Zithromax ♣ ★) is a semisynthetic macrolide antibiotic with a narrow spectrum of activity that includes chlamydiae, mycoplasma, and some streptococci and staphylococci. The drug accumulates in tissue and has a prolonged elimination half-life. In human medicine, a single dose of azithromycin is used to treat uncomplicated venereal infection caused by *Chlamydia trachomatis*. Azithromycin combined with ethambutol and either ciprofloxacin or rifabutin is recommended for the prophylaxis and treatment of *Mycobacterium avium* complex infections in HIV patients.

The pharmacokinetics of azithromycin were studied in 7 ball pythons held at 30°C. Single doses of 10 mg/kg were administered orally and IV, and blood azithromycin levels were measured for up to 96 hours. The mean bioavailability after oral administration was 77%, and the mean terminal half-life was 51 hours. A mean peak plasma concentration of 1.04 µg/mL was reached at 8.4 hours. Azithromycin was found to have a wider volume of distribution in pythons than either amikacin or piperacillin, but this value was substantially lower than that described in mammals. Tissue concentrations of azithromycin were also measured at 24 and 72 hours in snakes given a single oral dose of 10 mg/kg and were 4 to 40 times greater than those in plasma. The authors concluded that an oral dose of 10 mg/kg, administered every 2 to 7 days (depending on organism susceptibility and site of infection), was appropriate for treatment of ball pythons.

ADVERSE AND COMMON SIDE EFFECTS: In humans, the presence of food in the stomach decreases the rate and extent of gastrointestinal absorption. Azithromycin is eliminated principally via the liver; therefore, caution is recommended in treating humans with hepatic disease.

SUPPLIED AS HUMAN PRODUCTS:
Tablets containing 200 mg ★, 250 mg ♣, and 600 mg ♣ (Zithromax)
Powder (oral suspension base) to be reconstituted to 100 mg ♣, 200 mg ★, and 500 mg ♣/5 mL (Zithromax)
For injection, containing 500 mg/vial (Zithromax ♣ ★)

BARIUM SULFATE

INDICATIONS: Barium sulfate ♣ ★ is an inert radiopaque material that provides positive contrast during x-ray or fluoroscopic examination. Barium sulfate is not absorbed or metabolized and is eliminated intact from the body through the feces as a function of gastrointestinal transit time.

Barium sulfate is commonly used in reptiles for GIT contrast studies. The rate of passage will vary with species, ambient temperature, and the presence of anesthetic or sedative agents. It is likely that the appropriate volume to be administered will vary among species (based on gastric volume); however, this has not been specifically determined for most species. One study using green iguanas recommended a volume of 25 mL/kg of a 25% w/v suspension for best gastric filling and contrast.

ADVERSE AND COMMON SIDE EFFECTS: The most common side effects reported in humans are constipation or diarrhea and cramping. The use of barium sulfate is contraindicated when the possibility of gastric or intestinal perforation exists. Aspiration of barium sulfate can lead to significant pneumonia and possibly death.

SUPPLIED AS HUMAN PRODUCTS:
Numerous barium sulfate suspensions from 1.2% to 98 % w/w and 4.9% to 220 % w/v (♣ ★)

BUPRENORPHINE

INDICATIONS: Buprenorphine hydrochloride (Buprenex ★) is a partial opiate agonist with analgesic properties. It is used for the management of mild pain. For more information, see BUPRENORPHINE HYDROCHLORIDE in the Small Animal section.

Buprenorphine has been suggested for use as an analgesic in reptiles. Although there is almost no work investigating the effectiveness of analgesics in reptiles, it is assumed that their use is appropriate in situations where pain might be occurring, and that drugs used in other species should have similar effects.

BUTORPHANOL

INDICATIONS: Butorphanol (Torbugesic ♣ ★, Torbutrol ♣ ★) is a narcotic agonist/antagonist analgesic that is also used as a preanesthetic. See BUTORPHANOL in the Small Animal section for further information.

Butorphanol has been suggested for use as an analgesic in reptiles. Although there is almost no work investigating the effectiveness of analgesics in reptiles, it is assumed that their use is appropriate in situations where pain might be occurring, and that drugs used in other species should have similar effects.

ADVERSE AND COMMON SIDE EFFECTS: Butorphanol has minimal cardiovascular effects and causes only slight respiratory depression. When it is used alone butorphanol causes little sedation.

CALCITONIN SALMON

INDICATIONS: Calcitonin (Calcimar ♣ ★) inhibits bone resorption and antagonizes parathormone (PTH), lowering circulating calcium and phosphorous levels. Osteoclast activity is inhibited, while that of osteoblasts is increased. Urinary calcium excretion is increased in the presence of calcitonin.

In reptiles, calcitonin is used in the treatment of metabolic bone disease in conjunction with calcium and vitamin D_3 supplementation and husbandry changes. Blood calcium levels should be stabilized before treatment is initiated. Most case reports refer to use in the green iguana. For more information, see CALCITONIN SALMON in the Small Animal section.

ADVERSE AND COMMON SIDE EFFECTS: The use of calcitonin can precipitate acute hypocalcemia in animals with low blood calcium levels.

CALCIUM BOROGLUCONATE
CALCIUM GLUBIONATE
CALCIUM GLUCONATE
CALCIUM GLUCONATE/CALCIUM LACTATE

INDICATIONS: Calcium products are used for the treatment of hypocalcemia and metabolic bone disease, and for the pretreatment of uterine inertia and egg binding prior to the administration of oxytocin or vasotocin. The management of animals with metabolic bone disease should also include vitamin D_3 supplementation and diet and husbandry correction.

Calcium glubionate (also known as calcium glucono-galacto gluconate) syrup (Calcionate ★, Neo-Calglucon ★, Calcium Sandoz ♣) is the most favored product for oral use. Calcium glubionate should be given before feeding to enhance calcium absorption. Other liquid calcium products contain calcium carbonate ★ (oral suspension); calcium citrate ★, calcium lactate-gluconate ♣, and calcium carbonate ♣ (tablets for oral solution), calcium gluceptate and calcium gluconate ♣ (oral solution). Capsules and tablets are available containing calcium carbonate, citrate, gluconate, lactate, and calcium phosphate. These should be compared on the basis of elemental calcium, rather than the "strength" of the tablet as some calcium salts have more elemental calcium than others. Published dosages for oral calcium supplementation range from 20 to 500 mg/kg. The lower end of the dosage range, equating to approximately 1 mL/kg of the most commonly used oral products, is most frequently cited.

Calcium gluconate and calcium glycerophosphate/lactate combinations can be administered IV or in a diluted form (<5%), IM or SC. Intramuscular or SC injection is often preferred to avoid too rapid changes in blood calcium levels and when venous access is unavailable. Intravenous calcium chloride produces higher and more predictable levels of ionized calcium in plasma. Calcium gluconate/lactate combinations are used for IM injection. Parenteral administration is used most commonly for the treatment of hypocalcemic tetany and for reproductive management. Animals with metabolic bone disease should be switched to oral therapy as soon as possible. For more information, see CALCIUM GLUCONATE or CALCIUM LACTATE in the Small Animal section and CALCIUM BOROGLUCONATE in the Large Animal section.

ADVERSE AND COMMON SIDE EFFECTS: Parenteral calcium can rarely be administered IV, while IM and SC injection of calcium products can result in inflammation, necrosis, and sloughing. This is especially true with large volumes and high concentrations of solution. Intracoelomic administration may result in mild peritonitis and precipitation of calcium onto the peritoneal surfaces.

SUPPLIED AS HUMAN PRODUCTS:
Oral syrup containing 115 mg calcium glubionate per 5 mL (Calcionate ★, Neo-Calglucon ★) and 1.2 g calcium lactobionate and 530 mg calcium gluconate (110 mg of calcium ion)/5 mL (Calcium-Sandoz ♣)

SUPPLIED AS VETERINARY PRODUCTS:
Calcium glycerophosphate/lactate: solution containing 5 mg/mL of each element for IM and SC use (Calphosan Solution ★), and IM, SC, and IV use (Cal-Pho-Sol solution SA ★)

Calcium gluconate or borogluconate: numerous solutions for IV, SC, IP use containing 230 mg/mL (23% solution ✤ ★) and ~267 mg/mL (~26 % solution ✤ ★)

See CALCIUM BOROGLUCONATE in the Large Animal section.

CALCIUM EDTA

INDICATIONS: Calcium disodium EDTA (Calcium Disodium Versenate ✤ ★) is a favored chelating agent for the treatment of lead toxicity in a variety of species. This medication was successfully used in a snapping turtle with elevated blood lead levels and clinical signs consistent with lead poisoning. A dose of approximately 2 mg/kg was administered every 6 to 13 days for four treatments. For more information, see CALCIUM EDTA in the Small Animal section.

SUPPLIED AS HUMAN PRODUCT:
For injection containing 200 mg/mL (Calcium Disodium Versonate ✤ ★)

CARBARYL

INDICATIONS: Carbaryl (Sevin ✤, Zodiac Flea and Tick Powder ✤, and many others) is a carbamate insecticide and cholinesterase inhibitor used in the eradication of arthropod ectoparasites, including mites and ticks. A 2.5% w/v solution in alcohol can be used as a topical wipe. Care should be taken to avoid the eyes and mouth. The 5% w/w powder can be applied to environmental surfaces with which the animal has no direct contact, and has been used topically with caution. The powder should be thoroughly rinsed off after approximately 30 minutes of skin contact. For more information, see CARBAMATE INSECTICIDES in the Small Animal section.

ADVERSE AND COMMON SIDE EFFECTS: Toxicity results in miosis, salivation, frequent urination and defecation, vomiting, bronchoconstriction, ataxia, incoordination, muscle tremors, convulsions, respiratory depression, paralysis, and possibly death. Atropine (0.2 mg/kg) is given to effect as the antidote. In dogs, one fourth of the total dose is given intravenously, and the balance is given intramuscularly or subcutaneously. Diazepam has been used to augment the effects of atropine, hastening recovery.

The safety of carbaryl was evaluated in leopard tortoises. Twice the recommended mammalian dosage was dusted over all accessible skin surfaces and experimental animals were observed for side effects for 72 hours. This treatment was carried out 3 times at weekly intervals. Several minor side effects lasting for under 1 hour were observed and included: decreased food consumption, reduced defecation, diarrhea and skin irritation. Eye irritation occurred and was of longer duration, with a mean of 2 hours. In a second *in vitro* portion of the same study, carbaryl was found to be ineffective in killing *Amblyomma marmoreum* ticks.

CARBENICILLIN

INDICATIONS: Carbenicillin (Geopen ✻ ★, Geocillin ★, Pyopen ✻) is an extended spectrum, penicillinase-sensitive, semisynthetic penicillin used for the treatment of a variety of bacterial infections. It is effective against *Pseudomonas* and *Aeromonas* spp. For more information, see CARBENICILLIN and PENICILLIN ANTIBIOTICS in the Small Animal section.

In an experimental study in snakes (individuals of various species) held at 30°C, carbenicillin administered IM at 400 mg/kg reached peak blood levels in 1 hour. Therapeutic blood levels (defined as >50 to 60 µg/mL) persisted for at least 12 hours after drug administration. The authors suggested that previously recommended dosages of approximately 100 mg/kg would not provide effective blood levels and suggested treatment with 400 mg/kg once daily. In a similar study performed in Greek and Hermann's tortoises, also held at 30°C, carbenicillin was rapidly absorbed from the IM injection site. Thirty-seven hours after injection blood antibiotic levels began to rise again. This was attributed to reabsorption of unchanged drug from the bladder, where urine can be held for long periods of time. Although maintenance of therapeutic blood levels could be erratic, the authors recommended carbenicillin as a clinically effective drug in tortoises and suggested a dose of 400 mg/kg every 48 hours. The pharmacokinetics of carbenicillin absorption and excretion did not appear to be affected by the site of IM injection (i.e., cranial versus caudal portion of body) in carpet pythons.

A study carried out in red-eared slider turtles kept at 28°C compared the pharmacokinetic parameters resulting from the IM administration of 200 mg/kg carbenicillin in either the forelimb or hindlimb. Significant differences in the drug's relative bioavailability were noted; however, these were not thought to be clinically significant. The mean elimination half-lives were 12.76 and 12.08 hours, and the maximum plasma concentrations were 796 and 623 µg/mL for injection into the forelimbs and hindlimbs, respectively. It was determined that in order to maintain a steady-state concentration of carbenicillin between a peak of 400 µg/mL and a trough of 100 µg/mL, doses of 115 mg/kg every 24 hours in the forelimb and 120 mg/kg every 24 hours in the hindlimb would be appropriate.

Carbenicillin has been suggested for long-term treatment (i.e., 2 to 6 months) of osteomyelitis.

ADVERSE AND COMMON SIDE EFFECTS: Pain upon injection has been noted in snakes and in tortoises. Skin rashes have developed after administration to desert tortoises.

DRUG INTERACTIONS: Carbenicillin is used primarily in combination with aminoglycosides to reduce the rate of development of bacterial resistance. Carbenicillin may have a deactivating effect on aminoglycoside antibiotics; therefore, the two drugs should not be mixed *in vitro* (i.e., in the syringe). Treatment with carbenicillin is sometimes delayed until 48 hours after the initiation of aminoglycoside administration.

CARPROFEN

INDICATIONS: Carprofen (Rimadyl ❋ ★) is a carboxylic acid non-steroidal anti-inflammatory agent with analgesic, anti-inflammatory, and antipyretic properties. Carprofen has been suggested for use as an analgesic and anti-inflammatory agent in reptiles. Although there is no work investigating the physiology and effectiveness of nonsteroidal analgesics in reptiles, it is assumed that their use is appropriate in situations where pain might be occurring, and that drugs used in other species should have similar effects. For more information, see CARPROFEN in the Small Animal section.

CEFOPERAZONE

INDICATIONS: Cefoperazone (Cefobid ★) is a third-generation cephalosporin with increased resistance to β-lactamase–producing bacteria. The drug has an expanded spectrum of activity against gram-negative bacteria including *Pseudomonas, Proteus, Enterobacter,* and *Citrobacter* spp., and anaerobes, compared with first- and second-generation cephalosporins. Cefoperazone has less activity against many gram-positive organisms than first-generation drugs. Although cefoperazone is registered for IV and IM use in humans, it is most often used IV. In reptiles, doses for cefoperazone have been described in tegu lizards and false water cobras.

ADVERSE AND COMMON SIDE EFFECTS: In humans, cefoperazone is combined with lidocaine for intramuscular injection to prevent pain upon injection. Reported side effects in humans include hypothrombinemia and diarrhea. As cefoperazone is primarily excreted via the liver, hepatic disease will likely reduce elimination of the drug.

DRUG INTERACTIONS: Cefoperazone can be combined with an aminoglycoside antibiotic, particularly for the treatment of *P. aeruginosa* infection. Concurrent administration of vitamin K has been suggested to prevent or reduce the occurrence of hypothrombinemia.

SUPPLIED AS HUMAN PRODUCTS:
For injection containing 20 mg/mL and 40 mg/mL (Cefobid ★)

CEFOTAXIME

INDICATIONS: Cefotaxime (Claforan ❦ ★) is a third-generation cephalosporin used in the treatment of bacterial infections, including those by *Pseudomonas aeruginosa*. For more information, see CEFOTAXIME and CEPHALOSPORIN ANTIBIOTICS in the Small Animal section.

CEFTAZIDIME

INDICATIONS: Ceftazidime (Fortaz ❦ ★) is a third-generation, broad-spectrum cephalosporin with similar activity to cefotaxime against gram-negative bacteria and greater activity against *Pseudomonas aeruginosa*. It is used as an alternative to or in conjunction with the aminoglycoside antibiotics. Ceftazidime is a drug of choice for initial antimicrobial therapy while awaiting culture results. For more information, see CEFTAZIDIME and CEPHALOSPORIN ANTIBIOTICS in the Small Animal section.

In an experimental study in a variety of snakes (mangrove, boa constrictor, reticulated and Burmese pythons, yellow rat snakes) held at 30°C, ceftazidime administered IM at 20 mg/kg reached peak blood levels between 1 and 8 hours; therapeutic levels (defined as >8 µg/mL) persisted for at least 96 hours after drug administration. The recommended dosing interval was 72 hours. The snakes used in this work were clinically ill patients, pharmacokinetic studies were not carried out in healthy animals. Ceftazidime has been suggested for long-term treatment (i.e., 2 to 6 months) of osteomyelitis, and for prophylactic antibiotic therapy in green iguanas before surgery for egg-binding.

The pharmacokinetics of ceftazidime were studied in juvenile loggerhead sea turtles held at approximately 24°C. Experimental groups of four animals were administered doses of 20 mg/kg ceftazidime either IV or IM. Maximum plasma concentrations (69.74 ± 11.14 µg/mL and 69.90 ± 8.53 µg/mL, IV and IM respectively) and elimination half-lives (20.6 ± 3.2 hours and 19.1 ± 0.8 hours, IV and IM respectively) were almost identical for the two routes of administration. The resulting plasma concentrations were compared to minimum inhibitory concentration (MIC) values for two strains of *Pseudomonas* spp. and in all animals remained above 4 and 8 µg/mL for 72 and 60 hours, respectively. The dosage suggested for the treatment of *Pseudomonas* infections in this species was 20 to 22 mg/kg each 72 hours.

ADVERSE AND COMMON SIDE EFFECTS: Ceftazidime is less nephrotoxic than other cephalosporins; however, renal damage can occur at high-dose levels. The drug is poorly absorbed after oral administration. Some variability in half-life was seen in the above study, but it could not be determined whether this was due to variability in dosing technique or species response.

CEFTIOFUR

INDICATIONS: Ceftiofur (Excenel ✤ ★, Naxcel ★, Excenel RTU ✤) is a third-generation, broad-spectrum cephalosporin active against gram-positive and gram-negative bacteria, including β-lactamase–producing strains. The drug is marketed for use in a variety of domestic animal species. For more information, see CEFTIOFUR in the Large Animal section and CEPHALOSPORIN ANTIBIOTICS in the Small Animal section.

Ceftiofur has been recommended for general antibiotic therapy in a variety of reptiles, and for long-term treatment (i.e., 2 to 6 months) of osteomyelitis.

ADVERSE AND COMMON EFFECTS: Thrombocytopenia and anemia, which may be reversible, can occur in mammals given 3 to 5 times the recommended dose of ceftiofur.

SUPPLIED AS VETERINARY PRODUCTS:
For injection containing 50 mg/mL ceftiofur sodium (Excenel ✤, Naxcel ★)
For injection containing 50 mg/mL ceftiofur hydrochloride (Excenel RTU ✤, Excenel ★)

CEFUROXIME

INDICATIONS: Cefuroxime (Zinacef ✤ ★, Ceftin ✤ ★, Kefurox ✤) is a broad-spectrum cephalosporin antibiotic used for treatment of gram-positive and gram-negative infections. Cefuroxime axetil is intended for oral use and cefuroxime sodium for parenteral administration. For more general information, see CEPHALOSPORIN ANTIBIOTICS in the Small Animal section.

ADVERSE AND COMMON SIDE EFFECTS: The concomitant administration of aminoglycosides and some cephalosporins has resulted in nephrotoxicity in humans. In humans, pseudomembranous colitis has been reported in association with treatment with cefuroxime.

DRUG INTERACTIONS: Cefuroxime has been used for the treatment of gram-negative infections in snakes at a dosage of 100 mg/kg daily for 10 days, in combination with gentamicin.

SUPPLIED AS HUMAN PRODUCTS:
For oral medication tablets containing 125 (Ceftin ★), 250, and 500 mg (Ceftin ✤ ★)

Oral suspension containing 125 mg/5 mL (Ceftin ✤ ★) and 250 mg/ 5 mL (Ceftin ✤)
For injection containing 750 and 1,500 mg/vial (Cefuroxime ★, Zinacef ✤ ★, and Kefurox ✤)

CEPHALEXIN

INDICATIONS: Cephalexin (Keflex ✤ ★, Keftab ★, Novo-Lexin ✤, Nu-Cephalex ✤) is a broad-spectrum first-generation cephalosporin antibiotic available for oral use. Cephalexin is used for the treatment of bacterial infections. First-generation cephalosporins are active against gram-positive bacteria, including penicillin-resistant staphylococci, and against some gram-negative bacteria, including *E. coli*, *Proteus*, and *Klebsiella* spp. For more information, see CEPHALEXIN and CEPHALOSPORIN ANTIBIOTICS in the Small Animal section.

Cephalexin has been recommended for prophylactic antibiotic therapy in green iguanas before surgery for egg-binding.

CEPHALOTHIN

INDICATIONS: Cephalothin (Keflin ✤, Ceporacin ✤) is a broad-spectrum first-generation cephalosporin antibiotic for parenteral use. First-generation drugs are active against gram-positive bacteria, including penicillin-resistant staphylococci, and against some gram-negative bacteria, including *E. coli*, *Proteus*, and *Klebsiella* spp. For more information, see CEPHALOSPORIN ANTIBIOTICS in the Small Animal section.

In reptiles, cephalothin has been suggested for long-term treatment (i.e., 2 to 6 months) of osteomyelitis at a dose of 30 mg/kg (IM; q 12 hours).

ADVERSE AND COMMON SIDE EFFECTS: Cephalothin is irritating; large or repeated IM injection may cause pain and result in local inflammatory reactions or sterile abscesses. Thrombophlebitis has been associated with IV use in humans. In humans, cephalothin is potentially nephrotoxic and should not be used in conjunction with an aminoglycoside. This parenteral product is not acid stable and should not be given orally.

CHLORAMPHENICOL

INDICATIONS: Chloramphenicol (Azramycine ✤, Chlor Palm ✤, Chlor Tablets ✤, Chloromycetin ✤ ★, Karomycin Palmitate ✤, Viceton ★, and many others) is a bacteriostatic antibiotic with activity against a number of pathogens including gram-positive and gram-negative bacteria, most anaerobes, chlamydiae, rickettsiae, coxiellae, mycoplasmas, and some protozoa. In reptiles, chloramphenicol is used for the treatment of superficial and systemic bacterial diseases, including septicemic cutaneous ulcerative disease in aquatic turtles. For more information, see CHLORAMPHENICOL in the Small Animal section.

In experimental work with gopher snakes, oral chloramphenicol at a dosage of 12 mg/kg was slowly absorbed and resulted in blood levels of only 10 μg/mL (therapeutic blood levels were defined as blood concentrations of >20 to 40 μg/mL). Clinical recommendations range from 50 to 100 mg/kg once daily PO.

The pharmacokinetics of parenteral chloramphenicol have also been studied in snakes. In one study involving 16 different species held at 26°C, there was erratic absorption of chloramphenicol after SC injection, a wide variation in the rate of elimination among the various species, wide standard deviations within species, and a difference in mean plasma concentrations between two commercial preparations. To maintain plasma concentrations above a trough level of 5 μg/mL, IM injection of 50 mg/kg at the following hourly intervals was recommended: gray rat snake—7.7; indigo snake—9.8; boa constrictor—27.6; Burmese python—29.6; hog-nose snake—30.7; copperhead—36.5; cotton mouth—39.1; Indian rock python—49; eastern diamond back rattlesnake—51; timber rattlesnake—53.4; red-bellied watersnake—61.3; Midland water snake—69.2. In another study in gopher snakes kept at 29°C, a SC injection of 40 mg/kg resulted in peak blood levels of 26 μg/mL in just over 3 hours after drug administration, and a plasma elimination half-life of 5.25 hours. The authors suggested once-daily administration of the drug.

ADVERSE AND COMMON SIDE EFFECTS: Although mammalian side effects such as blood dyscrasias have not been reported in reptiles, one snake in a pharmacokinetic study became anemic and had green discolored plasma. Chloramphenicol in propylene glycol and benzyl alcohol base may cause focal indurated lesions at sites of injection.

DRUG INTERACTIONS: Lizards and tortoises have been reported to be cleared of enteric *Salmonella* spp. after oral administration of 250 mg chloramphenicol combined with 75 mg ampicillin daily for 10 days. Chloramphenicol inhibits hepatic cytochrome P-450 enzymes; and therefore, therapy with chloramphenicol may affect the levels of a variety of other therapeutic agents.

CHLORHEXIDINE

INDICATIONS: Chlorhexidine (ChlorhexiDerm ★, Hibitane ♣, Nolvadent ★, Nolvasan ★, Savlon ♣, and others) is a chemical used for disinfection and as a base for a variety of antiseptic products. Diluted chlorhexidine solutions are used topically and orally, and the compound is also formulated into a number of topical creams. Diluted chlorhexidine has been used topically for superficial mycotic dermatitis and, in combination with systemic antibiotics, for the treatment of mouth rot in snakes and shell infections in chelonians. For more information, see CHLORHEXIDINE in the Small Animal section.

ADVERSE AND COMMON SIDE EFFECTS: Two red-bellied short-necked turtles developed flaccid paralysis and corneal opacity after 45 minutes of immersion in 0.024% v/v chlorhexidine (12 mL of 2% solution/L of water) at a temperature of 30°C. Both animals eventually died. On necropsy, keratitis, tracheitis, pharyngitis, and myocardial necrosis were described.

SUPPLIED AS VETERINARY PRODUCTS:
Numerous products containing 0.1% to 5% w/v as udder washes and teat dip solutions, lavage solutions, skin cleansers, shampoos, and ointments (✤ ★)

CHLORTETRACYCLINE

INDICATIONS: Chlortetracycline (Aureomycin ✤ ★, Fermycin Soluble ★, Aureomix ★, and others) is a broad-spectrum bacteriostatic antibiotic with activity against gram-positive and gram-negative organisms, chlamydiae, rickettsiae, mycoplasmas, and many anaerobes. For more information, see TETRACYCLINE ANTIBIOTICS in the Small Animal section.

ADVERSE AND COMMON SIDE EFFECTS: Tetracyclines, especially chlortetracycline, inhibit protein synthesis and are immunosuppressive in mammals and birds.

DRUG INTERACTIONS: Oral absorption is inhibited by calcium, magnesium, and iron-containing substances.

SUPPLIED AS VETERINARY PRODUCTS:
Water-soluble powders and agricultural feed additives containing various concentrations of chlortetracycline (Aureomycin ✤ ★, Fermycin Soluble ★, Aureomix ★, and many others)
Tablets containing 25 mg (Aureomycin Tablets ★)

CIMETIDINE

INDICATIONS: Cimetidine (Novo-Cimetine ✤, Tagamet ✤ ★), a histamine (H_2)-receptor blocking agent, reduces gastric acid secretion and is used in the management of gastric and duodenal ulceration that does not result from the administration of nonsteroidal anti-inflammatory drugs (NSAIDs). Cimetidine also increases caudal esophageal sphincter tone and promotes gastric emptying in mammals. The drug is available as both an oral and injectable formulation. For further information, see CIMETIDINE in the Small Animal section.

In reptiles, cimetidine has been suggested to treat gastritis and gastric ulceration.

DRUG INTERACTIONS: By interfering with hepatic microenzyme systems, cimetidine affects the metabolism of many drugs. For further information, see CIMETIDINE in the Small Animal section.

CIPROFLOXACIN

INDICATIONS: Ciprofloxacin (Cipro ♣ ★) is a fluoroquinolone antibiotic with activity against a range of gram-negative and gram-positive bacteria (e.g., *Escherichia coli, Klebsiella, Proteus, Pseudomonas, Staphylococcus, Salmonella, Shigella, Yersinia, Campylobacter,* and *Vibrio* spp.) and some spirochetes. The drug is available for oral, IV, and ophthalmic use and is produced *in vivo* as a metabolite after the administration of enrofloxacin.

In reptiles, ciprofloxacin is a drug of choice for initial antimicrobial therapy while awaiting bacterial culture results. Although recommendations exist in the literature for formulation of an oral suspension using ciprofloxacin tablets, the stability of the formulation may be short-lived; and therefore, it may be only appropriate for immediate administration. For more information, see CIPROFLOXACIN and FLUOROQUINOLONE ANTIBIOTICS in the Small Animal section.

CISAPRIDE

INDICATIONS: Cisapride (Propulsid ★, Prepulsid ♣) was marketed in North America for the treatment of heartburn in humans, but has been removed from general access due to its association with cardiac arrhythmias. The drug had been used in Small Animal Practice to stimulate GIT motility in cases of primary motility disorders and in cases of gastroesophageal reflux. The drug generally is given 15 minutes before a meal. For more information, see CISAPRIDE in the Small Animal section.

Cisapride has been used in reptiles when improvement in gastrointestinal motility was desired. Metoclopramide would be a possible alternative. In desert tortoises, daily oral dosing with cisapride at 1 mg/kg did not significantly affect, and may have even slowed, the gastrointestinal passage of plastic markers in tortoises with normal gastrointestinal function.

DRUG INTERACTIONS: Concurrent therapy with drugs that inhibit cytochrome P-450 enzymes, e.g., clarithromycin, erythromycin, fluconazole, itraconazole, and ketoconazole, will result in elevated blood cisapride levels. These interactions have led to fatalities in humans.

CLARITHROMYCIN

INDICATIONS: Clarithromycin (Biaxin ✤ ★) is a semisynthetic β-lactamase resistant macrolide antibiotic used to treat a variety of bacterial infections in people, including respiratory infections caused by *Mycoplasma* spp. The drug is well absorbed orally and reaches high intracellular concentrations, accumulating in certain tissues, including the respiratory tract. For more information, see CLARITHROMYCIN in the Avian section.

Wild caught gopher tortoises maintained at 30°C to 33.3°C were used for single- and multiple-dose pharmacokinetic studies to evaluate the potential use of clarithromycin against *Mycoplasma agassizii*. Clarithromycin was administered orally to experimental groups of tortoises at doses of 7.5 and 15 mg/kg once, and 15 mg/kg once daily for 9 days. Based on the results of these studies and using several different mathematical modeling systems, a dosage of 15 mg/kg each 2 to 3 days was predicted to maintain blood levels of 2 to 7.5 μg/mL, the therapeutic target concentration in humans. Significant variation in GIT absorption was postulated, based on the very low serum antibiotic levels obtained in several animals.

ADVERSE AND COMMON SIDE EFFECTS: In humans, infrequent side effects include diarrhea, nausea, and abnormal taste.

DRUG INTERACTIONS: A number of drug interactions exist as clarithromycin inhibits cytochrome P-450 enzymes. Concurrent treatment with cisapride is contraindicated.

SUPPLIED AS HUMAN PRODUCTS:
Pediatric granules for suspension at 125 mg/5 mL and 250 mg/5 mL (Biaxin ✤)
Tablets containing 125 mg and 500 mg (Biaxin ✤, Biaxin BID ✤ ★, Biaxin XL Filmtab Tablets ★)
Oral suspension containing 125 mg/5 mL, 187.5 mg/5 mL, 250 mg/5 mL after reconstitution (Biaxin ★)

CLINDAMYCIN

INDICATIONS: Clindamycin (Antirobe ✤ ★, Cleocin ★) is a lincosamide antibiotic with activity against a wide range of gram-positive, gram-negative, and anaerobic bacteria, and some sporozoan organisms. Oral administration of clindamycin to reptiles has been described in the literature. For more information, see CLINDAMYCIN in the Small Animal section.

CLOTRIMAZOLE

INDICATIONS: Clotrimazole (Canesten ✤, Lotrimin ★, Mycelex ★) is a topical imidazole antifungal agent useful in the treatment of localized dermatophytosis, candidal stomatitis, and nasal aspergillosis in small animals. For more information, see CLOTRIMAZOLE in the Small Animal section. Clotrimazole has been suggested for the topical treatment of localized fungal infections in reptiles.

CYFLUTHRIN

See PYRETHRIN-CONTAINING PRODUCTS

DEXAMETHASONE

INDICATIONS: Dexamethasone (Azium ✤ ★, Azium SP ✤ ★, Dex-5 ✤) is a glucocorticoid that has been used in small animal medicine for its anti-inflammatory effects and in the treatment of a variety of disease conditions. Dexamethasone sodium phosphate does not require hepatic biotransformation and is active immediately upon injection. In reptiles, it is used in the treatment of septic shock and acute head trauma. In one report, dexamethasone appeared to stimulate appetite in a Ridley's sea turtle. For more information, see DEXAMETHASONE in the Small Animal section.

ADVERSE AND COMMON SIDE EFFECTS: The routine use of glucocorticoids in reptiles is not recommended because of immunosuppressive effects.

DIAZEPAM

INDICATIONS: Diazepam (Valium ✤ ★, Valrelease ★) is a benzodiazepine used as an anticonvulsant for the control of seizures. It is also used as a sedative and preanesthetic, sometimes in combination with butorphanol to increase analgesia, and in combination with ketamine for anesthesia. Diazepam is formulated for oral and intravenous use. A similar benzodiazepine compounded for intramuscular use is midazolam. For more information, see DIAZEPAM in the Small Animal section.

Diazepam has been described for use in alligators but should also be effective for a variety of reptilian species. The drug was administered IM at a mean dose of 0.37 mg/kg (range 0.22 to 0.63 mg/kg) to adult female American alligators to reduce stress and the dose of succinylcholine required to facilitate artificial insemination. Within 20 minutes of administration of diazepam, aggressive behaviors were markedly reduced, although not eliminated.

In agamid lizards, the addition of 0.15 mL of diazepam IM (calculated from the report to equate to 15 to 37.5 mg/kg) to a dose of 30 mg/kg ketamine IM reduced both induction time and time to full recovery. The authors commented that muscle relaxation was not improved, and that cardiopulmonary responses were "erratic."

DICHLORVOS IMPREGNATED RESIN STRIPS

INDICATIONS: Dichlorvos (Vapona No Pest Strip and others ✤ ★) is a cholinesterase-inhibitor anthelmintic and insecticide. Dichlorvos impregnated resin strips are used for the treatment of ectoparasites including mites, ticks, and fleas. Sections of strip should be placed inside the cage within a ventilated container, such as a perforated plastic vial, to prevent direct contact or ingestion. The animal's water bowl should be removed during treatment to prevent ingestion of dichlorvos. The dose or length of strip used is empirical. Some "doses" are used to eliminate ectoparasites in the cage environment without animals being present. Dichlorvos resistance has been described in both snake mites and ticks. For more information, see DICHLORVOS and CHLORINATED HYDROCARBONS in the Small Animal section.

ADVERSE AND COMMON SIDE EFFECTS: This product may be hazardous for humans as headache and nausea have been reported after breathing Vapona-laden air. Persons handling the strips should wear gloves. In addition, the strips should be allowed to breathe outside for several hours before use. Some lizards, including anoles, may develop hind leg paralysis on exposure to this chemical. See CHLORINATED HYDROCARBONS in the Small Animal section for more information on clinical signs and treatment of toxicity in mammals.

SUPPLIED AS COMMERCIAL PRODUCTS:
Impregnated resin strips containing 20% w/w dichlorvos (Vapona No Pest Strip ✤ ★, Black Flag Insect Strip, and many others)

DIETHYLCARBAMAZINE

INDICATIONS: Diethylcarbamazine (DEC) (Carbam ★, Decacide Tabs ✤ ★, Diethylcarbamazine Citrate ★, Filaribits ✤ ★, Nemacide ★) is an antiparasitic agent that has been used for the treatment of ascarids and microfilaria in reptiles. For more information, see DIETHYLCARBAMAZINE in the Small Animal section.

DIHYDROSTREPTOMYCIN

INDICATIONS: Dihydrostreptomycin (Ethamycin ✤) is an aminoglycoside antibiotic used parenterally for the treatment of bacterial infections and topically for the treatment of abscesses and necrotic stomatitis in snakes. For more information, see DIHYDROSTREPTO-MYCIN and AMINOGLYCOSIDE ANTIBIOTICS in the Small Animal section.

ADVERSE AND COMMON SIDE EFFECTS: During treatment, it is essential to maintain hydration by ensuring the availability of fresh water or by administration of oral, intracoelomic, or SC isotonic fluids. For prolonged therapy, monitoring of plasma or serum uric acid levels may be appropriate. Streptomycin should not be used in the presence of impaired renal function or dehydration.

DILOXANIDE

INDICATIONS: Diloxanide furoate is an anti-infective agent that has been used for the treatment of amebiasis.

SUPPLIED AS HUMAN PRODUCT:
Diloxanide furoate is available in the United States by special request from the Centers for Disease Control and Prevention (Furamide ★).

DIMETRIDAZOLE

INDICATIONS: Dimetridazole (Dimetridazole ❦, Emtryl ❦) is a water-soluble antimicrobial agent effective against anaerobic bacteria and protozoa, and used for the treatment of amebiasis and trichomoniasis in snakes.

ADVERSE AND COMMON SIDE EFFECTS: Several species of snakes are considered sensitive to the use of metronidazole and dimetridazole as deaths have occurred after treatment with doses greater than 100 mg/kg. These include tricolor king snakes, milk snakes, indigo snakes, and Uracoan rattlesnakes. A lower dose of 40 mg/kg is recommended in these animals. Other species of snakes may react similarly.

SUPPLIED AS VETERINARY PRODUCTS:
Water-soluble powder with 40% w/w (Dimetridazole 40% ❦, Emtryl Soluble ❦)
Feed additives (Dimetridazole 30% w/w Premix ❦, Emtryl Premix ❦)

DOXAPRAM

INDICATIONS: Doxapram (Dopram-V ❦ ★) is a central respiratory stimulant that has been recommended for use in reptiles to stimulate respiration in patients with postanesthetic respiratory depression or apnea. Doxapram is intended for intravenous use, but will have an effect when given by other parenteral routes if venous access cannot be obtained. For more information, see DOXAPRAM in the Small Animal section.

DRUG INTERACTIONS: Halothane and enflurane may precipitate arrhythmias. It is recommended that doxapram use be delayed about 10 minutes after discontinuation of these anesthetic agents.

DOXYCYCLINE

INDICATIONS: Doxycycline (Vibramycin ✤ ★, Vibra-Tabs ✤ ★, and others) is a second-generation, long-acting, lipid-soluble tetracycline antibiotic used in the treatment of bacterial, rickettsial, chlamydial, and mycoplasmal infections. Doxycycline has been used to treat respiratory syndrome in desert tortoises. The MIC for doxycycline against *Mycoplasma alligatoris* isolated from American alligators was <1 µg/mL, making it an appropriate option for the treatment of infection by this agent. For more information, see DOXYCYCLINE and TETRACYCLINE ANTIBIOTICS in the Small Animal section.

Experimental pharmacokinetic work on doxycycline has been carried out in spur-tailed tortoises held at 27°C in conjunction with investigations into the MIC values for bacteria isolated from reptiles. After IM injection of 25 and 50 mg/kg into the gluteal muscles, therapeutic serum concentrations (defined as 8 µg/mL) were maintained for 36 and 70 hours, respectively. These dosages were considered appropriate for the treatment of infections by sensitive strains of *Klebsiella* and *Staphylococcus* spp., but not *Salmonella* spp. The author suggested a dosage of 50 mg/kg would provide adequate blood concentrations for 78 hours (this time interval was also described as 8 days later in the same paper), after which a second dose of 25 mg/kg could be administered if necessary. Drug elimination half-lives were not described.

The IM administration of most IV preparations results in severe muscle damage due to the acid pH of these solutions. Vibravenos or specially compounded formulations must be used for this route of administration.

As with all tetracyclines, doxycycline should be protected from light to prevent formation of toxic oxidation by-products.

DRUG INTERACTIONS: In birds, minerals including calcium and zinc in the intestinal tract may bind to excreted or orally administered doxycycline and block enterohepatic cycling, thus increasing the drug's overall clearance. Dietary iron decreases absorption by 80% to 90%, whereas the presence of organic acids such as citric acid increases absorption by 2 to 5 times. The absorption of oral doxycycline was reduced by the presence of grit in the diet of pigeons.

SUPPLIED AS VETERINARY PRODUCTS:
Avian product: for injection containing 20 mg/mL (Vibravenos—not registered for use in North America at present)

Water-soluble powder containing 50 mg/g (Vibravet 5% ✹)
Oral suspension containing 5 mg/mL after reconstitution (Vibravet ✹)

SUPPLIED AS HUMAN PRODUCTS:
Tablets and capsules containing 50 mg (Monodox ★), and 100 mg (Monodox ★, Alti-Doxycycline ✹, Apo-Doxy ✹, Doxycin ✹, Doxytec (lactose) ✹, Novo-Doxylin ✹, Nu-Doxycycline ✹, Vibramycin ✹, Vibra-Tabs ✹ ★)
Oral suspension containing 5 mg/mL after reconstitution (Vibramycin ★)
Oral suspension containing 50 mg/5 mL (Vibramycin calcium syrup ★)
For injection in 100 mg and 200 mg vials (Vibramycin ★)
For IV injection in vials of 100 and 200 mg (Doxy 100 ★, Doxy 200 ★, Vibramycin hyclate ★, doxycycline hyclate ★, Vibramycin-IV ✹)

EMETINE HYDROCHLORIDE

INDICATIONS: Emetine hydrochloride ✹ ★ is a tissue amebicide that acts within the intestinal wall and at extra-intestinal sites such as the liver and lungs. It is not effective against intraluminal parasites. The drug has been used in the treatment of amebiasis and trematode infections. In human medicine, metronidazole is considered the treatment of choice for both intestinal and extra-intestinal forms of *Entamoeba histolytica*.

ADVERSE AND COMMON SIDE EFFECTS: Emetine should be administered by deep subcutaneous or intramuscular injection and may cause abscesses at the site of injection. The drug is erratically absorbed after oral administration. It must not be administered intravenously. Emetine has a variety of serious side effects in humans including cardiotoxicity, neuromuscular abnormalities, diarrhea, and dermatoses.

DRUG INTERACTIONS: Emetine should be used in combination with an intraluminal amebicidal drug such as metronidazole.

SUPPLIED AS HUMAN PRODUCTS:
Emetine hydrochloride powder ✹ ★

ENROFLOXACIN

INDICATIONS: Enrofloxacin (Baytril ✹ ★) is a fluoroquinolone antibiotic with activity against a range of gram-positive and gram-negative bacteria, mycoplasmas, chlamydiae, rickettsiae, and atypical mycobacteria. Enrofloxacin has limited activity against anaerobes. The drug is used commonly for the treatment of bacterial infections in reptiles, including *Pseudomonas aeruginosa* infections and middle ear infections in box turtles. Enrofloxacin is a drug of choice for initial antimicrobial therapy while awaiting bacterial culture results. Parenteral administration, combined with nasal flushing, is the treatment of choice for upper respiratory tract disease in tortoises due to the drug's effectiveness against *Mycoplasma* spp. and *Pasteurella testudinis.* The MIC for enrofloxacin against *M. alligatoris* isolated from American alligators was <1 µg/mL, making it an appropriate option for the treatment of infection by this agent. A portion of the enrofloxacin dose is metabolized to ciprofloxacin *in vivo;* therefore, both drugs are involved in the therapeutic effect. The injectable formulation of enrofloxacin can be administered orally in suspensions formulated in sweet or flavored syrups to mask the bitter taste of the drug. The enrofloxacin liquid concentrate licensed for use in poultry can also be diluted with a sweet liquid such as Karo syrup for treatment of individual animals. Oral tablets can be formulated into a suspension by a compounding pharmacy. For general information, see ENROFLOXACIN and FLUOROQUINOLONE ANTIBIOTICS in the Small Animal section.

Pharmacokinetic studies have been carried out in juvenile Burmese pythons held at 26°C. Single and multiple dose trials using 5 mg/kg IM resulted in mean peak plasma levels of 1.66 and 2.78 µg/mL, respectively. Plasma elimination half-lives were also different between the two trials, with the single dose producing a 6.37 hour half-life and the multiple dose producing a half-life ranging from 12.4 to 31.9 hours during the 4-week period of administration. Levels of ciprofloxacin increased steadily during this period to a peak of 1.11 µg/mL. Administration of an initial IM dose of 10 mg/kg, followed by 5 mg/kg every 48 hours was considered adequate to provide blood concentrations of enrofloxacin greater than the MIC (0.1 µg/mL) for relatively susceptible gram-negative organisms, such as *Escherichia coli, Klebsiella,* and *Proteus,* but a dose of 10 mg/kg every 48 hours was recommended to attain an MIC considered suitable for treatment of *Pseudomonas* (0.5 µg/mL).

Experimental work has also been carried out in gopher, Indian star, and spur-tailed tortoises using single and multiple dose IM administration of 5 mg/kg and single dose IM administration of 10 mg/kg. In gopher tortoises held at 30°C, plasma concentrations remained above 0.75 µg/mL for 24 hours and above 0.32 µg/mL for 48 hours. Doses of 5 mg/kg every 24 to 48 hours were recommended for the treatment of respiratory pasteurellosis and other bacterial infections in these tortoises. In Indian star tortoises held at 26°C to 30°C and given a single injection of 5 mg/kg, plasma levels remained above 0.2 µg/mL for at least 12 hours in most tortoises. The suggested dosing regimen was 5 mg/kg every 24 hours for susceptible species, or every 12 hours for *Pseudomonas* and *Citrobacter* spp. Single-dose pharmacokinetics of dosages of 5 and 10 mg/kg were evaluated in spur-tailed tortoises held at 27°C. Twelve hours after the administration of enrofloxacin at 5 mg/kg, serum levels were undetectable. After a dose of 10 mg/kg therapeutic concentrations, defined as 3.5 µg/mL, were maintained for 12 hours. When a second injection of 10 mg/kg was administered 24 hours after the first, therapeutic blood levels were maintained for an additional 16 hours.

A preliminary investigation of the pharmacokinetics of enrofloxacin was carried out in green iguanas (ambient temperature not specified). Enrofloxacin was administered to small numbers of animals at 5 mg/kg either PO or IM. The drug was absorbed rapidly with mean maximal plasma concentrations of 1.16 and 2.03 µg/mL after PO and IM administration, respectively. The mean elimination half-lives were 22.3 hours after PO administration and 26 hours after IM administration. Plasma concentrations remained above therapeutic levels (defined as >0.2 µg/mL) for a mean of 31.7 hours for PO and 16 hours for IM administration; however, there was considerable variability in pharmacokinetic parameters after PO administration.

The efficacy of enrofloxacin against sensitive strains of *Salmonella* has been studied in green iguanas. All 20 animals dosed with 10 mg/kg PO every 24 hours for 14 days were cleared of infection. The presence or absence of the organism was based on culture of cloacal samples every 5 days for 15 days and on culture and PCR evaluation of necropsy samples of liver, gallbladder, colon, small intestine, spleen, and blood. In a follow-up study, 65% of treated animals were negative for *Salmonella* 70 days after cessation of treatment. *Salmonella* isolates from animals that remained positive were still sensitive to enrofloxacin, suggesting that development of resistance was not responsible for failure of clearance. In a second study, 1 of 9 iguanas continued to shed *Salmonella* organisms after 14 days of oral treatment with enrofloxacin at 10 mg/kg every 24 hours. It appears that treatment with enrofloxacin does not reliably eliminate carriage of *Salmonella* spp. in green iguanas.

Preliminary pharmacokinetics of a single dose of 5 mg/kg enrofloxacin administered IV were carried out in five American alligators held at 27°C. Plasma enrofloxacin levels were maintained above 1 µg/mL, the target MIC for *Mycoplasma lacerti,* an organism that had been identified in an outbreak of disease, for an average of 31 hours. A dosing interval of 36 hours was recommended for the treatment of this organism.

ADVERSE AND COMMON SIDE EFFECTS: Enrofloxacin may cause discoloration of the skin or tissue necrosis in some animals if given by SC administration. Muscular necrosis after injection has been described in many species and probably also occurs in reptiles. Oral administration is generally recommended for long-term therapy. For parenteral injection, the largest available and appropriate muscle mass should be used. Local pain or inappetence may be noted after administration. Long-term usage in desert tortoises, boas and pythons, and green iguanas has been associated with increased uric acid levels. Maintenance of normal hydration through ensuring the availability of fresh water or the administration of oral, intracoelomic, or SC isotonic fluids as required is suggested. Monitoring of serum or plasma uric acid levels may also be appropriate.

FEBANTEL + PRAZIQUANTEL

See PRAZIQUANTEL

FENBENDAZOLE

INDICATIONS: Fenbendazole (Panacur ✤ ★) is an anthelmintic recommended for the treatment of gastrointestinal nematodes including ascarid, strongyle, and strongyloides infections in snakes, lizards, and tortoises. Tortoises may require 2 to 3 weeks to expel the worms. For more information, see FENBENDAZOLE in the Small Animal section.

A head to head fenbendazole versus ivermectin efficacy study was carried out in ball pythons positive for nematode ova on fecal examination. Fenbendazole was administered at 10, 25, 50, and 100 mg/kg orally every 14 days. All snakes were cleared of infection after four treatments while 95.6% were clear after three treatments. All doses were equally effective. Efficacy of fenbendazole treatment at each weekly evaluation was slightly greater than for ivermectin, which was administered orally at 200 µg/kg every 14 days, for the first through third treatments. After the fourth treatment the efficacy of both compounds was the same, with all animals cleared of infection.

In another study, fenbendazole was used via cloacal administration in Greek, Kleinmann's, and Indian star tortoises to treat oxyurid infestations. Treatment resulted in immediate expulsion of adult worms, and fecal flotations were negative for parasite ova 2 and 4 weeks later. Efficacy was greater than had been previously experienced using the oral route. This was attributed to the achievement of higher levels of fenbendazole within the lower intestine, the actual location of the worms.

ADVERSE AND COMMON SIDE EFFECTS: Fenbendazole toxicity has been described in four juvenile Fea's vipers given single oral doses of 428 to 1064 mg/kg before a quarantine period. Snakes were inappetent and lost weight after treatment. All snakes died within 71 days of treatment. Segmental thickening and reddening of the entire small intestine due to moderate to severe necrosis of mucosal epithelium and sepsis were found at necropsy.

SUPPLIED AS VETERINARY PRODUCTS:
Granules (222 mg fenbendazole/gram) to be mixed with food (Panacur ✤ ★)
Oral paste containing 10% fenbendazole (Panacur ✤ ★, Safe-Guard ★)
Oral suspension containing 10% fenbendazole (Panacur ✤ ★, Safe-Guard ✤ ★)

FIPRONIL

INDICATIONS: Fipronil (Frontline ★, Top Spot ★) is a phenyl pyrazole pesticide which acts as an insecticide by disruption of the insect central nervous system via the γ-aminobutyric acid (GABA) regulated chloride channel. Fipronil has been marketed to control fleas, ticks and mites on domestic animals and as a pour-on or dip for cattle to control ticks.

Fipronil has been suggested for the control of mites and ticks on reptiles by topical spray. In an *in-vitro* study evaluating the effectiveness of various acaricides against *Amblyomma marmoreum* ticks from leopard tortoises, fipronil was found to be much less effective than permethrin or cyfluthrin.

ADVERSE AND COMMON SIDE EFFECTS: Toxicity testing has been carried out in lizards as part of evaluation protocols for the use of fipronil as an agricultural pesticide. The LD50 for fringe-toed lizards fed fipronil-treated prey was estimated at 30 μg active ingredient/g body weight (i.e., 30 mg/kg) in laboratory tests. The authors classified fipronil as "highly toxic" when ingested by this species. Animals died during a 4-week period after treatment. Reduced locomotor activity and prey consumption and reduction in body weight, as compared to controls, have been described in the same species of lizard after treatment. Given the toxicity of ivermectin in some reptilian species, fipronil should be used with caution.

SUPPLIED AS VETERINARY PRODUCTS:
Spray containing 0.29% w/v (Frontline Spray Treatment ★)
Solution containing 9.7% w/v (Frontline Top Spot for Cats and Kittens ★, Frontline Top Spot for Dogs and Puppies ★)

FLUCONAZOLE

INDICATIONS: Fluconazole (Diflucan ✲ ★) is a synthetic azole derivative fungistatic antimycotic agent. Fluconazole has greater water solubility, better oral bioavailability, higher plasma and extravascular levels, and a longer plasma elimination half life than ketoconazole. Fluconazole is only recommended if topical treatment (e.g., enilconazole) is not feasible. Fluconazole penetrates well into the brain, cerebrospinal fluid, and eyes. For more information, see FLUCONAZOLE in the Small Animal section.

The pharmacokinetics of fluconazole were studied in juvenile loggerhead sea turtles held between 23°C and 26.5°C. An initial single dose trial looked at the pharmacokinetic parameters for IV and SC administration of 2.5 mg/kg. Route of administration did not significantly affect the maximum plasma concentration or the elimination half-life (132.5 and 139.5 hours, IV and SC respectively). A dosage regimen of 10 mg/kg SC every 5 days following a loading dose of 21 mg/kg was suggested, and administered to four juvenile sea turtles for 10 days. Plasma fluconazole concentrations ranged from approximately 8 to 19 µg/mL, above the 8 µg/mL target concentration used for the treatment of a variety of fungal infections in humans. Diluting the IV product in saline for SC injection did not result in local irritation.

FLUNIXIN MEGLUMINE

INDICATIONS: Flunixin meglumine (Banamine ♣ ★, Flunixamine ★, and others) is a potent nonsteroidal antiprostaglandin agent with anti-inflammatory and antipyretic properties that make it useful in the treatment of inflammation and pain associated with musculoskeletal disease. For more information, see FLUNIXIN in the Small Animal section. Flunixin has been suggested for use as an analgesic in reptiles. Although there is no work investigating the physiology and effectiveness of nonsteroidal analgesics in reptiles, it is assumed that their use is appropriate in situations where pain might be occurring, and that drugs used in other species should have similar effects.

ADVERSE AND COMMON SIDE EFFECTS: Nephrotoxicity has been associated with the use of flunixin in birds. In reptiles it is likely also important to avoid the use of flunixin in animals that are dehydrated or have renal disease, and to supplement hydration. Flunixin can cause necrosis at the site of injection. For more information, see FLUNIXIN in the Avian section.

FUROSEMIDE

INDICATIONS: Furosemide (Lasix ♣ ★) is a potent loop diuretic that is effective in reducing edema of cardiac origin and promoting diuresis. For more information, see FUROSEMIDE in the Small Animal section. Furosemide has been suggested for use in reptiles.

GENTAMICIN SULFATE

INDICATIONS: Gentamicin (Gentocin ♣ ★, Gentasul ♣, Garagen ★) is an aminoglycoside antibiotic used in the treatment of bacterial infections, especially those caused by gram-negative organisms. Gentamicin was one of the most commonly used drugs for treating gram-negative infections in reptiles, especially in snakes. However, the nephrotoxicity of gentamicin and the development of newer antibiotics have decreased the popularity of this drug. Amikacin is now the most commonly used aminoglycoside in reptile medicine. For more general information, see GENTAMICIN and AMINOGLYCOSIDE ANTIBIOTICS in the Small Animal section.

Pharmacokinetic and toxicity studies have been performed in several species of snakes and turtles and in juvenile American alligators. Despite this, specific doses and dosage intervals are difficult to state conclusively. These studies have demonstrated significant variation in drug distribution and excretion relating to animal to animal variation, species, dosage amount, and ambient/body temperature. For example, in Florida broad-banded water snakes administered 4 mg/kg of gentamicin IM, the clearance of the drug at 30°C was twice that at 15°C. At a dosage of 16 mg/kg, clearance was 3 times faster at the higher temperature. In juvenile American alligators, the gentamicin elimination half-life was significantly shorter for a dose of 1.25 as compared to 1.75 mg/kg. Route of administration did not appear to affect pharmacokinetic parameters when IM injections were administered into the fore or hind legs of Eastern box tortoises. This variation in drug pharmacodisposition makes overdosage, leading to accumulation of serum gentamicin and nephrotoxicity, or underdosage, resulting in prolonged periods of subtherapeutic blood levels, quite possible.

In gopher snakes kept at 15°C, dosage with 2.5 mg/kg every 72 hours maintained adequate therapeutic levels (defined as 8 to 12 µg/mL) without reaching toxic concentrations (defined as >15 µg/mL). However, an elimination half-life of approximately 80 hours and the fact that blood levels did not drop below the recommended trough of 2 µg/mL between injections suggests that the dosing interval was too short. The same dose and dosing interval applied to a single Burmese python resulted in excessively high serum gentamicin concentrations (>17 µg/mL). In blood pythons held at 28°C to 30°C, the recommended treatment regimen was for a first dose of 2.5 or 3 mg/kg (depending on the MIC desired), then 1.5 mg/kg every 96 hours, based on an elimination half-life, which ranged from 32 to 110 hours. Peak serum gentamicin levels were initially reached in 6 to 10 hours, and were between 5 and 6 µg/mL for the 2.5 mg/kg initial dose, and between 5 and 6 µg/mL for the 3 mg/kg initial dose.

Two studies have looked at the effect of site of injection (i.e., forelimb versus hindlimb) in chelonians. In eastern box turtles kept at 29°C and administered a single dose of 3 mg/kg IM, site of injection had no significant effect on plasma concentrations or pharmacokinetics. The mean plasma elimination half-life was 41.9 hours. Plasma gentamicin concentrations remained above 2 µg/mL throughout the 96-hour period of evaluation, resulting in the authors' speculation that the dose of gentamicin used might have been higher than necessary for this species.

A second study carried out in red-eared slider turtles kept at 28°C compared the pharmacokinetic parameters resulting from the IM administration of 10 mg/kg gentamicin in either the forelimb or hindlimb. There were no significant differences in the drug's relative bioavailability related to location of administration. The mean elimination half-lives were 28.78 and 26.39 hours, and the maximum plasma concentrations were 54.4 and 55.9 μg/mL for injection into the forelimbs and hindlimbs, respectively. The half-lives obtained in this study were of the same level of magnitude but lower than those determined in chelonians in previous studies using doses of gentamicin from 2.5 to 20 mg/kg (31.3 to 56.8 hours). It was determined that in order to maintain a steady-state concentration of gentamicin between a peak of 10 μg/mL and a trough of 2 μg/mL, doses of 2.5 mg/kg every 72 hours in the forelimb and 2.3 mg/kg every 72 hours in the hindlimb would be appropriate.

Gentamicin has been used extensively as a dip for red-eared slider turtle eggs to reduce the prevalence of *Salmonella* carriage in animals destined for the pet trade. Treatment of eggs over 2 days of age substantially reduced the shedding of bacteria from hatching turtles to a prevalence rate of 0.15%, as compared to 40% in untreated controls. This practice has raised concerns over the development of resistant bacterial strains.

ADVERSE AND COMMON SIDE EFFECTS: Gentamicin is nephrotoxic in reptiles and has a low margin of safety. Due to interspecies variation in drug absorption and clearance, a dosage safe in one species may be toxic in another. In 2 boid snakes, gentamicin administered at 4.4 mg/kg twice daily for 2 days, then once daily for 5 days, resulted in nephrotoxicity and death. Nephrotoxicity, with a range of morphologic changes ranging from cloudy swelling to frank tubular necrosis, has been created in gopher snakes and banded water snakes with doses as low as 5 mg/kg once daily. Toxicity increased with increased dosage and decreased dosing interval and was greater in banded water snakes held at 30°C as compared to 15°C. Toxicity may not be evident until after therapy has ceased.

Administration of supplemental isotonic fluids orally, SC, or intracoelomically is recommended during the course of treatment and for several days afterward. Plasma or serum uric acid levels should be monitored during treatment and for 2 weeks afterward. Fasting, to lower the protein load on the kidneys, may reduce the occurrence of renal damage. Therapeutic drug monitoring of blood gentamicin levels would be valuable whenever possible.

Ototoxicity has been described in lizards that received more than 100 mg/kg for up to 3 weeks duration.

DRUG INTERACTIONS: Gentamicin is often used in combination with penicillins and cephalosporins for treatment of severe gram-negative infections. Cefuroxime has been given at 100 mg/kg once daily, in combination with gentamicin, for 10 days to treat *Proteus* infections in snakes. Gentamicin loses antimicrobial action in the presence of carbenicillin and cephalothin; therefore, these drugs should not be combined before administration. In mammals with decreased renal function, *in vivo* inactivation may also occur. Because of this, some authors have suggested delaying carbenicillin administration until 48 hours after initial treatment with gentamicin. If renal function is unaltered, this precaution is probably unnecessary.

GENTIAN VIOLET

INDICATIONS: Gentian violet ♣ ★ is a topical antifungal agent used in human medicine for the treatment of cutaneous *Candida* infections. In reptiles, gentian violet has been used topically to treat fungal shell infections in chelonians.

ADVERSE AND COMMON SIDE EFFECTS: Gentian violet is a messy product to use and leaves a purple stain on most objects it comes into contact with.

SUPPLIED AS HUMAN PRODUCTS:
Topical solution containing 1% w/v (Generic ★) and 2% w/v (Generic ★)
Topical wound spray (Gentian Violet Purple Spray ★, generic ♣)

GLUCOSE

INDICATIONS: Glucose ♣ ★ is used for the oral treatment of fasting- and stress-induced hypoglycemia in crocodilians. D-Glucose and dextrose are equivalent products.

SUPPLIED AS VETERINARY PRODUCTS:
Parenteral solutions containing 50% dextrose (Dextrose 50% ★, Glucose ♣)

SUPPLIED AS HUMAN PRODUCTS:
50 g (166.6 mg/mL), 75 g (250 mg/mL), 100 g (333.3 mg/mL) (Glucodex ♣)

GLYCOPYRROLATE

INDICATIONS: Glycopyrrolate (Robinul-V ★, Robinul ♣ ★) is an anticholinergic agent used as an alternative to atropine in preanesthetic regimens to prevent or treat vagally induced bradycardia and reduce oral and upper respiratory secretions. The drug has also been used to reduce oral mucus in conjunction with systemic antibacterial therapy in snakes with necrotic stomatitis or respiratory tract infections. For more information, see GLYCOPYRROLATE in the Small Animal section.

GRISEOFULVIN

INDICATIONS: Griseofulvin (Fulvicin U/F ♣ ★) is used for the treatment of dermatophyte infections in mammals. The drug is fungistatic, binding to keratin and disrupting fungal growth by inhibiting mitosis. Griseofulvin is detectable in the skin within 4 to 8 hours of oral administration. Absorption of griseofulvin is enhanced by dietary fat and is affected by the particle size of the product. Treatment is usually continued for at least 2 to 4 weeks. Griseofulvin has been suggested for the treatment of fungal dermatitis in reptiles.

ADVERSE AND COMMON SIDE EFFECTS: A variety of toxic effects are described in mammals. For more information, see GRISEOFULVIN in the Small Animal section. Griseofulvin is teratogenic and should not be used in breeding animals.

IODINE

INDICATIONS: Iodine is used orally for the treatment and prevention of iodine deficiency, or goiter, in tortoises fed a goitrogenic diet. Dietary correction should be instituted once a diagnosis of goiter is made. Topical iodine preparations have also been used for the treatment of fungal infections of the skin or shell in reptiles either swabbed directly on the lesion or by soaking.

DRUG INTERACTIONS: Iodine products oxidize when exposed to light and should be stored in dark bottles.

SUPPLIED AS HUMAN PRODUCTS:
Tincture of iodine containing 2.5% iodine and 2.5% potassium iodide ♣ ★
Lugol's iodine containing approximately 50 mg/mL iodine and 100 mg/mL potassium iodide ♣ ★
Sodium iodine containing 100 µg elemental iodide (118 µg sodium iodide) per mL (Iodopen ★)

SUPPLIED AS VETERINARY PRODUCTS:
Solution containing 1% titratable iodine (10,000 ppm) (Xenodine ★, Xenodine Spray ★), 1.9% (Bexblis ♣), 2% U.S.P. (Briodine ♣), 3.5% (Ultra-Dyne ★), and 4.5% (Theratrate ★)
Topical containing 2% (Generic ★) and 7% (Generic ★)
Spray containing 2.4% (Gentle Iodine Wound Spray ★)
Shampoo containing 1% (Aloedine Medicated Shampoo ★)

ISOFLURANE

INDICATIONS: Isoflurane (Aerrane ♣ ★, Forane ♣ ★, IsoFlo ♣ ★, Iso-Thesia ★) is a halogenated inhalant anesthetic agent with a low blood:gas partition coefficient, which results in rapid induction and recovery periods. Cardiovascular status is better maintained with isoflurane than halothane, and isoflurane does not sensitize the heart to epinephrine-induced cardiac arrhythmias, as does halothane. For more information, see ISOFLURANE in the Small Animal section.

Isoflurane is the inhalant of choice for reptilian anesthesia. Animals can be mask or chamber induced, although breath-holding may result in significant delays, manually intubated and "bagged" until anesthetized, or placed on isoflurane after induction with an injectable agent. Commencing induction with a lower percentage of isoflurane, as compared to 4% to 5 %, may reduce initial breath-holding in some animals.

ITRACONAZOLE

INDICATIONS: Itraconazole (Sporanox ♣ ★) is a triazole antifungal drug active against many topical and systemic fungal pathogens. The drug is used orally and is best absorbed with a fatty meal. Itraconazole is partially converted by hepatic biotransformation to hydroxyitraconazole, which is also fungicidal. In humans, treatment duration from 6 months to a year is recommended. For more information, see ITRACONAZOLE in the Small Animal section. See ITRACONAZOLE in the Avian section for information on compounding formulations for small patients.

The pharmacokinetics of itraconazole have been studied in spiny lizards held at ambient temperature (exact temperature not stated) with a basking lamp. The animals were dosed orally with 23.5 mg/kg once daily for 3 days. Sporanox capsules were opened and the individual beads counted for each animal. The drug was well absorbed; plasma levels considered to be therapeutic were obtained within 24 hours. Based on the elimination half-life, it was predicted that steady-state blood concentrations would be reached within 10 days. The drug was present in high levels in liver within approximately 90 hours; however, drug levels in muscle were minimal. Blood levels persisted within reported minimal inhibitory concentrations of common fungal pathogens for 6 days after peak concentration. The parent molecule had an elimination half-life of 48 hours. A specific dosing interval was not recommended.

The pharmacokinetics of orally administered itraconazole capsules were studied in juvenile Kemp's ridley sea turtles under treatment for cold shock and held at ambient temperatures of 25°C to 28°C. In order to maintain trough plasma itraconazole concentrations above 0.5 μg/mL, considered a therapeutic concentration based on human studies, a dosage of 5 mg/kg every 24 hours was recommended. A dose of 15 mg/kg every 72 hours produced equally consistent (among turtles) but somewhat lower plasma concentrations. At this dosage, the elimination half-life was 75 hours for itraconazole and 55 hours for the active metabolite, hydroxyitraconazole. Based on results from one turtle that died, itraconazole concentrations in tissues were much greater than those in plasma.

ADVERSE AND COMMON SIDE EFFECTS: The capsular formulation of itraconazole makes accurate dosing, especially of small patients, very difficult. Itraconazole should be used with caution in conjunction with drugs that affect the cytochrome P-450 enzyme system.

SUPPLIED AS HUMAN PRODUCTS:
Capsules containing 100 mg (Sporanox ✤ ★)
Oral solution containing 10 mg/mL (Sporanox ✤ ★)
For IV injection containing 10 mg/mL (Sporanox ★)

IVERMECTIN

INDICATIONS: Ivermectin (Heartgard ✤ ★, Ivomec ✤ ★, Eqvalan ✤ ★, and others) is used to treat reptiles infested with nematodes and/or by arthropod ectoparasites including ticks and skin mites in snakes. The drug may have some effect against pentastomes and subcutaneous dracunculosis. For more information, see IVERMECTIN in the Small Animal section.

Ivermectin has been widely recommended for the elimination of enteric nematode parasites in reptiles; however, several case reports describe poor results and/or suggest that the efficacy of fenbendazole or febantel/praziquantel is greater. In a study comparing the efficacy of fenbendazole (various doses) and ivermectin (200 µg/kg; PO) in ball pythons positive for nematode ova on fecal examination, the two drugs were administered every 14 days and fecal egg counts performed. The efficacy of fenbendazole was superior to ivermectin until the fourth treatment at which point all animals ceased to shed eggs.

Ivermectin has been highly successful for the treatment of cutaneous mites in snakes, either by systemic administration or as a topical spray. Concentrations of ivermectin used topically generally range from 5 to 20 mg/L water. Environmental clean-up is also required during mite treatment.

Two reports describe the oral use of ivermectin, administered once or twice at a 14- to 16-day interval, at a dose of 1,000 µg/kg in Tokay and Standing's day geckos. All animals treated ceased to shed pentastome eggs. Necropsies were not performed to determine whether adult worms were in fact killed. Ivermectin used at standard dosage was felt to have been effective to treat pentastome infection in a Bosc's monitor, in conjunction with antibiotics and a variety of supportive care. Dexamethasone was administered concurrently (0.2 mg/kg q 48 hours for 6 days; IM) to reduce adverse effects relating to the presence of dead worms.

ADVERSE AND COMMON SIDE EFFECTS: Flaccid paresis, paralysis, and death have resulted from administration of ivermectin to chelonians. After IM administration of 400 µg/kg, ivermectin resulted in the death of 4 of 5 red-footed tortoises, an experimental trial was conducted in red-footed, leopard, and box tortoises and red-eared slider turtles. Neurologic signs were seen in leopard tortoises given 25 µg/kg, in some eastern box tortoises given 100 µg/kg, in some red-footed tortoises given 50 µg/kg, and in red-eared sliders given 150 µg/kg. Cumulative toxicosis was also noted after two red-footed tortoises were given a second dose 72 hours after the first. A separate study also described toxicity and death in red-eared slider turtles given 200 µg/kg orally. In red-footed tortoises, a dosage of 50 µg/kg at 7-day intervals was found to be safe; however, elimination of parasites was not complete. Two spurred tortoises administered ivermectin at 220 and 190 µg/kg SC did not show clinical signs of toxicity.

Neurologic signs have also been reported in ball pythons and a rough-necked monitor. Transitory and mild, but significant, tremors and stupor were noted in 6 of 98 ball pythons that had received 200 µg/kg orally. Seizure-like activity was described in the rough-necked monitor. One author has also described aggressive behaviors in king snakes after ivermectin therapy. Caution has also been advised in skinks and indigo snakes.

In chameleons, skin discoloration may result at the site of injection. Lethargy and complete inactivity lasting for 7 days occurred 24 hours after a Senegalese chameleon was treated for infestation by the filarid nematode *Foleyella furcata* with a single dose of ivermectin at 200 µg/kg SC. It was not determined whether this adverse reaction was in response to the ivermectin or to endotoxin release from dying microfilaria.

DRUG INTERACTIONS: Concurrent administration of diazepam may potentiate the toxic effects of ivermectin as both act on the γ-aminobutyric acid–benzodiazepine receptor complex.

SUPPLIED AS VETERINARY PRODUCTS:
Commercial ivermectin for injection can be diluted 1:10 or 1:100 in propylene glycol for administration to small patients.

KANAMYCIN

INDICATIONS: Kanamycin (Kantrim ★) is an aminoglycoside antibiotic used for the treatment of gram-negative bacterial infections, especially *Pseudomonas* spp. For more information, see KANAMYCIN in the Small Animal section.

ADVERSE AND COMMON SIDE EFFECTS: Published dosages are empirical since no pharmacokinetic/pharmacodynamic work has been done with this drug. Kanamycin is potentially nephrotoxic and should not be used in the presence of impaired renal function or dehydration. During treatment, it is essential to maintain hydration by ensuring the availability of fresh water or by administration of oral, intracoelomic, or SC isotonic fluids. For prolonged therapy, monitoring of plasma or serum uric acid levels may be appropriate.

KETAMINE

INDICATIONS: Ketamine (Ketalean ♣, Ketaject ★, Ketaved ★, Rogarsetic ♣, Vetaket ★, Vetamine ★, Vetame ★, Ketaset ♣ ★, Vetalar ♣ ★) is a nonbarbiturate anesthetic used for chemical restraint or anesthesia. In mammals, the drug is characterized by a rapid onset of action, good somatic analgesia, maintenance of normal muscle tone and laryngeal reflex, mild cardiac stimulation, and respiratory depression. Recovery generally is smooth and uneventful. For more information, see KETAMINE in the Small Animal section.

Ketamine has been used extensively and at a wide range of dosages for sedation and anesthesia in reptiles. Induction of anesthesia with intramuscular administration occurs within 10 to 30 minutes; however, duration of anesthesia and time until full recovery vary markedly according to dose, ambient temperature, species, and individual. As a general trend, the levels of dosage required to achieve similar depth of effect increase from lizards to snakes to chelonians. When ketamine has been used alone at doses high enough for surgical procedures, recoveries could take more than a day. Ketamine is currently used at the low end of the dose range to facilitate tracheal intubation and induction of inhalant anesthesia, or in combination with sedatives or tranquilizers including diazepam, midazolam, medetomidine, and xylazine for shorter or less painful procedures. The drug has also been used to facilitate "milking" of venomous snakes.

ADVERSE AND COMMON SIDE EFFECTS: Ketamine should not be used in debilitated animals. Prolonged apnea and extremely delayed recoveries may occur at high doses. Hypertension, tachycardia, and reduced respiration and ventilation have been described in snakes anesthetized with ketamine. Snakes may also respond violently to ketamine injection. Uncompensated metabolic acidosis occurred in gopher snakes receiving 75 mg/kg IM. It was hypothesized that this resulted from an increase in activity immediately after injection.

KETOCONAZOLE

INDICATIONS: Ketoconazole (Nizoral ♣ ★) is an antifungal agent active against a range of dimorphic fungi, yeasts, and dermatophytes. Ketoconazole is fungistatic at low concentrations and fungicidal at higher levels. Absorption of ketoconazole is enhanced in an acid environment and with a high-fat meal. High levels of dietary carbohydrate reduce gastrointestinal absorption in humans. For more information, see KETOCONAZOLE in the Small Animal section. In reptiles, ketoconazole has been used for the treatment of superficial and systemic fungal infections, including dermatitis, shell rot, and pneumonia.

Single-dose and multidose pharmacokinetic studies in gopher tortoises have indicated that ketoconazole is absorbed orally and that therapeutic levels of the drug can be obtained and maintained in blood and tissue without evidence of toxicity. At an ambient temperature of 27°C, a dose of 15 mg/kg PO once daily was recommended to maintain plasma levels of ketoconazole above 1 µg/mL. Much higher empirical doses are described in the literature for general usage without reports of toxicity.

ADVERSE AND COMMON SIDE EFFECTS: Because hepatotoxicity is described in mammals, caution should be used in prescribing ketoconazole to reptiles with hepatic dysfunction. Presumptive ketoconazole toxicity was described in a Greek tortoise undergoing treatment for a pulmonary infection by *Candida albicans*. By day 9 after the initiation of treatment with 15 mg/kg orally every 12 hours, the tortoise was depressed and anorexic with green urates. Plasma aspartate aminotransferase (AST), alanine aminotransferase (ALT), and bile acids were elevated while creatine phosphokinase (CPK) remained normal. Clinical signs resolved within several days of cessation of therapy.

DRUG INTERACTIONS: Ketoconazole has been used in combination with thiabendazole (each dosed at 50 mg/kg PO once daily) for the treatment of mycotic pneumonia in juvenile green turtles. The drug is synergistic with 5-flucytosine and amphotericin B.

KETOPROFEN

INDICATIONS: Ketoprofen (Anafen ♣, Ketofen ★) is an NSAID with potent analgesic and antipyretic properties. The drug inhibits the cyclooxygenase and lipoxygenase inflammatory pathways. Ketoprofen is used in the management of fever and acute, subacute, and chronic pain associated with musculoskeletal disease. Onset of activity of the drug occurs within 30 minutes of parenteral administration and 1 hour after oral use in mammals. The duration of action in dogs and cats is approximately 12 hours. For more information, see KETOPROFEN in the Small Animal section.

Ketoprofen has been suggested for use as an analgesic in reptiles. Although there is no work investigating the physiology and effectiveness of nonsteroidal analgesics in reptiles, it is assumed that their use is appropriate in situations where pain might be occurring, and that drugs used in other species should have similar effects.

LEVAMISOLE

INDICATIONS: Levamisole (Levasole ★, Ripercol ♣, Tramisol ♣ ★, Prohibit ★, Totalon ★) is an anthelmintic used for the treatment of nematode infestations. Levamisole may also help restore immune function by increasing the number and function of T lymphocytes and macrophages. It has also been reported to stimulate antibody production, increase phagocytosis by macrophages, inhibit tumor growth, and stimulate suppressor cell activity.

Levamisole has been used to treat reptiles infested by nematodes, acanthocephalans, and pentastomes, and for pulmonary rhabdiasis in snakes. For more information, see LEVAMISOLE in the Small Animal section.

ADVERSE AND COMMON SIDE EFFECTS: Do not use levamisole in debilitated animals. The margin of safety may be narrow, particularly in tortoises.

LEVOTHYROXINE

INDICATIONS: Levothyroxine (Eltroxin ❋ ★, Synthroid ❋ ★) is a synthetic form of T_4 used in the treatment of hypothyroid disease. For more information, see LEVOTHYROXINE in the Small Animal section. Levothyroxine has been suggested for the treatment of hypothyroidism in tortoises.

LINCOMYCIN

INDICATIONS: Lincomycin (Lincocin ❋ ★, Lincomix ★) is a lincosamide antibiotic primarily active against gram-positive cocci, particularly *Staphylococcus* and *Streptococcus* spp., and anaerobes. It can also be used to treat infections by *Clostridium tetani* and *C. perfringens,* and *Mycoplasma* spp.

In reptiles, lincomycin has been used to treat conditions including peptostreptococcal wound infections in snakes and infections by anaerobic organisms. For more information, see LINCOMYCIN in the Small Animal section.

ADVERSE AND COMMON SIDE EFFECTS: Lincomycin should not be used in the presence of impaired renal or hepatic function or dehydration.

SUPPLIED AS VETERINARY PRODUCTS:
See also Small and Large Animal sections.
Oral solution containing 50 mg/mL (Lincocin Aquadrops ★) and 100 mg/mL (Lincocin Sterile Solution [Lincomix] ★)
Water-soluble powder containing 16 g/40-g packet and 32 g/80-g packet (Lincomix ❋ ★, Lincomycin ❋ ★)

MEBENDAZOLE

INDICATIONS: Mebendazole (Telmin ❋ ★, Vermox ❋ ★) is an anthelmintic used for the elimination of a variety of gastrointestinal nematode infestations. A broad range of dosages can be found in the literature. For more information, see MEBENDAZOLE in the Small Animal section.

ADVERSE AND COMMON SIDE EFFECTS: Although adverse effects are rare in mammals, toxicity has been described in a number of avian species. Mebendazole should not be used in animals with liver disease.

SUPPLIED AS VETERINARY PRODUCTS:
Tablets containing 100 mg (Wormaway IV ✤)
Powder containing 40 and 166.7 mg mebendazole/g (Telmin Equine Wormer ★, Telmintic Powder ★)
Oral suspension containing 33.3 mg/mL (Telmin ★)
Oral paste containing 200 mg mebendazole (Telmin Syringe Wormer ★, Telmin Syringe Formula ✤)

SUPPLIED AS HUMAN PRODUCT:
Tablets (chewable) containing 100 mg (Vermox ✤ ★)

MEDETOMIDINE

INDICATIONS: Medetomidine (Domitor ✤ ★) is an α_2-receptor agonist with sedative and analgesic properties. For more information, see MEDETOMIDINE and ATIPAMEZOLE in the Small Animal section. Medetomidine has been used as a sedative agent and for anesthesia in combination with ketamine in chelonians and crocodilians.

The cardiopulmonary effects of medetomidine were evaluated in desert tortoises administered a single dose of 150 µg/kg IM in the forelimb. This dose was selected on the basis of a preliminary trial comparing administration of 50, 100, 150, and 200 µg/kg. Tortoises were housed at 30°C to 34°C, but during the experimental period the ambient temperature was 24°C. Sedation, varying in depth from light to heavy, was achieved within 20 minutes and was accompanied by significantly reduced heart rate and cardiac blood pressure, severe bradypnea, and a reduction in ventricular PO_2. Paradoxically, PCO_2 did not increase. Animals were still sedated 2 hours after medetomidine administration. Atipamezole was administered to five animals (0.75 mg/kg; IM) 60 minutes after the medetomidine injection. Sedation was reversed within 30 minutes and heart rate and ventricular PO_2 returned to baseline; however, ventricular blood pressure and respiratory rate remained depressed. The authors recommended provision of supplemental oxygen for procedures longer than 120 minutes, and continued cardiopulmonary monitoring after reversal of sedation.

Medetomidine plus ketamine was evaluated at two dosage levels in red-eared slider turtles: 100 µg/kg medetomidine + 5 mg/kg ketamine, and 200 µg/kg medetomidine + 10 mg/kg ketamine; IM. Anesthesia sufficient for minor clinical procedures and endotracheal intubation was obtained at both dosages; the higher dosage was adequate for skin incision and suture placement. Administration of this combination did not affect heart rate. Sixty minutes after induction atipamezole was administered at 5 times the medetomidine dose (in mg) and all turtles were swimming within 60 minutes.

Medetomidine (100 µg/kg) + ketamine (5 mg/kg) was administered IV to six adult gopher tortoises held at 30°C to 35°C, and their subsequent cardiopulmonary function evaluated in detail. During the resulting period of immobilization, heart rate was stable; however, there was a moderate transient increase in arterial blood pressure. Moderate hypoventilation, which peaked 15 minutes after induction, resulted in hypercapnia, hypoxemia, and respiratory acidosis. It was thus recommended that supplemental oxygen and/or assisted ventilation be provided with this drug combination. Thirty minutes after administration of medetomidine-ketamine, atipamezole was used to accelerate recovery. Medetomidine + ketamine was also used in gopher tortoises at 50 µg/kg + 5 mg/kg, and 75 µg/kg + 7.5 mg/kg. The lower dose induced light anesthesia in 11/15 tortoises, with a mean time to peak anesthesia of about 20 minutes. At the higher dose, 5/5 tortoises reached the same level of anesthesia in a mean of 23 minutes. The tortoises given the higher doses required longer to recover after atipamezole (5 times mg:mg dose) was administered: 33.5 (range 17 to 60) and 93.4 (range, 30 to 180), minutes, respectively. Profound bradycardia was noted in all tortoises, although an initial increase in heart rate was seen 5 to 15 minutes after drug administration in the higher-dose group.

Three species of tortoises were immobilized with a combination of medetomidine and ketamine for various minor clinical purposes. Leopard and yellow-footed tortoises, held at 29.5°C, received doses of 100 µg/kg medetomidine + 5 mg/kg ketamine IV. Aldabra tortoises, held between 24°C and 29.5°C, received 25 to 80 µg/kg medetomidine + 3 to 8 mg/kg ketamine IV. Induction, defined as the point when the head of the tortoise could be pulled from the shell and its mouth opened, occurred within 4 to 16 minutes for the leopard and yellow-footed, and within 15 to 45 minutes for the Aldabra tortoises. Heart rates in most leopard and yellow-footed tortoises dropped between injection and induction times, but never below 8 beats/minute. One Aldabra tortoise prolapsed its penis during two of three immobilizations, and transient hindlimb paresis, unaffected by anesthetic reversal with atipamezole, occurred in one yellow-footed and three Aldabra tortoises. As the drugs were administered into the dorsal coccygeal vein, the epidural anesthetic injection was considered as a possible cause of these adverse effects. Immobilizations were rapidly reversed (median time 5 minutes) with atipamezole, administered IV at doses of 4 to 4.5 times the dose of medetomidine (mg:mg basis).

Medetomidine (50 µg/kg; IV) and ketamine (5 mg/kg; IV) were used for anesthetic induction in loggerhead sea turtles. Induction times ranged from 2 to 40 minutes, with a mean of 11 minutes. Heavy sedation and profound muscle relaxation were achieved, permitting endotracheal intubation and transfer to inhaled sevoflurane for a range of clinical and surgical procedures. Bradycardia was noted soon after induction; however, heart rates remained within the wide physiologic range seen in these aquatic turtles. Additional medetomidine (25 to 50 µg/kg) was administered intraoperatively to several animals for additional analgesia. Atipamezole was used at the end of the procedure to reverse any continuing effects of medetomidine.

A combination of medetomidine plus ketamine was used to anesthetize juvenile and adult American alligators. Juvenile animals required significantly larger doses of both medetomidine (220.1 ± 76.9 versus 131.1 ± 19.5 µg/kg; IM) and ketamine (10.0 ± 4.9 versus 7.5 ± 4.2 mg/kg; IM) to achieve anesthesia. The mean induction time for juvenile animals was 19.6 minutes (range 5 to 27 minutes) and for adults was 26.6 minutes (range 10 to 65 minutes). Significant decreases in heart rate were noted within 30 to 60 minutes after administration of the medetomidine plus ketamine combination, and cardiac arrhythmias were seen in two of 16 animals. After 61 to 250 minutes of anesthesia (supplementary isoflurane was utilized after 120 minutes) atipamezole, administered in equal volumes to medetomidine (equivalent to 5 mg atipamezole to 1 mg medetomidine), effectively reversed the effects of medetomidine. Mean recovery time for juvenile animals was 35.4 minutes (range 10 to 88 minutes) and for adults was 37.9 minutes (range 19 to 94 minutes).

ADVERSE AND COMMON SIDE EFFECTS: Medetomidine can significantly depress both cardiovascular and pulmonary function, although the effect may vary with species. In American alligators, medetomidine used alone at doses of 150 to 160 µg/kg IM resulted in profound bradycardia (4% to 96% decrease) and respiratory depression (7% to 100% decrease).

DRUG INTERACTIONS: In mammals, atropine and glycopyrrolate given at the same time as or after medetomidine may induce bradycardia, heart block, premature ventricular contraction, and sinus tachycardia.

MELOXICAM

INDICATIONS: Meloxicam (Metacam ❖, Mobic ★, Mobicox ❖) is a nonsteroidal anti-inflammatory agent with analgesic and antipyretic properties. The drug inhibits prostaglandin synthesis and is primarily a COX-2 inhibitor. Meloxicam is indicated for the relief of inflammation and pain in acute and chronic musculoskeletal disease, including postoperative pain. For more information, see MELOXICAM in the Small Animal section.

Meloxicam has been suggested for use as an analgesic in reptiles. Although there is no work investigating the physiology and effectiveness of nonsteroidal analgesics in reptiles, it is assumed that their use is appropriate in situations where pain might be occurring, and that drugs used in other species should have similar effects.

SUPPLIED AS VETERINARY PRODUCTS:
For injection containing 5 mg/mL (Metacam ♣)
Oral suspension containing 1.5 mg/mL (Metacam ♣)

SUPPLIED AS HUMAN PRODUCTS:
Tablets containing 7.5 mg (Mobic ♣, Mobicox ★) and 15 mg (Mobicox ♣)

MEPERIDINE

INDICATIONS: Meperidine (Demerol ♣ ★) is a short-acting narcotic analgesic used for the relief of moderate to severe pain and as a pre-anesthetic. It has minimal sedative effects. For more information, see MEPERIDINE in the Small Animal section.

A controlled study of the responsiveness of juvenile Nile crocodiles to a hot plate indicated that the intraperitoneal administration of meperidine increased the latency of the response, with a plateau effect reached at doses of 2 to 4 mg/kg. This work suggests that crocodiles are very sensitive to the antinociceptor effects of this drug. It is likely that this drug would be useful in providing analgesia in a variety of other reptilian species.

METOCLOPRAMIDE

INDICATIONS: Metoclopramide (Reglan ★, generics ♣ ★) is an antiemetic agent with central (chemoreceptor trigger zone) and peripheral activity. It contributes to lower esophageal sphincter competence and promotes gastric emptying. It is useful in the management of vomiting, gastroesophageal reflux, and gastric motility disorders. For more information, see METOCLOPRAMIDE in the Small Animal section. Metoclopramide has been suggested to improve gastric motility and emptying in tortoises. In desert tortoises, daily oral dosing with metoclopramide at 1 mg/kg did not significantly alter the gastrointestinal passage of plastic markers.

METRONIDAZOLE

INDICATIONS: Metronidazole (Flagyl ♣ ★) is a synthetic antibacterial and antiprotozoal agent with activity against anaerobic bacteria, *Giardia*, trichomonads, amebae, balantidiae, and trypanosomes. The drug also may have immunosuppressive or immunostimulatory properties. For more information, see METRONIDAZOLE in the Small Animal section.

In reptiles, metronidazole has been used in the treatment of amebiasis, trichomoniasis, and infection by other flagellates. Metronidazole is also a drug of choice for anaerobic bacterial infections. In a study of the antimicrobial sensitivities of bacteria isolated from clinically affected reptiles, 19 of 19 anaerobic organisms cultured were sensitive to metronidazole. Reported dosage regimens vary considerably with the most common being 40 to 100 mg/kg PO once, then repeated in 2 weeks. Dosage with 75 to 275 mg/kg has been recommended as a single dose, once daily for up to 10 days, or once weekly administration. Oral metronidazole has been suggested for long-term treatment (i.e., 2 to 6 months) in cases of osteomyelitis at a dose of 20 mg/kg every 24 hours PO. Juvenile spurred tortoises were treated with metronidazole benzoate suspension at 100 mg/kg PO every 24 hours for 2 doses, then every 48 hours for 10 doses without signs of toxicity.

The 5 mg/mL metronidazole preparation intended for IV administration has been used in small chelonians (<1 kg in weight) at a dosage of 60 to 80 mg/kg SC once daily for three treatments. Administration of the formulation was SC in the axial area.

A preliminary investigation of the pharmacokinetics of metronidazole was carried out in yellow rat snakes (ambient temperature not specified). In two animals given a single dose of 20 mg/kg PO, peak plasma metronidazole levels were greater than the MIC for many anaerobic bacterial pathogens (2 to 4 µg/mL). In five snakes administered the same dose of metronidazole 6 times at 48-hour intervals, mean plasma levels of the drug remained above 4 µg/mL for 24 hours after initial treatment and for 48 hours following the last treatment. A dosage of 20 mg/kg PO each 48 hours was recommended for treatment of anaerobic bacterial infections in this species.

The pharmacokinetics of metronidazole were also investigated in five green iguanas held at 31°C to 34°C. Metronidazole was administered once at an oral dosage of 20 mg/kg, and then after 48 hours had passed, the same dosage was administered each 24 hours for an additional 10 doses. Tablets were crushed and suspended in sterile water. The predicted peak plasma concentration of metronidazole was 7.6 ± 1.3 µg/mL between 3 and 4 hours after drug administration. The elimination half-life was calculated to be 12.7 ± 3.7 hours, with mean plasma metronidazole levels remaining above 4 µg/mL (the target level for infections by many anaerobic bacteria) for 12 hours following the initial single treatment and for 24 hours following the final treatment in the multidose experiment. The recommended dosages based on this study were 20 mg/kg every 48 hours to treat infections by highly sensitive anaerobic bacteria, or every 24 hours for more resistant organisms.

Metronidazole is formulated as a tablet base, which is bitter and poorly soluble in water, and as a benzoate powder, which has a bland taste. Use of metronidazole benzoate formulation in humans results in substantially lower plasma levels (i.e., by 30%) than with the tablet base. Similar results have been found in reptiles.

ADVERSE AND COMMON SIDE EFFECTS: Several species of snakes are considered sensitive to the drug, and deaths have occurred after treatment with doses greater than 100 mg/kg. These include tricolor king snakes, milk snakes, indigo snakes, and Uracoan rattlesnakes. A lower dose of 40 mg/kg is recommended in these animals. Other species of snakes may react similarly.

In one report, metronidazole was inadvertently administered once daily at a dose of 142 mg/kg PO, for 8 days to a loggerhead musk turtle. From days 10 to 12 after the initiation of treatment, the turtle became progressively weaker and anorectic and partial paralysis was noted. Supportive care was initiated and clinical signs gradually resolved over a period of 8 weeks. Anecdotal reports of snakes developing neurologic signs after administration also exist. Treatment with metronidazole may result in faunal imbalance in herbivorous species.

OTHER USES: Metronidazole has been used to stimulate the appetite of anorectic snakes. The mechanism of this effect is unclear.

MICONAZOLE

INDICATIONS: Miconazole (Conofite ♣ ★, Micazole ★, Monistat ♣ ★, Micatin ♣, and others) is a synthetic imidazole-derived antifungal agent active against most pathogenic fungi, gram-positive bacteria, and some *Acanthamoeba* spp. In human medicine, miconazole products are used topically for fungal infections of skin and mucous membranes (e.g., candidiasis). For more information, see MICONAZOLE in the Avian section.

In reptiles, miconazole has been suggested for the topical treatment of localized fungal infections.

SUPPLIED AS HUMAN PRODUCTS:
Several topical spray and cream gynecologic preparations (Micatin ♣, Miconozone ♣, Monistat ♣)

SUPPLIED AS VETERINARY PRODUCTS:
Cream containing 20 mg/g (Conofite ♣ ★)
Lotion and spray containing 1% (Conofite ★, Miconosol ★)
Shampoo containing 2% (Dermaxzole ★)

MIDAZOLAM

INDICATIONS: Midazolam (Versed ✤ ★) is a short-acting, parenteral, benzodiazepine CNS depressant, with sedative-hypnotic, anxiolytic, muscle-relaxing, and anticonvulsant properties. The drug is 2 to 3 times more potent than diazepam and has a shorter elimination half-life. Midazolam is formulated for intramuscular use, unlike diazepam. Midazolam can be used in combination with butorphanol to increase analgesia, and with ketamine for anesthesia. The effects of midazolam can be reversed with flumazenil. For more information, see MIDAZOLAM in the Small Animal section.

The sedative effects of midazolam, alone and in conjunction with ketamine, have been studied in red-eared slider, painted, and snapping turtles. In snapping turtles housed at 21°C, mild sedation inadequate for procedural manipulation was achieved using midazolam alone at 2 mg/kg. However, this dose combined with 20 or 40 mg/kg of ketamine resulted in sedation and chemical restraint adequate for extensive manipulation. Onset of effect was within 5 minutes, duration of sedation was 5 to 20 minutes, and all animals completely recovered within 210 minutes after drug administration. In red-eared slider turtles held at 24°C to 27°C, a dose of 1.5 mg/kg IM resulted in sedation with an onset of 4 to 28 minutes, a duration of 3 to 114 minutes, and a recovery of 20 to 60 minutes. Wide individual variation was noted, and one animal died. Midazolam has been recommended in this species to provide relaxation enabling the head to be withdrawn from the shell for clinical manipulations. In contrast to this, in painted turtles doses of midazolam ranging from 2 to 20 mg/kg IM did not result in sedation. In red-eared slider turtles anesthetized with ketamine at a dose of 60 mg/kg, combination with midazolam at 2 mg/kg reduced respiratory rate, although blood gas parameters did not change significantly from ketamine only controls, but did not alter the degree of anesthesia.

ADVERSE AND COMMON SIDE EFFECTS: Myositis and edema developed at the thoracic inlet near the injection sites into the forelimbs in 3 of 12 red-eared slider turtles dosed with midazolam. Two of the 3 turtles gradually recovered but the third died. The study in which these turtles were involved included repeated doses of midazolam, and the volume of individual injections may have been high for these animals.

MILBEMYCIN

INDICATIONS: Milbemycin oxime (Interceptor ✤ ★) is an anthelmintic, insecticidal, and acaricidal compound. For more general information, see MILBEMYCIN in the Small Animal section.

Milbemycin has been administered to red-eared slider turtles at dosages of 0.2, 0.5, and 1.0 mg/kg orally, and to the same species and

Gulf coast box and ornate box turtles at a dose of 0.5 mg/kg SC with no adverse reactions. Milbemycin has been effective in eliminating shedding of nematode eggs at a dose of 0.25 mg/kg SC once or twice at an 8-day interval. The drug was not effective against acanthocephalan parasites.

ADVERSE AND COMMON SIDE EFFECTS: Milbemycin has a mode of action and potential toxicity similar to that of ivermectin. The safety of milbemycin has been evaluated in only a small number of animals and in a limited number of species.

NEOMYCIN

INDICATIONS: Neomycin (Biosol ✿, Mycifradin ✿ ★) is an aminoglycoside antibiotic used topically and, less commonly, orally for the treatment of bacterial enteritis. It is not absorbed from the gastrointestinal tract and is, therefore, active only against enteric bacteria when administered by this route. For more information, see NEOMYCIN in the Small Animal section.

ADVERSE AND COMMON SIDE EFFECTS: Neomycin is generally less effective than amikacin and gentamicin, and when used systemically, is the most toxic aminoglycoside.

DRUG INTERACTIONS: Oral neomycin has been used in combination with systemic gentamicin and oral administration of live lactobacillus for treatment of severe enteritis and septicemia.

SUPPLIED AS VETERINARY PRODUCT:
Oral liquid containing 140 mg/mL (Biosol Liquid ✿ ★)

SUPPLIED AS HUMAN PRODUCTS:
Tablets containing 500 mg (Mycifradin ✿, Generic ★)
Oral suspension containing 125 mg/5 mL (Mycifradin ✿ ★)

NYSTATIN

INDICATIONS: Nystatin (Mycostatin ✿ ★, Nilstat ✿ ★) is a polyene macroline antifungal agent related to amphotericin B. Nystatin is fungistatic and fungicidal. The drug is primarily used for the treatment of gastrointestinal yeast infections, including oral candidiasis. For more information, see NYSTATIN in the Small Animal section.

Nystatin has been used empirically to treat oral and GIT mycotic conditions in reptiles, particularly snakes. Although published recommendations are for once-daily treatment, the activity of nystatin is based on topical contact; therefore, more frequent administration may be more efficacious. For more information, see NYSTATIN in the Small Animal section.

OIL, OLIVE OR VEGETABLE OIL SPRAY PRODUCT

INDICATIONS: Olive oil and spray vegetable oil products such as PAM have been used in reptiles as topical treatments to kill skin mites. The mites are suffocated by the oil.

ADVERSE AND COMMON SIDE EFFECTS: Keep away from the animal's eyes and mouth to avoid irritation or inhalation of the oil.

OXFENDAZOLE

INDICATIONS: Oxfendazole (Benzelmin ❧ ★, Synanthic ★) is a benzimidazole antiparasitic agent licensed for use in cattle, sheep, and horses. Oxfendazole is also a metabolic product of the breakdown of fenbendazole, which is in turn a metabolite of the prebenzimidazole, febantel. Oxfendazole is effective against lungworms and a variety of gastrointestinal nematodes, and has activity against cestodes. Since absorption and time to peak blood levels are slower for oxfendazole versus many of the older benzimidazoles, effective concentrations are maintained for a longer period of time in both the serum and the intestinal tract. These absorption parameters seem to impart greater efficacy, particularly against immature and inhibited larvae. For more information, see OXFENDAZOLE in the Large Animal section.

Oxfendazole is considered the benzimidazole of choice for treating roundworm infections in tortoises.

ADVERSE AND COMMON SIDE EFFECTS: Toxic effects involve the gastrointestinal tract and bone marrow, and would be expected to be similar to those of fenbendazole.

SUPPLIED AS VETERINARY PRODUCTS:
Oral paste containing 4.5 g/12 g of paste (Benzelmin ★), 5.4 g/14.4 g of paste (Benzelmin ❧), and 185 mg/g (18.5%) (Synanthic Bovine Dewormer ★)
Oral suspension containing 90.6 mg/mL (9.06%) (Benzelmin ❧, Synanthic ❧, Synanthic Bovine Dewormer ★) or 225 mg/mL (22.5%) (Synanthic ❧, Synanthic Bovine Dewormer ★)

OXYTETRACYCLINE

INDICATIONS: Oxytetracycline (Liquamycin ❧ ★, Terramycin ❧ ★) is a short-acting, water-soluble tetracycline with activity against a broad range of gram-positive and gram-negative organisms as well as chlamydiae, rickettsiae, and mycoplasmas. For more information, see OXYTETRACYCLINE and TETRACYCLINE ANTIBIOTICS in the

Small Animal section. In reptiles, oxytetracycline has been used for the treatment of bacterial infections, including *Aeromonas* spp. septicemia and ulcerative stomatitis in turtles and tortoises. The MIC for oxytetracycline against *M. alligatoris* isolated from American alligators was <1 µg/mL, making it an appropriate option for the treatment of infection by this agent.

Preliminary pharmacokinetics of a single dose of 10 mg/kg oxytetracycline administered IV were evaluated in two American alligators held at 27°C. The mean plasma level 96 hours after administration was 6.53 µg/mL, which exceeded the target MIC of 1.0 µg/mL for *Mycoplasma lacerti,* an organism that had been identified in an outbreak of disease. An accurate dosing interval could not be recommended based on the limited data collected.

ADVERSE AND COMMON SIDE EFFECTS: Oxytetracycline may cause inflammation at sites of injection.

OXYTOCIN

INDICATIONS: Oxytocin (Pitocin ★, Syntocinon ♣ ★) is a hormone of the posterior pituitary gland used to treat dystocia resulting from uterine inertia. For more information, see OXYTOCIN in the Small Animal section.

Oxytocin is not the hormone primarily responsible for oviposition in reptiles, which probably explains the variable results obtained with its use. Oxytocin appears to work best in chelonians. It is not known whether estrogens are required to sensitize the reptilian uterus before oxytocin administration. Medical stabilization and concurrent or prior treatment with calcium is usually recommended. It has been suggested that slow IV or intraosseous infusion over several hours may be more effective than a single IM injection. Oviductal contractions usually occur in 30 to 60 minutes after oxytocin administration, although not all animals respond. Provision of environmental conditions conducive to oviposition, such as the correct nesting area and ambient temperature, are essential. If green iguanas treated with oxytocin do not produce eggs within 24 hours, surgical intervention has been recommended. Promising results have been obtained using vasotocin, a more appropriate but not readily available compound.

ADVERSE AND COMMON SIDE EFFECTS: Uterine rupture may occur if underlying uterine pathology prevents egg passage. Mortality has been reported after treatment with oxytocin, although the significance of the drug in directly causing death is unknown. Some animals will pass only a portion of the egg clutch after oxytocin administration.

PAROMOMYCIN

INDICATIONS: Paromomycin (Humatin ♣ ★) is an aminoglycoside antibiotic with a broad spectrum of activity against bacteria, protozoa, and cestodes. In humans, paromomycin is used for the treatment of intestinal amebiasis and, in HIV patients, cryptosporidiosis.

Paromomycin has been used to treat amebiasis in snakes and acts primarily in the intestinal lumen, against trophozoite and encysted forms. Doses are empirical. Paromomycin administered orally to snakes was effective in reducing the magnitude of clinical signs and decreasing or eliminating shedding of cryptosporidial oocysts; however, on necropsy, large numbers of organisms were present on the gastric epithelium.

ADVERSE AND COMMON SIDE EFFECTS: Paromomycin is poorly absorbed from the intestinal tract. The drug is potentially nephrotoxic and ototoxic and may have neuromuscular blocking effects. Other adverse effects in humans include gastrointestinal upset.

SUPPLIED AS HUMAN PRODUCT:
Oral capsules containing 250 mg (Humatin ✤ ★)

PENICILLIN G
PENICILLIN, BENZATHINE
PENICILLIN, PROCAINE

INDICATIONS: Procaine penicillin G and the combination of benzathine and procaine penicillin G are the repository forms of penicillin G. Penicillin compounds have been used for the treatment of bacterial infections in reptiles; however, antibacterials with a broader spectrum of activity, particularly against gram-negative organisms, are more appropriate in most situations. Penicillin G is also used to lavage open wounds. For more information, see PENICILLIN ANTIBIOTICS in the Small Animal section.

PERMETHRIN

See PYRETHRIN-CONTAINING PRODUCTS.

PIPERACILLIN

INDICATIONS: Piperacillin (Pipracil ✤ ★) is a third-generation, broad-spectrum, semisynthetic penicillin with activity against most aerobic gram-negative bacteria and some gram-positive and anaerobic organisms. It is used to treat bacterial infections, including those caused by *Pseudomonas aeruginosa*. Piperacillin has been suggested for long-term treatment (i.e., 2 to 6 months) of osteomyelitis. For more information, see PENICILLIN ANTIBIOTICS in the Small Animal section.

The pharmacokinetics of piperacillin have been studied in five blood pythons held at 28°C to 30°C. Initial IM doses of 100 mg/kg and

200 mg/kg, followed by 100 mg/kg after 24 hours, were evaluated. Peak blood concentrations were achieved within 4 hours of injection, and blood piperacillin concentrations well above the MIC for a series of bacteria isolated from the glottises of snakes (0.25 to 4 µg/mL) were reached. The elimination half-life was approximately 12 to 17 hours. A dose of 100 mg/kg IM every 48 hours was recommended in this species. There was no elevation of serum uric acid levels in the one animal in which renal function was assessed.

ADVERSE AND COMMON SIDE EFFECTS: Thrombophlebitis and pain on injection have been noted in human patients. No such response was noted in the study described above.

DRUG INTERACTIONS: Piperacillin has been used in combination with amikacin or tobramycin for septic patients. Under these circumstances the low end of the dosage range has been recommended. Piperacillin and aminoglycosides may be inactivated if mixed *in vitro;* therefore, administer each medication separately.

SUPPLIED AS HUMAN PRODUCT:
For injection in vials containing 2, 3, and 4 g (Pipracil ✤ ★)

PIPERAZINE

INDICATIONS: Piperazine (Hartz Once-a-Month ★, Once-a-Month Roundworm Treatment ✤, Pipa-Tabs ★, Purina Liquid Dog Wormer ★) is an anthelmintic used for the treatment of gastrointestinal nematodes, particularly roundworms. For more information, see PIPERAZINE in the Small Animal section.

ADVERSE AND COMMON SIDE EFFECTS: Piperazine may be toxic in debilitated reptiles.

POLYMYXIN B

INDICATIONS: Polymyxin B (Aerosporin ✤ ★, Neosporin ✤ ★) is a basic polypeptide antibiotic derived from *Bacillus polymyxa* (*B. aerosporus*). Polymyxin B has a bactericidal action against almost all gram-negative bacilli except the *Proteus* group, and is a treatment of choice for *Pseudomonas* infections in humans. Polymyxin B is particularly used in the treatment of gram-negative infections, especially those resistant to aminoglycosides. The drug is available in combination with other agents for topical and ophthalmic use. For more information, see POLYMYXIN B in the Small Animal section.

In reptiles, polymyxin B has been used in the treatment of bacterial infection, especially when caused by gram-negative organisms.

ADVERSE AND COMMON SIDE EFFECTS: Nephrotoxicity and neurotoxicity are described in humans. Some renal tubular damage occurs at therapeutic dosage in humans. The drug should be used with extreme caution in reptiles.

SUPPLIED AS HUMAN PRODUCTS:
For injection containing 500,000 U/20-mL vial, equivalent to 50 mg polymyxin (Polymyxin B ★)
Numerous products for topical use ❧ ★

PRAZIQUANTEL

INDICATIONS: Praziquantel (Droncit ❧ ★, Prazarid ❧) is the anthelmintic drug of choice for treating trematode and cestode infections, especially extra-intestinal forms. For more information, see PRAZIQUANTEL in the Small Animal section.

Praziquantel was used with 100% efficacy to clear wild-caught green sea turtles of cardiovascular spirorchid fluke infestations. A very high dose was used (150 mg/kg, administered as 50 mg/kg 3 times in one day, orally). It is probable that lower doses would also be effective. The pharmacokinetics of praziquantel were studied in juvenile loggerhead sea turtles held at 27°C to 30°C. Plasma concentrations of the drug were measured after administration of single oral doses of 25 and 50 mg/kg, and of 3 doses of 25 mg/kg at 3-hour intervals. Maximum plasma concentrations of 109 and 342 ng/mL were reached 10 and 14 hours after administration of the 25 and 50 mg/kg doses, respectively. However, large variations in plasma praziquantel concentrations occurred among animals. Plasma levels were undetectable more than 24 hours after administration, in comparison with turtles receiving the three doses where plasma concentrations of 90 ng/mL were measured 48 hours after administration. The efficacy of these doses against spirorchid parasites was not assessed.

ADVERSE AND COMMON SIDE EFFECTS: Increased AST and ALT levels were seen in the green sea turtles described above. These elevations were thought to be a response to the death of the flukes, rather than to the drug itself. One loggerhead sea turtle that received an oral dose of 50 mg/kg developed necrotizing skin lesions resembling a drug reaction within 48 hours of administration.

DRUG INTERACTIONS: Oral praziquantel plus febantel (Vercom ★) has been used successfully to clear nematode eggs from the feces of prehensile-tailed skinks. Efficacy was felt to be better than that of ivermectin.

SUPPLIED AS VETERINARY PRODUCTS:
PRAZIQUANTEL
See Small Animal section

PRAZIQUANTEL PLUS FEBANTEL
Paste containing 3.4 mg praziquantel plus 34 mg febantel per g (Vercom ★)
Tablets containing 22.7 mg praziquantel plus 113.4 mg febantel plus 22.7 mg pyrantel pamoate (Drontal Plus for Small Dogs ✤) and 68 mg praziquantel plus 340.2 mg febantel plus 68 mg pyrantel pamoate (Drontal Plus for Medium and Large Dogs ✤)

PREDNISONE
PREDNISOLONE

INDICATIONS: Prednisolone (Delta-Cortef ★) and prednisone (Deltasone ✤, Meticorten ★) are intermediate-acting glucocorticoid agents. Prednisone is converted by the liver to prednisolone. Except for cases of liver failure, the drugs can essentially be used interchangeably. For more information, see PREDNISOLONE and GLUCOCORTICOID AGENTS in the Small Animal section. Prednisolone sodium succinate has been recommended in the treatment of septic shock, and prednisolone for its anti-inflammatory effects.

ADVERSE AND COMMON SIDE EFFECTS: Routine use of glucocorticoids in reptiles is not recommended because of immunosuppressive effects.

PROPOFOL

INDICATIONS: Propofol (Rapinovet ✤ ★, Diprivan ✤ ★, Propoflow ★) is a sedative/hypnotic IV anesthetic agent used for the induction and maintenance of general anesthesia. In mammals, it is indicated to provide general anesthesia for procedures lasting less than 5 minutes and for induction and maintenance of general anesthesia using incremental doses to effect. It is particularly useful for cases in which a short recovery is desired. For more information, see PROPOFOL in the Small Animal section.

Propofol has been used for the induction of anesthesia in a variety of lizards, snakes, and chelonians, and is considered by many to be the induction agent of choice. Induction is rapid, taking from less than a minute to 3 to 5 minutes, depending on whether the drug is truly injected intravenously and the size and body temperature of the patient. Although results are somewhat dose dependent, anesthesia generally lasts 10 to 30 minutes, with full recovery requiring from 20 to 40 minutes. When propofol was used to anesthetize brown tree snakes, agitated and obese animals had shorter durations of anesthesia than other snakes in the experimental group. Intraosseous administration has been used as well as the recommended IV route. Smooth induction and recovery, with minimal excitation, are seen. Low doses of ketamine or sedative agents can be used to sedate animals to assist in venous access. An inhalant anesthetic is generally used to continue anesthesia beyond the time obtained by the initial propofol injection, although both repeated boluses and constant rate infusion are possible.

ADVERSE AND COMMON SIDE EFFECTS: Propofol administration often results in initial hypoventilation or apnea in reptiles as it does in mammals and birds. Slower rates of infusion may reduce the severity of this initial respiratory depression. In a study of the anesthetic and cardiopulmonary effects of propofol in green iguanas, apnea was seen for 1 to 4 minutes after induction with 10 mg/kg intraosseously. Although animals were breathing spontaneously by 5 minutes after induction, respiration was significantly reduced for up to 25 minutes. Intubation and provision of oxygen by intermittent positive-pressure ventilation (IPPV) was recommended to prevent hypoxia. In a second portion of the study iguanas were given an initial dose of 5 mg/kg and then maintained with a dose rate of 0.5 mg/kg per minute via the intraosseous route. It was concluded that this dose rate was too high and propofol accumulation was occurring, based on the development of bradycardia, apnea, hypoventilation, hypoxemia, and hypercapnia as the anesthetic period progressed.

Six of nine brown snakes became apneic for 30 to 60 seconds after an intracardiac injection of 5 mg/kg propofol. A reduction in respiratory rate was noted for the first 6 minutes of anesthesia, but blood gas parameters were not significantly altered from baseline. Dosages greater than 6 mg/kg, used during a pilot trial, produced erratic results with apnea in some animals lasting over an hour.

PROPRANOLOL

INDICATIONS: Propranolol (Inderal ✤ ★) is a nonselective β_1- and β_2-receptor blocking agent whose use in veterinary medicine is primarily in the management of cardiac disease. In reptiles, propranolol has been used to induce oviposition. For more information, see PROPRANOLOL in the Small Animal section and VASOTOCIN in this section.

DRUG INTERACTIONS: The striped plateau lizard was used as an experimental subject to investigate the hypothesis that adrenergic inhibition of uterine muscular activity exists in reptiles. The relative success in inducing oviposition was studied using single doses of 1 mg/kg of propranolol (as an adrenergic blocking agent), 0.5 mg/kg arginine vasotocin, and 25 µg/kg prostaglandin $F_{2\alpha}$. Administration of these compounds resulted in oviposition in 4 of 8 lizards (2 of the clutches were partial), 2 of 3 lizards (1 partial clutch), and 0 of 4 lizards, respectively. When animals were pretreated with propranolol, subsequent administration of arginine vasotocin or prostaglandin $F_{2\alpha}$ resulted in oviposition in 3 of 3 and 6 of 7 lizards (1 partial clutch). Only animals that had received prostaglandin exhibited nesting or nest-guarding behavior. Tunneling and nest-building behavior have also been seen in a green iguana that received 7.5 mg/kg of propranolol followed by 18.5 µg/kg of prostaglandin $F_{2\alpha}$. This animal did not pass eggs, which may have been due to the much lower dose of propranolol or to prior treatment with oxytocin and passage of a portion of the clutch.

PROSTAGLANDIN $F_{2\alpha}$, E_2

INDICATIONS: Prostaglandin $F_{2\alpha}$ (Lutalyse ✤ ★), or dinoprost, is an abortifacient and is used for the management of reproductive conditions in mammals. The drug causes contraction of the myometrium and relaxation of the cervix. Prostaglandin $F_{2\alpha}$ has been used to induce oviposition in some species of viviparous lizards. The drug also appears to stimulate nesting behavior in some species of lizards.

Prostaglandin E_2 (Prepidil ✤ ★, Prostin E_2 ✤) gel is used to "ripen" the cervix and induce parturition in humans. The drug has also been used in birds to stimulate relaxation of the uterovaginal junction of dystocic birds and aid in oviposition. Prostaglandin E_2 was used in a spotted python that retained two eggs after oviposition. The gel was applied intracloacally near the cervix, and 20 minutes later an IM injection of 0.6 mg/kg prostaglandin $F_{2\alpha}$ was administered. The snake passed the remaining two eggs within 8 hours. Prostaglandin E_2 is available in a gel formulation for single dose in humans, which can be divided into aliquots of an appropriate dose and then frozen for subsequent use. For more information, see PROSTAGLANDIN $F_{2\alpha}$ in the Small and Large Animal sections, PROSTAGLANDIN E_2 in the Avian section, and PROPRANOLOL in this section.

ADVERSE AND COMMON SIDE EFFECTS: In humans, side effects of prostaglandin E_2 include stimulation of smooth muscle in the GIT and hypotension as a result of changes in vascular smooth muscle. Caution should be taken to avoid contact of the product with the skin of the person administering the drug.

DRUG INTERACTIONS: In humans, it is recommended that oxytocin not be administered until 6 to 12 hours after prostaglandin E_2 is used.

SUPPLIED AS VETERINARY PRODUCT:
Prostaglandin $F_{2\alpha}$: See Small and Large Animal sections

SUPPLIED AS HUMAN PRODUCTS:
Prostaglandin E_2 (Dinoprostone)
Gel formulation containing 0.5 mg/3.0 g (0.5 mg/2.5 mL) (Prepidil ✤ ★), 1 mg/3 g (1 mg/2.5 mL) and 2 mg/3 g (2 mg/2.5 mL) (Prostin E_2 ✤)

PYRETHRIN-CONTAINING PRODUCTS

INDICATIONS: Pyrethrin-containing products (Happy Jack ★, Mycodex ★, Ovitrol ♣, Zodiac ♣, and others) are naturally occurring insecticides derived from the plant *Chrysanthemum cinerariae-folium*. These drugs are GABA agonists, which stimulate the insect's CNS causing muscular excitation, convulsions, and paralysis. Insect mortality is enhanced when these products are combined with piperonyl butoxide. For more information see PYRETHRIN-CONTAINING PRODUCTS in the Small Animal section.

Pyrethrin-containing topical insecticides, in either dip or shampoo formulations, are used most frequently for the treatment of ectoparasites in lizards and snakes. Products should be applied, left for short periods of time (e.g., 5 minutes), and then rinsed off thoroughly to prevent systemic absorption and toxicity.

An *in-vitro* study evaluating the effectiveness of various acaricides against *Amblyomma marmoreum* ticks from leopard tortoises found pyrethrin products to be much less effective than permethrin or cyfluthrin, broad-spectrum synthetic pyrethroid insecticides. Permethrin is available in a 0.5% spray formulation (Provent-a-Mite) registered for premise use against mites and ticks on snakes. Proventic is another commonly listed product. Permethrins are well tolerated in snakes and lizards at doses of 0.05 and 0.1 mg active ingredient/kg (1% pour-on solution) when used for the control of ticks and mites.

ADVERSE AND COMMON SIDE EFFECTS: Avoid contact of the chemical with the eyes and mouths of animals. Pyrethrin products may be too toxic for neonatal reptiles. Pyrethrins act rapidly; therefore, animals can be blotted to remove excess product and/or rinsed thoroughly within a few minutes of application. Clinical pyrethroid toxicity, with signs including lethargy, depression, muscle tremors, hyperesthesia, weakness, ataxia, and dyspnea, has been reported. Do not use pyrethrins or pyrethroids with other cholinesterase inhibitors as toxicity may result. For example, toxicity was reported in a green tree python after being sprayed with permethrin, a synthetic pyrethroid. The animal had been treated with an organophosphate 10 days earlier.

The safety of permethrin and cyfluthrin was evaluated in leopard tortoises. Twice the recommended mammalian dosage was applied by pipette to the base of the legs, anal area, and neck, and experimental animals were observed for side effects for 72 hours. This treatment was carried out 3 times at weekly intervals. For both products, minor side effects lasting for under 1 hour included reduced defecation and diarrhea. In a second *in-vitro* portion of the same study, permethrin and cyfluthrin killed all ticks within 24 hours at dilutions of up to 1:10,000. Cyfluthrin should not be considered safe for general use in reptiles as toxicity has been recorded in snakes and lizards even at very low doses.

SUPPLIED AS VETERINARY PRODUCTS:
Powder, spray, and shampoo formulations containing varying percentages of pyrethrin and piperonyl butoxide; some products also contain carbaryl and other insecticidal compounds.

PERMETHRIN
Spray containing 0.5% (Provent-a-Mite ★)

SELENIUM

See VITAMIN E + SELENIUM.

SILVER SULFADIAZINE

INDICATIONS: Silver sulfadiazine (Flamazine ♣, Silvadene ★, SSD ★, Thermazene ★) is a water-miscible cream with bactericidal activity against a broad range of gram-positive and gram-negative bacteria, including *Pseudomonas* and *Aeromonas* spp., and some yeasts. It has been used most commonly for topical treatment of mouth rot and burns but is also effective for other cutaneous injuries and bacterial infections.

SUPPLIED AS HUMAN PRODUCTS:
1% topical cream (Flamazine ♣, Silvadene ★, SSD ★, Thermazene ★, Silver sulfadiazine cream ★)

SPIRAMYCIN

INDICATIONS: Spiramycin (Rovamycine ♣) is an antibacterial agent with antiprotozoal activity. In human medicine, spiramycin is used to treat infections by a variety of gram-positive bacteria and to treat toxoplasmosis in pregnant women. The drug has been investigated for the treatment of cryptosporidiosis in patients with HIV infection.

Spiramycin administered orally to snakes was effective in reducing the magnitude of clinical signs and decreasing or eliminating shedding of cryptosporidial oocysts; however, on necropsy, large numbers of organisms were present on the gastric epithelium.

SUPPLIED AS HUMAN PRODUCTS:
Capsules containing 250 mg (Rovamycine 250 ♣) and 500 mg (Rovamycine 500 ♣)

STREPTOMYCIN

See DIHYDROSTREPTOMYCIN

SUCRALFATE

INDICATIONS: Sucralfate (Carafate ★, Sulcrate ✤, generics), a complex of sucrose sulfate, accelerates the healing of oral, esophageal, gastric, and duodenal ulcers through several mechanisms. Sucralfate may be useful for the prevention of NSAID-induced ulceration. Sucralfate normalizes serum phosphorous levels, which makes it of potential benefit in cases of secondary hyperparathyroidism associated with renal failure in small animals. For more information, see SUCRALFATE in the Small Animal section.

Sucralfate has been suggested for use in reptiles as a gastric protectant. Its effects on blood phosphorous levels in reptiles have not been evaluated.

SULFONAMIDE DRUGS

INDICATIONS: The sulfonamides are antibacterial and antiprotozoal drugs that have been used for the treatment of intestinal and biliary coccidiosis. They are not effective against gastric cryptosporidiosis. For more information, see SULFONAMIDE ANTIBIOTICS and SULFADIMETHOXINE in the Small Animal section, or SULFONAMIDES in the Large Animal section.

ADVERSE AND COMMON SIDE EFFECTS: Sulfonamide drugs should not be used in the presence of dehydration or renal disease.

SUPPLIED AS VETERINARY PRODUCTS:

SULFADIAZINE
See TRIMETHOPRIM-SULFADIAZINE

SULFADIMETHOXINE
Various formulations for oral use in drinking water (Albon, Di-Methox, and others ★)
Oral suspension containing 250 mg/5 mL (Albon Oral Suspension-5% ★)
Tablets containing 125 mg (S-125 ✤, Albon ★) and 250 mg (S-250 ✤, Albon ★)
For injection containing 400 mg/mL (Albon Injection-40% ★, Di-Methox ★, Sulfadimethoxine Injection ★)

SULFAMETHAZINE
Various formulations for oral use in drinking water (Sulmet ★, Purina Sulfa ★, Sulfamethazine ★, Sulfamethazine 25 ✤, Sulfa-25 ✤, and others)

SULFACHLORPYRIDAZINE
For injection containing 200 mg/mL (Vetisulid ★, Prinzone Injection ★, Pyradan Injection ★)
Oral suspension containing 50 mg/mL (Prinzone Oral Suspension ★, Pyradan Oral Suspension ★, Vetisulid Oral Suspension ★)

Oral powder containing 50 g/54 g powder (Vetisulid ★)

SULFAQUINOXALINE PRODUCTS
Liquid concentrate for use in drinking water at 19% (Sulfaquinoxaline 19.2% Liquid Concentrate ✹), 20% (20% Sulfaquinoxaline Sodium Solution ★, Sulfa Q 20% Concentration ★), and 31.92% (31.92% Sul-Q-Nox ★)

TETRACYCLINE

INDICATIONS: Tetracycline (Panmycin Aquadrops Liquid ★, Tetrachel-Vet Syrup ★, Novo-tetra suspension ✹) is a bacteriostatic antibiotic effective against many aerobic and anaerobic gram-positive and gram-negative bacteria, spirochetes, mycoplasmas, and rickettsial organisms. It is used to medicate drinking water or for direct oral administration. For more information, see TETRACYCLINE ANTIBIOTICS in the Small or Large Animal sections.

In reptiles, tetracycline has been used for the treatment of bacterial infections, including *Aeromonas* spp. septicemia in crocodilians and osteomyelitis in snakes.

ADVERSE AND COMMON SIDE EFFECTS: Tissue damage may occur at the site of IM injection. Calcium, magnesium, and iron chelate tetracycline resulting in formation of insoluble complexes. Long-term use in birds may predispose to yeast infections; therefore, antifungal agents are often administered concurrently.

SUPPLIED AS VETERINARY PRODUCTS:
For oral administration containing 25 mg/mL (Tetrachel-Vet Drops ★) and 100 mg/mL (Panmycin Aqua-drops liquid ✹ ★, Tetrachel-Vet Syrup ★)
Numerous liquid and powder formulations for use in drinking water (✹ ★)

SUPPLIED AS HUMAN PRODUCT:
Oral suspension containing 125 mg/5 mL (Novo-tetra suspension ✹)

THIABENDAZOLE

INDICATIONS: Thiabendazole (Equizole ★, Mintezol ★, Thibenzole ★) is a broad-spectrum anthelmintic drug that also has antipyretic and anti-inflammatory effects and fungicidal activity. It is used for the elimination of gastrointestinal nematodes, including strongyloides. The drug is reported to be more effective against ascarids in tortoises than mebendazole or diethylcarbamazine citrate, although it may only reduce the worm burden. Thiabendazole also has antifungal activity, and has been used topically and systemically for mycotic infections. For more information, see THIABENDAZOLE in the Small Animal section.

DRUG INTERACTIONS: Thiabendazole has been used in combination with ketoconazole for the treatment of mycotic pneumonia in juvenile green turtles.

TICARCILLIN

INDICATIONS: Ticarcillin (Ticar ★) is an extended spectrum parenteral penicillin antibiotic with activity similar to, but more potent than, carbenicillin. In humans, the drug is active against gram-negative bacteria, including *Klebsiella pneumoniae, Proteus mirabilis* and *vulgaris, E. coli, Enterobacter aerogenes, Serratia marcescens, Pseudomonas aeruginosa,* and *Bacteroides fragilis,* and gram-positive organisms, including *Staphylococcus aureus,* coagulase-positive staphylococci, enterococci, and streptococcal organisms. Bacterial susceptibility is similar in veterinary medicine. The antibiotic is available in combination with clavulanic acid (Timentin ✤ ★) that is effective against many penicillinase-producing strains of bacteria. For more information, see TICARCILLIN and PENICILLIN ANTIBIOTICS in the Small Animal section.
In reptiles, ticarcillin has been used as an alternative drug to piperacillin.

DRUG INTERACTIONS: Ticarcillin is physically and/or chemically incompatible with aminoglycosides and can inactivate the drug *in vitro.*

TILETAMINE ZOLAZEPAM

INDICATIONS: Tiletamine plus zolazepam (Telazol ★) is an injectable dissociative anesthetic/tranquilizer combination useful for sedation and restraint and for anesthetic induction or anesthesia of short duration requiring mild to moderate analgesia. For more information, see TILETAMINE ZOLAZEPAM in the Small Animal section.
Telazol has been used in a variety of reptilian species for sedation and chemical restraint for minor procedures and to assist with IV access or tracheal intubation before anesthetic induction using other agents, or as an anesthetic agent itself. Reported doses fall into two main groupings: under 5 mg/kg, and between 10 and 30 mg/kg. Use of higher doses may delay recovery considerably. The ability to reconstitute Telazol at high concentration makes it useful dealing with large species or specimens to reduce the volume of drug to be injected.

DRUG INTERACTIONS: Premedication with atropine or glycopyrrolate has been recommended. Because the half-life of tiletamine is shorter than that of zolazepam, one should administer ketamine rather than additional Telazol as a top-up to prolong sedation or anesthesia. Flumazenil, a reversal agent for benzodiazepine tranquilizers, will help reverse the effects of zolazepam.

ADVERSE AND COMMON SIDE EFFECTS: A dose of 55 mg/kg has been reported as toxic in snakes. Recoveries requiring over 24 hours have been reported.

TOBRAMYCIN

INDICATIONS: Tobramycin (Nebcin ✣ ★) is an aminoglycoside antibiotic closely related to gentamicin used for the treatment of bacterial infections, especially those caused by *Pseudomonas* spp., against which it has better activity than gentamicin. For more information, see TOBRAMYCIN in the Small Animal section.

ADVERSE AND COMMON SIDE EFFECTS: Tobramycin is less nephrotoxic than gentamicin but may be more nephrotoxic than amikacin. Standard precautions for using any aminoglycoside antibiotic apply.

DRUG INTERACTIONS: Tobramycin's activity is potentiated by β-lactam antibiotics.

TOLNAFTATE

INDICATIONS: Tolnaftate (Tolnoxequine ✣, Pitrex ✣, Tinactin ✣ ★, Zeasorb ✣ ★, Ting ★, NP-27 ★, Aftate ★) is a topical fungicidal agent used for the treatment of superficial fungal infections. Tolnaftate has been described for the topical treatment of mycotic dermatitis in snakes, after the affected areas were soaked in dilute organic iodine, and for chronic dermatitis in Solomon Island prehensile-tailed skinks.

SUPPLIED AS VETERINARY PRODUCT:
Cream containing 1% tolnaftate (Tolnoxequine Thrush Treatment ✣)

SUPPLIED AS HUMAN PRODUCTS:
Cream and liquid containing (1%) 10 mg/g tolnaftate (Pitrex ✣, Tinactin ✣ ★, Zeasorb ✣ ★, Ting ★, NP-27 ★, Aftate ★)

TRIMETHOPRIM-SULFADIAZINE
TRIMETHOPRIM-SULFADOXINE
TRIMETHOPRIM-SULFAMETHOXAZOLE

INDICATIONS: Trimethoprim plus sulfadiazine (or sulphadiazine), sulfadoxine, and sulfamethoxazole (Tribrissen ✣ ★, Trivetrin ✣, Borgal ♣, Septra ♣ ★, Bactrim ♣ ★, and many others) are bactericidal antibiotic combinations commonly used for the treatment of bacterial infections in reptiles, including pneumonia, osteomyelitis in snakes, and middle ear infections in box turtles. Trimethoprim-sulfa combinations have also been used as anticoccidial agents. These drugs have been used safely for long-term therapy, i.e., 90 days or more, for the treatment of chronic infections. Despite the frequency of use of these drugs, and perhaps because of their safety, no pharmacokinetic evaluations have been performed. For more information, see TRIMETHOPRIM-SULFADIAZINE in the Small Animal section and SULFONAMIDES: POTENTIATED in the Large Animal section.

It has been reported that long-term therapy with trimethoprim-sulfa combinations may help reduce shedding and eliminate gastric cryptosporidiosis in snakes when combined with appropriate husbandry and supportive measures. A treatment regimen of 30 mg/kg PO once daily for 4 weeks, then 60 mg/kg PO once daily for 2 months has been described. Snakes given 30 mg/kg once daily for 14 days, then 1 to 3 times/week for several months were negative on gastric biopsies after treatment, but necropsies were not performed. Treatment with this drug combination is felt to improve but not clear infection.

SUPPLIED AS VETERINARY PRODUCTS:

For injection containing 40 mg/mL trimethoprim and 200 mg/mL sulfadiazine (Tribrissen 24% ♣)

For injection containing 40 mg/mL trimethoprim and 200 mg/mL sulfadoxine (Bimotrin ♣, Borgal ♣, Trimidox ♣, Trivetrin ♣)

For injection containing 80 mg/mL trimethoprim and 400 mg/mL sulfadiazine (Tribrissen 48% ♣)

Tablets containing trimethoprim plus sulfadiazine in the following combinations: 5 + 25, 20 + 100, 80 + 400 (DiTrim ★, Tribrissen ♣ ★)

Oral suspension containing approximately 10 mg trimethoprim and 50 mg sulfadiazine/mL (Tribrissen ★, Tribrissen Piglet Suspension ♣)

Oral paste containing 67 mg/g trimethoprim and 333.3 mg/g sulfadiazine (Tribrissen 400 Oral Paste ★)

SUPPLIED AS HUMAN PRODUCTS:

Oral suspensions containing 8 mg trimethoprim and 40 mg sulfamethoxazole/mL (Bactrim ♣ ★, Coptin ♣, Septra ♣ ★, and others)

TYLOSIN

INDICATIONS: Tylosin (Tylan ♣ ★, Tylocine ♣, Tylosin ♣ ★) is a bacteriostatic macrolide antibiotic active against gram-negative and some gram-positive bacteria, spirochetes, chlamydiae, and mycoplasmas. Tylosin has been used for the treatment of bacterial infections, especially pneumonia in snakes and chelonians. Treatment with tylosin may help to alleviate the clinical signs of respiratory syndrome of desert tortoises. The MIC for doxycycline against *M. alligatoris* isolated from American alligators was <1 µg/mL, making it an appropriate option for the treatment of infection by this agent. For more information, see TYLOSIN in the Small Animal section.

VASOTOCIN

INDICATIONS: Arginine vasotocin has been used experimentally and in small numbers of clinical reports to stimulate oviposition in reptiles. Experimental work on three species of lizards showed vasotocin to be 10 times more potent for this purpose than oxytocin. Another report describes a success rate of over 70% in inducing oviposition in a variety of snakes, lizards, and chelonians as compared to only 19% with oxytocin. A response is expected within 10 minutes to 24 hours after intracoelomic or IV injection. A repeat in dosing may be necessary to produce clinical effect. Pretreatment with calcium is recommended by some authors.

ADVERSE AND COMMON SIDE EFFECTS: Precautions are similar to those for oxytocin (i.e., underlying uterine pathology may result in failure to pass eggs or in uterine rupture). Arginine vasotocin is poorly stable and small aliquots should be frozen after reconstitution from powder. No adverse responses were seen in individual reptiles given up to 50 µg/kg.

DRUG INTERACTIONS: The striped plateau lizard was used as an experimental subject to investigate the hypothesis that adrenergic inhibition of uterine muscular activity exists in reptiles. The relative success in inducing oviposition was studied using single doses of 1 mg/kg of propranolol (as an adrenergic blocking agent), 0.5 mg/kg arginine vasotocin, and 25 µg/kg prostaglandin $F_{2\alpha}$. Administration of these compounds resulted in oviposition in 4 of 8 lizards (2 of the clutches were partial), 2 of 3 lizards (1 partial clutch), and 0 of 4 lizards, respectively. When animals were pretreated with propranolol, subsequent administration of arginine vasotocin or prostaglandin $F_{2\alpha}$ resulted in oviposition in 3 of 3 and 6 of 7 lizards (1 partial clutch). Only animals that had received prostaglandin exhibited nesting or nest-guarding behavior.

SUPPLIED AS CHEMICAL PRODUCT:
Arginine vasotocin (Sigma Chemicals)

VITAMIN A

INDICATIONS: Vitamin A (Aquasol A ❧ ★, Aquasol A Parenteral ★) is used as a supplement for sick reptiles and for the treatment of vitamin A deficiency, especially in pet turtles and tortoises. Published dosages include single, daily, and weekly treatment with doses ranging from 200 to 50,000 IU/kg. Parenteral dosages above 2,000 IU/kg should probably be avoided. Oral administration is recommended by some authors to decrease the risk of overdosage, whereas others prefer the parenteral route.

ADVERSE AND COMMON SIDE EFFECTS: Overdose by parenteral routes in terrestrial chelonians may result in subacute xeroderma followed by severe necrotizing dermatitis, epidermal lifting, and ulceration. These lesions have been seen in 3 box turtles administered 5,000 IU/kg per week for 2 to 3 weeks, but have not been experimentally re-created. Another report states that lesions can be produced in chelonians with a single dose of >10,000 IU/kg IM. An anecdotal report describes similar and extremely severe sloughing of the skin in a snake that had received extensive supplementation with injectable vitamin A. Oral treatment is not thought to result in xeroderma; however, caution should be taken in assessing both the dose administered and the frequency of administration. Herbivorous species often receive adequate vitamin A in their diet and should not be treated before dietary evaluation.

SUPPLIED AS HUMAN PRODUCTS:
Capsules containing 10,000, 25,000 or 50,000 IU (Aquasol A ❧ ★, Natural Source Vitamin A [retinol] ❧, and others)
Oral solution containing 50,000 IU/mL (Aquasol A ★)
For injection containing 50,000 USP units/mL (15 mg retinal/mL) (Aquasol A Parenteral ★)
In gel formulation containing 10,000 IU Pro-Vitamin A (ACES Antioxidant Soft Gels ★)

VITAMIN B COMPLEX

INDICATIONS: Vitamin B ❧ ★ complex injections are used as a nutritional supplement for sick reptiles and to stimulate appetite, especially in chelonians and lizards. Dosages are usually listed by volume; however, products differ in their vitamin content. Dosing by thiamine level can be used to compensate for this.

SUPPLIED AS VETERINARY PRODUCTS:
For injection containing various vitamin levels and combinations (multiple products ❧ ★)

Oral to add to drinking water (Vitamin B Complex ✤, Liquid B Complex ★)
Oral syrup (V.A.L. Syrup ★)

VITAMIN B₁ (THIAMINE)

INDICATIONS: Thiamine (Vitamin B₁ ✤ ★, B-1 ★, T-Dex ✤, Thiamine HCl Injection ✤ ★, T Sol ✤, Ultra-B₁ ✤) is used for the treatment of thiamine deficiency and as a dietary supplement, especially in fish-eating animals. Dietary correction for the patient should also be undertaken. For more information, see THIAMINE in the Small and Large Animal sections.

DRUG INTERACTIONS: Injectable thiamine is also available in multiple B complex.

VITAMIN B₁₂ (CYANOCOBALAMIN)

INDICATIONS: Vitamin B₁₂ or cyanocobalamin (Vitamin B-12 ✤ ★, Am-Jet ★, Am-Tech ★, Am-Vet ★) is used in the treatment of general nutritional debility, and may act as an appetite stimulant.

SUPPLIED AS VETERINARY PRODUCTS:
For injection containing:
1,000 and 5,000 µg/mL (Vitamin B-12 ✤)
1,000, 3,000, and 5,000 µg/mL (Vitamin B12 ★, AmTech Vitamin B₁₂ ★, AmJec Vitamin B12 ★, and others)
1,000 and 3,000 µg/mL (Vita-Jec B-12 ★)

VITAMIN C

See ASCORBIC ACID.

VITAMIN D₃

INDICATIONS: Vitamin D₃ (Hydro-Vit D₃ ✤, Solu-Vit D₃ ✤, Vita-D ✤, High-D Dispersible ★, Poten-D ✤, Downer-D ✤) (cholecaliciferol, colecalciferol) is used orally as a general supplement to ensure proper absorption and utilization of calcium and phosphorus, and parenterally for the treatment of nutritional secondary hyperparathyroidism and metabolic bone disease. Suggested dosages in the literature vary 10-fold, but administration at no less than weekly intervals is generally recommended. Vitamin D₃ therapy should occur in conjunction with calcium supplementation and, in some cases, administration of calcitonin. Parenteral treatment is generally discontinued when serum calcium/phosphorus ratios return to normal and dietary corrections are instituted. For more information, see VITAMIN D in the Large Animal section.

ADVERSE AND COMMON SIDE EFFECTS: Excess vitamin D_3 administration may result in vascular and/or renal calcification.

DRUG INTERACTIONS: Vitamin D_3 is more commonly supplied in combination with vitamins A and E or for oral use with calcium and phosphorus.

SUPPLIED AS HUMAN PRODUCTS:
1 IU = 0.025 µg of vitamin D_3
For injection containing 1 µg/mL of calcitriol (Calcijex ✚ ★) and 400 IU/mL (Di-Vi-Sol ✚)

VITAMIN E + SELENIUM

INDICATIONS: Vitamin E + selenium (BO-SE ★, E-SE ✚, Myosel ★, Dystosel ✚, and others) combinations are indicated for the prevention and treatment of vitamin E and/or selenium deficiency, particularly in large animal practice. A single case report describes a green iguana with muscular weakness, limb contractions, and fasciculations that apparently disappeared after treatment with vitamin E and selenium. The clinical presentation resembled hypocalcemia. Vitamin E is also used for treatment of steatitis in aquatic turtles and crocodilians. Dosages and frequency of dosing to clinical cases are empirical. For more information, see VITAMIN E in the Small Animal section, and VITAMIN E + SELENIUM in the Large Animal section.

DRUG INTERACTIONS: Vitamin E is commonly used in combination with selenium.

SUPPLIED AS VETERINARY PRODUCTS:
Vitamin E for injection containing 200 IU/mL (DL Alpha ★) and 300 IU/mL (Vitamin E-300 ★)
Multiple products for injection containing various levels of vitamin E + selenium
1 mg selenium and 68 IU vitamin E per mL (BO-SE ★)
2.5 mg selenium and 50 mg vitamin E per mL (E-SE ✚)
2.5 mg selenium and 68 IU mg vitamin E per mL (E-SE ★)
3 mg selenium and 136 IU vitamin E per mL (E-SEL ✚, Dystosel ✚)
5 mg selenium and 68 IU vitamin E per mL (MU-SE ★, Mu-Se Injectable ✚)
6 mg selenium and 136 mg vitamin E per mL (Dystosel DS ✚)
51 mg selenium and 68 IU vitamin E per mL (Myosel-B ★)
52.5 mg selenium and 68 IU vitamin E per mL (Myosel-E ★)

55 mg selenium and 68 IU vitamin E/mL (Myosel-M ★, Velenium ★) Chewable Tablets containing 10 IU vitamin E and 10 µg selenium (MultiVed Comfort Antioxidant Chewable Tablets ★)
Feed supplements and oral powders

VITAMIN K

INDICATIONS: Vitamin K_1 or phytonadione (Aqua-Mephyton ★, Mephyton ★, Veta-K1 ✽ ★) is used to treat coagulopathies due to vitamin K deficiency and vitamin K antagonism caused by salicylates, coumarins, and indanediones, including warfarin poisoning. Vitamin K deficiency as a result of fat-soluble vitamin malabsorption may occur with long-term use of antibacterial agents. For more information, see VITAMIN K_1 in the Small Animal section.

In reptiles, vitamin K_1 is used for the treatment of vitamin K deficiency in crocodilians and as a supplement in debilitated animals to assist in the formation of coagulation factors.

XYLAZINE

INDICATIONS: Xylazine (Anased ✽ ★, Rompun ✽ ★, and others) is an α_2-adrenergic sedative agent characterized by a rapid induction, good to excellent sedation, excellent analgesia, and a smooth recovery. For more information, see XYLAZINE in the Small Animal section.

In reptiles, xylazine has been used in combination with ketamine for anesthesia; however, some authors question its efficacy. Medetomidine is a more commonly used alternative.

Handbook of Veterinary Drugs, Third Edition, edited by Dana Allen,
Lippincott Williams & Wilkins, Baltimore. © 2005

Section 17

The Use of Chemotherapeutic Agents in Avian Medicine

CHOICE OF MEDICATION

The majority of drug dosage and safety recommendations for pet birds are still empirical and based on clinical experience, although increasing numbers of pharmacokinetic and controlled studies are being undertaken. Most published information relates to the common caged bird species, raptors, and domestic poultry. Extrapolation from these reports and from mammalian dosage regimens is common practice. Unfortunately for the practitioner, increasing pharmacokinetic data further highlight the considerable differences in uptake, distribution, metabolism, and excretion of some drugs among various species of birds. This is not surprising given the diversity in body size, physiology, and habits present in the class Aves. Metabolic scaling has been used to help tailor drug dosage and dosage intervals to varied body size; this technique does not take into account, however, the innate differences among various types of birds. With the increasing importance of pediatric medicine in psittacine species, patient age has become an important factor about which we know very little.

Very few drugs are specifically licensed for use in birds, and most of these are for domestic poultry. In almost all cases, therefore, the veterinarian is prescribing "extralabel" based partially on his or her own experience and knowledge. The compounds listed in this text are those described in the literature and currently marketed or used in Canada or the United States. Dosages that are based on pharmacokinetic or controlled efficacy trials or are licensed for use in a particular avian species are noted with an asterisk in the table. It is essential that the veterinarian remain current with the literature in order to be aware of new medications or recently determined contraindications.

ROUTES OF ADMINISTRATION

Drugs are usually administered to avian patients via the standard routes: PO, IM, SC, and IV. Often, treatment is initiated via the parenteral route and then continued orally. Patient factors, such as species, size and age, personality, diet and husbandry, and medical conditions, and drug factors, such as formulation, pharmacokinetics, and possible drug interactions, influence the selection of route of administration. Liquid oral medications can be administered directly into the oral cavity or, more commonly, into the esophagus or crop with a metal or rubber tube. Many antibiotics are available in flavored syrups that are palatable to birds and can be placed in or on a favorite food item, thus avoiding stressful capture at frequent intervals. Few avian patients can be "pilled"; a small number of tablet formulations, however, are marketed for use in pigeons. Factors relating to gastrointestinal anatomy and function (i.e., the presence of a crop, the degree of ventricular grinding) will particularly influence the uptake of medications in tablet or capsular form. Medications can easily be mixed into formulas used to hand-raise baby birds.

Although medication of drinking water is common practice in the poultry industry, it is not routinely used in most other avian species. Maintenance of adequate and consistent dosage depends on total water consumption, drinking patterns, and palatability, bioavailability, absorption, and stability in solution of a given drug. Water consumption patterns vary widely among different types of birds; many birds do not drink at night. Illness may result in increased or decreased water consumption, thereby affecting the dose of medication ingested. Taste preferences and sensitivities also vary; sweeteners such as aspartame or fruit drink crystals can be used to mask the taste of unpleasant or bitter compounds. Most medications must be changed on at least a daily basis. Medications that are not intended for use in drinking water may not dissolve or remain well in solution. Most pet avian species will not drink adequate amounts of water to self-medicate when they are ill. Despite these drawbacks, medication of drinking water is sometimes the most practical way to treat birds in aviary or quarantine situations or when prolonged treatment is necessary.

Medication-impregnated feeds are used primarily in aviary situations and for the treatment of chlamydiosis. Millet and pellets containing chlortetracycline are commercially available. Medicated mash diets can be specially formulated for the treatment of individuals or groups of birds. The amount of medication absorbed depends on its concentration in the feed, the amount of feed eaten, and the bioavailability of the drug. The amount of feed eaten depends on the palatability and energy content of the diet. Most birds will not readily accept an abrupt change in diet, especially when it consists of a switch from seed mix to pelleted diet. Ill birds often have reduced food intakes.

Intramuscular injection is the most common form of parenteral administration. The pectoral muscles are generally the best developed and most easily accessed. When treating young birds, it is important not to penetrate the poorly developed pectoral muscle and thin sternum. Ratites do not have adequate pectoral musculature and the legs or epaxial muscles must be used for injection. Because birds have a renal portal system, injection into the hind legs is not recommended when drugs are nephrotoxic or excreted or metabolized by the kidneys. Experimental studies have not proven whether these precautions are necessary. Repeated intramuscular injections may result in myonecrosis; many compounds are irritating. With repeated or large volume injections, multiple sites must be used.

Subcutaneous injections are less frequently recommended but may be appropriate for larger volumes of injection or in pediatric patients with little pectoral muscle mass. The rate of absorption via the subcutaneous route may be slower than that achieved intramuscularly. Injections should not be made in the cervical area in order to avoid penetration into the subcutaneous air sac extensions. The shoulder, inguinal, or cranial thigh regions are most frequently used.

Intravenous injections are most commonly used for initiation of treatment in seriously ill birds. Continued intravenous therapy is not practical, especially in small species, because of difficulties in obtaining repeat venipuncture in small and often uncooperative patients. The frequency of hematoma formation often precludes making multiple injections into the same vein. Intraosseous injection is an alternative route for the administration of sterile, nonirritating compounds. Continued infusion or repeated injections are possible in this manner. Little information is available on the rate of absorption of medications administered by this technique; it is assumed to be rapid.

Topical products can be applied to the integument; potential adverse effects, however, include soiling of the feathers, loss of thermal insulation, and, if products are ingested during preening, toxicity. Flushing of the nasal passages and sinuses is often incorporated into therapy for chronic sinus infections. Nebulization (using particles of <3 μm in size) and direct intratracheal or air sac administration of drugs have been used to treat respiratory disease. Higher local drug levels may be reached by these methods than by standard parenteral or oral routes. Concurrent parenteral therapy is advised.

This book does not address concerns regarding the treatment of birds intended for, or laying eggs for, human consumption. The issue of drug residues should be further investigated by veterinarians treating those patients.

Handbook of Veterinary Drugs, Third Edition, edited by Dana Allen,
Lippincott Williams & Wilkins, Baltimore. © 2005

Section 18

Common Dosages in Avian Medicine

Drug	Dosage	Indication/Species
Acetic acid (5% apple cider vinegar)	5 to 15 mL/L of drinking water	To help control mild GI yeast infections
	15 mL/50 mL of hand feeding formula	To help control mild GI yeast infections in hand-fed neonates or juvenile birds
Acetylcysteine 10%	2 to 5 drops in sterile saline per treatment	For nebulization or intranasal flushing; may also be combined with other medications including antibiotics or aminophylline
	0.25 mL acetylcysteine in 5 mL sterile water	As above
Acetylsalicylic acid	5 mg/kg tid to qid; PO	Analgesia and anti-inflammatory effects
	325 mg/250 mL drinking water	Analgesia and anti-inflammatory effects
ACTH (corticotropin)	*15 to 25 U/bird; IM	Various psittacines

(continued)

Drug	Dosage	Indication/Species
ACTH (cosyntropin)	*0.125 mg/bird; IM	ACTH stimulation test, various psittacines, bald eagle, Andean condor
Acyclovir	*80 mg/kg tid; PO	Pacheco's disease, Quaker parakeets
	*40 mg/kg tid; IM	Pacheco's disease, Quaker parakeets
	25 to 80 mg/kg tid; PO, IM, IV	General recommendation for herpesviral infections
	423 mg to 2.2 g/L drinking water	Range of recommended doses for flock medication during a Pacheco's outbreak
	24 mg/bird bid; PO in food	Large psittacines
	6 mg/bird bid; PO in food	Small psittacines
	*400 mg capsular drug per 2 quarts (2.2 L) parrot seed plus 1 mg (IV form)/mL drinking water	Quaker parakeets
Allopurinol	10 mg/kg tid to qid; PO initially; reduce frequency to bid to tid as required	Psittacines
	10 mg/30 mL drinking water; change solution several times per day	Budgerigars
Amikacin	10 to 20 mg/kg bid to tid; SC, IM, IV	General range of recommendations
	*10 to 20 mg/kg bid to tid; IM, IV	African gray parrots
	*15 to 20 mg/kg bid to tid; IM	Cockatiels
	*20 mg/kg tid; IM	Chickens
	*7.6 mg/kg tid; IM	Ostriches
	1 mL (50 mg/mL product)/5 mL sterile saline for nebulization	Treatment of respiratory disease

Drug	Dosage	Indication/Species
Aminopentamide hydrogen sulfate	0.05 mg/kg bid to tid for 1 day, then reduce frequency of dosage for 2 additional days; SC, IM	To control acute vomiting in psittacines
Aminophylline (25 mg/mL product)	0.5 mL/5 mL sterile saline for nebulization	Treatment of respiratory disease in combination with nebulized antibiotic or acetylcysteine
Amoxicillin	*150 mg/kg q 4 hours; IM	Pigeons
	*150 mg/kg qid; PO	Pigeons
	150 to 175 mg/kg once daily to tid; PO, SC, IM	General recommendations in the literature
	300 to 500 mg/kg of soft food	Canaries and small passerines
	200 to 400 mg/L in drinking water	Canaries and small passerines
Amoxicillin + clavulanate	*125 mg/kg once daily; PO	Pigeons
	*125 mg/kg tid; PO	Blue-fronted Amazon parrots
	50 to 100 mg/kg bid to qid; PO	General range of recommended dosage
Amphotericin B	*1.5 mg/kg tid; IV	Turkeys, great horned owls, red-tailed hawks
	1.5 mg/kg once daily to tid; IV	Raptors, psittacines; recommendations from 3 to 14 days of treatment
	1 mg/kg once, bid to tid for up to 1 month; intratracheally	Dilute in sterile water
	1 to 7 mg/mL; nebulize for 15 minutes once daily to bid	Diluted in sterile water
	Once daily to bid; topically	Oral candidiasis

(continued)

Drug	Dosage	Indication/Species
Amphotericin B (cont.)	*5 mg bid; PO	"Megabacteriosis" in budgerigars
	*1 mg/mL in drinking water for 22 days	"Megabacteriosis" in budgerigars
	100 mg/kg bid; PO	"Megabacteriosis" in budgerigars
Ampicillin	*15 to 20 mg/kg bid; IM	Emus, cranes
	*15 mg/kg bid; IM	Hawks
	*25 mg/kg tid; IM	Gallinules, pigeons
	*25 to 120 mg/kg once daily to bid; PO (capsule form)	Pigeons
	*100 mg/kg bid; IM	Pigeons, sensitive organisms
	*50 mg/kg tid to qid; IM	Amazon and blue-napped parrots, localized infections
	*100 mg/kg q 4 hours; IM	Amazon and blue-napped parrots, systemic disease
Amprolium	0.5 mL of 9.6% solution/L drinking water for a minimum of 5 days	Enteric coccidiosis
	1.25 mL of 20% powder/L of drinking water for 5 to 7 days	Enteric coccidiosis in pigeons
	2 to 4 mL of 9.6 % solution/gallon (3.8 L) drinking water for 5 to 7 days	Enteric coccidiosis in finches
	30 mg/kg once daily for 6 days; PO	Enteric coccidiosis in falcons
Ascorbic acid (see vitamin C)	20 to 40 mg/kg once daily to once weekly; IM	General supportive care
Atipamezole	5 times dosage of medetomidine on a milligram to milligram (mg:mg) basis; IM	Reversal agent for medetomidine

Drug	Dosage	Indication/Species
	Equivalent volume of Antisedan to volume of Domitor used	Reversal agent for medetomidine
Atracurium	*0.25 mg/kg; slow IV	Chickens, used for muscle relaxation during surgery
Atropine	0.1 to 0.5 mg/kg q 3 to 4 hours as needed; ¼ dose can be given IV, the remainder IM or SC	Organophosphate or carbamate toxicity
	0.02 to 0.1 mg/kg once; SC, IM	Preanesthetic or to reduce vagal bradycardia during anesthesia
	0.01 to 0.02 mg/kg; IV	Preanesthetic or to reduce vagal bradycardia during anesthesia
Azithromycin	50 to 80 mg/kg once daily for 3 consecutive days in each week; PO	For chlamydiosis (6-week treatment) and mycoplasmosis (3-week treatment)
	*40 mg/kg once per week; PO	For chlamydiosis in cockatiels
BAL (dimercaprol)	25 to 35 mg/kg bid 5 days/week for 3 to 5 weeks; PO	Lead poisoning
Barium sulfate	25 mL/kg; PO	Psittacine birds
Bismuth subsalicylate (Pepto-Bismol)	2 mL/kg bid; PO	Gastrointestinal irritation
Buprenorphine	0.01 to 0.05 mg/kg; IM	Analgesia (see description of drug use in Section 19)
Butorphanol	0.4 to 3 mg/kg q 2 to 8 hours, as needed; SC, IM	Analgesia, possibly for feather picking in psittacine birds
	0.02 to 0.04 mg/kg; IV	Analgesia

(continued)

Drug	Dosage	Indication/Species
Calcium borogluconate/ glubionate	1 mL/30 mL drinking water	Calcium supplementation (115 mg Ca per 5 mL product)
	1 mL/kg once daily; PO (115 mg Ca per 5 mL)	
Calcium EDTA	20 to 50 mg/kg once daily to tid; PO, SC, IM, IV	Lead or zinc poisoning (see description of drug use for duration of therapy)
Calcium gluconate	50 to 300 mg/kg slowly to effect; IM (diluted to <5%); IV	Hypocalcemic tetany, convulsions
Calcium gluconate/ calcium lactate/calcium glycerophosphate	5 to 10 mg/kg once daily to bid; SC, IM; can be repeated weekly for longer term therapy	Calcium deficiency
Carbaryl (5% powder)	Topical application, as needed	Arthropod ectoparasites
Carbenicillin	100 to 200 mg/kg bid to qid; IM, IV	Psittacines
	100 to 200 mg/kg once daily to bid; PO	Psittacines, ground tablets mixed in food
	100 mg/kg once daily to bid; intratracheally	Pneumonia in psittacines; in combination with parenteral aminoglycosides
	200 mg/10 mL saline for nebulization	
Carnidazole	*10 mg single dose; PO	Trichomoniasis in pigeons
	*5 mg single dose; PO	Newly weaned pigeons
	20 to 35 mg/kg single dose; PO	Empirical dosage in species other than pigeons
Carprofen	*1 mg/kg; SC	Analgesia in chickens
	1 to 4 mg/kg once daily to tid; PO; IM	Analgesia, anti-inflammatory

Drug	Dosage	Indication/Species
	2 to 10 mg/kg once daily; IM	Analgesia, anti-inflammatory
Cefazolin	50 to 100 mg/kg bid; IM	Raptors
Cefotaxime	50 to 100 mg/kg tid to qid; IM	General antibiotic use
Cefoxitin	50 to 75 mg/kg; IM, IV	General antibiotic use
Ceftazidime	100 mg/kg tid; IM	General antibiotic use
Ceftriaxone	*100 mg/kg at least tid; IV	Blue-fronted Amazon parrots
	75 to 100 mg/kg q 4 to 8 hours; IM, IV	
Celecoxib	10 mg/kg once daily; PO	Anti-inflammatory
Cephalexin	*35 to 50 mg/kg q 2 to 3 hours; PO	Bobwhite quail, hybrid rosybill ducks
	*35 to 50 mg/kg qid; PO	Pigeons, cranes, emus
	50 mg/kg tid; PO	Empirical dose
Cephalothin	*100 mg/kg q 2 to 3 hours; IM, IV	Bobwhite quail, hybrid rosybill ducks
	*100 mg/kg qid; IM, IV	Pigeons, cranes, emus
Cephradine	As for cephalexin	
Chloramphenicol	*102 mg/kg qid; IM, IV	Chinese spot-billed ducks
	*50 mg/kg qid; IM	Macaws, conures
	*50 mg/kg bid; IM	Budgerigars, turkeys, chickens, Egyptian geese, *Buteo* hawks, barred owls
	*50 mg/kg once daily; IM	Peafowl, bald eagles
	200 mg/15 mL saline for nebulization	
	80 mg/kg bid to tid; IM	Commonly recommended dosage
	50 mg/kg tid to qid; IV	
Chloramphenicol palmitate	75 to 100 mg/kg bid to qid; PO	Psittacines
	50 mg/kg qid; PO	Chickens, turkeys

(continued)

Drug	Dosage	Indication/Species
Chlorhexidine	10 to 30 mL of 2% solution/gallon (3.8 L) drinking water	Oral candidiasis, prevention or treatment during therapy for chlamydiosis
Chloroquine phosphate	10 mg/kg loading dose, then 5 mg/kg at 6, 18, and 24 hours; PO + 0.03 mg/kg primaquine once daily for 3 days; PO	*Plasmodium* spp. malaria in penguins; in combination with primaquine phosphate
	25 mg/kg loading dose, then 15 mg/kg at 12, 24, and 48 hours; PO + 0.75 to 1 mg/kg primaquine once; PO	*Plasmodium* spp. malaria in pigeons; in combination with primaquine phosphate
	10 mg/kg of chloroquine + 1 mg/kg primaquine, 1 day weekly; PO in drinking water	To prevent seasonal malaria in budgerigars, canaries, and finches; in combination with primaquine phosphate
Chlortetracycline	*0.5% impregnated millet for 30 days (5,000 mg/kg of diet)	Budgerigars, canaries, finches, parakeets (previously available as Keet Life)
	*1% impregnated pellets or mash for 45 days (10,000 mg/kg of diet)	AVMA general recommendation for treatment of chlamydiosis
	*95 mg/kg qid **OR** 190 mg/kg tid; PO	Pigeons with calcium in diet
	*30 mg/kg qid **OR** 95 mg/kg tid; PO	Pigeons with no calcium in diet
	*40 to 50 mg/kg tid; PO	Pigeons with grit in diet
	*40 to 50 mg/kg bid; PO	Pigeons with no grit in diet
	*0.5% to 1% in diet for 45 days (5,000 to 10,000 mg/kg of diet)	Canary-winged parakeets

Drug	Dosage	Indication/Species
	0.5% in soft mixed diet for 45 days (5,000 mg/kg)	Alternate general recommendation for most psittacines
	0.2% to 0.25% in diet for 45 days (2,000 to 2,500 mg/kg of diet)	Macaws, lovebirds, grass parakeets, rosellas, *Brotogeris* spp.
	0.15% in soft diet for 30 days (1,500 mg/kg of diet)	Finches and other small passerines
	1,000 to 1,500 mg/L of drinking water for 30 days	Finches and other small passerines
Chorionic gonadotropin	1,000 IU/kg IM single dose or repeated as necessary	To stop ovulation and egg laying and for behavioral feather picking in psittacine birds that may have a hormonal association
Cimetidine	5 mg/kg tid; PO, IM, IV	Gastric ulceration and gastritis in psittacines
Ciprofloxacin	*50 mg/kg bid; PO	Red-tailed hawks
	20 to 40 mg/kg bid; PO	Psittacines, including pediatrics
	15 to 30 mg/kg once daily to bid; PO, IM	Common range of empirical dosage
	80 mg/kg once daily; PO combined with ethambutol (30 mg/kg once daily; PO) + rifampin (45 mg/kg once daily; PO) or rifabutin (15 mg/kg once daily; PO) for a minimum of 6 months	Combination treatment regimen for mycobacteriosis

(continued)

Drug	Dosage	Indication/Species
Ciprofloxacin (cont.)	20 mg/kg bid; PO combined with clofazimine (1.5 mg/kg once daily; PO) + cycloserine (5 mg/kg bid; PO) + ethambutol (20 mg/kg bid; PO) for a minimum of 6 months 793 mg/L drinking water, for 7 days	Combination treatment regimen for mycobacteriosis
Cisapride	0.5 to 1 mg/kg bid; PO	To stimulate GI motility
Cisplatin	*1 mg/kg in 0.9% NaCl infused over 1 hour; IV	Sulfur-crested cockatoos, chemotherapeutic agent
Clarithromycin	55 mg/kg once daily; PO combined with enrofloxacin (30 mg/kg once daily; PO) + ethambutol (30 mg/kg once daily; PO) + rifabutin (6 mg/kg once daily; PO) for a minimum of 6 months; drugs were compounded with powdered sugar and water to create a combined oral medication of practical volume	Budgerigar, combination treatment regimen for mycobacteriosis
	85 mg/kg once daily; PO	For mycobacteriosis (must be combined with other antimycobacterial drugs)
Clazuril	*2.5 mg single dose; PO	Coccidiosis in pigeons
Clindamycin	100 mg/kg once daily; PO	Pigeons, parrots

Drug	Dosage	Indication/Species
	50 to 100 mg/kg bid; PO	Psittacines, raptors
Clofazimine	1.5 mg/kg once daily; PO + ciprofloxacin (20 mg/kg bid; PO) or enrofloxacin (15 mg/kg bid for 10 days; PO or IM; then PO) + cycloserine (5 mg/kg bid; PO) + ethambutol (20 mg/kg bid; PO) for a minimum of 6 months	Combination treatment regimen for mycobacteriosis
	6 mg/kg bid; PO + ethambutol (30 mg/kg once daily; PO) + rifampin (45 mg/kg once daily; PO) for a minimum of 6 months	Combination treatment regimen for mycobacteriosis
Clomipramine	0.5 to 1 mg/kg once daily to bid; PO (adjust dosage as required)	Psittacines for psychological feather picking
	3 mg/kg bid; PO	Cockatoos for psychological feather picking
Clotrimazole (1% product)	2 to 3 mL diluted; nebulize for 30 to 60 minutes once daily to qid as needed; some protocols rotate 3 days on treatment, 2 days off treatment for several months	Psittacines and raptors for respiratory aspergillosis
Colchicine	0.04 mg/kg once daily to bid; PO	For hyperuricemia or treatment of hepatic fibrosis, efficacy poorly documented

(continued)

Drug	Dosage	Indication/Species
Cycloserine	5 mg/kg bid; PO + ciprofloxacin (20 mg/kg bid; PO) or enrofloxacin (15 mg/kg bid for 10 days; PO) + clofazimine (1.5 mg/kg once daily; PO) + ethambutol (20 mg/kg bid; PO) for a minimum of 6 months; bird needs intact immune system	Combination treatment regimen for mycobacteriosis
Deferiprone	*50 mg/kg bid; PO	Chickens and pigeons, to chelate excess iron
	*100 mg/kg once daily; PO	Chickens and pigeons, to chelate excess iron
Deferoxamine	100 mg/kg once daily; SC	Hepatic hemochromatosis in a channel-billed toucan
Dexamethasone	1 to 4 mg/kg as needed; IM, IV	Shock, head trauma, anti-inflammatory
	0.25 mg/kg; IM, IV as needed	Anti-inflammatory
Diazepam	0.1 to 2 mg/kg bid to tid; IM, IV	Sedation, for convulsions
	0.2 to 0.5 mg/kg; IV	Sedation
	2.5 to 4 mg/kg as needed; PO	Psittacines
	0.5 to 0.6 mg/kg bid to tid; IM, IV	Psychogenic feather picking in psittacines
Diclazuril	0.0001% in medicated feed	Coccidiosis prevention in broiler chickens
	10 mg/kg on day 0, 1, 2, 4, 6, 8, and 10; PO	Presumptive toxoplasmosis in a Hawaiian crow
Diethylstilbestrol	0.025 to 0.083 mg/kg once; IM	To treat estrogen-responsive problems

Drug	Dosage	Indication/Species
	1 drop of 0.25 mg/mL solution per 30 mL drinking water	
Digoxin	*0.02 mg/kg once daily; PO	Budgerigars, sparrows
	*0.05 mg/kg once daily; PO	Quaker parakeets
	*0.019 mg/kg bid; IV	Male Pekin ducks
	*0.0035 mg/kg once daily; IV	Male turkeys
	*0.0049 mg/kg bid; IV	Roosters
	*0.01 mg/kg once daily; PO	Indian hill mynah, secretary bird
Dimetridazole	*0.02% to 0.04% in drinking water, 5 days treatment, 5 days rest, 5 days treatment	Giardiasis in budgerigars
	50 mg/kg once daily for 5 days; PO	Trichomoniasis in pigeons and doves
	1.25 to 2.5 mL powder per 4 L drinking water for 3 days (Emtryl powder)	Trichomoniasis in pigeons
	1 teaspoon/gallon drinking water (182 g/ 6.42 ounces powder) for 5 days	Most species (see comments in text)
	100 mg/L drinking water	Canaries and small passerines (see text concerning adverse effects)
	0.5 teaspoon/gallon drinking water (182 g/ 6.42 ounces powder) for 5 days	Mynahs and lories
Diphenhydramine	2 to 4 mg/kg bid; PO, deep IM	Antihistamine, sedation, treatment of feather picking in psittacines

(continued)

Drug	Dosage	Indication/Species
Diphenhydramine (cont.)	0.5 mg/8 ounces drinking water = 2.2 mg/L drinking water 0.013 to 0.065 mg/mL drinking water; this equals 0.06 to 0.1 mL of pediatric Benadryl per 10 mL of drinking water	
DMSA (2,3-dimercaptosuccinic acid)	25 to 35 mg/kg bid or for 5 days/week for 3 to 5 weeks; PO	Lead and zinc toxicosis
	*40 mg/kg bid for up to 21 days; PO	Lead poisoning in cockatiels
Doxapram	5 to 10 mg/kg once; IM, IV	Respiratory stimulant
Doxycycline (oral)	*40 to 50 mg/kg once daily for 45 days; PO	Cockatiels, Senegal parrots, blue-fronted and orange-winged Amazon parrots
	*25 mg/kg once daily for 45 days; PO	African gray parrots, Goffin's cockatoos, blue and gold and green-winged macaws
	*25 mg/kg once daily **OR** 7.5 mg/kg bid; PO	Pigeons with no calcium in diet
	*150 mg/kg once daily **OR** 25 mg/kg bid; PO	Pigeons with calcium in diet
	25 to 30 mg/kg once daily for 45 days; PO	Cockatoos and macaws
	25 to 50 mg/kg once daily for 45 days; PO	Other psittacine species
	10 to 15 mg/kg bid; PO	Cockatiels with pharyngitis due to a spiral bacterium

Drug	Dosage	Indication/Species
Doxycycline (injectable)	75 to 100 mg/kg q 5 to 7 days for 4 weeks, then every 5 days for the remainder of a 45-day treatment; IM; some sources suggest a 30-day course for small psittacines	Psittacines (Vibravenos or specially compounded formulations only) for chlamydiosis
	*80 mg/kg at intervals of 7, 7, 7, 6, 6, 6, 5 days; SC, IM	Houbara bustards
	10 to 50 mg/kg once or twice; IV	Initial aggressive therapy (Vibramycin hyclate)
	*100 mg/kg every 6 days for 3 injections; IM	Pigeons (formulated doxycycline hyclate)
Doxycycline (in feed)	300 to 440 mg/kg food for 45 days	
	*0.1% (1 g/kg) in corn diet, feed 100 g twice daily for 45 days	Blue and gold and scarlet macaws
	*500 mg/kg wet weight of seeds for 45 days	Cockatiels
	*240 to 300 mg/kg impregnated into hulled seeds	Budgerigars and small parakeets
	0.1% (1 g/kg) in soft food for 30 days	For finches, canaries and small passerines
Doxycycline (in water)	*800 mg/L in drinking water for 42 days	African gray parrots and Goffin's cockatoos
	*400 mg/L in drinking water for 42 days	Orange-winged Amazon parrots and Goffin's cockatoos
	*280 to 830 mg/L in drinking water for 45 days	Cockatiels
	250 mg/L in drinking water for 30 days	Finches, canaries and small passerines, for chlamydiosis

(continued)

Drug	Dosage	Indication/Species
Doxycycline (in water) (cont.)	250 to 800 mg/L drinking water	Pigeons, for *Mycoplasma*, *Pasteurella*, chlamydiosis
Enilconazole	Topical use	Fungal infections
	Aerosol treatment with Clinifarm smoke (per product instructions)	Respiratory aspergillosis, facility disinfection
	6 mg/kg bid; PO	Eclectus parrot with glossal candidiasis
	200 mg/L drinking water	Canary with cutaneous dermatophytosis
Enrofloxacin	*15 mg/kg bid; PO, IM	African gray parrots
	*7.5 to 15 mg/kg bid; PO, IM	Orange-winged and blue-fronted Amazons, African gray parrots, and Goffin's cockatoos
	*15 mg/kg once daily; PO, IM, or IV with caution	Red-tailed hawks
	*15 mg/kg once daily; PO, IM	Great horned owls
	*5 mg/kg bid; PO, SC, IM	Pigeons
	*10 mg/kg bid; PO	Houbara bustards
	*15 mg/kg bid to tid; PO, IM	Senegal parrots
	*2.2 mg/kg bid; IV	Emus
	*10 mg/kg once daily; PO	Chickens
	5 to 30 mg/kg bid; PO, SC, IM	Commonly recommended range of dosage
Enrofloxacin (in drinking water)	*100 to 200 mg/L drinking water for 7 days	Pigeons
	*190 to 750 mg/L drinking water	African gray parrots

Drug	Dosage	Indication/Species
	*50 mg/L drinking water for 5 days	*Mycoplasma iowae* in turkey poults
	*50 mg/L drinking water on day 1, 25 mg/L in water on subsequent days	Domestic ducklings
	*50 mg/L drinking water	Chickens and turkeys
	200 mg/L drinking water	Canaries, finches, small passerines; treat for 20 days for chlamydiosis
Enrofloxacin (in food)	250 to 1,000 mg/kg food	Psittacines, range of published dosage
	200 mg/kg of soft food	Canaries, finches, small passerines; treat for 21 days for chlamydiosis
	100 to 200 mg/kg food	Pigeons, for chlamydiosis
Enrofloxacin (anti-mycobacterial protocols)	30 mg/kg once daily; PO + ethambutol (30 mg/kg once daily; PO) + rifabutin (15 mg/kg once daily; PO) or rifampin (45 mg/kg once daily; PO) for a minimum of 6 months	Combination treatment regimen for mycobacteriosis
	15 mg/kg bid; PO or IM for 10 days then switch to oral formulation + clofazimine (1.5 mg/kg once daily; PO) + cycloserine (5 mg/kg bid; PO) + ethambutol (20 mg/kg bid; PO) for a minimum of 6 months	Combination treatment regimen for mycobacteriosis

(*continued*)

Drug	Dosage	Indication/Species
Enrofloxacin (cont.)	30 mg/kg once daily; PO + clarithromicin (55 mg/kg once daily; PO) + ethambutol (30 mg/kg once daily; PO) + rifabutin (6 mg/kg once daily; PO) for 6 months; drugs were compounded with powdered sugar and water to create a combined oral medication of practical volume	Budgerigar, combination treatment regimen for mycobacteriosis
Epinephrine	0.1 mg/kg; IV, intracardiac, intratracheal, intraosseous	For nonanesthetic-related cardiac arrest
	0.01 to 0.02 mg/kg; IV, intracardiac, intratracheal, intraosseous	For anesthetic-related cardiac arrest; use lower dosage for halothane than isoflurane
	0.5 to 1 mL/kg of epinephrine 1:1,000; intratracheally, IV, or intraosseously	For cardiac arrest
	0.07 mg/kg once; IM	To stimulate egg expulsion
Ergonovine maleate		
Erythromycin	10 to 20 mg/kg bid; PO	Psittacines
	44 to 88 mg/kg bid; PO for 5 to 7 days	Psittacines
	100 mg/kg bid to tid; PO	
	20 mg/kg once daily; IM	
	200 mg/kg of soft food	Finches, canaries, small passerines

Drug	Dosage	Indication/Species
	125 mg/L drinking water	Finches, canaries, small passerines
	500 mg/gallon drinking water, 10 days on, 5 days off, 10 days on	
	100 mg in 250 mL saline for nasal flush	Sinusitis
	100 to 200 mg in 10 mL saline, nebulize for 15 minutes q 8 to 12 hours	Respiratory disease
Ethambutol	30 mg/kg once daily; PO + rifabutin (6 mg/kg once daily; PO) + enrofloxacin (30 mg/kg once daily; PO) + clarithromycin (55 mg/kg once daily; PO) for 6 months; drugs were compounded with powdered sugar and water to create a combined oral medication of practical volume	Budgerigar, combination treatment regimen for mycobacteriosis
	20 mg/kg bid; PO + clofazimine (1.5 mg/kg once daily PO) + ciprofloxacin (20 mg/kg bid; PO) or enrofloxacin (15 mg/kg bid for 10 days; PO or IM; then PO) + cycloserine (5 mg/kg bid; PO) for a minimum of 6 months	Combination treatment regimen for mycobacteriosis

(continued)

Drug	Dosage	Indication/Species
Ethambutol (cont.)	30 mg/kg once daily; PO + ciprofloxacin (80 mg/kg once daily; PO) or enrofloxacin (30 mg/kg once daily; PO) + rifampin (45 mg/kg once daily; PO) or rifabutin (15 mg/kg once daily; PO) for a minimum of 6 months	Combination treatment regimen for mycobacteriosis
	30 mg/kg once daily; PO + clofazimine (6 mg/kg bid; PO) + rifampin (45 mg/kg once daily; PO) for a minimum of 6 months	Combination treatment regimen for mycobacteriosis
	30 mg/kg once daily; PO + rifampin (45 mg/kg once daily; PO) + isoniazid (30 mg/kg once daily; PO) for a minimum of 6 months	Combination treatment regimen for mycobacteriosis
Fenbendazole	5 to 15 mg/kg once daily for 5 days; PO	Anseriformes
(See comments concerning toxicity in drug description)	10 to 50 mg/kg once daily for 3 to 5 days; PO	Finches
	50 mg/kg bid for 5 days; PO	Various columbiformes, for ascarids, tetramerids
	20 to 50 mg/kg once, repeat in 10 to 14 days; PO	Ascarids
	20 to 50 mg/kg once daily for 5 to 7 days; PO	Capillaria

Drug	Dosage	Indication/Species
	20 to 50 mg/kg once daily for 3 days; PO	Microfilaria, trematodes
	10 mg/kg directly into air sac + 25 mg/kg once daily for 3 days; PO	After surgical removal of *Serratospiculum seurati* from air sacs of Middle Eastern falcons
	125 mg/L drinking water for 5 days	Pigeons, ascarids
	20 to 100 mg/kg seed	Note toxicity in some species of finch
Fluconazole	2 to 10 mg/kg once daily for 7 to 10 days or longer as needed; PO	*Candida* spp. infection of the digestive system
	15 mg/kg bid; PO	Candidal dermatitis, nasal and respiratory aspergillosis
	50 mg/L drinking water for 5 to 10 days	Oral candidiasis in pigeons
Flucytosine	*75 to 120 mg/kg qid; PO	Turkeys, great horned owls, red-tailed hawks
	50 to 250 mg/kg bid; PO for up to several months	Psittacines, raptors, finches
	18 to 40 mg/kg qid; PO	Raptors
	50 mg/kg bid for 2 to 4 weeks; PO	Prophylactic treatment for aspergillosis in swans
Flumazenil	0.05 mg/kg; IM, or half IV and the remainder IM or SC	Reversal of sedation by midazolam or diazepam
Flunixin	1 to 10 mg/kg once daily as needed; IM	Analgesic, anti-inflammatory
Furosemide	0.15 to 2.2 mg/kg once daily to bid; PO, SC, IM	Diuretic

(continued)

Drug	Dosage	Indication/Species
Gentamicin	*2.5 mg/kg tid; IM	Red-tailed hawks, great horned owls, golden eagles
	*3 mg/kg bid; IM	Turkeys
	*5 mg/kg tid; IM	Pheasants, cranes
	*10 mg/kg qid; IM	Quail
	*5 to 10 mg/kg bid; IM	Cockatiels
	10 mg/kg bid; IM	Blue and gold macaws
	10 mg/kg tid; IM	African gray parrots
	2 to 5 mg/kg bid to tid; IM	See note on toxicity in Section 19
	40 mg/kg once daily to tid for 2 to 3 days; PO	Enteric infections
	50 mg/10 mL saline bid to tid; nebulize for 15 minutes	Sinusitis, air sacculitis
	50 mg in 250 mL saline for nasal flush	Sinusitis
	5 to 10 mg/kg once daily; intratra-cheally	Pneumonia, combined with IM carbenicillin or tylosin
Glycopyrrolate	0.01 to 0.02 mg/kg; IM, IV	Preanesthetic or to reduce vagal brady-cardia during anesthesia
Haloperidol	0.08 to 0.2 mg/kg once daily to bid; PO; start low and adjust dose to individual	Psittacines, feather picking and self-mutilation
	1 to 2.5 mg/kg q 2 to 3 weeks; IM; start low and adjust dose to individual	Psittacines, feather picking and self-mutilation
Hyaluronidase	150 U/L of fluids; SC	To enhance subcuta-neous absorption of fluids
Hydrocortisone	10 mg/kg; IV	Short-acting glucocorti-coid agent

Drug	Dosage	Indication/Species
Hydroxyzine	2.2 mg/kg tid; PO	Red-lored Amazon parrot for feather picking
Ibuprofen (pediatric suspension)	10 mg/kg q 4 to 6 hours; PO	Analgesia, anti-inflammatory
Interferon	1,500 IU/kg once daily; PO	Psittacines
	1 IU/mL (3,800 IU/gallon) drinking water for 14 to 28 days	Pigeons for circoviral infection
Iodine	1 drop of stock solution per 30 to 250 mL drinking water; stock solution contains 2 mL Lugol's (Strong) iodine in 30 mL water	Iodine deficiency goiter in budgerigars; daily for treatment, 2 to 3 times weekly for prevention
	20% sodium iodine in saline for injection; 0.01 mL/budgerigar once; IM	For initiation of therapy
	122 mg/kg of diatrizoate sodium (37% iodine); IM	
Iohexol	25 to 30 mL/kg PO, either undiluted or diluted 1:1	Psittacines, for radiographic GI contrast studies
	*25 to 30 mL/kg either undiluted or diluted 1:1; PO	GI contrast series in 4 Amazons and a cockatoo
	5 mL intranasally	Used for a sinogram in a scarlet macaw
Iron dextran	10 mg/kg once, repeat in 7 to 10 days if needed; IM	Iron deficiency anemia, after hemorrhage
Isoflurane	3% to 5% for induction, 0.5% to 2% or as required for maintenance	Inhalant anesthetic of choice

(continued)

Drug	Dosage	Indication/Species
Isoniazid	30 mg/kg once daily; PO + rifampin (45 mg/kg once daily; PO) + ethambutol (30 mg/kg once daily; PO) for a minimum of 6 months	Combination treatment regimen for mycobacteriosis
Itraconazole	*6 mg/kg bid; PO	Pigeons
	*5 to 10 mg/kg once daily; PO	Blue-fronted Amazon parrots
	*10 mg/kg once daily; PO	Red-tailed hawks
	5 to 10 mg/kg once daily to bid; PO	Raptors, psittacines, waterfowl; aspergillosis or systemic candidiasis
	2.5 to 5 mg/kg once daily; PO	African gray parrots
	26 mg/kg bid; PO	Pigeons
Ivermectin	0.2 to 0.4 mg/kg once, repeat in 10 to 14 days if necessary; PO, IM	Nematode and arthropod parasites including *Knemidokoptes* and air sac mites
	0.2 mg/kg or 1 drop of 1% solution topically; repeat in 14 days (take caution not to overdose)	Finches, canaries, small passerines
	0.4 mg/kg once monthly; SC	Spirurid nematodes of the proventriculus in African jacanas
	1 mg/kg; SC, repeat in 10 days	*Serratospiculum seurati* in air sacs of falcons and falcon-hybrids
	0.05 mg once; topically in the eye	Ocular oxyspirurids in crested wood partridges and chickens
	0.8 to 1 mg/L in drinking water	For canaries and small passerines

Drug	Dosage	Indication/Species
	1 mg/L drinking water for 24 hours	Pigeons
	0.4 mg/L drinking water	Aviary treatment
Kanamycin	50 to 250 mg/gallon (11 to 55 mg/L) drinking water for 3 to 5 days	Enteric infections
Kaolin and pectin products	2 mL/kg bid to qid; PO	Antidiarrheal agent
Ketamine	5 to 75 mg/kg; IM	Common range of dosage
Ketamine + diazepam	5 to 30 mg/kg + 0.5 to 2 mg/kg diazepam; IM	Common range of dosage
	2.5 to 5 mg/kg + 0.5 to 2 mg/kg diazepam; IV	Common range of dosage
Ketamine + medetomidine (see Medetomidine + ketamine)		
Ketamine + xylazine	5 to 30 mg/kg; IM + 1 to 4 mg/kg xylazine; IM	Common range of dosage
	2.5 to 5 mg/kg + 0.25 to 2 mg/kg xylazine; IV	Common range of dosage
Ketoconazole	20 to 30 mg/kg bid; PO	Candidiasis, other mycotic infections
	200 mg/L drinking water for 7 to 14 days	Finches, canaries, small passerines
	20 mg/kg of soft food	Finches, canaries, small passerines
Ketoprofen	*5 mg/kg; IM	Mallard ducks
	2 to 4 mg/kg once daily to tid; IM, PO	Analgesia, anti-inflammatory
Lactulose	0.1 to 0.3 mL of 667 mg/mL suspension per kg once daily to bid; PO	Hepatic dysfunction, laxative

(continued)

Drug	Dosage	Indication/Species
Leuprolide acetate	50 to 150 µg/kg per day calculated for 28 days (single injection of 1 month depot formulation); IM	Reversibly stops ovulation in cockatiels
	200 to 800 µg/kg (depot formulation) each 3 to 6 weeks; IM	To stop egg laying
	100 µg/kg per day multiplied by number of days for which dose in intended (depot formulation); IM	Sexual feather picking
Levamisole	*20 mg/bird single dose; PO	Anthelmintic dose for pigeons (Spartakon)
	15 mg/kg once, repeat in 10 days; PO	Anthelmintic dose, Australian parakeets
	20 to 50 mg/kg once, repeat in 10 days; PO	Anthelmintic dose, waterfowl
	4 to 8 mg/kg once, repeat in 10 to 14 days; SC, IM	Anthelmintic dose, general use
	5 to 15 mL of 13.65% injectable solution per gallon (1.1 to 3.3 mL/L) drinking water for 1 to 3 days, repeat in 10 days	Anthelmintic dose; do Not use in debilitated finches
	2 mg/kg 3 times at 14-day intervals; IM, SC	As an immunostimulant
	0.3 mL of 13.65% injectable solution per gallon (0.03 mL/L) drinking water for several weeks	As an immunostimulant

Drug	Dosage	Indication/Species
Levothyroxine	15 to 20 µg/kg once daily to bid; PO	Hypothyroidism, to stimulate a moult
	30 µg to 2 mg in 113 to 120 mL drinking water	Range of published dosage
	15.4 µg/kg bid initially, then once daily for maintenance; PO	Hypothyroidism in a scarlet macaw
	0.1 mg tablet/30 mL drinking water daily	Budgerigars, birds who drink little water
	0.1 mg tablet dissolved in 100 to 300 mL drinking water	Other species
	For both doses, stir water, offer for 15 minutes, then remove	
Lidocaine	Do not exceed a dose of 4 mg/kg	Local anesthesia
Lincomycin	1 drop of 50 mg/mL suspension bid for 7 to 14 days; PO	Budgerigars
	75 to 85 mg/kg bid for 7 to 14 days; PO	Amazon parrots
	167 mg/kg once daily for 7 to 14 days; PO	Amazon parrots
	100 mg/kg once daily; PO	Raptors
	*16.9 mg/L drinking water for 7 days	Necrotic enteritis in chickens
Lincomycin + spectinomycin	2.5 mg lincomycin + 5 mg spectinomycin per chick; SC	Day-old poultry chicks to reduce early mortality
	1 part lincomycin + 2 to 3 parts spectinomycin in drinking water at 2 g/gallon (3.8 L) for 10 days	Mycoplasmosis in turkeys

(continued)

Drug	Dosage	Indication/Species
Lincomycin + spectinomycin (cont.)	⅛ to ¼ teaspoon LS-50 powder per pint (0.5 L) of drinking water for 10 to 14 days	Chronic respiratory disease
	100 to 200 mg/L in drinking water	For canaries and small passerines (Linco-Spectin)
	200 mg/kg of soft food	For canaries and small passerines (Linco-Spectin)
Magnesium sulfate	0.5 to 1 g/kg once daily; PO	Oral cathartic and chelating agent
Mebendazole	25 mg/kg bid for 5 days; PO	Raptors and psittacines
	5 to 15 mg/kg once daily for 2 days; PO	Waterfowl
	20 mg/kg PO once daily for 14 days	*Serratospiculum seurati* (air sac filarial worm) in falcons
Medetomidine + ketamine	100 µg/kg medetomidine + 25 mg/kg ketamine; IM	Anesthesia in psittacines, chickens, pigeons
	75 to 100 µg/kg medetomidine + 3 to 7 mg/kg ketamine; IM	Psittacines
	50 to 100 µg/kg medetomidine + 2 to 5 mg/kg ketamine; IV	Psittacines
	80 µg/kg medetomidine + 5 mg/kg ketamine; IM	Minor sedation in pigeons
	50 to 100 µg/kg medetomidine + 3 to 5 mg/kg ketamine; IM	Raptors
	25 to 75 µg/kg medetomidine + 2 to 4 mg/kg ketamine; IV	Raptors

Drug	Dosage	Indication/Species
	100 to 200 µg/kg medetomidine + 5 to 10 mg/kg ketamine; IM, IV	Geese
	*80 µg/kg medetomidine + 2 mg/kg ketamine; IM	Moderate to heavy sedation in young ostriches
Medetomidine + midazolam	80 µg/kg medetomidine + 0.5 mg/kg midazolam; IM	Minor sedation in pigeons
Medroxyprogesterone	18 to 50 mg/kg (according to size) once q 4 to 12 weeks; IM, SC 150 g = 50 mg/kg 150 to 300 g = 40 mg/kg 300 to 700 g = 30 mg/kg 700 g = 25 mg/kg Umbrella cockatoo = 18 mg/kg	To suppress ovulation, possibly to reduce feather picking
	5 to 50 mg/kg once or repeated in 4 to 6 weeks; SC, IM	Suppress reproductive behavior, feather picking
	0.1% in feed	To suppress ovulation in pigeons
Meloxicam	0.2 to 0.3 mg/kg once daily to bid; PO, IM; reduce as soon as possible to an effective maintenance dose	Analgesia, anti-inflammatory
Meperidine	1 to 5 mg/kg as needed; IM	Analgesia; psittacines
	1 to 3 mg/kg as needed; IM	Analgesia; raptors
Methylprednisolone	0.5 to 1 mg/kg; IM	Anti-inflammatory
	Stock solution of 1.4 mL of 40 mg/mL product in 7.5 mL lactulose;	To prevent seasonal recurrence of "Amazon foot necrosis" syndrome

(continued)

Drug	Dosage	Indication/Species
Methylprednisolone (cont.)	1 drop/week in problem month, 1 drop/month for remainder of year; PO	
Metoclopramide	0.5 mg/kg once daily to tid; IM, SC	Promote gastric motility
Metronidazole	10 to 50 mg/kg once daily to bid for up to 10 days; PO	Range of oral dosage—anaerobic, bacterial, and protozoal infections, psittacines, pigeons, raptors
	10 to 20 mg/kg bid **OR** 10 to 50 mg/kg once daily for 2 to 5 days; IM	Range of parenteral dosage—anaerobic, bacterial, and protozoal infections
	50 mg/kg once daily for 5 days; PO	Trichomoniasis in pigeons and doves
	*30 mg/kg once; PO	*Cochlosoma* infections in finches
Metronidazole (in food)	100 mg/kg of soft food	For canaries and small passerines
Metronidazole (in drinking water—product dissolves poorly)	100 mg/L in drinking water	For canaries and small passerines
	*40 mg/L drinking water for 3 days	*Cochlosoma* infections in finches
	1.5 g/gallon (330 mg/L) of drinking water for 7 days	Finches, canaries, small passerines for crop and sinus trichomoniasis
	40 mg to 2 g/L of drinking water for 3 days	*Cochlosoma* infections in finches
	4 g/gallon (800 mg/L) drinking water for 5 days	Trichomoniasis in pigeons
	200 to 400 mg/L drinking water for 5 days	Giardiasis in budgerigar nestlings
Mibolerone	10 µg/kg once; PO	To stop oviposition
Miconazole	10 mg/kg once daily for 6 to 12 days; IM	Aspergillosis in raptors and Humboldt penguins

Drug	Dosage	Indication/Species
	20 mg/kg tid; IV (slowly)	Systemic mycotic infections in psittacines
	Topically bid to tid	Mycotic infections of skin and mucous membranes
	2 mg IV formulation in 300 mL of acetylcysteine; via nebulization	Red-lored Amazon parrot
Midazolam	*2 to 6 mg/kg; IM	Bobwhite quail
	0.1 to 0.5 mg/kg; IM	Sedation
	1 to 2 mg/kg; IM, IV	Sedation in psittacines, swans
	2 to 4 mg/kg; IM	Geese
Minocycline	0.5% impregnated millet	Chlamydiosis in small psittacines, canaries
Monensin	90 g/ton feed	Poultry, quail; disseminated visceral coccidiosis in crane chicks
Moxidectin	0.2 mg/kg; PO, IM	Capillariasis in pigeons, parasites in raptors and owls
Naloxone	0.05 to 0.25 mg/kg; IM or slow IV	Opioid reversal (human dose)
Naltrexone	1.5 mg/kg bid	Psychological feather picking, psittacines
Neomycin	1 to 8 drops of the 50 mg/mL preparation per 28 mL of drinking water	Enteric infections
	1 to 4 drops/ounce (30 mL) drinking water (Biosol liquid)	
	5 g/gallon of drinking water	
Nortriptyline	2 mg/110 mL drinking water	Feather picking in psittacine birds
Nystatin	300,000 U/kg once daily to tid for 7 to 14 days; PO	Candidiasis of the oral cavity and gastrointestinal system

(continued)

Drug	Dosage	Indication/Species
Nystatin (cont.)	200,000 IU/kg of soft food	Candidiasis; canaries and small passerines
	100,000 IU/L in drinking water, for 3 to 6 weeks (canaries)	Candidiasis; canaries and small passerines, pigeons
	5,000 IU/bird bid; by gavage	"Megabacteriosis" in goldfinches
Oxacillin	100 mg/kg tid for 4 to 6 weeks; PO	Bacterial dermatitis
Oxfendazole	*10 mg/kg praziquantel + 10 mg/kg oxfendazole once, repeat each 6 to 8 weeks (commercial tablet formulation)	Nematodes and cestodes in pigeons and poultry
	40 mg/kg once daily; PO	
	10 to 40 mg/kg single dose; PO	Finches
Oxytetracycline	*50 to 100 mg/kg q 48 to 72 hours for 30 to 45 days; SC, IM (long-acting formulation)	Goffin's cockatoos, blue-fronted and orange-winged Amazon parrots, blue and gold macaws; for chlamydiosis
	*43 mg/kg once daily; IM	Ring-necked pheasants
	*16 mg/kg once daily; IM	Great horned owls
	*58 mg/kg once daily; IM	Amazon parrots
	152 mg/kg q 72 hours; SC (long-acting formulation)	*Pasteurella multocida* infection in turkeys
	1 to 1.5 g/gallon (263 to 396 mg/L) drinking water for 7 to 14 days	Chlamydiosis in pigeons
Oxytocin	0.2 to 2 IU/bird once; IM	Egg binding, uterine hemorrhage
	5 to 10 IU/kg single dose; IM	Egg binding

Drug	Dosage	Indication/Species
Pancreatic enzyme replacements	⅛ to ½ teaspoon/kg food or use as directed	Pancreatic insufficiency, maldigestion
Paromomycin	100 mg/kg for 5 days; PO in food	Cryptosporidiosis in Lady Gouldian finches
	100 mg/kg once daily for 7 days; PO	Cryptosporidiosis
Penicillamine	50 to 55 mg/kg bid; PO	Lead and zinc poisoning
Penicillin G	*50 mg/kg bid to tid; IM (potassium penicillin G)	Turkeys
	*100 mg procaine + 100 mg benza-thine penicillin/kg once daily or every second day; IM	Turkeys
Phenobarbital	1 to 5 mg/kg bid; PO	Seizure control
	1 to 7 mg/kg as needed; IV	Seizures due to 4-aminopyridine toxicity in pigeons
Phenylbutazone	3.5 to 7 mg/kg bid to tid; PO	Psittacines
	20 mg/kg tid; PO	Raptors
Piperacillin	*50 mg/kg tid; IV	Blue-fronted Amazon parrots
	*100 mg/kg tid; IM	Blue-fronted Amazon parrots
	*100 mg/kg q 4 to 6 hours; IM	Red-tailed hawks and great-horned owls (suggested for medium-sized raptors)
	50 to 200 mg/kg bid to qid; IM, IV	General range of recommendations
	100 mg/10 mL saline for nebulization; bid to qid for 10 to 30 minutes	Respiratory disease
	4 mg/macaw egg, 2 mg/smaller eggs, days 14, 18, and 22; into the air cell	To reduce embryo mortality

(continued)

Drug	Dosage	Indication/Species
Piperazine	100 to 500 mg/kg once, repeat in 10 to 14 days; PO	Ascarid nematodes in gallinaceous birds
	45 to 200 mg/kg once, repeat in 10 to 14 days; PO	Ascarid nematodes in waterfowl
	300 mg/gallon (79 mg/L) drinking water	Finches
Polymyxin B	333,000 IU (33.3 mg) in 5 mL saline, nebulize for 15 minutes; tid	Pneumonia and air sacculitis
	50,000 IU/kg of soft food or /L drinking water	For canaries and small passerines
Polysulfated glyco-saminoglycans	100 mg once weekly for 3 mo; IM	King vulture, frostbite and amputation of digits
	12.5 to 25 mg once; intra-articularly	Osteoarthritis in Palawan peacock pheasant, demoiselle crane
Pralidoxime chloride	10 to 30 mg/kg once, do not repeat; IM	Organophosphate toxicity in conjunction with atropine
Praziquantel	*10 mg/kg (tablet form) or 25 mg/kg (aqueous form); PO	*Raillietina tetragona* in chickens
	*8.5 mg/kg; IM or 11 mg/kg; SC	*R. tetragona* in chickens
	*10 mg/kg praziquantel + 10 mg/kg oxfendazole once, repeat each 6 to 8 weeks; PO	Nematodes and cestodes in pigeons and poultry
	10 to 20 mg/kg once, repeat in 10 to 14 days; PO	General recommendation, including finches
	5 to 9 mg/kg once, repeat in 10 to 14 days; IM	Psittacines

Drug	Dosage	Indication/Species
	9 to 10 mg/kg once daily; IM for 3 days, then PO for 11 days	Hepatic trematodes in a toucan, general recommendation
	10 to 20 mg/kg once daily for 10 to 14 days; PO	Hepatic parasites
	0.06 mg/bird (0.05 mL of suspension of 23 mg tablet in 20 mL water); PO	Enteric cestodes in Lady Gouldian finches
Prednisolone	2 to 4 mg/kg once; IM, IV	Shock, trauma, endotoxemia (immuno-suppressive)
	0.5 to 1 mg/kg once; IM	Anti-inflammatory
Prednisolone sodium succinate	0.5 to 1 mg/kg; IV, IM	Anti-inflammatory, for shock and head trauma at the upper dose
Prednisone	0.5 to 1 mg/kg bid; PO; decrease dose to a minimum effective level	Anti-inflammatory
Primaquine	0.03 mg/kg primaquine once daily for 3 days; PO + 10 mg/kg chloroquine loading dose, then 5 mg/kg at 6, 18, and 24 hours; PO	*Plasmodium* spp. malaria in penguins; in combination with chloroquine
	0.75 to 1 mg/kg primaquine once; PO + 25 mg/kg chloroquine initial dose, then 15 mg/kg at 12, 24, and 48 hours; PO	*Plasmodium* spp. malaria in pigeons; in combination with chloroquine

(continued)

Drug	Dosage	Indication/Species
Primaquine (cont.)	1 mg/kg primaquine + 10 mg/kg of chloroquine 1 day each week; in drinking water	To prevent seasonal malaria in budgerigars, canaries, and finches; in combination with chloroquine
Propofol	*Loading dose of 5 mg/kg and constant infusion of 0.5 mg/kg per minute; IV	Anesthesia; wild turkeys
	*Loading dose of 7 to 11 mg/kg and constant infusion of 0.7 to 1.1 mg/kg per minute; IV	Anesthesia; chickens
	*Loading dose of 3 mg/kg and constant infusion of 0.2 mg/kg per minute; IV	Anesthesia in juvenile ostriches previously sedated with medetomidine + ketamine
	*Loading dose of 8 to 10 mg/kg, boluses of 1 to 4 mg as required; IV	Mallard ducks
	14 mg/kg; IV	Anesthesia; pigeons
Prostaglandin E_2	0.2 mg/kg topically to the uterovaginal junction, once	To facilitate oviposition
Pyrantel pamoate	4.5 mg/kg once, repeat in 10 to 14 days; PO	Intestinal nematodes; general recommendation including finches
	20 to 25 mg/kg once; PO	Ascarids, tetramerids in pigeons
Pyrethrin products	Topical, light mist or dusting as needed	Ectoparasites, especially lice
Pyrimethamine	0.5 mg/kg bid for 30 days; PO	Sarcocystosis, toxoplasmosis, plasmodial malaria; in combination with a trimethoprim/sulfonamide combination

Drug	Dosage	Indication/Species
	0.5 mg/kg pyrimethamine bid; PO for 14 to 30 days + - trimethoprim-sulfamethazole or trimethoprim-sulfadiazine (30 mg/kg bid; PO for 14 or 30 days)	*Sarcocystis falcatula* in psittacines
	0.5 to 1 mg/kg pyrimethamine bid for 2 to 4 days, then decreased to 0.25 mg/kg bid for 30 days; PO + a trimethoprim/sulfonamide combination (5 mg/kg bid; IM or 30 to 100 mg/kg bid for 7 days; PO)	*Sarcocystis falcatula* in psittacines
Ranitidine	3 mg/kg bid to tid; PO	Treatment of gastric ulceration
Rifabutin	6 mg/kg once daily; PO + enrofloxacin (30 mg/kg once daily; PO) + clarithromycin (55 mg/kg once daily; PO) + ethambutol (30 mg/kg once daily; PO) for 6 months; drugs were compounded with powdered sugar and water to create a combined oral medication of practical volume	Budgerigar, combination treatment regimen for mycobacteriosis

(continued)

Drug	Dosage	Indication/Species
Rifabutin (cont.)	15 mg/kg once daily; PO + ethambutol (30 mg/kg once daily; PO) + ciprofloxacin (80 mg/kg once daily; PO) or enrofloxacin (30 mg/kg bid; PO) for a minimum of 6 months	Combination treatment regimen for mycobacteriosis
Rifampin	45 mg/kg once daily; PO + ethambutol (30 mg/kg once daily; PO) + isoniazid (30 mg/kg once daily; PO) for a minimum of 6 months	Combination treatment regimen for mycobacteriosis
	45 mg/kg once daily; PO + ethambutol (30 mg/kg once daily; PO) + clofazimine (6 mg/kg bid; PO) for a minimum of 6 months	Combination treatment regimen for mycobacteriosis
	45 mg/kg once daily; PO + ethambutol (30 mg/kg once daily; PO) + ciprofloxacin (80 mg/kg once daily; PO) or enrofloxacin (30 mg/kg bid; PO) for a minimum of 6 months	Combination treatment regimen for mycobacteriosis
	10 to 20 mg/kg once daily to bid; PO	Mycobacteriosis, must be in combination with other antimycobacterial drugs

Drug	Dosage	Indication/Species
Ronidazole	*1 g of 6% w/w product/L drinking water for 7 days	Motile protozoal infections of GIT in pigeons, budgerigars, canaries, and finches
	*10 mg/kg once daily for several days	Trichomoniasis in falcons
	*60 mg/L drinking water for 7 days	*Cochlosoma* in various finches
	6 to 10 mg/kg once daily; PO for 10 days	Protozoal infections in finches
	400 mg/kg of soft food	Canaries and small passerines
	50 to 400 mg/L of drinking water for 10 days	Flagellated protozoa of crop and GIT in tropical finches
Selenium (see Vitamin E + selenium)		
Sevoflurane	3% to 5% for induction, 0.5% to 2% or as required for maintenance	Inhalant anesthetic
Spectinomycin	*11 to 22 mg/kg; SC, q 5 days	*Pasteurella multocida* in turkeys
	*1 g powder (500 mg drug)/L drinking water	Mycoplasmosis in turkeys and chickens
	400 mg/kg of soft food	Finches and small passerines
	200 to 400 mg/L of drinking water	Finches and small passerines
	20 mL/gallon drinking water for 5 to 10 days	Gram-negative enteric infections
	200 mg/15 mL saline for nebulization	Pneumonia and air sacculitis
Stanozolol	25 to 50 mg/kg once or twice weekly; IM	Anabolic steroid
	2 mg tablet/120 mL drinking water	

(continued)

Drug	Dosage	Indication/Species
Streptomycin	10 to 50 mg/kg bid to tid; IM	Galliformes, pigeons, large birds; do not use in pet birds
Sucralfate	25 mg/kg q 8 hours; PO	Gastric protectant, psittacines
Sulfachlorpyridazine	¼ to ½ teaspoon/L drinking water for 5 to 10 days	*Escherichia coli* and other enteric infections
	300 mg/L drinking water for 7 to 10 days	Coccidiosis in pigeons
	400 mg/L drinking water for 7 to 10 days	To control secondary infections during circovirus outbreaks in pigeons
	0.25 to 1 teaspoon Vetisulid powder per U.S. gallon (3.8 L) drinking water	Enteric coccidiosis in finches
Sulfadimethoxine	25 to 50 mg/kg once daily, 3 days on, 3 days off, 3 days on	Coccidiosis in raptors
	312 to 375 mg/L drinking water for 1 day, then 188 mg/L for 4 days	Coccidiosis in pigeons
	200 mg/mL saline for nebulization	Pneumonia and air sacculitis
Sulfadimidine	150 mg/L in drinking water	Coccidiosis in canaries and small passerines
Sulfamethazine	0.1% to 0.2% in drinking water for 5 days; or for 3 days on, 3 days off, 3 days on	Coccidiosis in budgerigars
	0.5% in drinking water for 4 days	Coccidiosis in pigeons
	375 mg/L drinking water for 1 day, then 188 to 250 mg/L for 4 days	Coccidiosis in pigeons

Drug	Dosage	Indication/Species
	30 mg/30 mL drinking water	Small psittacines
Sulfaquinoxaline	500 mg/L drinking water for 6 days, off 2 days, on 6 days	Coccidiosis in pigeons
Terbinafine	10 to 15 mg/kg once daily to bid for up to 4 months; PO	Antifungal in psittacines
	1 mg/mL by nebulization for 20 minutes tid	Respiratory mycosis in psittacines
Testosterone	8 mg/kg once, repeat weekly for anemia as needed; IM	Increase male libido, anemia, feather problems, debilitation
	2.5 mg/kg weekly for 6 weeks; IM	Canaries
	Stock solution of 2 × 10 mg tablets **OR** 100 mg of injectable formulation in 30 mL water; 5 drops of this per 30 mL drinking water, provide daily for 6 weeks; if no response is seen after 2 weeks, double the dose	To induce male canaries to sing
Tetracycline	200 to 250 mg/kg once daily to bid; PO	Initial therapy for chlamydiosis
	50 mg/kg tid; PO	Psittacines (empirical)
	250 mg of syrup/cup (237 mL) of soft food	In conjunction with switching to medicated pelleted feed

(continued)

Drug	Dosage	Indication/Species
Tetracycline (cont.)	1 teaspoon powder (10 g/6.4 ounces)/ gallon (3.8 L) drinking water for 5 to 10 days, change water 2 to 3 times daily	
Thiabendazole	250 to 500 mg/kg once, repeat in 10 to 14 days; PO	Ascarids
	100 mg/kg once daily for 7 to 10 days; PO	*Syngamus trachea*
Tiamulin	*100 g/360 L drinking water (125 mg/L, 278 mg/L) for 3 to 5 days (Rodotium 45% water-soluble granules)	Prevention of chronic respiratory disease in chickens and turkeys
	*100 g/180 L drinking water (250 mg/L, 556 g/L) for 3 to 5 days (Rodotium 45% water-soluble granules)	Treatment of chronic respiratory disease in chickens and turkeys
	250 mg powder/L drinking water	Mycoplasmosis in pigeons
	1 g powder/kg of feed	Mycoplasmosis in pigeons
Ticarcillin	150 to 200 mg/kg bid to qid; IM, IV	Systemic antibiotic therapy
Ticarcillin + clavulanate	200 mg/kg bid; IM	Part of supportive care in a Buffon's macaw
Tiletamine + zolazepam	2 to 10 mg/kg; IM	Sedation and anesthesia in ratites
(Telazol)	1 to 3 mg/kg; IV	Sedation and anesthesia in ratites
Tobramycin	2.5 to 10 mg/kg bid; IM	Pheasants, cranes, psittacines, raptors

Drug	Dosage	Indication/Species
Toltrazuril	75 mg/L of drinking water for 2 days each week, 4-week treatment	Atoxoplasmosis in canaries
	10 mg/kg once daily for 4 days; PO	*Caryospora neofalconis* infection in raptors
Trimethoprim + sulfonamide (parenteral)	15 to 30 mg/kg bid; IM	
	50 to 100 mg/kg bid; SC, IM	
Trimethoprim + sulfonamide (oral)	10 to 30 mg/kg bid to qid; PO (sulfamethoxazole)	Psittacines
	50 to 100 mg/kg bid; PO	
	60 mg/kg bid; PO	Pigeons
	1 × 30 mg tablet/ pigeon bid for 7 to 10 days (sulfadiazine)	Pasteurellosis in pigeons
	25 mg/kg once daily for 5 days; PO	Coccidiosis in mynahs and toucans
Trimethoprim + sulfonamide (in drinking water)	360 mg/L drinking water for 10 to 14 days (sulfamethoxazole)	Pigeons; to prevent secondary abscesses around pox lesions
	450 to 900 mg/L drinking water for 10 to 14 days (sulfamethoxazole)	Pasteurellosis in pigeons
	1,800 to 3,600 mg/ U.S. gallon (476 to 951 mg/L) drinking water (Sulfatrim)	Pasteurellosis in pigeons
	50 to 100 mg/L drinking water (dosage described both as trimethoprim portion and as total dose)	Finches, canaries, small passerines

(continued)

Drug	Dosage	Indication/Species
Trimethoprim + sulfonamide (in feed)	100 mg/kg of soft food (dosage described as trimethoprim portion and as total dose)	Finches, canaries, small passerines
Trimethoprim + sulfonamide + pyrimethamine	30 mg/kg bid; IM + pyrimethamine (0.5 mg/kg bid; PO) for 2 weeks (sulfadiazine)	Sarcocystosis in parrots
	30 mg/kg bid; PO + pyrimethamine (0.5 mg/kg bid; PO) for 30 days (sulfamethoxazole)	Sarcocystosis in parrots
	30 to 100 mg/kg bid; PO, bid for 7 days or longer pyrimethamine (0.5 to 1 mg/kg bid; PO for 2 to 4 days, then 0.25 mg/kg bid; PO for 30 days	Sarcocystosis in parrots
Tylosin	*15 mg/kg tid; IM	Cranes
	*25 mg/kg qid; IM	Bobwhite quail, pigeons
	*25 mg/kg tid; IM	Emus
	10 to 40 mg/kg bid to tid; IM	General range of dosage
	*1 g in 50 mL DMSO, nebulize for 1 hour	Bobwhite quail, pigeons
	100 mg in 10 mL saline; nebulize for 10 to 60 minutes bid	For nebulization
	400 mg/kg of soft food	Finches, canaries and small passerines
	Up to 300 g/ton of feed	*Mycoplasma synoviae* in poultry
	250 g/8.8 ounces powder; 1:10 in water as eye spray; bid to tid	Conjunctivitis

Drug	Dosage	Indication/Species
	250 to 400 mg/L drinking water	Finches, canaries, and small passerines
	0.5 mg/mL drinking water for 4 to 8 days	*Mycoplasma* spp. in poultry
	1 mg/mL drinking water for more than 21 days	*Mycoplasma gallisepticum* conjunctivitis in house finches
	250 g/8.8 ounces powder; ¼ teaspoon/8 ounces, or 2 teaspoon/gallon (3.8 L) of drinking water; 10 days on, 5 days off, 10 days on	Chronic respiratory disease
Vecuronium	0.2 mg/kg; IM	Skeletal muscle relaxant for detailed ophthalmic evaluation under isoflurane anesthesia
Vitamin A	50,000 U/kg twice during the first week, then weekly as needed; IM	Vitamin A deficiency
Vitamin A, D_3, E (Injacom 100)	0.3 to 0.7 mL/kg; IM; can double dose first treatment, then treat once weekly as required	Vitamin deficiency, supportive care
Vitamin B complex	Dose by thiamine content, 10 to 30 mg/kg once per week; IM	
Vitamin B_1 (thiamine)	1 to 2 mg/kg daily in food	Raptors, penguins, cranes
	50 mg/kg IM	Falcons with lead poisoning, supportive care
Vitamin B_{12}	250 to 500 µg/kg once per week; SC, IM	General supportive care
	125 mg/kg IM	Supportive care; falcons

(*continued*)

Drug	Dosage	Indication/Species
Vitamin C	20 to 40 mg/kg once daily to once weekly; IM	General supportive care
Vitamin D (see Vitamin A, D₃, E)		
Vitamin E	200 to 400 IU/day; PO	Great blue heron
Vitamin E + selenium	0.06 mg/kg selenium q 72 hours; IM	Myopathy
	0.06 mg/kg selenium every 3 to 14 days; IM	Neuropathy in cockatiels
	0.05 to 0.1 mg selenium/kg q 14 days; IM	
	0.1 mL/kg of preparation containing 1 mg selenium + 50 mg vitamin E/mL; IM	0.01 mL for cockatiel 0.03 mL for African gray parrot 0.05 mL for eclectus parrot 0.1 mL for macaw
Vitamin K	0.2 to 5 mg/kg 1 to 3 times or as needed; PO, IM	Coagulopathies
	10 to 20 mg/kg bid; PO, IM	Psittacines
	10 to 12.5 mg/kg bid for 4 days; PO, SC	Coagulopathy in pelicans
Xylazine	See ketamine	Anesthesia combined with ketamine
Yohimbine	0.1 to 1 mg/kg; IV, IM	Reversal agent for xylazine

AVMA, American Veterinary Medical Association.
*indicates dosages based on pharmacokinetic or controlled efficacy trials or licensed for use in a particular species.

Handbook of Veterinary Drugs, Third Edition, edited by Dana Allen,
Lippincott Williams & Wilkins, Baltimore. © 2005

Section 19

Description of Drugs for Birds

ACETIC ACID/VINEGAR

INDICATIONS: Acetic acid (5% apple cider or white vinegar) is used
in avian practice to lower the pH of drinking water or hand-feeding
formulas to prevent gastrointestinal overgrowth of *Candida* spp., particularly in birds that are stressed or undergoing concurrent antibiotic
therapy. Provision of treated water or food may also reduce the number of yeast in birds that are positive for organisms on fecal Gram
stain but are not showing clinical signs of overt disease.

ACETYLCYSTEINE

INDICATIONS: Acetylcysteine (Mucomyst ✽ ★) is a mucolytic agent
used to help liquefy abnormal viscous or inspissated mucous secretions of the respiratory tract and eye. The drug has been used in birds
by nebulization and direct nasal and sinus flushes. Acetylcysteine may
be used combined with an antibiotic, e.g., amikacin, and aminophylline
(for nebulization). For more information, see ACETYLCYSTEINE in
the Small Animal section.

ADVERSE AND COMMON SIDE EFFECTS: Dyspnea, lethargy,
tachycardia, and edema of the eyelids have been described in neonatal birds after nebulization with acetylcysteine.

DRUG INTERACTIONS: Formation of a precipitate or a change in the color or clarity of the drug mixture may occur when acetyl-cysteine is combined with tetracycline, oxytetracycline, chlortetracycline, or hydrogen peroxide, suggesting incompatibility of these drugs.

ACETYLSALICYLIC ACID

INDICATIONS: Acetylsalicylic acid (ArthriCare ★, Entrophen ♥, and many others) has been used empirically in birds for its analgesic and anti-inflammatory properties. A pharmacokinetic study using sodium salicylate in young ostriches showed that after intravenous injection of 25 mg/kg the drug was rapidly cleared, with a plasma elimination half-life of only 1.32 hours. A therapeutic plasma concentration above 50 μg/mL was present at only the 15-minute assessment point after drug administration. Sodium salicylate has been used in poultry to reduce lameness and associated pain. For more information, see ASPIRIN in the Small Animal section.

ACTH

INDICATIONS: ACTH, or corticotropin (ACTH ♥, A.C.T.H. ♥, Cortrosyn ♥ ★), is a polypeptide hormone secreted by the anterior pituitary. Cosyntropin is a synthetic analog that is preferred for use in testing for adrenocortical insufficiency. Each 0.25 mg of cosyntropin is equivalent to 25 U (25 mg) of corticotropin. Cosyntropin is injected IM to stimulate a rise in serum corticosterone levels. In birds, serum cortisol does not elevate in response to exogenous ACTH administration.

ADVERSE AND COMMON SIDE EFFECTS: Hypersensitivity reactions occur rarely in humans.

DRUG INTERACTIONS: Patients should not receive pretest doses of cortisone or hydrocortisone as these will interfere with diagnostic testing.

SUPPLIED AS HUMAN PRODUCTS: COSYNTROPIN
For injection containing 0.25 mg/mL (Cortrosyn ♥ ★)
1.0 mg/mL (Synacthen ♥)
For injection containing 1 mg/ampule cosyntropin/zinc hydroxide (Synacthen Depot ♥)

SUPPLIED AS VETERINARY PRODUCTS: CORTICOTROPIN
For injection containing 40 and 80 U ACTH in a repository preparation (A.C.T.H. ♥, A.C.T.H. I.U. ♥)

ACYCLOVIR

INDICATIONS: Acyclovir (Avirax ✤, Zovirax ✤ ★) is an antiviral drug with activity against various herpes viruses and cytomegalovirus. In birds, the drug is used to reduce mortality during outbreaks of Pacheco's disease, a herpes viral infection. Treatment is most effective in birds that are not yet showing clinical disease. The oral form of acyclovir, available in capsules, is relatively insoluble in water. It is best administered by direct oral gavage, although in large aviaries treatment of drinking water and feed has been used. The water-soluble sodium salt intended for IV use has been given IM. Birds should be treated for a minimum of 7 days.

ADVERSE AND COMMON SIDE EFFECTS: An IM injection of the sodium salt can result in hemorrhage and muscle necrosis. Phlebitis commonly follows IV administration. The reconstituted solution is unstable and should be divided into aliquots and frozen for future treatments. The drug has not produced toxic effects even at 240 mg/kg administered 3 times daily. In humans, headaches, vomiting, and diarrhea are the most common adverse reactions reported. Nephrotoxicity and, rarely, neurologic signs can occur with parenteral administration. Because acyclovir is incompletely absorbed from the gastrointestinal system, oral overdosage and toxicity is unlikely.

DRUG INTERACTIONS: Amphotericin B and ketoconazole increase the effectiveness of acyclovir against some viral diseases in humans.

SUPPLIED AS HUMAN PRODUCTS:
Capsules containing 200 mg (Acyclovir ★, Zovirax ★)
Tablets containing 200 mg (Avirax ✤, Gen-Acyclovir ✤, Nu-Acyclovir ✤, Zovirax ★, Zovirax Oral ✤), 400 mg (Acyclovir ★, Apo-Acyclovir ✤, Avirax ✤, Gen-Acyclovir ✤, Nu-Acyclovir ✤, Zovirax ★, Zovirax Oral ✤), and 800 mg (Acyclovir ★, Apo-Acyclovir ✤, Gen-Acyclovir ✤, Nu-Acyclovir ✤, Zovirax Oral ✤)
Suspension containing 200 mg/5 mL (Zovirax ✤ ★)
For injection containing 500 mg or 1 g of acyclovir sodium (Zovirax ✤ ★)
Cream containing 50 mg/g (Zovirax ✤)
Ointment containing 50 mg/g (Zovirax ✤ ★)

ALLOPURINOL

INDICATIONS: Allopurinol (Aloprim ★, Purinol ✤, Zyloprim ✤ ★) inhibits the enzyme xanthine oxidase and blocks the formation and urinary excretion of uric acid. For more information, see ALLOPURINOL in the Small Animal section.

Allopurinol has been used in birds to reduce circulating uric acid levels and treat articular gout. Improvement may be seen after 2 to 3 days of treatment; however, not all patients respond. The drug is well absorbed after oral administration. Clinical success with allopurinol has been described using direct oral administration and medication of the drinking water. Allopurinol tablets can be crushed and made into suspension with sterile water or simple syrup.

ADVERSE AND COMMON SIDE EFFECTS: Allopurinol was administered to red-tailed hawks to prevent postprandial hyperuricemia; however, in three of six birds marked increases in serum uric acid and visceral gout occurred. The other three birds showed no effect of the drug. This suggests there may be considerable species and individual variability in efficacy and toxicity.

DRUG INTERACTIONS: A number of significant drug interactions exist. See ALLOPURINOL in the Small Animal section.

AMIKACIN

INDICATIONS: Amikacin (Amiglyde-V ✿ ★, Amikin ✿ ★, Amiject D ★) is an aminoglycoside antibiotic indicated in the treatment of infections caused by many gram-negative bacteria including susceptible strains of *Escherichia coli, Klebsiella* spp., *Proteus* spp., and *Pseudomonas* spp. For more information, see AMIKACIN and AMINOGLYCOSIDE ANTIBIOTICS in the Small Animal section.

Amikacin is the aminoglycoside of choice in avian medicine and is often recommended for initial therapy when urgent antimicrobial therapy is required. It is commonly used in pediatric patients where it may be injected SC. In a pharmacokinetic study in African gray parrots, amikacin given IM was rapidly absorbed with a peak serum level reached by 45 minutes after injection. The plasma elimination half-life was similar to that found in other vertebrates. Almost all detectable serum amikacin was eliminated by 8 hours after injection. Based on pharmacokinetic calculations, no accumulation was predicted at an IM or IV dosage of 10 to 20 mg/kg every 8 to 12 hours. Similar pharmacokinetic data were recorded in a study in cockatiels. At a dosage of 15 mg/kg IM every 12 hours, peak and trough levels of 27.3 and 0.6 μg/mL, respectively, were reached. Human guidelines for peak and trough amikacin levels are 15 to 30 μg/mL and 5 to 10 μg/mL, respectively. In ostriches, 2.12 mg/kg of amikacin injected subcutaneously resulted in lower blood levels than did IM injection into the muscles of the axial or thigh regions.

ADVERSE AND COMMON SIDE EFFECTS: Amikacin is generally considered less nephrotoxic than gentamicin; however, toxic effects have been described in birds. Although some sources recommend dosages up to 40 mg/kg, an Amazon parrot given 40 mg/kg twice daily IM developed polydipsia and polyuria on the second day of treatment. These signs persisted for 3 weeks after treatment ended. Mild polyuria and polydipsia and elevated creatinine phosphokinase (CPK) and aspartate aminotransferase (AST) levels were also noted in orange-winged Amazon parrots given a dose of 13 mg/kg IM every 8 hours, or 20 mg/kg IM every 12 hours. Concurrent administration of balanced electrolyte fluids is recommended to reduce the chance of renal damage, especially in neonates. Measurement of peak and trough blood antibiotic concentrations would help prevent toxicity. Pain on injection, transient lameness after injection, and elevated CPK levels have been described in ostriches. The toxicity of amikacin is enhanced under a number of conditions. See AMINOGLYCOSIDE ANTIBIOTICS in the Small Animal section for information on specific drug interactions.

DRUG INTERACTIONS: Amikacin is often used in combination with penicillins (e.g., carbenicillin, piperacillin, and ticarcillin) and with cephalosporins (e.g., ceftazidime and cefotaxime). Amikacin plus enrofloxacin has been used in the treatment of avian mycobacteriosis, although more complex combination drug therapy is recommended for long-term treatment.

AMINOPENTAMIDE HYDROGEN SULFATE

INDICATIONS: Aminopentamide hydrogen sulfate (Centrine ★) is an anticholinergic drug indicated for the treatment of acute abdominal visceral spasm, pylorospasm, nausea, vomiting, and diarrhea in dogs and cats. The actions of this drug are similar to those of atropine, with lesser mydriatic and salivary effects.

Aminopentamide hydrogen sulfate has been used to control acute vomiting in psittacines.

ADVERSE AND COMMON SIDE EFFECTS: Aminopentamide hydrogen sulfate delays gastric emptying and should not be used in cases of pyloric obstruction. Use of this drug may mask clinical signs indicative of gastrointestinal blockage.

SUPPLIED AS VETERINARY PRODUCTS:
For injection containing 0.5 mg/mL (Centrine ★)
Tablets containing 0.2 mg (Centrine ★)

AMINOPHYLLINE

INDICATIONS: Aminophylline (Phyllocontin ✽ ★ and generics) is a bronchodilator principally used for the management of cough due to bronchospasm. It has mild inotropic properties and mild, transient diuretic activity. For more information, see AMINOPHYLLINE in the Small Animal section.

In birds, aminophylline has been used for nebulization in combination with antibiotics and/or acetylcysteine. Because aminophylline solutions are alkaline, they may be incompatible with and precipitate other medications.

ADVERSE AND COMMON SIDE EFFECTS: A variety of side effects and drug interactions have been described in small animals. For more information, see AMINOPHYLLINE in the Small Animal section.

SUPPLIED AS HUMAN PRODUCTS:
For injection containing 25 mg/mL (19.7 mg/mL theophylline) and 50 mg/mL (39.4 mg/mL theophylline)

AMOXICILLIN

INDICATIONS: Amoxicillin (Amoxi-Tabs ★, Amoxi-Drop ★, Amoxi-Inject ★, Amoxil ♣ ★, Moxilean ♣, Robamox-V ★) is indicated for the treatment of superficial and systemic bacterial infections. For more information, see AMOXICILLIN in the Small Animal section.

Pharmacokinetic studies have been carried out in a number of species of birds, including pigeons, chickens, and ducks. Parenteral amoxicillin administration provided higher and more predictable antibiotic levels than did oral administration. In pigeons, oily parenteral formulations resulted in a lower peak plasma level, but were more slowly excreted and, therefore, longer lasting as compared to the sodium salt. Tissue levels were greater than those in extravascular fluids. Using an IM dose of 100 mg/kg of the aqueous formulations, amoxicillin had a greater bioavailability (57%) and tissue penetration than similar dosages of ampicillin (bioavailability 26%). In pigeons the use of oral tablets did not produce reliable antibiotic levels; greater bioavailability was seen with capsular formulations.

In canaries given amoxicillin in feed (500 mg/kg food) or water (300 mg/L) mean blood levels of 1.8 and 1.09 µg/mL were reached.

General recommendations in the literature often recommend much lower dosages and less frequent administration than those suggested by pharmacokinetic studies. For example, the elimination half-life of oral amoxicillin in pigeons in one study was only 0.9 hours, and in canaries it was 0.5 hours.

AMOXICILLIN + CLAVULANATE

INDICATIONS: Amoxicillin combined with clavulanate (Clavamox ♣ ★), a β-lactamase inhibitor, extends the bactericidal spectrum of amoxicillin to include many β-lactamase–producing organisms. The combination diffuses readily into most body tissues with the exception of brain and spinal fluid. For more information, see CLAVAMOX and PENICILLIN ANTIBIOTICS in the Small Animal section.

A multiple dose pharmacokinetic trial in blue-fronted Amazon parrots suggested a dosage of 125 mg/kg (combined amoxicillin + clavulanate) at approximately 8 hour intervals would result in plasma levels effective against many bacteria. The elimination half-life for the amoxicillin portion of the drug was similar to that described in pigeons in a previous study.

An experimental trial evaluated the safety and efficacy of amoxicillin + clavulanate in pigeons. Ten birds were given a 125 mg tablet PO once daily for 7 days. The only clinical abnormalities noted were 9 episodes of regurgitation and pink or red-brown discoloration of the feces. After 7 days of treatment no bacteria were isolated from the feces of 4/10 birds, in comparison with the isolation of *Escherichia coli* and or *Streptococcus faecalis* from all 10 birds before treatment commenced, and from the 10 control birds. Treatment did not seem to affect the development of lesions resulting from the inoculation of *Staphylococcus aureus* into the foot pad of 5 birds receiving antibiotics. Pharmacokinetic parameters for the drug were not evaluated.

AMPHOTERICIN B

INDICATIONS: Amphotericin B (Amphocin ★, Fungizone ✿ ★) is an effective fungicidal agent that has been the traditional first-line treatment for a variety of systemic mycotic infections, including "megabacterial" (avian gastric yeast) infection. For more information, see AMPHOTERICIN B in the Small Animal section.

Amphotericin B is used for the treatment of aspergillosis and other systemic fungal infections in many species of birds, particularly raptors, penguins, and psittacines. The drug can be administered IV, intratracheally, or by nebulization. The intraosseous route has been suggested when venous access is not available; however, its efficacy has not been proven. When used via nebulization, amphotericin B is poorly absorbed by the respiratory epithelium and has a primarily topical effect. It has been suggested that fluconazole and clotrimazole may be more effective than amphotericin B for nebulization. Amphotericin B can also be used topically for oral candidiasis that is refractory to nystatin. Protocols for the treatment of systemic or severe fungal infections often include initial intravenous treatment with amphotericin B, followed or combined with oral itraconazole and nebulization with compounds such as clotrimazole. One case report describes the combined use of systemic fluconazole and nebulized clotrimazole for the apparently successful treatment of cryptococcal lesions in the air sacs of a sulfur-crested cockatoo.

Plasma levels above the minimal inhibitory concentration for *Aspergillus fumigatus* were reached in turkeys, great horned owls, and red-tailed hawks given IV amphotericin B; however, clearance of the drug from the bloodstream was extremely rapid suggesting multiple daily dosing was required. Intratracheal injection of 1.5 mg/kg did not produce measurable plasma levels.

Orally administered amphotericin B appears to be one of the more effective drugs for the treatment of "megabacteriosis" (avian gastric yeast infection). Thirty budgerigars positive on fecal smears for "megabacteria" were administered 5 mg/kg of amphotericin B twice daily by crop gavage for 10 days. Nineteen birds (63%) were fecal negative after 5 days of treatment and 28 (93%) were negative after 10 days. In a second study, 98% effective treatment was obtained administering amphotericin B in the drinking water (1 g/L for 22 days) in two large budgie aviaries. In both studies, the percentage of "megabacteria" positive birds increased after treatment was completed, suggesting either reinfection or reemergence of the disease. The possibility of amphotericin-resistant strains was also considered.

Crystalline amphotericin B is insoluble in water. The drug is combined with sodium desoxycholate to form a mixture that provides a colloidal dispersion for intravenous infusion following reconstitution. The drug is reconstituted using sterile water into a 3% suspension with a pH of 6 to 8. Reconstituted amphotericin B is sensitive to light and is inactivated at low pH. Once reconstituted, amphotericin B has a shelf life of only a few hours at room temperature and approximately 1 week if refrigerated. The drug can be reconstituted with sterile water and frozen in aliquots, then diluted in 5% dextrose or water as necessary for IV use or nebulization, respectively. More stable water-based suspensions have been compounded using products such as cellulose gum. Amphotericin B should not be combined with saline or other electrolyte solutions to prevent precipitation and crystal formation. Intratracheal and intranasal administration of improperly prepared product has been associated with severe tissue reactions. Liposomal formulations are also available.

ADVERSE AND COMMON SIDE EFFECTS: Amphotericin B may be nephrotoxic and may induce bone marrow suppression; however, there have been no reports of these problems occurring in birds. No evidence of renal toxicity was seen in turkeys given IV amphotericin B at the following doses: 1.5 mg/kg once, 1 mg/kg once daily for 3 days; and in great horned owls and red-tailed hawks given three IV injections of 1.5 mg/kg at 2-hour intervals. Rapid IV injection of doses above 1.0 mg/kg resulted in transitory incoordination and mild convulsions. The use of amphotericin B as a nasal flush for 14 days in an African gray parrot resulted in severe inflammation and necrosis of the sinuses and adjacent muscle and led to the bird's death. Improper reconstitution and crystal formation may have been responsible for these reactions. Concern was also raised that the drug may have been absorbed through inflamed tissue, creating a risk for systemic (i.e., renal) toxicity.

DRUG INTERACTIONS: Amphotericin B can be used in combination with other antifungal agents such as itraconazole or flucytosine.

SUPPLIED AS HUMAN PRODUCTS:
For IV injection containing 50 mg/vial (Amphocin ★, Fungizone ✤ ★)
For IV injection (liposome formulation) containing 50 mg/vial (AmBisome ★)
For IV injection containing 2.5 mg/mL (Fungizone ✤) and 5 mg/mL (Albelcet ✤ ★)

AMPICILLIN

INDICATIONS: Ampicillin (Omnipen ★, Polyflex ✤ ★, Principen ★) is indicated in the treatment of bacterial diseases, including some *Pasteurella* spp. infections. For more information, see AMPICILLIN in the Small Animal section.

Pharmacokinetic parameters vary among species, based on studies carried out in pigeons, Amazon parrots, blue-napped parrots, emus, and chickens. After intravenous injection of ampicillin, elimination half-lives of 0.65 hours and 10 to 15 minutes were obtained from pigeons (100 mg/kg) and chickens (dose not specified). Half-lives obtained from studies using the IM route ranged from 0.5 hour in chickens (25 mg/kg) to 1.67 hours in emus (dose not specified). Sodium ampicillin injected IM at 100 mg/mL produced substantially lower peak plasma levels in pigeons (13.7 µg/mL) than in Amazon parrots (58.3 µg/mL).

The formulation of parenteral products also influences absorption and blood concentrations. In pigeons, the bioavailability of sodium ampicillin administered IM at 100 mg/kg was low (26%). The use of oily ampicillin suspensions resulted in greater bioavailability and longer persistence in plasma, but lower peak plasma concentrations than did administration of the sodium salt. The authors of these studies concluded that amoxicillin is preferable to ampicillin for IM use in pigeons.

Although dosages for oral administration of ampicillin are commonly found, variable or poor absorption reduces the usefulness of this drug. The absorption and subsequent bioavailability of ampicillin is highly dependent on drug formulation: capsule formulations provided similar pharmacokinetic results to administration of oral solutions; whereas tablets were unlikely to provide predictable blood ampicillin levels. It has been recommended that ampicillin should only be administered orally to pigeons to treat infections within the digestive tract. Despite these concerns, ampicillin was found to be more effective than erythromycin, enrofloxacin, or trimethoprim (all drugs administered in the drinking water) in preventing morbidity in pigeons experimentally infected with *Streptococcus bovis*.

AMPROLIUM

INDICATIONS: Amprolium (Amprol ♣, Corid ★) is an antiprotozoal agent and coccidiostat. For more information, see AMPROLIUM in the Small or Large Animal sections.

Amprolium is used for the treatment of enteric coccidiosis in a variety of avian species. Drug resistance has been described in several groups of birds after repeated use, and for some coccidia found in mynahs and toucans.

ADVERSE AND COMMON SIDE EFFECTS: Thiamine-responsive seizures were reported in a juvenile merlin with enteric *Caryospora neofalconis* that was treated orally once a day with amprolium for a total of 16 consecutive days: 6 days at 22 mg/kg, then 10 days at 7.5 mg/kg.

ASCORBIC ACID

INDICATIONS: Ascorbic acid or vitamin C (Apo-C ♣, Redoxon ♣, generics, and many others) is essential for the synthesis and maintenance of collagen and intercellular ground substance of body tissues, blood vessels, bone, cartilage, tendons, and teeth. It is also important in wound healing and resistance to infection. It may influence the immune response. For more information, see ASCORBIC ACID in the Small Animal section.

Ascorbic acid has been used in the general supportive care of debilitated avian patients.

SUPPLIED AS VETERINARY PRODUCTS:
For injection containing 250 mg/mL (Ascorbic Acid Injection ♣, Ascorbic Acid Inj. U.S.P. ♣, Centravite-C ♣, Sodium Ascorbate ♣)

SUPPLIED AS HUMAN PRODUCTS:
Tablets containing 100, 250, 500, or 1,000 mg (♣ ★)
For injection containing 222 mg/mL (Generic ★), 250 mg/mL (Generic ★), and 500 mg/mL (Generic ★, Cecore 500 ★, Cee-500 ★, Mega-C/A Plus ★)

ATIPAMEZOLE

INDICATIONS: Atipamezole (Antisedan ♣ ★) is a synthetic α-adrenergic antagonist marketed for the reversal of the sedative and analgesic effects of medetomidine hydrochloride. It has been used to reverse medetomidine in a wide variety of avian species including psittacines, chickens, ostriches, and mallard ducks. Atipamezole (as Antisedan) is generally given on a volume-per-volume basis (milliliter for milliliter) of medetomidine (as Domitor) administered, which is equivalent to a dosage of 5 times the medetomidine given on a milligram to milligram basis. In dogs, calculated dosages of atipamezole are based on body surface rather than body weight. The recommended route of administration is intramuscularly, but in an anesthetic study in ostriches the dose of atipamezole was divided and half given subcutaneously and half intravenously. Rapid recoveries are reported. For more information, see ATIPAMEZOLE in the Small Animal section.

ATRACURIUM

INDICATIONS: Atracurium (Atracurium Besylate ♣, Atracurium Besylate Injection ★, Tracrium ♣ ★) is a nondepolarizing neuromuscular blocking agent used in conjunction with general anesthesia to produce muscle relaxation during surgery. In avian medicine, atracurium has been recommended to eliminate ocular and periocular movement during ophthalmic surgery. In chickens, slow intravenous administration of 0.25 mg/kg resulted in a substantial depression of the twitch response and clinically useful relaxation lasting for an average of 20 minutes. Reversal was obtained using slow intravenous injection of edrophonium at a dose of 0.5 mg/kg. For more information, see ATRACURIUM in the Small Animal section.

ATROPINE

INDICATIONS: Atropine ♣ ★ is an anticholinergic, antispasmodic, and mydriatic drug also used to treat organophosphate toxicity. For more information, see ATROPINE in the Small Animal section.

In birds, atropine can be used as a preanesthetic agent or during an anesthetic protocol to prevent or treat bradycardia, although it may cause thickening of tracheal secretions and therefore predispose to blockage of an endotracheal tube. Atropine is used for the treatment of organophosphate and carbamate toxicity, to control vomiting, and as an antispasmodic. Atropine is not effective for inducing mydriasis in birds as the iris is composed of striated rather than smooth muscle.

ADVERSE AND COMMON SIDE EFFECTS: Thickening of tracheal secretions during anesthesia may result in the development of mucous plugs within the endotracheal tube. Gastrointestinal paralysis or stasis may become worse after treatment with atropine.

AZITHROMYCIN

INDICATIONS: Azithromycin (Zithromax ♣ ★) is a semisynthetic macrolide antibiotic with a narrow spectrum of activity that includes chlamydiae, mycoplasmas, and some streptococci and staphylococci. The drug accumulates in tissue and has a prolonged elimination half-life. In human medicine, a single dose of azithromycin is used to treat uncomplicated venereal infection caused by *Chlamydia trachomatis*. Azithromycin combined with ethambutol and either ciprofloxacin or rifabutin is recommended for the prophylaxis and treatment of *Mycobacterium avium* complex infections in HIV patients.

Azithromycin has been used in birds to treat chlamydial and mycoplasmal infections and may be useful for treating mycobacteriosis. Clinical concerns exist as to its effectiveness in eliminating *Chlamydophila psittaci* organisms from infected birds. Lactulose and water have been used as the base for compounding oral suspensions. Veterinarians differ in their willingness to treat avian mycobacteriosis due to the difficulty in ensuring that the infection is fully eliminated and concerns over the potential for zoonotic spread of the disease under certain conditions.

Preliminary pharmacokinetic trials have been carried out in mealy Amazon parrots and cockatiels. In the parrots, large differences in some pharmacokinetic parameters suggested individual variations in crop emptying time and thus irregular absorption of the drug. In some birds, enterohepatic recycling of the drug appeared to be occurring. In cockatiels, azithromycin levels, which should be inhibitory for *Chlamydophila psittaci*, were reached and sustained for at least a week in lung, kidney, and liver following a single oral dose of 40 mg/kg. Tissue levels were 10 to 100 times higher than in plasma.

ADVERSE AND COMMON SIDE EFFECTS: In humans, the presence of food in the stomach decreases the rate and extent of gastrointestinal absorption. Azithromycin is eliminated principally via the liver; therefore, caution is recommended in treating humans with hepatic disease.

SUPPLIED AS HUMAN PRODUCTS:
Tablets containing 200 mg ★, 250 mg ✤, and 600 mg ✤ (Zithromax)
Powder (oral suspension base) to be reconstituted to 100 mg ✤, 200 mg ★, and 500 mg ✤/5 mL (Zithromax)
For injection, containing 500 mg/vial (Zithromax ✤ ★)

BAL (DIMERCAPROL)

INDICATIONS: BAL ✤ ★, or dimercaprol, is a sulfhydryl-containing compound that chelates arsenic. It is principally used for the treatment of arsenic toxicity and occasionally for toxicity caused by lead, mercury, and gold. BAL is not very effective in advanced cases of heavy metal toxicity. It is, therefore, best to administer the drug shortly after exposure. For more information, see BAL-DIMERCAPROL in the Small Animal section.

Dimercaprol has been used to treat lead toxicosis in birds. The drug can be given orally. It may be more effective than calcium EDTA for removing lead from the central nervous system and decreasing blood lead levels.

ADVERSE AND COMMON SIDE EFFECTS: See BAL-DIMER-CAPROL in the Small Animal section. IM injection is painful.

BARIUM SULFATE

INDICATIONS: Barium sulfate ✤ ★ is an inert radiopaque material that provides positive contrast during x-ray or fluoroscopic examination. Barium sulfate is not absorbed or metabolized and is eliminated intact from the body through the feces as a function of gastrointestinal transit time. The rate of gastrointestinal emptying will vary with the presence of anesthetic or sedative agents.

In birds, the dose of barium must be adjusted according to species in order to match anatomic features such as the presence or absence of a crop.

ADVERSE AND COMMON SIDE EFFECTS: The most common side effects reported in humans are constipation or diarrhea and cramping. The use of barium sulfate is contraindicated when the possibility of gastric or intestinal perforation exists. Aspiration of barium sulfate can lead to significant pneumonia and possibly death.

SUPPLIED AS HUMAN PRODUCTS:
Numerous barium sulfate suspensions from 1.2% to 98% w/w and 4.9% to 220% w/v (✤ ★)

BETAMETHASONE

INDICATIONS: Betamethasone (Betasone ★) is a long-acting injectable glucocorticoid agent, which has been used in birds for its anti-inflammatory properties. For more information on the use of glucocorticoids in birds, see DEXAMETHASONE in this section. For general information, see GLUCOCORTICOID AGENTS in the Small Animal section.

ADVERSE AND COMMON SIDE EFFECTS: As birds are extremely sensitive to the immunosuppressive effects of glucocorticoids, the use of short-acting agents in avian patients is recommended. See also DEXAMETHASONE in this section.

BISMUTH SUBSALICYLATE

INDICATIONS: Bismuth subsalicylate (Pepto-Bismol ✤ ★) is used in the treatment of gastritis and diarrhea. It inhibits the synthesis of prostaglandins responsible for gastrointestinal tract hypermotility and inflammation. The drug may also have antibacterial and anti-secretory properties. Bismuth subsalicylate relieves indigestion by forming insoluble complexes with offending noxious agents and by forming a protective coating.

ADVERSE AND COMMON SIDE EFFECTS: See BISMUTH SUB-SALICYLATE and ASPIRIN in the Small Animal section.

DRUG INTERACTIONS: The antimicrobial action of tetracyclines may be reduced if these drugs are used concurrently. It is advised that oral tetracycline be given at least 2 hours before or after bismuth administration.

BUPRENORPHINE

INDICATIONS: Buprenorphine hydrochloride (Buprenex ★) is a partial opiate agonist with analgesic properties. It is used for the management of mild pain. For more information, see BUPRENORPHINE HYDROCHLORIDE in the Small Animal section.

Although buprenorphine has been suggested as an analgesic for avian patients, African gray parrots administered buprenorphine at dosages of 0.1 and 0.5 mg/kg IM did not show changes in the threshold of response to a noxious electrical stimulus as compared to a saline control. Physiologic work in chickens and pigeons suggests that opioid drugs active at kappa sites (such as butorphanol) would be more effective than those affecting mu sites (buprenorphine).

BUTORPHANOL

INDICATIONS: Butorphanol (Torbugesic ❋ ★, Torbutrol ❋ ★) is a narcotic agonist/antagonist analgesic with potent antitussive activity in some species. For more information, see BUTORPHANOL in the Small Animal section.

In birds butorphanol is most commonly used as an analgesic for situations involving acute pain, but has also been suggested as a treatment for feather plucking in psittacine birds.

Little experimental work has been done on analgesia in birds. In chickens, butorphanol decreased isoflurane anesthetic concentrations in a dose-dependent manner. A similar response was seen in cockatoos and African gray parrots, but not in blue-fronted Amazon parrots, given 1 mg/kg of butorphanol (IM). In African gray parrots, butorphanol administered at 1 and 2 mg/kg significantly decreased the responses to a noxious electrical stimulus in a dose dependent manner. Doses of 1 and 3 mg/kg had similar effects in Hispaniolan Amazon parrots. Because butorphanol has a short elimination half-life, the need for frequent redosing is expected; sedation has been described with repeated use, however, at doses as low as 1 mg/kg IM every 12 hours.

ADVERSE AND COMMON SIDE EFFECTS: Severe sedation, recumbency, and possibly respiratory depression would be expected as evidence of dosages that are too high. In experimental trials in budgerigars given 0.1 mg IM (approximately 3 to 4 mg/kg), half of the birds showed motor deficits and were unable to perch tightly for 2 to 4 hours after drug administration. The birds remained alert and had stable heart and respiratory rates. Dosages of greater than 1 mg/kg can result in recumbency in some raptors. Some Hispaniolan Amazon parrots dosed with 6 mg/kg showed hyperalgesia. Treatment with naloxone should reverse the effects of the drug.

CALCIUM BOROGLUCONATE
CALCIUM GLUBIONATE
CALCIUM GLUCONATE
CALCIUM GLUCONATE/CALCIUM LACTATE

INDICATIONS: Calcium products are used for the treatment of hypocalcemia and for calcium supplementation. Calcium glubionate (also known as calcium glucono-galacto gluconate) syrup (Calcionate ★, Neo-Calglucon ★, Calcium Sandoz ✤) is the most favored product for oral use in avian patients. Calcium glubionate should be given before feeding to enhance calcium absorption. Other liquid calcium products contain calcium carbonate ★ (oral suspension); calcium citrate ★, calcium lactate-gluconate ✤, and calcium carbonate ✤ (tablets for oral solution); calcium gluceptate and calcium gluconate ✤ (oral solution). Capsules and tablets are available containing calcium carbonate, citrate, gluconate, lactate, and calcium phosphate. These should be compared on the basis of elemental calcium, rather than the "strength" of the tablet as some calcium salts have more elemental calcium than others.

Calcium gluconate and calcium glycerophosphate/lactate combinations can be administered IV or, in a diluted form (<5%), IM or SC. Intramuscular or SC injection is often preferred to avoid too rapid changes in blood calcium levels and when venous access is unavailable. Intravenous calcium chloride produces higher and more predictable levels of ionized calcium in plasma. Calcium gluconate/lactate combinations are used for IM injection. For more information, see CALCIUM GLUCONATE or CALCIUM LACTATE in the Small Animal section and CALCIUM BOROGLUCONATE in the Large Animal section.

In birds, calcium products are used for the treatment of clinical calcium deficiency including hypocalcemic tetany and egg binding, for the pretreatment of uterine inertia and egg binding before the administration of oxytocin, and for supplementation of birds with mineral deficiency. Initial administration is usually by the parenteral route; oral supplementation is used for long-term therapy.

DRUG INTERACTIONS: Oral calcium supplements should not be given to birds being treated with tetracycline-medicated feed because uptake of the medication is significantly reduced. Injectable supplementation is recommended if tetracycline is being administered concurrently.

SUPPLIED AS HUMAN PRODUCTS:
Oral syrup containing 115 mg calcium glubionate/5 mL (Calcionate ★, Neo-Calglucon ★) and 1.2 g calcium lactobionate and 530 mg calcium gluconate (110 mg of calcium ion)/5 mL (Calcium-Sandoz ✢)

SUPPLIED AS VETERINARY PRODUCTS:
Calcium glycerophosphate/lactate: solution containing 5 mg/mL of each element for IM and SC use (Calphosan Solution ★), and IM, SC, and IV use (Cal-Pho-Sol Solution SA ★)
Calcium gluconate or borogluconate: numerous solutions for IV, SC, IP use containing 230 mg/mL (23% Solution ✢ ★) and ~ 267 mg/mL (~ 26% solution ✢ ★). See CALCIUM BOROGLUCONATE in the Large Animal section.

CALCIUM DISODIUM EDETATE (EDTA)

INDICATIONS: Calcium disodium EDTA (Calcium Disodium Versenate ✢ ★) is the most common chelating agent used for the treatment of heavy metal toxicity. Before administration, calcium EDTA is diluted to a 1% solution using 5% dextrose in water. For more information, see CALCIUM EDTA in the Small Animal section.

In birds, calcium EDTA is used in the treatment of heavy metal poisoning, particularly lead and zinc. The drug also chelates, but to a much lesser extent, cadmium, copper, iron, and manganese. Calcium disodium EDTA chelates lead in the bone and plasma, creating insoluble complexes that are excreted by the kidneys. There is less risk of blood calcium chelation with disodium EDTA than with EDTA-acid or sodium EDTA. Oral administration will result in chelation of lead and zinc in the gastrointestinal tract. Other drugs used in the treatment of lead poisoning in birds include dimercaprol, DMSA, and penicillamine.

Calcium EDTA has been used IM or IV for the complete treatment period, or for initial therapy followed by oral treatment. Some authors recommend DMSA as an alternative for long-term oral therapy. Treatment should continue for 5 to 7 days, until no lead is visible radiographically, or until clinical signs abate. Monitoring of blood lead levels allows the best assessment of when to discontinue therapy. Treatment of large or chronic lead burdens may require weeks of treatment. It is sometimes recommended that for long-term therapy "rest periods" be interspersed between 3 to 7 day periods of treatment. Once therapy is discontinued, patients should be watched carefully for the reappearance of clinical signs as lead in tissues continues to leach into the circulation.

ADVERSE AND COMMON SIDE EFFECTS: Calcium EDTA is nephrotoxic in mammals. Although nephrotoxicity associated with the use of this drug has not been documented in birds, calcium EDTA should be used with caution in avian patients with impaired renal function or dehydration. Concurrent fluid therapy may be appropriate. There was no evidence of nephrotoxicity in cockatiels administered 40 mg/kg IM every 12 hours for 21 days. In dogs, vomiting, diarrhea, and depression have also been described. Polydipsia has been reported in psittacines. Although some authors have described the use of calcium EDTA PO, it has been suggested that this may actually increase absorption of lead from the gastrointestinal tract. Because IM injection of the drug is painful, diluting with sterile water and combining with an equal volume of 1% procaine hydrochloride has been described. Despite successful chelation therapy, clinical signs referable to peripheral neuropathy may not completely resolve, and birds may die of persistent gizzard impaction and stasis. Long-term treatment (i.e., several weeks) could result in chelation and depletion of normal blood cations; however, this has not been reported despite the frequency of long-term use of this product in birds.

DRUG INTERACTIONS: Do not use calcium EDTA in combination with nephrotoxic drugs. Renal toxicity may be enhanced by concurrent administration of glucocorticoids. Oral administration of fiber laxatives such as psyllium, or peanut butter may assist in passage of lead particles from the gastrointestinal tract.

SUPPLIED AS HUMAN PRODUCT:
For injection containing 200 mg/mL (Calcium Disodium Versonate 🍁 ★)

CARBARYL

INDICATIONS: Carbaryl dusting powder (Sevin 🍁, Zodiac Flea and Tick Powder 🍁, and many others), a carbamate insecticide and cholinesterase inhibitor, is used for the eradication of arthropod ectoparasites. For more information, see CARBAMATE INSECTICIDES in the Small Animal section.

In birds, 5% w/w carbaryl dust is used either by direct application to the bird or by addition to nest box litter. Approximately 1 teaspoon

(5 mL) is required for a cockatiel nest, 2 tablespoons (30 mL) for a large macaw nest box. Carbaryl may also be used to reduce ant infestations of the cage or nest box.

SUPPLIED AS VETERINARY PRODUCTS:

Dusting powder containing 5% w/w carbaryl (Dusting Powder ✤, Sevin ✤, Zodiac Flea and Tick Powder ✤, Happy Jack Flea Powder II ★, Prozap Garden & Poultry Dust ★) and 50% w/w carbaryl (Sevin ✤)

CARBENICILLIN

INDICATIONS: Carbenicillin (Geopen ✤ ★, Geocillin ★, Pyopen ✤) is an extended-spectrum, penicillinase-sensitive, semisynthetic penicillin used for the treatment of a variety of bacterial infections. It is effective against *Pseudomonas* and *Aeromonas* spp. and in abscesses. For more information, see CARBENICILLIN and PENICILLIN ANTIBIOTICS in the Small Animal section.

In birds, carbenicillin is used IM, IV, and PO. Ground carbenicillin tablets can be mixed in food for oral administration. Although the drug has been placed in drinking water, the ground tablets are not water-soluble and form a suspension with uneven distribution. Respiratory disease can be treated by nebulization or by direct intratracheal injection.

ADVERSE AND COMMON SIDE EFFECTS: Carbenicillin is unstable once reconstituted. Some authors have suggested freezing the reconstituted drug in aliquots for subsequent treatments; however, subsequent stability has not been investigated. Ground tablets have an objectionable taste and odor that must be camouflaged with sweeteners or flavored compounds for use in drinking water.

DRUG INTERACTIONS: Carbenicillin is frequently used in combination with aminoglycosides, particularly amikacin. Separate syringes should be used to avoid *in vitro* inactivation of the aminoglycoside. Amikacin is more resistant to this inactivation than gentamicin. Intratracheal administration of carbenicillin has been used in combination with parenteral gentamicin for the treatment of *Pseudomonas* spp. pneumonia.

CARNIDAZOLE

INDICATIONS: Carnidazole (Carnidazole ✤ ★) is an antiprotozoal drug licensed for the treatment of trichomoniasis in pigeons that are not intended for human consumption. It is also effective against hexamitiasis and histomoniasis. The drug is administered as a single oral dose in tablet form. Newly weaned birds are given half the adult dose. Investigations into experimental and natural infections have shown efficacy rates of between 75% and 100% after a single oral treatment. The drug is also marketed under the trade name of Spartrix.

ADVERSE AND COMMON SIDE EFFECTS: Carnidazole was administered to pigeons in single doses of 40, 160, 320, and 640 mg/kg and at 40 mg/kg once daily for 7 days without adverse effects. No drug-related adverse reactions were observed in newly weaned pigeons administered up to 10 times the recommended dose of 5 mg, or in adult birds treated with up to 32 times the recommended therapeutic dose of 10 mg. At 64 times the therapeutic dose, 4 out of 6 birds exhibited slight vomiting.

DRUG INTERACTIONS: None described.

SUPPLIED AS VETERINARY PRODUCT:
Tablets containing 10 mg (Carnidazole ♣ ★)

CARPROFEN

INDICATIONS: Carprofen (Rimadyl ♣ ★) is a carboxylic acid nonsteroidal anti-inflammatory agent with analgesic, anti-inflammatory, and antipyretic properties. Carprofen has been described anecdotally for the treatment of both acute postoperative pain and chronic arthritic or painful conditions in birds. Carprofen has been used experimentally in chickens by SC injection and orally in feed to reduce lameness in broiler chickens; pain thresholds appeared to remain raised for at least 90 minutes after a dose of 1 mg/kg SC. For more information, see CARPROFEN in the Small Animal section.

CEFAZOLIN

INDICATIONS: Cefazolin (Ancef ♣ ★, Kefzol ♣ ★) is a rapidly acting, first-generation cephalosporin. Of the cephalosporins, it achieves the greatest serum concentrations at equal doses on a mg/kg basis, has the longest elimination half-life, and is the most active against *Escherichia coli, Klebsiella,* and *Enterobacter.* For additional information, see CEFAZOLIN and CEPHALOSPORIN ANTIBIOTICS in the Small Animal section.

Cefazolin has been recommended for the treatment of osteomyelitis, especially in raptors. Use of the drug by nebulization has also been described.

ADVERSE AND COMMON SIDE EFFECTS: Administration of cefazolin IM to great horned owls, red-tailed hawks, brown pelicans, and great blue herons has resulted in extensive hemorrhage in the pectoral muscles at the site of injection. One great horned owl had a hematocrit of 10% after treatment. In humans, thrombocytopenia is a recognized adverse effect, and therefore, this could possibly occur in birds as well.

CEFOTAXIME

INDICATIONS: Cefotaxime (Claforan ✚ ★) is a third-generation, broad-spectrum cephalosporin used in the treatment of bacterial infections, especially by gram-negative organisms. For more information, see CEFOTAXIME and CEPHALOSPORIN ANTIBIOTICS in the Small Animal section.

Cefotaxime is often recommended for initial parenteral antibiotic therapy for seriously ill birds. Terminal half-lives of less than 45 minutes were obtained following single doses (50 mg/kg IV or 100 mg/kg IM) of cefotaxime administered to blue-fronted Amazon parrots. Rapid absorption was seen after intramuscular administration. Dosage at least 3 times daily was recommended at the conclusion of this study, particularly when treating organisms of only moderate susceptibility.

Reconstituted cefotaxime is stable for 10 days under refrigeration or can be frozen in aliquots for up to 6 months. Greater dilution of the drug is necessary for IV, as compared to IM, administration.

ADVERSE AND COMMON SIDE EFFECTS: Treatment with cefotaxime may result in an elevation in AST in some birds.

DRUG INTERACTIONS: Cefotaxime potentiates the antibacterial effects of aminoglycosides.

CEFOXITIN

INDICATIONS: Cefoxitin (Mefoxin ✚ ★) is a semisynthetic broad-spectrum, second-generation cephalosporin antibiotic. Cefoxitin has some activity against gram-positive cocci, good activity against many strains of *Escherichia coli* and *Klebsiella* and *Proteus* organisms, and is highly effective against many anaerobic infections. For more information, see CEFOXITIN and CEPHALOSPORIN ANTIBIOTICS in the Small Animal section.

Reconstituted cefoxitin is stable for 10 days under refrigeration or can be frozen in aliquots for up to 6 months. Greater dilution of the drug is necessary for IV, as compared to IM, administration.

DRUG INTERACTIONS: Synergistic effects are seen against some organisms when cefoxitin is used in conjunction with the penicillins or chloramphenicol. Cefoxitin should not be used at the same time as aminoglycoside antibiotics because of possible incompatibility. Nephrotoxicity is of concern in mammals when cefoxitin is used in conjunction with aminoglycosides, vancomycin, polymyxin B, or diuretics. Pain may occur on IM injection.

CEFTAZIDIME

INDICATIONS: Ceftazidime (Fortaz ✚ ★) is a third-generation, broad-spectrum cephalosporin antibiotic similar to cefotaxime, with activity against gram-negative bacteria and greater activity against *Pseudomonas aeruginosa*. Ceftazidime is the third-generation cephalosporin of choice in avian medicine, particularly when treating *Pseudomonas* infections. For more information, see CEFTAZIDIME and CEPHALOSPORIN ANTIBIOTICS in the Small Animal section.

ADVERSE AND COMMON SIDE EFFECTS: The most common adverse effects in humans include local reactions after injection (phlebitis, thrombophlebitis, pain), fever, pruritus, diarrhea, nausea, and transient elevations in serum urea, creatinine, and hepatic enzymes.

DRUG INTERACTIONS: Concurrent use with aminoglycosides may cause an additive nephrotoxic effect. For more information, see CEFTAZIDIME and CEPHALOSPORIN ANTIBIOTICS in the Small Animal section.

CEFTRIAXONE

INDICATIONS: Ceftriaxone (Rocephin ✚ ★, generics ✚ ★) is a semisynthetic, third-generation cephalosporin antibiotic with expanded activity against gram-negative organisms. The drug's spectrum of activity is similar to those of cefotaxime, ceftazidime, and ceftizoxime. For more general information, see CEPHALOSPORIN ANTIBIOTICS in the Small Animal section.

In a single-dose pharmacokinetic study in blue-fronted Amazon parrots given 100 mg/kg ceftriaxone IV, an initial plasma concentration of approximately 175 μg/mL was measured, and a terminal half-life of less than 45 minutes obtained. Dosage at least 3 times daily was recommended at the conclusion of this study, particularly when treating organisms of only moderate susceptibility.

In chickens, after a single IM injection of 100 mg/kg, serum antibiotic levels had peaked (18.03 μg/mL) by 30 minutes after injection, and were undetectable by 4 to 6 hours. Peak blood concentrations were above the minimal inhibitory concentration values for *Escherichia coli*, enterobacteria, and *Salmonella* spp. isolated from psittacine cloacal swabs, but not for *Proteus, Pseudomonas,* or *Klebsiella* spp. Birds were also nebulized with 40 mg/mL in sterile water, and with 40 and 200 mg/mL in sterile water and DMSO. Ceftriaxone was detectable in the serum of only one bird immediately after the cessation of nebulization. Level of drug in the respiratory tissues was not assessed.

Reconstituted ceftriaxone is stable for 10 days under refrigeration or can be frozen in aliquots for up to 6 months. Greater dilution of the drug is necessary for IV than IM administration.

ADVERSE AND COMMON SIDE EFFECTS: Adverse effects reported for ceftriaxone in humans are similar to those of other cephalosporins.

DRUG INTERACTIONS: The antibacterial action of ceftriaxone and the aminoglycosides, amikacin, gentamicin, and tobramycin, may be additive or synergistic against some strains of Enterobacteriaceae and *Pseudomonas aeruginosa. In vitro* inactivation has occurred with these combinations; therefore, separate syringes should be used for administration.

SUPPLIED AS HUMAN PRODUCTS:
For injection containing 0.25, 1, and 2 g/vial (Rocephin ✦); 0.25 g, 0.50 g, 1 g, 2 g, and 10 g (Rocephin Injectable Vials ★)

CELECOXIB

INDICATIONS: Celecoxib (Celebrex ✦, Celebrex Capsules ★) is a nonsteroidal anti-inflammatory drug (NSAID) with specific COX-2 inhibition. In humans, the drug is used for osteoarthritis and rheumatoid arthritis. Celecoxib has been used to treat psittacine birds with proventricular dilation disease. Improvement in gastrointestinal function and body condition has been reported in some cases with therapy for up to 24 weeks. The drug was made into an aqueous suspension, kept refrigerated, and used for 14 days.

ADVERSE AND COMMON SIDE EFFECTS: In humans, celecoxib has a lower incidence of adverse effects on the stomach than many other anti-inflammatory drugs. Because celecoxib is metabolized in the liver to inactive compounds, care should be taken in treating birds with hepatic dysfunction.

DRUG INTERACTIONS: Celecoxib should not be used in conjunction with other anti-inflammatory drugs or with corticosteroids.

SUPPLIED AS HUMAN PRODUCT:
Capsules containing 100 and 200 mg (Celebrex ✦ ★)

CEPHALEXIN

INDICATIONS: Cephalexin (Keflex ✦ ★, Keftab ★, Novo-Lexin ✦, Nu-Cephalex ✦) is a broad-spectrum, first-generation cephalosporin available for oral use. For more information, see CEPHALEXIN and CEPHALOSPORIN ANTIBIOTICS in the Small Animal section.
    Cephalexin has been recommended as a drug of choice for the treatment of dermatitis in psittacine birds. In a pharmacokinetic

study involving pigeons, bobwhite quail, hybrid rosybill ducks, emus, and greater sandhill cranes given oral cephalexin, the elimination half-life was 36 to 126 minutes and varied directly with body weight. No difference in pharmacokinetic parameters was seen in fasted as compared to nonfasted quail.

CEPHALOTHIN

INDICATIONS: Cephalothin (Keflin ♣, Ceporacin ♣) is a broad-spectrum, first-generation cephalosporin antibiotic for parenteral use. First-generation drugs are active against gram-positive bacteria, including penicillin-resistant staphylococci, and against some gram-negative bacteria, including *E. coli, Proteus,* and *Klebsiella* spp. For more information, see CEPHALOTHIN and CEPHALOSPORIN ANTIBIOTICS in the Small Animal section.

In a pharmacokinetic study involving pigeons, bobwhite quail, hybrid rosybill ducks, emus, and greater sandhill cranes given cephalothin IM, the elimination half-life ranged from 16 to 54 minutes and varied directly with body weight in all species except the ducks. The high frequency of dosing made use of this drug impractical in many situations.

ADVERSE AND COMMON SIDE EFFECTS: Cephalothin is irritating; large or repeated IM injection may cause pain and result in local inflammatory reactions or sterile abscesses. Thrombophlebitis has been associated with IV use in humans. Cephalothin is potentially nephrotoxic, which may be enhanced when used in conjunction with an aminoglycoside. This parenteral product is not acid stable and should not be given orally.

CEPHRADINE

INDICATIONS: Cephradine (Velosef ★) is a first-generation, semi-synthetic cephalosporin with a spectrum of activity similar to that of cephalexin. The drug is available in oral as well as an injectable formulation. For further information, see CEPHRADINE and CEPHALO-SPORIN ANTIBIOTICS in the Small Animal section.

No pharmacokinetic work has been carried out in birds; however, it is assumed that treatment should parallel that with cephalexin.

CHLORAMPHENICOL

INDICATIONS: Chloramphenicol (Azramycine ♣, Chlor Palm ♣, Chlor Tablets ♣, Chloromycetin ♣ ★, Karomycin Palmitate ♣, and many others) is a bacteriostatic antibiotic with activity against a number of pathogens including gram-positive and gram-negative bacteria, most anaerobes, chlamydiae, rickettsiae, coxiellae, mycoplasmas, and some protozoa. For more information, see CHLORAMPHENICOL in the Small Animal section.

In pharmacokinetic studies using various doses and routes of administration of chloramphenicol in 18 species of birds, elimination half-lives ranged from 26 minutes in the pigeon to 288 minutes in the bald eagle. Oral administration resulted in low and inconsistent blood chloramphenicol levels, with considerable variation in absorption among species. In chickens, oral absorption of chloramphenicol was slow; administration of 50 mg/kg resulted in minimally adequate blood levels. In pigeons, elimination was so rapid that frequency of administration would be impractical. IV or IM injection of the succinate ester resulted in plasma concentrations 1.5 times less than those produced by the ethanol, benzyl alcohol, or propylene glycol formulations.

In Chinese spot-billed ducks, oral absorption was also variable. Blood levels resulting after 55 mg/kg was orally administered did not reach therapeutic levels. Peak blood levels were reached within an hour of an IM injection of 22 mg/kg. It was suggested that, due to the high volume of distribution, tissue levels may be greater than those in plasma.

In chickens, therapeutic blood levels could be reached by oral administration of 50 mg/kg; however, there was considerable individual variation. Increasing the dose to 200 mg/kg PO increased the apparent half-life, but not the peak serum level.

Because of its high palatability, chloramphenicol palmitate has been administered orally in food, particularly in mixtures for hand-fed neonates. However, for a number of reasons including its erratic absorption and concerns over risks to humans exposed to the drug, chloramphenicol has generally been replaced with newer antibacterial agents in avian practice. Parenteral administration of chloramphenicol should be used for serious infections. Chloramphenicol succinate has been used for the treatment of respiratory disease by nebulization. Chloramphenicol powder from capsules has been mixed with seed or mash diets to medicate entire flocks, especially for infections by *Salmonella* spp. The drug is insoluble in drinking water at doses used clinically.

ADVERSE AND COMMON SIDE EFFECTS: Reversible, dose-dependent anemia, anorexia, and depression have been described in chickens, turkeys, and ducks; however, large doses are required to induce toxicity. Vomiting and diarrhea may also occur. Temporary infertility has been described in male pigeons. Owners of pet birds should be warned about the potential risks to humans from this drug.

DRUG INTERACTIONS: Chloramphenicol inhibits hepatic cytochrome P-450 enzymes; and therefore, therapy with chloramphenicol may affect the levels of a variety of other therapeutic agents.

CHLORHEXIDINE

INDICATIONS: Chlorhexidine (ChlorhexiDerm ★, Hibitane ✤, Nolvadent ★, Nolvasan ★, Savlon ✤, and others) is a chemical used for disinfection and as a base for a variety of antiseptic products. Diluted chlorhexidine solutions are used topically and orally, and the compound is also formulated into a number of topical creams. For more information, see CHLORHEXIDINE in the Small Animal section.

Two percent chlorhexidine solution (nonscented formulation) in drinking water is used to prevent and treat candidiasis, especially in birds receiving long-term therapy with chlortetracycline-impregnated feed. Chlorhexidine is not absorbed from the intestine. Washing and misting with chlorhexidine was used to reduce saphrophytic fungal growth on soiled or "greased" feathers in psittacine birds.

ADVERSE AND COMMON SIDE EFFECTS: Chlorhexidine may not be palatable to canaries, especially in the drug's scented form. Reduced water consumption, possibly to a fatal degree, can result from offering treated drinking water. Chlorhexidine has been reported as toxic to finches.

SUPPLIED AS VETERINARY PRODUCTS:
Numerous products containing 0.1% to 5% w/v as udder washes and teat dip solutions, lavage solutions, skin cleansers, shampoos, and ointments (✤ ★)

CHLOROQUINE PHOSPHATE

INDICATIONS: Chloroquine (Aralen ✤ ★) is a synthetic antimalarial agent available for oral administration as the phosphate salt. It is effective against the circulating forms of many strains of *Plasmodium* spp. and as a tissue amebicide, and has anti-inflammatory actions that are used against some auto-immune conditions in human medicine. Preerythrocytic and exoerythrocytic forms of *Plasmodium* spp. are not affected by the drug.

Chloroquine combined with primaquine has been used for the initial therapy of *Plasmodium* spp. malaria in penguins, and prophylactically, in drinking water, to prevent seasonal malaria in outdoor budgerigars, canaries, and finches. The tablets can be dissolved in water (up to a concentration of 1 g/15 mL) and dosed based upon estimated daily water intake.

ADVERSE AND COMMON SIDE EFFECTS: The bioavailability of chloroquine phosphate is greater, and adverse gastrointestinal effects lesser, in humans when the drug is administered with food. A number of significant side effects have been described in humans. Overdosage may lead rapidly to cardiovascular collapse. Depression and vomiting have been seen with overdosage in penguins.

DRUG INTERACTIONS: Therapy should be combined with primaquine phosphate.

SUPPLIED AS HUMAN PRODUCTS:
Tablets containing 250 mg and 500 mg (Aralen ❦ ★)

CHLORTETRACYCLINE

INDICATIONS: Chlortetracycline (Aureomycin ❦ ★, Fermycin Soluble ★, Aureomix ★, and others) is a broad-spectrum bacteriostatic antibiotic with activity against gram-positive and gram-negative organisms, chlamydiae, rickettsiae, mycoplasmas, and many anaerobes. For more information, see TETRACYCLINE ANTIBIOTICS in the Small Animal section.

Chlortetracycline-impregnated feed has historically been the most common compound used to treat birds infected with *Chlamydophila psittaci*, especially in aviaries and quarantine facilities. Birds are provided with only treated feed for 30 to 45 days to maintain blood chlortetracycline levels greater than 1 µg/mL. Blood levels drop rapidly if consumption of medicated feed is interrupted. Medication of water does not provide consistent blood levels. Doxycycline is the treatment of choice for individual patients.

A commercial product consisting of millet impregnated with 0.5% w/w chlortetracycline (Keet Life) was widely recommended for the treatment of budgerigars, canaries, and finches, but is no longer commercially available. With this product, therapeutic blood levels were reached within 24 hours.

In North America, the recommended level of chlortetracycline for mash or pelleted diets is 1%. In Europe, 5% is the general recommendation; however, 2.0% to 2.5% is used for some psittacines including large macaws, lovebirds, rosellas, and parakeets. In one report, canary winged parakeets developed higher blood levels than other psittacine birds in the same study, including other *Brotogeris* spp. Use of 0.5% to 1% chlortetracycline in the diet was recommended for this species. Impregnated pellets are available from a number of commercial suppliers. Compared to specially formulated mash diets, pellets have a longer shelf life, are easier to feed, and have more consistent nutritional and therapeutic values. Mash diets must be made fresh daily.

Nectar solutions for nectar-feeding birds should contain 0.5% chlortetracycline.

Oral, compared to IV, administration of chlortetracycline to chickens and turkeys results in much lower bioavailability. This may be due to a number of reasons, including first-pass hepatic excretion into the bile immediately after intestinal absorption.

ADVERSE AND COMMON SIDE EFFECTS: Many birds are reluctant to eat new foods; therefore, pelleted diets must be introduced carefully to ensure adequate food intake. Direct medication with oxytetracycline or doxycycline may need to be carried out during the transition period. Long-term chlortetracycline therapy may predispose birds to fungal and yeast overgrowth, especially oral and gastrointestinal candidiasis, and to gastrointestinal upset due to disruption of normal flora. Tetracyclines, especially chlortetracycline, inhibit protein synthesis and are immunosuppressive.

DRUG INTERACTIONS: Dietary grit and minerals, particularly calcium, reduce absorption of chlortetracycline and, therefore, potentially reduce therapeutic effect. Diets should contain no more than 0.7% calcium. A decrease in dietary calcium from 1% to 0.5% increased chlortetracycline absorption by 2.5 times in one study.

SUPPLIED AS VETERINARY PRODUCTS:
Water-soluble powders and agricultural feed additives containing various concentrations of chlortetracycline (Aureomycin ♣ ★, Fermycin Soluble ★, Aureomix ★, and many others)
Tablets containing 25 mg (Aureomycin Tablets ★)
Pellets impregnated with 1.0% chlortetracycline (Avi-Sci Inc ★, Pretty Bird International, Inc ★, Rolf C. Hagen ♣, Roudybush ★, Ziegler Brothers, Inc. ★, Wings of Life ♣, and others)

CHORIONIC GONADOTROPIN

INDICATIONS: Human chorionic gonadotropin (HCG) (Veterinary Products: A.P.L. ♣, Chorionad ♣, Chorionic Gonadotropin ★, Chorulon ♣ ★; Human Products: Follutein ★, Progon 10,000 ♣) is produced in the human placenta and the commercial product is obtained from the urine of pregnant women. The action of HCG is virtually identical to that of pituitary luteinizing hormone (LH), although HCG appears to have a small degree of follicle-stimulating hormone (FSH) activity as well.

In birds, HCG has been used to inhibit ovulation and egg laying and in the treatment of feather picking in psittacine birds, which may have an underlying hormonal stimulus. A treatment interval from 3 to 7 days has been suggested to halt egg laying, but the frequency of administration will vary among birds. HCG is considered safer than medroxyprogesterone but has a shorter duration of action. For more information, see CHORIONIC GONADOTROPIN in the Large Animal section.

ADVERSE AND COMMON SIDE EFFECTS: Chorionic gonadotropin is a foreign protein and can cause anaphylaxis when administered parenterally. Continued administration may result in antihormone antibody production and loss of effectiveness. As androgens may cause fluid retention, HCG should be used with caution in patients with cardiac or renal disease. Other side effects described for humans include headache, irritability, restlessness, fatigue, edema, and pain at the site of injection.

DRUG INTERACTIONS: Dexamethasone is sometimes used in conjunction with HCG for the treatment of egg-related peritonitis and to repress subsequent egg laying. It is postulated that dexamethasone may reduce yolk-related inflammation and delay the development of an anti–HCG immune response.

CIMETIDINE

INDICATIONS: Cimetidine (Novo-Cimetine ♣, Tagamet ♣ ★), a histamine (H_2)-receptor blocking agent, reduces gastric acid secretion and is used in the management of gastric and duodenal ulceration that does not result from the administration of NSAIDs. Cimetidine also increases caudal esophageal sphincter tone and promotes gastric emptying in mammals. The drug is available for oral use and for injection. For further information, see CIMETIDINE in the Small Animal section.

DRUG INTERACTIONS: By interfering with hepatic microenzyme systems, cimetidine affects the metabolism of many drugs. For further information, see CIMETIDINE in the Small Animal section.

CIPROFLOXACIN

INDICATIONS: Ciprofloxacin (Cipro ♣ ★) is a fluoroquinolone antibiotic with activity against a range of gram-negative and gram-positive bacteria (e.g., *Escherichia coli, Klebsiella, Proteus, Pseudomonas, Staphylococcus, Salmonella, Shigella, Yersinia, Campylobacter,* and *Vibrio* spp.) and some spirochetes. The drug is available for oral, IV, and ophthalmic use and is produced *in vivo* as a metabolite after the administration of enrofloxacin. For more information, see CIPROFLOXACIN and FLUOROQUINOLONE ANTIBIOTICS in the Small Animal section.

Ciprofloxacin has been recommended for oral gavage in individual birds or for use in drinking water for the treatment of flocks. Tablets dissolve well in water once the protective outer coating is removed; however, the duration of activity once in suspension may be very short. Ciprofloxacin has been used in combination with several other drugs for the treatment of avian mycobacteriosis. In human medicine, clarithromycin or azithromycin combined with ethambutol and either ciprofloxacin or rifabutin is recommended for the prophylaxis and treatment of *Mycobacterium avium* complex infections in HIV patients. Veterinarians differ in their willingness to treat avian mycobacteriosis due to the difficulty in ensuring that the infection is fully eliminated and concerns over the potential for zoonotic spread of the disease under certain conditions.

A pharmacokinetic trial using a single oral dose of 50 mg/kg in fasted red-tailed hawks revealed the drug to be rapidly absorbed from the gastrointestinal tract. Mean peak serum concentration was 3.64 μg/mL; dosage with 50 mg/kg every 12 hours was recommended to maintain blood levels above 1.38 μg/mL, the minimal inhibitory concentration for many susceptible bacteria.

A series of wild house finches infected with *Mycoplasma gallisepticum* were treated topically with ciprofloxacin ophthalmic ointment for 5 to 7 days and systemically with tylosin in the drinking water (approximately 1 mg/mL water) for at least 21 days. This combined therapy was highly effective in eliminating clinical signs and preventing relapses, but the presence of a continued carrier state could not be ruled out. Birds treated with ciprofloxacin ophthalmic drops alone had a high rate of recurrence of conjunctivitis.

ADVERSE AND COMMON SIDE EFFECTS: Ciprofloxacin in water has a salty, bitter taste that should be masked by a sweetener or flavored compound. There is one report of an Amazon parrot that became aggressive while being treated. Similar behavior has been reported in birds treated with enrofloxacin.

CISAPRIDE

INDICATIONS: Cisapride (Propulsid ★, Prepulsid ✤) was marketed in North America for the treatment of heartburn in humans, but has been removed from general access due to its association with cardiac arrhythmias. The drug was used in Small Animal Practice to stimulate GI motility in cases of primary motility disorders and in cases of gastroesophageal reflux. The drug generally is given 15 minutes before a meal. For more information, see CISAPRIDE in the Small Animal section.

In birds, cisapride has been used to stimulate gastrointestinal motility in conditions including proventricular dilation disease. Metoclopramide would be an alternative drug.

DRUG INTERACTIONS: Concurrent therapy with drugs that inhibit cytochrome P-450 enzymes (e.g., clarithromycin, erythromycin, fluconazole, itraconazole, and ketoconazole) will result in elevated blood cisapride levels. These interactions have led to fatalities in humans.

CISPLATIN

INDICATIONS: Cisplatin (Platinol ★ and generics ✤) is a platinum-containing chemotherapeutic agent that has modest efficacy in the treatment of some adenocarcinomas, squamous cell carcinomas, and osteosarcomas. For more information, see CISPLATIN in the Small Animal section.

An experimental study in sulfur-crested cockatoos evaluated the safety of cisplatin at a dose of 1 mg/kg intravenously in 0.9% sodium chloride over a period of one hour. All birds recovered well from the anesthesia and infusion, but regurgitation and abnormalities in urine and feces were noted during the first 24 hours. Based on levels of cisplatin in blood, urine, and tissue, the study concluded that the pharmacokinetic disposition of the drug in these cockatoos was similar to that reported previously in rodents, dogs, and humans, and that levels should be within the therapeutic range to treat neoplasia.

A small number of case reports describe the use of cisplatin in birds, but no conclusions can yet be made as to its efficacy against avian neoplasms.

ADVERSE AND COMMON SIDE EFFECTS: Significant nephrotoxicity and death occurred in one of two sulfur-crested cockatoos given a dose of 6.4 mg/kg IV in a pilot study. Posttreatment regurgitation, yellowing of urates, and loose lime/dark green feces were noted in both groups but were more pronounced in birds treated with 6.4 mg/kg than in birds treated with 1 mg/kg.

CLARITHROMYCIN

INDICATIONS: Clarithromycin (Biaxin ♣ ★) is a semisynthetic macrolide antibiotic used to treat a variety of bacterial infections in people. It is particularly marketed for respiratory infections in adults and children, *Helicobacter pylori* gastritis, and prevention and therapy of *Mycobacterium avium* complex disease in HIV patients in combination with ethambutol plus ciprofloxacin or rifabutin. It may also be useful alone or in combination with azithromycin for the prevention and treatment of toxoplasmosis.

ADVERSE AND COMMON SIDE EFFECTS: In humans, infrequent side effects include diarrhea, nausea, and abnormal taste.

DRUG INTERACTIONS: A number of drug interactions exist as clarithromycin inhibits cytochrome P-450 enzymes. Concomitant use of rifabutin and clarithromycin may cause decreased clarithromycin levels and increased rifabutin levels. Concurrent treatment with cisapride is contraindicated.

SUPPLIED AS HUMAN PRODUCT:
Pediatric granules for suspension at 125 mg/5 mL and 250 mg/5 mL (Biaxin ♣)
Tablets containing 125 mg and 500 mg (Biaxin ♣, Biaxin BID ♣ ★, Biaxin XL Filmtab Tablets ★)

Oral suspension containing 125 mg/5 mL, 187.5 mg/5 mL, 250 mg/ 5 mL after reconstitution (Biaxin ★)

CLAZURIL

INDICATIONS: Clazuril (Appertex) is an anticoccidial drug licensed for use in non–food pigeons in Europe against *Eimeria labbeana* and *E. columbarum*. The drug was previously marketed in North America. For information on similar compounds, see TOLTRAZURIL and DICLAZURIL in this section.

ADVERSE AND COMMON SIDE EFFECTS: At 125 times the recommended dose, pigeons developed mild, transient vomiting and watery diarrhea. Clazuril is safe to use during the breeding season. No adverse effects were noted in cranes given 5 times the recommended dose. Clazuril was suggested as a treatment for *Caryospora neofalconis* in juvenile merlins instead of sulfadimidine or amprolium.

SUPPLIED AS VETERINARY PRODUCT:
Tablets containing 2.5 mg (Appertex—not marketed in North America at this time)

CLINDAMYCIN

INDICATIONS: Clindamycin (Antirobe ♣ ★, Clindrops ★) is a lincosamide antibiotic with activity against a wide range of infectious organisms, including many anaerobes and some sporozoan organisms. The drug is widely distributed in most body tissues and may penetrate the cerebrospinal fluid and ocular tissue if inflammation is present. For more information, see CLINDAMYCIN in the Small Animal section.

Clindamycin has been recommended for the treatment of conditions such as osteomyelitis where long-term therapy is required. Treatment with clindamycin has been effective in several reports describing enteric clostridial infections in psittacine chicks and adults.

ADVERSE AND COMMON SIDE EFFECTS: Renal and hepatic function should be monitored during long-term use. Overgrowth of gastrointestinal yeasts may also occur.

CLOFAZIMINE

INDICATIONS: Clofazimine (Lamprene ★) is an anti-infective drug used in human medicine for the treatment of conditions including *Mycobacterium avium* complex (MAC) and leprosy. For first-line treatment of MAC infections, a recommended protocol includes either clarithromycin or azithromycin combined with at least one other drug, usually ethambutol plus clofazimine, ciprofloxacin, or rifabutin.

In birds, clofazimine has been included in multidrug combination treatment protocols for mycobacteriosis. However, in humans, the drug is not recommended for use in disseminated infections such as are often present in avian patients. Veterinarians differ in their willingness to treat avian mycobacteriosis due to the difficulty in ensuring that the infection is fully eliminated and concerns over the potential for zoonotic spread of the disease under certain conditions.

ADVERSE AND COMMON SIDE EFFECTS: Clofazimine should be taken with food. In humans, side effects include: discoloration of skin, feces, sputum, sweat, and tears; intestinal problems; dizziness; and photosensitization.

SUPPLIED AS HUMAN PRODUCT:
Capsules containing 50 and 100 mg (Lamprene ★)

CLOMIPRAMINE

INDICATIONS: Clomipramine (Clomicalm ❋ ★) is a tricyclic antidepressant and antiobsessional human medication that has been used in psittacine birds to try and control psychological feather picking and self-mutilation. Tricyclic antidepressants also have powerful antihistamine-like activity, which may assist in treating birds where pruritus is a stimulus for feather picking. The drug has been effective in some birds in some case reports; however, the response of each patient is highly unpredictable. Birds should be started on a low dose that can be adjusted over several days according to the clinical response. One controlled study in five species of cockatoo suggested that a dose of 3 mg/kg PO every 12 hours should be safe.

ADVERSE AND COMMON SIDE EFFECTS: Adverse effects described in psittacine birds include drowsiness, occasional regurgitation, and an episode of ataxia in a cockatoo. There have been anecdotal reports of deaths of birds being treated with clomipramine. A variety of anticholinergic, psychiatric, neurologic, and cardiovascular adverse effects are described in humans. Cardiac function should be assessed in patients before commencing and during treatment, including evaluation of EKGs. The effects of long-term treatment have not been systematically evaluated.

DRUG INTERACTIONS: In humans, clomipramine should not be given with or within 14 days of treatment with a monoamine oxidase (MAO) inhibitor, e.g., Amitraz, as this combination may predispose to hypertension. Clomipramine may potentiate the cardiovascular effects of sympathomimetic drugs, e.g., epinephrine.

SUPPLIED AS VETERINARY PRODUCT:
Tablets containing 20, 40, and 80 mg (Clomicalm ✤ ★)

CLOTRIMAZOLE

INDICATIONS: Clotrimazole (Canesten ✤, Lotrimin ★, Mycelex ★) is a topical imidazole antifungal agent useful in the treatment of localized dermatophytosis, candidal stomatitis, and nasal aspergillosis in dogs. For more information, see CLOTRIMAZOLE in the Small Animal section.

Clotrimazole is used topically and to treat fungal respiratory disease (e.g., aspergillosis) by nebulization and by direct endoscopic placement on air sac lesions. A widely adopted protocol involves the initial use of amphotericin B and concurrent treatment with oral itraconazole and clotrimazole by nebulization. Frequency and duration of the period of nebulization vary greatly among reports.

In one report describing the successful treatment of 5 psittacines and raptors with confirmed respiratory aspergillosis, treatment was initiated with systemic therapeutic agents, including amphotericin B, flucytosine, or itraconazole, and nebulization began once the birds were out of respiratory distress. The clotrimazole was solubilized in polyethylene glycol with a resulting pH of 6 to 6.5, and nebulized at a particle size of 0.5 to 5 microns. Clinical improvement was seen within a week in several cases. Treatment was continued for 2 to 4 months and could be carried out by the owners at home. Birds were monitored closely during treatment and showed no evidence of renal or hepatic dysfunction.

ADVERSE AND COMMON SIDE EFFECTS: Two of the three psittacines in the above report showed mild discomfort during nebulization, perhaps because of the dense fog produced. One Amazon parrot regurgitated during the first few minutes of a treatment. A white film developed in the nares of one bird after 3 months of treatment; however, this film was manually removed without difficulty. Ophthalmic lubricant should be used to reduce ocular irritation. Repeated nebulization with clotrimazole may result in the accumulation of a film of drug on the bird's feathering. Hepatic function should be monitored during therapy as toxicity might occur if there is systemic absorption.

COLCHICINE

INDICATIONS: Colchicine (generic products ✤ ★) is an alkaloid prepared from the dried corns and seeds of *Colchicum autumnale*, the autumn crocus, which is used in human medicine to reduce inflammation and pain associated with gout, and in familial Mediterranean fever. The main anti-inflammatory mechanism of this drug is to inhibit granulocyte migration into the inflamed area.

In birds, colchicine has been recommended for the treatment of hyperuricemia and gout. In chicken livers, colchicine reversibly inhibits xanthine dehydrogenase and hence could have some effect on uric acid levels. There have been no controlled studies indicating efficacy of colchicine in the treatment of gout in birds, although some authors have suggested improvement in clinical cases with therapy. In humans, because of the toxicity of colchicine in high doses, NSAIDs are preferred to treat acute gout. However, colchicine at lower doses is very effective in preventing recurrent attacks of gout.

Colchicine has also been suggested for the treatment of hepatic fibrosis in birds, based on evidence that it may be helpful in humans and dogs. As well as its anti-inflammatory actions, colchicine inhibits microtubular assembly and blocks transcellular movement of procollagen fibers. Colchicine also increases collagenase activity, which may promote degradation of existing collagen.

ADVERSE AND COMMON SIDE EFFECTS: Colchicine inhibits mitosis thus affecting tissues with high cell turnover (e.g., GI tract, bone marrow). In humans, there is a narrow margin of safety with symptoms of overdosage similar to those of radiation poisoning. There is usually a latent period between overdosage and the onset of symptoms, regardless of the route of administration.

SUPPLIED AS HUMAN PRODUCTS:
Tablets containing 0.5 mg and 0.6 mg (Colchicine Tablets USP ✤ ★)

CYCLOSERINE

INDICATIONS: Cycloserine (Seromycin ★) is an antibacterial drug used in human medicine to treat infectious conditions including active pulmonary and extrapulmonary tuberculosis, usually in conjunction with other therapeutic agents. It is also used for acute urinary tract infections caused by susceptible strains of gram-positive and gram-negative bacteria, especially *Enterobacter* species and *E. coli.* Cycloserine acts by inhibiting cell wall synthesis in susceptible strains of bacteria.

In birds, cycloserine has been included in multidrug combination treatment protocols for mycobacteriosis. Treatment should continue for a minimum of 6 months; response is dependent on integrity of the host's immune system.

ADVERSE AND COMMON SIDE EFFECTS: In humans, common side effects include headaches and changes in attitude and mentation. Convulsions, skin rash, and changes in sensation of the hands and feet are less commonly described.

DRUG INTERACTIONS: Cycloserine may interfere with the absorption of calcium, magnesium, folic acid, vitamin B_6, and vitamin B_{12}.

SUPPLIED AS HUMAN PRODUCT:
Capsules containing 250 mg (Seromycin ★)

DEFERIPRONE

INDICATIONS: Deferiprone (Ferriprox) is the first oral iron chelator used clinically in human medicine, mainly in thalassemia patients. Deferiprone is an α-ketohydroxpyridine, with high affinity for binding iron, including protein-bound forms being transported and stored in the body. Deferiprone removes excess iron from a variety of locations, including the liver and particularly the heart, in iron-loaded patients.

Deferiprone may prove useful in treating birds with excessive iron storage and hemochromatosis, particularly as it is intended for oral use. Pharmacokinetic and efficacy studies using deferiprone in pigeons and chickens found that an oral dose of 50 mg/kg maintained plasma concentrations effective for iron chelation for at least 8 hours. When administered at this dose twice daily, deferiprone eliminated the hemosiderotic state induced by experimental iron-loading within a 30 day treatment period. A dose of 100 mg/kg once daily would likely also be effective in these species.

ADVERSE AND COMMON SIDE EFFECTS: The most significant adverse effect in humans is neutropenia and agranulocytosis, but transient musculoskeletal and joint pain, gastric intolerance, and zinc deficiency have also been reported. Regular monitoring of neutrophil counts is recommended.

In pigeons and chickens treated orally twice daily for 30 days, there was a significant decline in serum zinc levels as chelatable iron stores decreased. Zinc levels should be monitored during therapy, and supplemented if indicated. Daily prophylactic use of deferiprone is not recommended due to the potential for toxicity associated with inhibition of enzymes requiring iron for normal function.

DRUG INTERACTIONS: Interactions have not been reported. The potential exists for interactions between deferiprone and trivalent cation-dependent medicinal products, such as aluminum-based antacids. Based on adverse interactions that can occur with desferrioxamine (another iron-chelating medication), caution should be used when administering concurrent deferiprone and vitamin C.

SUPPLIED AS HUMAN PRODUCTS:
Not currently marketed in North America.
Tablets or capsules containing 500 mg (Ferriprox: Europe, Australia)
Capsules containing 150 and 500 mg (Kelfer: India)

DEFEROXAMINE

INDICATIONS: Deferoxamine (Desferal ❧ ★, Desferrioxamine Mesilate for Injection BP ❧, PMS-Deferoxamine ❧) is a chelating agent that complexes primarily with trivalent iron and aluminum ions. It is used in humans to treat acute or chronic iron intoxication. The drug forms complexes with free iron or iron-binding proteins such as ferritin and hemosiderin. The resulting complex, ferrioxamine, is excreted in the urine and feces. Deferoxamine is poorly absorbed orally as it is rapidly hydrolyzed in the gastric environment, but is well absorbed after IM or SC injection.

Deferoxamine was effective in a channel-billed toucan with iron storage disease. While under treatment, the bird's condition was monitored closely with chemical and image analyses for iron levels on monthly liver biopsies. With treatment, the bird improved clinically and its liver iron levels decreased to within the reference range for poultry. It died of severe cardiac fibrosis several months after treatment was discontinued. There was no speculation as to the cause of the cardiac disease. Liver iron levels were unremarkable at that point.

ADVERSE AND COMMON SIDE EFFECTS: A variety of adverse effects are described in humans including gastrointestinal upset, disturbances of hearing and vision, increased coagulability, and decreased serum glucose, calcium, and sodium.

DRUG INTERACTIONS: In humans with ascorbic acid deficiency, supplementation with vitamin C enhances the excretion of iron complexes. Patients receiving high amounts of vitamin C, however, may be predisposed to cardiac impairment as a result of toxic levels of labile iron within tissues. Vitamin C supplements should not be given to patients with cardiac disease.

SUPPLIED AS HUMAN PRODUCTS:
For injection containing 500 mg/vial (Desferrioxamine Mesilate for Injection ♣, PMS-Deferoxamine ♣, Desferal ♣ ★) and 2 g/vial (PMS-Deferoxamine ♣, Desferal ♣ ★)

DEXAMETHASONE

INDICATIONS: Dexamethasone (Azium ♣ ★, Azium SP ♣ ★, Dex-5 ♣) is a glucocorticoid used in small animal medicine for its anti-inflammatory effects and in the treatment of a variety of disease conditions. Dexamethasone sodium phosphate does not require hepatic biotransformation and is active immediately upon injection. For more information, see DEXAMETHASONE in the Small Animal section.

In birds, dexamethasone is used for the treatment of acute head trauma, shock, and at a lower dose as an anti-inflammatory agent. It may be helpful in reducing the inflammation associated with egg yolk peritonitis, and in the treatment of goiter in budgerigars in combination with iodine. For long-term therapy, a decreasing dose schedule is recommended. Dexamethasone has been used in combination with antibiotics for the treatment of the "Amazon foot necrosis" syndrome. Despite evidence of the strong immunosuppressive effects of corticosteroids in birds (see below), many published dosages are very high. For many of the conditions described above, nonsteroidal anti-inflammatory agents may be more appropriate as they are not immunosuppressive.

ADVERSE AND COMMON SIDE EFFECTS: Concern is frequently expressed regarding the high sensitivity of birds to the immunosuppressive effects of glucocorticoids. This has been supported by experimental work in pigeons, which showed the hypothalamic-pituitary-adrenal system to be more sensitive to suppression by glucocorticoids than that of mammals, and that suppression is dose dependent. The minimum intravenous dose required to suppress plasma corticosterone levels was 50 µg/kg. Administration of 1 mg/kg IM once daily for 6 weeks resulted in complete suppression of the pituitary–adrenal system. When administration of dexamethasone was discontinued, 6 to 7 weeks were required for basal plasma corticosterone levels to return to normal range. The duration of suppression by dexamethasone was greater than that of prednisolone, which was also evaluated in these studies. In another study, dexamethasone was administered orally at 50 µg/kg, ophthalmically at approximately 8 µg/kg, topically to bare skin at approximately 10 µg/kg, and topically in combination with DMSO to bare skin at doses of 0.05 to 50 µg/kg. Suppression of corticosterone levels occurred for up to 28 hours in the groups given oral, ophthalmic, and topical dexamethasone with DMSO at 50 µg/kg. An oral dose of 3 drops of Azium (2 or 4 mg/mL, strength not stated) per gallon of drinking water was found to be immunosuppressive in another study. Elevations in liver enzymes, polydipsia, polyuria, and diarrhea can occur secondary to treatment.

Barred owls and red-tailed hawks given 3 mg/kg dexamethasone IV or IM had elevated plasma dexamethasone levels for 3 to 4 hours postinjection, and decreased plasma corticosterone levels for 24 and 18 hours after treatment, respectively. In red-tailed hawks given 4 mg/kg of dexamethasone as a single dose IM, elevations in AST and alanine aminotransferase (ALT) occurred. Levels peaked at 3.2 times baseline levels between 24 and 36 hours, and were still elevated at 72 hours after injection.

DIAZEPAM

INDICATIONS: Diazepam (Valium ✽ ★, Valrelease ★) is a benzodiazepine used in birds as an anticonvulsant for the control of seizures, as a sedative, preanesthetic, or in combination with anesthetic agents such as ketamine. It is also used for the treatment of acute hyperexcitability and seizures as occur with 4-aminopyridine toxicity in pigeons. Diazepam has also been suggested for the treatment of psychogenic feather picking in psittacine birds; however, response to treatment is extremely variable among birds and may be negligible. Diazepam can be administered orally or by injection. Parenteral diazepam is formulated for intravenous use only, although dosages for IM delivery are sometimes reported. An equivalent benzodiazepine product for intramuscular use is midazolam. The effects of diazepam can be reversed with flumazenil. For more information, see DIAZEPAM in the Small Animal section.

DICLAZURIL

INDICATIONS: Diclazuril (Clinicox ♣ ★) is licensed for the prevention of coccidiosis in broiler chickens. A related drug, clazuril, was previously commercially available in tablet formulation for use in pigeons.

Diclazuril was administered orally over an 11-day period to treat a Hawaiian crow that presented with lethargy, weight loss, and an elevated titer to *Toxoplasma gondii*. By the end of therapy the bird's clinical presentation had returned to normal. Paired plasma samples collected at the beginning of therapy and 3 days after its conclusion revealed a 50% decrease in the antibodies to *T. gondii*. The authors felt that diclazuril may be an effective drug to treat toxoplasmosis in birds.

SUPPLIED AS VETERINARY PRODUCTS:
Premix for medicated feed, containing 0.5% w/w diclazuril (Clinicox ♣) and 0.25% w/w diclazuril (Clinacox ★)

DIETHYLSTILBESTROL

INDICATIONS: Diethylstilbestrol or DES (Stilboestrol ♣, Stilbestrol ♣, Stilphostrol ★, Honvol ♣) is used in the management of estrogen-responsive reproductive problems in female birds and plumage problems in both sexes. Tablets are insoluble (diethylstilbestrol) or sparingly soluble (diethylstilbestrol diphosphate) in water, but soluble in alcohol. For more information, see DIETHYLSTILBESTROL in the Small Animal section.

ADVERSE AND COMMON SIDE EFFECTS: Overdose may result in anemia. Diethylstilbestrol is not recommended for use in humans with liver or cardiovascular disease.

SUPPLIED AS VETERINARY PRODUCT:
Tablets containing 1 mg DES (Stilboestrol ♣)

SUPPLIED AS HUMAN PRODUCTS:
Tablets containing 0.1, 0.5, and 1 mg DES (Stilbestrol ♣), 5 mg (Diethylstilbestrol ★), 50 mg (Stilphostrol ♣ ★), and 100 mg (Honvol ♣) For injection containing 250 mg/5 mL (Honvol ♣) and 50 mg/mL (Stilphostrol ★)

DIGOXIN

INDICATIONS: Digoxin (Lanoxin ★, Cardoxin ✤ ★) is a positive inotropic and negative chronotropic agent used in the treatment of congestive heart failure. For more information, see DIGOXIN in the Small Animal section.

The pharmacokinetic properties of digoxin have been studied in a number of avian species, including chickens, turkeys, ducks, Quaker parakeets, sparrows, and budgerigars. Digoxin elixir is rapidly absorbed after oral administration. The elimination half-life varied among the species tested, from 6.67 hours in roosters to 25.9 hours in Quaker parakeets. In turkeys, pharmacokinetic variables changed with age of the bird and distribution with dosage levels. In budgerigars 0.02 mg/kg (approximately 0.0005 mg) produced blood levels in the therapeutic range for mammals. The digoxin elixir was diluted 1:4 to draw a measurable dose. A dose of 0.05 mg/kg per day was recommended as a safe initial dose in Quaker parakeets.

Digoxin has been used clinically to treat birds in congestive heart failure, but little investigative work has been done on the efficacy of digoxin in avian species. In a trial involving chickens, a dose of 0.1 mg/kg daily reduced the incidence of ascites. When possible, measurement of blood plasma levels should be undertaken. In an Indian hill mynah with congestive heart failure, digoxin administered at 0.01 mg/kg once daily improved cardiac function and the trough digoxin levels measured 1.6 ng/mL. Dosage of 0.01 mg/kg once daily to a secretary bird with dilative cardiomegaly resulted in a trough level of 1.4 ng/mL. The bird improved clinically for a short period but was eventually euthanized.

ADVERSE AND COMMON SIDE EFFECTS: In chickens, roosters, turkeys, and ducks, no toxic effects were seen at high plasma levels. In the Indian hill mynah described above, dosage with 0.02 mg/kg resulted in second-degree heart block. Trough levels of digoxin were 2.4 ng/mL and well above the therapeutic reference range in cats of 1 to 2 ng/mL. Dosage with 0.1 mg/kg in pigeons induced cardiac arrhythmias.

DIHYDROSTREPTOMYCIN

See STREPTOMYCIN.

DIMETRIDAZOLE

INDICATIONS: Dimetridazole (Dimetridazole ✤, Emtryl ✤) is a water-soluble antimicrobial agent effective against anaerobic bacteria and protozoa.

In birds, dimetridazole has been dosed orally or in the drinking water to treat trichomoniasis in pigeons, doves, cockatiels, and budgerigars; giardiasis in budgerigar nestlings; and histomoniasis and hexamitiasis. In homing pigeons, medicated water containing 400 mg/L had to be provided for at least 3 days to suppress infection by *Trichomonas gallinae*. Treatment once daily for 2 days using 20 mg tablets was ineffective in fasted and fed pigeons. The absolute bioavailability of the tablet in fasted pigeons was 83.8%, and was decreased by 20% if the drug was administered with food. After intravenous administration of 20 mg dimetridazole, the mean elimination half-life was 3.9 hours.

Dimetridazole has also been suggested for the treatment of infections by anaerobic bacteria.

ADVERSE AND COMMON SIDE EFFECTS: In situations where water intake is increased, birds may ingest toxic quantities of dimetridazole. These include periods of hot weather, when parents are feeding young, and during the breeding season when males increase their activity level. Extended therapy with dimetridazole may result in toxicity or overgrowth of *Candida*. Cockatiels, budgerigars, and pigeons have been reported to have developed incoordination and acute seizures and to have died after receiving 1 teaspoon (182 g dimetridazole per 6.42-ounce product) per gallon of drinking water. Dimetridazole is toxic or lethal in Pekin robins, and possibly in other passerine birds, even at therapeutic levels. Acute hepatitis has been reported in cockatiel chicks. B vitamins may help resolve clinical signs of toxicity.

SUPPLIED AS VETERINARY PRODUCTS:
Water-soluble powder with 40% w/w (Dimetridazole 40% ✤, Emtryl Soluble ✤)
Feed additives (Dimetridazole 30% w/w Premix ✤, Emtryl Premix ✤)

DIPHENHYDRAMINE

INDICATIONS: Diphenhydramine (Benadryl ✤ ★) is an antihistamine also used as an antiemetic. For more information, see DIPHENHYDRAMINE and ANTIHISTAMINES in the Small Animal section.

Diphenhydramine is used in psittacine birds for its antihistamine properties, as a mild sedative, and to try and control feather picking. Results with feather picking birds are extremely variable, with no improvement in many cases.

ADVERSE AND COMMON SIDE EFFECTS: Birds become sleepy if the dosage is too high; thus, tailoring treatment to each individual patient is necessary. Caution must be taken when the dosage recommendations are phrased simply as a volume (i.e., mL, tsp). The adult Benadryl elixir contains twice the concentration of the pediatric product that is commonly used (12.5 versus 6.25 mg/mL) and is formulated in an alcohol base. Veterinarians must ensure that clients are clear about which preparation they should use.

DMSA (MESO-2,3-DIMERCAPTOSUCCINIC ACID)

INDICATIONS: DMSA, or Succimer (DMSA ❧, Chemet ★), is an oral chelating agent with a high affinity for lead used in the treatment of lead poisoning in children. Children with blood lead levels greater than 70 µg/mL, or with clinical signs of encephalopathy, receive initial or concurrent therapy with parenteral calcium EDTA (CaEDTA) and dimercaprol. In humans, the initial dosage is 10 mg/kg every 8 hours for 5 days, then every 12 hours for an additional 14 days. Repeated treatment courses at a minimum of 14-day intervals may be appropriate.

DMSA chelates lead from soft tissues more rapidly than does CaEDTA, without an initial increase in CNS lead levels. Water-soluble complexes are formed that are excreted in the urine. DMSA is less effective at removing lead from bone than is CaEDTA. DMSA is fairly specific for lead, mercury, and arsenic, and has been described as having only a limited effect on zinc. DMSA has not been reported to cause nephrotoxicity.

DMSA has been used orally for the treatment of lead and zinc poisoning in birds. An experimental study comparing the ability of DMSA and CaEDTA to lower blood lead levels in lead poisoned cockatiels found DMSA administered at 40 or 80 mg/kg (q 12 hours for 21 days; PO) was more effective in lowering blood levels and increasing survival (compared to experimental control birds) than CaEDTA administered at 40 mg/kg (q 12 hours for 21 days; IM). There was no difference between groups administered the higher dose of DMSA and CaEDTA, or the higher dose of DMSA alone.

Because DMSA is administered orally, it may be rational to consider the concurrent use of parenteral CaEDTA if a patient is showing evidence of regurgitation or other abnormalities in gastric motility. It has been suggested that DMSA is more effective than CaEDTA for the treatment of zinc poisoning, but there are no scientific comparisons available and this theory runs counter to general information on the chelating ability of DMSA for zinc.

ADVERSE AND COMMON SIDE EFFECTS: DMSA was highly toxic to cockatiels at a dose of 80 mg/kg (q 12 hours for 21 days; PO) in the study described above. Four of 12 experimental birds (i.e., with lead administered) and 8/12 control birds (i.e., with no lead administered) that received this dose of DMSA died during the treatment period. Regurgitation and significant weight loss were also noted in treated birds. All birds receiving the lower dose of DMSA (40 mg/kg q 12 hours for 21 days; PO) survived and did not show adverse effects.

SUPPLIED AS HUMAN PRODUCT:
Capsules containing 100 mg (Chemet ★)

DOXAPRAM

INDICATIONS: Doxapram (Dopram-V ♣ ★) is a central respiratory stimulant used to stimulate respiration in patients with postanesthetic respiratory depression or apnea and to encourage the return of laryngopharyngeal reflexes in patients with mild to moderate respiratory and central nervous system depression due to anesthetic overdose. For more information, see DOXAPRAM in the Small Animal section.

DOXYCYCLINE

INDICATIONS: Doxycycline (Vibramycin ♣ ★, Vibra-Tabs ♣ ★, and others) is a second-generation, long-acting, lipid-soluble tetracycline antibiotic used in the treatment of bacterial, rickettsial, chlamydial, and mycoplasmal infections. As compared to other tetracyclines, doxycycline and minocycline are rapidly and almost completely absorbed by the gastrointestinal system and have greater activity against anaerobes and facultative intracellular bacteria. The elimination half-life of doxycycline is almost 3 times that of chlortetracycline. For more information, see DOXYCYCLINE and TETRACYCLINE ANTIBIOTICS in the Small Animal section.

Doxycycline is the treatment of choice for chlamydiosis in individual birds. In addition, recent studies suggest the drug can be used as an alternative to chlortetracycline for medication of feed and water. Doxycycline has also been used successfully to treat finches with hepatitis due to *Campylobacter* infection, and cockatiels with pharyngitis caused by an uncharacterized spiral shaped bacterium.

For the treatment of infection by *Chlamydophila psittaci,* doxycycline can be administered by the IV, IM, and PO routes. Intravenous injection has been recommended for the initial treatment of severely ill birds; however, the IM route is more practical. To avoid severe necrosis of muscle at the site of injection only neutral pH solutions can be injected. Vibramycin hyclate, reconstituted for intravenous use according to the manufacturer's instructions, cannot be used for intramuscular injection. Because Vibravenos, the formulation recommended for IM use, has not been available in the United States and has recently become unavailable in Canada, veterinarians have had compounding pharmacists create neutral sodium phosphate-buffered solutions of doxycycline for IM injection. However, severe muscle damage has been reported in some birds after use of some compounded products. Veterinarians must, therefore, use caution when using untested compounded formulations.

Once clinical signs begin to resolve, a switch is often made to oral therapy, either directly or through medication of the food. Treatment should continue for a period of 45 days, regardless of the method of administration. Pharmacokinetic studies have been performed in a variety of avian species. The therapeutic goal is to have minimum inhibitory concentrations greater than 1 µg/mL in plasma for the treatment period.

In psittacine birds, single IM doses of 80 to 100 mg/kg provide adequate blood levels for 5 to 6 days; however, the rate of elimination of the drug increases over time. A reduction in the time interval between injections is, therefore, recommended. Two recommended treatment schedules are 1) eight injections given at intervals of 7, 7, 7, 7, 6, 5, and 5 days; 2) six injections at 5-day intervals followed by four injections at 4-day intervals. Effective blood levels are reached within a few hours and shedding of chlamydiae usually stops within 24 hours of commencement of treatment. Species that require lower amounts of chlortetracycline for treatment, such as the large macaws; lovebirds (*Agapornis*); eastern, western, and pale-headed rosellas; Bourke's, red-winged, turquoise, and mulga parrots; and red-fronted, canary-winged, and gray-cheeked parakeets, can be treated with doxycycline at 75 mg/kg on the same schedule. Elimination half-lives of doxycycline in psittacines are species specific, ranging from 10 to over 20 hours. Intramuscular injection with formulated doxycycline hyclate at 100 mg/kg every 6 days for 3 injections was shown to maintain therapeutic plasma concentrations for 44 days in pigeons.

Houbara bustards injected IM or SC with 100 mg/kg of Vibravenos 7 times over a 38-day period maintained plasma levels greater than 1 µg/mL. With SC compared to IM injection, absorption was slightly slower and apparent elimination more rapid. SC was preferred to deliver the large volume of the drug. Mild irritation was noted at the sites of injection. Over 250 bustards were treated based on these results.

In a separate study, once-daily administration of 25 to 50 mg/kg in seven psittacine species produced therapeutic blood levels. In chickens given 10 mg/kg once daily orally, blood concentrations peaked at over 50 µg/mL and remained above 1 µg/mL for at least 12 hours. Oral absorption of doxycycline was erratic in growing chickens fed a liquid diet, which may be of relevance to the administration of doxycycline in hand-feeding formulas to psittacine chicks.

Doxycycline can be formulated into pelleted or mash diets. Seeds impregnated with 250 to 300 mg/kg fed to budgerigars resulted in therapeutic blood levels. Blood levels of doxycycline in birds fed mash diets containing 0.1%, 0.2%, and 0.4% for 6 weeks varied among birds and within individual birds from day to day. In one study, blue and gold and scarlet macaws were fed 100 g of a corn diet medicated with 0.1% doxycycline hyclate daily for 45 days. Blood levels greater than 1 µg/mL were obtained by day 3 and maintained throughout the treatment period. Although absorption of oral doxycycline is less affected by calcium levels than is chlortetracycline, dietary calcium levels should probably be kept below 0.7%.

Several pharmacokinetic trials have investigated the use of doxycycline in drinking water. In one such study, doxycycline hyclate from generic capsules used at 800 mg/L was given to 7 African gray parrots and 8 Goffin's cockatoos for 42 days. Mean doxycycline levels, and levels in almost all individual samples, were >1 µg/mL when measured on multiple occasions between days 4 and 42. In a pilot study that also included orange-winged Amazon parrots, a lower dosage of 400 mg/L doxycycline in drinking water resulted in plasma doxycycline concentrations of approximately 1 µg/mL in the Amazon parrots, >1 µg/mL in the Goffin's cockatoos, and <1 µg/mL in the African gray parrots, based on samples collected between days 4 and 42. In this pilot study, Amazon parrots given the 800 mg/L doxycycline had lower plasma levels than those that received 400 mg/L of the drug. This was assumed to be due to a reduction in water intake when birds were provided with water containing the greater concentration of medication. Chickens medicated with 20 mg/L in the drinking water did not attain serum levels of 1 µg/mL; however, levels in kidney and lung were greater than in serum.

A large pharmacokinetic study compared the results of administering doxycycline hyclate to cockatiels by intramuscular injection (100 mg/kg IM every 10 days for 5 injections) or by mixing with drinking water (0.28 or 0.83 mg/mL), seeds (500 mg/kg wet weight), or mash (1,000 mg/kg) over a 45-day period. Birds receiving doxycycline by intramuscular injection had variable, localized tissue reactions including mild to moderate swelling, bruising, hemorrhage, and occasional leakage of doxycycline from the injection site, and did not obtain the desired therapeutic concentration (i.e., mean plasma concentration of >1 µg/mL). Birds that received doxycycline in mash had high plasma doxycycline concentrations and showed severe clinical illness (e.g., weight loss, anorexia, lethargy), suggestive of doxycycline toxicosis. Drug administration was; therefore, discontinued on day 3. The birds that received doxycycline in drinking water and in seeds maintained group mean doxycycline concentrations of >1 µg/mL. It was concluded from the clinical and pharmacokinetic results of this study that the drinking water and seed formulations were the safest and most effective.

ADVERSE AND COMMON SIDE EFFECTS: Clinical signs of doxycycline toxicity include: lethargy, inappetence, inactivity, yellow or green urates or urine, and elevated AST, lactate dehydrogenase (LDH), and bile acids. These adverse effects may be seen in some birds at therapeutic drug levels. The oral lethal dose in 50% (LD_{50}) of week-old chickens was 2,500 mg/kg. In Goffin's cockatoos fed a corn- and bean-based diet containing 1,000 mg doxycycline hyclate per kg diet, plasma AST and LDH levels increased during treatment. Mild transient elevations in AST, LDH, and bile acids were noted in the same species given 800 mg doxycycline per L drinking water, and in cockatiels given doxycycline orally in the drinking water at 0.28 and 0.83 mg/mL and in seeds at 500 mg/kg of diet (wet weight). Treatment with doxycycline may halt oviposition in hens and has been associated with bone deformities in toucans, especially young toucans. One report describes hemorrhages and delays in blood coagulation associated with repeated doxycycline injections. Vitamin K administered at the same time appeared to partially protect against this coagulation abnormality. Red discoloration of the feces may occur in treated birds.

Vomiting has been reported in blue and gold macaws after both IM and oral administration of the drug at generally recommended dose levels. Reducing the overall dosage in this species has been suggested, as has halving the dose and administering it every 12 hours, as compared to every 24 hours. Because of its more complete absorption and enteric secretion as an inactive conjugate, doxycycline has less disruptive effects on gastrointestinal flora than does chlortetracycline. Birds should, nevertheless, be monitored for the overgrowth of gastrointestinal yeasts such as *Candida* spp.

The IM administration of most IV preparations results in severe muscle damage due to the acid pH of these solutions. Vibravenos or specially compounded formulations must be used for this route of administration; however, even then muscle necrosis and accompanying changes in clinical chemistry values will still occur.

As with all tetracyclines, doxycycline should be protected from light to prevent formation of toxic oxidation by-products.

DRUG INTERACTIONS: The effect of dietary calcium on reducing oral absorption of doxycycline is less pronounced than with chlortetracycline. In pigeons without calcium in the diet, the apparent elimination half-life was 6.25 hours while the presence of calcium in the diet decreased the elimination half-life to 3.81 hours. Calcium and zinc in the intestinal tract may bind to excreted doxycycline and block enterohepatic cycling, thus increasing the drug's overall clearance. Dietary iron decreases absorption by 80% to 90%, whereas the presence of organic acids such as citric acid increases absorption by 2 to 5 times. The absorption of oral doxycycline was reduced by the presence of grit in the diet of pigeons.

SUPPLIED AS VETERINARY PRODUCTS:
Avian product: for injection containing 20 mg/mL (Vibravenos—not registered for use in North America at present but available through special permits)
Water-soluble powder containing 50 mg/g (Vibravet 5% ♣)
Oral suspension containing 5 mg/mL after reconstitution (Vibravet ♣)

SUPPLIED AS HUMAN PRODUCTS:
Tablets and capsules containing 50 mg (Monodox ★) and 100 mg (Monodox ★, Alti-Doxycycline ♣, Apo-Doxy ♣, Doxycin ♣, Doxytec (lactose) ♣, Novo-Doxylin ♣, Nu-Doxycycline ♣, Vibramycin ♣, Vibra-Tabs ♣ ★)

Oral suspension containing 5 mg/mL after reconstitution (Vibravet
♣, Vibramycin ★)
Oral suspension containing 50 mg/5 mL (Vibramycin calcium syrup ★)
For injection in 100 mg and 200 mg vials (Vibramycin ★)
For IV injection in vials of 100 and 200 mg (Doxy 100 ★, Doxy 200 ★)

ENILCONAZOLE

INDICATIONS: Enilconazole (Imaverol ♣) is an imidazole antifungal agent that has activity against *Penicillium* and the dermatophytes and marketed as a topical preparation for the treatment of
dermatophytosis. For more information, see ENILCONAZOLE in the
Small Animal section.

Although enilconazole solution is marketed for topical use, there
are several reports of the drug being used orally against candidiasis
and in the drinking water to prevent and treat pulmonary aspergillosis in chicks.

Enilconazole is also available as a spray and a smoke bomb used to
fumigate poultry hatcheries and chick rooms infected with *Aspergillus
fumigatus,* with or without the birds present in the rooms. Clinafarm
smoke has also been used for the aerosol treatment of respiratory aspergillosis, particularly in ratites, by setting off the "bomb" in an enclosure
containing the affected bird(s).

ADVERSE AND COMMON SIDE EFFECTS: Some birds reduce consumption of drinking water medicated with enilconazole. In some
reported cases alternate day therapy was efficacious. An elevation in
AST was seen in an eclectus parrot treated orally with 6 mg/kg twice
daily for 7 days. The undiluted Clinafarm spray may be irritating to
the skin or the eyes. The diluted emulsion is well tolerated.

SUPPLIED AS VETERINARY PRODUCTS:
Solution containing 100 mg/mL (Imaverol ♣)
Smoke generator containing 5 g/generator (Clinafarm Smoke)
Emulsifiable liquid containing 150 mg/mL (Clinafarm Spray)

ENROFLOXACIN

INDICATIONS: Enrofloxacin (Baytril ♣ ★) is a fluoroquinolone antibiotic active against a range of gram-positive and gram-negative
bacteria, mycoplasmas, chlamydiae, rickettsia, and atypical mycobacteria. Enrofloxacin has limited activity against anaerobes. For
more information, see ENROFLOXACIN and FLUOROQUINOLONE
ANTIBIOTICS in the Small Animal section.

Enrofloxacin is one of the most commonly used antibiotics in avian
medicine; hence, some bacterial resistance is developing. Oral sus-

pensions formulated from the injectable product are commonly used as an alternative to long-term therapy by injection. A sweet or flavored syrup must be used to mask the bitter taste of the drug. The oral concentrate licensed for use in poultry has also been diluted appropriately and used to treat individual birds. Enrofloxacin has been used to treat infection by *Chlamydophila psittaci*, but insufficient research is available to supplant doxycycline as the recommended therapeutic agent. As well, clinical experience suggests that enrofloxacin is less effective than doxycycline for this purpose. Enrofloxacin is partially metabolized by the liver to ciprofloxacin, also an effective antibacterial agent.

Enrofloxacin has been included in drug regimens for combination treatment of avian mycobacteriosis. These have been derived from human regimens that often include ciprofloxacin. Veterinarians differ in their willingness to treat avian mycobacteriosis due to the difficulty in ensuring that the infection is fully eliminated and concerns over the potential for zoonotic spread of the disease under certain conditions.

Several pharmacokinetic studies have been carried out in African gray parrots. In a single-dose trial, enrofloxacin was administered at 15 mg/kg IM and at 3, 15, and 30 mg/kg PO. Peak plasma concentrations were reached 1 hour after IM injection and 2 to 4 hours after oral administration. The relative bioavailability of the oral medication was 51% of that of the IM dose. IM injection resulted in a higher peak plasma concentration than the oral dose; however, 2 hours after administration there was no difference between the two. In a multidose trial, birds were given 30 mg/kg orally twice daily for 10 days. Based on the results of this trial, the authors suggested an increase in dosage might be necessary for prolonged treatment.

In another study in African gray parrots, enrofloxacin in the drinking water produced lower plasma levels than the previous two routes of drug administration. Birds given 0.09, 0.19, 0.38, and 0.75 mg/mL enrofloxacin in drinking water had similar serum levels of enrofloxacin (mean values from 0.10 to 0.15 µg/mL) and showed no significant differences in mean daily water consumption or weight loss as compared to control birds. Based on mean body weight and mean daily water consumption, these birds consumed 4.0, 8.5, 16.9, and 33.4 mg enrofloxacin per kg, respectively, daily. Birds administered enrofloxacin in water at 1.5 and 3.0 mg/mL became depressed, lost weight, and exhibited polyuria and polydipsia, although no biochemical abnormalities were detected. Adverse signs resolved within 3 days of ending treatment. Birds had poor acceptance of water containing more than 0.75 mg/mL. In this study, mean plasma ciprofloxacin concentrations were lower than but paralleled those for enrofloxacin. At all dosages studied, these African gray parrots had lower serum levels of enrofloxacin than broiler chickens and turkeys given the drug at a dosage of 0.1 mg/mL drinking water, suggesting that interspecies generalizations may not be accurate.

A single-dose pharmacokinetic study compared 15 mg/kg of enrofloxacin administered by PO, IM, and IV routes in red-tailed hawks and great horned owls. After oral administration in both species, peak concentrations were reached after 4 to 8 hours, and plasma levels remained above 1 µg/mL for at least 18 hours. After IM administration peak plasma levels were reached after 0.5 to 2 hours, and were maintained above 1 µg/mL for at least 15 hours, as they did in red-tailed hawks treated IV. Two owls showed acute weakness, bradycardia, and peripheral vasoconstriction during IV injection; this mode of administration was not evaluated further in this species. In red-tailed hawks, the absolute bioavailability as compared to IV administration was 76% for PO and 87% for IM administration. Similar values were estimated for owls on the basis of more limited data. The dosages recommended on the basis of this study were 15 mg/kg every 24 hours, PO or IM, for the two species. Intravenous injection of enrofloxacin is contraindicated in great horned owls and caution is suggested for IV use in red-tailed hawks.

Protection trials were performed in Muscovy ducks challenged with intratracheal *Escherichia coli* and in canaries challenged with *Yersinia pseudotuberculosis*. Birds were experimentally infected then treated with enrofloxacin in the drinking water. Good therapeutic efficacy was described in ducks who had access to water containing 12.5 or 25 mg/mL for 4 hours daily for 5 days and in the canaries who were treated with 150 mg/L (150 ppm). Enrofloxacin provided in drinking water at 150 mg/L is recommended for the treatment of enteric *Campylobacter* spp. infections in Lady Gouldian finches.

ADVERSE AND COMMON SIDE EFFECTS: Myonecrosis at injection sites can be severe. In a study in which 102 birds were given 100 or 200 mg/mL enrofloxacin in drinking water or 10 mg/kg IM once daily for 10 days, 22 birds developed polyuria and polydipsia that resolved after the trial ended, 19 had reduced food intake, and 8 had infections due to mycotic overgrowth in the gastrointestinal tract (GIT). Depression, polyuria, and polydipsia were also seen in African gray parrots given enrofloxacin in the drinking water at concentrations of 1.5 and 3.0 mg/mL. Renal damage was identified in a Senegal parrot treated for 10 days with enrofloxacin and ketoconazole. Vomiting and inappetence have also been described in birds receiving enrofloxacin. Agitation and aggression have been recorded in a yellow-napped and a red-headed Amazon parrot being treated with enrofloxacin.

In an experimental trial in racing pigeons given 200, 400, or 800 mg/L in drinking water over a long term, no abnormalities were noted in the birds themselves; however, there was a dose-related increase in embryo mortality in eggs from treated parents. Chicks raised by parents given 800 mg/mL had a slightly delayed increase in body weight and growth of long feathers, and in some birds joint lesions occurred. There was no long-term effect on growth or fertility of the chicks. It has been suggested that treatment with enrofloxacin may cause joint problems in some young psittacines and pigeons; however, the drug is widely used in pediatric patients.

Two great horned owls showed significant acute weakness, bradycardia, and peripheral vasoconstriction during IV administration of enrofloxacin. These signs resolved within 1 to 3 hours of supportive therapy.

SUPPLIED AS VETERINARY PRODUCTS:
See also Small Animal section
Liquid concentrate containing 32.3 mg/mL (Baytril 3.23% Concentrate Antimicrobial Solution ★)

EPINEPHRINE

INDICATIONS: Epinephrine ♣ ★ is indicated in cardiac arrest associated with ventricular asystole. It accelerates atrial and ventricular contraction rates. It has been suggested that the avian heart is more sensitive to norepinephrine. For more information, see EPINEPHRINE in the Small Animal section.

ERGONOVINE MALEATE

INDICATIONS: Ergonovine maleate (Ergonovine Maleate Solution ♣) is an oxytocin principle of ergot that has been used in conjunction with calcium and vitamin A injections to aid in egg expulsion. The drug should be diluted for use in small birds. Oxytocin is more frequently described for the same purpose. For more information, see ERGONOVINE in the Large Animal section.

ADVERSE AND COMMON SIDE EFFECTS: The use of ergonovine is contraindicated where there is physical obstruction to the passage of an egg. In humans, hypertension may follow IV administration. Ergonovine overdose results in a variety of clinical signs including gangrene and seizures in humans. Ergonovine should not be used in patients with cardiovascular disease.

SUPPLIED AS HUMAN PRODUCTS:
For injection containing 0.2 mg/mL (Ergotrate Maleate ★) and 0.25 mg/mL (Ergonovine Maleate ♣)
Tablets containing 0.2 mg (Ergotrate ★, Ergotrate Maleate ♣)

ERYTHROMYCIN

INDICATIONS: Erythromycin (Erythro-100 ★, Gallimycin ✦ ★) is a macrolide antibiotic with primary activity against gram-positive bacteria. The drug also has activity against *Campylobacter fetus*, mycoplasmas, chlamydiae, rickettsiae, spirochetes, and some atypical mycobacteria, leptospires, and amebae. For more information, see ERYTHROMYCIN in the Small Animal section.

In birds, erythromycin is primarily used by oral administration or by nebulization with the injectable formulation for the treatment of chronic respiratory disease, especially air sacculitis and sinusitis, when mycoplasmas are suspected. Most psittacine gram-negative infections are resistant to the drug. Erythromycin has been used in the drinking water at a concentration of 300 mg/L for the treatment of enteric *Campylobacter* spp. infections in Lady Gouldian finches. Erythromycin has also been used for the treatment of hepatic *Campylobacter* infections in small passerines.

ADVERSE AND COMMON SIDE EFFECTS: The injectable solution given IM may result in severe muscle necrosis. During oral therapy, some birds may develop gastrointestinal signs, including regurgitation and diarrhea that resolve when erythromycin administration is stopped.

DRUG INTERACTIONS: Erythromycin inhibits hepatic cytochrome P-450 enzymes, and therefore, therapy with erythromycin may affect the levels of a variety of other therapeutic agents.

ETHAMBUTOL

INDICATIONS: Ethambutol (Myambutol ✦ ★) is a bacteriostatic antimycobacterial drug used in human medicine for the treatment of mycobacterial infections. Clarithromycin or azithromycin combined with ethambutol and either ciprofloxacin or rifabutin is recommended for the prophylaxis and treatment of *Mycobacterium avium* complex infections in HIV patients. Resistance to ethambutol has rarely been observed. Ethambutol is administered orally and is well absorbed through the intestine and is excreted unchanged in the urine and feces. Ethambutol is not used for the treatment of ocular or renal mycobacteriosis.

In birds, ethambutol has been used in combination drug regimens for the treatment of mycobacteriosis. Veterinarians differ in their willingness to treat avian mycobacteriosis due to the difficulty in ensuring that the infection is fully eliminated and concerns over the potential for zoonotic spread of the disease under certain conditions.

ADVERSE AND COMMON SIDE EFFECTS: In humans, a range of adverse effects are described including decreased visual acuity and color sensitivity, anaphylactoid reactions, pruritus, joint pain, gastro-intestinal disturbances, vertigo, headache, and peripheral neuritis. It is recommended that renal function be monitored during treatment as elevations in serum uric acid levels have been reported and acute gout episodes precipitated.

DRUG INTERACTIONS: In humans, administration of 10,000 IU vita-min A per day for 30 days is recommended as prophylactic treatment of the visual side effects. Ethambutol is always used in combination with other antimycobacterial agents.

SUPPLIED AS HUMAN PRODUCT:
Tablets containing 100 mg and 400 mg (Myambutol ✤ ★)

FENBENDAZOLE

INDICATIONS: Fenbendazole (Panacur ✤ ★) is an anthelmintic rec-ommended for the elimination of nematodes and some tapeworms. It is also effective against *Giardia* and some trematodes and micro-filaria. For more information, see FENBENDAZOLE in the Small Ani-mal section.

In birds, fenbendazole is used for the treatment of nematode infec-tions, including ascarids, capillariasis, and *Syngamus* spp. infection. It is not effective against gizzard worms in finches. The drug has been used by direct oral administration or mixed in feed. In a pharmaco-kinetic study in white Pekin ducks given 5 mg/kg orally or IV, no significant abnormalities were noted in complete blood cell counts, serum biochemistry, corticosterone levels, or thyroid function. Fen-bendazole was not effective against hepatic trematodes in cockatoos at doses up to 100 mg/kg every 8 hours for three days.

ADVERSE AND COMMON SIDE EFFECTS: Several recent reports warn of toxicity and death in birds associated with the use of benzimi-dazole anthelmintics, namely fenbendazole and albendazole. These drugs inhibit microtubule function and hence cell division. There appears to be an increased susceptibility to toxicity in some orders of birds, as well the severity of toxicity appears to be dose related. Reports most frequently involve birds in the order Columbiformes, including domestic pigeons; however, toxicity has also been reported in solitary lories, keas (with albendazole), and painted storks. Clini-cal signs include weight loss and lethargy, a marked initial leuko-penia due to a profound heteropenia (e.g., WBC < 1,000/μL), severe progressive anemia, and possibly thrombocytopenia. Some birds have recovered with supportive care. On necropsy severe bone mar-row necrosis and depletion, intestinal crypt cell necrosis, and over-whelming sepsis appear to be the most consistent findings. Dosing with fenbendazole at 50 and 100 mg/kg once daily PO for periods of

5 to 10 days has resulted in toxicosis in columbiformes, and with 34 to 35 mg/kg once daily PO for 5 days in painted storks. Clinical signs of illness are often apparent as early as 5 days after initiation of treatment, although the exact number of days of treatment necessary to induce toxicity is not known. In a retrospective study of the medical and necropsy records of 402 pigeons and doves from a large zoological collection that were treated with fenbendazole as part of routine quarantine or arrival processing, adverse effects appeared to be more severe in birds treated with 100 mg/kg as compared to 50 mg/kg.

In one report, a preparation of 200 mg fenbendazole impregnated into 1 kg of finch seed and fed for 6 to 7 days was toxic to long-tailed, blue-faced parrots, and diamond fir-tail finches, and chestnut-breasted mannikins. Deaths in birds have been reported 3 to 5 days after administration of 1,000 mg/L in drinking water. Ataxia, mydriasis, and depression have also been described in canaries at this dose. Fenbendazole should not be used during periods of feather growth as stunting of feathers may result.

SUPPLIED AS VETERINARY PRODUCTS:

Granules (222 mg fenbendazole/gram) to be mixed with food (Panacur ✤ ★)
Oral paste containing 10% fenbendazole (Panacur ✤ ★, Safe-Guard ★)
Oral suspension containing 10% fenbendazole (Panacur ✤ ★, Safe-Guard ✤ ★)

FLUCONAZOLE

INDICATIONS: Fluconazole (Diflucan ✤ ★) is a synthetic azole derivative fungistatic antimycotic agent. Fluconazole has greater water solubility, better oral bioavailability, higher plasma and extravascular levels, and a longer plasma elimination half-life than ketoconazole. Fluconazole is only recommended if topical treatment (e.g., enilconazole) is not feasible. Fluconazole penetrates well into the brain, cerebrospinal fluid, and eyes. For more information, see FLUCONAZOLE in the Small Animal section.

In birds, fluconazole has been used primarily to treat and is the drug of choice for mucosal and systemic infections with *Candida* spp. Absorption of the drug is not affected by gastric pH. This feature is useful in the treatment of pediatric patients whose gastric pH is relatively high. Fluconazole has been successfully used to reduce the number of candidal organisms in oral and fecal smears from psittacines at doses of 2, 5, and 10 mg/kg every 24 hours for 2 to 4 days. Umbrella cockatoos and blue-fronted Amazon parrots required 5 mg/kg to reduce numbers of organisms in feces to normal within 48 hours. Tablets were dissolved in water and the resulting suspension administered orally.

Fluconazole has also been used in the treatment of *Aspergillus* spp. infections. Outbreaks of mycotic respiratory disease in hummingbird colonies, caused by *Aspergillus* spp. and *Alternaria* spp., were successfully controlled by providing the birds with a 9% protein-supplemented nectar containing 25 mg/L of fluconazole for up to 2 weeks. One case report describes the combined use of systemic fluconazole and nebulized clotrimazole for the apparently successful treatment of cryptococcal lesions in the air sacs of a sulfur-crested cockatoo.

ADVERSE AND COMMON SIDE EFFECTS: Transient regurgitation has been reported after treatment with fluconazole, especially in cockatoos and cockatiels. Inappetence and depression have also been listed as adverse effects. Increases in AST and LDH were seen during treatment; however, enzyme levels returned to normal by 2 weeks after treatment.

FLUCYTOSINE (5-FLUOROCYTOSINE)

INDICATIONS: Flucytosine (Ancobon ★) is a fluorinated pyrimidine antifungal agent often used in combination with amphotericin B, with which it is synergistic. Combined drug therapy also reduces the development of resistance. For more information, see FLUCYTOSINE in the Small Animal section.

In birds, flucytosine has been used for the treatment of severe candidiasis of the digestive system, systemic candidal infections, and for the prevention and treatment of respiratory aspergillosis. *In vitro* work has shown that significant numbers of these organisms are resistant to the drug. Preventive treatment has been especially recommended for high-risk patients such as immunosuppressed birds, birds with severe chlamydial infections, and stressed birds, particularly raptors, accipiter hawks, some falcons, and swans.

In a pharmacokinetic study involving turkeys, great horned owls, and red-tailed hawks, oral administration of flucytosine at doses of 75 to 120 mg/kg was recommended at 6-hour intervals to maintain plasma levels above the minimum inhibitory concentration for *Aspergillus fumigatus*. Published dosing regimens are broad and range from 50 to 250 mg/kg every 12 hours, which differs tremendously from the pharmacokinetic study described above. Flucytosine appears to have been used safely at various dosages within this range in a variety of species including raptors, psittacines, and finches for periods up to several months in duration. Some authors suggest lower doses for larger birds (i.e., >500 g, use 60 mg/kg; and <500 g, use 150 mg/kg) but this is by no means consistent.

ADVERSE AND COMMON SIDE EFFECTS: Gastrointestinal irritation has been described in some birds. Because of potential bone marrow toxicity, hematologic parameters should be monitored in birds on long-term therapy. Concerns have been expressed regarding the possibility of hepatotoxicity.

DRUG INTERACTIONS: Flucytosine can be used in combination with amphotericin B.

FLUMAZENIL

INDICATIONS: Flumazenil (Anexate ✤ ★) is a specific benzo-diazepine receptor antagonist, which is used to reverse the effects of benzodiazepines such as diazepam and midazolam by competitive inhibition. In humans, flumazenil is rapidly metabolized by the liver. Depending on the initial dose of benzodiazepine, resedation could occur as the flumazenil is metabolized. Ideally, the dose of flumazenil is titrated to the desired effect. The use and efficacy of flumazenil have not been well described in birds.

ADVERSE AND COMMON SIDE EFFECTS: A variety of adverse effects are described in humans.

SUPPLIED AS HUMAN PRODUCT:
For injection containing 0.1 mg/mL (Anexate ✤ ★)

FLUNIXIN MEGLUMINE

INDICATIONS: Flunixin meglumine (Banamine ✤ ★, Flunixamine ★, and others) is a potent nonsteroidal antiprostaglandin agent with anti-inflammatory and antipyretic properties that make it useful in the treatment of inflammation and pain associated with musculoskeletal disease. For more information, see FLUNIXIN in the Small Animal section.

Flunixin has been recommended for use in pediatric patients with intestinal pain and anorexia and for birds in shock or with traumatic injuries. Newer NSAIDs, such as meloxicam, appear to have less potential for adverse effects in avian patients than does flunixin.

A study in mallard ducks to evaluate the effect of flunixin on thromboxane levels found ducks given single doses of 5 mg/kg had significant suppression of thromboxane levels for 4 hours after administration; and for approximately 12 hours more, levels were decreased compared with baseline samples. At necropsy, there was no evidence of GI bleeding but muscle necrosis was present at the sites of injection. This work suggests that flunixin has anti-inflammatory and analgesic effects in waterfowl; however, parenteral administration is not recommended.

In young ostrich chicks given flunixin at 1.1 mg/kg IV, the mean plasma elimination half-life was only 0.17 hours and tissue distribution was limited based on a calculated volume of distribution of only 0.13 L/kg.

ADVERSE AND COMMON SIDE EFFECTS: Significant glomerular pathology was produced in bobwhite quail held off water for 24 hours (to simulate clinical dehydration) and then administered doses of flunixin ranging from 0.1 to 32 mg/kg IM every 24 hours for 7 days. Renal damage was not mirrored by plasma biochemistry: uric acid levels were not increased. Lesions were present in all groups but were more severe at higher doses. Renal disease and death have been reported in psittacine birds and cranes receiving flunixin. Flunixin should likely not be used in cranes. Many clinicians avoid flunixin as a result of concerns about renal function or use flunixin only in conjunction with fluid supplementation. The drug is contraindicated in birds with preexisting renal disease or dehydration.

In an experimental trial in budgerigars given 10 mg/kg (route not stated but assumed to be IM), five of six birds vomited between 2 and 5 minutes after administration but appeared normal thereafter. Diarrhea, tenesmus, and frank blood in the feces have also been reported with the use of flunixin in birds. In a study in mallard ducks, intramuscular injection of flunixin resulted in myonecrosis at the sites of injection. Severe myonecrosis was also noted in bobwhite quail given a very high dose of 32 mg/kg IM.

FUROSEMIDE

INDICATIONS: Furosemide (Lasix ❦ ★) is a potent loop diuretic that is effective in reducing edema of cardiac origin and promoting diuresis. For more information, see FUROSEMIDE in the Small Animal section.

Furosemide has been used in birds to reduce ascites and pulmonary edema of cardiac origin.

ADVERSE AND COMMON SIDE EFFECTS: Overdosage may result in dehydration and electrolyte abnormalities. Neurologic signs and death have also been reported. Some species, such as lories, are very sensitive to furosemide and are easily overdosed. The therapeutic index in birds appears to be low.

GENTAMICIN

INDICATIONS: Gentamicin (Gentocin ❦ ★, Gentasul ❦, Garagen ★) is an aminoglycoside antibiotic used in the treatment of bacterial infections, especially those caused by gram-negative organisms. For more information, see GENTAMICIN and AMINOGLYCOSIDE ANTIBIOTICS in the Small Animal section.

Gentamicin has been used widely in avian medicine, but nephrotoxicity is a real concern. Pharmacokinetic parameters vary widely among avian species; therefore, direct application of dosage recommendations from one species to another may be inappropriate. In recent years, amikacin has replaced gentamicin as a less toxic alternative when an aminoglycoside antibiotic is desired.

In pharmacokinetic studies carried out in bobwhite quail, pheasants, and greater sandhill cranes given from 5 to 20 mg/kg IM, peak plasma concentrations varied with increasing drug dose. The mean plasma elimination half-life ranged from approximately 40 minutes in quail to 165 minutes in cranes. In another study involving red-tailed hawks, great horned owls, and golden eagles given 10 mg/kg IV, significant differences in serum half-life and total body clearance were seen among the different species. This dose resulted in peak and trough levels greater than those associated with nephrotoxicity and ototoxicity in humans.

In a study in quail, cranes, and ducks, levels of gentamicin in lung and leg muscle paralleled those in plasma while levels in liver and kidney were greater than plasma. Movement and elimination of the drug differed among the species examined. Similar findings were described for hawks, owls, chickens, and turkeys. Gentamicin was present in renal tissue for 3 to 4 weeks after cessation of treatment in chickens and turkeys.

A pharmacokinetic study in cockatiels concluded that a dosage of 5 to 10 mg/kg IM 2 to 3 times daily was appropriate. A plasma elimination half-life of 71 minutes was calculated in this species based on an IM dose of 5 mg/kg twice daily. The mean peak and trough levels were 4.6 µg/mL and 0.2 µg/mL, respectively. In human medicine, the desired peak and trough levels of gentamicin are 8 to 10 µg/mL and less than 2 µg/mL, respectively.

Gentamicin has been used to treat sinusitis and air sacculitis by nebulization where it has a primarily topical effect due to poor absorption from the respiratory epithelium. Sinusitis can also be treated by direct intranasal administration of gentamicin ophthalmic solution. Direct intratracheal injection has also been suggested for the treatment of respiratory disease. Gentamicin is not absorbed through intact intestinal mucosa; therefore, oral therapy is limited to treatment of infections confined to the gut.

ADVERSE AND COMMON SIDE EFFECTS: Gentamicin is nephrotoxic, especially in birds that are dehydrated or suffering from pre-existing renal disease. Concurrent administration of balanced electrolyte solutions may help reduce renal damage. Measurement of blood antibiotic concentrations should be carried out whenever possible.

Renal toxicity has been described in a wide variety of avian species, including psittacines and raptors, given gentamicin at a total dose of 10 mg/kg per day and greater. Polyuria and polydipsia were commonly seen; however, neither clinical signs nor serum biochemical parameters were considered good indicators of the degree of renal damage. Renal function did not return to normal for up to several weeks after cessation of treatment. Recent work suggests that less frequent administration of aminoglycoside antibiotics (allowing trough levels to drop to 1 µg/mL) reduces the likelihood of toxicity. Deaths have occurred in birds given daily doses of 20 mg/kg or greater. Lories may be particularly susceptible to the toxic effects of gentamicin. Weakness, apnea, and sudden death attributed to neuromuscular blockade have been described in hawks and great horned owls. Some birds also showed ataxia after gentamicin administration, which was presumed to result from vestibular damage.

DRUG INTERACTIONS: Gentamicin is inactivated *in vitro* if mixed with carbenicillin or ticarcillin. Some cephalosporins potentiate the nephrotoxic effect of gentamicin.

GLYCOPYRROLATE

INDICATIONS: Glycopyrrolate (Robinul-V ★, Robinul ✚ ★) is an anticholinergic agent used in preanesthetic regimens to reduce salivary, tracheobronchial, and pharyngeal secretions, to reduce the volume and acidity of gastric secretion, and to inhibit cardiac vagal inhibitory reflexes during anesthetic induction and intubation.

In birds, glycopyrrolate can be used as a preanesthetic agent or during an anesthetic protocol to prevent or treat bradycardia, although it may cause thickening of tracheal secretions and therefore predispose to blockage of an endotracheal tube. In an emergency situation, atropine may provide a stronger and more rapid response.

ADVERSE AND COMMON SIDE EFFECTS: Thickening of tracheal secretions during anesthesia may result in the development of mucous plugs within the endotracheal tube. In mammals, excretion of the drug may be prolonged in animals with impaired renal or gastrointestinal function. Refer also to ADVERSE AND COMMON SIDE EFFECTS of ATROPINE in the Small Animal section.

DRUG INTERACTIONS: A variety of drug interactions exist, although most listed drugs are not commonly used in avian medicine. Glycopyrrolate may antagonize the activity of metoclopramide. For more information, see ATROPINE and GLYCOPYRROLATE in the Small Animal section.

HALOPERIDOL

INDICATIONS: Haloperidol (Haldol ✚ ★, Novo-Peridol ✚, and others) is an antipsychotic drug, similar in structure to droperidol, which is used to treat human psychiatric disorders. Both oral and long-acting (decanoate) IM formulations are available and have been used in birds.

In birds, haloperidol has been used for the treatment of feather picking and self-mutilation. There is tremendous variability in response; therefore, treatment should be initiated with the oral formulation and carefully adjusted to each individual patient. The repository injectable formulation may be appropriate for birds that have responded to haloperidol but are difficult to medicate on a daily basis. The doses of the two formulations are not equivalent on an mg/kg basis; therefore, the correct dosage must be reestablished if the patient is switched to the long-acting formulation. Better success has been reported treating self-mutilation, including Amazon foot necrosis, than treating feather picking. Cockatoos, Quaker parakeets, and lovebirds appeared to respond more favorably than other psittacines, including African gray parrots. Two cases have been reported where birds have remained on therapy for 7 and 9 years. Attention to environmental and other factors is an important component of therapy.

ADVERSE AND COMMON SIDE EFFECTS: In humans, there is a narrow range between the effective therapeutic dose and that causing extrapyramidal neurologic symptoms. Adverse effects related to other body systems are also described. In birds, appetite suppression is likely to be the first adverse effect observed. Other side effects, including depression, anorexia, agitation, and excitability, may follow. If these occur, treatment should be stopped immediately. Administration of haloperidol can be resumed at a lower dose once the patient has returned to normal. African gray parrots and Quaker parakeets have shown disorientation or abnormal behaviors with treatment. Quaker parakeets and Moluccan and umbrella cockatoos may require a lower dose than other psittacine species. An anecdotal report describes the deaths of a hyacinth macaw and a red-bellied macaw within several days of oral haloperidol administration. The exact circumstances were not described. In an unusual report, a Quaker parakeet developed bilateral hock joint dislocations shortly after haloperidol therapy was initiated. The dislocations were successfully reduced after the drug was discontinued. However, upon readministering haloperidol, the joints again dislocated.

DRUG INTERACTIONS: Haloperidol may be additive with or potentiate the effects of central nervous system depressants, including opiates and other analgesics, and anesthetics.

SUPPLIED AS HUMAN PRODUCTS:
Tablets containing 0.5, 1, 2, 5, 10, and 20 mg (Novo-Peridol ✚, Haldol ★, Haloperidol ★)
Oral solution containing 2 mg/mL (Apo-Haloperidol ✚, Haldol Concentrate ★, Haldol Oral Solution Concentrate ★)
For injection containing 5 mg/mL (Haldol ✚ ★, Haloperidol ✚, Haloperidol Injection ★), 50 mg/mL and 100 mg/mL (Apo-Haloperidol LA ✚, Haloperidol LA ✚)

HYALURONIDASE

INDICATIONS: Hyaluronidase (Wydase ★) is an enzyme used to enhance fluid absorption from subcutaneous tissue. Hyaluronidase temporarily lyses the normal interstitial barrier, which consists mainly of hyaluronic acid, decreasing the viscosity of the connective tissue for about 24 to 48 hours. The increased rate of absorption of fluids given subcutaneously is effective as long as there is sufficient interstitial pressure, and this mechanical impulse is usually initiated by the injected solution. In human medicine, hyaluronidase is either injected directly into the SC site, added to the fluids to be infused, or both.

In birds, hyaluronidase is used to increase the rate of SC fluid absorption, particularly in small species or dehydrated patients where venous access is not possible or desirable. The drug has also been used by direct injection into the phallus to reduce paraphimosis in waterfowl.

ADVERSE AND COMMON SIDE EFFECTS: The SC administration of hyaluronidase in humans has been associated with very few adverse reactions. Allergic reactions (urticaria) are rare and the intravenous administration of as much as 75,000 U (500 times the therapeutic dose) of hyaluronidase in animals caused no tissue changes. Subcutaneous injection of hyaluronidase may cause local discomfort.

SUPPLIED AS HUMAN PRODUCTS:
For injection (lyophilized) in vials containing 150 USP units/mL (Wydase ★)
For injection (in solution) containing 150 USP units/mL (Wydase ★)

HYDROCORTISONE

INDICATIONS: Hydrocortisone (Uni-Cort ✤, Cortef Tablets ✤, Hydrocortone Tablets ★) is a short-acting glucocorticoid agent. For more information, see GLUCOCORTICOID AGENTS in the Small Animal section.

Because birds are extremely sensitive to the immunosuppressive effects of glucocorticoids, the use of short-acting agents in avian patients is recommended.

ADVERSE AND COMMON SIDE EFFECTS: See DEXAMETHA-SONE in this section for further information on the effects of glucocorticoids in birds.

DRUG INTERACTIONS: Corticosteroids and NSAIDs should not be used concurrently.

SUPPLIED AS VETERINARY PRODUCT:
For injection containing 200 μg/mL (Uni-Cort ✤)

SUPPLIED AS HUMAN PRODUCTS:
Tablets containing 5 mg (Cortef ★), 10 mg (Cortef ✤ ★, Hydrocortone ✤), and 20 mg (Cortef ✤ ★)
Oral suspension containing 10 mg/5 mL (Cortef ★)
For injection containing 25 mg/mL and 50 mg/mL (Generic ★)

HYDROXYZINE

INDICATIONS: Hydroxyzine (Atarax ✤ ★, Vistaril ★, and others) is a piperazine derivative antihistamine agent with sedative and tranquilizing effects. The drug is used in humans primarily for the symptomatic management of anxiety and the management of pruritus caused by allergy.

In birds, hydroxyzine has been used to treat feather picking. There is tremendous variability in response and the dosage must be carefully adjusted for each individual patient. Attention to environmental and other factors is also an essential component of therapy.

ADVERSE AND COMMON SIDE EFFECTS: The most common adverse effects in humans are drowsiness and dry mouth. A variety of other reactions are described.

DRUG INTERACTIONS: Hydroxyzine may be additive with or potentiate the effects of central nervous system depressants including opiates and other analgesics, anesthetics, and anticholinergic agents.

SUPPLIED AS HUMAN PRODUCTS:
Tablets containing 10 mg (Apo-Hydroxyzine ✤, Novo-Hydroxyzine ✤), 25 mg (Apo-Hydroxyzine ✤, Atarax ✤, Multipax ✤, Novo-Hydroxyzine ✤), and 50 mg (Apo-Hydroxyzine ✤, Multipax ✤, Novo-Hydroxyzine ✤)
Capsules containing 10 mg (Novo-Hydroxyzine ✤), 25 and 50 mg (Novo-Hydroxyzine ✤, Vistaril ★) and 100 mg (Vistaril ★)
Oral syrup containing 2 mg/mL (Atarax ✤ ★)
Oral suspension containing 25 mg/5 mL (Vistaril ★)
Oral solution containing 25 mg/mL and 50 mg/mL (Vistaril ★)
For injection containing 25 mg/mL (Vistaril ★) and 50 mg/mL (Atarax ✤, Hydroxyzine HCI ★, Vistaril ✤ ★)

IBUPROFEN

INDICATIONS: Ibuprofen (Advil ✤ ★, Motrin ✤ ★) is an NSAID with antipyretic and analgesic properties that is used in small animal practice particularly for the management of joint pain secondary to degenerative joint disease. For more information, see IBUPROFEN in the Small Animal section.

In avian medicine, ibuprofen is sometimes selected as an anti-inflammatory agent because it is readily obtained by clients from a human pharmacy. Meloxicam is more commonly used in general avian practice.

ADVERSE AND COMMON SIDE EFFECTS: In small animals, the frequency of GI side effects is greater than that seen with other NSAIDs such as aspirin or meloxicam. For more information, see IBUPROFEN in the Small Animal section.

SUPPLIED AS HUMAN PRODUCTS:
Oral suspension containing 20 mg/L (Children's Motrin Suspension ♣, Children's Advil ★, Motrin ★, Ibuprofen ★), 40 mg/mL (Advil Pediatric Drops ♣, Infant's Motrin Suspension Drops ♣)

INTERFERON

INDICATIONS: Interferon (Roferon A ♣ ★) has immunomodulating and antiproliferative capabilities as well as antiviral activity. For more information, see INTERFERON in the Small Animal section.

Interferon has been used in birds infected or exposed to the putative virus that causes psittacine proventricular dilation disease (PDD). In a preliminary study, the drug appeared to halt the spread of PDD virus through a psittacine breeding nursery when administered orally once daily for 6 weeks and may have some effect on slowing the progress of disease in infected birds. Interferon has also been suggested for the treatment of pigeons with circoviral infection.

IODINE

INDICATIONS: Iodine is used for the treatment and prevention of iodine deficiency, or goiter, in budgerigars. The drug is usually provided in a dilute form in the drinking water; however, in birds that are vomiting, injectable use of sodium iodide is possible as is cutaneous application. Supplementation is not necessary for birds fed iodine treated seed mixes.

DRUG INTERACTIONS: Iodine products oxidize when exposed to light and should be stored in dark bottles. Medicated drinking water should be replaced daily.

SUPPLIED AS HUMAN PRODUCTS:
Tincture of iodine containing 2.5% iodine and 2.5% potassium iodide ♣ ★
Lugol's iodine containing approximately 50 mg/mL iodine and 100 mg/mL potassium iodide ♣ ★

Sodium iodine containing 100 μg elemental iodide (118 μg sodium iodide) per mL (Iodopen ★)

IOHEXOL

INDICATIONS: Iohexol (Omnipaque 🍁 ★) is a nonionic, iodinated contrast medium with low osmolality (as compared to diatrizoate Na and diatrizoate meglumide [Gastrograffin]), which is extensively used in human clinical radiology and considered essentially free from side effects. Like other iodine-containing contrast media, it is eliminated from the body by excretion in the urine, when used parentally.

A study compared the quality of contrast radiographs obtained using barium sulfate and iohexol orally in Amazon parrots and a cockatoo. Iohexol was administered undiluted and diluted 1:1 at a volume of 25 to 30 mL/kg. Iohexol provided adequate opacification of the gastrointestinal tract lumen to allow all portions to be adequately evaluated. The transit time from crop to cloaca was on average at least 55 minutes faster with iohexol than barium. All birds had contrast material still present in the crop by the time it reached the cloaca. Iohexol did not obscure material in the GI tract (e.g., grit) as does barium.

Iohexol has also been used for contrast studies of other anatomic locations. One report describes its use for a sinogram in a scarlet macaw.

ADVERSE AND COMMON SIDE EFFECTS: After each iohexol study, birds expelled large volumes of clear watery droppings assumed to be iohexol. Dilution of iohexol at ratios greater than 1:1 is not recommended as it results in poor opacification of gastrointestinal structures.

SUPPLIED AS:
Sterile solution for IV injection containing 180, 240, 300, and 350 mg/mL (Omnipaque [veterinary product ★, human product 🍁])

IRON DEXTRAN

INDICATIONS: Iron dextran (Ferrodex ★, Ironol-100 🍁, and others) is used for the treatment of iron deficiency anemia and after hemorrhage. For more information, see IRON DEXTRAN in the Small Animal section.

ADVERSE AND COMMON SIDE EFFECTS: Iron dextran should be used with caution in avian species that are predisposed to hemochromatosis.

DRUG INTERACTIONS: Iron dextran is reported to be incompatible with chlortetracycline and sulfadiazine sodium.

ISOFLURANE

INDICATIONS: Isoflurane (Aerrane ❋ ★, Forane ❋ ★, IsoFlo ❋ ★, Iso-Thesia ★) is a halogenated inhalant anesthetic agent with a low blood:gas partition coefficient that results in rapid induction and recovery. Cardiovascular status is better maintained with isoflurane than with halothane, and isoflurane does not sensitize the heart to epinephrine-induced cardiac arrhythmias as does halothane. For more information, see ISOFLURANE in the Small Animal section.

Isoflurane is currently the standard inhalant anesthetic agent used in birds due to its relative safety and rapid induction and recovery times. The results of one study suggest that anesthesia with isoflurane does not affect the rate of barium sulfate transit through the gastrointestinal tract in psittacine birds; however, some anecdotal evidence would debate this.

ADVERSE AND COMMON SIDE EFFECTS: Isoflurane depresses respiration, particularly at high concentrations and during long procedures. Cardiac depression, hypotension, and arrhythmias can also occur.

ISONIAZID

INDICATIONS: Isoniazid (Dom-Isoniazid ❋, Isotamine ❋ ★, Isoniazid ❋ ★, Nydrazid ★, Laniazid ★, PMS-Isoniazid ❋) is an antimicrobial agent active only against organisms of the genus *Mycobacterium*. The drug is bacteriostatic or bactericidal depending on concentrations in tissue and the susceptibility of the organism. It is only active against replicating organisms. Humans are treated with the drug for a minimum of 6 months. Isoniazid is also used prophylactically in high-risk situations, but recent work in HIV patients infected with *M. avium* suggests that most strains of the organism are resistant to this drug.

Isoniazid has been used to treat birds infected with mycobacterial organisms. Veterinarians differ in their willingness to treat avian mycobacteriosis due to the difficulty in ensuring that the infection is fully eliminated and concerns over the potential for zoonotic spread of the disease under certain conditions.

ADVERSE AND COMMON SIDE EFFECTS: In humans, administration with food reduces absorption and peak plasma concentrations. A variety of adverse effects are reported, including hepatic dysfunction, hypersensitivity, and peripheral neuritis.

DRUG INTERACTIONS: In humans, isoniazid is used alone or, more commonly, in combination with drugs such as rifampin and pyrazinamide.

SUPPLIED AS HUMAN PRODUCTS:

Syrup containing 10 mg/5 mL (Isotamine ♣) and 50 mg/5 mL (Isotamine ♣, Isoniazid syrup ★)

Tablets containing 50 (Isoniazid ♣), 100 (Isoniazid ♣ ★), and 300 mg (Isoniazid ♣ ★, Isotamine ♣)

Syrup containing 50 mg/5 mL (Isotamine ♣, PMS-Isoniazid ♣, Laniazid ★)

Tablets containing 50 mg (PMS-Isoniazid ♣, Laniazid ★), 100 mg (PMS-Isoniazid ♣, Laniazid ★), and 300 mg (PMS-Isoniazid ♣, Laniazid ★, Isotamine ♣)

For injection containing 100 mg/mL (Nydrazid ★)

ITRACONAZOLE

INDICATIONS: Itraconazole (Sporanox ♣ ★) is a triazole antifungal agent active against histoplasmosis, blastomycosis, aspergillosis, cryptococcosis, dermatophytosis, and candidiasis. Unlike ketoconazole, itraconazole reaches adequate levels in the central nervous system at therapeutic doses. The drug is used orally and is best absorbed with a fatty meal. Itraconazole is partially converted by hepatic biotransformation to hydroxyitraconazole, which is also fungicidal. In humans, treatment from 6 months to a year is recommended. For more information, see ITRACONAZOLE in the Small Animal section.

A 10 mg/mL liquid formulation of itraconazole is also available for the treatment of oral and esophageal candidiasis in humans. The human absorption profile of this and the capsule formulation differ. Sporanox liquid should not be taken with food. The two drugs are not considered interchangeable in humans. In humans, the relative bioavailability is as follows: capsules with empty stomach 0.5; capsules with food 1.0; liquid with food 1.25; liquid with empty stomach 1.6. Sporanox capsules contain lactose granules coated with itraconazole. In the past, dosage was determined by the laborious process of counting the number of granules in a capsule and then dividing the total milligrams of drug in the capsule by this number, or by solubilizing the contents of a capsule in 0.1 N HCl (50 mg/mL) by sonication, and then diluting it in orange juice to a final concentration of 5 mg/mL. The new oral formulation eliminates the need to solubilize Sporanox capsules; however, it may still be more convenient to use individual granules for treatment in food.

There has been considerable interest in the use of itraconazole to treat respiratory aspergillosis in birds, and there have been pharmacokinetic studies using the capsule formulation. Minimal inhibitory concentration (MIC) values for aspergillus have been reported to range from 0.01 to 1.0 µg/mL. It is likely that higher blood levels are required for the treatment of active infection, as compared to prevention against infection. Maximum blood and tissue concentrations have been reached in pigeons 4 hours after a single oral dose of 10 mg/kg. After 12 treatments at 6-hour intervals, steady-state plasma concentrations of 3.6 µg/mL and an elimination half-life of 13.3 hours were recorded in the same birds. A dosage of 6 mg/kg twice daily was recommended to maintain plasma fungicidal concentrations and reduce fluctuations in the concentration of the drug. Levels of itraconazole in pulmonary parenchyma were much lower than in plasma. It was suggested that a dosage as high as 26 mg/kg twice daily might be necessary to maintain an MIC of greater than 1 µg/mL in the lung; however, concern was expressed that this dose might be toxic.

In another study in pigeons, itraconazole was administered orally at a dosage of 5 mg/kg either once or once daily for 14 consecutive days. Birds received the drug as is from the capsules or solubilized in acid. Plasma and tissue levels were measured. By day 14 of treatment the group receiving the acid formulation had higher plasma levels. This was attributed to better gastrointestinal absorption. Concentrations of itraconazole and hydroxyitraconazole were measured in the tissues of these pigeons. It was found that their concentrations increased in the lungs and air sacs over the 14 days of treatment. Concentration values for the two drugs combined were above the MIC for most strains of *Aspergillus*.

Blue-fronted Amazon parrots were treated with 5 or 10 mg/kg every 24 hours; PO for 14 consecutive days. The itraconazole was dissolved in acid and diluted in orange juice before administration. Plasma concentrations were up to 10 times greater in these parrots than in the pigeons in the previous study. It is not known whether this relates to a species difference or if there is was greater bioavailability of the acid formulation used in the parrot study. The plasma elimination half-life after 14 days of treatment was 6 to 7 hours, which was shorter than that of the pigeons. Bioaccumulation of itraconazole was noted at the 10 mg/kg dosage. Based on these results, a dosage of 5 mg/kg once daily was expected to be effective in most cases of aspergillosis. A dosage of 10 mg/kg was recommended for *Candida* spp. and when there was not good clinical response at 5 mg/kg. Amazon parrots have been treated for up to 3 months at the higher dose without adverse effects.

Plasma and tissue levels of itraconazole and hydroxyitraconazole were evaluated in red-tailed hawks given 5 mg/kg or 10 mg/kg orally once daily for 15 consecutive days. Itraconazole beads were acid solubilized and diluted in orange juice to a concentration of 5 mg/mL. Birds were gavaged with the preparation and then this was followed with several milliliters of canine or feline A/D diet. Results suggested that steady-state plasma concentrations of itraconazole and hydroxyitraconazole would be reached by 14 days with the 10 mg/kg dosage. Plasma levels of itraconazole were similar to those in pigeons and much less than those obtained in Amazon parrots using similar dosage regimens. There were also differences in tissue distribution among species of birds. Blood and tissue levels in most hawks were considered adequate for the treatment of most fungal infections, but there was considerable variability among birds. The authors have used the dosage of 10 mg/kg every 24 hours for 3 to 6 months of treatment in red-tailed hawks and bald eagles without signs of toxicity.

The pharmacokinetics of itraconazole were investigated in two Gentoo penguins that received 10 and 20 mg/kg once daily for 6 consecutive days. Trough serum itraconazole levels were 2.5 times greater at day 6 than on day 3 but were not substantially different between the two doses.

Blood levels of itraconazole were measured in a silky chicken being treated at a dosage of 10 mg/kg every 12 hours. On day 30 the blood itraconazole levels were 1.4 μg/mL and 0.7 μg/mL 5 and 9 hours after administration, respectively.

Case reports describe the use of itraconazole for the treatment of *Candida* and *Aspergillus* spp. infections in a range of species, including psittacines, raptors, and penguins. Doses of 8 to 10 mg/kg once daily resulted in serum trough levels above the MIC for the organism cultured in several of these cases. Itraconazole is also widely used for the prevention and treatment of aspergillosis in waterfowl. It may also have some effectiveness in treating avian "megabacterial" infections.

ADVERSE AND COMMON SIDE EFFECTS: Anorexia and depression have been reported in two African gray parrots given 8 and 10 mg/kg once daily; one of the birds subsequently died. It is generally considered that African gray parrots are more sensitive to the adverse effects of itraconazole and that lower dosages and careful monitoring are required. Similar concerns have also been expressed regarding some other African parrots, e.g., *Poicephalus* spp. Amazon parrots have been treated at 10 mg/kg without evidence of toxicity; although in one report, an Amazon parrot became lethargic and anorectic after 1 year of treatment. The bird returned to normal demeanor once treatment was discontinued.

In a case report, one of two penguins that received itraconazole at 20 mg/kg showed moderately reduced appetite. Aspartate aminotransferase elevations were noted while on the drug.

SUPPLIED AS HUMAN PRODUCTS:
Capsules containing 100 mg (Sporanox ♣ ★)
Oral solution containing 10 mg/mL (Sporanox ♣ ★)
For IV injection containing 10 mg/mL (Sporanox ★)

IVERMECTIN

INDICATIONS: Ivermectin (Heartgard ♣ ★, Ivomec ♣ ★, Eqvalan ♣ ★, and others) is used for the eradication of endoparasites and ectoparasites. For more information, see IVERMECTIN in the Small Animal section.

In birds, ivermectin is the treatment of choice for cutaneous *Knemidokoptes* spp. and tracheal mites (*Sternostoma tracheacolum*), and is used for the eradication or control of a wide range of other parasitic infestations. The commercial bovine 10 mg/mL product is diluted 1:4 in propylene glycol for more accurate dosing. The equine injectable product (previously available) has sometimes been described as water-soluble; however, propylene glycol remains the best diluent. Ivermectin can be administered PO, in the drinking water for aviary situations, SC, or IM. Subcutaneous administration has been described as less irritating and providing better absorption, as compared to the IM route, and is the route of choice in small birds. In very small species, ivermectin has been used topically over the right jugular vein at the calculated dose or using 1 drop of a diluted product. Unfortunately, various concentrations of the diluted product have been described in the literature: 0.01% (which equals 0.1 mg/mL); 1 mg/mL (which equals 0.1 %); and a 10 mg/mL solution diluted by 1:20 (which equals 0.05%). There is a 10-fold range within these concentrations. It is essential to be fully aware of the mg/kg dose being administered.

In a study of the efficacy of ivermectin against ocular oxyspirurids in crested wood partridges and chickens, the parasite was eliminated by doses from 0.005 to 0.05 mg placed in the conjunctival sac, but not by a dose of 0.01 mg given orally or parenterally. Ocular toxicity was not noted in chickens treated with up to 1 mg ocularly once daily for 10 consecutive days. Systemic treatment with ivermectin, at the standard dosage, is useful in eradicating maggots from wounds.

Ivermectin was found to be effective at a high dose of 1 mg/kg SC to control *Serratospiculum seurati,* an air sac filarid worm, and *Capillaria* in various falcons and falcon hybrids. Oral administration of the same dose was completely ineffective.

Ivermectin was apparently successful in killing circulating and tissue microfilaria in a saddle-billed stork and a yellow-collared macaw, respectively.

ADVERSE AND COMMON SIDE EFFECTS: In aviaries treated with ivermectin for tracheal mites, mortalities of 3% to 12% have been reported. The cause of death has been attributed to tracheal occlusion with dead mites and inflammatory debris and exudate. The propylene glycol base of the ivermectin formulation may cause adverse effects when administered IM, especially in small birds. Toxicity has been reported in bullfinches and goldfinches that received a dose of 0.4 mg/kg topically. Deaths have occurred in budgerigars and finches after IM administration of the equine product at the standard dose of 0.2 mg/kg. Particular concern should be taken when administering ivermectin by the droplet technique to avoid accidental overdosage. In small passerine birds, ivermectin can be diluted to an appropriate dose in sterile saline but must be used immediately.

In falcon and falcon hybrids being treated for the air sac filarial worm *Serratospiculum seurati,* ivermectin dosages of 2 and 3 mg/kg IM resulted in adverse effects in 12/340 (3.5%) and 27/600 (4.5%) of birds, respectively. These adverse effects included temporary bilateral blindness, anorexia, vomiting, and ataxia that lasted for up to 48 hours in some cases. The effects were more severe at the higher dose.

KANAMYCIN

INDICATIONS: Kanamycin (Kantrim ★) is an aminoglycoside antibiotic used for the treatment of gram-negative bacterial infections, especially *Pseudomonas* spp. For more information, see KANAMYCIN and AMINOGLYCOSIDE ANTIBIOTICS in the Small Animal section.

Kanamycin has been recommended for use in drinking water to control enteric infections and as a preventive measure in stressed birds, especially finches.

KAOLIN-PECTIN

INDICATIONS: Kaolin-pectin (Kaopectate ✤ ★ and others) is a gastrointestinal protectant used in the management of diarrhea. It coats the surface of the gut and exerts a mild demulcent and absorbent effect. It is actually relatively ineffective in absorbing toxins produced by enteropathogenic bacteria. It appears to act by adding particulate matter to the feces, which improves consistency until the disease spontaneously resolves. Kaolin is a potent coagulation activator and may be of some benefit in treating diarrhea associated with mucosal disruption and hemorrhage. Some antidiarrheal products registered for use in humans, including Kaopectate Oral Suspension, contain attapulgite (magnesium aluminum silicate) rather than kaolin (aluminum silicate). For more information, see KAOLIN-PECTIN in the Small Animal section.

SUPPLIED AS VETERINARY PRODUCTS:
Oral suspension containing 197 mg kaolin and 4.33 mg pectin per mL (large animal preparation) (Kaopectate ✤), 5.85 g kaolin and 130 mg pectin per 30 mL (Kaopectolin ★, Kaolin Pectin ★, Kaolin-Pectin Plus ★, Kao-Pec ★), and 5.8 g kaolin and 268 mg pectin per 30 mL (Kaolin-Pectin Suspension ★)

SUPPLIED AS HUMAN PRODUCTS:
Oral suspension containing 5.2 g kaolin and 260 mg pectin per 30 mL (Kao-Spen ★), 5.85 g kaolin and 130 mg pectin per 30 mL (Kaopectolin ★), 7 g kaolin and 143 mg pectin per 30 mL (Donnagel-MB ✤)

Oral suspension containing attapulgite (Kaopectate Oral Suspension ✿ ★) in 600 mg/15 mL (Children's, Regular) and 750 mg/15 mL (Extra-strength)

KETAMINE

INDICATIONS: Ketamine (Ketalean ✿, Ketaject ★, Ketaved ★, Rogarsetic ✿, Vetaket ★, Vetamine ★, Vetame ★, Ketaset ✿ ★, Vetalar ✿ ★) is a nonbarbiturate anesthetic used for chemical restraint or anesthesia of short duration. In mammals, the drug is characterized by a rapid onset of action, good analgesia, maintenance of normal muscle tone and laryngeal reflex, mild cardiac stimulation, and respiratory depression. Recovery generally is smooth and uneventful. For more information, see KETAMINE in the Small Animal section.

Ketamine has been used widely as an anesthetic agent in many avian species in combination with a benzodiazepine tranquilizer (e.g., midazolam, diazepam) or α_2-adrenergic sedative (e.g., medetomidine, xylazine). The onset, duration, and physiologic changes during anesthesia will vary according to the dose of ketamine and the dose and nature of any drugs used in combination. In general, induction occurs within 1 to 5 minutes of IM administration, with anesthesia lasting 20 to 30 minutes.

ADVERSE AND COMMON SIDE EFFECTS: No specific adverse effects of ketamine have been noted in birds but general precautions should be taken to monitor cardiac and respiratory function as for any anesthetized patient. Muscle relaxation is poor. Considerable variation in effective dose occurs among avian species.

KETOCONAZOLE

INDICATIONS: Ketoconazole (Nizoral ✿ ★) is an antifungal agent used for the treatment of deep fungal and yeast infections. Ketoconazole is fungistatic at low concentration, and fungicidal at higher levels. Absorption of ketoconazole is enhanced in an acid environment and with a high fat meal. High levels of dietary carbohydrate reduce absorption in humans. For more information, see KETOCONAZOLE in the Small Animal section.

In birds, ketoconazole is used orally for the treatment of yeast infections, particularly *Candida albicans* infections that are refractory to nystatin therapy. Other *Candida* spp. may be more resistant to the drug. Ketoconazole is used less frequently to treat pulmonary aspergillosis. Ketoconazole is insoluble at neutral pH but readily soluble at pH <2. One fourth of a 200 mg tablet can also be dissolved in 0.2 mL 1 N HCl and 0.8 mL water. The liquid turns pink when the drug is dissolved. Orange juice and vinegar have also been suggested as acid environments for solubilization. Ground tablets have been suspended in methylcellulose and mixed 50:50 with cherry-based syrup by a compounding pharmacist. This suspension was stable for 6 months. Minimal pharmacokinetic information is available on the use of ketoconazole in birds. Pigeons given a single oral dose of 30 mg/kg attained peak serum levels in 0.5 to 4 hours and the plasma elimination half-life was 2.3 hours. In Moluccan cockatoos given the same dose the half-life was 3.8 hours. In the literature, recommended dosage ranges from 10 to 50 mg/kg every 12 hours. Treatment should be continued for at least a month to treat systemic fungal conditions. Ketoconazole does not appear to be effective in the treatment of gastric "mega-bacteriosis."

ADVERSE AND COMMON SIDE EFFECTS: Regurgitation has been described in psittacines receiving ketoconazole orally. No adverse effects were noted in pigeons given 30 mg/kg every 12 hours orally for 30 days. Serum alanine aminotransferase, aspartate aminotransferase, and uric acid were monitored as well as behavioral parameters. Because hepatotoxicity is described in mammals, caution should be used in prescribing ketoconazole to birds with hepatic dysfunction. Changes in adrenal or hormonal steroid production have not been noted in birds; however, the drug has not been studied in any detail in avian species.

DRUG INTERACTIONS: Ketoconazole has been used in birds in combination with amphotericin B. Ketoconazole inhibits hepatic cytochrome P-450 enzymes and; therefore, therapy with ketoconazole may effect the levels of a variety of other therapeutic agents.

KETOPROFEN

INDICATIONS: Ketoprofen (Anafen ♣, Ketofen ★) is an NSAID with potent analgesic and antipyretic properties. The drug inhibits the cyclooxygenase and lipooxygenase inflammatory pathways. Ketoprofen is used in the management of fever and acute, subacute, and chronic pain associated with musculoskeletal disease. Onset of activity of the drug occurs within 30 minutes of parenteral administration and 1 hour after oral use. The duration of action in dogs and cats is approximately 12 hours. For more information, see KETOPROFEN in the Small Animal section.

Several authors have suggested ketoprofen as an analgesic for birds. A study in mallard ducks to evaluate the effect of ketoprofen on thromboxane levels found that ducks given single doses of 5 mg/kg had significant suppression of thromboxane levels for 4 hours after administration. As well, levels were decreased as compared to baseline samples for an additional 12 hours. At necropsy, there was no evidence of GI bleeding.

DRUG INTERACTIONS: NSAIDs should not be used concurrently with corticosteroid agents.

LACTULOSE

INDICATIONS: Lactulose (Cephulac ♣ ★, Chronulac ♣ ★, and many others) is a synthetic nonabsorbable disaccharide. It acts as a mild osmotic laxative, increases the rate of passage of ingesta, and leads to the reduction of bacterial production of ammonia, which is useful in the management of hepatic encephalopathy. For more information, see LACTULOSE in the Small Animal section.

In birds, lactulose may also be effective as an appetite stimulant and to help reestablish natural enteric flora. It has been used as a component of supportive care for a variety of clinical conditions in a variety of avian species.

ADVERSE AND COMMON SIDE EFFECTS: Reduce dosage if diarrhea occurs.

LEUPROLIDE ACETATE

INDICATIONS: Leuprolide acetate (Lupron ♣ ★) is a synthetic gonadotropin-releasing hormone (GnRH) analog. The drug binds to GnRH receptors in the anterior pituitary with high specificity, affinity, and activity. It initially induces hormonal upregulation, but after prolonged exposure these receptors are downregulated. After administration of leuprolide acetate there is an initial stimulation of FSH and LH production and release, which may induce ovulation, and then a subsequent decrease in LH and, in some species, FSH. In humans, leuprolide acetate is used to treat prostate cancer, endometriosis, and central precocious puberty.

In birds, leuprolide acetate is used to stop persistent egg laying, for the treatment of psittacine feather picking, which may have an underlying hormonal stimulus, and for the treatment of cystic ovaries. Evaluation and manipulation of environmental factors is also critical in the treatment of repeated egg laying and feather picking.

Leuprolide acetate, intended for human use, is available in several injectable depot formulations with different durations of action. The drug can be reconstituted according to manufacturer's directions and then further diluted in sterile water for injection, often to a concentration of 0.5 to 1 mg/mL. Under sterile conditions, the final solution is divided into aliquots of appropriate dose (generally 0.1 mg) and kept frozen (freezing at −70°C is preferred; however, anecdotally −20°C appears adequate for periods of up to one year). When handled correctly, the product should remain effective until the manufacturer's expiry date. The choice of product and total dose are based on the number of days for which the clinical effect is intended. The

30-day depot formulation is most frequently used for the treatment of birds.

ADVERSE AND COMMON SIDE EFFECTS: A large number and wide range of effects have been reported in people to the extent that a "National Lupron Victims Network" has been established. There has been inadequate use of the drug in birds to determine what adverse effects might occur.

SUPPLIED AS HUMAN PRODUCTS:

LUPRON INJECTION
For daily use containing 5 mg/mL ★

LUPRON DEPOT FOR INJECTION
For monthly use containing 3.75 mg ❦ ★ and 7.5 mg ❦ ★ per vial
For use every 3 months containing 11.25 mg ❦ ★ and 22.5 mg ❦ per vial
For use every 4 months containing 30 mg ❦ ★ per vial

LEVAMISOLE

INDICATIONS: Levamisole (Levasole ★, Ripercol ❦, Tramisol ❦ ★, Prohibit ★, Totalon ★) is an anthelmintic used for the treatment of nematode infestations. Levamisole may also help restore immune function by increasing the number and function of T lymphocytes and macrophages. It has also been reported to stimulate antibody production, increase phagocytosis by macrophages, inhibit tumor growth, and stimulate suppressor cell activity. For more information, see LEVAMISOLE in the Small Animal section.

Tablets containing 20 mg levamisole (Spartakon) were previously available in North America and are still sold elsewhere for the treatment of *Ascaridia columbae* and *Capillaria obsignata* in nonfood pigeons. It was recommended that birds be fasted for 24 hours before and 3 hours after treatment.

Levamisole is also effective against tetrameriasis. The injectable form of the drug can be administered by IM or SC injection, orally in the drinking water, or by gavage. Microfilaremia in a marabou stork was cleared after treatment with 12 mg/kg of levamisole PO every 24 hours for 10 days. The effect on adult worms could not be assessed.

Levamisole has also been used to stimulate the immune system in immunosuppressed birds. Experimental work in chickens suggested that doses of 1.25 to 2.5 mg/kg orally or SC were effective for this purpose.

ADVERSE AND COMMON SIDE EFFECTS: Levamisole has a low therapeutic index in birds and should be used with caution, especially by the IM route. Published dosages are empirical and range from 2 to 50 mg/kg. The commercial pigeon product has a specified on-label dose. Levamisole should not be used in debilitated birds or lories. Doses of 2 to 4 times the recommended dosage may result in depression. The drug has also caused vomiting and neurologic signs including mydriasis, ataxia, and death. These adverse events have been described in cockatoos, budgerigars, and mynah birds at a dose of 40 mg/kg injected IM or SC. Hepatotoxicity in budgerigars has been associated with a dose of 25 mg/kg IM. Swelling at sites of injection has also been noted. Vomiting has been reported in pigeons treated with the tablet formulation. Lethal doses have included 35 mg/kg IM in pigeons, 66 mg/kg IM in peach-faced lovebirds, and 22 mg/kg IM in white ibis.

SUPPLIED AS VETERINARY PRODUCTS:
Avian product: Tablets containing 20 mg (Spartakon—not currently available in North America)
See also Small and Large Animal sections

LEVOTHYROXINE

INDICATIONS: Levothyroxine (Eltroxin ♣ ★, Synthroid ♣ ★) is a synthetic form of T$_4$ used in the treatment of hypothyroid disease. For more information, see LEVOTHYROXINE in the Small Animal section.

Levothyroxine has been used for the treatment of birds with thyroid insufficiency, for goiter in budgerigars, for thyroid-responsive syndromes including obesity, delayed molting and poor feathering, and to shrink subcutaneous lipomas and xanthomas. Response to therapy is extremely variable; therefore, caution should be taken to monitor treated birds carefully. Measurement of T$_4$ levels may be helpful. In a hypothyroid scarlet macaw, treatment with levothyroxine restored circulating thyroxine levels, and the bird's feathering and clinical condition returned to normal. Published dosages vary widely and all are empirical.

ADVERSE AND COMMON SIDE EFFECTS: Overdose may result in hyperthyroidism manifested by tachycardia, polyuria, polydipsia, hyperesthesia, vomiting, weight loss, and death.

LIDOCAINE

INDICATIONS: Lidocaine (Lurocaine ♣, Anthracaine ★, Lidoject ★) is licensed as a local anesthetic in small animals. For more information, see LIDOCAINE in the Small Animal section.

ADVERSE AND COMMON SIDE EFFECTS: The total dosage of lidocaine should not exceed 4 mg/kg to avoid seizures and possible cardiac arrest. Particular care must be taken not to overdose small birds; dilution of the drug to ensure accurate dosing is recommended.

LINCOMYCIN

INDICATIONS: Lincomycin (Lincocin ♣ ★, Lincomix ♣ ★) is a lincosamide antibiotic primarily active against gram-positive cocci, particularly *Staphylococcus* and *Streptococcus* spp. It can also be used to treat infections by *Clostridium tetani* and *C. perfringens,* and *Mycoplasma* spp. For more information, see LINCOMYCIN in the Small Animal section.

Lincomycin is not commonly used in psittacine medicine because of its poor activity agaisnt gram-negative organisms. It has been used for the treatment of necrotic enteritis caused by *C. perfringens* in chickens, and for the treatment of *Streptococcus bovis* and *S. zooepidemicus* in pigeons and canaries.

ADVERSE AND COMMON SIDE EFFECTS: Deaths have occurred after IV injection. Secondary yeast infections can occur after prolonged treatment.

DRUG INTERACTIONS: Lincomycin is used in combination with spectinomycin, especially for mycoplasmal infections. The minimal inhibitory concentration for the combination of these two drugs is lower than that for either used alone.

SUPPLIED AS VETERINARY PRODUCTS:
See also Small and Large Animal sections.
Oral solution containing 50 mg/mL (Lincocin Aquadrops ★) and 100 mg/mL (Lincocin Sterile Solution ★, Lincomix ★)
Injectable containing 100 mg/mL (Lincomix-100 ♣)
Water-soluble powder containing 16 g/40-g packet and 32 g/80-g packet (Lincomix ♣ ★, Lincomycin ♣ ★)
Containing lincomycin and spectinomycin:
Water-soluble powder containing 16.7 g lincomycin and 33.3 g spectinomycin per 75-g packet (L-S 50 Water Soluble ★)
Water-soluble powder containing 33.3 g lincomycin and 66.6 g spectinomycin per 150-g packet (Linco-Spectin 100 soluble powder ♣)
For injection containing 50 mg lincomycin and 100 mg spectinomycin/ mL (Linco-Spectin Sterile solution ♣ ★)
Various agricultural feed additives and premixes

MAGNESIUM SULFATE

INDICATIONS: Magnesium is essential for electrolyte balance across all membranes. Magnesium sulfate (Epsom salts) has been used in birds with heavy metal poisoning as an oral chelating agent and osmotic cathartic. Concurrent therapy with calcium EDTA is required.

ADVERSE AND COMMON SIDE EFFECTS: Magnesium sulfate must be diluted to prevent damage to the epithelium of the intestinal tract.

SUPPLIED AS:
Salts containing 98% to 100% magnesium sulfate heptahydrate (Epsom salts)

MEBENDAZOLE

INDICATIONS: Mebendazole (Telmin ♣ ★, Vermox ♣ ★) is an anthelmintic useful for the elimination of a variety of nematode parasites, including *Capillaria* spp. For more information, see MEBENDAZOLE in the Small Animal section.

Mebendazole has been used in a variety of avian species and toxicity has been reported in a number of these. Mebendazole is commonly placed in food to treat nematodes in waterfowl.

ADVERSE AND COMMON SIDE EFFECTS: Acute toxic hepatitis has been reported in raptors. A dose of 12 mg/kg has been reported to have caused death in *Columbiformes*. Toxicity is also described in cormorants and pelicans. Deaths secondary to intestinal obstruction with dead nematodes have been reported in heavily parasitized finches and psittacine birds.

SUPPLIED AS VETERINARY PRODUCTS:
Tablets containing 100 mg (Wormaway IV ♣)
Powder containing 40 and 166.7 mg mebendazole/g (Telmin Equine Wormer ★, Telmintic Powder ★)
Oral suspension containing 33.3 mg/mL (Telmin ★)
Oral paste containing 200 mg mebendazole (Telmin Syringe Wormer ★, Telmin Syringe Formula ♣)

SUPPLIED AS HUMAN PRODUCT:
Tablets (chewable) containing 100 mg (Vermox ♣ ★)

MEDETOMIDINE

INDICATIONS: Medetomidine (Domitor ♣ ★) is an α_2-receptor agonist with sedative and analgesic properties. For more information, see MEDETOMIDINE and ATIPAMEZOLE in the Small Animal section.

Medetomidine has been used alone as an anesthetic or sedative agent in birds, and in combination with ketamine or midazolam. Medetomidine alone provides dose-dependent sedation in a variety of avian species, but doses as high as 1 mg/kg may not eliminate the righting reflex.

In pigeons, doses of 80, 150, and 200 µg/kg IM resulted in only minor sedation, which was inadequate for restraint. Combining 80 µg/kg IM medetomidine with ketamine (5 mg/kg IM) or midazolam

(0.5 mg/kg IM) resulted in sedation, which was described as adequate for minor procedures; however, the degree of sedation in individual birds was unpredictable and recoveries were sometimes prolonged.

The sedative and cardiopulmonary effects of dosages of 1.5 mg/kg and 2 mg/kg IM were evaluated in pigeons and yellow-crowned Amazon parrots. All birds given 1.5 mg/kg showed signs of sedation: pigeons could be laid on their backs and the parrots were in sternal recumbency with their heads drooped. At the higher dose an increase in sedation was noted in the parrots, which could be laid on their backs, but not in the pigeons. In both species at both doses, heart and respiratory rates were lower than those taken as baseline controls; however, birds were manually restrained for the initial assessments. Smooth, rapid, and complete reversal of sedation was achieved with doses of atipamezole at 2.5 or 5 times the dose of medetomidine. The authors concluded that the degree of sedation obtained with doses as high as 2 mg/kg was not suitable for procedures usually performed under chemical restraint.

Medetomidine (80 µg/kg IM) and ketamine (2 mg/kg IM) were administered to juvenile ostriches. Six of the eight birds treated were profoundly sedated and in sternal recumbency within a mean time of 14.6 ± 10.0 minutes. Two birds remained standing but were moderately sedated. The birds were then induced with IV propofol and carefully monitored during anesthesia, where bradycardia was noted. Reversal with atipamezole (400 µg/kg, one half IV and one half SC) was smooth with a mean recovery time of 21.0 ± 7.3 minutes.

Mallard ducks were given medetomidine (0.05 µg/kg) + midazolam (2 mg/kg) + ketamine (10 mg/kg) IV in a study looking for a dosing regimen to provide analgesia and anesthesia suitable for a 30-minute invasive surgical protocol. The degree of anesthesia and analgesia was not consistent among birds, and in one group, birds showed significant respiratory depression, apnea, and acidosis.

ADVERSE AND COMMON SIDE EFFECTS: Bradycardia, vomiting, and twitching have been noted in pigeons given medetomidine. Cardiac arrhythmias have been noted in some pigeons given combinations of medetomidine and ketamine or midazolam. In the high-dose study described above, all pigeons opened and closed their beaks at short intervals during the first few minutes after receiving medetomidine. This could be interpreted as a sign of nausea.

DRUG INTERACTIONS: In mammals, atropine and glycopyrrolate given at the same time as or after medetomidine may induce bradycardia, heart block, premature ventricular contraction, and sinus tachycardia.

MEDROXYPROGESTERONE ACETATE

INDICATIONS: Medroxyprogesterone (Depo-Provera ✤ ★, Pro-vera ✤ ★) is a synthetic, prolonged-action, progestational compound that suppresses secretion of FSH and LH, thus arresting the development of graafian follicles and corpora lutea within the ovary. For more information, see MEDROXYPROGESTERONE ACETATE in the Small Animal section.

In birds, medroxyprogesterone has been used to stop egg laying in chronic layers. A single dose may be effective for up to 6 months in some birds. The drug has been used, with variable success, to suppress sexual activity, possessive aggression, and reduce feather picking and self-mutilation that are presumed to be hormonally influenced.

In a study in quail, a dose of 40 mg/kg IM did not consistently affect ovarian activity. In five of the seven birds the average duration of cessation of egg laying was 5.8 ± 2.3 days. In the remaining two birds, egg laying stopped for an extended time (19 and 49 days). Levo-norgestrel was more effective in this study.

ADVERSE AND COMMON SIDE EFFECTS: Caution should be taken when administering medroxyprogesterone as treatment may result in obesity, polyuria, polydipsia, lethargy, hepatic lipidosis, and diabetes. Cockatoos and Quaker parakeets should receive a lower dose than is generally recommended. Necrosis can occur at the site of IM injection.

MELOXICAM

INDICATIONS: Meloxicam (Metacam ✤, Mobic ★, Mobicox ✤) is a nonsteroidal anti-inflammatory agent with analgesic and antipyretic properties. The drug inhibits prostaglandin synthesis and is primarily a COX-2 inhibitor. Meloxicam is indicated for the relief of inflammation and pain in acute and chronic musculoskeletal disease, including postoperative pain. For more information, see MELOXICAM in the Small Animal section.

Meloxicam has been used empirically in avian practice and appears to be an effective drug. There is little experimental information concerning its effectiveness or pharmacokinetics in birds. In young ostrich chicks given meloxicam at 0.5 mg/kg IV, the drug was cleared rapidly from the blood. The mean plasma elimination half-life was only 30 minutes, and tissue distribution was limited as suggested by a calculated volume of distribution of only 0.58 L/kg. Meloxicam is not soluble in water but the oral liquid, tablet, and injectable formulations have all been diluted in methylcellulose for oral use in small birds. The methylcellulose-meloxicam suspension must be mixed well and shaken before use. The suspension made with the injectable product has a bitter taste, which should be masked with a sweetener or other flavored compound.

ADVERSE AND COMMON SIDE EFFECTS: Not specifically reported in birds at this date, although cockatoos may be less tolerant of the drug. Expected adverse effects would be similar to those seen with any NSAID.

DRUG INTERACTIONS: NSAIDs and corticosteroids should not be used concurrently.

SUPPLIED AS VETERINARY PRODUCTS:
For injection containing 5 mg/mL (Metacam ✦)
Oral suspension containing 1.5 mg/mL (Metacam ✦)

SUPPLIED AS HUMAN PRODUCTS:
Tablets containing 7.5 mg (Mobic ★, Mobicox ✦) and 15 mg (Mobicox ✦)

MEPERIDINE

INDICATIONS: Meperidine (Demerol ✦ ★) is a short-acting narcotic analgesic used for the relief of moderate to severe pain or as a pre-anesthetic. It has minimal sedative effects. For more information, see MEPERIDINE in the Small Animal section.

In birds, meperidine is used by the parenteral route. No information is available on blood levels or duration of activity; however, it appears that a single dose of the drug may have longer lasting effects than would be expected based on the elimination half-life in mammals.

METHYLPREDNISOLONE

INDICATIONS: Methylprednisolone (Medrol ✦ ★, Depo-Medrol ✦ ★) is an intermediate-acting glucocorticoid used in mammals for its anti-inflammatory properties to control autoimmune skin diseases, as adjunctive therapy in spinal cord trauma, and in the treatment of shock. For more information, see METHYLPREDNISOLONE and GLUCO-CORTICOIDS in the Small Animal section.

In birds, methylprednisolone has also been used to prevent the seasonal recurrence of "Amazon foot necrosis" syndrome in Amazon parrots. For further information on the immunosuppressive effects of corticosteroids in birds, see DEXAMETHASONE and PREDNI-SOLONE in this section.

METOCLOPRAMIDE

INDICATIONS: Metoclopramide (Reglan ★, generics ✦ ★) is an anti-emetic agent with central (chemoreceptor trigger zone) and peripheral activity. It contributes to lower esophageal sphincter competence and promotes gastric emptying. It is useful in the management of vomiting, gastroesophageal reflux, and gastric motility disorders. For more information, see METOCLOPRAMIDE in the Small Animal section.

In birds, metoclopramide has been used to stimulate motility of the crop, proventriculus and ventriculus, and intestines, particularly in pediatric medicine and for birds with delayed gastrointestinal motility as a result of proventricular dilation disease.

ADVERSE AND COMMON SIDE EFFECTS: Hyperactivity has been reported in psittacine birds treated with metoclopramide. Metoclopramide should not be used when there is mechanical blockage to the flow of ingesta or when there is gastrointestinal bleeding or perforation.

METRONIDAZOLE

INDICATIONS: Metronidazole (Flagyl ✤ ★) is a synthetic antibacterial and antiprotozoal agent with activity against anaerobic bacteria, *Giardia*, trichomonads, amebae, balantidiae, and trypanosomes. The drug may also have immunosuppressive or immunostimulatory properties. For more information, see METRONIDAZOLE in the Small Animal section.

In birds, metronidazole is used orally by gavage, in the drinking water, or by IM injection to treat protozoal infections such as trichomoniasis and giardiasis, or anaerobic bacterial infections. Commonly reported dosages range from 10 to 50 mg/kg once or twice daily with little specificity for species or condition being treated. All dosing strategies are empirical. Some authors report difficulty dissolving the tablet formulation resulting in inconsistent drug distribution through the drinking water.

In a preliminary study, two blue-fronted Amazon parrots were given a single 50 mg/kg oral dose of metronidazole base. Resulting plasma levels were reported as attaining 10 times the reported MIC levels for most anaerobes; therefore, a dose of 30 mg/kg was suggested for further investigation.

Metronidazole has been described as being toxic to finches but several reports discuss the successful use of the drug when placed in drinking water to treat small passerine birds. Over 1,000 birds were treated with drinking water containing 1.5 g metronidazole per gallon over a seven day period with no increase in mortality. This protocol was effective in limiting the progression of sinusitis due to an organism most consistent with *Trichomonas gallinae*. Birds with advanced sinusitis and extensive exudates did not respond well to treatment. This dosing regimen was also used to control crop trichomoniasis.

Metronidazole was effective against *Cochlosoma* sp. in a variety of finches at doses as low as 30 mg/kg body weight given once by crop gavage or at 40 mg/L of drinking water for 3 days. All birds ceased passing flagellates by 24 hours after a single oral dose and within 48 hours of commencing medication in the water.

ADVERSE AND COMMON SIDE EFFECTS: Metronidazole was not effective in clearing budgerigar aviaries of *Giardia* sp. at 200 mg/mL in one report, but in a second report, treatment with 200 to 400 mg/mL was successful. The IV product causes myonecrosis if used IM. Toxicity was not seen in a variety of finches given doses up to 179 mg/kg by gavage once daily for 4 days or 2 g/L of drinking water for 3 days.

MIBOLERONE

INDICATIONS: Mibolerone (Cheque Drops ★) is an androgenic, anabolic, antigonadotropic agent. For more information, see MIBOLERONE in the Small Animal section. Mibolerone has been used experimentally in birds to stop oviposition.

MICONAZOLE

INDICATIONS: Miconazole (Conofite ♣ ★, Micazole ★, Monistat ♣ ★, Micatin ♣, and others) is a synthetic imidazole-derived antifungal agent active against most pathogenic fungi, gram-positive bacteria, and some *Acanthamoeba* spp. In human medicine, miconazole products are used topically for fungal infections of skin and mucous membranes (e.g., candidiasis).

Miconazole has been used topically for the treatment of dermatophytosis and cutaneous candidiasis and for nebulization in psittacine birds. For nebulization, the drug has been either compounded as an aqueous solution or combined with acetylcysteine. IM administration of the IV formulation was used successfully for the treatment of aspergillosis in raptors in one report and in 16 Humboldt penguins in another; however, the same treatment regimen was not effective in two psittacine species. The authors of the psittacine work speculated that the dosage and frequency of dosage might not have been adequate to obtain therapeutic blood levels, and that inadequate tissue penetration might occur with parenteral miconazole.

Miconazole gel has been applied directly to the thoracic esophagus and crop of falcons with oral candidiasis twice daily for 5 consecutive days using cotton-tip applicators provided with long wooden handles. The progress of treatment was monitored by daily endoscopy. Mucosal improvement was noted within 12 hours after initiating treatment, by day 3 all diphtheritic membranes had disappeared, and most lesions were completely resolved by day 5. The authors concluded that this method of therapy was effective, rapid, and inexpensive.

ADVERSE AND COMMON SIDE EFFECTS: No safety or efficacy trials have been performed in birds. There was no evidence of muscle damage at the sites of IM injection of the IV product in 6 raptors that were necropsied after treatment. In humans, miconazole is less toxic than amphotericin B. Extreme caution should be taken using the product parenterally. Anaphylaxis, cardiac abnormalities, phlebitis, hepatitis, and pruritus have been recorded after IV injection, particularly with rapid infusion and possibly due to the castor oil diluent. Gastrointestinal upset, transient anemia, thrombocytopenia, and hyperlipidemia are some of the reported adverse effects in people.

DRUG INTERACTIONS: Miconazole enhances the activity of coumarin anticoagulants. Antagonism may exist between amphotericin B and miconazole.

SUPPLIED AS HUMAN PRODUCTS:
Several topical spray and cream gynecologic preparations (Micatin ♣, Miconozone ♣, Monistat ♣)

SUPPLIED AS VETERINARY PRODUCTS:
Cream containing 20 mg/g (Conofite ♣ ★)
Lotion and spray containing 1% (Conofite ★, Miconosol ★)
Shampoo containing 2% (Dermaxzole ★)

MIDAZOLAM

INDICATIONS: Midazolam (Versed ♣ ★) is a short-acting, parenteral, benzodiazepine central nervous system depressant with sedative, hypnotic, anxiolytic, muscle relaxant, and anticonvulsant properties. The drug is 2 to 3 times more potent than diazepam and has a shorter plasma elimination half-life. Midazolam is formulated for intramuscular use, unlike diazepam. Midazolam can be reversed with flumazenil. For more information, see MIDAZOLAM in the Small Animal section.

In birds, midazolam is used to provide sedation for diagnostic and nonpainful procedures, and as a preanesthetic. In a controlled trial in Canada geese given 2 mg/kg IM, maximum sedation was seen 15 to 20 minutes after injection. Minimal cardiovascular or respiratory changes occurred. Anesthesia and analgesia were produced in mallard ducks given a high dose of midazolam (5 mg/kg) + ketamine (50 mg/kg) IV, and birds remained moderately sedated for a considerable period of time, even after flumazenil was given IV. In bobwhite quail, midazolam was evaluated at doses of 2, 4, and 6 mg/kg.

Sedation was seen within 5 minutes of administration, peaking after 10 minutes in most birds. The degree of sedation reached was quite variable but was dose related, with 3/7 birds in the 2 mg/kg group and 9/10 birds in the 6 mg/kg group reaching heavy sedation (dorsal recumbency with wings outstretched). Cardiopulmonary function was unaffected. Sedation was rapidly and completely reversed by flumazenil administered at 0.1 mg/kg IM.

Midazolam is also used for the treatment of hyperexcitability and seizures such as occurs with 4-aminopyridine toxicity in pigeons.

ADVERSE AND COMMON SIDE EFFECTS: Ducks are poorly sedated by midazolam at doses up to 8 to 10 mg/kg IM.

MINOCYCLINE

INDICATIONS: Minocycline (Minocin ♣ ★) is a second-generation, long-acting, lipid-soluble tetracycline. It is more active against anaerobes and several facultative intracellular bacteria than other tetracyclines, with the exception of doxycycline. Minocycline is also more active against *Nocardia* spp. and staphylococci than other tetracyclines. For more information, see MINOCYCLINE and TETRACYCLINE ANTIBIOTICS in the Small Animal section.

In avian medicine, minocycline has been used primarily in the treatment of chlamydiosis. A dosage of 100 mg/kg of minocycline produces blood levels that are slightly higher, but more rapidly eliminated, than the same dose of doxycycline. Millet impregnated with 0.5% w/w minocycline was fed to yellow-napped, orange-cheeked, and blue-crowned parakeets. Blood levels greater than 5 µg/mL were achieved; levels greater than 1 µg/mL persisted for 48 hours after medicated feed was withdrawn. The authors commented that a lower concentration of drug would probably be adequate to maintain therapeutic blood levels greater than 1 µg/mL.

MONENSIN

INDICATIONS: Monensin (Coban ♣ ★, Rumensin ♣ ★, Rumensin CRC ♣) is an ionophore antibiotic used commonly as a feed additive in the poultry and livestock industries for control of coccidiosis and as a ruminant growth promotant. Coban 60 is also licensed for use in quail in the United States. For more information, see MONENSIN in the Large Animal section.

Monensin has been used to control coccidiosis in galliform birds and pigeons, and may be more effective than amprolium or clazuril. Monensin was a candidate drug for the control of visceral coccidiosis in whooping cranes; thus, a safety trial was conducted in sandhill cranes. Monensin was safe when fed at 1, 2, and 5 times the recommended poultry dose of 99 mg/kg (90 g/ton). Some reduction in appetite was noted in birds fed the highest concentration of medicated feed, but no abnormalities were noted on clinical and necropsy evaluations. An efficacy trial was not conducted, but coccidia were not noted in the feces or viscera of treated birds, in contrast to untreated control birds.

ADVERSE AND COMMON SIDE EFFECTS: Toxicity most frequently results from errors in mixing of the feed. Clinical signs of anorexia, dyspnea, ataxia, depression, recumbency, and death and pathologic lesions of skeletal and cardiac myodegeneration have been reported in a variety of species, including guinea fowl, chickens, and turkeys. The drug may be lethal to adult turkeys or guinea fowl. No toxicity was seen in crane chicks given 5 times the recommended poultry dose.

SUPPLIED AS VETERINARY PRODUCTS:
As a feed additive containing 132.2 g/kg (Coban 60 ★), 176 g/kg (Rumensin ★), and 200 g/kg (Coban ♣, Rumensin ★, Monensin ♣)

MOXIDECTIN

INDICATIONS: Moxidectin (ProHeart 6 ♣ ★, Guardian ♣, Cydectin ♣, Quest ♣ ★) is a new second-generation macrocyclic lactone parasiticide in the milbemycin family. Moxidectin is used orally or by injection in dogs for heartworm prevention and the treatment of hookworm infections, and by topical use in cattle and deer against sensitive gastrointestinal roundworms (including inhibited larvae of *Ostertagia ostertagi*), lungworm, biting and sucking lice, mange mites, and ticks. Moxidectin also appears to have macrofilaricidal activity, killing adult filarial worms in clinical trials. For more information, see MOXIDECTIN in the Small Animal section.

In pigeons, moxidectin has been found to be highly effective against the adult stages of *Capillaria* sp. at a dose of 0.2 mg/kg IM. This was based on evaluation of egg production per gram of feces. Moxidectin has also been used at the same dose, orally, to control parasites in birds of prey including sparrow hawks, European kestrels, peregrine falcons, and barn, tawny, and little owls.

SUPPLIED AS VETERINARY PRODUCTS:
For injection containing 3.4 mg/mL once reconstituted (ProHeart 6 Sustained Release Injectable for Dogs ♣ ★)
Oral paste containing 20 mg/mL (Quest 2% Equine Oral Gel ♣ ★)
Topical pour-on liquid containing 5 mg/mL (Cydectin Pour-On ♣ ★)
For injection containing 10 mg/mL (Cydectin ♣)

NALOXONE

INDICATIONS: Naloxone (Naloxone ♣ ★, Narcan ♣ ★) is a narcotic antagonist used to reverse general and respiratory depression induced by narcotic drugs including meperidine and butorphanol. One milliliter (0.4 mg) of P/M Naloxone counteracts 100 mg of meperidine. For more information, see NALOXONE in the Small Animal section. The use of naloxone has not been specifically described in birds.

NALTREXONE

INDICATIONS: Naltrexone (Trexonil ★, ReVia ✿ ★) is a narcotic antagonist used in human medicine for the treatment of opioid addictions and alcoholism. Naltrexone has shown some promise for the treatment of behavioral feather plucking in psittacine birds. The rationale for its use is based on the theory that feather plucking induces endorphin release, which becomes addictive. By blocking the effect of endorphins, naltrexone would remove the positive reinforcement for this behavior. For more information see NALTREXONE in the Small Animal section.

ADVERSE AND COMMON SIDE EFFECTS: Unknown in birds. Naltrexone is not addictive in people.

NEOMYCIN

INDICATIONS: Neomycin (Biosol ✿, Mycifradin ✿ ★) is an aminoglycoside antibiotic used topically and orally for the treatment of bacterial enteritis. Neomycin is not absorbed from the gastrointestinal tract; therefore, it is active only against enteric bacteria when administered by this route. For more information, see NEOMYCIN in the Small Animal section.

Neomycin has been administered to birds by direct oral gavage or in the drinking water.

ADVERSE AND COMMON SIDE EFFECTS: The drug is extremely toxic if administered systemically. Biosol M, which also contains methscopolamine bromide, can be toxic in birds.

SUPPLIED AS VETERINARY PRODUCT:
Oral liquid containing 140 mg/mL (Biosol Liquid ✿ ★)

SUPPLIED AS HUMAN PRODUCTS:
Tablets containing 500 mg (Mycifradin ✿, Generic ★)
Oral suspension containing 125 mg/5 mL (Mycifradin ✿ ★)

NORTRIPTYLINE

INDICATIONS: Nortriptyline (Aventyl ✿ ★, Norventyl ✿, and generics) is an oral tricyclic antidepressant drug used in humans.

Nortriptyline has been used, with very limited success, to treat feather picking in psittacine birds. In humans, it is suggested that the dosage should be initially low and gradually adjusted for each individual. Maximal antidepressant effects may require 2 weeks or more of therapy. Once symptoms are controlled, the dose is gradually reduced to the lowest effective level.

ADVERSE AND COMMON SIDE EFFECTS: Hyperactivity has been reported in treated birds. If this occurs, the dosage should be reduced, or if the bird does not return to normal activity patterns, the treatment with nortriptyline should be discontinued. Withdrawal symptoms are seen in humans after abrupt withdrawal of the drug.

SUPPLIED AS HUMAN PRODUCTS:
Capsules containing 10 and 25 mg (Alti-Nortriptyline ✹ ★, Alti-Nortriptyline Hydrochloride ✹, Aventil ✹, Gen-Nortriptyline ✹, Norventyl ✹, Novo-Nortriptyline ✹, Nu-Nortriptyline ✹, PMS-Nortriptyline ✹) and 10, 25, 50, and 75 mg (Nortriptyline Hydrochloride ★, Nortriptyline HCl ★, Pamelor ★)
Oral solution containing 10 mg/5 mL in 4% alcohol (Aventyl ★, Pamelor ★)

NYSTATIN

INDICATIONS: Nystatin (Mycostatin ✹ ★, Nilstat ✹ ★) is a polyene macroline antifungal agent related to amphotericin B. Nystatin is fungistatic and fungicidal. The drug is primarily used for the treatment of gastrointestinal yeast infections, including oral candidiasis. For more information, see NYSTATIN in the Small Animal section.

In birds, nystatin is used for the prevention and treatment of oral and gastrointestinal candidiasis, especially in hand-fed neonates and birds on long-term antibiotic therapy. Nystatin has generally been found to be ineffective against gastric "megabacteriosis," although in one small study in European goldfinches efficacy was reported using the drug via crop gavage (5,000 U/bird twice daily for 10 days) or in the drinking water (5,000,000 U/L).

Nystatin is effective topically and is not systemically absorbed across intact epithelium. Oral lesions must be treated by direct contact with the medication. When treating hand-fed neonates it is probably better to administer nystatin separately from formula to maximize nystatin's concentration and epithelial contact time. Doses are empirical and vary widely in the literature. There are a number of recommendations for treatment of drinking water; however, some authors suggest that nystatin is poorly soluble and does not remain homogenous in solution.

ADVERSE AND COMMON SIDE EFFECTS: Regurgitation is seen infrequently.

OXACILLIN

INDICATIONS: Oxacillin (Bactocill ★, Prostaphlin ★) is a penicillin antibiotic used in the treatment of gram-positive infections, including staphylococcal infections and infections caused by β-lactamase–producing bacteria. The drug has been used in the treatment of pyoderma, bacterial endocarditis, and blepharitis in dogs and cats. For more information, see OXACILLIN and PENICILLIN ANTIBIOTICS in the Small Animal section.

In birds, oxacillin has been recommended for the treatment of bacterial dermatitis.

OXFENDAZOLE

INDICATIONS: Oxfendazole (Benzelmin ✹ ★, Equi-Cide ★, Synanthic ★) is a benzimidazole anthelmintic agent licensed for use in cattle, sheep, and horses. Oxfendazole is also a metabolic product of the breakdown of fenbendazole, which is in turn a metabolite of the prebenzimidazole, febantel. Oxfendazole is effective against lungworms and a variety of gastrointestinal nematodes, and has activity against cestodes. Because absorption and time to peak blood levels are slower for oxfendazole versus many of the older benzimidazoles, effective concentrations are maintained for a longer period of time in both the serum and the intestinal tract. These absorption parameters seem to impart greater efficacy, particularly against immature and inhibited larvae. For more information, see OXFENDAZOLE in the Large Animal section.

In birds, oxfendazole has been recommended for the treatment of gastric spiruroid parasites and *Capillaria* sp. in small passerines. A commercial tablet formulation containing praziquantel and oxfendazole (20 mg each, 1 tablet/2 kg) is available to treat enteric nematodes and cestodes in pigeons and poultry in some parts of the world.

SUPPLIED AS VETERINARY PRODUCTS:
Oral paste containing 4.5 g/12 g of paste (Benzelmin ★), 5.4 g/14.4 g of paste (Benzelmin ✹), and 185 mg/g (18.5%) (Synanthic Bovine Dewormer ★)
Oral suspension containing 90.6 mg/mL (9.06%) (Benzelmin ✹, Synanthic ✹, Synanthic Bovine Dewormer ★) or 225 mg/mL (22.5%) (Synanthic ✹, Synanthic Bovine Dewormer ★)

OXYTETRACYCLINE

INDICATIONS: Oxytetracycline (Liquamycin ✹ ★, Terramycin ✹ ★) is a short-acting, water-soluble tetracycline with activity against a broad range of gram-positive and gram-negative organisms as well as chlamydiae, rickettsiae, and mycoplasmas. For more information, see OXYTETRACYCLINE and TETRACYCLINE ANTIBIOTICS in the Small Animal section.

In birds, oxytetracycline has been used IM or SC in the treatment of bacterial infections and chlamydiosis. Doxycycline is now the preferred drug for the treatment of *Chlamydophila psittaci* infections in individual birds. Oxytetracycline is eliminated through the bile and the kidneys. In chickens given oxytetracycline IM, the highest tissue levels were found in liver, then gluteal muscle, heart, kidney, and pectoral muscle. In a pharmacokinetic study involving ring-necked pheasants, great horned owls, and several species of Amazon parrots, no correlation was noted between half-life and the body weights of the various species. In a study of Goffin's cockatoos given single doses of oxytetracycline at 50, 75, and 100 mg/kg IM and SC, increased dosage resulted in increased blood levels. Comparison of the two routes of administration at different doses showed a significant difference in plasma blood levels at only one time versus dose point. There was no accumulation of drug in the plasma of birds given 100 mg/kg SC every 72 hours for 30 days. No adverse effects, other than injection site reactions, were noted. The elimination half-life of oxytetracycline in these cockatoos was shorter than that in the three species previously mentioned and in turkeys.

In turkeys given the long-acting oxytetracycline formulation at 152 mg/kg SC, the plasma elimination half-life of the drug was 12 hours and blood concentrations remained greater than 1 µg/mL (the target therapeutic MIC for *C. psittaci* and *Pasteurella multocida*) for 72 hours. In a study using the standard formulation of oxytetracycline, 12-week-old turkeys received 200 mg/bird SC. Blood levels had dropped below 1 µg/mL by day 2 after injection.

In Pekin ducks infected with *Salmonella* spp., oral oxytetracycline fed at 50 and 200 mg/kg of feed decreased the duration of shedding of oxytetracycline-sensitive bacterial strains but increased the duration of shedding of resistant strains.

ADVERSE AND COMMON SIDE EFFECTS: Irritation and necrosis occur at the sites of both SC and IM injections. In cockatoos, injection site damage was dose related, more severe at IM sites, and increased in severity after multiple injections. Concurrent elevations in aspartate aminotransferase, creatinine kinase, and lactate dehydrogenase were also noted in the same study.

OXYTOCIN

INDICATIONS: Oxytocin (Pitocin ★, Syntocinon ✚ ★) is a hormone of the posterior pituitary gland. For more information, see OXYTOCIN in the Small Animal section.

In avian medicine, oxytocin is used to stimulate uterine contractions in egg-bound birds. Concurrent administration of injectable calcium has been recommended. The drug has also been used to control uterine hemorrhage. Oxytocin is preferable to prostaglandin $F_{2\alpha}$, which may cause systemic reactions when used parenterally. Oxytocin receptors are located only in the uterus.

ADVERSE AND COMMON SIDE EFFECTS: Because oxytocin does not relax the uterovaginal sphincter, shell rupture can occur. Oxytocin is contraindicated where physical reasons prevent passage of the egg. Oxytocin may not be effective in hypocalcemic birds.

DRUG INTERACTIONS: The topical application of prostaglandin E_2 to the oviductal opening (via the cloaca) 20 to 30 minutes before instituting oxytocin therapy is highly recommended to relax the uterovaginal sphincter, allowing easier passage of the egg.

PANCREATIC ENZYME REPLACEMENT

INDICATIONS: These products (Pancrease-V ✤, Pancrezyme ★, Creon ✤ ★, Ultrase ✤ ★, Viokase ✤ ★) are mixtures containing standardized activities of the pancreatic enzymes lipase, amylase, and protease used for the management of pancreatic exocrine insufficiency. For further information, see PANCREATIC ENZYME REPLACEMENT in the Small Animal section.

In birds, pancreatic enzyme products are used for the treatment of pancreatic insufficiency, delayed crop emptying, and maldigestion. The compounds are mixed with moistened food or given by gavage. Food should be incubated for 15 minutes before feeding. Viokase-V is the product described more commonly in clinical reports.

PAROMOMYCIN

INDICATIONS: Paramomycin (Humatin ✤ ★) is an aminoglycoside antibiotic with a broad spectrum of activity against bacteria, protozoa, and cestodes. In humans, paromomycin is used for the treatment of intestinal amebiasis and, in HIV patients, cryptosporidiosis. A case report describes the use of paromomycin to reduce morbidity and mortality in a flock of Lady Gouldian finches with cryptosporidiosis. The dose of the drug was calculated for the flock weight of all birds and administered in food. The amount of treated food provided was doubled for wastage. In another report, the contents of a 250 mg capsule was dissolved in 10 mL of water to create a solution for gavage.

ADVERSE AND COMMON SIDE EFFECTS: Paromomycin is poorly absorbed from the intestinal tract. The drug is potentially nephrotoxic and ototoxic and may have neuromuscular blocking effects. Other adverse effects in humans include gastrointestinal signs.

SUPPLIED AS HUMAN PRODUCT:
Oral capsules containing 250 mg (Humatin ✤ ★)

PENICILLAMINE

INDICATIONS: Penicillamine (Cuprimine ✤ ★, Depen ✤ ★) is a thiol compound that chelates cystine, lead, and copper and promotes their excretion in the urine. For more information, see PENICILLAMINE in the Small Animal section.

Penicillamine has been used orally in birds to treat lead and zinc poisoning once the patient is stabilized using CaEDTA.

ADVERSE AND COMMON SIDE EFFECTS: Regurgitation severe enough to require cessation of therapy is commonly recorded in birds receiving oral penicillamine. The therapeutic index in mammals is low. For more information, see PENICILLAMINE in the Small Animal section.

PENICILLIN G

INDICATIONS: For more information, see PENICILLIN ANTI-BIOTICS in the Small Animal section. Penicillin is not used commonly in pet bird medicine; however, there are several reports of the drug's use in ratites (e.g., an emu with *Erysipelothrix rhusiopathiae* infection, a rhea with GI disease attributed to *Toxoplasma gondii* infection). Penicillin G is acid labile, hence oral administration results in poor absorption and low blood levels.

In a pharmacokinetic study in turkeys, a combination of procaine and benzathine penicillins was better absorbed than the potassium salt or either penicillin formulation alone (IM administration). The calculated elimination half-life for potassium penicillin G was 30 minutes. In chickens, aqueous penicillin was absorbed more rapidly than procaine penicillin after IM administration; however, serum concentrations were undetectable 4 hours after injection of 6 to 50 mg/kg. At IM doses of 12 mg/kg, the half-life of procaine penicillin in chickens is 10 times longer than that of penicillin-G (5.8 hours and 0.55 hours, respectively); however, peak levels are much lower. Procaine penicillin may maintain therapeutic blood levels for up to 48 hours in some species. The drug is most commonly used in gallinaceous birds and waterfowl that are difficult to treat on a daily basis.

Equivalency of milligram and United States Pharmacopeia units:

Penicillin G sodium—1 mg = 1,500 to 1,750 USP units

Penicillin G sodium powder—1 mg = 1,420 to 1,667 USP units

Penicillin G procaine—1 mg = 900 to 1,050 USP units

Penicillin G benzathine—1 mg = 1,090 to 1,272 USP units

ADVERSE AND COMMON SIDE EFFECTS: Adverse reactions to the injection of the procaine/benzathine combination have been reported in small birds even at doses of 1 mg/kg, probably due to procaine toxicity. Other reactions include vomiting and acute collapse in a South American black-collared hawk and regurgitation and trembling in pigeons given 500 mg/kg (833,500 IU/kg). No reactions were seen in pigeons given 100 or 200 mg/kg, or in chickens and turkeys given 100 mg/kg.

PHENOBARBITAL

INDICATIONS: Phenobarbital ♣ ★ is the drug of choice for the control of seizure activity in small animals. It has been used for this purpose in psittacine birds as well as to treat pigeons poisoned with 4-aminopyridine. Monitoring of serum levels is important in determining optimum long-term dosage requirements. For more information, see PHENOBARBITAL and BARBITURATES in the Small Animal section.

PHENYLBUTAZONE

INDICATIONS: Phenylbutazone (Butasone ♣, Butazone ♣, Bizolin 200 ★ Phenylbutazone ♣ ★, and many others) has analgesic, antipyretic, and anti-inflammatory properties that make it useful in the treatment of osteoarthritis and inflammation of the skin and soft tissue. For more information, see PHENYLBUTAZONE in the Small or Large Animal sections.

Phenylbutazone has been used orally in psittacines and raptorial birds for its anti-inflammatory properties.

PIPERACILLIN

INDICATIONS: Piperacillin (Pipracil ♣ ★) is a broad-spectrum, semisynthetic penicillin with activity against most aerobic gram-negative bacteria and some gram-positive and anaerobic organisms. It is used to treat bacterial infections, including those caused by *Pseudomonas aeruginosa* and *E. coli*. For more information, see PENICILLIN ANTIBIOTICS in the Small Animal section.

A single-dose pharmacokinetic study of piperacillin in blue-fronted Amazon parrots measured initial plasma concentrations of approximately 50 µg/mL (<0.5 hour after administration of 50 mg/kg IV) and 150 µg/mL (approximately 0.5 hour after administration of 100 mg/kg IM). The elimination half-life was short, less than 45 minutes. Dosage at least 3 times daily was recommended at the conclusion of this study, particularly when treating organisms of only moderate susceptibility.

In red-tailed hawks and great horned owls administered a single dose of 100 mg/kg piperacillin IM, mean maximum plasma piperacillin concentrations were 204 µg/mL and 221 µg/mL, respectively. Absorption was very rapid with maximum concentrations reached at 15 minutes (hawks) and 30 minutes (owls). The elimination half-lives were 77 minutes in the hawks and 118 minutes in the owls. A maximum dosing interval of 4 to 6 hours was recommended for medium sized raptors using a MIC of 8 µg/mL as a goal.

Piperacillin has also been administered through nebulization, intranasally, and by injection into the air cell of the egg to increase egg hatchability.

ADVERSE AND COMMON SIDE EFFECTS: Piperacillin is unstable once reconstituted. Some authors have suggested freezing the reconstituted drug in aliquots for subsequent treatments; however, subsequent stability has not been investigated. Adverse effects are similar to those of other extended-spectrum penicillins.

DRUG INTERACTIONS: Piperacillin can be used synergistically in combination with the aminoglycosides, particularly amikacin and tobramicin in birds.

SUPPLIED AS HUMAN PRODUCT:
For injection in vials containing 2, 3, and 4 g (Pipracil ✚ ★)

PIPERAZINE

INDICATIONS: Piperazine (Hartz Once-a-Month ★, Once-a-Month Roundworm Treatment ✚, Pipa-Tabs ★, Purina Liquid Dog Wormer ★) is an anthelmintic used for the eradication of roundworms. For more information, see PIPERAZINE in the Small Animal section.

Piperazine has been used for the treatment of intestinal ascarids in birds.

POLYMYXIN B

INDICATIONS: Polymyxin B (Aerosporin ✚ ★, Neosporin ✚ ★, Pediotic Suspension ★) is a basic polypeptide antibiotic derived from *Bacillus polymyxa* (*B. aerosporus*). Polymyxin B has a bactericidal action against almost all gram-negative bacilli except the *Proteus* group, and is a treatment of choice for *Pseudomonas* spp. infections in humans. Polymyxin B is particularly used in the treatment of gram-negative infections, especially those resistant to aminoglycosides. The drug is available in combination with other agents for topical and ophthalmic use. For more information, see POLYMYXIN B in the Small Animal section.

Polymyxin has been used in topical ophthalmic preparations and by nebulization for the treatment of pneumonia and air sacculitis in birds. The drug is poorly absorbed by the respiratory epithelium and has primarily a topical effect.

ADVERSE AND COMMON SIDE EFFECTS: Weakness, incoordination, vomiting, and death have been reported in Amazon parrots receiving parenteral doses of 5 to 10 mg/kg.

SUPPLIED AS HUMAN PRODUCTS:
For injection containing 500,000 U/20-mL vial, equivalent to 50 mg polymyxin (Aerosporin ★)
Numerous products for topical use (✚ ★)

POLYSULFATED GLYCOSAMINOGLYCANS

INDICATIONS: Polysulfated glycosaminoglycans (Adequan IM ✚ ★, Cosequin ★) may be beneficial in the treatment of osteoarthritis through a variety of mechanisms. To maximize therapeutic benefit, treatment should begin soon after the inciting traumatic event. For more information, see POLYSULFATED GLYCOSAMINOGLYCANS in the Small Animal section.

The use of polysulfated glycosaminoglycans has been reported to treat arthritic lesions in a king vulture (IM), and intra-articularly in a demoiselle crane and a Palawan peacock pheasant.

PRALIDOXIME CHLORIDE

INDICATIONS: Pralidoxime chloride (Protopam Chloride ✚ ★) or 2-PAM chloride is a cholinesterase reactivator used to treat organophosphate toxicity. The drug is most effective when given within 24 hours of exposure and is usually not effective after 36 to 48 hours have passed. In humans, administration by slow IV injection is suggested; the IM and SC routes are alternates when venous access is not possible. The use of pralidoxime in the treatment of carbamate toxicity is controversial and generally not recommended.

ADVERSE AND COMMON SIDE EFFECTS: IM administration of pralidoxime may result in pain at the site of injection. There is an anecdotal report of death in a bald eagle after treatment.

DRUG INTERACTIONS: Pralidoxime has little effect on muscarinic activity; therefore, animals should be pretreated with atropine. Pralidoxime is contraindicated in cases of carbaryl exposure because toxicity appears to increase.

SUPPLIED AS HUMAN PRODUCT:
For injection containing 1 g/20-mL vial (Protopam chloride ✚ ★)

PRAZIQUANTEL

INDICATIONS: Praziquantel (Droncit ✚ ★, Prazarid ✚) is an anthelmintic used for the elimination of cestodes and some trematodes. For more information, see PRAZIQUANTEL in the Small Animal section.

In birds, praziquantel is used parenterally and orally for the elimination of cestodes. The injectable formulation can also be used for oral administration. A commercial tablet formulation containing praziquantel and oxfendazole (20 mg each, 1 tablet/2 kg) is available to treat nematodes and cestodes in pigeons and poultry in some parts of the world.

Several reports describe the use of praziquantel against hepatic trematodes. In toucans, an IM dose of 10 mg/kg once daily for 3 days, then once daily for 11 days PO halted the shedding of trematode eggs. In a Moluccan cockatoo given 10 mg/kg once daily for 3 days SC, there was a sharp decrease in shedding of eggs, but at necropsy adult flukes of abnormal appearance were still present in the liver.

ADVERSE AND COMMON SIDE EFFECTS: The injectable form of the drug may be toxic to finches. There is an anecdotal report of weakness, disorientation, and even deaths in baby and juvenile African gray parrots that were treated with 9 mg/kg IM in quarantine stations. Adults of the same species showed no adverse effects. Depression and death have been described in birds receiving doses of 100 to 250 mg/kg IM.

PREDNISOLONE
PREDNISOLONE SODIUM SUCCINATE
PREDNISONE

INDICATIONS: Prednisolone (Delta-Cortef ★) and prednisone (Deltasone ♣, Meticorten ★) are intermediate-acting glucocorticoid agents. Prednisone is converted by the liver to prednisolone. Except for cases of liver failure, the drugs can essentially be used interchangeably. For more information, see PREDNISOLONE and GLUCOCORTICOID AGENTS in the Small Animal section.

These drugs are used by parenteral administration for the treatment of shock, trauma, and endotoxemia, and PO as anti-inflammatory agents. Nonsteroidal anti-inflammatory agents may be more appropriate for inflammatory or chronic conditions as they are not immunosuppressive (see below). Despite evidence of the strong immunosuppressive effects of corticosteroids in birds, many published dosages are very high. Tablets can be suspended in water to make a solution of appropriate concentration. A decreasing dosage schedule should be used for long-term therapy. Prednisone has been used in the supportive care of birds with acute head trauma and after treatment of canaries for respiratory mites.

ADVERSE AND COMMON SIDE EFFECTS: Concern is frequently expressed regarding the high sensitivity of birds to the immunosuppressive effects of glucocorticoids. This has been supported by experimental work in pigeons that showed that the hypothalamic-pituitary-adrenal system is more sensitive to suppression by glucocorticoids than that of mammals. Suppression is dose dependent. The minimum intravenous dose of prednisolone required to suppress plasma corticosterone levels was 0.7 µg/kg. The duration of suppression by prednisolone was shorter than that of dexamethasone, which was also evaluated in these studies. In another study, prednisolone was administered orally at 350 µg/kg, topically to bare skin at approximately 500 µg/kg, topically in combination with DMSO to bare skin at a dose of 350 µg/kg, and ophthalmically at approximately 70 µg/kg. Suppression of corticosterone levels occurred in all groups except those treated topically without DMSO.

PRIMAQUINE

INDICATIONS: Primaquine ♣ ★ is a synthetic antimalarial agent used in combination with chloroquine for the therapy of malaria caused by *Plasmodium* spp., especially in penguins. The combination can also be used prophylactically, in drinking water, to prevent seasonal malaria in outdoor budgerigars, canaries, and finches. The tablets can be dissolved in water (up to a concentration of 1 g/15 mL) and a dosing regimen established based on estimated water intake. A medicated water formulation for this species can be made by dissolving one 500-mg chloroquine tablet and 75 mg of primaquine in 15 mL of water as a stock solution and placing 1 mL of stock solution in 480 mL of drinking water as treatment. Primaquine may also suppress the tissue stages of *Atoxoplasma* sp. in canaries.

DRUG INTERACTIONS: Primaquine is active against the exerythrocytic or tissue form of *Plasmodium* spp. but not the circulating parasite form; therefore, chloroquine is used concurrently.

ADVERSE AND COMMON SIDE EFFECTS: Depression and vomiting have been seen with overdosage in penguins.

SUPPLIED AS HUMAN PRODUCT:
Tablets containing 15 mg primaquine base ♣ ★

PROPOFOL

INDICATIONS: Propofol (Rapinovet ♣ ★, Diprivan ♣ ★, Propoflow ★) is a sedative/hypnotic IV agent used to provide general anesthesia for procedures lasting less than 5 minutes and for induction and maintenance of general anesthesia using incremental doses to effect. It is particularly useful for cases in which a short recovery is desired. For more information, see PROPOFOL in the Small Animal section.

The cardiopulmonary effects of propofol have been studied in a number of avian species, including chickens, pigeons, wild turkeys, barn owls, canvasback and mallard ducks, and ostriches. Dosages vary with species; however, apnea and hypoventilation are consistent concerns. Careful monitoring and ventilatory support is recommended in all species.

Propofol was found to have a low therapeutic index in canvasback ducks when administered at a 15 mg/kg loading dose IV, delivered over 1 minute, followed by a constant infusion rate of 0.8 mg/kg per minute to maintain anesthesia. One duck died during dose determination and another during the cardiopulmonary study. During the anesthetic period (1 to 30 minutes), body temperature and PaO_2 values decreased significantly while mean arterial pressure and $PaCO_2$ increased. The arterial pH decreased significantly at 5, 10, and 15 minutes after induction. Five minutes after propofol was discontinued (35 minutes), none of the physiologic values measured were significantly different from baseline values. The same authors found that administration of propofol to mallard ducks produced smooth induction and recovery (8 to 10 mg/kg initial dose; IV), excellent muscle relaxation, and short duration of anesthesia requiring additional boluses of 1 to 4 mg/kg IV to prolong and maintain anesthesia.

Propofol was used to induce (3 mg/kg IV) and maintain (0.2 mg/kg per minute constant rate infusion) anesthesia in juvenile ostriches that had been sedated with a combination of medetomidine and ketamine. This dose of propofol enabled intubation and provided muscle relaxation adequate for the 30-minute evaluation period. Apnea was observed after initial administration, but spontaneous ventilation resumed within 60 to 90 seconds after induction. By 5 minutes after induction, the respiratory rate had increased significantly and remained satisfactory. During the anesthetic period, systolic, diastolic, and mean blood pressures, as well as arterial pH, PaO_2, $PaCO_2$, and end tidal carbon dioxide partial pressure showed no significant changes. Arterial blood gas analysis indicated adequate arterial oxygenation.

ADVERSE AND COMMON SIDE EFFECTS: In birds, as in mammals, propofol induces dose dependent ventilatory depression resulting in periods of apnea, decreased tidal volume, and respiratory acidosis. In a controlled study in chickens, cardiac arrhythmias were common, likely due to hypoxia, hypercarbia, and perhaps catecholamine release. Other negative cardiovascular effects have been reported. Opisthotonus, muscle tremors, and temporary neurologic signs have been observed on recovery.

PROSTAGLANDIN E_2

INDICATIONS: Prostaglandin E_2 (Prepidil 🍁 ★, Prostin E_2 🍁) gel is used to "ripen" the cervix and induce parturition in humans. The drug is applied to the uterovaginal junction of dystocic birds to stimulate relaxation of this region and aid in passage of the egg. The egg will often pass within 5 to 10 minutes of application. Low doses of oxytocin may increase the strength of the contractions in the shell gland, which are responsible for expulsion of the egg.

The human gel product can be divided into aliquots of an appropriate dose for birds then frozen for subsequent use.

ADVERSE AND COMMON SIDE EFFECTS: Excessive doses of prostaglandin E_2 may result in smooth muscle relaxation. Caution must be taken to ensure that there are no mechanical obstructions to passage of the egg.

SUPPLIED AS HUMAN PRODUCTS:
Prostaglandin E_2 (Dinoprostone)
Gel formulation containing 0.5 mg/3.0 g (0.5 mg/2.5 mL) (Prepidil ✤ ★), 1 mg/3 g (1 mg/2.5 mL) and 2 mg/3 g (2 mg/2.5 mL) (Prostin E_2 ✤)

PYRANTEL PAMOATE

INDICATIONS: Pyrantel pamoate (Pyr-A-Pam ✤, Pyran ✤, Nemex ★) is an anthelmintic used for the eradication of intestinal nematodes in a variety of avian species. The drug has a high therapeutic index. In one report describing the treatment of an aviary containing large psittacines, pyrantel pamoate was more efficacious against ascarids than ivermectin. For more information, see PYRANTEL PAMOATE in the Small Animal section.

PYRETHRIN-CONTAINING PRODUCTS

INDICATIONS: Pyrethrin-containing products (Happy Jack ★, Mycodex ★, Ovitrol ✤, Zodiac ✤, and others) are naturally occurring insecticides derived from the plant *Chrysanthemum cinerariae-folium.* These drugs are γ-aminobutyric acid (GABA) agonists, which stimulate the insect's central nervous system causing muscular excitation, convulsions, and paralysis. Insect mortality is enhanced when these products are combined with piperonyl butoxide, which inhibits pyrethrin metabolism. For more information, see PYRETHRIN-CONTAINING PRODUCTS in the Small Animal section.

In birds, pyrethrin spray or powder products are used topically for the treatment of external arthropod parasites, especially lice. Care should be taken to spray the axillary area with the wings of the bird extended to contact all the parasites. Pyrethrins have a high therapeutic index but little residual activity.

ADVERSE AND COMMON SIDE EFFECTS: Avoid contact of the chemical with the eyes and oral cavity.

PYRIMETHAMINE

INDICATIONS: Pyrimethamine (Daraprim ♣ ★) is an antiparasitic drug that is highly selective against *Plasmodium* spp. and is used in combination with the sulfonamides (e.g., sulfadiazine) in the treatment of infections with *Toxoplasma gondii*. For more information, see PYRIMETHAMINE in the Small Animal section.

Pyrimethamine has also been used successfully in the treatment of *Sarcocystis* spp. infection in two Amazon and one eclectus parrots. Trimethoprim-sulfadiazine (30 mg/kg q 12 hours; IM) was administered concurrently for the first 7 days of the 30-day treatment. Pyrimethamine was made into an oral solution by suspending a 25 mg tablet in 21 mL of water, and adding 4 mL of a water-soluble lubricating jelly to create a 1 mg/mL suspension.

RANITIDINE

INDICATIONS: Ranitidine (Zantac ♣ ★) is a histamine (H_2)-receptor antagonist that is used for the treatment of GI ulceration. It is more potent in inhibiting gastric acid secretion than cimetidine, but clinically is no more effective. H_2-receptor antagonists do not prevent NSAID-induced gastric ulcers, although ranitidine may prevent NSAID-induced duodenal ulceration. In mammals, ranitidine increases the passage of ingesta through the gut by stimulating gastric, small intestinal, and colonic motility. It may also stimulate pancreatic exocrine secretion. For more information, see RANITIDINE in the Small Animal section.

In birds, ranitidine has been used in the treatment of gastric ulceration and gastritis, particularly in parrots.

ADVERSE AND COMMON SIDE EFFECTS: Adverse effects in dogs and cats appear rare. Dogs given dosages greater than 225 mg/kg per day exhibited muscle tremors, vomiting, and rapid respiration. In humans, nausea and bradycardia with IV injection are reported. Pain at the injection site may occur with IM use.

DRUG INTERACTIONS: Antacids decrease GI absorption; therefore, concurrently used medications should be spaced apart by at least 2 hours. Ranitidine interferes with the metabolism of drugs removed by hepatic cytochrome P-450 enzyme systems.

RIFABUTIN

INDICATIONS: Rifabutin (Mycobutin ♣ ★) is an antimycobacterial drug used in human medicine for the treatment of mycobacterial infections. In human medicine, clarithromycin or azithromycin combined with ethambutol and either ciprofloxacin or rifabutin is one of the drug combinations recommended for the prophylaxis and treatment of *Mycobacterium avium* complex infections in HIV patients. The resistance pattern to rifabutin and rifampin are similar.

In birds, rifabutin has been used in combination drug regimens for the treatment of mycobacteriosis. Veterinarians differ in their willingness to treat avian mycobacteriosis due to the difficulty in ensuring that the infection is fully eliminated and concerns over the potential for zoonotic spread of the disease under certain conditions.

ADVERSE AND COMMON SIDE EFFECTS: A variety of side effects are described in human medicine. Monitoring of hepatic enzymes is probably appropriate.

DRUG INTERACTIONS: Rifabutin induces hepatic cytochrome P-450 enzymes; therefore, therapy with rifabutin may affect the levels of a variety of other therapeutic agents.

AVAILABILITY: HUMAN PRODUCT
Capsules containing 150 mg (Mycobutin ♣ ★)

RIFAMPIN

INDICATIONS: Rifampin (Rifadin ♣ ★, Rimactane ★, Rofact ♣) is an antibiotic used alone or in combination with other agents in the treatment of actinomycosis, *Coxiella burnetii* (Q fever), feline leprosy, listeriosis, Rocky Mountain spotted fever, and tuberculosis. It is active against staphylococci and intracellular organisms (e.g., *Chlamydophila* spp.). The drug may also be useful in the treatment of chronic staphylococcal infection, such as severe pyoderma and chronic osteomyelitis, but it should always be used with another antibiotic because resistance develops rapidly. For more information, see RIFAMPIN in the Small Animal section.

In birds, rifampin has been used most frequently in multidrug combinations (e.g., isoniazid, ethambutol, clofazimine, ciprofloxacin, or enrofloxacin) to treat mycobacterial infections. The resistance pattern to rifabutin and rifampin are similar. Veterinarians differ in their willingness to treat avian mycobacteriosis due to the difficulty in ensuring that the infection is fully eliminated and concerns over the potential for zoonotic spread of the disease under certain conditions.

RONIDAZOLE

INDICATIONS: Ronidazole is a 5-nitroimidazole antiprotozoal agent that has been used to treat histomoniasis in turkeys. It is effective, and in some parts of the world licensed for use, against motile protozoa including *Trichomonas, Hexamita, Giardia,* and *Cochlosoma* spp. in caged and aviary birds and pigeons (water treatment) and

Trichomonas sp. in falcons (direct oral treatment). The drug is related to dimetridazole and carnidazole. Ronidazole has been banned for use in food-producing animals due to human health concerns related to residues in foods, and is being withdrawn in many countries. Ronidazole is frequently recommended for use in pigeons.

In pigeons, use of the prolonged release product resulted in very irregular absorption patterns, which did not allow prediction of a reliable dosing regimen. Absorption was more reliable when birds were dosed with an empty crop. A variety of finches subclinically infected with *Cochlosoma* sp. treated with ronidazole in the drinking water at 60 mg/L ceased shedding organisms within 24 hours of the onset of treatment and 10/10 birds were negative on fecal evaluation through 7 days of treatment.

ADVERSE AND COMMON SIDE EFFECTS: No toxic effects have been seen in finches at doses of 50 to 100 mg/L in drinking water, unlike dimetridazole, which has been described as toxic in passerine birds, even at therapeutic levels.

SUPPLIED AS VETERINARY PRODUCTS:
Not currently marketed in North America

SELENIUM

See VITAMIN E + SELENIUM in this section.

SEVOFLURANE

INDICATIONS: Sevoflurane (Sevoflurane ✤, Ultane ★) is a nonflammable, halogenated inhalation anesthetic agent for induction and maintenance of general anesthesia. In mammals, induction and recovery times are generally faster than for isoflurane; however, as sevoflurane is less potent than isoflurane, greater inspired concentrations will be required to maintain anesthesia. For more information, see SEVOFLURANE in the Small Animal section.

Sevoflurane is still being evaluated experimentally and in clinical practice to determine whether it is a better agent for the anesthesia of avian patients than is isoflurane.

SPECTINOMYCIN

INDICATIONS: Spectinomycin (Spectam ✤ ★, Prospec ★, Spectinomycin Hydrochloride Injectable ★) is an aminocyclitol broad-spectrum antibiotic effective against gram-negative bacteria including *Escherichia coli, Klebsiella, Salmonella, Proteus,* and *Enterobacter* spp. as well as gram-positive bacteria, including streptococci, and staphylococci. Spectinomycin is related structurally to the aminoglycosides and it shares many properties. For more information, see SPECTINOMYCIN in the Large Animal section.

Spectinomycin is registered for SC use in turkeys to reduce mortality resulting from infection by sensitive strains of *Pasteurella multocida* and for use in the drinking water to control mycoplasmal infections in chickens and turkeys. The drug has been used by nebulization for the treatment of pneumonia and air sacculitis and in drinking water for the treatment of gram-negative enteric infections.

ADVERSE AND COMMON SIDE EFFECTS: Spectinomycin has a low degree of toxicity. SC injections of up to 50 mg/turkey poult caused no adverse effects. Transient ataxia and coma, of up to 4 hours in duration, occurred after administration of 90 mg/poult. Some humans who handle spectinomycin develop serious cutaneous reactions.

DRUG INTERACTIONS: Spectinomycin is most frequently used in conjunction with lincomycin. See LINCOMYCIN in this section.

SUPPLIED AS VETERINARY PRODUCTS:
For injection containing 5 mg/mL and 10 mg/mL (Spectam Injectable ★) and 100 mg/mL (Adspec Sterile Solution ✿, Spectam Injectable ✿ ★, Spectinomycin Injectable ★)
Oral solution containing 50 mg/mL (Spectam Scour Halt ✿ ★, Spectinomycin Oral Liquid ★)
Water-soluble concentrate or powder containing 500 mg/g (Spectam ✿ ★)

STANOZOLOL

INDICATIONS: Stanozolol (Winstrol-V ✿ ★) is an anabolic steroid with strong anabolic and weak androgenic activity. For more information, see STANOZOLOL and ANABOLIC STEROIDS in the Small Animal section.

Stanozolol has been administered orally or by injection for anabolic therapy in birds that are debilitated, anemic, or anorectic to stimulate appetite and weight gain.

ADVERSE AND COMMON SIDE EFFECTS: Stanozolol should be used with caution in birds with hepatic or renal disease and in laying hens. Despite this caution, it is sometimes effective in waterfowl with severe hepatic amyloidosis.

STREPTOMYCIN (DIHYDROSTREPTOMYCIN)

INDICATIONS: Streptomycin and dihydrostreptomycin (Ethamycin ✿) are aminoglycoside antibiotics. For more information, see

DIHYDROSTREPTOMYCIN and AMINOGLYCOSIDE ANTIBIOTICS in the Small Animal section.

Streptomycin is used most commonly in the poultry industry. In chickens, streptomycin is absorbed rapidly and is excreted slowly after IM injection. After IM doses of 12 mg/kg and 100 mg/kg, elimination half-lives and maximum serum concentrations were 2.35 hours and 21 µg/mL, and 3.97 hours and 127 µg/mL, respectively. Oral absorption of streptomycin is poor. The drug has also been used in pigeons.

ADVERSE AND COMMON SIDE EFFECTS: Streptomycin should not be used in pet birds due to the risk of toxicity. Paralysis and death have been reported in some species.

SUCRALFATE

INDICATIONS: Sucralfate (Carafate ★, Sulcrate ♣, and generics), a complex of sucrose sulfate, accelerates the healing of oral, esophageal, gastric, and duodenal ulcers through several mechanisms. Sucralfate may be useful for the prevention of NSAID-induced ulceration. For more information, see SUCRALFATE in the Small Animal section.

Sucralfate has been recommended for use in psittacine birds for the above-mentioned conditions. The tablets can be ground and mixed with water for administration.

ADVERSE AND COMMON SIDE EFFECTS: Sucralfate can decrease the bioavailability of orally administered drugs, i.e., tetracycline antibiotics. Constipation can occur in small animals.

SULFACHLORPYRIZIDINE
SULFADIMETHOXINE
SULFADIMIDINE
SULFAMETHAZINE
SULFAQUINOXALINE

INDICATIONS: The sulfonamides are antibacterial and antiprotozoal drugs used for the treatment of bacterial diseases and intestinal and biliary coccidiosis. For more information, see SULFONAMIDE ANTIBIOTICS and SULFADIMETHOXINE in the Small Animal section.

Sulfamethazine is used primarily in the drinking water for the control of enteric coccidia. Sulfadimethoxine has also been used for this purpose, as well as by nebulization to treat pneumonia and air sacculitis. Sulfachlorpyridazine is used in the drinking water to treat enteric infections, including those caused by *Escherichia coli*. All the drugs in this section except sulfadimidine have been recommended for the control of coccidiosis in pigeons.

Sulfadimidine has been used to treat enteric *Caryospora neofalconis* infections in juvenile merlins in a breeding facility. Based on a recommended dose of 50 to 100 mg/kg once daily for 5 to 7 consecutive days, birds were treated with 50 mg/kg orally or IM for up to 10 days. The parenteral route was preferred because of concurrent vomiting. One bird received 25 mg/kg every 12 hours orally for 6 weeks without adverse effects. Clinical response was variable. Oocyst production declined after initial treatment but in some birds it increased again within 7 to 10 days. The authors concluded that the drug was effective but that clazuril or toltrazuril might be better choices. Sulfadimidine has also been suggested as a treatment for clostridial enteritis in psittacines.

SUPPLIED AS VETERINARY PRODUCTS:

SULFADIMETHOXINE
Various formulations for oral use in drinking water (Albon, Di-Methox, and others ★)
Oral suspension containing 250 mg/5 mL (Albon Oral Suspension-5% ★)
Tablets containing 125 mg (S-125 ♣, Albon ★) and 250 mg (S-250 ♣, Albon ★)
For injection containing 400 mg/mL (Albon Injection-40% ★, Di-Methox ★, Sulfadimethoxine Injection ★)

SULFADIMIDINE (SULFAMETHAZINE)
Various formulations for oral use in drinking water (Sulmet ★, Purina Sulfa ★, Sulfamethazine ★, Sulfamethazine 25 ♣, Sulfa-25 ♣, and others)

SULFACHLORPYRIDAZINE
For injection containing 200 mg/mL (Vetisulid ★, Prinzone Injection ★, Pyradan Injection ★)
Oral suspension containing 50 mg/mL (Prinzone Oral Suspension ★, Pyradan Oral Suspension ★, Vetisulid Oral Suspension ★)
Oral powder containing 50 g/54 g powder (Vetisulid ★)

SULFAQUINOXALINE
Liquid concentrate for use in drinking water at 19% (Sulfaquinoxaline 19.2% Liquid Concentrate ♣), 20% (20% Sulfaquinoxaline Sodium Solution ★, Sulfa Q 20% Concentration ★), and 31.92% (31.92% Sul-Q-Nox ★)

TERBINAFINE

INDICATIONS: Terbinafine hydrochloride (Lamisil ♣ ★ and generics) is a new, synthetic allylamine antifungal agent used in human medicine primarily for the treatment of dermatophyte infections, particularly when there is chronic nail involvement. Tablet, topical cream, and liquid formulations are available. Terbinafine is highly lipophilic and tends to accumulate in skin, nails, and fatty tissues. Terbinafine is considered more effective and significantly less toxic than griseofulvin, while requiring a shorter duration of therapy. Terbinafine has *in vitro* activity against a wide variety of dermatophytes, molds, and dimorphic fungi, including most *Candida* and *Aspergillus* spp.

Information on the use of terbinafine in birds consists primarily of case reports. It has been suggested as an alternative drug in species sensitive to the toxic effects of itraconazole, e.g., African gray parrots. In a series of cases it was concluded that terbinafine was safe and effective when administered to parrots orally or by nebulization. Terbinafine appeared to be at least as effective as standard antifungal agents. Nebulization appeared to be clinically effective in an African gray parrot with advanced respiratory mycosis in which conventional systemic therapy had not been effective. Oral tablets were crushed and suspended in distilled water to the desired concentration. The nebulization solution was composed of 500 mg terbinafine and 1 mL of acetylcysteine (Mucomyst) in 500 mL of distilled water. Terbinafine is freely soluble in methanol and methylene chloride, soluble in ethanol, and slightly soluble in water. In one of the cases described, terbinafine was used in combination with itraconazole and amphotericin B. No adverse effects, based on clinical appearance and biochemistry, were noted. One bird was treated for 4 months with terbinafine, initially twice daily and later once daily.

ADVERSE AND COMMON SIDE EFFECTS: The most commonly reported adverse effects in humans are skin rash, headache, and GI upset.

DRUG INTERACTIONS: Terbinafine has been used in combination with fluconazole to treat oropharyngeal infections due to fluconazole-resistant *Candida* spp. in humans.

SUPPLIED AS HUMAN PRODUCTS:
Tablets containing 125 mg (Novo-Terbinafine ♣) and 250 mg (Apo-Terbinafine ♣, Gen-Terbinafine ♣, Lamisil ♣, Novo-Terbinafine ♣, PMS-Terbinafine ♣, Lamisil Tablets ★)
Topical spray containing 10 mg terbinafine/g (Lamisil Spray ♣)
Topical cream containing 1% terbinafine (Lamisil Cream 1% ♣)

TESTOSTERONE

INDICATIONS: Testosterone is an androgenic steroid. For more information, see TESTOSTERONE and ANABOLIC STEROIDS in the Small Animal section.

In birds, testosterone has been used by injection or PO in the drinking water to increase male libido, to stimulate male canaries to sing, and to treat anemia, debilitation, and feather loss. The use of testosterone in birds that have stopped singing may discourage owners from investigating underlying health problems. Testosterone has also been used to break the cycle of hens in persistent lay.

ADVERSE AND COMMON SIDE EFFECTS: Long-term testosterone therapy will interfere with the normal hormonal feedback systems. Testosterone therapy is contraindicated in birds with hepatic or renal disease.

TETRACYCLINE

INDICATIONS: Tetracycline (Panmycin Aquadrops Liquid ★, Tetrachel-Vet Syrup ★, Novo-tetra suspension ✚) is a bacteriostatic antibiotic effective against many aerobic and anaerobic gram-positive and gram-negative bacteria, spirochetes, mycoplasmas, and rickettsial organisms. It is used to medicate drinking water or for direct oral administration. For more information, see TETRACYCLINE ANTIBIOTICS in the Small or Large Animal section.

The primary use of tetracycline in avian medicine has been as an initial treatment for chlamydiosis while birds acclimate to medicated diets. Syrup formulations are palatable to birds and can be added to soft food mixes. Birds may not consume adequate amounts of medicated water to ensure therapeutic blood levels of the drug. Doxycycline is now preferred by most veterinarians for the direct oral treatment of birds with chlamydiosis. Tetracycline has also been used to treat *Campylobacter fetus jejuni* enteric infections in finches.

ADVERSE AND COMMON SIDE EFFECTS: Calcium, magnesium, and iron chelate tetracycline resulting in formation of insoluble complexes. Long-term use may predispose to yeast infections; therefore, antifungal agents are often administered concurrently. Disruption of the enteric flora resulting in vitamin K deficiency is also of concern. Tetracycline is potentially nephrotoxic and may be immunosuppressive. Bone deformities may develop in toucans, especially young birds, after the use of tetracyclines.

SUPPLIED AS VETERINARY PRODUCTS:
For oral administration containing 25 mg/mL (Tetrachel-Vet Drops ★) and 100 mg/mL (Panmycin Aqua-drops liquid ✚ ★, Tetrachel-Vet Syrup ★)

SUPPLIED AS HUMAN PRODUCT:
Oral suspension containing 125 mg/5 mL (Novo-tetra suspension ✚)

THIABENDAZOLE

INDICATIONS: Thiabendazole (Equizole ★, Mintezol ★, Thibenzole ★) is a broad-spectrum anthelmintic drug that also has antipyretic and anti-inflammatory effects and fungicidal activity. For more information, see THIABENDAZOLE in the Small Animal section.

In birds, thiabendazole has been used orally for the treatment of nematode parasites, including ascarids and *Syngamus trachea*. A pharmacodynamic study in turkeys, red-tailed hawks, broad-winged hawks, and great horned owls evaluated the potential for use of thiabendazole in the treatment of pulmonary aspergillosis. Serum from birds that received oral doses of 20, 60, and 120 mg/kg did not inhibit the growth of *Aspergillus* spp. isolates *in vitro*. The drug was not recommended for this purpose.

ADVERSE AND COMMON SIDE EFFECTS: Thiabendazole may be toxic in ostriches, diving ducks, and cranes.

TIAMULIN

INDICATIONS: Tiamulin (Denagard ✿ ★ and generics) is a semisynthetic antibiotic of the diterpene group with activity against various gram-positive and gram-negative bacteria, mycoplasmas, and spirochetes. The drug is marketed for use in pigs (water soluble and parenteral formulations) and for the prevention and treatment of chronic respiratory disease in chickens and turkeys (water soluble formulation).

Tiamulin has been recommended for the treatment of mycoplasmosis in pigeons. Clinical signs should decrease after drug administration; however, the infection may not be completely eliminated.

DRUG INTERACTIONS: Tiamulin is incompatible with ionophore antibiotics.

SUPPLIED AS VETERINARY PRODUCTS:
For injection containing 100 mg/mL (Denagard [Tiamulin] Injection ✿)
Powder and liquid concentrates for use in drinking water containing various concentrations of tiamulin (Denagard [Tiamulin] Liquid Concentrate ✿, Denagard Liquid Concentrate ★, Denagard [Tiamulin] Soluble Antibiotic ✿, Denagard 10 ★)
For medicated premixes containing 17.8 g/kg (Denagard [Tiamulin] Medicated Premix ✿, Tiamulin 1.78% Premix ✿)

TICARCILLIN

INDICATIONS: Ticarcillin (Ticar ★) is an extended-spectrum parenteral penicillin antibiotic with activity similar to, but more potent than, carbenicillin. Ticarcillin is especially useful for the treatment of resistant gram-negative infections, including those by *Pseudomonas* spp. For more information, see TICARCILLIN and PENICILLIN ANTIBIOTICS in the Small Animal section.

ADVERSE AND COMMON SIDE EFFECTS: Reconstituted ticarcillin is stable for 14 days if refrigerated; however, according to label recommendation it should not be used for multidose purposes after 72 hours. Some authors have suggested freezing the reconstituted drug in aliquots for subsequent use, but the stability of this formulation has not been investigated. Hepatotoxicity was described in a rose-breasted cockatoo treated with the combination of ticarcillin and tobramycin.

DRUG INTERACTIONS: Ticarcillin is synergistic with aminoglycosides but may inactivate them *in vitro;* therefore, solutions should not be mixed. Ticarcillin in combination with clavulanic acid (Timentin ❧ ★) is effective against many penicillinase-producing strains of bacteria.

TILETAMINE ZOLAZEPAM

INDICATIONS: Tiletamine plus zolazepam (Telazol ★) is an injectable dissociative anesthetic/tranquilizer combination useful for sedation and restraint and for anesthetic induction or anesthesia of short duration (30 minutes) requiring mild to moderate analgesia. For more information, see TILETAMINE ZOLAZEPAM in the Small Animal section.

Telazol has been used IM and IV in ratites to induce anesthesia and for short, relatively nonpainful procedures such as radiography.

ADVERSE AND COMMON SIDE EFFECTS: Some reports describe violent recoveries from anesthesia with Telazol.

DRUG INTERACTIONS: Because the elimination half-life of tiletamine is shorter than that of zolazepam, one should administer ketamine rather than additional Telazol as a top-up to prolong sedation or anesthesia. Flumazenil, a reversal agent for benzodiazepine tranquilizers, will help reverse the effects of zolazepam.

TOBRAMYCIN

INDICATIONS: Tobramycin (Nebcin ❧ ★) is an aminoglycoside antibiotic closely related to gentamicin used for the treatment of bacterial infections, especially those caused by *Pseudomonas* spp., against which it has better activity than gentamicin. For more information, see TOBRAMYCIN and AMINOGLYCOSIDE ANTIBIOTICS in the Small Animal section.

ADVERSE AND COMMON SIDE EFFECTS: Tobramycin is less nephrotoxic than gentamicin with 40% to 65% less accumulation in the kidneys of red-tailed hawks, great horned owls, and barred owls. Hepatotoxicity was described in a rose-breasted cockatoo treated with the combination of ticarcillin and tobramycin.

DRUG INTERACTIONS: Tobramycin is potentiated by penicillins and cefotaxime; and, therefore, a lower dose should be used in combination.

TOLTRAZURIL

INDICATIONS: Toltrazuril (Baycox) is used for the prevention and/ or treatment of coccidiosis in broiler chickens and pigs, but is not currently licensed in North America. The drug is active against all intracellular stages of coccidia in poultry, as well as against mammalian coccidia, *Sarcocystis*, and *Toxoplasma* spp.

Toltrazuril has been administered in the drinking water to treat atoxoplasmosis in canaries and has been suggested for the treatment of *Caryospora neofalconis* in raptors. A related drug, clazuril, was previously available in tablet formulation for use in pigeons.

SUPPLIED AS VETERINARY PRODUCTS:
Not currently registered for use in North America
Liquid concentrate for use in drinking water containing 2.5% toltrazuril (Baycox 2.5%)
Oral suspension containing 5% toltrazuril (Baycox Suspension)

TRIMETHOPRIM-SULFADIAZINE
TRIMETHOPRIM-SULFADOXINE
TRIMETHOPRIM-SULFAMETHOXAZOLE

INDICATIONS: Trimethoprim-sulfadiazine, trimethoprim-sulfadoxine, and trimethoprim-sulfamethoxazole (Tribrissen ♣ ★, Trivetrin ♣, Borgal ♣, Septra ♣ ★, Bactrim ♣ ★ and many others) are bactericidal antibiotic combinations. For more information, see TRIMETHOPRIM-SULFADIAZINE in the Small Animal section or SULFONAMIDES: POTENTIATED in the Large Animal section.

Trimethoprim-sulfonamide combinations are widely used in avian medicine especially for respiratory and enteric infections and for the treatment of hand-fed baby psittacines. Many reports do not specify the specific drugs used and simply call the combination trimethoprim + "sulfa." Despite the frequency of use of trimethoprim-sulfa combinations in birds, there are virtually no pharmacokinetic data available. Oral bioavailability is, however, considered to be excellent. The elimination half-life of trimethoprim is 2.5 hours in geese.

Trimethoprim-sulfa combinations are effective against some protozoa, including coccidia of toucans and mynahs. A dose of 50 mg/kg twice daily IM for 9 consecutive days resulted in the clinical recovery of a cassowary with presumptive toxoplasmosis.

ADVERSE AND COMMON SIDE EFFECTS: Regurgitation has been reported after oral administration of trimethoprim-sulfonamide drugs to raptors and psittacines, especially macaws. Facial flushing and gastrointestinal stasis have also been reported in some species, again particularly in macaws. Pigeons tolerate the oral trimethoprim-sulfa medications well. Decreased food and water consumption and anemia have been described in 6-week broiler chickens given up to 4.4 times the recommended dose. Concerns have been expressed by clinicians regarding the potential for sulfonamide crystallization in glomeruli or renal tubules.

DRUG INTERACTIONS: Trimethoprim-sulfadiazine and trimethoprim-sulfamethazole have been used in combination with pyrimethamine for the treatment of sarcocystosis in parrots.

SUPPLIED AS VETERINARY PRODUCTS:
For injection containing 40 mg/mL trimethoprim and 200 mg/mL sulfadiazine (Tribrissen 24% ✹)
For injection containing 40 mg/mL trimethoprim and 200 mg/mL sulfadoxine (Bimotrin ✹, Borgal ✹, Trimidox ✹, Trivetrin ✹)
For injection containing 80 mg/mL trimethoprim and 400 mg/mL sulfadiazine (Tribrissen 48% ✹)
Tablets containing trimethoprim plus sulfadiazine in the following combinations (mg): 5 + 25, 20 + 100, 80 + 400 (DiTrim ★, Tribrissen ✹ ★)
Oral suspension containing approximately 10 mg trimethoprim and 50 mg sulfadiazine/mL (Tribrissen ★, Tribrissen Piglet Suspension ✹)
Oral paste containing 67 mg/g trimethoprim and 333.3 mg/g sulfadiazine (Tribrissen 400 Oral Paste ★)

SUPPLIED AS HUMAN PRODUCTS:
Oral suspensions containing 8 mg trimethoprim and 40 mg sulfamethoxazole/mL (Bactrim ✹ ★, Coptin ✹, Septra ✹ ★, and others)

TYLOSIN

INDICATIONS: Tylosin (Tylan ✹ ★, Tylocine ✹, Tylosin ✹ ★) is a bacteriostatic macrolide antibiotic. It is bacteriostatic against gram-negative and some gram-positive bacteria, spirochetes, chlamydiae, and mycoplasmas. For more information, see TYLOSIN in the Small Animal and Large Animal sections.

In avian medicine, tylosin is used primarily for the treatment of mycoplasmal infections, especially of the respiratory tract, and conjunctivitis. In pharmacokinetic studies in bobwhite quail, pigeons, sandhill cranes, and emus, IM tylosin was rapidly absorbed, attaining peak plasma levels within 30 to 90 minutes, and penetrated rapidly into tissues. The elimination half-life in emus was 4.7 hours, as compared to 1.2 hours in the other species evaluated. Tissue levels, especially kidney and liver, were higher than those of plasma. Six hours after administration, tylosin levels in lung, liver, and kidney were greater than 1 µg/mL, the minimal inhibitory concentration for many susceptible microorganisms, even though plasma levels were barely detectable. Nebulization for 1 hour resulted in effective antibiotic levels in the lungs and air sacs of pigeons and quail; however, in quail the drug levels in tissue were negligible by 1 (lungs) and 3 (air sacs) hours after nebulization was completed. Systemic absorption of the drug was minimal.

Tylosin was used to treat *Mycoplasma gallisepticum* conjunctivitis in house finches. The drug was placed in the drinking water at a concentration of 1 mg/mL for 21 to 77 days. The recommended dose in poultry is 0.5 mg/mL of drinking water for 4 to 8 days of therapy. The birds were treated concurrently with ophthalmic ciprofloxacin for 5 to 7 days. At the end of the treatment period, conjunctival cultures on all birds were negative; however 2 of 18 birds were positive on polymerase chain reaction. The carrier status could not be ruled out based on this research, but *M. gallisepticum* could not be isolated from necropsied birds.

Rheas with respiratory and ocular disease, from whose tracheal swabs *Mycoplasma synoviae* and *Escherichia coli* were isolated, responded rapidly to a combination treatment regimen including a single shot of long-acting doxycycline, medication of the drinking water with tylosin for 4 weeks, and direct ophthalmic therapy with tylosin powder diluted 1:10 in sterile water.

ADVERSE AND COMMON SIDE EFFECTS: Drinking water containing tylosin powder has a bitter taste that may need to be masked for adequate water consumption. In mammals, tylosin has a wide margin of safety and is relatively nonirritating on injection.

DRUG INTERACTIONS: In an experimental study, DMSO added to tylosin for nebulization resulted in a greater level and longer duration of antibiotic concentration in the lung and air sacs.

VECURONIUM BROMIDE

INDICATIONS: Vecuronium bromide (Vecuronium Bromide ✦, Norcuron ✦, Norcuron for Injection ★, Vecuronium Bromide for Injection ★) is a nondepolarizing neuromuscular blocking agent of intermediate duration that acts by competing for cholinergic receptors at the motor endplate. In humans, under balanced anesthesia, the time to recovery to 25% of control (clinical duration) is approximately 25 to 40 minutes after injection and recovery is usually 95% complete approximately 45 to 65 minutes after injection of a dose sufficient for intubation.

Vecuronium has been used in anesthetized birds to relax ocular skeletal muscle for detailed examination or manipulation. In pigeons, vecuronium results in complete mydriasis and areflexia with an average lag period of approximately 26 seconds and a duration of 256 minutes. Concurrent isoflurane concentration can be reduced by approximately 25%.

ADVERSE AND COMMON SIDE EFFECTS: The effect of vecuronium is prolonged in humans with liver failure. Hypoventilation and respiratory failure occur as a result of increasing muscle paralysis; and therefore, careful monitoring of respiratory parameters and ventilation are necessary. Neuromuscular block is reversed by acetylcholinesterase inhibitors such as neostigmine, edrophonium, and pyridostigmine in conjunction with atropine or glycopyrrolate.

DRUG INTERACTIONS: The neuromuscular blocking action of vecuronium is potentiated with inhalant anesthetics including isoflurane. Certain antibiotics may intensify or produce neuromuscular block on their own, including aminoglycosides (neomycin, streptomycin, kanamycin, gentamicin, and dihydrostreptomycin) and tetracyclines.

SUPPLIED AS HUMAN PRODUCTS:
For injection containing 10 mg/vial (Vecuronium Bromide ✤, Norcuron for Injection ★, Vecuronium Bromide for Injection ★) and 1 mg/mL after reconstitution (Norcuron ✤)

VITAMIN A

INDICATIONS: Vitamin A (Aquasol A ✤ ★, Aquasol A Parenteral ★) is used in the treatment of hypovitaminosis A and during the therapy of avian poxvirus infections, chronic sinusitis, and ophthalmic disorders. Long-term therapy may be required to replenish liver stores.

SUPPLIED AS HUMAN PRODUCTS:
Capsules containing 10,000, 25,000 or 50,000 IU (Aquasol A ✤ ★, Natural Source Vitamin A [retinol] ✤, and others)
Oral solution containing 50,000 IU/mL (Aquasol A ★)
For injection containing 50,000 USP units/mL (15 mg retinal/mL) (Aquasol A Parenteral ★)
In gel formulation containing 10,000 IU Pro-Vitamin A (ACES Antioxidant Soft Gels ★)

VITAMIN A, D₃, E

INDICATIONS: Vitamin A, D₃, and E combinations are used in the treatment of vitamin deficiencies and as a general supportive measure. Because they contain vitamin D₃, these products may help in the treatment of soft bones, soft eggs and egg-binding, and bone repair. Injacom 100 is an aqueous-based product for IM administration whose use is frequently mentioned in the literature.

ADVERSE AND COMMON SIDE EFFECTS: African gray parrots should be treated once only to avoid problems with calcium metabolism. Vitamin D toxicity is a potential hazard after repeated injection; however, it has not been reported in the literature. Injacom, a large animal formulation, is oil based and contains excess vitamin D.

SUPPLIED AS VETERINARY PRODUCTS:
CONTAINING VITAMIN A AND D₃
For injection containing 5,000,000 IU Vitamin A and 75,000 IU Vitamin D₃ per mL (Co-op A+D ✤, Vitamin A&D ✤, Vitamin AD-500 ✤)
CONTAINING VITAMIN A, D₃, AND E
For injection containing 100,000 IU Vitamin A, 10,000 IU Vitamin D and 300 IU Vitamin E per mL (Emulsi Vit E/A&D ★, Vital E-A+D ★, Vitamin E+AD ★, Vitamin E-AD300 ★)

VITAMIN B COMPLEX

INDICATIONS: Vitamin B complex ✤ ★ is administered as a supportive therapy in the treatment of diseases characterized by debility, anemia, peripheral neuropathy, and muscular weakness. It is also used to stimulate appetite and following long-term antibiotic therapy.

ADVERSE AND COMMON SIDE EFFECTS: Overdose may result in anaphylaxis. Dose calculations should be made by thiamine content.

SUPPLIED AS VETERINARY PRODUCTS:
For injection containing various vitamin levels and combinations (multiple products ✤ ★)
Oral to add to drinking water (Vitamin B Complex ✤, Liquid B Complex ★)
Oral syrup (V.A.L. Syrup ★)

VITAMIN B₁ (THIAMINE)

INDICATIONS: Thiamine (Vitamin B₁ ✤ ★, B-1 ★, T-Dex ✤, Thiamine HCl Injection ✤ ★, T Sol ✤, Ultra-B₁ ✤) is used orally as a nutritional supplement in birds on fish diets that may be deficient in thiamine due to dietary thiaminase. Thiamine powder or capsules can be added to the food. Thiamine may also be helpful in the treatment of heavy metal toxicosis in some species. For more information, see THIAMINE in the Small Animal and Large Animal sections.

DRUG INTERACTIONS: Injectable thiamine is also available in multiple B complex.

VITAMIN B$_{12}$ (CYANOCOBALAMIN)

INDICATIONS: Vitamin B$_{12}$ or cyanocobalamin (Vitamin B-12 ❦ ★, Am-Jet ★, Am-Tech ★, Am-Vet ★) is used for the treatment of anemia.

ADVERSE AND COMMON SIDE EFFECTS: Pink droppings may be observed after administration of vitamin B$_{12}$.

SUPPLIED AS VETERINARY PRODUCTS:
For injection containing:
1,000 and 5,000 µg/mL (Vitamin B-12 ❦)
1,000, 3,000, and 5,000 µg/mL (Vitamin B12 ★, AmTech Vitamin B$_{12}$ ★, AmJec Vitamin B12 ★, and others)
1,000 and 3,000 µg/mL (Vita-Jec B-12 ★)

VITAMIN C

INDICATIONS: Vitamin C, or ascorbic acid, is a water-soluble vitamin necessary for a variety of metabolic processes. For more information, see ASCORBIC ACID in the Small Animal section.

Although virtually all birds can produce vitamin C, research in poultry has shown that dietary supplementation has a protective effect against bacterial and viral diseases and that it can improve the immune response to certain stimulations. It also has been shown to reduce the impact of stressors such as high temperature in chickens. Vitamin C supplementation is suggested by some authors as part of supportive care for ill or debilitated birds.

VITAMIN D$_3$

INDICATIONS: Vitamin D$_3$ (Calcijex ❦ ★) (cholecalciferol, colecalciferol) is used as a supplement for birds with calcium deficiency, and, in combination with vitamins A and E, as a general nutritional supplement.

ADVERSE AND COMMON SIDE EFFECTS: Particular caution should be taken in treating young psittacine birds on heavily fortified diets. Clinical hypervitaminosis D was described in a nursery containing macaw chicks. The oral lethal dose in 50% (LD$_{50}$) of mallard ducks is >2,000 mg/kg. The dietary lethal concentrations in 50% (LC$_{50}$) are 4,000 mg/kg (mallard duck) and 2,000 mg/kg (bobwhite quail).

SUPPLIED AS HUMAN PRODUCT:
1 IU = 0.025 µg of vitamin D$_3$

For injection containing 1 µg/mL of calcitriol (Calcijex ✤ ★) and 400 IU/mL (Di-Vi-Sol ✤)

VITAMIN E + SELENIUM

INDICATIONS: Vitamin E (BO-SE ★, E-SE ✤, Myosel ★, Dystosel ✤, and others) has been used in the treatment of steatitis. Vitamin E and selenium are used in combination for the treatment of myopathies and muscular weakness. A syndrome of paralysis in cockatiels is vita-min E plus selenium responsive. Supplementation may assist in the treatment of limb dysfunction in chicks. One report describes a positive clinical response to vitamin E plus selenium therapy in mockingbirds that developed ascending paralysis while on a diet of cat food. Vitamin E plus selenium is often administered to large birds after severe muscular exertion to prevent the occurrence of or reduce the severity of capture myopathy. For more information, see VITAMIN E in the Small Animal or Large Animal sections.

ADVERSE AND COMMON SIDE EFFECTS: Selenium is teratogenic; chronic exposure results in increased embryonic and chick death. Acute toxicity is possible. Reports in waterfowl describe anasarca and pulmonary edema associated with a flaccid heart.

SUPPLIED AS VETERINARY PRODUCTS:
Vitamin E for injection containing 200 IU/mL (DL Alpha ★) and 300 IU/mL (Vitamin E-300 ★)
Multiple products for injection containing various levels of Vitamin E + selenium:
1 mg selenium and 68 IU vitamin E/mL (BO-SE ★)
2.5 mg selenium and 50 mg vitamin E/mL (E-SE ✤)
2.5 mg selenium and 68 IU mg vitamin E/mL (E-SE ★)
3 mg selenium and 136 IU vitamin E/mL (E-SEL ✤, Dystosel ✤)
5 mg selenium and 68 IU vitamin E/mL (MU-SE ★, MuSe Injectable ✤)
6 mg selenium and 136 mg vitamin E/mL (Dystosel DS ✤)
51 mg selenium and 68 IU vitamin E/mL (Myosel-B ★)
52.5 mg selenium and 68 IU vitamin E/mL (Myosel-E ★)
55 mg selenium and 68 IU vitamin E/mL (Myosel-M ★, Velenium ★)
Chewable Tablets containing 10 IU vitamin E and 10 µg selenium (MultiVed Comfort Antioxident Chewable Tablets ★)
Feed supplements and oral powders

VITAMIN K₁

INDICATIONS: Vitamin K₁ or phytonadione (Aqua-Mephyton ★, Mephyton ★, Veta-K1 ✤ ★) is used to treat coagulopathies due to fat-soluble vitamin malabsorption such as occurs with long-term use of antibacterial agents, and vitamin K antagonism caused by salicylates, coumarins, and indanediones, including warfarin poisoning. For more information, see VITAMIN K₁ in the Small Animal section.

In birds, vitamin K is used in the treatment of hemorrhagic disorders and as a preventive measure during long-term medication with amprolium or sulfonamide drugs. Decreased blood coagulability and hemorrhages have been seen in psittacine birds receiving the injectable doxycycline product Vibravenos. Concurrent treatment with vitamin K was partially protective. Vitamin K therapy is also used in combination with calcium in bleeding syndromes of undetermined etiology, such as occurs in conures. There is little information available on the oral use of vitamin K in birds. Based on human pediatric recommendations, more frequent administration would be required using the oral route rather than IM injection. The injectable formulation can be given orally at the same dose (mg/kg basis) when tablets or capsules are not available.

XYLAZINE

INDICATIONS: Xylazine (AnaSed ♣ ★, Rompun ♣ ★, and others) is an α₂-adrenergic sedative agent characterized by a rapid induction, good to excellent sedation, excellent analgesia, and a smooth recovery. For more information, see XYLAZINE in the Small Animal section.

In birds, xylazine is used in combination with ketamine for injectable anesthesia of a wide variety of species. This combination is not recommended for use in pet birds since the safety of inhalant agents such as isoflurane is considerably greater. Yohimbine can be used as a reversal agent.

ADVERSE EFFECTS: Adverse effects including bradycardia, bradyarrhythmias, hypotension, hypoxemia, and death have been reported with the use of xylazine in birds.

YOHIMBINE

INDICATIONS: Yohimbine (Yobine ♣ ★, Antagonil ♣ ★) is a competitive α₂-adrenergic blocking agent used to reverse the effects of xylazine and speed anesthetic recovery in a wide variety of avian species. Yohimbine is generally thought to have little effect on the cardiovascular system. For more information, see XYLAZINE in the Small Animal section or YOHIMBINE in the Large Animal section.

ADVERSE AND COMMON SIDE EFFECTS: Excitement and mortality have been described in mammals receiving doses of more than 1 mg/kg.

DRUG INTERACTIONS: Administration of yohimbine should be delayed for approximately 20 to 30 minutes if ketamine has been used in combination with xylazine. Otherwise, reversal of the xylazine will leave an animal under the influence of ketamine alone, and recovery from anesthesia may not be smooth.

SUPPLIED AS VETERINARY PRODUCTS:
For injection containing 2 mg/mL (Yobine ♣ ★) and 5 mg/mL (Antagonil ♣ ★)

INDEX